Diseases of Children in the Subtropics and Tropics

4th edition

C

Diseases of Children in the Subtropics and Tropics

4th edition

Edited by
Paget Stanfield, Martin Brueton, Michael Chan,
Michael Parkin and Tony Waterston

Edward Arnold
A division of Hodder & Stoughton
LONDON MELBOURNE AUCKLAND

First published in Great Britain 1958
Second edition 1970
Third edition 1978

British Library Cataloguing in Publication Data
Diseases of children in the tropics and
 tropics. – 4th ed
 1. Tropical regions. Children. Diseases
 I. Stanfield, J. Paget
 618.92'9883

 ISBN 0-340-50633-4

Whilst the advice and information in this book is believed to be
true and accurate at the data of going to press, neither the
author nor the publisher can accept any legal responsibility or
liability for any errors or omissions that may be made. In
particular (but without limiting the generality of the preceding
disclaimer) every effort has been made to check drug dosages;
however, it is still possible that errors have been missed.
Furthermore, dosage schedules are constantly being revised and
new side effects recognized. For these reasons the reader is
strongly urged to consult the drug companies' printed
instructions before administering any of the drugs
recommended in this book.

Typeset in 9½/10½ Baskerville by Colset Private Limited,
Singapore.
Printed and bound in Great Britain for Edward Arnold, a
division of Hodder and Stoughton Limited, Mill Road, Dunton
Green, Sevenoaks, Kent TN13 2YA by Butler and Tanner
Limited, Frome and London.

Foreword

Paediatrics is often thought of as following two main routes. One is that of ultratechnology and ever-narrower specialization. The other is recognition of child health in a community context, related to family circumstances (especially the health and welfare of mothers) and influenced by the environment, social stresses, economic limitations, cultural attitudes and practices, and policy decisions and priorities based on the political system.

Neither is right, but rather a balance is needed. Thus, preventive programmes, such as immunization, depend on refined technology to produce appropriate vaccines and devise workable equipment for effective 'cold-chains'. Curative paediatrics, especially simplified methods in appropriate technology, has to be underpinned by science – both by necessity and to achieve acceptance by orthodox members of the Establishment. Examples include the work of gastroenterologists on the intestinal 'sodium pump' and how this can be 'primed' and made more effective by glucose. In this way, essential scientific credence has been given to the seemingly simple methods of oral rehydration, using prepared ORS packets or home-made mixtures of sugar and salt or dilute rice (or other staple) gruels.

However, as always, it can be difficult to persuade physicians, including paediatricians, to acquire a community perspective, understanding and, still more, a truly active role. This is often in part because of their training which frequently remains predominantly clinical – 'we teach what we have been taught'. However, things are changing in some more enlightened training establishments, and the trend is certainly indicated in this Fourth Edition.

Sound clinical work, as in a hospital environment, is vital and will always remain a major need. This approach alone cannot begin to touch the major issues of child health. Some of these may be beyond the scope of the paediatrician or of medical science. Nevertheless, an awareness of the need for an advocacy role has to be cultivated. In this way, advice and guidance may begin to move those in power towards policies which can improve community child health.

The 'complete' paediatrician anywhere, but especially in less technically developed countries, often in tropical regions, needs to be much more than a blinkered 'vertical'/'horizontal' expert. Rather, there is a need for 'lateral' thinking, training and action. This implies realization of the wide range of factors needing consideration in child health work and also recognization of the value of a dove-tailed curative–preventive approach, as part of a team including paediatricians, nurses, community health workers and (importantly) parents, particularly mothers, in the community itself.

The present edition of *Diseases of Children in the Subtropics and Tropics* moves in this direction and will most certainly be valuable not only as a clinical reference text. My hope is that it will also persuade its readers that a paediatrician should not only be clinically sound, but also able to recognize the wider community issues involved in the causation of problems and the need for imaginative interdisciplinary programes to improve the outlook for life and health of mothers and children in the Third World.

D.B. Jelliffe, MD, FRCP.
Professor of Public Health and Pediatrics,
Director, International Health Program,
School of Public Health,
University of California,
Los Angeles, USA

Preface

The fourth edition of this book incorporates significant advances in technical knowledge and also takes into account the widening role of paediatricians in the health care of children in developing countries. As in earlier editions, it seeks to provide paediatricians with an up-to-date review of the diseases of children encountered in the tropics, together with their diagnosis and treatment, with particular reference to the practical management of difficult problems facing the busy doctor. Technically there have been spectacular advances since the last edition, for example oral rehydration and drugs for the treatment of schistosomiasis, neonatal septicaemia and malignant diseases in childhood. There have also been setbacks, such as increasing drug resistance in malaria and leprosy. The mechanisms of many nutritional, genetic and metabolic disturbances have been considerably clarified and means of early detection of disease and the identification of risk to health factors have been developed even though many need yet to be adequately applied.

The vital relationship of the health of the mother to the well-being of the child has become a major concern in developing countries since the last edition was published. A new section has been added to focus on practical care for pregnant women, the management of labour and delivery, the care of the newborn infant, and the organization of perinatal care.

Doctors are becoming increasingly aware of the limitations of a largely hospital and curative based medical education in preparing practitioners to play a leading part in child health. This edition is intended to prepare its readers for the task of improving the health care of children in the developing world.

The environment remains the major determinant of child health. The balance of influence changes in favour of the child wherever there is stability, education, economic growth, more equitable distribution of resources and a political will to improve the health of mothers and children. In contrast, national and international economic constraints and political conflicts have profoundly damaging effects on child health, both through diminished government budgets available for services and through decreased parental employment and income. Likewise, the grim consequences of natural and man-made disasters have highlighted the vulnerability of mothers and children, for example, among refugees.

Increasingly efficient and penetrating communication is also having its effects throughout the world. The shrinking globe has exposed traditional ways of life to the stimulus, advantages and distortions of other cultures. Extended family units, which have buffered the mother and child from severe physical and social deprivation, are tending to break up. There is a steady migration of people from country into city and agriculture to industry while urban unemployment continues to increase. The impact of modern, ecologically inappropriate advertising has adversely influenced many child-rearing practices such as breast-feeding, as well as the prescribing of drugs.

Alongside these potentially harmful developments there has been emerging a world-wide emphasis on the extension of primary health care to the community. This has been accompanied by a growing sense of the importance of local participation in the provision of community-based health care. There has been a new recognition of the enhanced role of community selected health volunteers, including trained indigenous healers and health attendants, not only in effecting changes of attitudes and behaviour towards health but also in gathering information about the incidence and causes of ill health within a community.

Those concerned with paediatrics need to become vigorous advocates of child health services and of legislation which favours mothers and children. This requires persistent education, persuasion and, in political terms, lobbying of those in control of budgetary priorities and national policy. New skills in communication and teaching methods are required. The complete paediatrician needs to know about critical pathway analysis, discreet education and persuasive presentation as well as about the murmurs of mitral stenosis and the clinical picture of malaria.

Against this background the present edition sets out to achieve a difficult but essential blend. Each section attempts to find a balance between clinical and applied paediatrics; between curative and preventive medical care; between disease in the individual child and in the community; between maternal and child health, acknowledging that mother and child are biologically and psychologically an inseparable dyad throughout the reproductive life of the one and the prenatal, neonatal and early pre-school life of the other. A balance has to be struck between the assembly of information and instruction needed by the paediatrician in the reference centres of excellence and the study and practice of management at the level of primary care.

The book therefore aims to be a readable specialized reference source appropriate to the care of children in well-equipped hospitals. In addition, it describes explicitly the presentation and management of child-hood disease problems in a way relevant to the practice of primary and preventive health care of the children in their communities. Furthermore, the perspectives of this edition are intended not only for those dealing with the practice and problems of child health now but also for medical students who will be the practitioners and leaders of health care in the future. It is very important that we share our hopes and ideals with those to whom they will become realities. The present publication is therefore geared to the training of medical students as well as offering a resource for general practitioners,

primary health centre doctors, paediatricians and those responsible for the planning and administration of maternal and child health services in the developing world.

The sudden and unexpected death of Michael Parkin, as this edition has gone to press, is a grievous loss to us all. It has been a great privilege to have worked with him as a member of our team in editing and writing parts of this edition. In spite of his many commitments he joined us gladly and his contribution to its production has been substantial. Michael was dedicated to family life in the North East of England, where he was known and loved by many parents and children. Sheila, Michael's wife, shared his commit-ments to the well-being of children throughout the world. She would join us in the hope that this book will enable many to appreciate and share Michael's care for mothers and children and the ways in which he practised this care. In his wide travels he made it clear, as he writes in his introduction, that the principles and practice he learned and taught in Newcastle were rele-vant to all parts of the world. It was characteristic of Michael that he introduced the section on growth and development with a verse from the Bible. We are grate-ful that he was able to complete this task.

Paget Stanfield
Michael Chan
Martin Brueton
Tony Waterston
1991

Acknowledgements

The editors acknowledge with thanks a number of colleagues and publishing houses who have contributed figures, tables and photographs which have helped to illustrate the text. The origins of these contributions are acknowledged individually as they appear in the book and we sincerely hope that no omissions have occurred.

It has been a privilege to work with such a ready, willing and patient team of contributors whose experience and knowledge are broadening and deepening the care of mothers and children throughout the world.

The editors would also like to thank Paul Price and the editorial staff at Edward Arnold for all their support, encouragement and advice.

In all, we hope readers of this book will benefit as much from its study as we have from its production.

Contents

Section 4 Infectious Diseases Paget Stanfield

Section 5 Diseases of the Systems Martin Brueton

Contributors

SD Adeyemi, MB BS(Lagos), FRCS(C), FMCS, FWACS, CSCPS.
Associate Professor and Consultant Paediatric Surgeon, Department of Surgery, College of Medicine, and Lagos University Teaching Hospital, Lagos, Nigeria.

Peter J Aggett, MSc, MB ChB, FRCP, DCH(Eng.).
Senior Lecturer in Child Health and Nutrition, Department of Child Health, University of Aberdeen, UK.

Suresh Rao Aroor, MB BS, DCH, MD, DM.
Associate Professor of Paediatric Neurology, National Institute of Mental Health and Neurosciences, Bangalore, India.

JD Baum, MA, MSc, MD, FRCP.
Professor of Child Health, Department of Child Health, University of Bristol, Royal Hospital for Sick Children, Bristol, UK.

FJ Bennett, MB ChB, DPH, FFCM.
Formerly Director, Department of Community Health, African Medical and Research Foundation, Nairobi, Kenya.

I Bhargava, MB BS, MS, DSc, FIAP, FAMS.
Formerly Deputy Director General, Ministry of Health and Family Welfare, Government of India, New Delhi, India.

SK Bhargava, MB BS, DCH, MD, FIAP.
Consultant Paediatrician, Gouri Hospital, New Delhi and formerly Professor and Head of Department of Paediatrics, Safdarjung Hospital, New Delhi, India.

SG Browne, MD, FRCP, FRCS, FKC, CMG, OBE.
Formerly International Consultant in Leprosy; Director of the Leprosy Study Centre, and Medical Consultant to the Leprosy Mission, London, UK.

Martin Brueton, MD, MSc, FRCP, DCH.
Reader in Child Health, Department of Child Health, Westminster Children's Hospital, London, UK.

J Burn, B Med Sci(Hon), MB, FRCP.
Consultant Clinical Geneticist and Clinical Lecturer, Department of Human Genetics, University of Newcastle upon Tyne, UK.

Nimrod Bwibo, MB ChB, MPH, FAAP, MRCP.
Deputy Vice-Chancellor and Professor of Paediatrics, College of Health Sciences, University of Nairobi, Kenyatta National Hospital, Kenya.

Michael Chan, MD, FRCP, FRACP.
Senior Lecturer, Department of Tropical Paediatrics and International Child Health and Honorary Consultant Paediatrician, Liverpool School of Tropical Medicine, UK.

Ranjit Kumar Chandra, MD, FRCP(C), PhD, DSc(Hon), DPhil(Hon).
Professor of Paediatric Research and Medicine, Director of Immunology, Memorial University of Newfoundland, Newfoundland, Canada.

SN Chaudhuri, MB BS(Rgn), MD(AIIMS).
Director, Child In Need Institute, Vill. Daulatpur, PO Pailan, Via-Joka, 24 Parganas South, 743512, West Bengal, India.

C Chintu, MD, LMCC, FRCP(C), DABP.
Professor of Paediatrics and Child Health, Consultant Haematologist and Oncologist, University Teaching Hospital, Lusaka, Zambia.

Tan Chongsuphajaisiddhi, MD, PhD, DTM & H.
Dean, Faculty of Tropical Medicine, Mahidol University, Bangkok, Thailand.

Badrul Alam Chowdhury, MD, PhD.
Resident, Department of Internal Medicine, Wayne State University School of Medicine, Detroit, Michigan, USA.

Zafrullah Chowdhury, MB BS.
Projects Coordinator, Gonoshasthaya Kendra (Peoples' Health Centre), PO Nayarhat; via Dhamrai, Dhaka, Bangladesh.

MA Church, MB B Chir, FFCM, DTPH.
Medical Advisor, Scottish Health Education Group, Health Education Centre, Edinburgh, UK.

AJ Clarke, BSc, MD, MRCP.
Senior Lecturer in Medical Genetics, University Hospital of Wales, Cardiff, UK.

CJ Clements, MSc, MB BS, MFPHM(NZ), MCCM, DCH, Dip Obst.
Medical Officer, Expanded Programme on Immunization, WHO, Geneva, Switzerland.

William AM Cutting, MB ChB, FRCPE, DCH, DObst RCOG.
Senior Lecturer and Honorary Consultant Paediatrician, Department of Child Life and Health, University of Edinburgh, UK.

Jan Desmyter, PhD, MD, Dip Trop Med.
Professor of Microbiology and Epidemiology, University Hospital and Rega Institute for Medical Research, University of Leuven, Belgium.

MA de Souza, PhD.
Professor of Community Medicine, Department of Community Health, Federal University of Ceara, Brazil.

M Elizabeth Duncan, MD(Hons), FRCSE, FRCOG.
Consultant to the WHO, Ethiopia and Associate Research Worker, Department of Bacteriology, Edinburgh University Medical School, Edinburgh, UK.

Roger Eeckels, MD, Dip Trop Med.
Professor of Paediatrics, University of Leuven, Belgium.

HG Egdell, MB ChB, FRCP, FRC Psych, DPM.
Clinical Lecturer, Department of Psychiatry, University of Liverpool, UK.

Katherine Elliott, MRCS, LRCP, FFCM.
Formerly Director of Appropriate Health Resources and Technology Action Group (AHRTAG), 1 London Bridge Street, London SE1 9SG, UK.

Olive Frost, MB ChB, MSc, MFCM, FRCOG.
Consultant in Public Health Medicine, Clinical Lecturer, Department of Paediatrics and Child Health, University of Liverpool and Honorary Senior Lecturer, Department of Tropical Paediatrics, Liverpool School of Tropical Medicine, UK.

David Goodall, MB BS, MRCS, LRCP, MRCOG.
Consultant in Gynaecology and Obstetrics, Queens Park Hospital, Blackburn and Honorary Senior Lecturer, Department of Tropical Paediatrics, Liverpool School of Tropical Medicine, UK.

Janet Goodall, FRCPEd, DCH, DObst RCOG.
Formerly Consultant Paediatrician, City General Hospital, Stoke on Trent, UK.

Patrick Goubau, MD, Dip Trop Med.
Senior Registrar, Department of Virology, University Hospital, Leuven and Lecturer, Institute of Tropical Medicine, Antwerp, Belgium.

RJ Hay, DM, FRCP, MRCPath.
Professor of Cutaneous Medicine, Department of Dermatology, United Medical and Dental Schools of Guy's and St Thomas' Hospitals, University of London, UK.

Christopher Holborow, OBE, TD, MD, FRCS, FRCSEd.
Consultant ENT Surgeon, Westminster Hospital, London, UK.

RL Huckstep, CMG, FTS, MA, MD(Cantab.), Hon.MD(NSW), FRCS, FRCSE, FRACS.
Professor and Head, Department of Traumatic and Orthopaedic Surgery and Chairman of the School of Surgery, University of New South Wales, Prince of Wales Hospital, Sydney, Australia.

Andrew Hughes, MA, BM BCh, MRCP, MRCPath.
Consultant Haematologist, Harold Wood Hospital, Romford, UK.

Stella Imong, MD, MRCP.
Clinical Lecturer in Paediatrics, Department of Child Health, University of Leicester, UK.

Dorothy A Jackson, D Phil.
Research Fellow in Child Health, Department of Child Health, University of Bristol, Royal Hospital for Sick Children, Bristol, UK.

F Jaiyesimi, MB BS(Ibadan), FRCP(Lond.), DCH, FMCPaed, FWACP.
Professor of Paediatrics, University of Ibadan and Consultant Paediatrician and Paediatric Cardiologist, University College Hospital, Ibadan, Nigeria.

MA Kibel, FRCP(Edin), DCH(Lond.).
Professor of Child Health, Department of Paediatrics and Child Health, University of Cape Town, South Africa.

Valerian P Kimati, MB ChB, FRCPE, FRCP(Glasg.), MRCPI, DCH.
Chief of Health, UNICEF, Lagos, Nigeria.

WH Lamb, MB BS, MD, MRCP.
Consultant Paediatrician, Bishop Auckland General Hospital, Durham, UK.

Michael C Latham, OBE, MB, FFCM, MPH, DTM&H.
Professor of International Nutrition and Director, Program of International Nutrition, Cornell University, New York, USA.

Philippe Lepage, MD.
Head, Department of Paediatrics, Centre Hospitalier de Kigali, Kigali, Rwanda.

WEK Loening, MB ChB, FCP(Paed.).
Professor of Maternal and Child Health, Department of Paediatrics and Child Health, University of Natal, Durban, South Africa.

David Mabey, MA, BM BCh, MRCP, MSc.
Senior Lecturer, Department of Clinical Sciences, London School of Hygiene and Tropical Medicine and Honorary Consultant Physician, Hospital for Tropical Diseases, London, UK.

JW Mak, MB BS, MD, MPH, MRCPath, DAP & E.
Head, Malaria and Filariasis Research Division, Institute for Medical Research, Kuala Lumpur, Malaysia.

DD Murray McGavin, MD, FRCSEd, FCOphth, DCH.
Associate Senior Lecturer, Department of Preventative Ophthalmology, Institute of Ophthalmology, London, UK.

A Miller, PhD, MS, BS.
Formerly Associate Professor of Medical Entomology, School of Public Health and Tropical Medicine, Tulane University, New Orleans, Louisiana, USA.

K Minde, MD, FRCP(C).
Chairman of the Division of Child Psychiatry, McGill University, Director of Psychiatry, Montreal Children's Hospital and Professor of Psychiatry and Pediatrics, McGill University, Montreal, Canada.

P Morrell, MB ChB, MRCP.
Consultant Paediatrician, South Cleveland Hospital, Cleveland, UK.

S Musisi, MB ChB, FRCP(C).
Consultant Psychiatrist, York Central Hospital, Ontario, Canada.

Indira Narayanan, MD, MNAMS.
Formerly Head of Department of Neonatology and Senior Consultant in Paediatrics, Shri Mool Chand Kharaiti Ram Hospital, New Delhi, India.

AD Nikapota, MB BS(Ceylon), DPM(Lon), MRC Psych(UK).
Consultant Child and Adolescent Psychiatrist,

Brixton Child Guidance Unit and Senior Lecturer, Institute of Psychiatry, London, UK.

AN Okoro, MB ChB, MRCP, FRCP.
Consultant Dermatologist, University of Nigeria Teaching Hospital, Enugu, Nigeria.

CLM Olweny, MB ChB, MMed, MD, FRACP.
Professor, University of Manitoba, and Co-Director, WHO Collaborating Centre for Quality of Life in Cancer Care, St. Boniface General Hospital, Manitoba, Canada.

PES Palmer, MD, FRCP, FRCR.
Emeritus Professor of Radiology, University of California, Sacramento, California, USA.

Michael Parkin, MD, FRCP.
Formerly Professor of Clinical Paediatrics, Department of Child Health, Royal Victoria Infirmary, Newcastle upon Tyne, UK.

AA Paul BSc.
Scientist, MRC Dunn Nutrition Unit, University of Cambridge, UK.

AS Paynter, MB BS(Madras), MRCP, DCH.
Consultant Paediatrician, Community Child Health, West Cumberland Hospital, Cumbria, UK.

Michel Pechevis, MD.
Consultant Paediatrician and Head, Training Department, Centre Internationale de L'Enfance, Paris, France.

S Ramji, MB BS, MD.
Associate Professor, Department of Paediatrics, Maulana Azad Medical College, New Delhi, India.

John P Ranken, BA, MIPM, LHA.
Senior Lecturer, Tropical Child Health Unit, Institute of Child Health, University of London, UK.

V Reddy, MD, DCH, FIAP.
Director, National Institute of Nutrition, Indian Council of Medical Research, Hyderabad, India.

MGM Rowland, MB BS, FRCP(UK), MCFM, DCH, DTM&H.
Consultant Epidemiologist, East Anglian Regional Health Authority, Cambridge, UK.

David Sanders, MB ChB, MRCP, DCH, DTPH.
Associate Professor and Consultant Paediatrician, Department of Community Medicine, University of Zimbabwe, Harare, Zimbabwe.

John Seaman, MB BS, DCH.
Senior Overseas Medical Officer, Save The Children Fund, London, UK.

Kusum P Shah, BSc, MD, DGO.
Formerly Associate Professor of Obstetrics and Gynaecology, Grant Medical College, Bombay, India.

DH Shennan, MD, DPH, DCH, DTCD.
Tuberculosis Officer, Department of Health, Ciskei, South Africa.

Ruth Sidel, PhD.
Professor of Sociology, Hunter College, City University of New York, USA.

Victor W Sidel, MD.
Professor of Social Medicine, Montifiore Centre, Albert Einstein College of Medicine, New York, USA.

Nigel Speight, MB BChir, DCH, FRCP.
Consultant Paediatrician, Dryburn Hospital, Durham, UK.

Paget Stanfield, MD, FRCP, FRCPS, DCH.
Director, Department of Community Health, African Medical and Research Foundation, Nairobi, Kenya.

H Taelman, MD, Dip Trop Med.
Head, Department of Internal Medicine, Centre Hospitalier de Kigali, Kigali, Rwanda.

Gill Tremlett, B Nurse, MSc.
Nurse, midwife and health visitor, London, UK.

John Vince, MD, FRCP.
Specialist Medical Officer in Paediatrics, Port Moresby Hospital and Honorary Lecturer in Child Health, University of Papua New Guinea.

Tony Waterston, MD, MRCP, DCH, DRCOG.
Consultant Paediatrician, Community Child
Health, Newcastle General Hospital, Newcastle
upon Tyne, UK.

J KG Webb, OBE, MA, BM BCh, FRCP.
Emeritus Professor, University of Newcastle upon
Tyne, UK.

RG Whitehead, MA, PhD, FI Biol, Hon. MRCP.
Director, MRC Dunn Nutrition Unit, University of
Cambridge, UK.

HA Wilkins, MA, MB BChir, DTM&H, DObst
RCOG.
Director, Medical Research Council Laboratories,
Fajara, The Gambia.

Wong Hock Boon, MB BS, FRCP(Lond.),
FRCP(Ed), FRACP, FRCP, DCH, PJG, PPA.
Senior Fellow and Emeritus Professor, Department
of Paediatrics, National University of Singapore,
Singapore.

MW Woolridge, PhD.
Research Fellow in Child Health, Department of
Child Health, University of Bristol, Royal Hospital
for Sick Children, Bristol, UK.

Yap Hui Kim, MB BS, MMed(Paed.).
Associate Professor and Head, Department of
Paediatrics, Division of Paediatric Nephrology,
Immunology and Urology, National University
Hospital, Singapore.

P Zinkin, MB ChB, FRCP, DCH.
Senior Lecturer, Department of International Child
Health, Institute of Child Health, London, UK.

SECTION I

Maternal and Child Health

Tony Waterston

CHAPTER 1

Introduction

Tony Waterston and Paget Stanfield

There must be very few doctors working with children in the closing years of the twentieth century who do not accept two cardinal statements about child health: first, that children cannot be considered apart from their family and society; and second, that doctors treating sick children in hospital have a wider responsibility for those outside who fail to reach their wards. It has taken time for these messages to penetrate into medical education, and to a wider public, through the efforts of prescient thinkers in developing and developed countries. The concepts of integrated health care, of health promotion, of a group approach in addition to individual care, and of the political content of health are now widely accepted and have been well-publicized both by the World Health Organization and by UNICEF in its annual reports on *The State of the World's Children*.

It might with logic be asked, why have a section on mother and child health in a textbook on children's diseases? To answer this question, we need first to define health. Many doctors find the World Health Organization definition (a sense of complete physical, mental and social well-being) tendentious and illusory; such a state is unlikely to be achieved in most parts of the world, even if it is the ideal, and progress towards such a state is impossible to measure. However, measurement of health is essential if we are to use the more positive term health promotion in addition to the rather negative 'disease prevention'. Indices are now available to measure health.[1] This section is entitled 'maternal and child health' because the health of the mother is intimately bound up with that of the child, and because similar approaches are needed in the delivery of paediatric and obstetric care. But perhaps in the future, family health will become the more correct term. Its use would not only encourage the inclusion of fathers, but also of grandparents, uncles and aunts. Fathers are essential to families and the recent spate of publications on fatherhood[2,3] is a sign of the times. The fact that in many families, the father is absent or contributes little to child care does not negate this – there is a trend towards more paternal involvement and we hope that paediatricians will encourage this. Children need fathers too.

However, the above concepts have tended to suffer from excessive rhetoric and require illumination by detailed examples; they also require the application of a scientific approach. Health workers should not assume that public participation in health is an easy aim to achieve, nor that prevention in the community can succeed without special skills and long effort. In this section of the book we hope to provide the evidence for the effectiveness of the Primary Health Care approach (further defined on p. 26ff.) by giving the reader access to the basic sciences of preventive medicine: epidemiology, anthropology, psychology and sociology among others. A good grasp of politics is also needed but perhaps, like medicine, politics is more of an art than a science. The political content of medicine has long been recognized: it was Virchow who stated in the nineteenth century, 'Politics is nothing more than medicine on a grand scale'.

The world situation

Globally, the annual death toll of mothers and children is still appalling and despite improved delivery of health care there is little light on the horizon because of the overall socio-economic depression affecting most developing countries. Experience in Western Europe has shown that health inputs alone contribute little to mortality reduction – improved nutrition and hygiene are more important factors. However, health measures which are appropriately targeted and which are integrated with initiatives from other sectors are effective, as some very poor countries have shown (see Fig. 1.1.1).

Improved care has barely touched the 'gap' area between the last antenatal visit and the first postnatal contact. Upwards of 80 per cent of women in developing countries deliver at home, attended by older female family members or traditional midwives. Both mother and child pass this perilous time hidden and effectively out of reach from any health facility. The recent unveiling of the magnitude of neonatal tetanus mortality by dint of retrospective surveys has emphasized the high and, for the most part, unrecorded maternal and perinatal mortality and morbidity rates in these countries.

Figures 1.1.2–1.1.7 illustrate the problems. In most developing countries children make up 50 per cent of the population and this proportion is not decreasing. The world figures for death rates and causes of death at different ages are shown, as well as comparisons from high, middle and low-mortality countries. It is important to remember that there are differences within, as well as between, developing countries and this is illustrated by an example from Asia (Fig. 1.1.6). Such disparities are the result of the 'dual economy'

which exists in many low-resource countries and which is further discussed below.

It is now well-known that the most common causes of death in these countries are malnutrition, infectious diseases and (for mothers and children) childbirth. It should be remembered, however, that child morbidity and disability also form an increasing burden, particularly in situations where medical services prevent child deaths but do not combat their causes. Some of these conditions (for which accurate figures are rarely available) are outlined in Table 1.1.1. The burden these conditions present to the community is enormous, yet they are highly amenable to prevention. If preventable, why not prevented?

Causes of high mortality and morbidity

The multiple origins of child and maternal deaths are now well understood. Detailed analysis of causes will be found under the various disease sections but we will examine more closely here two of the fundamental factors: the socio-economic background, and the structure of medical services.

Socio-economic background

Most of the diseases of developing countries are poverty-associated rather than purely tropical diseases and the spectrum is very similar to that seen in Europe in the nineteenth century, as shown in Table 1.1.2. There remains a close association between economic status and child deaths as illustrated by Fig. 1.1.8 comparing economic development and infant mortality. Poverty contributes to child deaths for

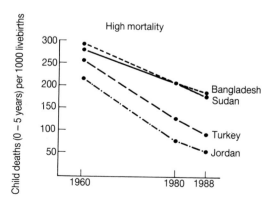
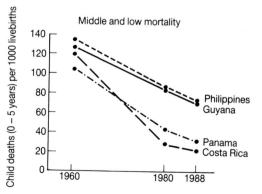

Fig. 1.1.1   Mortality reduction among children under five in some developing countries. (Reproduced from *State of the World's Children 1990*, by permission of the Oxford University Press.)

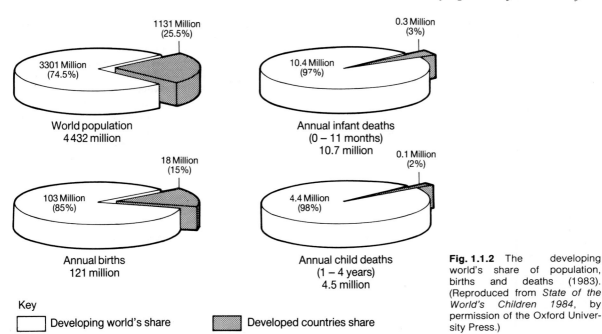

Fig. 1.1.2 The developing world's share of population, births and deaths (1983). (Reproduced from *State of the World's Children 1984*, by permission of the Oxford University Press.)

Table 1.1.1 Causes of child morbidity and disability

Disease	Disability
Recurrent diarrhoea	Malnutrition; time off school
Malnutrition	Mental and physical stunting; infections; blindness
Measles	Malnutrition; blindness; cancrum oris
Whooping cough	Mental retardation; respiratory impairment
Polio	Paralysis and deformity
Tuberculosis	Respiratory impairment; chronic bone disease; mental retardation; deafness
Malaria	Anaemia
Helminth infections; hookworm; ascaris	Anaemia; mental and physical stunting
Bilharzia	Liver disease; renal disease
Trachoma; vitamin deficiencies	Blindness
Neonatal jaundice; birth asphyxia	Deafness, cerebral palsy
Accidents	Physical handicap

various reasons, some of which are listed in Table 1.1.3. It is always worth asking the fundamental question 'Why?' when a child is admitted to hospital with a problem. Werner has shown the value of this approach well (see Fig. 1.1.9).

'Development' has a harmful effect on particular sectors of the population within low resource countries as a result of the so-called 'dual economy'. This phenomenon is also recognized within industrialized countries for the same reasons. In the very high-mortality countries this disparity is less noticeable, since the population is almost entirely rural and dependent on subsistence. Urbanization is occurring less rapidly in these countries and everyone remains poor. However, in the medium-mortality countries poverty is more and more an urban phenomenon. The rural population suffers relative poverty but, except when affected by drought or war, are able to live at sub-sistence level. It is the drift to the cities, the result of national and international development, which leads to the dual economy whereby a relatively well-off élite is dependent for its servicing on the poverty-stricken masses living in the slums and shanty towns. Table 1.1.4 illustrates the degree of urbanization in develop-ing countries. To some extent, urbanization is encouraged by patterns of agricultural development which favour capital-intensive cash crops such as

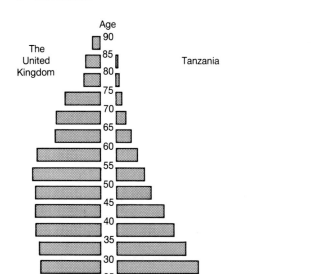

Fig. 1.1.3 Population age structure in developed and developing countries.

off – which includes food marketing, personal services and petty crime. The environment in which such families are forced to rear their children in the peri-urban and inner-city ghettos is appalling, with inadequate housing, poor sewage and water supplies, limited health services and an absolute dependence on the cash sector for food and resources. It is hardly surprising that in these circumstances there is a shift to bottle-feeding (copying the habits of the well-off), weaning diets are inadequate, malnutrition and diarrhoea are rife, and families break up as the mother and often older children are forced to work – yet no appropriate child-care facilities are available. It is the exception for urban 'development' funds to trickle down to the inhabitants of the inner-city or periurban slums.[4]

This picture of gloom is hardly lightened when we look at the overall relationship between spending on health and on other sectors of the economy. World Bank figures show that the 43 countries with the highest infant mortality rates (over 100 deaths per 1000 livebirths) are currently spending three times as much on defence as on health. Yet at the same time, aid from industrialized countries has fallen from 0.51 per cent of their combined GNP in 1960 to 0.37 per cent in 1982. During this period (see Fig. 1.1.10) arms spending has increased world-wide and we now have a situation where the more developed countries spend 20 times as much on the military as on development assistance, while developing countries spend twice as much on arms as on the health of their children. In a significant number of countries, war (either internally or externally mediated) is a major cause of death of children.

These grim statistics illustrate the interdependence of health and development and show that political factors lie at the root of the major health problems affecting mothers and children. Only a redistribution of national resources, both within countries and between rich and poor countries will begin to affect the balance in

tobacco, cotton, tea and coffee and, more recently, exotic fruit and vegetables intended for the luxury markets of the richer countries. For those moving to the cities, the only work to be found in the informal sector is in ministering to the needs of, or robbing, the well-

Table 1.1.2   Death rates (per million) in 1848/54 and 1971 in England and Wales

	1848/54	1971	Percentage of reduction attributable to each category
Conditions attributable to micro-organisms (communicable)			
Airborne diseases	7259	619	40
Water- and food-borne diseases	3562	35	21
Other conditions	2144	60	13
Total	12 965	714	74
Conditions not attributable to micro-organisms	8891	4070	26
All diseases	21 856	5384	100

Reproduced with permission from Sanders, D. *The Struggle for Health*, 1985, Macmillan.

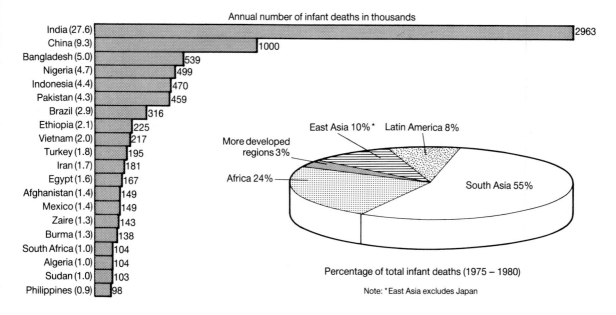

Annual number of infant deaths in thousands

Note: Figures in parentheses are the percentages of the world total

Percentage of total infant deaths (1975 – 1980)

Note: *East Asia excludes Japan

Fig. 1.1.4 Countries with the greatest number of infant deaths (1975–1980). (Reproduced from *State of the World's Children 1984*, with permission from the Oxford University Press.)

Table 1.1.3 Poverty and child death

Underlying factor	Cause of death
Poor land; urbanization and migrant labour; low income; low parental education	Malnutrition
Overcrowding; lack of water/latrines; lack of appropriate health services	Infectious diseases
Maternal malnutrition; lack of health services; low parental education	Maternal/neonatal deaths

Table 1.1.4 Proportion of urban population and projected increase in 109 developing countries (1980–2000)

Proportion urban population (%)	1980 No. (%) countries	2000 No. (%) countries
0–25	41 (37)	19 (17)
26–50	38 (35)	32 (29)
51–75	22 (20)	42 (38)
Over 75	8 (7)	16 (15)

Reproduced from Ebrahim GJ, *Social and Community Paediatrics in Developing Countries*, 1985, Macmillan.

favour of the disadvantaged. The countries which have attempted this have achieved a measure of success, as outlined below.

Effect of development on the environment

'Development' affects health not only through urbanization but by its effect on the land. Population pressure and the lack of national energy policies leads to a shrinking of forested land as trees are cut down for firewood. This not only makes the women's tasks heavy (for who collects wood but the women ?) but also causes soil erosion and makes the land less productive. Land policies which encourage the production of cash crops by commercial farmers cause malnutrition in at least three ways: less food is grown for local consumption; small farmers stop producing and become labourers, so entering the cash sector (but farm workers are often very poorly paid); and the land requires expensive fertilizer to grow crops to international standards, with consequent diversion of scarce foreign exchange. There are many complex interrelationships between agriculture and health which merit deeper study by thoughtful paediatricians.

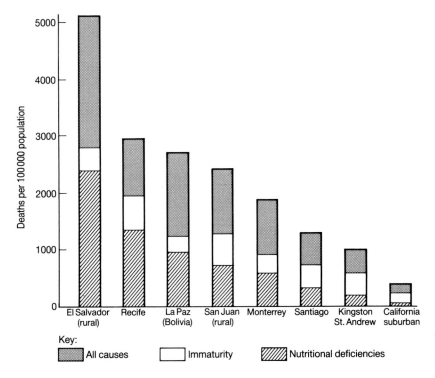

Fig. 1.1.5 Mortality in children under five years of age from all causes and from nutritional deficiency and immaturity. (Reproduced with permission from Sanders, D. *The Struggle for Health*, 1985, Macmillan.)

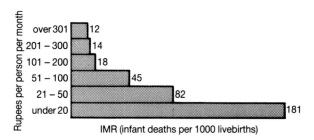

Fig. 1.1.6 Income and infant mortality, New Delhi (1969–74). (Reproduced from *State of the World's Children 1984*, with permission from the Oxford University Press.)

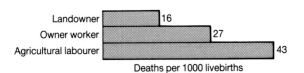

Fig. 1.1.7 Occupation of household head and child death rate, Matlab, Bangladesh (1974–7). (Reproduced from *State of the World's Children 1984*, with permission from the Oxford University Press.)

Health service delivery

Any discussion on methods of prevention must take into account the past role of the health services in its effect (or lack of it) on the pattern of disease in children. Writers such as Cicely Williams, Morley, Illich and McKeown have analysed the over emphasis of these services on disease, on the curative approach and on high-technology medicine practised in large hospitals, to the detriment of health, prevention and community-based medicine. Two memorable statistics tell us that the cost of one bed in a major teaching hospital in Africa would pay for the upkeep of a rural health centre, while 250 such centres could be built for the same price as that large hospital. The historical evolution of curative care for the individual has made this situation inevitable. Doctors are trained to treat sick people, ill people desperately want help, and the well-off are better at finding help than the poor. Criticisms of this situation are less helpful than attempted solutions, and it is essential to remember that adequate curative services provided appropriately at primary, secondary and sometimes tertiary level are a necessary part of any primary health care programme.

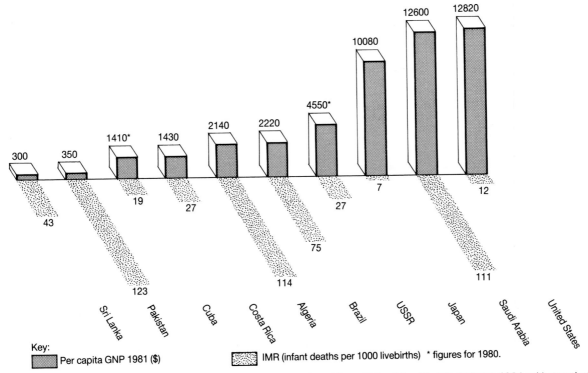

Fig. 1.1.8 Economic development and infant mortality. (Reproduced from *State of the World's Children 1984*, with permission from the Oxford University Press.)

A further constraint in the health sector in addition to the maldistribution of services is the professional attitude of many medical personnel which again Werner illustrates well (Fig. 1.1.11).

Health workers in the past were taught not to disclose information to patients as this might cause anxiety and confusion and would not be understood. Sanders considers[5] that doctors deliberately withheld health knowledge in order to retain their control over the health care system. Whatever the reason, the fact is that doctors have tended to play little part in effective health education or promotion. Since they set an example and teach many of the other cadres in the service, this deficiency is soon replicated throughout the system; hence the importance of improving training as a way of improving the system (see pp. 114–28).

A third factor in the health services which more positively contributes to ill health is iatrogenesis, or medically-induced sickness. Two areas where this is particularly obvious are bottle-feeding and the misuse of potent drugs. The reasons for harm are not positive intent but the increasing technological orientation of

the system, as well as the intervention of the commercial sector in health. Doctors have been passive partners in this process, perhaps failing to recognize its side-effects. Thus, the swing to artificial feeding is influenced by hospital practices (e.g. separation of mother and baby after birth) and by commercial promotion of breast-milk substitutes (see p. 100). Drug misuse is accelerated by opportunist sales tactics, by excessive medical prescribing, by a demand for injections (at first doctor-induced), and by the lack of government controls over the sale of potent drugs on the open market. A single example illustrates the tragedies which may result from the unrestricted commercial sale of drugs in poor countries:

As the boat drew into the shore we heard a strange sound from the bank. A woman was crying. We found her with a dead baby in her arms and a collection of medicine bottles beside her. She had spent all her money on these expensive drugs. She could not understand why they had not saved her baby. This Bangladeshi woman had never been told what was obvious to the doctor who found her. The baby had become severely dehydrated from diarrhoea. Her death could have

Q: What caused Luis's illness?
A: Tetanus – the tetanus bacterium.

Q: BUT WHY did the tetanus bacteria attack Luis and not someone else?
A: Because he got a thorn in his foot.

Q: BUT WHY did that happen?
A: Because he was barefoot.

Q: BUT WHY was he barefoot?
A: Because he was not wearing sandals.

Q: BUT WHY not?
A: Because they broke and his father was too poor to buy him new ones.

Q: BUT WHY is his father so poor?
A: Because he is a sharecropper.

Q: BUT WHY does that make him poor?
A: Because he has to give half his harvest to the landholder.

Q: BUT WHY?
A: (A long discussion can follow, depending on conditions in your particular area.)

Q: Let us go back for a minute. What is another reason why the tetanus bacteria attacked Luis and not someone else?
A: Because he was not vaccinated.

Q: BUT WHY was he not vaccinated?
A: Because his village was not well covered by the vaccination team from the larger town.

Q: BUT WHY was the village not covered?
A: Because the villagers did not cooperate enough with the team when it did come to vaccinate.

Q: What is another reason?
A: The doctor refused to let the midwife give vaccinations.

Q: BUT WHY did he refuse?
A: Because he did not trust her. Because he thought it would be dangerous for the children.

Q: WHY did he think that way? Was he right?
A: (Again a whole discussion.)

Q: BUT not all children who get tetanus die. WHY did Luis die while others live?
A: Perhaps it was God's will.

Q: BUT WHY Luis?
A: Because he was not adequately treated.

Q: WHY NOT?
A: Because the midwife tried first to treat him with a tea.

Q: WHY ELSE?
A: Because the doctor in San Ignacio could not treat him. He wanted to send Luis to Mazatlan for treatment.

Q: BUT WHY?
A: Because he did not have the right medicine.

Q: WHY NOT?
A: Because it is too expensive.

Q: BUT WHY is this life-saving medicine so expensive?
A: (A whole discussion can follow. Depending on the group, this might include comments on the power and high profits of international drug companies, etc.)

Q: BUT WHY did Luis's parents not take him to Mazatlan?
A: They did not have enough money.

Q: WHY NOT?
A: Because the landholder charged them so much to drive them to San Ignacio.

Q: WHY did he do that? (A whole discussion on exploitation and greed can follow.)
A: Because they were so poor.

Q: BUT WHY are they so poor? (This question will keep coming up.)

Fig. 1.1.9 A group discussion is presented with a story about the death of a boy called Luis. To help the group recognize the complex chain of causes that led to Luis's death they play the game 'But why . . .?'. Everyone tries to point out different causes. Each time an answer is given, the question 'But why . . .?' is asked. This way, everyone keeps looking for still other causes. If the group examines only one area of causes, but others exist, the discussion leader may need to go back to earlier questions, and rephrase them so that the group explores in new directions. The question game might develop as shown above. (Reproduced from Werner D, Bower B, *Helping Health Workers Learn*, 1982.)

been prevented with a simple home-made solution of water, salt and sugar. No amount of medicine could have kept her alive. (Melrose D. *Bitter Pills*. Oxford, Oxfam, 1984.)

It is because some doctors are too closely associated with such tactics, that they are sometimes seen more as a part of the problem of under-development, than as a part of its solution.

Primary health care

It is heartening to see from UNICEF figures (Fig. 1.1.1) that some countries are succeeding in improving their children's health, and these examples should be proclaimed by paediatricians everywhere. There is no reason now for any country to fail to show progress on the child health front – even though major improvements will depend on reforms in international trade, aid and finance. Within poor countries WHO and UNICEF have shown unquestionably that primary health care can improve the lot of the poor but a strong commitment to its implementation is essential, as well as an understanding of its radical nature. Governments practising primary health care need to have close contact with their people; it would be hard indeed for a

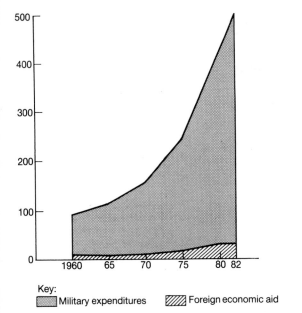

Key:
▓ Military expenditures ▨ Foreign economic aid

Fig. 1.1.10 Military and aid expenditures, industrialized nations (1960–82). (Reproduced from *State of the World's Children 1986*, with permission from the Oxford University Press.)

country which neglects human rights and which gives its people no political or economic power to practise true primary health care.

Primary health care depends on:

- health workers at grass-roots level;
- integration of prevention with cure;
- recognition in secondary/tertiary care of the priority of primary health care;
- integration of health with other sectors of the economy;
- involvement of people in their own care, including planning.

There is an increasing recognition that health care at primary level is a synthesis between health care delivery and community-based health care (which people generate for themselves). Such programmes require considerable skill and experience and are better organized locally ('horizontal') than through national or international directives ('vertical'). The community is encouraged to identify and select some of its own members for a short training in health care. Training will include 'awareness developing' or 'conscientization' as described by Paulo Freire in Brazil[6] and further discussed by Werner.[7] Shaffer[8]

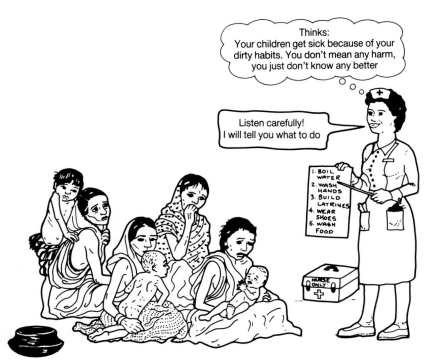

Fig. 1.1.11 Attitude of medical personnel. (Adapted from Werner op. cit.) This teacher assumes ignorance among those being taught and gives advice which is inappropriate for the moment and impractical. Health education to parents should relate to their immediate needs and build on their considerable knowledge of children, child care and the constraints under which they live.

has summarized the training required in mnemonic form as LePSA: Learner-centred, Problem-posing, Self-awareness-creating and Action-demanding. The learners are encouraged to answer their own questions: what are our problems and their causes, how do we measure their importance, what can we do about them and how, or where do we find help? The job of the health service then becomes one of helping to start the process and planning, providing knowledge and some technical resources and monitoring and encouraging progress.

The role of traditional medicine

The need for cooperation between Western and traditional medical systems is increasingly accepted in both developed and developing countries, mainly as a result of a greater emphasis on the 'whole person approach' and the recognition of the cultural connections of health. The traditional healer does assess the patient in the context of his/her family, culture and environment. However, the difficulties of cooperation between doctors and traditional healers should not be underestimated and more research in this area is much needed. Traditional healers are sometimes quacks, may overcharge their patients and can cause iatrogenesis just as much as private medical practitioners do. Each side needs to learn how the other works and traditional healers will need to modify their knowledge and practice if cooperation is to develop fruitfully. Such cooperation has developed faster in the field of traditional midwifery and we hope that the next decade will show similar experiments in a wider field of traditional medicine.

Women and children in primary health care

Several critical constituents of a primary health care programme identified by UNICEF as pertaining particularly to children are:

- **G**rowth monitoring
- **O**ral rehydration
- **B**reast-feeding
- **I**mmunization.

These are presently organized as vertical programmes and ignore the 'community participation' component as well as economic factors (e.g. pure water supplies are just as important as oral rehydration).[9] However, they do serve to highlight key preventive techniques. To the acronym GOBI are added three Fs which are directed at women's health: female education, family spacing and food supplementation. The grudging acceptance of the

place of women in development was one of the side-effects of the UN Decade of Women. It is now perceived, at least by the aid agencies, that women's influence in agriculture, in rural businesses, in health and in the domestic environment is pre-eminent and must be recognized in political and economic planning. Where this has happened, the success has been remarkable. An example is Kerala, one of the poorest states of South India which now has the lowest population growth rate in the country – seemingly because of its emphasis on female education (see p. 91).

In the long run, socio-economic advances are likely to make a greater contribution to disease reduction than specific medical interventions (with the possible exception of immunization).

Children's rights

It is only in the last three decades that political recognition has been given to the rights of children – though major religions have, for a long time, done the same. The United Nations has drawn up a Charter of Children's Rights now formulated as a convention. Yet child abuse, which includes neglect, abandonment, sexual exploitation and torture, is becoming common all over the world. It could be said that malnutrition of early childhood amongst the young of the Third World is an example of child abuse by the developed world.

Accompanying the recognition of the rights of the child, is the realization of the way children can join in their own health care and that of their siblings. The child to child approach[10] makes use of this capacity of children to influence society at large and is evidence of new enlightened attitudes in those delivering childcare.

The role of doctors in primary health care

Even though most preventive work in maternal and child health will be carried out by health workers other than doctors, the medical role in primary health care is extremely important. Doctors are seen as leaders in health care who set an example for others to follow; they are responsible for writing the textbooks and teaching the teachers of many grades of health worker. They are enormously respected by most patients who are at the same time members of the general public. It is doctors who advise government on the priorities and whose voices are close to the centre of power. Can they rise to the challenge?

Increasingly, doctors are learning to temper the excitement of diagnosis in a sick person with the interest of a community survey; to alternate a postgraduate lecture on coronary bypass, with a talk on training the general public in techniques of coronary resuscitation; to devote resources to haemoglobinometers in place of a computerized scanner. The pace of change is slow but accelerating. It will be up to medical schools to adapt their curriculum to ensure that students are taught in rural areas as well as in the city; are taught about group medicine as well as about care of the individual, and the politics of immunization as well as about measles management. Many medical schools are proceeding in this direction. We hope that readers of this book will see themselves taking on the role of primary health care promoters – described by Mahler as requiring 'sagacity, scientific and technical knowledge, social understanding, managerial acumen and political persuasiveness, and become 'leaders in the social revolution for people's health'.[14]

References

1. Teeling Smith G. *Measurement of Health*. London, Office of Health Economics, 1985.
2. Jackson B. *Fatherhood*. London, George Allen and Unwin, 1983.
3. Yogman MW. The father's influence on child health. In: Macfarlane A. ed. *Progress in Child Health*, Vol 1. Edinburgh, Churchill Livingstone, 1984. pp. 130–56.
4. WHO. *Urbanization and Its Implications for Child Health*. Geneva, World Health Organization. 1988.
5. Sanders D. *The Struggle for Health*. London, Macmillan, 1985.
6. Freire P. *Pedagogy of the Oppressed*. London, Penguin Books, 1972.
7. Werner D, Bower B. *Helping Health Workers Learn*. Palo Alto, Hesperian Foundation, 1982.
8. Shaffer R. *Beyond the Dispensary*. Nairobi, African Medical and Research Foundation, 1983.
9. Rifkin S, Walt G. Selective or comprehensive primary case? *Social Science and Medicine* 1988; **26** (9): 877–977.
10. Aaron A, Hawes H, Gayton J. *Child to Child*. London, Macmillan, 1979.
11. Grant JP/UNICEF. *The State of the World's Children 1984*. Oxford University Press, 1983.
12. Grant JP/UNICEF. *The State of the World's Children 1986*. Oxford University Press, 1985.
13. Ebrahim GJ. *Social and Community Paediatrics in Developing Countries*. Basingstoke, Macmillan, 1985.
14. Mahler H. Primary health care: health for all and the role of doctors. *Tropical Doctor*. 1983; **13**: 146–8.

CHAPTER 2

Cultural aspects of common childhood diseases

Valerian Kimati

Introduction

In reality, traditionalism, fatalism, an overwhelming illiteracy, crushing poverty and a sheer lack of alternatives guarantee the predominant reliance of the people on the practice of traditional medicine in Asia, Africa and Latin America where the majority of the poor Third World population resides. Some of the traditions in the Third World countries do seem similar, although there are large distances between the areas where these traditions exist. The practice of extended families and the concept of 'hot' and 'cold' foods with regard to disease found in South America and India[1], demonstrate surprising similarities in cultures of people living thousands of miles apart.

The means used to cure disease and avoid calamities in infancy and childhood are usually consistent with people's concept of their causes. For example, to placate spirits, gods and goddesses in India, people have used sympathetic and homoeopathic magic, sacrifices, grandmother prescriptions, ordeals, vows, rites, ceremonies, prayers and often extensive ritualistic procedures. It is not only medicine but also blessings which blended together form the curing practices. Consequently, in many instances in India, a sick person not only needs the attention of a medical professional but also the assistance of soothsayers, priests, sadhus (holy men) and other local traditional healers.

Children everywhere can be said to be born into three worlds. The first world is that of culture – customs, ideas and behaviour created for them by their elders and ancestors (traditional KAP = knowledge, attitudes and practices). The children are affected by culture even before they are born. The second world is that of physical environment (desert, snow, mountains, etc.). The third world is that of people, i.e. parents and members of the immediate family (responsible for care of children), witches and sorcerers (responsible for harming children) and traditional healers (responsible for promoting health, preventing illnesses and curing children when diseases strike).

The local cultural pattern is of great importance for child health workers for the following reasons.[2]

- It leads to an understanding of cultural factors underlying disease patterns in the community.
- It gives an insight into people's values, knowledge of and attitudes to health and disease.
- It suggests how to ensure from a population the best cooperation, participation and appreciation of health work carried out by personnel trained in foreign scientific medicine.
- It may enable scientific medicine to become enriched by new ideas, methods and teachings.

Cultural knowledge, attitudes and practices can be classified[2] as those that are good, harmless, uncertain and harmful. It is always advisable to conduct a KAP study before embarking on health education, because only the messages and means of communication which are shaped according to the culture will have beneficial impact. Furthermore, good cultural practices can be utilized by health workers to encourage trust and confidence in their health care provisions.

In this chapter, Africa and Asia are used as typical examples where culture deeply affects child health and childhood disease patterns, as well as management of these diseases. Indian and Tanzanian cultures have been selected to represent Asian and African cultures respectively.

Traditional KAP in relation to culture and childhood diseases

Concept of causes of disease and cure

Both in Africa and Asia, the causes of disease as understood by the majority of rural people fall into two groups; supernatural and physical.

The supernatural causes of diseases such as smallpox, chickenpox and measles, include the wrath of gods and goddesses. In India and neighbouring countries, such as Bangladesh and Pakistan, when a child has measles it is believed that a goddess has visited the home. The goddess has to be propitiated and no medical or other treatment is allowed, to avoid making her angry! As a result of this belief, the child with measles is kept inside the house and visitors are not allowed. The house is kept meticulously clean inside and out, and leaves of the neem tree (which have a bactericidal effect) are exhibited at the front door indicating that there is a child with measles in the house. The child is also bathed with water that has been boiled with leaves of the neem tree. When the skin rash dries out the goddess is believed to have left the house. The child is then sent to the temple where thanksgiving and offerings are made. It is because of this practice that India became virtually the last country in South East Asia to introduce measles vaccine into its immunization programme in 1985.[3]

Cultural patterns and childhood diseases

The five aspects of cultural patterns that are of particular and direct relevance to childhood disease are now considered.

Preparation for parenthood, mating, pregnancy and childbirth

Circumcision   Female circumcision has been practised in a number of African countries but is now declining rapidly. Female circumcision has led to difficulties at delivery (because of extensively scarred external genitalia) and this may affect the newborn child.

A variety of operations, ranging from clitoridectomy to extensive mutilation of labia minora and majora of the female genitalia, have been reported. In many instances the operation is performed by non-skilled practitioners under unhygienic conditions. Serious complications such as surgical shock, bleeding, infection, tetanus and retention of urine, which may lead to death, are not uncommon.

In Sudan and Somalia, the so-called 'Pharaonic circumcision' has been practised on females. In this, the entire clitoris and labia minora and at least the anterior two-thirds of the medial part of the labia majora are removed. The two sides of the vulva are then stitched together by silk or catgut sutures (in the Sudan) or by thorns (in Somalia), thus obliterating the vaginal introitus except for a very small opening posteriorly to allow exit of urine and menstrual blood. Complete occlusion of the introitus is prevented by the insertion of a small piece of wood, usually a matchstick.[4]

Early marriages and preferences for boys   In India, traditionally, boys and girls grow up to look upon marriage as a bond which should not be broken. This has had the effect of making Indian marriages very stable; a good positive cultural aspect which contributes to good child-care and child health development. However, in recent years there have been some suicidal maternal deaths and broken marriages because wives have been unable to settle high dowry demands from their husbands and/or from their husband's relatives. This is mainly an urban phenomenon due to a recent trend towards 'conspicuous consumerism'. This trend if left to increase will adversely affect children of suicidal mothers or broken marriages.

Early marriage has been practised within some communities in India. However, traditionally, girls who were married at a young age stayed with their parents and were allowed to join their husbands when they reached the age of puberty and slightly beyond. In recent years there has been a tendency to let married girls join their husbands before they are old enough to lead a married life. Girls below the age of 20 years who bear children tend to produce low-birth-weight babies, and indeed, 30 per cent of children born in India belong to this category. Early marriage is one cause of the high rate of low-birth-weight infants.

Early childhood and teenage marriages occur in several other Third World countries like Oman, Ethiopia and Sudan.[4] Obvious disadvantages of child marriages include:

- high infant mortality rate;
- high incidence of low-birth-weight infants;
- early interruption of the education of girls;
- necessity of operative surgery during birth.

In Tanzania, circumcision among males and females is practised among some tribes just before marriage. Until recently, male and female circumcision was compulsory by tribal traditions. Female circumcision is rapidly going out of fashion among educated communities in these tribes. Circumcision of males is done during childhood, particularly among the Muslim communities. Among a few tribes, however, circumcision of males takes place when they are about to marry and is supposed to prepare young men to marry and have children. Some tribes in South Tanzania practise circumcision in the bush away from homes. Tetanus, sepsis and meningitis are the complications which await some of the circumcised young people. Those undergoing circumcision also receive sex education. In North East Tanzania, specially nutritious feeds are given to circumcised males and females to make them look attractive to the opposite sex. Whereas circumcision has the possible beneficial effect of protecting males from cancer of the penis, circumcision of females (clitoridectomy) leads to scarring of the vaginal orifice, with the later risk of obstructed labour.

Indian culture has a strong preference for boys. Parental neglect of female children has led to higher morbidity and mortality among female infants and children than among the boys. Female infanticide, until recently, was practised among some Indian communities. At present, the male to female ratio in India is 1000:935; cultural preference for boys directly contributes to this sex ratio.

Marriage among relatives Choice for mating is very important. Marriage among brothers, sisters, first and second cousins leads to a high transmission of genetic diseases. In some parts of India marriage among first cousins is practised, especially among the Muslims and Parsees. Among Muslims and South Indian Hindus, uncles and nieces marry. However, among North Indian Hindus, cousins are regarded as brothers and sisters and do not marry. Sickle-cell disease is common in Tanzania and in some tribal areas in India while β-thalassemia is widespread in India. These two diseases are hereditary and if near relatives marry, the chances of their offspring suffering from either disease will be very high.

In India and Tanzania, pregnant women are encouraged to eat less so that the child in the womb does not become too big and cause obstructed delivery. This practice may contribute to low birth weight and its associated higher mortality.

Childbirth – a dirty process Childbirth in India is regarded as a 'dirty process' in which 'dirty substances' like blood, faeces and urine are involved. Both the child and mother are 'dirty' after birth. In India, the delivery work is traditionally done by the lowest caste, the untrained birth attendant, with consequent high infant morbidity and mortality rate. In Nepal, up to 90 per cent of mothers in some areas deliver babies at home by themselves without assistance. It is also customary not to touch the mother and the baby until 40 days have elapsed after delivery. Such cultural trends have harmful effects on the newborn. In many places in India immunization cannot start earlier than three months because the baby and mother are regarded as dirty during this period and should not be touched. This may lead to some children contracting whooping cough or tuberculosis before they receive DPT or BCG at three months.

Indigenous medical systems

In India and the neighbouring states of Sri Lanka, Bangladesh, Pakistan, Afghanistan and Nepal, traditional, formal, indigenous medical systems exist beside the Western allopathic medical system. Ayurveda, Unani, Siddha, Homoeopathy and Naturopathy are medical systems that have existed in India for centuries.[5] Most of these systems have training and research institutions all over the country. The Government of India manages these indigenous medical systems side by side with allopathic medicine. It is worth noting that these 'scientific' systems have a 'scientific' basis just like the Chinese acupuncture system. However, there are also other non-formal traditional systems of illness management which have a deep cultural basis but lack a scientific background. While these practices may have some marginal beneficial psychological effect on the sick or may be harmless, some can be extremely harmful. Examples of such systems in India are bone-setters, herbalists, and a large group of people generally known as 'quacks'.

The indigenous traditional medical systems are well known to the people who have deep-rooted faith in them. The practitioners of these systems are found in rural as well as in urban areas (although practitioners of allopathic medicine are mostly found in urban areas). Most people use traditional systems of cure first, or side by side with Western medicine. The Indian government has been trying to integrate the Western and indigenous medical systems by running two different directorates of these systems within the Health Ministry.

In Tanzania, the traditional healers do not have systematized, indigenous medical systems. Most of the traditional indigenous practitioners have learned their art from their parents or near-relatives. Some of their skills are useful in the field of mental health, psychological problems, and chronic illnesses and some herbs have positive pharmacological effects. A recent study done by anthropologist Raimo Harjula in Tanzania[6], indicated that a local traditional medicine man managed diarrhoea in children according to the following format.

- Symptoms: toddler's diarrhoea with flatulence but without blood in stools
- Aetiology: dirty or unsuitable food
- Remedy: 'Mamiso' – a local name of a local plant (*Bidens pilosah*)
- Usage: the flowers of this plant are boiled and the solution is administered as the remedy – 15–20 flowers are needed for one dose taken twice a day

The plant has been chemically analysed and its extracts have shown antibacterial activity against a variety of microorganisms, including five enteric pathogens. One merit of the remedy is that the child gets some sort of oral rehydrant which may be beneficial, although the rehydrant may not have the amount of salts required.

Each practitioner has his or her own methods. Some of their treatments have no scientific basis and are often harmless, but some can, at times, be harmful. There is a traditional healers association which is largely a trade union rather than a professional body. The Government of Tanzania has set up a research unit[7] to study cures that might have a scientific basis and to attempt to integrate them into the national health system.

Food habits and taboos

Food habits have deep psychological roots and are associated with love, affection, warmth, self-image and social prestige. Diet is influenced by local conditions (soil, climate) and religious customs and beliefs. Vegetarianism is given a place of honour in Hindu society[5]. Hindus (over 75 per cent of India's population) do not eat beef. Children of a pure vegetarian society do not

get access to animal protein, except milk. Animal protein is abundant in most parts of India and the cultural taboo in giving animal protein (beef) to children may contribute to iron and folate deficiency. However, it is important to note that pure vegetarianism (no milk and milk products) may protect against metabolic diseases such as gout and hypercholesterolaemia. Muslims abhor pork for religious reasons. Eggs (which are excellent animal protein) are forbidden in some parts of India among pure vegetarians and among pregnant women. Women and children are forbidden to eat eggs in most African cultures, including Tanzania. Eating and drinking from common utensils is considered a sign of brotherhood among Indians and Tanzanians, but diseases such as oral and gastro-intestinal infections can be spread easily in this way. Hindus, especially those from the South, do not eat from a common plate. They will not put their lips to a glass of water, but rather pour water into the mouth so that the glass remains clean for somebody else to use. Men are served the best part of the food; children and women take whatever remains, usually quantitatively smaller amounts and qualitatively inferior with adverse nutritional consequences on the mother and child.

In India, high-protein foods like meat and milk are considered 'hot' foods and not given in diseases such as diarrhoea, fever and measles. Pregnant and nursing women are not given eggs, meat or even some legumes and vegetables because they are considered 'hot'. In winter, 'cold' things are eaten. Whereas milk is considered 'hot', buttermilk (which also has a high protein content) is considered 'cold' and can be given in diarrhoea.

Child-rearing practices

The cultural practices of rearing children may be classified as good, harmless, uncertain and harmful.[2]

Prolonged breast-feeding which is prevalent in Asia and Africa is good for infant nutrition and is an effective contraceptive in areas where family planning facilities are not available.[8] The habit of abandoning breast-feeding following an episode of diarrhoea in the child (the mother's milk being pinpointed as the cause of the diarrhoea) results in more diarrhoea and increasing malnutrition (see Fig. 1.2.1.).

In India, application of oil or paste of turmeric on the anterior fontanelle is harmless. The practice of applying black soot mixed with oil to the eyelids, partly for beautification and partly warding off the effects of 'evil eye', has uncertain effects on the child which cannot yet be said to be a good or bad practice. Usually it is

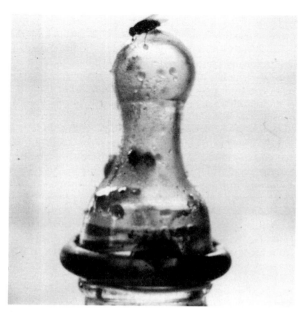

Fig. 1.2.1   A dirty milk bottle teat used to feed an infant with artificial milk in India.

harmless medicated carbon oil, but if it contains lead could lead to poisoning (see Fig. 1.2.2).

However, certain practices in child-rearing have deleterious effects on the health of children. For example, the practice in India (and in Tanzania) of applying cow dung to the umbilicus of the newborn is a cause of annual deaths of up to a quarter of a million infants with neonatal tetanus. The practice of late introduction of weaning food contributes to the prevalence of childhood malnutrition both in India and in Tanzania. The practice of leaving infants with younger children or of the mother taking the child to the fields, leads to the infants being fed less frequently with bad nutritional consequences. The well-known custom, in some parts of India and Tanzania, of not giving colostrum to newborns is responsible for the neonatal marasmus sometimes seen. In Tanzania, cases of neonatal marasmus have been reported as a result of the child being given only water after birth until the milk is 'clean'.

Patterns of household authority

The man is the head of the family and has absolute and final authority in the home among the major tribes in Tanzania, wives being completely subservient. This long-standing cultural pattern seems to have created an atmosphere of relative marriage stability, ensuring stable child-care by both parents. However, among the educated and Western-oriented couples, families are run more democratically, with the wife sharing home management authority with the husband, although the husband still remains the functional head of the family. Development of an 'anti-cultural' women's liberation movement among the educated class in Tanzania, has led to family arguments and disputes as to who should have the final say on home management. This trend seems to have led to rather unstable marriages, with adverse consequences for child-care and child health among the educated élite.

In India, the male is usually the head of the family. However, in southern India, and elsewhere among more tribal communities, the head of the family is sometimes the female. This partly explains why, in the Kerala state of India, women are so highly literate with high status in the community. Kerala today enjoys a far lower infant mortality rate than the Government of India's goal set for the year 2000! The female family headship has contributed to this.[9]

Physical environment and geographical surroundings

Sanitary habits are influenced by climate, topography, level of education, economy, culture and religious customs and beliefs. Lack of sanitation leads to common diseases such as diarrhoea, respiratory infections and intestinal worms.

Disposal of excreta

In Tanzania, about 30 per cent of homes have latrines for disposal of human waste. However, intestinal worms are one of the main reasons for attendance at government health units, second only to malaria. The Muslim population in Tanzania, for religious reasons, clean the anus with fingers and water after defaecation. In India, most of the population use water and hands to wash the anus after defaecation. Where water is not available, stones or leaves are used. Long finger nails and improper cleaning of fingers after defaecation makes it possible for ova to remain on the hands and so contaminate food. Others who use paper to clean the anus after defaecation may also contaminate their fingers, and if they eat with the unclean fingers are liable to infect others or themselves.

About 90 per cent of the people in rural India use the open fields for defaecation. This practice is time-honoured and considered to be harmless. The average

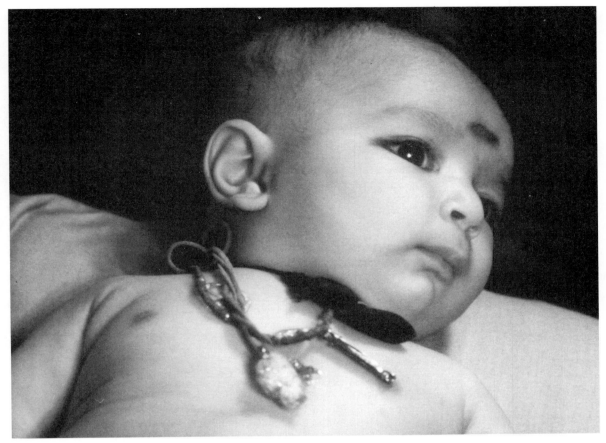

Fig. 1.2.2 An Indian child with black paste on her face and eyelids and wearing 'protective' charms.

Indian villager is averse to the idea of latrines. He considers that latrines are meant for city dwellers, where there are no fields for defaecation. He is unaware that faeces are infectious, pollute water and soil and promote fly breeding. Thus, the problem of excreta disposal is bound up with beliefs and habits based on ignorance.[8] Indiscriminate defaecation pollutes rivers or man-made furrows and canals, or contaminates vegetables and fruits which, if not properly cleaned or cooked, can be a source of intestinal helminth infections.

Disposal of wastes

In Tanzania and India, the average villager is affected by mosquitoes that breed where there is a collection of waste water, and as a result malaria is endemic. In rural homes, as well as in urban slums, the solid refuse

from the house is allowed to accumulate in front of the houses leading to housefly breeding. This is a common source of diarrhoea and other infections.

Water supply

In India, the well occupies a pivotal place in the villages. It is a place where animals are washed and allowed to drink. Such practices pollute the well water. Some rivers are considered holy and pilgrims go to these rivers to have a dip and to drink the raw water, which they consider sacred. Samples of holy water are bottled and carried over long distances for distribution among friends and relatives. Epidemics of cholera and gastroenteritis have resulted from these cultural practices. Step-wells in the states of Rajasthan and Madhya Pradesh of India are associated with guinea-worm disease (dracunculiasis), as the water is highly infested with the cyclops which carry guinea-worms (see p. 649).

Housing and animals

Normal rural houses in India are usually ill-lit, ill-ventilated (without windows for security reasons), small and often overcrowded. This encourages spread of respiratory diseases like tuberculosis. The same pattern of housing appears in Tanzania. Indians love animals and cows are considered sacred. Cows and buffaloes are important and economically valuable. Infrequently human beings and animals live under the same roof. Dogs are also considered sacred in some parts of India and live in the houses with human beings. The practice of living with animals encourages zoonotic diseases. Some home-kept pet dogs in New Delhi, India have been found to be carriers of rabies. In Tanzania, some tribal cultures involve living under the same roof with cows and this leads to frequent contact with cow dung which usually carries tetanus bacilli. Both in India and Tanzania neonatal tetanus is very common and contributes to 25–50 per cent of neonatal deaths.

The family

In India as well as in Tanzania the extended family system is common; more so in rural agricultural areas than in urban, where gradual erosion by education and industrialization is occurring. Extended families consist of a married couple or married couples, children, sisters, brothers, cousins, parents and even grandparents. The merit of the extended family system is based on the motto 'union is strength'. There is sharing of responsibilities in almost all matters, thus giving the family greater economic security and social support for the old, the helpless and the unemployed. The family pools its income to help the young through school, to pay for marriage, or to begin a commercial venture. It offers many of the services and advantages which an industrial society offers through more impersonal governmental, educational and financial agencies.

Because of a common environment, diseases such as tuberculosis, scabies, measles, mumps and diarrhoea spread rapidly in families.

Among broken families, separation of the child from one or both parents is an important factor in child development. Children who are victims of broken families early in their childhood, sometimes display in later years, psychopathic behaviour, immature personality, and retardation of growth, speech and intellect. Not infrequently, children from these families drift into prostitution, crime and vagrancy.[8]

People: roles in childhood diseases

Role of parents

The mother usually takes absolute care of infants and children up to a certain age, while the father provides education and teaches the children about traditions and customs with regard to feeding, nutrition, hygiene, sleep, clothing, discipline, etc. The role of the parents is to provide physical care of their young in order that they may reach adulthood, perpetuate the family and take care of the parents in their old age. Some childhood diseases are derived from deficiency of parental care, lack of education and harmful traditions. Many parents are unable to fulfil their proper role, particularly urban migrants. They are very poor and cannot provide for even the minimum physical and emotional needs of their children. Some underlying factors such as poverty, illness, mental and emotional instability and marital disharmony, undermine the ability of parents to bring up children and lead to a high risk of malnutrition and disease. Later these children become victims of child labour, prostitution, crime and vagrancy. This situation exists in both India and Tanzania.

Parents are responsible for seeking help for their sick children, but the person they consult depends very much on the customs and beliefs discussed earlier. The extended family in rural India and Tanzania provides support to handicapped children (as well as to aged and infirm adults). The husband takes care of the pregnant wife (and the unborn child). Some tribes in Tanzania provide special care and rest to pregnant women during the last trimester, and after the birth the mother is confined to the house for three to six months being 'fattened' by specially nutritious food (meat and milk diets). A man who fails to provide such a service to his wife (and unborn child), is liable to be accused in a family or community court and be fined if found guilty. This is a good tradition which should decrease the low-birth-weight rate as well as improving breast-feeding and child nutrition. The preference for a male child in Indian culture[10] as well as in Tanzanian culture[11] tends to lead to parental neglect of girls, and hence greater morbidity and mortality among girls than among boys.

Role of witches

In Tanzania, witches are believed to exist and are regarded as enemies to the community. Witches both here and in India, are regarded as supernatural beings who unpredictably and malevolently bring sickness, cause accidents and kill. Some tribes in Tanzania allege that community disasters (like epidemics, drought and famine) derive from the action of witches, and sometimes communities hunt for the witches, banish them to far areas and even take justice into their hands and kill the suspected witches. Both in India and Tanzania, children are protected from witches' 'evil eyes' by wearing charms (see Fig. 1.2.2) and amulets, etc. If a child is thought to have been bewitched, the local medicine man (traditional healer) is summoned to cure her by propitiation and by a wide variety of magical manipulations. The belief in witches is common even among élitist Tanzanians and seeking a traditional fortune teller or healer is popular even among civil servants and politicians in India. The cultural belief in witches is a common cause of late referral to hospitals of ill children, resulting in high mortality and disability, because parents consult the traditional healer first.

Role of traditional healers

Vaids

Among the many thousands of traditional health practitioners in rural India are the vaids, whose practice is based upon knowledge found in ancient texts of Hindu literature, and the Hakims who practice a form of medicine that was brought in with the Muslims and Persian scripts. There are also traditional healers whose actions have a psychological rather than scientific basis, such as sellers of magic charms which ward off sickness; the snake-bite curer who usually comes from the lower castes, and the exorcist who is the Eastern counterpart of the faith healer in the West.

Tanzania has a mixture of herbalists, magic curers, fortune tellers and 'devil chasers'. Some traditional herbalists claim to cure various illnesses. There is no system for documenting traditional healers' knowledge and practices.

Dais

The dai in India is a midwifery practitioner who operates on the basis of age-old traditions and customs. She inherits her caste occupation (as most people do in rural India) and generally comes from the lowest caste. She is not socially welcome in the higher caste homes, except when a prospective mother goes into labour. Her work of delivering a child is considered menial because during and immediately after delivery the mother and newborn are believed to be in a condition of pollution

and defilement. Delivery by untrained dais in India has been one of the major causes of a high infant mortality rate. The dais, because of their special position in the community, are being trained by the Government (1 per 1000 people) so that they can carry out deliveries in a safer way.[10] (See also pp. 94–5)

Registered medical practitioners (RMPs) in India

There are two types of RMP – the formally trained and those without formal training. The Ayurvedic and Unani practitioners are officially registered as RMPs and most of these have formal training in respective medical institutions. The Ayurvedic, Unani, Siddha and Homoeopathic medical systems were discussed earlier. The second type of RMPs have been trained as assistants to allopathic doctors or have had experience under allopathic doctors, and have undergone an examination to become RMPs in villages where no officially recognized doctor is available. The official recognition of these paraprofessionals, with some practical knowledge of Western medicine but limited formal education, was part of the Government effort to provide health services to the rural areas. There are also rural medical practitioners who are not registered and known as 'quacks'. RMPs are traditionally acceptable and accessible in all parts of remote rural India, as they come from the communities they work in and in most cases are the only medical help available in such areas. Remembering that formal allopathic health services only reach 30 per cent of the populations, RMPs have a great role in providing health services to the remaining 70 per cent of the population (including about 10 per cent coverage by registered private practitioners and recognized doctors).

Concluding remarks

It is appropriate to conclude by repeating the comments at the beginning of this chapter: that children everywhere are born into three worlds, ie. the worlds of culture, physical environment and people. These are responsible for many of the causes as well as the outcomes of major childhood diseases occurring in Asia and Africa, as exemplified here by India and Tanzania respectively. The relationship between believed causes of some major diseases, the treatment given by the traditional healer and the possible efficacy or harmful effects of such treatment is shown in Table 1.2.1; only a few examples are listed. Table 1.2.2 lists some cultural practices that can lead to morbidity and mortality in India and Tanzania; while Table 1.2.3 lists some

Table 1.2.1   Examples of possible effects of cultural knowledge, attitude and practices with regard to some childhood diseases in Tanzania

Childhood disease problem	'Cause'	Treatment or prevention through traditional healer or by standard medicines	Possible efficacy or harmful effects of treatment
Measles	Bad air	Treatment aims to encourage the skin rash to come out. Skin applicants can be red soil, ashes of banana leaves, water boiled with sugar-cane leaves or with leaves of other plants. Oral drink may be given in some cultures e.g. chicken soup (chicken must have a black colour), fish soup, water boiled with sugar-cane leaves	The results may be beneficial e.g. the skin applicants may have a soothing effect The soup serves as oral rehydrant with some nutritive values. In allopathic medicine, after all, there is no treatment against the virus and treatment is conservative
Tapeworms	Meat given to children (whether cooked or uncooked)	Some traditional cultures do not allow meat to be given to children under 2–5 years. Symptoms are treated by giving a bush herb which has positive pharmacological effect in expelling the worm	Eating the herb, results in visible expulsion of the worm
Convulsions	Demons or spirits	(a) Smoke inhalation administered as dry burning faeces of elephant. (b) Charms are worn. (c) Vigorous traditional dances and other rituals are performed to expel the demon or the spirit	Convulsions occur in serious diseases, e.g. cerebral malaria, meningitis, tetanus, encephalitis. Any time wasted without hospitalization will lead to almost 100% mortality
Pneumonia/ body swelling	Bad circulating blood	Blood-letting performed by making surgical incisions on the chest and upper abdomen (in pneumonia) or on top of the body swelling	Can lead to anaemia and tetanus
Diarrhoea	Recurrent diarrhoea said to be caused by bad breast-milk	Stopping breast-feeding is prescribed by healers and grandmothers; artificial milk replaces breast-feeding	Leads to further diarrhoea and malnutrition
Chronic cough/ tuberculosis	Elongated uvula said to cause chronic cough	Traditional uvulectomy is done	Harmful effects include anaemia, septicaemia, aspiration pneumonia and tetanus

cultural practices that can prevent childhood diseases and promote child health.

It is important for Western medical practitioners to be familiar with the knowledge, attitude and practices of communities with regard to major diseases before they embark on health education. Health education for behavioural change is a highly specialized field not to be tackled by amateurs. A thorough KAP study is necessary in communities, so that its results can be used to construct appropriate messages which have both a cultural slant and a scientific basis. Appropriate means must be used, which are known traditionally in the community, to achieve the desired impact (or behavioural change). Health messages are best designed by experts such as advertising agencies and market research agencies, rather than by health professionals who have no training in communication. The most suitable media for health education can also be determined from a KAP study. The people who convey messages of health education must be people from the community who are well trusted. Use of community health workers (volunteers), local youth organizations, local religious leaders, local opinion leaders and local elected councillors, will produce a better impact than the use of foreign health-care workers. Harmful practices will be the main concern of the child health worker, and will require modification by friendly persuasion in the form of personal or group discussion

Table 1.2.2　Cultural practices that can lead to morbidity and mortality in India and Tanzania

Cultural practice	Cultural reasons	Countries where practised	Morbidity/mortality
Colostrum not given to infants	Believed to be dirty and bad milk	In some parts of India and Tanzania	Colostrum gives extra immunity to child, lack of which makes children more susceptible to infectious disease and death
Late weaning	Child unable to digest food before walking	Widely practised in India and Tanzania and many Third World countries	After 6 months, mothers milk alone is insufficient to supply enough calories to the child. Lack of introduction of weaning food at 4–6 months leads to protein energy malnutrition and its sequelae
Cow dung, soil or ashes applied to umbilical cord after birth	Believed to stop bleeding. Cow dung from the sacred cow in India is believed to have healing and blessing effects	India, Tanzania and many Third World countries	Likely to give rise to neonatal tetanus whose case fatality rate may be up to over 90% even with medical treatment. In UP*, neonatal tetanus contributes over 50% of neonatal mortality rate
Starvation in diarrhoea	To let all dirt in the stomach be washed out	In some parts of India and other Asian countries	Results in dehydration leading to malnutrition and even death
Administration of various herbs in health and disease	E.g. herbs to relieve constipation or herbs to cure disease (no dosage standard of these herbs)	India and Tanzania	Toxic doses may be administered, sometimes leading to death
Female circumcision	Believed to prevent woman being too sexual and hence becoming unfaithful after marriage	Tanzania, Sudan and some other African countries	Causes obstructed labour in pregnancy because of scarring. Can lead to sepsis, anaemia and tetanus when done under unhygienic conditions
Traditional uvulectomy	Prevents and cures respiratory diseases	Tanzania, Ethiopia	Can cause anaemia, sepsis, pneumonia and tetanus
Extreme dietary restriction in pregnancy and disease	Fetus will be small enough not to obstruct labour	Tanzania, Uganda, India and Burma	Leads to low birth weight with high mortality
Preference for male children	Useful to continue propagating name of the family, more useful in supporting parents	India (with direct evidence) and Tanzania (with only indirect evidence, see Ref. 11)	Cause of higher morbidity (including malnutrition) among female children. Neglect of ill female child leads to premature and unnecessary death. In old days infanticide was practised in some parts of India
Consultation of traditional practitioners first and hospitals later	This is because of cultural attitude and placing more faith in traditional medicine than in Western medicine	Tanzania, India and in most Third World countries	Delays management of severe diseases leading to high mortality rate and disability

*UP = Uttar Pradesh – the most populous (110 million) of the 22 states and union territories in India.

Table 1.2.3   Cultural practices that can lead to prevention of childhood diseases and promotion of health

Cultural items	Reasons	Countries where practised	Possible advantages in disease prevention and promotion of health
Performance of various rituals as done or prescribed by traditional medicine man	Person with mental disease or psychological conditions	India and Tanzania	Can lead to relief of symptoms and possible cure
Prolonged breast-feeding	Believed to be best food for infants and children	India, Tanzania and nearly all Third World countries (except in some urban areas)	True, breast-feeding is best. Besides good physical growth, it provides immunity against most common killing diseases like diarrhoea and acute respiratory infections
Vigorous mouth washes	Mouth is dirty after meals	India (Hindus)	Prevents dental caries
Vegetarianism	Animals are generally regarded as sacred among Hindus	India	Provided enough plant proteins are consumed, this practice prevents intestinal worms and may protect against future coronary heart disease
Extra feeding and rest of mother after birth	To enable mother to have enough milk	Some parts of Tanzania	Ensures enough breast-milk for the child
Administration of galactogogues to mothers who fail to lactate or to women who have to breast-feed an orphaned infant		India, Tanzania	Enables motherless infants in the families to survive
Mother who has just given birth and child not to be touched for 40 days or so after birth	They are supposed to be dirty	Some parts of India and Nepal	Prevents bacterial contamination of mother and child from other people
Use of leaves of neem tree	Used to put in front of house door or to boil in bathing water for the child with measles	Widely used in India	Neem leaves have bactericidal effects and may perhaps prevent secondary bacterial infections in measles
Practice of wide utilization of indigenous systems of medicine, i.e. Ayurveda, Siddha and Unani	People have strong faith in these systems through tradition. Considered to be useful and curative during disease	India, Sri Lanka, Pakistan, Bangladesh, Nepal, Afghanistan	These systems of medicine have a 'scientific' basis and they are as useful as allopathic systems of medicine

and convincing demonstration. The ill-effects of a particular custom may then be modified, while at the same time the essence of the culturally accepted practice is retained. For example, cow's milk, which is classified as 'hot' should not be given to children recovering from diarrhoea in the state of West Bengal in India. However, buttermilk which is classified as 'cold' can be given. By advising the child to have buttermilk after diarrhoea, an increased protein intake can be achieved within the cultural framework of the Bengali village.

The following examples illustrate what can happen when the wrong means of communication is used. In Pakistan, a media campaign was launched some years ago to encourage the consumption of iodized salt. The posters used during this campaign portrayed unveiled women afflicted with goitre. Shortly after the campaign had begun not a single poster could be found intact. They had all been torn down by the conservative Muslim community which strongly disapproved of women revealing themselves in this way.[12] During a family planning programme in a remote Asian community, bamboo poles were used in demonstrating to men how condoms were to be used. Several months later, the trainers were confronted by groups of angry young women who were pregnant. Investigations revealed that the men had kept their condoms at the end of the bamboo poles![13]

The target audience can effectively receive a message through an appropriate means if we know something about their knowledge, attitude and practices.

The traditional healers and practitioners have the trust of the local population. If we are serious about reducing morbidity, mortality and disabilities due to diseases related to cultural beliefs, attitudes and practices, we must use the traditional healers as potential allies in carrying and disseminating health education messages for behavioural change and health promotion. A positive behavioural change becomes the new and beneficial cultural practice.

References

1. Romney K, and Romney R. The Kixtecans of Just-lahuanca Mexico. In: Whiting BB ed. *Six Cultures: Studies of Child Rearing*. New York, John Wiley and Sons, 1963. pp. 619.

2. William CD, Jelliffe DB. *Mother and Child Health: Delivering the Services*. Oxford, Oxford University Press, 1989.

3. The Ministry of Health and Family Welfare, Government of India. *Towards Universal Immunization*, 1985.

4. WHO/EMRO. *Traditional Practices Affecting the Health of Women and Children*. (Report of a seminar, Khartoum, 10–15 February 1979 – WHO Regional Office for Eastern Mediterranean, Alexandria). Technical Publication No. 2, 1979.

5. Nandi PK. Cultural constraints on professionalization. In: Giri Raj Gupta ed. *Social and Cultural Context of Medicine in India*. New Delhi, Vikas Publishing House, 1981. pp. 151–4.

6. Raimo Harjula. *Mirau and His Practice: A Study of the Ethnomedicinal Repertoire of a Tanzanian Herbalist*. London, Trimed Books, 1978.

7. WHO. *The Traditional Medicine and Health Care Coverage*. Bannerman RH, Chen wen Chieh eds, Geneva, WHO 1983.

8. Park JE, Park K. *Textbook of Preventive and Social Medicine*. 10th edn. India, M/s Banarsidas Bhanot, 1985.

9. Grant JP/UNICEF. *The State of the World's Children 1984*. Oxford University Press, 1983.

10. UNICEF *An Analysis of the Situation of Children in India*. New Delhi, UNICEF Regional Office for South Central Asia. 1984: 32.

11. Kimati VP, Scrimshaw NS. The nutritional status of under fives in Tanzania: anthropometric approach. *East African Medical Journal*. 1985; **62**: 105–17.

12. Mason D, Azhar R. Don't just say salt. *UNICEF News*. 1982; **114/4**.

13. Okwesa A. How the message does not get through. *UNICEF News*. 1982; **114/4**.

CHAPTER 3

Primary health care

F. J. Bennett

Introduction

Many of the major illnesses and causes of death in children are preventable by simple measures or changes in the personal behaviour of parents. Similarly, disability could easily be reduced from its present level of one in ten and growth and development of children enhanced, so that malnutrition would be less common. All this can be achieved not by medical care in institutions but by health care within the family or community. And yet where are most doctors and nurses content to expend their energy? Are their knowledge and skills directed only to the benefit of the sick or also to keeping individuals and families healthy? In fact, every doctor and nurse can be a health worker as well as a medical worker – it is a question of motivation and orientation. Primary health care (PHC) requires this reorientation of all health workers to see their role in relation to individuals, families, communities the district and the nation; but with the focal point being individuals within family and community. This also entails a change in horizon, from bedside clinical medicine to an epidemiological vision of wider problems requiring solution, with participation of the affected people in the places where most needed and at the times when most relevant.

Alma-Ata and the definition of primary health care

The International Conference on Primary Health Care held in Alma-Ata in 1978, which provided a new blueprint for health care, came as the result of accumulating evidence that existing health policies throughout the world were not proving adequate – that there were options for improvement. The most disturbing aspect of health services, especially in developing countries, was that they were unable to arrest the deteriorating national health status. These trends included, firstly, spending more and more on expensive, high-technology, hospital-based specialized activities for a minority, to the detriment of cheaper more widely applicable and effective technology for priority problems. Secondly, there was the increasing concentration of resources (financial, material and manpower) in urban areas, largely catering for the better-off urban residents, leaving the rural majority poorly served. Thirdly, there was greater emphasis on curative work and on disease, rather than on preventive and promotive aspects related to individuals within their family and community environments. Fourthly, there was an emphasis on what could be done by services, rather than on what could be done by individuals and families. These trends were especially noticed at the independence of countries from colonization, when there was a realization that the hospital-based systems they had been left with were providing health care which could not reach the people. In the 1960s and early 1970s, there had continued to be a downward trend in infant mortality rate but this decelerated and stagnated in the late 1970s. The socio-economic causes of ill health then came more clearly into focus. Some countries started experimenting with a new system which allowed for the development of resources and self-reliance within communities and which cast the national services in a more supportive role. *Health by the People*,[1] published in 1975, describes those new initiatives and also heralded an awareness of the great strides that China had made in improving health for a considerable proportion of the world's population.

The Alma-Ata Conference in 1978 provided a set of definitions and guidelines which has proved to be comprehensive. The 22 recommendations formulated are all very relevant for the development of PHC. Unfortunately, the language used in the conference report is often regarded as difficult because it is so condensed and uses terms that have more meaning for social scientists than for the average doctor or nurse. Within the definition lie four crucial new elements which make PHC different from previous attempts at providing basic services. These are:

- Political will to assure equity of resource distribution.
- Community participation and involvement.
- Intersectoral cooperation for health.
- Appropriate technology for health at family and community levels with these levels becoming the focal point of the health system.

For reference purposes, the full definition of PHC follows. It should be studied repeatedly and provides a 'minimum' statement of what PHC includes.

The Declaration of Alma-Ata states that:

Primary health care is essential health care based on practical, scientifically sound and socially acceptable methods and technology made universally accessible to individuals and families in the community through their full participation, and at a cost that the community and country can afford to maintain at every stage of their development in the spirit of self-reliance and self-determination. It forms an integral part both of the country's health system, of which it is the central function and main focus, and of the overall social and economic development of the community. It is the first level of contact of individuals, family and community with the national health system, bringing health care as close as possible to where people live and work, and constitutes the first element of a continuing health care process.

Primary Health Care:

1. reflects and evolves from the economic conditions and socio-cultural and political characteristics of the country and its communities and is based on the application of the relevant results of social, biomedical and health services research and public health experience;
2. addresses the main health problems in the community, providing promotive, preventive, curative and rehabilitative services accordingly;
3. includes at least: education concerning prevailing health problems and the methods of preventing and controlling them; promotion of food supply and proper nutrition; an adequate supply of safe water and basic sanitation; maternal and child health care, including family planning; immunization against the major infectious diseases; prevention and control of locally endemic diseases; appropriate treatment of common diseases and injuries; and provision of essential drugs; (the eight essential elements of PHC).
4. involves, in addition to the health sector, all related sectors and aspects of national and community development, in particular agriculture, animal husbandry, food, industry, education, housing, public works, communications and other sectors; and demands the coordinated efforts of all those sectors;
5. requires and promotes maximum community and individual self-reliance and participation in the planning, organization, operation and control of primary health care, making fullest use of local, national, and other available resources; and to this end develops through appropriate education the ability of communities to participate;
6. should be sustained by integrated, functional and mutually supportive referral systems, leading to the progressive improvement of comprehensive health care for all, and giving priority to those most in need;
7. relies, at local and referral levels, on health workers, including physicians, nurses, midwives, auxiliaries and community workers as applicable, as well as traditional practitioners as needed, suitably trained socially and technically, to work as a health team and to respond to the expressed health needs of the community.

(Adapted by permission from *Primary Health Care*. Report of the International Conference on Primary Health Care, Alma Ata, USSR. Geneva, WHO, 1978.)

Embodied within this definition and statement can be discerned certain principles (equity, health as part of social and economic development, self-reliance) and also certain important new or newly emphasized strategies. Besides the four crucial new elements previously mentioned (which are also strategies) there is also now an emphasis on the 'essential elements' of PHC. Restructuring of the health services with improved management is also implicit if the principles and strategies are to be put into practice.

Progress in defining primary health care

Since Alma-Ata, a series of publications have come from WHO (*Health for All*)[3] which have further elaborated the PHC strategy at both national and global levels. PHC has become, in quite a short time, the accepted key to reaching the social target of attainment by all people of the world by the year 2000, of a 'level of health that will permit them to lead a socially and economically productive life'. The series of publications on managerial process, indicators and global strategy, are filled with terms that need interpretation and so a glossary has been produced which defines, for example, community involvement, community participation, self-care, community health worker and self-reliance.

In many countries, however, workshops have had to be convened to enable workers from different sectors to come to their own definitions within their own context.

In Kenya, for example, the word 'community' has been debated and the following is an example of a definition which indicates some of the important features to be considered when starting the training of community health workers:

A community is a group of *families* falling into a small administrative area – they share common goals and problems and a common system of communication. They are sociologically and psychologically linked and recognize themselves as a community. They have common traditions and leadership and fall into a geographical area where a census can be taken to form a 'denominator' for health work.[2]

In many societies in Africa, there is a local term which fits the above concept.

Other words and phrases in the original PHC definition which have had their implications explored are 'universally accessible', 'full participation', 'cost that community and country can afford', 'self-reliance' and 'central function and main focus'.

'Availability' is defined as the ratio of population to health facilities and personnel, whilst 'accessibility' is measured by the proportion of population that can be expected to use a facility or service. Access can be thought of in terms of physical access, economic access or cultural access and would vary for different types of service. For example, how accessible would a maternity service be, which charges fees and is staffed largely by males, for women who come from a poor Muslim community two hours away on foot? Many countries are now trying to establish norms of at least physical accessibility for their primary and referral services.

'Participation' in the past has often been equated, by health workers, with compliance but the term 'community involvement' comes closer to what is intended: active involvement in some form of organization in the planning, operation and control of PHC using local, national and other resources. In this concept there is also an implication that individuals and families assume, in an informed way, responsibility for their own health and welfare and that of the community. As the end of the century approaches and the target 'health for all by the year 2000' becomes less and less realistic, the concept of involvement of people in their health makes 'all for health by the year 2000' a much more realistic and meaningful target.

The inclusion of the words 'self-reliance' and 'affordability' in the PHC definition, means that people use measures that they can apply themselves and which are closely linked to the viability of the technology for health.

The reorientation of health services to make PHC the central function and main focus has, however, been slow, as the perspective in many countries is still dominated by hospital and Ministry of Health functions. However, efforts at decentralization of services to the district in many countries have now helped to focus more on the community and health centre levels.

Politics and equity of resource distribution

A joint study by UNICEF and WHO of national decision-making for primary health care[4], coined the phrase that decisions on equitable resource allocation for health care are the 'litmus-test' of political commitment to PHC. Careful appraisal of resources provided by level of care, geographical area, degree of urbanization and social class should thus show a swing towards greater equity of distribution if the principles of PHC are being accepted by a country. Perhaps this problem is best illustrated by figures from Zambia, where the teaching hospital in the capital city used 40 per cent of the recurrent allocation for health, so that expenditure per capita in health in that city is 12.27 K (53 cents USA) as compared with 0.6 K (2.6 cents USA) spent per capita in rural areas served by health centres. Some countries, in the early enthusiasm for restructuring their health services, were able to demonstrate such a swing – with increased funds for rural health centres, more community nurses, essential drugs and immunization programmes, and slower increases in hospital expenditure. Increasing population and spiralling inflation, national debts, greater expenditure on defence and foreign exchange problems, coupled with increased costs of hospital care, have slowed or even reversed this process. Greater political commitment, sustained and loud advocacy for the underserved and further strategies for giving renewed emphasis to PHC are required.

Many countries are decentralizing the management of health and other services to the district level. This step, if it is accompanied by adequate financial resources, will facilitate planning for priority problems and stimulate community-based health activities. Unfortunately, the growth of cities with their louder political voice continues to require more hospitals and specialists. The money spent on health care per capita in urban areas is many times that spent in rural areas.

It is clear that the solution to this problem of resources is to be found in people becoming more aware of what they themselves can do to develop healthier life-styles, and of how they can take essential preventive measures and become involved in community-based health care. Another source of resources, till now little tapped, is the contribution that other sectors could make to health if they defined their roles more clearly.

Many countries, e.g. Tanzania, have a national document on PHC which sets out guidelines and clearly demonstrates the national commitment. These documents are very useful in defining the policy from which more local projects of community-based activities can derive their support. In the final analysis, the only real indicator of acceptance of PHC as a national strategy is the reallocation of resources on an equitable basis.

Community involvement

If community involvement in health care can be considered to have occurred only when people are empowered to take an active role in planning, management and evaluation of activities, then it differs considerably from mere participation in some programme organized by a health service. Much has been written about the oppressive, inhibiting effects of both donors and imposed or authoritarian committees on community involvement and on the delicate role of outsiders in stimulating or catalysing real involvement.

David Werner and Bill Bower in their book *Helping Health Workers Learn*[5] have developed this theme with numerous telling illustrations and anecdotes, and the text is almost a short cut to the process of reorientation of health workers for working and learning together with communities. The very title of this book deserves careful thought, as it is the basis of an internal change that is a prerequisite for any health worker attempting

to be an agent of change. All too often this process of gaining insight into the need to observe and listen to a community takes many years of sobering experience.

Factors which inhibit involvement are lack of sensitivity on the part of the initiating agency, frequent transfers of staff, expecting results in less than 3–5 years, doing things *for* people rather than *with* them, and not enough effort being given to listening to people's own ideas. Factors which promote community involvement, on the other hand, are the creation of awareness and providing support to existing community structures and resources. The process known as social mobilization aims at increasing people's awareness, knowledge and ability to organize themselves and mobilize available resources. It helps people to know what they can and must do for their families and increases their demands for satisfaction of their needs. Social mobilization as initiated by governments or other agencies requires very detailed analysis of behaviour, ideas, beliefs, social organization and channels of communication.

There is often some conflict between community demands and needs, and the programme priorities of a supporting institution or agency. For example, people may say that they need drugs and a clinic when the health service thinks that they need latrines and immunizations. One way to sort out these differences in perception and interest is through a community assessment by or with community participation and then through ongoing dialogue.

Sensitizing a community to PHC implies creating an awareness of the PHC strategy and its relevance for existing problems, and assisting communities to recognize and diagnose their problems and to assess their own powers and resources. The first is often done in multisectoral meetings at different levels – district, division, ward, village. In those countries where decentralization is a policy, this dialogue may have already been started and been supplemented by a media programme.

Creating awareness of existing problems can be achieved by assisting the community in self-diagnosis or in a community diagnosis done with community participation (see pp. 103–13). Awareness of the community's own strengths and resources will come to them through discussions, visits to other villages, and committee experience perhaps improved by management training. The use of appropriate technology manageable within the village, and a process of demystifying or simplifying essential health care can enable communities to take scientifically correct measures themselves.

Socialist countries have often developed mass

organizations and a social organization which involves groups of families in 'cells' or in cooperatives. Under these circumstances participation is much more easily obtained as there is a structure. Use of political party structures to initiate health activities works well in one-party states, but in countries with two or more parties it may cause polarization of the community with some participating and some antagonistic. Communities which have development committees or health committees have a structure suitable for involvement with planning, budgeting, implementation, supervision and evaluation as part of their duties. Mass organizations (women, youth), political party organizations and religious organizations can also facilitate involvement in some communities. This brief list of community organizations shows the need for careful assessment of groups which can become involved in PHC.

Intersectoral cooperation for health

PHC has as one of its essential pillars the cooperation for health and development of different sectors such as education, agriculture, water development, local government, social services and women's affairs, and information. Their contribution to health and the survival of children is seldom made explicit but coordinating committees at different levels could do so. Interministerial national health councils and health development networks are coordinating mechanisms which have perhaps existed more on paper than in practice. Fortunately, it is not so difficult to coordinate sectors at the district and village levels, where development committees can do just this. Often there are sub-committees for health which can then specify the main health problems and identify with different extension workers the role of each sector in the control of a problem.

Two examples of areas which need coordination are nutrition and information/communication. Nutrition becomes a visible problem in times of drought or emergency, when it is mandatory that all sectors cooperate – transport, marketing, health, information, water, education. More often, nutrition is a little recognized problem, perhaps most marked in cash crop or commercial farming areas or perhaps seasonal (at the onset of the rains). In such instances there are so many causative factors and prevention and control are so difficult, that it is not possible for the health sector alone to achieve any results. This is often the case when social, economic and cultural factors underlie a health problem.

An information–education–communication approach to community mobilization for health action (e.g. for achieving universal coverage of immunization) is also doomed to failure if it utilizes only the health education section or staff of the Ministry of Health. Local administration, the press and radio, the non-government organizations, adult literacy classes, school teachers, women's and youth organizations, church groups, local 'folk media' and the political party, should all play a part in communication and mobilization for health action.

Perhaps some of the best examples of social mobilization using all available community groups, leadership, multiple methods and channels of communication, have been the accelerated immunization campaigns assisted by UNICEF. Colombia, Turkey and Mogadishu (the capital of Somalia) have all used this strategy to achieve a situation where almost all mothers know about and demand immunization and obtain it for their children at points made more readily accessible to them.

Appropriate technology for health at family and community level

Intrinsic in the concept of PHC is the requirement that health technologies must be used which are available, affordable and manageable at the level closest to those who need them. This will also make it possible for individuals, families or communities to take measures themselves that are scientifically correct. The areas in which appropriate technology is most needed are food production and nutrition; maternal, neonatal and infant care; immunization; water and sanitation; and information/education/communication. There are still many as yet unrecognized or unpublicized forms of appropriate technology existing in communities that can be explored, developed and disseminated. There also exist organizations working in this field, e.g. PATH (Programme for Appropriate Technology for Health) and AHRTAG (Appropriate Health Resources and Technologies Action Group) which have produced many useful tools for health improvement. UNICEF too, for many years, has provided assistance and technical advice in appropriate technology.

Many procedures in areas of health and development which were previously considered too specialized and complex except for use by trained health workers are now to be found at village level. Growth monitoring, routine antenatal care, normal childbirth, preparation of weaning foods, protection of water supplies and safe disposal of excreta, can all take place at family or village level far more efficiently and correctly than ever before using appropriate technology. Immunization and family planning can be brought to the village level and it is often only legal considerations which prevent them from being undertaken by trained village or family members.

The concept of appropriate technology as enabling people to do things themselves with their own resources is, of course, also linked to considerations of cost or savings. It is unfortunate that the high-cost, high-technology saving of the life of one case of kidney or heart failure, has more political value than the saving of a thousand babies' lives with a salt and sugar mixture accurately made up using locally produced measures costing a few pence (see Fig. 1.3.1).

Essential elements of child survival and development

The World Health Organization has produced a matrix[6], by level of service, for the essential elements of PHC and given details of tasks, persons responsible, competence and knowledge required, supplies, equipment and logistics and support needed to the community. This comprehensive view is an ideal for which there are often insufficient resources – not all activities can be covered and inevitably some are more effective and acceptable than others. UNICEF[7], in a world view of the existing high infant and child mortality rates in developing countries, has formulated a package of priority activities which are synergistic, cost-effective and simple. They are growth monitoring, oral rehydration, breast-feeding, immunization, family spacing, female education

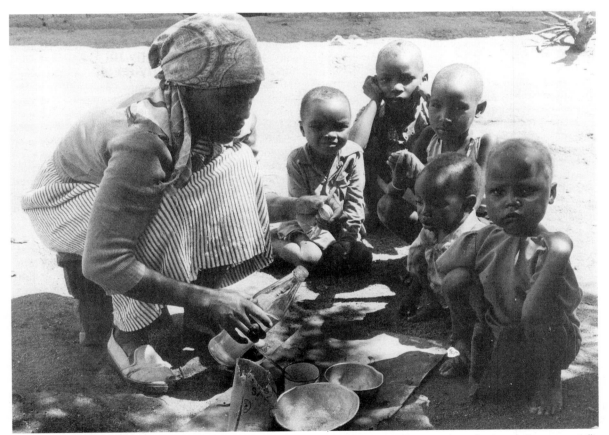

Fig. 1.3.1 Salt and sugar for oral rehydration – an appropriate technology for families to reduce diarrhoeal disease mortality. Photo: UNICEF.

and food supplementation (acronym GOBI-FFF). This combination of activities has been widely publicized as constituting the basis for a 'child survival and development revolution', which will receive political support and help change the world's response to the plight of children from one of resignation, to one of refusal to allow the present state to continue. The daily unnecessary loss of 40 000 children from measles, diarrhoea and malnutrition (the continuous quiet emergency as opposed to the loud emergencies of drought, famine and war) must be placed on people's consciences and nations must make accessible to all parents the simple interventions that prevent not only death of their infants but also a heavy burden of morbidity, retarded development and disability. The difference between the expressions 'child survival' and 'child health' should be noted. The UNICEF package labelled 'child survival' is intended to emphasize the magnitude of child mortality in the Third World in order to sensitize political and organizational wills to the urgency of increasing survival. To those delivering the services, the term fits uneasily into their activity which seeks to emphasize child health and quality of life. UNICEF have recognized this. Expanding the term to 'child survival and development' seems an ineffective attempt at getting the best out of both worlds, and is even more inappropriate at the level of intervention. One suggestion has been made which seems to fit both the needs of the donors and those delivering the services, namely the 'Expanded Programme of Child Health', in short, EPOCH. Twelve global indicators for monitoring progress towards health for all by the year 2000, were adopted by the World Health Assembly in 1981[8] and they included amongst others the following indicators of child survival and development:

Primary Health Care is available to the whole population with at least the following:

- safe water in the home or within 15 minutes walking distance and adequate sanitary facilities in the home or immediate vicinity;
- immunization against diphtheria, tetanus, whooping cough, measles, poliomyelitis and tuberculosis;
- local health care including availability of at least 20 essential drugs within one hour's walk or travel;
- trained personnel for attending pregnancy and childbirth and caring for children up to at least one year of age.

The nutritional status of children is adequate in that:

- at least 90% of newborn infants have a birth weight of at least 2500 g;
- at least 90% of children have a weight for age corresponding to the reference values given.

The infant mortality rate for all identifiable subgroups is below 50 per 1000 livebirths.

The adult literacy rate for both men and women exceeds 70%.

A target date, 1990, was set for universal coverage of immunization and this added to the urgency of this component of the GOBI package. Immunization has been seen as the 'cutting edge' of GOBI and GOBI as the 'spearhead' of PHC.

To achieve universal coverage that is sustainable and which facilitates other activities, a new strategy of social mobilization and communication is required. This, like the social marketing techniques of household products, aims to create a demand or an internalization of the need by parents to have their children immunized and to have them grow at optimal rates. By using modern techniques of information, education and communication, it is possible to make parents aware of what is necessary for the survival and development of their children and to motivate them to adopt the necessary behaviour.

Going parallel with social communication aimed at families is the need for mobilization of national political will and involvement of all sections of the health bureaucracy and of other sectors. This entails advocacy and the generation of interest and concern through the use of a carefully orchestrated set of targeted messages and events using all possible communication channels and social situations.

In many countries the government made a public commitment to Universal Coverage of Immunization by the Year 1990. President Rawlings of Ghana, for example, actually took part in immunizing children with a jet injector at the start of a national campaign – and women queued to have their children receive a presidential immunization shot.

Other priority interventions for child survival and development may be management of malaria and acute respiratory infections through primary health care. These would require training of health staff, community health workers and mothers in early recognition of the conditions and in correct therapy and referral. Correct therapy would be possible and assured if there were an essential drugs programme.

A national essential drugs programme assures that scarce foreign exchange is spent on the most useful drugs for priority conditions and at the same time it should provide for equitable distribution and for adequate training of staff and population in the correct use of drugs.

The prevention and management of neonatal deaths (including the problem of low birth weight) is another priority which should be given consideration in the PHC approach. There are many other activities which can be effectively done within families with community support. An example is rehabilitation of the disabled and special training modules have been prepared for this.

The increased flow of donor funds for the specific 'child survival' interventions has helped to develop the PHC infrastructure with improved management, training, information systems, logistics and supply as well as more involvement of communities. The combination of interventions in improving child health which this has made possible, far from fostering a vertical approach, has actually stimulated integration at the local level.

Training: trainers, community health workers and traditional birth attendants

Training for PHC should start with curriculum review for all cadres of development workers and especially those in the health sector. However, the implementation of any training programme is also dependent on the correct orientation of the tutors. Trained staff already working in health institutions or in other development sectors need reorientation if they are to be a supportive resource for communities rather than retaining an institution-based perspective.

Many communities, after becoming aware of their health problems, will wish to have one of their members trained as a local health worker to transmit health knowledge and skills and change attitudes and behaviour. There is then a need for staff close to the communities to be able to train community health workers and traditional birth attendants using a learner-centred, problem-solving, action-oriented type of training rather than a didactic classroom method. Training should provide social skills (such as working with groups, motivating people, or starting a process of self-discovery) and also should provide technical skills (e.g. building a latrine, making up an oral rehydration solution).

Werner's book *Where there is no Doctor*[9] has now been translated into many languages and has become widely used as a text for community health workers (CHWs)*. Many countries have also been working hard to produce useful and relevant training material in their local languages – often many agencies are involved, such as different Ministries, non-government organizations, university departments, and research centres. A few countries, such as Ethiopia, have set up a PHC network to facilitate interchange of ideas amongst those working in PHC.

*CHWs are also referred to as village health workers (VHWs). See p. 41.

This brief list of the training needed for PHC indicates that it must be a national process requiring considerable planning. On the other hand many non-government organizations (NGOs) may have started training CHWs alone and on a small scale, in which case this forms an isolated community-based series of projects without support from the national system. Liaison between government and NGO training is then required to bring all these projects together within the district development programmes.

Community health workers are workers both selected and supported by the community. If these two criteria are not present, then the worker probably merely represents another lower level of auxiliary belonging to the health service. Selection should, however, be an informed selection. For example, a community might, if left to itself without discussion, choose only men or might choose young and highly educated candidates for training. Through dialogue with the health service or the agency that will assist with training, the existence of priority maternal and child health problems requiring a woman worker may be brought into focus, and also the problem of young workers leaving the community after training may be pointed out. The community might then perhaps opt for training mature married women. Literacy is seldom really a criterion, as illiterates can learn as fast as literates if the methods of training are suitable for adults.[5,10] (See Fig. 1.3.2.)

Support of the CHWs by the community could mean different things – if they are part-time voluntary workers then it might only include recognition, continued interest and supervision by a committee and minimum supplies. If, on the other hand, they are full-time workers with a job description covering a variety of duties, then they will need some form of remuneration as determined and agreed upon by the community. All CHWs need supportive supervision and continuing education.

Much has been written about the training of traditional birth attendants (TBA) but there is less experience of them being trained for a wider range of activities. Were it not for age many might be trained further in antenatal care, postnatal care, family planning and child-care and nutrition. A good rapport between health service midwives and TBAs facilitates referral of high-risk cases and can also ensure that all women receive full tetanus immunization during pregnancy. TBAs are traditionally remunerated by the families they help and so there is usually no problem created by demands for remuneration from the health service.

In a few countries or communities the training of individuals as CHWs is not seen as a priority and group training for health committee members or women's groups is preferred.

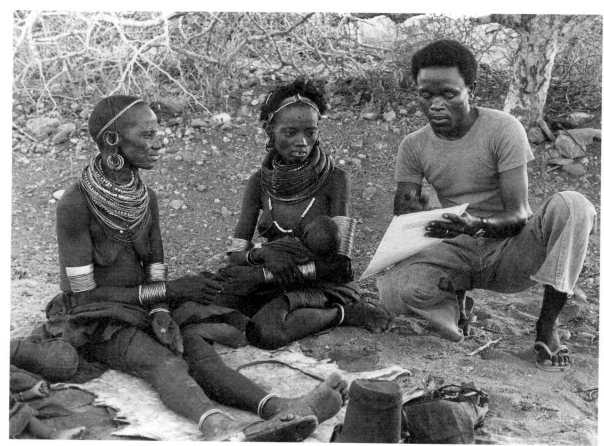

Fig. 1.3.2   A village health worker in Kenya doing a census of children for immunization. Photo: UNICEF.

Supportive role of professional staff and institutions

Many general duty doctors and nurses, as well as specialist paediatricians working in hospitals, may wonder what their role is in primary health care. For many, primary health care perhaps merely means a level of care, i.e. the first contact for illness or prevention with health care (which could be with a community health worker, a shopkeeper, a dispensary, a mobile or outreach clinic, a health centre or the outpatient department of a hospital). For some, it means the interface linking what is done by the community and what is done by the health service. For others, it is only what happens 'beyond the dispensary'.

If PHC is the central function and main focus of a country's health system then all health workers

(including nurses, doctors and paediatricians) have a role. No health centre or hospital is an island. It always has a catchment area with a population which it should know. Whatever the perspective the doctors or nurses have initially, their rightful concern must be to support the population's efforts at self-reliance. This might mean assisting referrals, providing outreach and follow-up, assisting with training of CHWs, providing feedback to community workers, supervision and continuing education of CHWs, TBAs and health committees, and possibly providing assistance with some essential supplies and equipment.

Initial work within a community could prove to be a 'community orientation' for the hospital or clinic. Getting to know the population in the area and assisting with community diagnosis is a process which enables both the community to determine its needs and the hospital to see how it can support the community.

Supervision of community health workers by hospital or clinic staff may be limited to technical aspects, while a community health committee provides administrative supervision and remuneration (if any). Supervision is best seen as a form of continued education and motivation and it reinforces the link between CHWs and health units. As there are always many communities there is a limit to the number of CHWs that one health unit can supervise and so this is best done from the nearest unit. The role of supervision thus falls more on the more numerous health centres than on hospitals. Hospitals, however, can set up a primary health care section with a community nurse and a public health technician and if provided with suitable transport (e.g. bicycles, motor cycles or small vehicles) they can assist in supervision and training in the communities.

The doctor in developing countries is usually part of a team – perhaps the leader. Leader does not imply the apex of a hierarchy but rather the coordination of a group with different skills – skills that are urgently needed to assist the community in training, investigating, analysing, informing, motivating and evaluating.

Evaluation of PHC is complex and the WHO has developed a set of questionnaires that are applied at different levels – national, provincial, district hospital, rural health centre, community and family. In these instruments, the eight essential elements of PHC are examined and also the degree of community involvement and intersectoral coordination. Certainly, doctors and nurses should take part in these national evaluations but also more modest monitoring and evaluation can be done at district or community level with participation of the population concerned.

No paediatrician should be satisfied with an infant mortality between 50 and 150 per 1000 in his district or province – nor with high levels of malnutrition or preventable disability. However, there is no way of knowing these rates unless the hospital or clinic seeks or assists with acquiring population-based data and is concerned with using relevant indicators. It is unfortunate that there are numerous instances of doctors and health professionals not being supportive of PHC or of appropriate activities – the world-wide delay in advocacy for getting oral rehydration therapy for diarrhoea to community and family level is an example.

Does primary health care work?

Almost all developing countries have adopted the primary health care approach. The visible evidence might lie in a better distribution of the essential elements of health care (immunization, maternal and child health services, essential drugs) but the participation of the community might be less evident. National PHC programes should start with management change within the Ministry of Health (as in Botswana) before commencing training of community health workers (and perhaps also traditional birth attendants). Training might be nation-wide from commencement, as in Zimbabwe. Many countries, however, start on a piecemeal or district approach, as in Kenya, or on a provincial (regional) approach with donor support, as in Somalia. Evaluations have shown that there have been considerable gains in accessibility and in community involvement. National programmes should by now have very detailed policy and strategy statements as in Zambia's 'Health by the People' document. (The examples, all from Eastern and Southern Africa, give an idea of the variability of PHC progress within even one region of a continent.)

PHC works well where the community, the area, the zone or the district decide the priorities. In this way, seasonal variations and endemic disease can also be given resources when needed. Schistosomiasis, trachoma, vitamin A deficiency, malaria and guinea-worm, to name but a few conditions, are often localized and major problems in only parts of a country. There are, nevertheless, always certain universal priorities in developing countries: immunization, oral rehydration, growth monitoring and nutrition, maternal care, sanitation and provision of safe water. These priorities also fit in very well with district programmes, where all sectors can be involved in the necessary social communication for participation. Some examples of the district or area approach are to be found in Kenya, Lesotho, Zambia and Zimbabwe.

Urban primary health care has its most obvious application in reaching the poorest of the poor in slum areas.[11] However, there are whole cities which are in the process of having community health workers trained for every neighbourhood – Addis Ababa is an example. Here, the city is divided into 'kebele' and each will have one or two trained community health workers assisted by street-level volunteers from the women's and youth organizations. This system, with support from the Party, the City Council and the Ministry of Health, has led to almost every child having a growth and immunization card and the majority being fully immunized. Urban PHC has priority areas of water, sanitation, and nutrition in the poorer areas of cities – in Lusaka, Zambia, there is even a place for 'urban agriculture'. Day-care centres, women's income generating groups, adult literacy classes and school feeding programmes are also aspects which can be developed through PHC. Cities that now have a PHC infrastructure have proved that they are able to cope with serious outbreaks such as cholera much more rapidly than previously when there was little community involvement.

Refugee and drought emergency camps have often found that the training of community health workers is one of the best ways of ensuring good sanitation, orderly feeding and high immunization coverage (see pp. 78, 996) and that these workers often can initiate the transition from relief to rehabilitation – from dependency to self-reliance.

Community-based health care can be, and has been, developed in almost all types of community – nomadic groups (in Sudan and Somalia), urban slums, sparsely populated rural areas, religious communities, and plantation workers. The essentials are increased awareness amongst the community members, some management structure within the community, and supportive and PHC-oriented health and other sectors with a referral system which can link levels of health care.

PHC as a strategy can be said to exist if all the four pillars are in place:

- Political will to assure equity of resource distribution.
- Community participation and involvement.
- Intersectoral cooperation for health.
- Appropriate technology for health at family and community levels with these levels becoming the focal point of the health system.

There is evident movement towards universal accessibility of essential health care.

UNICEF in producing its annual *State of the World's Children*[7] has tried to document on a global scale changes in infant mortality rate and other demographic, economic health and nutrition indicators. Perusal of these statistics, however, shows that the developing world still has a long way to go and that the economic situation of many countries is grim. PHC, drawing on the strengths of communities and the working together of all sectors, does offer hope of improvement.

Problems of primary health care

Primary health care is faced with problems often concealed behind a facade of rhetoric implying that it is being adopted, when study of the allocation of resources shows that only the words are adopted. Another problem is the lack of any change in the management within the Ministry of Health and lack of real reorien-

tation of workers which could allow for community involvement. Much of the health care is still health services provided to the people and not with them. Lack of supplies, inertia in providing supportive supervision, inadequate funds for transport and vertical top-down services, still frustrate the development of true PHC. The stifling of a spirit of self-reliance has led in many countries to lack of community support for community health workers so that there is a constant demand for payment by government or donors. Wars and (in Southern Africa) destabilization, drought, foreign debts and inflation, are all making it increasingly difficult to prevent actual deterioration in health status but the UNICEF report *Within Human Reach*[12] emphasizes some lines of action which all fit in with the PHC approach:

- emphasis on food security;
- improving women's economic role and capacity for food production;
- protecting the environment and managing land and water;
- strengthening local organizations and involving local communities.

It can thus be seen that PHC with its emphasis on self-reliance and community involvement is an approach suitable for countries in difficult circumstances but that it has to be an intersectoral approach to rise to the challenges of the next 20 years.

References

1. Newell KW (ed). *Health by the People*. Geneva, WHO, 1975.
2. WHO/UNICEF. *Primary Health Care* (Report of the International Conference on Primary Health Care, Alma-Ata, USSR). Geneva, WHO, 1978, pp. 49.
3. WHO. *Health for All Series* 1–8. Geneva, WHO, 1978–82.
4. WHO/UNICEF. *National Decision-making for Primary Health Care*. Geneva, WHO, 1981.
5. Werner D, Bower B. *Helping Health Workers Learn*. Palo Alto, Hesperian Foundation, 1982.
6. WHO. *Analysis of the content of the eight essential elements of primary health care*. PHC/PHC/REP/81.1 Geneva, WHO, 1981.
7. Grant J/UNICEF. *The State of the World's Children*. Oxford University Press, 1984–90.
8. WHO. *Development of Indicators for Monitoring Progress Towards Health for All by the Year 2000*. Geneva, WHO, 1981.
9. Werner D. *Where There is No Doctor*. Palo Alto, The Hesperian Foundation, 1977.
10. World Federation of Public Health Associations/UNICEF. *Training Community Health Workers*. New York, UNICEF, 1983.

11. WHO/UNICEF. *Primary Health Care in Urban Areas: Reaching the Urban Poor in Developing Countries*. Geneva, WHO SHA/84.4, 1984.
12. UNICEF. *Within Human Reach – A Future For Africa's Children*. New York, UNICEF, 1985.

Further reading

Morley D, Rohde J, Williams G. *Practising Health for All*. Oxford, Oxford University Press, 1983.
UNICEF. Community Participation: current issues and lessons learned. *Assignment Children*. 1982; **59/60**.
WHO Regional Office for SE Asia. Evaluating Primary Health Care in South-East Asia. *SEARO Technical Publication*. 1984; **4**.

WHO. *Primary Health Care: The Chinese Experience*. Geneva, WHO, 1983.
Contact – a bimonthly publication of the Christian Medical Commission World Council of Churches, Geneva, Switzerland.
PATH – Health Technology Directions (Program for Appropriate Technology for Health) published three times a year by PATH, Canal Place, 130 Nickerson Street, Seattle WA 98109, USA.
TALC – Teaching Aids at Low Cost, Box 49, St Albans, Herts., UK.
World Health Forum – An International Journal of Health Development, WHO, Geneva.
Salubritas – information exchange in PHC issued by the American Public Health Association and World Federation of Public Health Associations.

CHAPTER 4

Delivering the services

HOSPITAL AND CLINIC

W. E. K. Loening

Health for all means . . . that people will use much better approaches than they do now for preventing disease and alleviating unavoidable illness and disability, and that there will be better ways of growing up, growing old and dying gracefully. And it means that health begins at home and at the work place, because it is there, where people live and work, that health is made or broken. And it means that essential health care will be accessible to all individuals and families in an acceptable and affordable way, and with their full participation. *Halfdan Mahler, 1983.*[1]

Introduction

Health care 'delivery' is somewhat of a misnomer as it suggests that health is a commodity which can be brought to people. Health care should rather be seen as the care that people take of their health in their lifestyle. Health professionals can obviously make a positive contribution to this by providing their technical expertise and by ensuring that the structure within which they are operating is reaching its goals, in that it is medically effective and having a beneficial social impact.

As doctors, nurses and other professionals provide health care, it is important that they have a clear understanding of the issues involved, lest they fall into the trap of perpetuating past errors. By virtue of their professional status they can have an appreciable impact on shaping policy at national, regional, local and insti-tutional levels. Workers may find themselves in a situation where they are over extended, without making a substantial contribution to reducing mortality rates or improving life expectancy in the community. This unfortunate state of affairs is found where doctors are preoccupied with the diagnosis and management of diseases. Admittedly, curative care is one of the cornerstones of a health service. However, a far more comprehensive perspective is called for, which includes, amongst others, consideration of the factors undermining the health of mothers and children.

The health care service in a country is commonly but erroneously evaluated by the size and quality of hospitals. Health care is not ideally provided in static structures such as hospitals and clinics but by people and hence we need to focus on them principally. Regrettably, institutions usually confine themselves to secondary and tertiary care at the expense of primary health care, again making no appreciable contribution to the overall health of the community. Thus, whilst accepting that hospitals play a significant role in the delivery of health care services, we usually see them with a strong bias towards disease. As health care must be 'delivered' where the people are and preferably before disease has set in, a people-orientated primary health care approach is used in this section.

It would be foolhardy to assume, however, that preventive measures at a primary level will resolve most of a country's health problems: while poverty and inequitable distribution of resources prevail, the common diseases resulting therefrom will continue to undermine the health of the community.[2]

Principles of health care delivery

The health care service must be provided to the whole community

Whilst nobody will find any serious argument with this simple principle it frequently remains empty rhetoric, with no commitment to universal access and equitable distribution of health care resources. One of the main reasons for this may well be that very few health professionals are appropriately trained and orientated.

To ensure that health care corresponds to the needs of people, it is they rather than health professionals and bureaucrats who should make decisions regarding service programmes. To achieve as wide and as effective a cover as possible, priority must be given to the needs of the poor and others at high risk. Provision must be made for the disadvantaged as well as the privileged minority, for the healthy and for those that are sick. Furthermore, those that do not avail themselves of health services will require particular attention; accessibility or availability may be contributing factors here. In the case of the former, the aim should be to provide service points near the people (in schools, factories and shopping malls) and within easy travelling or walking distance of everyone in the community. For optimal availability, it is often necessary to introduce flexible working schedules to facilitate utilization of the service in the evenings and over weekends.

The temptation must be resisted to meet the demands of the most vociferous by providing costly, high-technology care for the élite. Whilst this undoubtedly enhances the prestige of the professionals, it makes grossly disproportionate demands on funds and staff.

Lastly, it must be emphasized that community enlightenment and participation is one of the best ways of securing a broad base for health care and improving coverage.

Comprehensive care must be given to every mother and child

Integration must replace fragmentation in preventive and curative services as well as in maternal and child health care. The Western model with preventive/promotive care divorced from curative services, regrettably, has been accepted by many countries in the Third World. Specialization has caused a further break

in the link between mother and child, even though the biological needs of the mother are very rarely in conflict with those of her child: for instance, antenatal care reduces the risk of maternal mortality and morbidity as well as the prevalence of low-birth-weight babies; the optimal birth interval will preserve the mother's resources and at the same time ensure that her infant obtains her full attention during the most delicate and formative years; breast-feeding is ideal for the baby and will help the mother to lose the excess adipose tissue accumulated during pregnancy and probably help to protect her against breast cancer.

Ideally antenatal clinics are combined or run concurrently with an under-fives clinic so that mother and child can obtain care simultaneously.

Health care planning and delivery need to go hand in hand with development in other sectors

The customary competition for budget allocation should be replaced by integrated planning with careful consideration and priority ranking of the needs of the community as a whole. Where malnutrition prevails, it indicates to the agricultural and transport sectors that improved food production and distribution must enjoy the highest priority.[3] Similarly, potable water for rural families is as important as, if not more so than, water for the industrial sector. The prevalence of diseases spread by the faecal–oral route gives a clear indication of the urgency of such a programme.

The ministries of health and education should cooperate in drawing up a syllabus which will promote a life-style conducive to physical, mental and spiritual well-being. Clearly the information on which this will be based must be obtained from doctors and nurses guided by the prevailing health problems.

Community group development must always receive high priority when dealing with the disadvantaged, as ill-health, one of the features of the syndrome of poverty, goes hand in hand with an inability to organize group efforts. As health care provides an acceptable entry point for social upliftment, workers in this field can make valuable contributions here.

The service must be adapted to prevailing social and economic circumstances and to the culture of the community

Poverty, illiteracy and other socio-economic factors are universal determinants of disease patterns amongst children. The health care service must thus be geared to manage the problems arising from these factors in the first instance. That will mean enteric infections, acute respiratory infections and protein energy malnutrition as emphasized elsewhere in this text.

Cultural attitudes to women, traditional healing practices and dietary and other taboos will all have a considerable bearing on the pattern of disease and consequently the character of the desirable health care service.

Finally, one must bear in mind that health professionals rarely, if ever, commence work in a community where no form of health care has been established. An evaluation of the available service *and* resources is a difficult but nevertheless essential task. Cognizance must be taken of the dynamic nature of most of the factors which determine health and consequently the necessary adjustments need to be made. For instance, the demography is constantly altered by urbanization, industrialization and other Western influences. The advent of commercial enterprises and the influence of various media may alter or eliminate traditional practices which previously appeared well entrenched.

A firm structure which will provide continuous support must underpin every aspect of a health service

It is relatively easy to establish a new service but unfortunately many a programme falters because there is little thought for an ongoing commitment. Planning should thus always ensure that the funding, staffing and equipment required to maintain a firm infrastructure are secured before a programme is launched. This applies as much to community group development as it would to the training of a new category of health worker.[4]

Administrative structure

The management of primary health care is commonly subordinated to the hospital administration. Consequently this has kept the former in a secondary or Cinderella role, as the demands of the hospital always appear to be more urgent. Furthermore, the training of health professionals is generally geared to secondary, if not tertiary care, leaving them somewhat uncomfortable in the role of a primary health care worker. It is thus essential that staff with a degree of authority from both the medical and nursing profession are set aside for primary health care. Whilst maternal and child health care will constitute the bulk of the work, other components of primary health care such as occupational health and vector control must not be overlooked.

It is essential, however, that close cooperation is maintained with those responsible for the hospital in order to integrate the levels of care maximally. Rotation of personnel obviates the 'them and us' attitude and improves channels of communication.

Planning and management need to be decentralized and flexible to allow for adaptations to local variations and needs.

The workers

It is customary to begin at the top of the professional pyramid when discussing the personnel hierarchy and gradually work down to the lower echelons as time and space permit. For reasons which will become obvious the order has been reversed in this text.

The mother

When we consider the provision of health care for the child it is surely the mother who should receive top priority. It is she who spends more time with the child than anyone else and it is she who will inevitably be the one to provide health care in the first instance. It is the mother who ultimately decides how to space her pregnancies, how long to breast-feed, when to have her child immunized, whether to opt for traditional or 'Western' healing methods, etc.

Thus, as the principal care-giver of her family, the mother must have the necessary knowledge and skills to enable her to give her children the best that is available under the prevailing circumstances.

The objectives are to empower the mother to:

- recognize the need and create a suitable environment for fully breast-feeding her infant;
- provide a domestic environment free of human and animal excreta;
- provide potable water sufficient for the child's needs;
- provide optimal nutrition at all times but particularly during periods of ill-health;
- initiate oral rehydration as soon as the child develops diarrhoea;
- distinguish between upper and lower respiratory infections so that she can deal appropriately with the former and call for more skilled assistance for the latter;
- recognize potential hazards for children which could result in accidents and take appropriate preventive action;
- recognize the need for intellectual stimulation of the under five-year-old and enrich the child's life with

simple toys fashioned from material available in the home;
- recognize the need for regular attendance at the under-fives clinic for weighing and immunization;
- recognize the value of the Road to Health Card;
- deal with minor injuries to avoid sepsis;
- protect the low-birth-weight infant against hypothermia and common infections;
- determine the optimal birth interval and use measures to control fertility;
- recognize the importance of skilled antenatal supervision.

Where it is not possible to provide the above for everyone in a family the needs of the most vulnerable must be given priority. It is constantly necessary to reinforce and update the mother's knowledge and skills at every contact with other health care workers.

Ideally training for motherhood is integrated into the school curriculum providing a foundation for primary child care.

The father must also be seen as a key figure in the welfare and nurturing of his children (Fig. 1.4.1). Ideally he should be considered already during the prenatal phase so that he enters parenthood with a well-adjusted attitude. The traditional exclusion of fathers from the day-to-day care of their children is changing rapidly, as the nuclear family replaces the extended family where these duties and responsibilities were shared by the females in the home. The mother was chosen by nature to be the initial carer of the infant but there is nothing to say that in due course the father cannot take over this function quite adequately. Health workers thus need to be reminded that the father must be included in the health care of his children whenever possible, but especially whenever any important decision must be made.

There are, of course, many cultural barriers to overcome, as in many communities the care of infants is regarded as unmanly. However, an altered role identity of the mother and father will be more readily accepted as the nuclear family becomes the predominant unit in society. The agent of change will be the mother, as health workers are more likely to be in touch with her. School curricula and entertainment media can play an important role here by introducing these new concepts. Nevertheless, it will be up to the mother to make room for the father in this process of child rearing. The milieu within the family must be such that a bond can form between the father and his child and it is the mother who is usually in a position to facilitate this. Physical contact and the responses of the infant to her father's approaches are probably the two most important factors in shaping this intimate relationship.

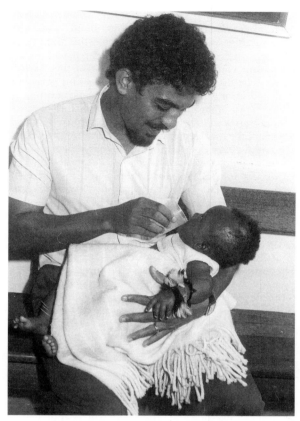

Fig. 1.4.1 Father giving oral rehydration therapy in the primary health care of his child.

The village health worker

The next category of worker who is in constant contact with the community is the Village Health Worker (VHW). As discussed in Chapter 3 (p. 26ff) this worker is best chosen by and is in the main accountable to the community. The title notwithstanding, there is as great a need for a health worker within the community of the urban poor as there is in rural areas. VHWs form a vital link in the total health care scheme and unless their position is given appropriate recognition projected goals will not be achieved. Health professionals can provide technical expertise and knowledge but it requires someone from within the community to interpret this into operational terms at the workface.

The functions of VHWs as health scouts and promoters and their relationship to other workers are outlined in detail in Chapter 3, but a few important principles with regard to their service responsibilities must be laid down here:

- VHWs are the mainstay for the mother. Their training must therefore equip them with the knowledge and skills necessary for this important task.
- Certain clinical skills beyond those of the mother must be displayed by VHWs: signs and stages of dehydration; recognition of loss of consciousness of an infant, of lower respiratory infection and of other common and life-threatening conditions; first-aid care of the convulsing child. Furthermore, they need to be aware of their limitations in the management of the sick child.
- VHWs must have some therapeutic measures at their disposal. This varies from one region to another and is largely determined by the availability of health workers with a more sophisticated training. It is very important, however, that the latter fully accept the principle that, given the knowledge, attitude and skills, VHWs can be trusted to use a considerable range of drugs efficiently. Table 1.4.1 gives a list of suggested drugs, which obviously needs to be adjusted to the prevailing disease pattern. Treatment of patients suspected of suffering from tuberculosis or leprosy is ordinarily not initiated by VHWs but the drugs are included here to make the medication for long-term therapy readily accessible.
- A well-functioning communication and transport system is essential for efficient two-way referral, as has been demonstrated by the 'barefoot doctor' system.[5] Prestige and self-esteem will be appreciably enhanced when patients are referred to VHWs for follow-up in the community. Similarly, defaulters can be traced and underlying reasons for this ascertained by the community worker.
- The activities of VHWs must be well integrated with those of the nearest static structure, whether a dispensary, clinic or hospital. They can be involved in the weighing of infants, in health education and in the discussion of those at risk. Health professionals can also use this opportunity to obtain information regarding current trends and beliefs in the community.

Table 1.4.1 Drugs for use by village health workers (VHWs)

Oral rehydration salts
Aspirin or paracetamol
Penicillin
Sulphonamides
Drugs for malaria, tuberculosis and leprosy
Anthelmintics
Antibiotic eye ointment
Diazepam (used p.r. in convulsions)

- VHWs can play an important role in community development. Group organization, critical analysis of problems and decision-making are skills which VHWs will find very useful in this process.[6] It is of considerable advantage if VHWs have the ear of local decision-makers, as programmes such as water and sanitation improvement require their cooperation. VHWs using tact and diplomacy can bring about significant political change, as the problems of maternal and child health provide an entry point which is generally not threatening and thus acceptable.
- Maintaining a record of births and deaths is an essential function and must be regarded as the barest minimum of data collection.

The medical assistant, auxiliary or nurse/midwife

Health workers at this level will have obtained a formal training course, the nature and extent varying considerably from one region to another. In some countries there may well be several categories of worker at this level, but for the sake of simplicity we will confine ourselves to one. Similarly, their skills and functions will differ from place to place, depending to some extent on disease prevalence and available resources. With regard to maternal and child health, however, certain generalizations can be made concerning the essential functions of these workers. It is assumed that the workers are based at a static structure, such as a clinic, the service function of which is described in greater detail below.

To be effective the workers must be able to identify with the mother of the most disadvantaged group in the community and be sensitive to people's interpretation of health problems. Together with the VHWs they develop schemes which address poverty in the community as a whole. Health workers need to recognize that poverty and lack of appropriate knowledge are the ultimate causes of ill-health amongst the disadvantaged. Hence, they must learn to help people towards a critical analysis of their health problems in order to find some fundamental solutions.[5] Over and above that, the impoverished mother needs to be given practical advice which will help her to cope with her immediate dilemma.

Job description

Clinical expertise The following are essential skills:

- diagnosis and management of common and life-threatening childhood infections: pneumonia, otitis media, measles, pertussis, meningitis and impetigo amongst others;

- management of the child with diarrhoea, including intravenous resuscitation but recognizing the importance of the oral route;
- knowledge of the nutritional requirements of the neonate through to childhood, with particular skills in coping with all the problems occurring in breast-feeding as well as the diagnosis and management of protein energy malnutrition;
- management of the child with fever and in particular the dangers and management of malaria;
- primary care for the child with asthma;
- primary care for the unconscious and the convulsing child;
- knowledge of the indications for and skills for performing a lumbar puncture where more skilled personnel is not available and initial therapy for septic meningitis and cerebral malaria;
- recognition and participation in the management of the abused child and where necessary forming the nucleus of a child protection team;
- simple laboratory procedures (in the absence of a technician) such as urine and CSF microscopy, Pandy's test and haemoglobin estimation.

Under-fives clinic   The workers must take the initiative and responsibility for establishing and maintaining these clinics. Although this is generally seen as a pre-dominantly preventive/promotive activity, a high degree of clinical acumen is required to detect minor ailments and deviations from normal. Furthermore, sensitivity for the skills and potential of the VHWs are called for, as the VHWs should be involved in the functions of this clinic.

Maternal health   Workers need to maintain a steady awareness of the mother's needs and refer her for nutritional supplementation, antenatal supervision and fertility control where necessary. Many a young mother will require moral support and possibly even protection when faced by domestic violence. Where this is a common phenomenon there may be a need for a women's refuge to provide shelter in times of crisis.

At-risk register   Constant vigilance must be maintained for those at risk so that they may benefit from this service. Workers can play a vital role in case discussions which are held at the clinic at regular intervals and assist in the review of risk criteria.

Data collection   The workers are responsible for keeping the databank up to date by ensuring regular input from

VHWs and their own field of work. For further details see 'The functions of the clinic' later.

Health education   The importance of promoting literacy and basic knowledge pertaining to health cannot be overemphasized. This will require constant updating of their own knowledge as well as practising a wide variety of communication skills. Above all, the workers must bear in mind that they constantly serve as role models. Hence, whenever possible the message must be reinforced by living it out in one's personal life.

Surgical skills   Where these skills fulfil a supportive function in maternal and child health care (e.g. tubal ligation) they must be promoted. On the other hand, workers at this level may have been trained to perform surgical procedures (e.g. herniotomy) which enhance the workers' prestige, but are neither urgent nor do they make any impression on the overall welfare of the community. Therefore, this aspect of the work must be reviewed critically, particularly with regard to evaluating whether staff time and expertise are used effectively in relation to presenting problems.

The doctor

The main responsibility for delivering the service usually falls on doctors. Yet the training they receive rarely equips them with skills other than those pertaining to clinical intervention. Fortunately, several medical faculties have recognized that if their graduates are to have a palpable effect on the goal of 'health for all by the year 2000', they require considerably more than diagnostic and therapeutic skills. Students from these universities are no longer confined to academic hospitals but are encouraged to move out to smaller institutions and the community. Formal training can be provided by health professionals in peripheral units where students experience a wider spectrum than can be offered in tertiary-level hospitals. It is hoped that there they will be encouraged to learn from those with a less sophisticated training than their own. This requires a degree of humility which is rarely imbued in an academic environment. This may also engender the flexibility necessary to adjust to Third World conditions from the sophisticated atmosphere of most medical faculties.

   Doctors commonly find that the demands made on them exceed their time and energy, hence it is wise to learn at an early stage to make equitable allocations to the three main components of the work, clinical, managerial and educational.

Clinical skills

In spite of having had exposure to some of the common tropical diseases in their training, doctors not uncommonly experience difficulty, initially, in coping with many of the presenting problems and recognizing their manifestations with ease. As the rest of the team is likely to be well-acquainted with these problems, this demands a willingness to learn from others.

Usually, it comes as a surprise to young graduates that they have to work within the constraints of limited resources and that they have to rely largely on clinical judgement by using their eyes, ears, hands and noses. On the other hand, being well acquainted with the latest diagnostic tools and modalities of therapy, young graduates may well be in a position to make this contribution to the pool of local knowledge.

As doctors, we need to remind ourselves that each one of our patients is a member of a family and a community. Prevailing attitudes and beliefs and the dynamics within the family may have a marked bearing on the severity and outcome of presenting problem. Each contact provides an opportunity to impart knowledge which is likely to have a ripple effect in the community. One has a better chance of dispelling taboos and beliefs which hinder development by gradually chipping away at them in this manner, rather than by open confrontation.

Life-saving procedures   As the most highly trained health workers, doctors are expected to perform life-saving procedures, particularly when working in isolated posts. Therefore, anyone in this type of situation should be competent to carry out the procedures mentioned in Table 1.4.2 on infants and small children.

GOBI   The four measures identified by UNICEF as the most effective means of bringing about a 'childhood survival and development revolution' are: growth charts, oral rehydration therapy, breast-feeding and immunization (GOBI). They require careful study. There are many aspects of these apparently simple tools which have a bearing on the medical profession, who tend to regard them with some disdain.

Table 1.4.2   Life-saving procedures

Laryngoscopy
Endotracheal intubation
Tracheostomy
Cardio-pulmonary resuscitation
Intravenous fluid replacement
Lumbar puncture
Intercostal drainage

Growth charts   These are also known as Road to Health Charts (RTHC). (See Fig. 1.4.2.) This home-based health record which every child should possess has been designed for and is recommended by WHO. As the child's total health record, it contains vital information and needs to be maintained meticulously and protected both in the hospital or clinic and the home.

The RTHC is an important instrument in the hands of the mother as it is easy to grasp the significance of her child's weight record in relation to the standard percentile curves. It reflects the effect of illnesses and other important life events, demonstrating the need for an adjustment to the diet. Provision is made on the card for perinatal data, immunization dates and fertility control measures.

In itself the RTHC is of considerable clinical value,[7] but when doctors are seen to use the chart and make appropriate entries thereon, only then will it be regarded as a document of some significance by the community.

From the clinical point of view, it alerts doctors at an early stage to malnutrition as the weight curve flattens out before clinical features become apparent. Full convalescence from an infection can be gauged by the weight curve regaining its position in relation to the centile lines.

Oral rehydration therapy (ORT)   Diarrhoea is unquestionably the most serious single child health problem in any disadvantaged community. Dehydration is responsible for the high mortality, whereas subsequent malnutrition results in chronic ill-health and susceptability to further infections. It thus follows that all doctors working in the subtropics and tropics must be well acquainted with all issues impinging on ORT.

From the clinical viewpoint the value of ORT, in preference to intravenous fluids, must be appreciated and the dangers of antidiarrhoeal mixtures and undesirable side-effects of antibiotics acknowledged. There is a distinct risk that this great life-saver is brought into disrepute by incorrect practices, such as prolonged ORT or administering clear fluids to the exclusion of all feeds. As incorrect mixing is one of the most serious mistakes, constant warnings must be issued regarding the dangers of using excessive salt.

Alternatives to the generally accepted formula may have to be used in many situations where sachets are not readily available in every home. The well-recognized sugar and salt home brew, or even rice-water, may have to be promoted where conditions demand it.[8,9] In their capacity as managers, doctors must ensure that a continuous supply of the preparation is available at all peripheral units, as well as of the necessary

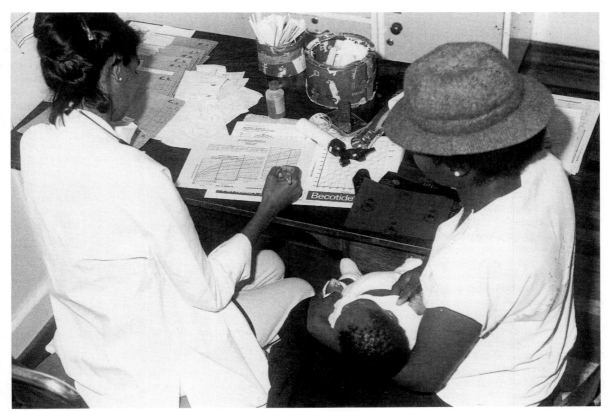

Fig. 1.4.2 Medical Officer making entries on the baby's Road to Health Card.

elements for the manufacture where the mixture is being prepared locally.

There is room for further research on this subject and what better place than a unit in the field, where the problems are being encountered?

Breast-feeding Infective diarrhoea and malnutrition, the two big infant killers, can largely be prevented by breast-milk in the first half year of life. Although doctors generally pay lip service to the value of breast-milk as the ideal infant food, there are still many obstacles to be overcome. Unfortunately several of these are iatrogenic in nature, calling for careful scrutiny of one's own practice and of the routines of the unit as a whole. Some of the common procedures which interfere with establishing and maintaining satisfactory breast-feeding are listed in Table 1.4.3.

Unless health professionals are well acquainted with all the common problems associated with breast-feeding, particularly during the first days and weeks, they are not in a position to give the mother the

Table 1.4.3 Practices which interfere with breast-feeding

Separation of mother and baby at birth
Delay of the first feed
Heavy sedation or analgesia during labour
Operative or assisted delivery
Disregard of reflexes associated with lactation and breast-feeding
Offering bottle feeds of any nature
Promotion of breast-milk substitutes

necessary advice to establish her confidence, which is essential for satisfactory lactation. The International Code of Marketing Breast-milk Substitutes[10] should be available for reference and guidance at every unit offering maternal or child health services. The recommendations contained in this document are very sound and practical and should be observed carefully.

Immunization Details of the WHO Expanded Programme for Immunization are discussed elsewhere (see p. 78). Suffice it to say that doctors must be aware that the complications of the various vaccines pale into insignificance when one considers the immense benefit derived from immunization. The unfortunate pre-occupation with these complications results in poor coverage and persistent and unacceptably high prevalence of the common childhood infections.

To obtain the minimum of 80 per cent coverage necessary to achieve an effective herd immunity, every doctor who deals with children must constantly be aware of the need to promote immunization. At every contact the immunization record of the child should be scrutinized and where necessary brought up to date. This applies not only to the under-fives clinic but more especially to the child presenting with an illness. Waiting areas and wards of hospitals and clinics are a dangerous source of infectious diseases and vigilance with regard to providing protection against these killers at points of contact is very important. Once again it must be stressed that, as a general rule, illness is not a contra-indication to immunization.

Goals need to be set with reasonable target dates to achieve the overall objective of herd immunity. Even when one has reached satisfactory coverage there may be pockets of unimmunized children who will act as a persistent nidus of infection. Annual mass immunization campaigns have been mounted in several countries over and above the regular vaccination programme to overcome this deficiency.

Three Fs   In addition to GOBI, UNICEF has recommended the three Fs, Female education, Food supplementation and Fertility regulation.

Female education This has been demonstrated to be one of the most powerful factors in improving the quality of life of a community. Mothers' literacy has a direct bearing on infant mortality with other factors (including poverty) being equal. Whilst it may not be within the power of clinicians to influence national policy on this matter, it is possible to ensure that every mother is kept well informed of her child's and her own state of health. It is advisable to involve her in the nursing of her child, should admission become essential; apart from giving her the satisfaction of active participation, it helps her to understand the disease and healing process. Factors promoting health and healing, such as nutrition, and those undermining health, such as the faecal–oral contact, require special emphasis and elaboration.

Food supplementation Supplementation for mothers should be considered, particularly at antenatal clinics: mothers weighing less than 45 kg and those with poor weight gain during pregnancy, are at considerable risk of progressive ill-health and of giving birth to a low-birth-weight baby. In certain circumstances, feeding programmes at day-care centres and schools may be indicated. Before embarking on a scheme of this nature one has to weigh up whether the necessary food supplies and community support and involvement are available to sustain it. The people must also determine whether such a project will put the available resources to optimal use.

Fertility control This is a sensitive subject which is not dealt with here, but it must be stressed that child health workers are in an ideal situation to offer advice regarding natural methods of fertility regulation and contraception. In the under-fives clinic or at the time of a medical consultation, the mother is especially receptive to any information which will enable her to give her child undivided attention during the first two years of life. The birth interval can be prolonged by encouraging the mother to suckle her baby day and night, thereby suppressing ovulation and reducing the risk of conception during lactational amenorrhoea to only five per cent. With the mother's approval the fertility control measure which is being used can be entered on the RTHC and will serve as a reminder for health workers to make the appropriate enquiries.

Respiratory infections   The fact that respiratory infections are the second most common precipitator of death of infants and young children calls for a clear understanding of the aetiological factors involved. Viral infections, which usually run a benign course in adults and in children of advantaged parents, are common precursors of these lethal infections. There is a pressing need for research, which could be initiated in the field, into host, agent and environmental factors involved in this serious problem (see pp. 706–24).

It is advisable for doctors in consultation with the rest of the team to draw up a management protocol for each level of health care: the mother is capable of caring for her child with an upper respiratory infection without referring to any other health worker, as she can readily learn to recognize the early features of obstructive and/or lower airway disease; the VHW can give her support in this, assist her with physiotherapeutic techniques to clear secretions and can refer her for antibiotic therapy when necessary; at the level of the medical assistant, there must be a clear understanding of indications for antibiotics, disadvantages of suppressing a productive cough and of features of respiratory distress requiring referral for more intensive treatment. The role of measles, mumps, tuberculosis and asthma as precursors or predisposing elements should be evaluated locally and appropriate measures introduced.

The doctor in the management role

Data collection This is an integral part of efficient management. As doctors have usually received some instruction in basic epidemiology they are in a position to make valuable contributions here. This can be done during the routine visits to the clinic helping the local staff to see a purpose in keeping statistics. Systematic recording of information in the hospital is of immeasurable benefit to the unit.

The infrastructure of the unit However small the unit is, its infrastructure requires careful attention if the health programme is to be successful. Coordination and liaison of the various components need to be fostered to avoid wastage and to promote efficiency. Although doctors are generally not expected to take full responsibility for this, it is important that they are aware of the significance of each aspect and serve as resource persons for the unit. Components of the infrastructure include communication, transport, supplies, maintenance, lighting and refrigeration.

Contact with the more isolated members of the team is vital. Weekly visits to the clinics are important but radio or telephone contact (the life-line of the team) is of far greater value, as the possibility to consult must be available at all times. A two-way referral system enhances efficiency of the service, particularly if the outward limb is fully utilized. Doctors are often reluctant to part with their patients until therapy has been completed. It is frequently in the interest of all parties concerned, however, to refer the patient to a peripheral worker for supervision of the remainder of the treatment. This not only reduces the duration of hospital stay but also improves compliance and enhances team spirit as the workers in the community begin to appreciate the importance of their role in the scheme.

Responsibility for the supply of drugs and domestic provisions must rest with a senior staff member at the base hospital and at peripheral units. Doctors may have to participate in this element of the infrastructure, particularly during visits to clinics. All items with limited life-span need to be regularly rotated to ensure that those approaching expiry date are used first. Professionals are often in a position where they recognize the need for, and can initiate, repair or maintenance of some component to avoid a breakdown.

The immunization programme depends to a large extent for its effectiveness on the 'cold chain'. Efficient refrigeration facilities are thus of paramount importance. Mass immunization campaigns, on the other hand, call for considerable community participation: community leaders need to be involved to get their support and cooperation; volunteers need to be recruited and trained for motivation of parents, arranging venues and assisting at assembly points.

Personnel matters These are a further issue preferably avoided by doctors, as team work and human relationships do not commonly form part of the medical curriculum. By virtue of their professional status, however, a certain degree of leadership is almost always expected of them. A few basic guidelines are recommended. Regular meetings of various staff categories are useful for airing views and ironing out problems before they become insuperable. Responsibility can be devolved, to a certain extent, if the staff share in decision-making. Rotation of staff from peripheral units through the hospital is mutually beneficial as previously mentioned and obviates the 'them and us' attitude. Doctors unfortunately have to accept as a fact of life that they serve as role models. This applies to attitudes as much as it does to life-style, choice of phraseology and even mannerisms.

Evaluation All the facets of the service must be evaluated to ensure effectiveness. This becomes a relatively simple task by setting goals and using recorded data to the best advantage.

Doctors commonly experience difficulty in delegating duties and consequently become overextended. Considerable judgement is required when allocating duties which carry responsibility, as an error in judgement may have disastrous consequences. Objectivity in evaluation of achievements and in assessment of potential is essential for this delicate matter.

Determination of coverage is a valuable and often sobering exercise, which may require home visits by field workers. In some countries school children have filled this slot admirably by reporting illnesses occurring in the home and how often health services are being used over a specific time period. Maps and population data are essential adjuncts when dealing with coverage and utilization of services.

The doctor as educator

As the most highly trained health workers, doctors will want to share their knowledge rather than regard it as a professional secret. There are, however, two major obstacles: their knowledge may not be relevant and skills to communicate may be lacking. Unless the doctor is of the same cultural group as the community, a staunch effort to study the local vernacular and customs will need to be made to bridge the gap.

Continuing medical education is as important as

imparting knowledge. Several centres throughout the world provide a wide variety of material specifically for health professionals in Third World countries. This includes skills in presenting scientific information in a medium comprehensible to less highly trained individuals. Regular journal club meetings with other health professionals help to keep pace with recent developments and stimulate discussion and further reading. Workers at neighbouring stations can participate in this where there are two-way radio facilities, thus preventing isolation and intellectual stagnation.

Those involved in training programmes for workers at other levels will be considerably encouraged if doctors show an interest in their work. In the absence of this important activity such a project should be initiated.

Health-related activities involving motivation of the community must receive priority. As has been mentioned previously, the overall health profile will not improve until the community as a whole can organize itself to break out of the vicious cycle of poverty. Existing structures such as church and women's groups are useful nuclei for further development. Health education in schools and the child-to-child programme[11] are other channels for fruitful dissemination of knowledge.

Every day-care centre can be regarded as an epicentre from which health care can emanate into the community. As day-care centres are in great demand in urban areas they should be used to full advantage in promoting maternal and child health. Play centres in remote rural regions of Zimbabwe, for example, have been effective in raising the health level of the whole community. The standard of care at these centres is often greatly enhanced by the interest shown and the expertise shared by the doctor. Particular attention, however, must be paid to the very real danger of the day-care centre as a source of common infections: faecal–oral contact and crowding are factors which need to be watched diligently.

The doctor's role in local health education programmes is discussed in detail on p. 114ff.

The structures

The clinic/health centre

The clinic is unquestionably the main structure in delivery of primary health care. Ideally, it is surrounded by a series of subclinics each serving a population of about 5000 with the main centre caring for a total of about 50 000. Furthermore, birth and limited lying-in facilities should be available. If primary health care workers in the community are functioning as outlined earlier, the work-load on professionals at the clinic should not be excessive.

Five to six medical assistants/nurses assisted by as many nurse aides form the core group. The number of births at the clinic is an important determinant of the total staff complement as maternity services demand round-the-clock attendants. A laboratory technician is a valuable member of the team, but where these are not available one of the above-mentioned should learn the basic skills. Maintenance and other ancillary staff members are essential to take care of the infrastructure as outlined above.

VHWs are a vital link in the health care of the community, as previously emphasized. To integrate their services into the clinic activities it is advisable that one of the professional workers takes on this task as a primary focus. This incorporates continuing education of the field workers in order to maintain a high level of competence and effectiveness. Similarly a nurse/midwife takes on the care of any traditional birth attendants attached to the clinic.

If we see the mother–child dyad as a single entity it follows that an integrated health service must be provided for them: for example, the midwife attending the mother prenatally should be conversant with routine child-care and some of the common problems. Similarly, those responsible for the child in the first instance must recognize the needs of the mother and be in a position to advise on fertility control, etc.

The functions of the clinic

These can be conveniently grouped as: clinical, database, resource centre, and outreach.

Clinical Child health care is provided at the under fives clinic and ambulatory care is available for those that are ill (see Table 1.4.4). Maternal care is given at the ante- and postnatal clinics and obviously during and immediately following delivery of the baby. The at-risk register is a function which straddles the clinical and other functions of the clinic. All clinics should offer their services at those times which are most convenient to mothers, e.g. in the late afternoon and over weekends. This may involve unpopular duty rosters but is unavoidable if the service is to be effective.

Under-fives clinics Such clinics can operate as one of two models: (a) well-baby clinic almost exclusively for promotive and preventive work; (b) a clinic for all comers. Both have advantages and disadvantages: it can be assumed in model (a) that mothers are more

Table 1.4.4 Functions of the clinic

Activity	Main objectives
Under-fives clinic	Immunization
	Nutritional assessment by weighing, etc.
	Developmental screening
	Fertility control advice
	Health education
	Selection of those at risk
Ambulatory clinic	Diagnostic and curative care
	Management of ongoing problems
	Incidental health education
	Selection of those at risk
Antenatal clinic	Examination for: general health, nutrition and anaemia; hypertension and proteinuria; diabetes mellitus
	Screening for obstetrical problems
	Monitoring fetal growth
	Immunizing against tetanus
	Issuing iron and folate supplements
	Preparation for breast-feeding

open to health education as they are not preoccupied with an ill child. Furthermore, VHWs can readily be involved, especially if the mothers from their particular area attend on specific days. On the other hand, separation of curative from preventive/promotive activities is a disadvantage. It must be stressed, however, that children are vulnerable and need to be nurtured. They warrant a clinic in their own right. The obvious advantage of model (b) is the integration of all the components of health care. This is probably outweighed by the high risk of cross-infection and the slow through-flow as the sick children require considerably more attention. A proposed clinic structure is shown in Fig. 1.4.3 and a flow-through scheme is suggested in Fig. 1.4.4.

The Road to Health Chart is presented by the mother on entering the clinic; the child is then weighed by a VHW or an aide, who also ascertains whether there is a specific problem warranting ambulatory care. If the child is essentially well they move through to the waiting area and play corner. Group health education is provided here before they are seen by the health professional responsible for the under-fives for that day. At this point the mother has another opportunity to voice any special concern. The chart is carefully scrutinized and the child is checked for developmental progress, nutritional state and any obvious abnormality. Maternal health matters are seen to and advice is offered on fertility control. Where risk criteria call for action, appropriate steps are taken. From here, mother and child are referred for immunization, food supple-

mentation or specific health education (e.g. management of the family with scabies).

Ambulatory clinic Most of the busy health centres offer this service in several rooms simultaneously with medical assistants/nurses being in charge. With an efficient health care network the children will have been screened peripherally and on arrival here need a professional opinion. As a rule, each staff member can cope with 40 to 60 children a day but anything in excess of that makes serious inroads on efficiency. Usually 80 to 90 per cent of presenting problems can be dealt with at this level. Some of the remainder will require urgent transfer, while the rest can be seen in consultation with the doctor on the weekly visit or referred as 'cold cases' to special clinics at the base or regional hospital. The flow of patients through the clinic can be enhanced by nurse-aides or auxiliaries assisting with health education, ushering, undressing children, etc.

A lock-up cabinet with stocks of the limited range of drugs required should be within easy reach (see Fig. 1.4.5) so that medication is dispensed at this point rather than at a central pharmacy. It is relatively easy for the attending professional to explain the purpose of the drug thus improving compliance. Furthermore, this reduces the chances of the mother receiving conflicting instructions and it smooths the way to a trusting relationship. This is really only possible if the mother sees the same attendant on a return visit, which is facilitated by a coloured sticker on the Road to Health Chart.

Each room must be equipped with a functioning auroscope and stethoscope, both of which can now be obtained in a light-weight format at low cost. Without these simple tools management of common ear and chest problems is based on pure guess-work!

Referral for immunization, additional health education or food supplementation improves the flow as indicated on the flow diagram in Fig. 1.4.4.

The at-risk register The purpose of this register is to identify those that require special attention. These are the most vulnerable and the ones least likely to avail themselves of services. Without further intervention they will almost certainly present with advanced disease if they come at all.

The register can operate fairly simply by earmarking the relevant card and entering the name in a diary for a return visit, as well as in a special register kept for this purpose. At times an immediate home visit is necessary to give support and advice where it is most effective. When the mother and child are seen on a subsequent visit, a new return date is given or, if appropriate, the name is removed from the register. A further home visit is called for should they fail to return.

All those on the register are discussed at a weekly

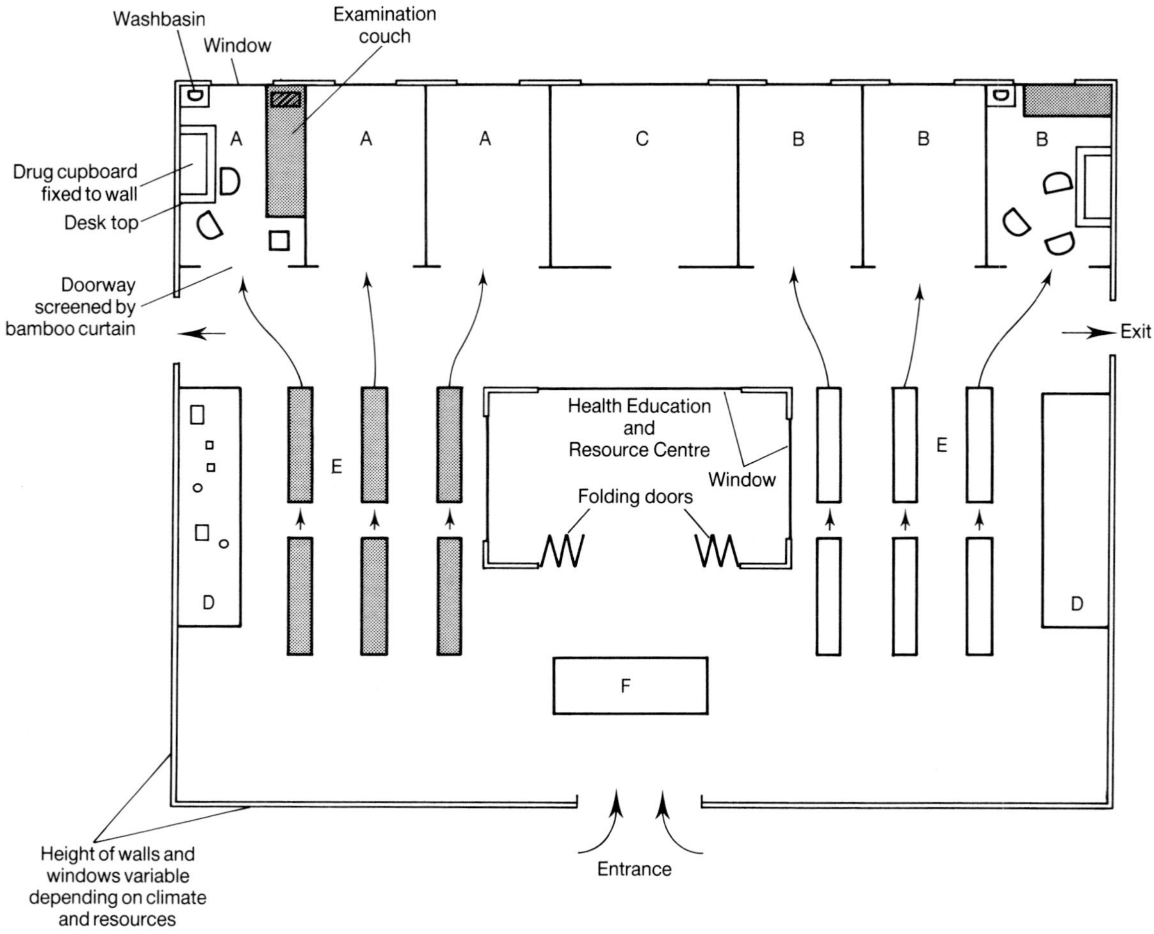

Fig. 1.4.3   Plan of clinic; A – examination cubicles (also for adults); B – examination cubicles (mainly for children); C – injection and dressing room; D – play area with low-cost constructive toys; E – waiting area; F – reception, weighing, issue of Road to Health Charts.

meeting with the visiting doctor. A senior member of the clinic personnel is responsible for maintaining the register and revising at-risk criteria from time to time (see Table 1.4.5). These vary from one region to another and often also within a region, depending on prevailing socio-economic circumstances. An excessive number of criteria will put an undue load on frontline workers and fail to single out the most vulnerable. On the other hand, one must ensure that those who need this special care do not slip through the health care net. Efficient functioning of the at-risk system depends largely on the training and reliability of those in contact with the community (i.e. the VHWs) and on the awareness of staff members.

Trauma register It is advisable to keep a register in addition to the above-mentioned, of all children under the age of five years presenting with trauma, as they are at risk of child abuse. Sufficient data need to be recorded so that they can be readily identified should they return with further injuries, thus appreciably raising the likelihood of abuse. All workers caring for children must maintain a high index of suspicion for various forms of abuse. This is particularly important where violence is part of daily life and where injuries generally are common. In that type of environment children are more liable to abuse and the non-accidental nature of the problem is likely to be missed. The aim of the register is to detect those who present with repeated

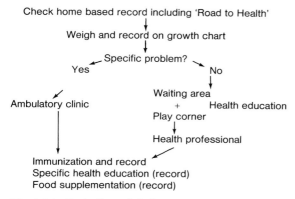

Check home based record including 'Road to Health'

↓

Weigh and record on growth chart

↓

Specific problem?

Yes ← → No

↓ ↓

Ambulatory clinic Waiting area

\+ Health education

Play corner

↓

Health professional

↓

Immunization and record
Specific health education (record)
Food supplementation (record)

Fig. 1.4.4 Under-fives clinic flow.

episodes of trauma and are thus possibly victims of non-accidental injuries or of neglect.

The clinic as a database From the outset this needs to be goal-directed with clear objectives spelled out to all members of the team. Accurate statistics play a fundamental role in evaluation of the health status of the region and in monitoring effectiveness. Furthermore, data are essential when seeking support for initiating or maintaining programmes.

The tally system is a simple and yet efficient method of recording, particularly where one is dealing with large numbers or for semiliterate members of the team. In the case of the latter, pictorial representations have been used very successfully.[12]

The range of data to be collected should be a team

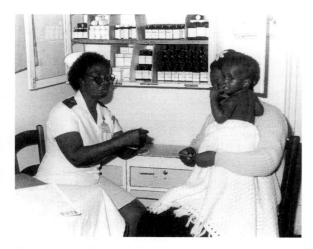

Fig. 1.4.5 Health professional dispensing medicine after discussing the problems at the time of the consultation.

Table 1.4.5 Suggested criteria for at-risk selection

Mother
    Weight <45 kg
    Height <150 cm
    Mid upper arm circumference <22.5 cm
    Age <15 and >40
    1st or >4th pregnancy
    Previous stillbirth or obstetric problem
Child
    Low birth weight
    Birth interval <24 months
    Birth order >4
    One of twins
    Off breast <6 months
    No weight gain × 2 months
    Physical/mental handicap
    Trauma (see text)
    Preventable death or illness of sibling
Social
    Abandoned
    Fostered, adopted or stepchild
    Single, unsupported parent
    Parent(s) victim(s) of child abuse
    Chronic illness in parent
    Violence and/or alcohol in family
    Member of deprived subgroup

decision; vital statistics clearly form the foundation of any health database, hence births and deaths take pride of place. Further suggestions together with a recommended priority rating are given in Table 1.4.6. Age-specific and, as far as is feasible, disease-specific mortality rates can be calculated readily from these data, which form the basis of regional health statistics.

Regular review and analysis of data at each unit, serve to remind team members of the aims which they have set themselves and whether goals are being achieved. The perinatal mortality rate is the best indicator of the quality of antenatal, obstetric and early neonatal care. Furthermore, it reflects the care given to mothers in the community. This review process helps to identify problem areas which require additional support.

Continuous evaluation of the utilization of health services is a further broad objective of data collection. Indicators of utilization and preventable disease

Table 1.4.6 Items for data collection (in suggested order of priority)

All deaths, including age at death and cause where possible
All births, including stillbirths >500 g
Infectious diseases preventable by immunization
Birth weights <2500 g
Diagnosis of patients admitted and duration of stay
Ambulatory problem presentation

prevalence are the number of children dying without having been attended to by a health worker.

Lastly, compiled data must be suitable for submission to the relevant authorities. Here one must bear in mind that their priorities are likely to be reducing expenditure and boosting national or regional prestige. Hence, it is to mutual advantage if material is prepared in a manner which suggests that these objectives are being supported.

The clinic as a resource centre   Trained health care workers owe it to the community to be agents for information on all matters impinging on health, as they have access to knowledge and media not generally available to people. It is especially important that professionals accept this challenge and help people to lift themselves out of the morass of poverty. One of the main objectives is to make appropriate technology available, using local material and decreasing dependence on complicated, imported equipment. The clinic can serve as a model where this principle can be put into practice (see Table 1.4.7).

Wherever feasible the clinic personnel must endeavour to demonstrate that these methods are acceptable even to them. This requires a degree of commitment but not undue sacrifice, as a fairly sophisticated home can be created using locally available material resourcefully.

As the clinic also serves as a centre for the training of VHWs, a range of audiovisual aids must be based here. With some imagination innovative techniques can put these media to maximal use making health education an exciting venture. Anything from puppets to video-tapes will be of great value. The Indian Children's Development Scheme provides an excellent example of how truly comprehensive care can be provided at one centre.[13] All the above-mentioned functions of the clinic can be found at centres of this scheme making a considerable contribution to the welfare of some of the poorest communities in India.

Outreach   Although most of the aspects of this function have already been covered, it is necessary to make

Table 1.4.7   Examples of applied technology at the clinic

Collection and storage of roof water
Spring protection
Ventilated, improved pit latrine
Food storage
Hot box
Home ventilation
Backyard vegetable garden
Compost from degradable refuse

special mention of the responsibility that the clinic personnel have for the welfare of the community as a whole. This takes on particular significance where there are no VHWs who can provide this all-important link. It is then advisable to delegate the responsibility of exploring channels of communication with the community to a senior staff member. For instance, mobile clinics can temporarily fulfil some of these functions, albeit a poor substitute for VHWs.

Consideration must be given to bringing community representatives in to the running and administration of the clinic. This requires courage and innovation but is essential if the clinic is not to be 'foreign' territory for the people.

The subclinic (dispensary)

Whereas the term 'dispensary' has found fairly widespread acceptance, it should probably be discouraged as it suggests that medicines are dispensed here. Whilst this may be one of its functions the subclinic should rather be seen as a point from where knowledge is disseminated.

Staffing of this structure depends largely on who is available in the region. It is desirable to have at least one, if not two, of the medical assistant/nurse category or, alternatively, one of the latter together with an auxiliary nurse. It is envisaged that these centres cater for a population of about 5000 with a cadre of VHWs caring for the immediate needs of the community. The nature and extent of activities thus also depend on available personnel and are determined by the team of health professionals responsible for peripheral work.

A great deal of what is outlined above for the main clinic applies to the subclinic suitably scaled down to prevailing circumstances.

The mobile clinic

These are in use in several regions where it has not been possible to establish static subclinics. The great advantage of this type of service is that coverage is extended to a relatively large population with limited staff. It must be strongly emphasized, however, that the coverage is very restricted, in that there is no continuous health care. Workers cannot develop a confidential relationship with individuals nor with the community as a whole. An added disadvantage is that a mother may delay seeking help for an acutely ill child for days or weeks in anticipation of arrival of the mobile clinic. The practice of itinerant health professionals providing an intermittent curative service under a tree or in the back of the village trading store is deprecated.

The hospital

Historically, the hospital has provided far more than a bed for the sick. As the name suggests it is an institution which provides shelter for the afflicted. Its function in the community extends well beyond medical care, as it is a place where expert care-givers are available throughout the day and night. Hence, it becomes a place of refuge for not only those with a physical ailment but also the destitute who are in social, mental or spiritual distress. And this is by no means confined to city hospitals as those who work in rural areas are experiencing, where the extended family no longer functions as the buffer for misfortune. This then is a care-giving function which health professionals render freely but we must ensure that the supportive and protective image does not become tarnished. Where the hospital is seen in this light by the community it can clearly bestow far more on people than mere secondary or tertiary medical care. The forbidding appearance of large edifices with stark corridors and austere wards is unlikely to foster a warm relationship with the staff unless a concerted effort is made to allow people to feel at home there. In the rush to complete daily chores and deal with a flood of emergencies it is difficult to sustain an amiable frame of mind. Nevertheless, that is what is required of the front-line workers, particularly if the hospital is to have a favourable impact on the welfare of the community.

How do we bridge the gap?

The principles of health care delivery apply to the hospital as much as they do to the peripheral limb of the service but are appreciably more difficult to apply here. Most workers in hospitals see their main task in caring for the sick as determining the immediate cause of the disease and effecting a cure or symptomatic relief. In the first place, the expectations of the people and secondly, the demands of the principles we have set ourselves go well beyond that. It therefore presents the hospital team with a challenge to close this gap lest they be accused of operating in a disease palace.

Where there are no representatives of the people on the board or on hospital committees, this is a good place to set the ball rolling. One must take care, however, that their voices are heard and their opinions sought and that it does not become a mere token gesture to democracy. Inviting a senior class from a neighbouring school to visit the hospital and then to write an essay on their impressions can be a sobering exercise. It may also provide an opportunity for teachers to comment on their view of the hospital as a resource for the community. A further spin-off from this may be an invitation for the staff to provide health education at the school. This offers almost unlimited scope for sowing seeds of the elements of good health by involving both students and teaching staff in analytical discussions concerning the fundamental causes of disease.

There is also considerable good-will within the community which the hospital team often does not utilize sufficiently. Doctors, in particular, are frequently unaware of voluntary organizations and groups that are anxious to participate in caring for the sick and suffering and that may be frustrated by lack of opportunity. Contact with such groups provides a rich potential for outreach where one can possibly assist members in defining their objectives.

Formal training programmes

The importance of the role of health professionals in training co-workers bears repetition. Regular evaluation of what is provided and what is required will help to determine direction and to set new goals. In the absence of VHWs or their equivalent, serious consideration must be given to establishing such a scheme. Even in countries with a sophisticated health care network, such as New Zealand (Aotearoa), community health workers have recently been introduced to assist in bridging the gap.

Nurses' training colleges attached to hospitals have helped beyond measure to raise the standard of care of the sick. Although there is a tendency to transfer this training to institutions for tertiary education, hospitals must continue to play a significant part.

As has been mentioned previously there is a welcome trend to decentralize medical student training so that staff in peripheral hospitals carry a responsibility in shaping the calibre of the doctor of tomorrow.

Doctors have to remind themselves when they are involved in a training programme to keep primary health care in the forefront as there will be a tendency to allow second-level care to predominate. The UNICEF 'tools' provide a useful framework on which to build.

Ambulatory care

The out-patient department can be seen as the most important point of contact with the people: regrettably it is commonly given a rather low profile and, furthermore, its potential for primary health care training is not realized. There is also an unfortunate tendency to allow the most junior members of the team to man this important section, where serious decisions based on clinical judgement must be made. It stands to reason that senior staff are in a better position to make these critical appraisals and to provide primary care training at this venue. Not only will the community appreciate the upgrading of their interface with the hospital but also unnecessary admissions will be reduced to a minimum.

Both ambulatory care and the under-fives clinic can function in a similar way to that outlined for the clinic.

The primary health care 'tools'

The strategy identified by UNICEF for achieving a 'childhood survival and development revolution', i.e. GOBI FFF, should be regarded as the main avenue of approach to primary health care even within the hospital setting. Although these items were discussed in some detail earlier it is necessary to look at them from a hospital perspective.

The growth chart (RTHC) This is of considerable value to the clinician as it provides a wealth of relevant information: perinatal data, weight and immunization records, notable family history and a summary of past illnesses. This document can become part of the hospital file for the duration of the child's stay in the ward, provided steps are taken to ensure that the card is updated as part of the discharge procedure. The mother's understanding of the need for the recovery of the weight curve during convalescence needs particular emphasis at this point.

The RTHC has found wide acceptance throughout the world but certain aspects, which provide scope for research, await validation. Any of the major Institutes of Child Health would be in a position to provide guidelines for this.

ORT This must be seen to be the treatment of choice for the child with acute infective diarrhoea, even though many doctors and nurses still prefer parenteral fluid therapy. Not only has it proved to be of greater benefit to the child but because it is an ideal 'tool' in the hands of the mother as a first resource in the home, the concept must be reinforced at this level. This situation further lends itself to demonstrating the dietary adjustments required during such an illness and convalescent phase, using the RTHC as suggested above. Before discharge from hospital, be this the ambulatory section or ward, the source of infection needs to be pinpointed, e.g. a contaminated feeding bottle, which should be abandoned, or cross-infection at a day-care centre. The hospital can serve as a resource centre for preparation of ORS sachets.[14]

Breast-feeding This was dealt with in some detail earlier but as hospital practices tend to set the trend in the community it is particularly important that it is given the attention which it warrants. The recom-

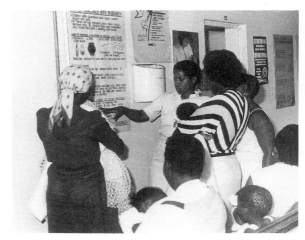

Fig. 1.4.6   Health education in a hospital setting.

mendations contained in the International Code of Marketing of Breast-milk Substitutes[10] require application to the local scene. This is one of the issues ideally suited to community involvement as those mothers who have breast-fed successfully are by far the best motivators. Wherever feasible, pressure groups should be encouraged to correct malpractices affecting the consumer. Lay members of the hospital personnel have a far reaching effect on feeding practices outside and can be drawn into setting up a local code.

Immunization This is customarily regarded as the task of the peripheral team, obviously not appreciating that a great deal of cross-infection takes place in hospital wards and waiting areas. Hence, it is important to have a strict vaccination protocol for all infants and children entering the hospital precincts. Prompt action by the hospital staff in response to a resurgence of an infectious disease will prevent the problem from reaching epidemic proportions. At times authorities need to be prodded into a mass immunization campaign where staff members could play a supportive role.

Female education One of the three Fs, this requires special emphasis. A conscious effort needs to be made to involve the mother in the management of her child's problem. To obtain her full cooperation she must be enlightened about the illness, known causative factors and therapeutic programme indicating to her where she can participate. It becomes obvious that the mother has a key role in the management of most of the diseases of childhood, e.g. infective diarrhoea, malnutrition, malaria, pneumonia, asthma and convulsive disorders (see Fig. 1.4.6).

There may be room for a 'court interpreter', i.e. a

member of the team who is particularly skilled in translating technical jargon to lay terms, as doctors are generally not good communicators and parents are commonly hesitant to voice their perplexity.

Lay members of the staff Very valuable contributions on a wide front of health related matters can be made by individuals from within the community. Special health education programmes directed at these 'agents' will encourage them to become active participants in the childhood survival revolution rather than passive cogs in a machine. Low birth weight is a problem admirably suited for this purpose, as it is responsible for a large proportion of neonatal and infant deaths. The delicate infant places a considerable strain on the ill-equipped and often over-burdened mother, not to mention the extra load on scant hospital resources. The team must therefore ensure that preventive measures, such as good prenatal supervision and nutritional supplementation, are available and promoted. The mother of a low-birth-weight infant needs to be counselled and supported in her home to empower her to use the resources at her disposal to best advantage and *secure an optimal environment for her baby.

Research

A great deal of expertise centred at hospitals could be put at the disposal of research. Medical science, and primary health care in particular, would be rendered a great service if peripheral hospitals could see themselves as research units. If this sounds like a daunting task, we can take courage from the *Lancet* editorial which heralded the humble ORT as one of the most important advances in medical science of this century.[8] Institutes of Child Health can be called upon to render assistance with regard to suitable projects and drawing up protocols. Generally it is advisable to concentrate on those problems which are peculiar to that area and yet not uncommon.

Criteria for the at-risk register are frequently in need of revision and a rich source for research. Not only will this throw the focus on those in greatest need of care but also involve workers in the community, who can derive great benefit from it provided they are fully informed with regard to objectives and envisaged outcome.

References

1. Mahler H. Primary health care: health for all and the role of doctors. *Tropical Doctor.* 1983; **13**: 146–8.
2. Klouda A. 'Prevention' is more costly than 'cure': health problems for Tanzania, 1971–81. In: Morley D, Rohde J, Williams G eds. *Practising Health for All.* Oxford, Oxford University Press, 1983. pp. 49–63.
3. Amartya Sen. Food Battles: conflicts in the access to food. *Food and Nutrition Bulletin.* 1984; **10**: 81–4.
4. Ebrahim GJ. Crucial issues in reaching the poor with health services. In: Ebrahim GJ ed. *Social and Community Paediatrics in Developing Countries.* Basingstoke, Macmillan, 1985. pp. 168–79.
5. Rohde J. Health for all in China: principles and relevance for other countries. In: Morley D, Rohde J, Williams G eds. *Practising Health for All.* Oxford, Oxford University Press, 1983. pp. 5–16.
6. Werner DB. Looking at how human relations affect health. In: Werner DB, Bower BL eds. *Helping Health Workers Learn.* Palo Alto, Hesperian Foundation, 1982.
7. Tremlett G, Lovel H, Morley D (1983). Guidelines for the design of national weight-for-age growth charts. *Assignment Children.* 1983; **61/62**: 143–75.
8. Editorial. Water with sugar and salt. *Lancet.* 1978; **ii**: 300–1.
9. Mehta MN, Subramaniam S. Comparison of rice water, rice electrolyte solution and glucose electrolyte solution in management of infantile diarrhoea. *Lancet.* 1986; **i**: 843–5.
10. WHO. *The International Code of Marketing Breast-milk Substitutes.* Geneva, WHO, 1981.
11. Aaron A, Hawes H, Gayton J. *Child to Child.* Basingstoke, Macmillan, 1979.
12. Morley D. Under fives clinic. In: Morley D ed. *Paediatric Priorities in the Developing World.* London, Butterworth, 1973.
13. Integrated Child Development Service. A co-ordinated approach to children's health in India. *Lancet.* 1981; **i**: 650–3.
14. WHO. Guidelines for the production of oral rehydration salts: *Program for Control of Diarrhoeal Diseases.* WHO/CDD/SER/80.3. Geneva, 1980.

CASE STUDIES IN PRIMARY HEALTH CARE
Zimbabwe: the children's supplementary feeding programme

David Sanders

Background	Evaluation
Aims	Later developments and lessons for others
Organization	Summary
Progress	Further reading
Constraints	

Background

In 1980, soon after Independence, a number of nutrition surveys were undertaken in Zimbabwe. These revealed a high prevalence of malnutrition in the 1–5 year age group, with approximately 30 per cent being significantly under weight (below the third centile of expected weight-for-age) and up to 40 per cent having mid-upper arm circumference measurements of under 13.5 cm. There was also evidence that the prevalence of undernutrition in most areas related inversely to availability of food, assessed by examining food stocks.

The 1980 food crisis was due partly to an influx of refugees, displaced to neighbouring states by the liberation war, and partly to the war policies of the former regime, whose tactics included destruction of food and agricultural resources. These 'acute' factors aggravated a chronic food problem that was the result of historical inequities in land tenure, ownership of the means of agricultural production, and income distribution, to cite only the most important factors.

These food shortages prompted a massive food distribution programme which commenced in early 1980 and ended with the harvest of April 1981. Funded by the United Nations High Commission for Refugees (UNHCR), it was initially administered by local voluntary agencies and later by the Government's Department of Social Services. Although this programme provided food (1600 kcals per person per day) to 800 000 people, many living in remote areas were excluded and the foods provided were not ideal for young children – as evidenced by the nutrition surveys cited earlier. It was felt that the impending agricultural season (November 1980 to April 1981) was going to be a 'crisis period' in terms of the nutrition and health of young children, 150 000 of whom were estimated to be 'at risk'.

Aims

Discussions began in August 1980 between some voluntary agencies and relevant government departments about a nutrition intervention programme. Using information gathered in the various surveys it was possible to construct a 'map of undernutrition' which allowed for a more effective selection of areas where the programme should commence. Within these areas, one-to-five-year-olds 'at risk' were to be identified using the mid-upper arm circumference (MUAC) measure. It was recognized that the limiting dietary factor in protein–energy malnutrition (PEM) is usually energy, and that energy-rich foods are more important in correcting undernutrition than the traditionally used protein. The possible danger of creating dependence on convenience foods by the use of proprietary brand supplements was also recognized.

The final proposal submitted to the Ministry of Health stressed the dual nature of the programme – the immediate short-term relief exercise together with a long-term educational component. Secondly, it emphasized the importance of the use of locally available foods in the programme. The choice of the supplementary meal was based on the understanding that it is lack of energy, and not lack of protein *per se*, that underlies protein–energy malnutrition, and that locally cultivatable foods are more appropriate than artificial (often protein-rich) foods. Hence, the local staple food (maize meal), together with beans and energy-rich groundnuts (which also contain a high percentage of protein) and oil were chosen (see Fig. 1.4.7).

The meal was planned to be in addition to, and not a substitute for, the child's normal diet. The meal consisted of maize meal (66 g), beans (20 g), groundnuts (20 g), oil (12.5 ml) and salt. This provided 530 kcal and 16 g of protein which was approximately one half of the daily energy requirements of the one to two-year-olds and approximately one-third of the daily energy needs of the three to five-year-olds.

Organization

The importance of the involvement and cooperation of workers in the health and community development departments was stressed. However, most important of all was the active support of the local community. Local people and local workers were asked to identify with and become involved in the programme – to supervise the consumption of food and to teach the importance of energy-rich locally available foods.

Structurally the programme was conceived as one of cooperation between government and non-governmental agencies, operating under the umbrella and direction of the Ministry of Health. A national working group was set up with representatives from relevant ministries and voluntary organizations. Within the provinces, the Provincial Medical Officers of Health set up provincial committees.

The organization of the programme at district and village levels was both complex and unique. The administrative infrastructure developed during the liberation war was utilized to organize the measuring of the children, to establish the feeding points close to people's homes and fields, and the cooking and the feeding of the supplementary meal for the children registered. Any child whose arm measured less than 13 cm was registered for inclusion in the programme, this being explained not only to the parents of registered children but also to those whose arms measured more than 13 cm and who were deemed not 'at risk'. In the local committees were health workers, school teachers, community development workers and women's advisors. At village level the ongoing administration, involving the daily registration of attendances and the preparation and feeding of the meal, was often performed by the mothers of the at-risk children often organized through the political party structures.

Between November 1980 and January 1981, the organizational structure of the children's supplementary feeding programme was established. Provincial committees were set up to work with the national working group. District committees were established and district coordinators appointed. Village organization was utilized, with considerable party involvement at each of the levels. The transport of food was arranged, children were measured, registered and organized into feeding points chosen by the committees themselves. Supervisors were selected for each feeding point.

Food was packed and transported to each of the five main provincial towns, where storage points were set up. The cost of loading and transport to the provincial warehouses was met by the national office. Transport from provincial warehouses to local distribution centres and to feeding points was done by local transporters and van owners and was paid for by provincial committees.

To simplify the logistics, the food packs were organized in such a way that they were sufficient to feed 10 children for 20 days. Each pack contained 3 × 5 kg maize meal, 4 × 1 kg beans, 4 × 1 kg groundnuts, 2.5 litre oil and 250 g salt. Each feeding point was sent enough '10-child' packs to feed the number of children registered there for a period of 20 days.

Progress

The first feeding point opened in January 1981, and over the next three months feeding points became established all over the country. The number of children registered rose from 5824 in January to 56 200 in March: a 10-fold increase. It peaked at 95 988 in May with over 2000 feeding points, and dropped back gradually to 57 556 in August. Screening and remeasuring of children registered at feeding points was regularly performed by district coordinators and a turnover was thus ensured.

A poster in English and the local languages was produced and displayed and discussed at feeding points. It reinforced the message that high-energy foods that could be grown locally would provide a nutritious meal for young children if added to the staple maize meal porridge. Thus, the relief and rehabilitation exercise contained an educational message (see Fig. 1.4.7).

Constraints

At the end of July 1981 the programme administration changed. The Ministry of Health began funding the programme with a view to taking over direct responsibility for the feeding programme. The take-over period proved difficult, as the final decision about the nature of the take-over was not concluded until October. The less flexible and more complicated method of government funding led to problems in food purchasing, payment of transport costs and salaries. This resulted in breaks in the feeding and near bankruptcy at provincial level. However, the importance of the programme was recognized, and its continuation in critical areas accepted as necessary. It was decided to change the emphasis: with less focus on relief, more on education.

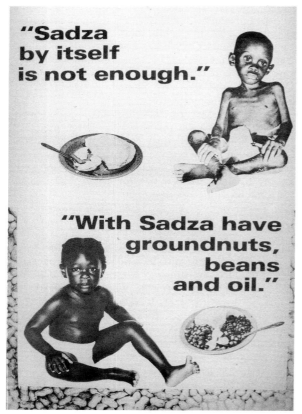

Fig. 1.4.7   The poster for the Children's Supplementary Feeding Programme. (Sadza = maize meal).

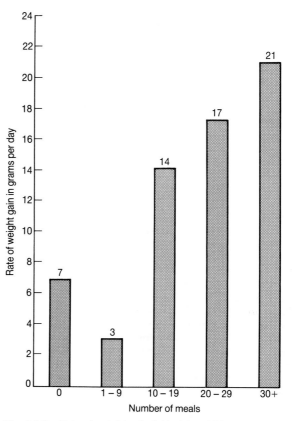

Fig. 1.4.8   Rate of weight gain (g/day) for children not attending supplementary meals and for those attending, divided into four groups according to the number of meals consumed.

Evaluation

An evaluation of the Children's Supplementary Feeding Programme (CSFP) was carried out in 1981. The first part involved weighing children in the programme and comparing them with a group of children of a similar age range, from the same area, but not attending the feeding programme, as their arm circumferences measured more than 13 cm. This showed that children in the feeding programme gained considerable weight, and that this could be attributed to the programme itself. On average, children attending for supplementary meals put on weight at twice the rate of the other children, while children attending 30 or more meals gained weight at three times the rate of the better nourished children (see Fig. 1.4.8). While these differences in weight gain are striking, other unmeasured effects may have been even more important. It has been noted in a major review of feeding programmes that increases in voluntary activity

and play may be the most significant changes induced.

The second part of the assessment was concerned with the perceptions of the programme of those involved. Mothers mostly reported improvement in their children's health, and in many areas the educational message had been accepted. Most found the timing of feeding convenient. One-third reported difficulty in participation due to the burden of housework, agricultural and child-care duties. Perhaps the most striking point that emerged was the geographical variation in food supply and usage. While some families were producing considerable amounts of crops, others had very little. Some of the constraints on production were described. The poverty of the people, measured in terms of food, was identified as one of the main causes of undernutrition. Another important finding was a change in intended production patterns, with a near doubling of the percentage of interviewees (48 to 80 per cent) who stated their desire to grow groundnuts in the following agricultural season.

The evaluation showed that the feeding programme had achieved much of what it set out to do. Its strength lay in having achieved its aims as a relief programme, and expanded into a programme with a different emphasis: education. Secondly, its strength lay in having sustained and built upon a grass-roots organization at district and village levels. To have local people in control of running a development project is perhaps the best indicator of the successful administration of a project.

Later developments and lessons for others

Following the evaluation, some committees approached the organizers of the programme and asked for groundnut seed to enable them to grow the crop for their children. It is known that in Zimbabwe, although groundnuts are widely cultivated, most of those produced in the peasant areas are sold: economic pressures have turned a nutritious food into a cash crop. Therefore, the CSFP Committee drew up a proposal suggesting the development of communal groundnut production plots: if production was collective it was far less likely that the crop would be sold. This proposal was accepted by the Ministry of Health which made available groundnut seed, gypsum and fertilizer to communities organized to cultivate collectively on a plot that was already, or soon would be, sited adjacent to a preschool centre. The harvest from these half-hectare plots was to be communally gathered and used as an important component of the daily meal given to preschool children attending that centre. Enough of the harvest would be retained to provide seed for the next year's planting. This scheme was launched in 1981 as a pilot, with a total of over 500 plots country-wide. It was intended that the successful plots would serve as demonstrations for communities not so far involved in this project.

By 1983/4 there were 292 supplementary food production units in 31 districts. Unfortunately, because of the severe and recurrent drought in Zimbabwe most of these failed. Together with substantial crop failures, it became necessary for government to mount a drought relief exercise which included a food distribution component. It also proved necessary to maintain and expand the CSFP whose infrastructure was, fortuitously, intact. During the next few years the total number of children qualifying for supplementary feeding increased, and during much of 1984 about a quarter of a million children were being fed.

Since the end of the drought the supplementary food production scheme has diversified with most plots now producing a mixture of maize and/or beans and/or groundnuts. In most cases these units are situated on land allocated by the District Council (a local government body) to village groups – usually female – who have come together to establish a supplementary food production plot. At district and provincial levels Supplementary Food and Nutrition Management Teams have been established. These are chaired by Agritex, the extension arm of the Ministry of Lands, Agriculture and Rural Resettlement, and are comprised of several government ministries, including Health and Community, Co-operative Development and Women's Affairs.

There are at present between two and three thousand supplementary food production plots distributed throughout all eight provinces of Zimbabwe. In some districts this scheme has been highly successful with the young child population in large areas being completely 'covered' by such units. Perhaps the best example is in the Musami area of Murewa District, some 80 km from Harare. Here there are over 50 food production plots and associated pre-school centres. Maize, groundnuts and beans are produced and in several centres a surplus exists even after the allocation for all pre-school children and retention for seed have taken place. These centres serve not only as activity and day care centres for all pre-school children but also as outreach points for the health service. When these places are visited each month immunization, health education and growth monitoring are performed. Those children attending the centre and any children from the 'catchment area' who are too young to be registered for day care are weighed. If growth faltering is detected the child's parents are counselled. If the child is not already attending the pre-school centre – usually because the child is too young – the parents are instructed to bring the child for daily weighing and supervised feeding. Thus, feeding points have been transformed into comprehensive child care centres and production units. The registers kept at Musami's Mission hospital indicate that the prevalence of young child undernutrition has declined markedly since the early 1980's and is considerably lower than the country average.

Summary

As a consequence of the war and several years of drought the background undernutrition in Zimbabwe had worsened. The relief side of the CSFP was therefore critical for a few years. As some district coordinators of the programme stated: 'Most children would have died without the CSFP'. However, the educational value of the CSFP was also noted: 'The programme has done a lot of good work to all malnourished children in the province. It has come to peoples' knowledge that local foods are very good to children, not food from stores only as people used to think'. In the 1981 evaluation of the CSFP, the structural constraints to better nutrition, health and living standards were identified. Clearly, the overcoming of these and the construction of a society based on social equity are necessary to solve the problem of undernutrition. Communal production and communal consumption of high energy, nutritious foods are only small steps in that direction.

Further reading

Beaton GH, Ghassemi H. Supplementary feeding programmes for young children in developing countries. *American Journal of Clinical Nutrition.* 1982; **35** (4): 864–916.

The Children's Supplementary Feeding Programme in Zimbabwe. Report presented to Ministry of Health, Zimbabwe, March 1982.

Dearden C, Harman P, Morley D. Eating more fats and oils as a step towards overcoming malnutrition. *Tropical Doctor.* 1980; **10**: 137–42.

Report on the Evaluation of the Child Supplementary Feeding Programme, Ministry of Health, Zimbabwe (undated and unpublished).

Sanders D. Nutrition and the use of food as a weapon in Zimbabwe and Southern Africa. *International Journal of Health Services.* 1982; **12** (2): 201–13.

Shakir A, Morley DC. Measuring malnutrition. *Lancet.* 1974; **i**: 758.

Tickner V. The food problem. *From Rhodesia to Zimbabwe,* No. 8. London, CIIR, 1979.

Waterlow JC, Payne PR. The protein gap. *Nature.* 1975; **258**: 113–17.

Brazil: oral rehydration therapy

M. A. de Souza

Gastroenteritis is a major cause of disease in children under five years of age and is responsible for 50 per cent of the infant mortality in north-east Brazil. Factors responsible include climatic characteristics, early weaning and scarce sanitation measures. In the period of 1978–81, a study was carried out in a rural area of the state of Ceara on the epidemiology of gastroenteritis in this particular age group. One of the results of that study was to show the 'itinerary' of mother with her sick child seeking resolution of his illness. During the first two days of his disease the mother herself treats her child with home remedies, such as different kinds of teas and infusions. Only if symptoms persist will she seek help from a traditional healer (rezadeira).

We decided to try to take advantage of the itinerary that the mother follows, as well as the confidence she places in the rezadeira. Thus, in 1984 we began an educational effort to involve the rezadeira in the rehydration of children with diarrhoea. The contact with the rezadeira was made through mothers who were asked which rezadeira they sought. Some were consulted more than others. After identifying two or three it was easy to locate the majority of the others.

One of the difficulties we had at the outset was that we were health 'professionals'. At first some traditional healers considered our presence as a kind of inspection of their work, since in the past physicians have criticized their work. With time, as we came to gain their confidence, this problem was resolved. In subsequent projects in other sites we have not identified ourselves at the beginning as health professionals, thereby avoiding this early barrier.

The rezadeira is generally a woman (although there are also some men), over 40 years old and mostly between 60 and 70 years old. She is frequently illiterate, humble and poor, and lives among others of the same condition. She talks simply and has a personality that inspires confidence in those who call on her. Often the traditional healer is also a midwife. The rituals of this traditional healer may vary but the attitude of confidence is always present. She performs her work voluntarily as an act of charity. As a class, rezadeiras do not have any organization representing them. We first observed that when a mother seeks the help of a traditional healer she will never say her child has 'diarrhoea' because this is considered to be only a symptom of another underlying common disease. These folk diagnoses (spell, fallen belly, evil-eye, teething, fright, etc.), of which there are around 20, are interesting since they are part of a dialect unknown to the official medical system. Furthermore, only the traditional healer is considered capable of 'curing' the child of certain of these folk illnesses.

Mothers consult the rezadeira during two periods of the day, early in the morning or at the end of the afternoon. At times, one will find a queue in front of her house. Some will attend each child separately, while others will fill the room and treat them collectively. It is interesting to note the touch of the rezadeira on the child. They will come to a folk diagnosis using, for

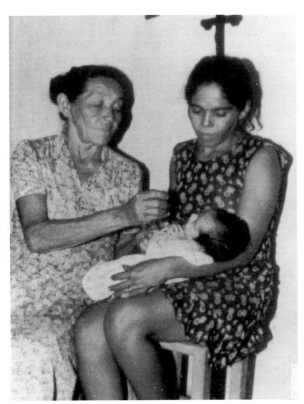

Fig. 1.4.9 Rezadeira giving oral rehydration solution.

example, measures of the limbs, giving great importance to differences between the arms or the legs. We also observed that the prayer, which constitutes the essential treatment, is the same for all cases, whether the child has diarrhoea or another illness. The prayer mentions all the internal organs in a sequence, to remove the ills from the body. A branch from a plant (each rezadeira having her specific preference) is repeatedly passed over the body of the child, especially the head and limbs. The process lasts about 10 minutes. She may also recommend various kinds of tea, but the most important element of the treatment is the prayer, and faith. Completing the prayer, she sends the mother and child home, always with the farewell 'God be with you'.

Once we learned the ritual of the rezadeira, the educational process began by trying to adapt to the folk language used and to support her work. During this phase it is important to be quick-minded, coherent, and above all, to renounce any attitude of superiority, to gain their support. It is also essential to learn to listen,

more than to speak. In this regard, time is the most important investment one can make when working with traditional healers or any other non-formal leaders.

We had numerous contacts with the rezadeiras, observing and trying to evaluate their reaction to oral rehydration solution (ORS). We would meet at one of their homes to listen to their opinions. Some of them were already familiar with ORS, but the difficulties we faced were to motivate them to actually distribute the packets to their clients, and to learn to teach the preparation of a sugar–salt–tea blend. Since most of them cannot read, all instructions had to be pictorial.

The specific orientation included preparation of the ORS from the packet, administration of it to the child, and the need to prepare a new litre of ORS every 24 hours. Two of the difficulties were the amount to be given to the child, and the discarding at 24 hours of the remaining volume. The mothers have the tendency to suspend the ORS as soon as the child begins to improve, and do not want to discard the excess, 'throwing away such a good treatment'.

Another difficulty is that a mother stops feeding her child when it has diarrhoea. She thinks that by giving foods to the infant she will be aggravating the diarrhoea. This concept was supported in the past by the medical community and, unfortunately, continues to be promoted to some extent.

Once we had solved the difficulties concerning our understanding of their language and the importance of distributing the ORS, we started an educational process about the risk of diarrhoea to children with the object of teaching recognition of the following risk symptoms: depressed fontanelle, pronounced skin creasing (tenting), sunken eyes and lethargy. Again, the difference in terminology was a problem because they had their own terms for each of these symptoms. We saw that they used the same risk criteria but with different phrases taken from popular terminology.

Following this period of discussion of the preparation of the ORS, and the identification of signs of risk, they began the distribution of ORS packets and with great enthusiasm. The rezadeira, after the prayer ritual, now showed the mother how to prepare and administer ORS and gave her packets to take home (see Fig. 1.4.9).

The great advantage of the participation of the rezadeira is that it permits introduction of ORS early in the illness, since the mother seeks her help at the outset of the illness, when dehydration is mild. Children with moderate or severe dehydration present among families who live further away, beyond the reach of this programme, are referred to the nearest health facility when necessary. Occasionally a mother may seek out a well-known rezadeira living in another community.

Supervision is provided by community health workers (CHWs) who maintain regular contact with the rezadeira, follow the child through home visits and refer the child for medical care if severe dehydration or other complications appear.

The participation of the CHW is fundamental because, in addition to serving as an intermediary between the rezadeira and the official health service, he/she is responsible for registering cases. Each CHW is capable of following five rezadeiras, and, ideally, will pay a visit when the rezadeira is receiving patients.

Normally the child will return to the rezadeira to repeat the prayer ritual several times, providing an opportunity for her to evaluate the evolution of the illness. Specific evaluation criteria, for example, based on weight loss, cannot be applied at this level, but the CHW will follow and care for complicated cases.

The first site where we began our work at the end of 1984 was a poor urban area with a population of 1000, including 180 children under five years of age. All the traditional healers are involved in actively distributing ORS. Assessment of the number of diarrhoea cases they attend is made by the number of packets distributed. In 1986 1920 packets were used and (estimating two packets per child per episode) roughly 960 episodes of diarrhoea in children were treated.

This specific project is being carried out in collaboration with the state government, through an agency responsible for social programmes in periurban areas of the capital (Programas de Assistencia as Favelas de Fortaleza – PROAFA).

The official health system, principally the physicians, is now beginning to discuss the idea of involving the rezadeira. The Federal University of Ceara, with support from the University of Virginia (USA) concluded, in 1987, a project in a rural community whose objective is the use of ORT by all traditional healers. It is hoped that this will facilitate the relationship between the official and the traditional health care systems. Discussion of this work has also been included in the curriculum of students of the health professions, and some are working directly with rezadeiras in other projects. This will certainly lead to greater integration between formal and non-formal health providers in the future.

We have learned from this work that the integration of modern and traditional healing is a necessity in this region of Brazil. The traditional healers are to be respected and supported as natural leaders in their communities.

China: primary health care

Victor W. Sidel and Ruth Sidel

Background
A policy for health
Recent developments in health services

Community participation – the 'one child' policy
Further reading

Background

China is the home of what is by far the world's largest population, over one billion people, unevenly distributed over an area approximately the same size as Australia, Canada or the United States. The vast majority of the people live in eastern China, with its three great river basins; western China, with its mountains and deserts, is exceedingly sparsely populated. Overall some 80 per cent of the Chinese people live in rural areas and only 20 per cent in cities and towns.

China is technologically a poorly developed country with a gross national product estimated at about $400 per capita. Great differences exist in material well-being between the cities and the countryside, between the areas in which the Han (Chinese) and the minority populations live, and among and even within cities and rural areas. The differences have been reduced in many ways and appear to be far less than the chasms that existed before 1949, although policies of the past few years may be perpetuating differences or even increasing some of them.

The people of China in the 1930s and 1940s suffered the consequences of widespread poverty, poor sanitation, continuing war and rampant disease. Most deaths in China were due to infectious diseases, usually complicated by some form of malnutrition. Preventive medicine was almost non-existent in most of China. Therapeutic medicine of the modern scientific type was almost completely unavailable in the rural areas and for most poor urban dwellers. What medical care was available to the vast majority of the Chinese people was provided by the roughly half-million practitioners of traditional medicine, who ranged from poorly educated pill peddlers to well-trained and widely experienced practitioners of the medicine the Chinese had developed over two millennia. These practitioners and those who practised Western medicine remained deeply mistrustful of each other and blocked each other's efforts in many ways.

Probably most important of all, three-quarters of the Chinese people were said to be illiterate. Cycles of flood and drought kept most of the people starving or, at the least, undernourished. And the limited resources that did exist were maldistributed, so that a few lived in comfort and the vast majority lived a life of grinding poverty. Feelings of powerlessness and hopelessness were widespread; individual efforts were of little avail, and community efforts were almost impossible to organize.

Yet today there is little evidence of the widespread malnutrition, disease and disability that accompanies poverty in most other poor countries of the world. Infant mortality, for example, has been sharply reduced, from approximately 200 deaths in the first year of life per 1000 livebirths in the 1940s to approximately 50 today and life expectancy at birth has increased from some 35 years to the high 60s today.

These changes in health status are certainly not solely the result of changes in medical care or even in what is usually narrowly defined as prevention; elements often included in primary health care, such as improvements in nutrition, sanitation, education and community organization are at least as important. Among those elements that are of special interest are: the society's fundamental redistribution of wealth and power, which made possible many of the other changes that have occurred; the system's emphasis on prevention, with its attempts to mobilize the mass of people to protect their own health and the health of their neighbours; its utilization of traditional Chinese medicine in combination with 'Western' medicine; and its training of part-time health workers who remain integral members of the community and until recently provided most of the primary health care.

A policy for health

In 1950, a new national policy for health services was established:

- Medicine should serve the needs of the workers, peasants and soldiers – those who previously had the least services were now to be the specially favoured recipients of services.
- Preventive medicine should be put first – where resources were limited, preventive medicine was to

take precedence over therapeutic medicine.
- Chinese traditional medicine should be integrated with Western scientific medicine – instead of competing, the practitioners of the two types of medical care should learn from each other.
- Health work should be conducted with mass participation – everyone in the society was to be encouraged to play an organized role in the protection of their own health and that of their neighbours.

In the 1950s, a number of new medical schools were established and class size in the older ones was vastly expanded. These efforts produced a remarkably large number of 'higher' medical graduates; it has been estimated that more than 100 000 doctors were trained over 15 years, an increase of some 500 per cent. But by 1965 China's population had also increased and the doctor/population ratio was still less than one per 5000 people. At the same time large numbers of 'middle' medical schools were established to train assistant doctors, nurses, midwives and other 'mid-level' health workers, but they too were still insufficient to meet the needs of China's vast population.

Changes after the cultural revolution

In 1965, in a written directive that was one of the forerunners of what came to be known as the Great Proletarian Cultural Revolution, Mao Zedong severely criticized the Ministry of Health for what he called its over-attention to urban problems and urged a series of changes in medical education, medical research and medical practice. As a result of his directive and of the first part of the Cultural Revolution, by the early 1970s much in medicine was markedly reorganized. Higher medical schools began to admit students who had had much less previous schooling but with considerable work experience and the curriculum was markedly shortened and altered to emphasize practice in the rural areas and the combination of Western and traditional Chinese medicine. Peasant health workers, known as 'barefoot doctors', were trained in large numbers and given responsibility for the provision of primary health care, including environmental sanitation, health education, family planning, immunization and first-level medical care. Although 'barefoot doctors' actually wore shoes most of the time and especially while performing their medical tasks, the term was used to emphasize the fact that these personnel were peasants who performed their medical work while maintaining their agricultural tasks.

Barefoot doctors, trained for relatively brief periods of time, generally worked in health centres provided at what was called the 'brigade' level (approximately 2000 people) of the communes (economic, political and social units of 10 000 to 50 000 people) into which China's rural areas were divided. The barefoot doctors provided treatment for 'minor and common illnesses', were skilled in first-aid and were available for medical emergencies. Barefoot doctors had a clear referral path, again imbedded in the commune structure; patients who needed more expert care were referred for primary and secondary care by physicians in the commune hospitals. If more specialized care was needed, the patient could be referred to a hospital at the county level, the third level of the 'three tier' system in the countryside.

The urban counterparts to the barefoot doctor were Red Medical Workers in the neighbourhoods and 'worker doctors' in the factories. They, like the barefoot doctor, were given responsibility for first-level care, for preventive medicine, for sanitation, for health education and for family planning at the local level.

During the late 1970s, following the end of the Cultural Revolution, there began to be open criticism of the barefoot doctors. Their training was said to be uneven, their supervision sometimes inadequate, and their practice at times incompetent. In keeping with the Chinese drive to improve technical quality, local departments of public health began to markedly upgrade the training of barefoot doctors: require the demonstration of their knowledge through examinations; define their role more narrowly; reduce their numbers; increase their supervision by more extensively trained medical personnel, and to some extent centralize the structure in which they work. Overall, Chinese estimates of the number of barefoot doctors in China fell from 1.8 million in 1975 to approximately 1.5 million in 1980 and to approximately 1.2 million in 1984.

Simultaneously, since the late 1970s, fundamental changes have taken place within Chinese society and particularly in the rural areas. As part of an attempt by the Chinese government to increase production, the 'contracted production responsibility system' has been introduced, giving individual households responsibility for production on assigned portions of the communally owned land. Peasants now receive direct financial rewards for individual or family output and, as a consequence, the economic structure of the communes has been significantly changed and their political role has been shifted to the 'township'. Almost 80 per cent of the brigades (now called 'villages') have shifted from a collective to a household-based system of production. Since the barefoot doctors and the cooperative medical services were largely financed by commune or brigade funds, the funding base of health care in most rural areas has shifted. For example, at its peak, some 80 to 90 per cent of China's rural population was covered by the cooperative medical care system (a medical insurance program at the brigade or commune level); as a result of the economic changes in the countryside, it is reported that only 40 to 50 per cent of the rural population is now covered.

Recent developments in health services

Even more recently, as part of the attempt to improve the technical quality of medical care in the countryside, the Ministry of Health has discontinued the use of the term 'barefoot doctors' (although some local areas continue to use it). According to the Ministry, those barefoot doctors who have received sufficient additional training and have passed qualifying examinations are to be called 'rural doctors'; those who fail to pass will either be required to give up their health work or will be called 'health aides'. Some recent visitors have reported instances of private fee-for-service practice by some rural or barefoot doctors; other observers note that less attention is being paid to public health matters such as sanitation, safe water supplies, and the pollution produced by new small factories being increasingly developed in the rural areas.

In the cities, the local primary health care workers called Red Medical Workers during the Cultural Revolution are now called Red Cross Health Workers. They work in what are now known as Red Cross Health Stations in the urban lanes, providing first-contact care. Patients with more serious problems (but those that would still fall in most countries under the heading of primary care) are referred, or are increasingly likely to go directly, to the neighbourhood hospitals or to the medical facilities in their factories. These are largely ambulatory care centres, usually including some inpatient beds, staffed by assistant doctors, doctors trained in Western-style medicine and doctors of traditional Chinese medicine. The Western-type doctors in the larger neighbourhood hospitals practice in the 'polyclinic' style, with different doctors concerned with pediatrics and with adult medicine and with a number of speciality clinics available. Most secondary and all tertiary-care patients are referred to the urban third tier, the district hospitals, and when necessary to municipal and specialized hospitals.

Community participation – the 'one child' policy

Community participation has been a central principle of the Chinese health care system since the early 1950s.

A key technique in controlling the rampant infectious disease, the participation of organized groups of workers and peasants continued to be encouraged during the 1960s and 1970s and continues to some extent to the present.

Community participation in health work has been instrumental in the massive efforts to lower the birth rate that began in the late 1960s. In 1979 a massive campaign was launched to limit families to one child. Elaborate and varied incentives and disincentives, health education techniques and intense persuasion by health workers and community leaders have convinced the vast majority of urban couples to have only one child, but appear to have had less success with rural couples. Over the past few years, the government seems to have accepted the virtual impossibility of limiting rural couples to only one child and criteria have been instituted under which it is permissible in rural areas (and in a few cities as well) for some couples to have two children.

Overall, enormous progress has been made over the past four decades, using principles of what now would be called 'primary health care'. Infectious disease, although causing a considerably smaller percentage of population morbidity and mortality than in comparably poor countries, remains at a higher level than in affluent countries. Death rates from cancer and cardio-vascular diseases are rising rapidly. Some regions, particularly in China's Western provinces and in areas in which minority people live, still lack access to adequate health care and medical technology is still primitive in many areas. Perhaps most important, the recent economic changes and the new drive toward high technology may be threatening the extraordinary efforts that have been made to eliminate the differences in the standard of living among China's people, to ensure equity of access to education, health and other human services, and to provide exemplary primary health care.

Further reading

Hsiao WC. Transformation of health care in China. *New England Journal of Medicine*. 1984; **310**: 932–3.

Sidel R, Sidel VW. *The Health of China: Current Conflicts in Medical and Human Services for One Billion People*. London, Zed Press, 1982.

Sidel VW. Medical care in China: equity vs modernization. *American Journal of Public Health*. 1982; **72**: 1224–5.

Sidel VW, Sidel R. *Serve the People: Observations on Medicine in the People's Republic of China*. Boston, MA, USA, Beacon Press, 1974.

Bangladesh: primary health care in the rural community

Zafrullah Chowdhury

Gonoshasthaya Kendra (People's Health Centre)

Gonoshasthaya Kendra (GK) was founded in 1972 in Savar Upazila*, 22 miles north-west of Dhaka, the capital of Bangladesh. It was started by a group of doctors and young people who had worked together in running a field-hospital for freedom fighters and refugees during the 1971 liberation struggle of Bangladesh. An extensive house-to-house survey by GK in the Savar area in October 1972 showed that only

*An upazila is an administrative unit with a population of 150 000–350 000; there are 460 upazilas in Bangladesh.

1.6 per cent of women and 8.4 per cent of men could read a local language (Bengali) newspaper. The group of workers from the field-hospital soon realized that high maternal mortality and death from diarrhoea and neonatal tetanus had little to do with the availability of drugs but a lot to do with the absence of education, adequate water supply and antenatal services. The excessively high infestation of intestinal parasites was due to inadequate sewage disposal. According to a government task force, maternal mortality in Bangladesh varied between 4.8 and 6.2 per 1000 pregnancies in 1982–3.[1] Another government survey[2] gave the average number of episodes of diarrhoea per child as 3.60 per annum. Of the children who died from diarrhoea, 41 per cent had received no treatment whatsoever and of the treated group 73 per cent were wrongly treated with methods other than oral rehydration therapy (ORT). Similarly, 41.4 per cent of women who died from pregnancy-related causes received no medical treatment.[3]

Poverty is a social disease which cannot be cured by medical treatment. For the first time doctors from the original group at GK were able to understand the full implications of this. The distribution of ill-health has an inverse relationship to income. Families with lower incomes have higher rates of morbidity and mortality. A survey[4] in Companyganj Upazila (population 120 000) in southern Bangladesh, showed that the crude death rate was markedly higher among landless families (Table 1.4.8).

Health problems are a consequence of underdevelopment. A strictly medical approach cannot achieve a healthy community. The community itself needs to be involved. But which community? 'The community' in rural Bangladesh is not a homogeneous entity. A small oppressive ruling élite live in close proximity with ordinary villagers and each class has different needs and priorities. The élite demand hospitals, while the poor need water for the crops (without which the crops will fail and the whole family starve). A health programme that ignores the conditions which produce ill-health must remain ineffective.

GK has responded over the years by helping in the formation of cooperatives for landless and marginal farmers. Vocational training centres for women have enabled them to learn skills and earn money. The centres have also provided basic education for women, concentrating on literacy and topics such as the value of immunization, birth spacing and preparation of oral rehydration solutions. There is also positive discrimination in favour of women in all project activities. Over 65 per cent of all workers at GK are women. The project has started primary schools, run entirely by women teachers, for the children of landless families. Health education is a part of the curriculum. Older children act as teachers for junior classes. The child to child teaching programme for health education has been very successful. It was noticed in some cases that children were more effective than the health workers in demonstrating the value of oral rehydration to their families. These activities give some idea of what is meant by an integrated approach to development and how the health work of GK is supported by other aspects of the centre's programme.

GK established a pharmaceutical factory in 1981 which produces low-cost but WHO-approved quality, essential drugs. The drugs are marketed under generic names. The advent of the factory has led to lower drug prices than those of multinational companies. The factory greatly influenced the Bangladesh government in the formulation of a National Drug Policy in 1982.

The GK health programme

The WHO declaration at Alma-Ata in 1978 emphasized that primary health care must be made accessible to all. The declaration also stressed the importance of community participation. Medical education, however, has often worked to prevent the provision of such primary care. Because of the inadequacy of the teaching and training in medical schools and because of their class background, doctors all over the world are unwilling to work where they are needed most. Doctors need help to provide primary health care in rural areas. A complementary cadre is required who will be trained in the special skills of communication and service delivery to villagers, areas in which a doctor is not trained. Such a person, who may be referred to as a 'paramedic', is not second-best to a doctor, any more than the primary school teacher is second-best to the university lecturer.

The GK health programme now covers a population of over 129 000 in Savar and another 50 000 in Sherpur.

Paramedics: their selection, training and duties

Selection

Ideally all paramedics should be recruited from the area where they work. This is not always feasible because not many girls with 10 years of education are available in places such as Savar. A community is consulted about the selection of the paramedics. But sole responsibility for selection of the candidate is not left with the community, as the rich and powerful villagers would

Table 1.4.8   Land holding and crude death rate

Acres of land per family	Crude death rate (per 1000 popn.)	Death rate in children (1–4 years/1000)
None	35.8	85.5
0.01–0.49	28.4	48.2
0.50–2.99	21.5	49.1
3 or more	12.2	17.5

always manage to get their sons and daughters appointed.

Criteria for selection are as follows:

- Preferably women, usually aged 16–25 years, but men are also employed.
- Candidates from poor families with 10 years of schooling are given preference.
- Smokers and/or betel nut chewers are not recruited.
- Candidates are interviewed and selected by senior paramedics.

Training

The training period is usually one year. During the first six months the trainee learns to ride a bicycle. She accompanies and assists a senior paramedic in village work and attends classes in the evening on subjects ranging from basic anatomy and physiology, to the problems of women and land distribution. The importance of breast-feeding, ORT, hygiene and sanitation is taught; also that children of non-smoking parents suffer less frequently from respiratory infections. The trainees also learn how to communicate the message of preventive health to people in the villages. The local language (Bengali) is the medium of instruction. The dangers and waste involved in unnecessary use of drugs, such as antibiotics and useless cough mixtures, are stressed. Paramedics are repeatedly reminded of the costs of curative care.

Much emphasis is placed on the causes of maternal mortality and its prevention. Overwork and inadequate diet contribute to the incidence of babies of low birth weight. Paramedics are taught to involve not only the pregnant woman but also her mother-in-law in antenatal care, since the latter is likely to be a key figure in deciding how much rest and food the pregnant woman needs.

Paramedics are taught immunization techniques, how to sterilize equipment, and how to do simple laboratory tests (haemoglobin estimation, blood count, ESR, acid-fast staining, etc.). They also learn the various methods of family planning, including menstrual regulation, and progress to learning how to undertake mini-laparotomy tubal ligation.[5]

Treatment of common diseases is included in the course with special emphasis on the social factors which lie at the root of many diseases. Thus, paramedics are taught not only how to treat skin diseases, pneumonia and diarrhoea but also about the association of these with poverty and malnutrition. A good paramedic will understand that malnutrition itself is not just a disease but a manifestation of inequality.

Besides specific health topics, paramedics are trained to be able to give advice on growing vegetables and other agricultural matters. Doctors and other workers at GK are involved in agriculture and work on the centre's own farm for an hour every morning to gain practical experience.

After the first six months, the paramedic is based at one of the subcentres where she starts working more independently. She is supervised and assessed by the senior paramedic in charge of the subcentre. Each trained paramedic is responsible for 3000–4000 people, depending on the distances between villages. Most of their work involves visiting households in the villages. Typically, the paramedic will sit on the verandah of one of the houses and can perform vaccinations and be consulted by anyone in the village with a health problem.

Duties

The duties of the paramedic include:

- Registration of births and deaths and enrolment for health insurance.
- Immunization.
- Identification of 'at risk' children, i.e. children with malnutrition and diarrhoea, chronic diarrhoea and night blindness, or persistent cough, fever, etc.
- Identification of pregnant women and 'at risk' pregnant women, who are given special antenatal checks in the village. Paramedics work in close liaison with traditional birth attendants (TBAs). More than 95 per cent of all rural deliveries are managed by TBAs. TBAs are given refresher courses at GK in safe birth care services and identification of high-risk women for referral.
- Health and nutrition education – breastfeeding, ORT, weaning food, etc.
- Motivation, supply and follow-up of family planning clients.
- Treatment of common diseases.

Paramedics are involved, in rotation, in curative care which is carried out through clinics at the main centre and subcentres. They are first to see and treat patients, referring difficult cases to one of the GK doctors. There is a 20 bed hospital in the main centre. Subcentres have facilities for two beds for obstetric and emergency patients.

Effects of the programme

Some of the most important changes resulting from the work of the paramedics are hard to quantify. They have

Table 1.4.9 Immunization rate (1985–6 and 1989–90) in the GK programme. (Numbers in brackets are percentages.)

	Year	
	1985–6	1989–90
DPT (6 weeks–2 years)	4806(68.02)	5902(73.5)
Polio (6 weeks–2 years)	4695(66.5)	5946(74.1)
Measles (9 months–2 years)	–	2984(88.1)
BCG (0–15 years)	45 441(83.3)	39 487(86.7)
TT (15–45 years; women)	19 709(83.5)	15 532(81.5)

DPT = diphtheria, pertussis, tetanus; TT = tetanus toxoid; BCG = Bacille Calmette-Guérin.

been able to build relationships of trust with local people through their regular visits to the villages. These visits are important since they provide the essential follow-up so often lacking from crash programmes – most notably in the areas of immunization and family planning. Immunization is undertaken, keeping the work schedule of the villagers in mind, and side-effects such as malaise and swelling which develop later can be dealt with on subsequent visits.

Quantitative justification is not lacking. Figures show much higher rates achieved for immunization in the population covered by GK compared with national figures. Tables 1.4.9 and 1.4.10 give figures for GK showing that over 66 per cent of infants and 83 per cent of married women of child-bearing age were fully immunized. Whereas for the country as a whole, 'by 1984 less than 2% of infants were fully immunized with BCG, DPT, polio (OPV) or measles vaccine'.[6]

Cost of the programme

These results have been achieved at a very low financial cost. WHO estimates[7] give the cost of full immunization of a child in the developing world against six EPI (Expanded Programme of Immunization) diseases as US$5–15. Full immunization of a child for DPT, polio and BCG in the GK programme costs taka 47.94 (US$1.60). This figure includes staff salaries, transport, electricity and administrative costs as well as the cost to the Government of imported vaccine.

In 1985–6 the cost of the whole GK health programme for Savar (population 129 000) was taka 1.8 million. This does not include the cost to the Government of vaccines and family planning supplies which were provided to GK free of charge by the authorities. Of the total cost of the programme, taka 0.8 million was spent on salaries: 4 doctors (13%); 47 paramedics (70%); 14 ancillary workers (17%). This shows that paramedics certainly give value for money.

Health insurance

The state has an essential role in the provision of health care and the ultimate responsibility. However, in the spirit of Alma-Ata the community (and this means all classes) must participate in the decisions and financing involved in health care.

The GK health insurance scheme was introduced in February 1973. Originally there was a uniform system of charging. This took no account of economic or class differences and so inevitably discriminated against the very poor – just those with the greatest health needs that GK was trying to help. The insurance scheme was changed. The population was divided into four groups. The poorest (Group A) consists of those who cannot afford two meals a day for the whole family throughout the year. For this priority group there are charges but they are minimal. Group B and C contains lower income and better-off families and Group D the rich; these groups pay correspondingly higher charges. Uninsured people can receive medical care but pay more for it.

Payment for services helps maintain a feeling of self-respect and self-reliance. People feel that they are benefiting from a service to which they are entitled because of payment – not just receiving charity. In particular, the very poor receive a similar level of service to the rich but a service they have paid for.

The insurance scheme has encouraged people to seek medical help early rather than delaying to the last possible moment because of cost. Though the sums collected from individuals are not large, the number of people taking up the scheme has meant that a substantial amount of money has been collected. Abel-Smith has pointed out that, 'Insurance contributions may be the crucial source of additional finance needed by many developing countries if they are to achieve

Table 1.4.10 Vital statistics of the Savar health programme area (1983–4 and 1989–90)

Year	Population	Total birth	CBR per 1000	Total death	CDR per 1000	Total infant live births	IMR per 1000 pregnancies	Total maternal deaths	MMR per 1000 pregnancies
1983–4	106 107	3403	32.1	929	8.76	324	95.2	6	1.76
1989–90	126 264	3062	24.3	819	6.5	303	98.9	4	1.3

CBR = Crude birth rate; CDR = Crude death rate; IMR = infant mortality rate; MMR = Maternal mortality rate.

health for all'.[8] Thus, about 45 per cent of the costs of the GK health programme have been met by the insurance scheme. This is not to say that the scheme is without flaws. The idea of medical insurance is new to most people in the rural community where GK works and it will take time before anywhere near universal coverage is achieved. Defaulters are a problem and, as with any insurance system, some people will make unnecessary claims for services in order to get their money's worth.

Lessons learned

Somewhere near the end of many standard textbooks on medicine there will usually be a short chapter on tropical diseases. Those very diseases crucially affect the life chances of three-quarters of the world's population. One lesson that has been learned at GK is that reversing this order of priorities is no easy matter. The development of the health programme has been a continuous learning process and involved change, often difficult and sometimes painful. Much has had to be unlearned too, as staff at GK have come to understand more about the needs of the range of people who make up the rural community.

Secondly, the staff at GK have had to realize that the conflict of interests between rich and poor in a rural community, as elsewhere, will inevitably spill over into every aspect of life. Health and the provision of health care can never be divorced from social and economic circumstances. For health workers and others at GK, ensuring that the programme reaches the poor and vulnerable has involved continuous struggle and sometimes very real sacrifice.

Workers at GK have learnt the importance of change and the need to be prepared for conflict in order to protect the interests of the needy. A few specific points that led to some rethinking may be of interest:

- An early plan to rely largely on voluntary workers was soon abandoned; few people can afford to work without pay, and those who can often have other motives for offering their labour.
- The barriers created by education – often based on a British model adopted in the colonial period – and differences in attitudes and ways of thinking, only disappear very slowly. Time had to be spent with local people, listening to them and learning to understand their problems.

- Constant vigilance is necessary if benefits are to reach the poorest. Members of the local hierarchy will always try and adapt any new service or system to their own advantage.

For the future, GK staff have been helping to plan a course for medical students which will focus on the needs of poor rural communities. Research being carried out into medicinal plants may help to provide an acceptable and readily available source of low-cost medicines.

Reflecting on the experiences of GK, it is possible to say that there is now a greater understanding of the needs and problems of the community which the centre serves. The health of women and children in the target population has shown a definite improvement, which suggests that GK is managing to reach and help these vulnerable groups.

References

1. Government of the People's Republic of Bangladesh. *Report of Maternal and Child Health Task Force*. Population Control Wing, Ministry of Health, 1985 Mimeograph.
2. Government of the People's Republic of Bangladesh. *Morbidity and Mortality Survey on Diarrhoeal Diseases in the Rural Areas of Bangladesh*. 1983. pp. 1–38.
3. Khan AR, Jahan FA, Begum SF. Maternal mortality in rural Bangladesh: the Jamalpur District. *Studies in Family Planning*. 1986; **17** (1): 7–12.
4. McCord C. *What's the use of a demonstration project?* Paper presented at the annual meeting of the American Public Health Association, Miami Beach, Florida, October, 1976 (Mimeograph).
5. Chowdhury S, Chowdhury Z. Tubectomy by paraprofessional surgeons in rural Bangladesh. *Lancet*. 1975; **2**: 567–9.
6. Government of the People's Republic of Bangladesh. *Universal Child Immunization in Bangladesh*. (An abridged version of the joint Government/UNICEF/WHO Plan of Action for Intensifying the Expanded Programme on Immunization in Bangladesh), 1985. pp. 2–31.
7. Henderson R H. *Providing immunization: the state of the art*. Paper presented at the Bellagio Conference, March, 1984. Quoted in *Population Reports* of the John Hopkins University, 1986; **XIV** (1): 154–92.
8. Abel-Smith B. Funding health for all: is insurance the answer? *World Health Forum*. 1986; **7** (1): 3–11.

MANAGEMENT IN PRIMARY HEALTH CARE

John P. Ranken

Need for management

Widespread concern with the implementation of primary health care (PHC) has highlighted the importance of management to support community-based health activities. In the past, PHC has suffered from a lack of adequate support services, highly centralized administrative structures, inadequate supervision, poor systems to manage and supply drugs, lack of funding, especially for day-to-day costs, lack of appreciation of the implications of community participation, unrealistic expectations of community health workers, and inadequate information systems for evaluation and control. In the face of such problems there is a clear need for those concerned to improve standards of mother and child health and to understand and get involved in management issues for which they may not necessarily have received much formal training.

Good management is concerned with planning, organizing, directing and controlling resources to achieve results. In the case of primary health care, these results are to do with improved health of communities, and frequently the most important resource is that of the community itself. Where there is effective community-based health care, communities themselves play a major part in identifying their own health needs, and organizing their own resources to meet them. This coordination of effort within the community through the activities of village health committees, community health workers, etc. forms the basis of a management system and infrastructure which is essential if effective primary health care is to be maintained.

Infrastructure and organization

Support for community-based activities may come from local political, religious, social or development institutions. For health matters there needs to be a health centre, dispensary or health post for first-level referrals and to provide continuing training and supervision. Such a facility may serve a population of 10 000 to 20 000 living in 8 or 10 distinct communities within a rural area. At a higher (district or area) level, planning, management and in-patient referral services are needed to serve populations of 100 000 or more. Establishing and maintaining such infrastructures to meet local needs is a key task for health managers. Factors which need to be taken into account include:

- ensuring that there is a reasonable spread of health facilities and workers throughout the area;
- ensuring that each level has ready access and contact with the levels immediately above and below it;
- obtaining necessary financial and other resources and ensuring that they are used as effectively as possible;
- building and supporting effective teams at each level, e.g. village health council, health centre team, district management team;
- defining the duties of workers clearly and ensuring that they are trained and motivated to carry them out;
- making provision for continuity, so that activities do not collapse if a key person is absent or leaves;
- ensuring that each person and group has a clear sense of purpose and idea of what they are trying to achieve;
- clearly identifying leaders and those with authority to make decisions;

- ensuring that necessary supplies, equipment, transport, etc. are available when needed;
- using and adapting appropriate systems for organizing and controlling work.

Devising a strategy

A plan of action is needed if anything significant is to be achieved in the field of health or any other field. Many countries have produced long-term strategic plans, which identify national health priorities and methods of implementation, but little is likely to be achieved unless there is effective local planning. Such planning integrates national priorities with local needs and is based on answering four key questions:

- Where are we now?   = situational analysis
- Where do we want to be?   = goals and objectives
- How do we get there?   = action plans
- How are we doing?   = evaluation

At the local level there is the opportunity to ensure that those who produce plans are the same people who have responsibility for implementing them. This ensures that whatever plans are produced are realistic because they are based on an accurate assessment of the local situation. Also the plans are more likely to be implemented, because the implementors have a real understanding and commitment to do something about them. Responsibility for producing local plans can be given to a District Health Management Team acting as a District Planning Team. Typical membership of such a team would be: medical officer, health administrator, senior nurse, environmental health officer, PHC coordinator. This team may have final responsibility for devising and implementing a plan but they need to involve many others, e.g. community and local political representatives, other health workers, representatives of other agencies and non-government organizations.

The planning process

Planning begins by recognizing problems and the need for action. This entails a basic epidemiological approach in identifying local health needs and problems, and also what resources and opportunities exist within the community and the health system to tackle them. National priorities need to be incorporated as these determine what resources may be made available locally, e.g. financial allocations, cold chain equipment and training opportunities to support an expanded programme of immunization. Priorities need to be set, by analysing needs in relation to their

importance, prevalence and manageability, and long-term goals and objectives set. Long-term objectives (e.g. in a five-year plan) are likely to be measured in terms of outcome, e.g. 5 per cent increase in life expectancy, 20 per cent decrease in infant mortality rate. At local level the planning emphasis is more short-term, (e.g. for one year) in which specific targets are important, e.g. increasing the annual number of vaccinations in a particular health centre by 50 per cent. Short-term targets then need to be broken down into specific tasks to be carried out, persons responsible at each level and part of the district, budgets and resources needed. A common problem at this stage is that plans are too ambitious, especially where there are few resources. This highlights the need for realism in planning, and to be flexible in adjusting plans in the light of whatever resources become available. Implementing plans entails allocating resources, setting up organization and training, supporting communities, and putting health staff to work. The final stage in planning is evaluation, or checking to see that what was planned is actually achieved. Evaluation needs to take place throughout implementation, so that changes can be immediately made, and also towards the end of the planning period, so that the results of evaluation can form an input for the next planning period. Fig. 1.4.10 sets out the main elements in a planning and implementation cycle.

For planning to be effective it needs to be built in at every level of the health infrastructure. Thus, each distinct village or community (level A) will have its own plan derived through community diagnosis and based on the particular needs and resources of that community. This means that each community needs to have an active health council which is able to plan for the needs of its own community. It is a prime function of the health centre (level B) to give support to each community within its area in preparing and implementing its plans. Similarly, each health centre also needs to prepare and implement its own plans which take into account the needs of the health centre itself, and of the communities it serves within its own area. These health centre plans are again taken into account as the district (level C) prepares and implements its own plans. This kind of 'bottom up' planning is needed to complement the 'top down' planning from national levels and requires effective coordination, particularly at the district level. In turn, as each district makes its own plans these are incorporated into national plans.

Planning and budgeting

Budgeting is normally done on an annual basis, i.e. in

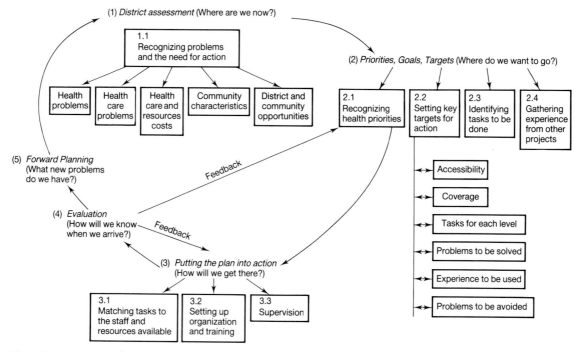

Fig. 1.4.10   The health planning and implementation cycle.

each district estimates of expenditure are made for the forthcoming year, based on the needs of the district, its plans, and a reasonable estimate of the resources (finance, manpower, etc.) likely to be available. Plans are modified once it is known more precisely what resources will be available, to become the district's annual programme of work. The annual programme of work then provides the framework for managing the district during the year. The annual programme of work needs to be broken down so that responsibilities for achieving results are clearly allocated to individuals. Those who have already been involved in producing plans thus become committed to achieving results based on those plans.

Management by objectives

This system translates plans into action by individual managers. It entails: reviewing the district's long-term and short-term plans; agreeing with each manager the 'key result areas' of their job, i.e. those aspects of the job which will achieve the results expected in the plan; specifying targets within each key result area, and detailed action plans to meet those targets; giving

support as needed; reviewing progress by use of appropriate control information.

Where much management of PHC falls down is in the lack of systematic support beyond central and district to health centre and community levels. This can be remedied where there is an ongoing system of targets, reports and reviews in operation throughout the district.

Targets, reports and reviews

A system for targets, reports and reviews requires a basic planning framework within the district. The important thing is to have the framework established. It may not be possible to have very elaborate plans and in fact too much planning (particularly at community levels) can distract attention from immediate things that need to be done. What is important is that health workers, community members and leaders in particular have a clear and agreed idea of what they are trying to achieve within reasonable periods of time; get practical help and support in trying to do it; and have the opportunity from time to time to review their achievements, correct any faults and reset their plans for the next period of time.

Clear accountability based on defined duties and targets for everyone in the district is necessary. Where people work with others in departments or teams, e.g. a hospital department, a health centre or immunization team, the responsibilities of the team as a whole need to be clear. The team leader, departmental head or supervisor must be held accountable for seeing that the team carries out its function and meets its targets. The task of managers, i.e. senior staff to whom team leaders, departmental heads and supervisors are accountable, is to see that those supervisors carry out their functions and meet their targets, and receive the help and support they need to do so.

A sensible and clear-cut organizational structure is required for the district as a whole. A common problem is that there is insufficient organizational support for PHC. In a large district it is impossible for the district medical officer of health and members of the district health team to give regular support to upwards of 100 or more villages and communities within the district. Such support can only realistically be given from the health centre level, which means that duties and responsibilities of health centre staff need to be defined in terms of giving support to community-based health care, and that the health centre superintendent is held accountable for providing such support. At the same time, the responsibilities of district level managers need to be defined in terms of supporting health centre superintendents in their PHC responsibilities. Frequently, however, the responsibilities of district and health centre managers are primarily defined in terms of providing curative services either directly themselves or through other health workers. One solution is to have a separate organizational structure for the district hospital whilst ensuring that there are effective links between the hospital and the PHC support organization.

A timetable for reports and reviews on a monthly cycle has many advantages. Various activities can be integrated so that, for example, monthly meetings are held in peripheral units at which salaries are paid, monthly supplies of drugs are issued, the previous month's work is discussed, problems sorted out, and priorities agreed for the following month.

Regular communication is the lifeblood of a PHC support system. In outlying rural areas its provision needs to be a high budget priority. Good systems are needed for scheduling, allocation, maintenance and use of vehicles. Appropriate transport may entail the provision of bicycles for community workers, motorcycles at health centres, and ensuring that full use is made of public transport by prompt reimbursement of money spent on fares.

Information has to be simple, easy to collect and of obvious use to those who collect it. A simple system is to have one-page weekly or monthly reports for each community, which are collated into monthly reports for each health centre, which are themselves collated into monthly district reports. Information will relate to activities carried out in communities and health centres, highlighting problems to be solved as against merely routine reporting.

Support and supervision

Support and supervision are key tasks for those in senior positions. Support is a better concept than supervision because it is a positive approach of helping and enabling workers to work well rather than negatively criticizing and inspecting them. Good supervisors build up an atmosphere of trust and helpfulness so that workers work well on their own. The key tasks of health centre supervisors are to plan the work of the health centre and the surrounding area; to allocate and coordinate the work of others; to set and encourage high standards of work; to instruct, train and support individual workers; to deal with problems that arise; to improve working methods and solve problems; and to encourage open communications by listening and explaining so that everyone is aware of what is going on. If supervisors are to do this task well they need to be carefully selected, given good training and have the authority to take full responsibility for the work of the health centre. This means that supervisors themselves must be able to rely on support from their own district managers in the form of clear guidance, trust, regular contact, backing for decisions, recognition and involvement in decision-making processes of the district as a whole.

The health centre supervisor has a key task of building and maintaining the staff of the health centre as an effective and hard-working team. For any team to be effective, it needs to have a clear purpose and task to which everyone is committed; each person needs to have a clear idea of their own job and how it relates to others; people need to be flexible so that they can help one another; there needs to be good leadership, loyalty and cooperation within the group; and the team must be successful in achieving its goals.

Discipline and standards

Managers need to set high standards for their own work, and maintain similar standards throughout the district. This means having clear work standards for each department, unit and individual worker, and encouraging supervisors to maintain them. Standards need to be reviewed from time to time, and lapses in discipline identified at an early stage. Disciplinary rules should define minimum standards of work behaviour concerned with timekeeping, carrying out instructions, use of money and other resources, e.g. drugs, transport. Where health workers are well motivated there should be few discipline problems but a clearly understood and agreed disciplinary procedure is needed to deal with lapses when they do occur. Such a procedure should provide for speedy action, proper investigation, warnings as necessary, rights of appeal, and backing for action, such as suspension or dismissal, where this is justified.

Particular problems arise with regard to unofficial practices, corruption, misappropriation of funds, etc. Such practices flourish where there is weak management and procedures for the use of funds and supplies, tendering of contracts, etc. are not clearly laid down or observed. Managers themselves need to set the highest standards of integrity and honesty, and to follow up reports of doubtful practice as a matter of priority and urgency.

Team-work

Because of the difficulties of managing large districts, successful managers try to ensure that their districts are made up of small groups of effective working teams. This is essential for PHC, with effective groups in every community, health centre, hospital ward and department. Linkages have to be established between teams, for no one team can work in isolation. This is particularly important in ensuring multisectoral collaboration. Many of the links between health workers and those in other agencies and departments such as agriculture and education will be established informally at first, but as joint projects are undertaken there will be need to work in various formal and informal groupings, making good use of a wide network of contacts throughout and beyond the boundaries of the district. To maintain these networks and groupings means that managers need to develop their social and interactive skills to a high degree, so that they can talk easily to people, make contacts, avoid disruptive conflicts, get agreement and cooperation, and maintain enthusiasm and commitment. Nowhere can this be more difficult than in planning and implementing changes, especially where those changes mean that someone else's interests or livelihood may be threatened.

Managing change

A positive approach to managing change (e.g. introducing a new drugs distribution system in a district) should entail the following:

- recognizing the need for change, e.g. faults in the existing system;
- identifying those who will be affected, e.g. pharmacist, medical assistants;
- explaining, winning the support, and incorporating the ideas of those affected, e.g. in agreeing contents of a basic drugs list;
- planning the details of the changeover, e.g. when, how and who;
- allocating new tasks and responsibilities to those involved;
- giving the new system a 'trial run';
- giving time to discuss and solve problems;
- monitoring the new system closely in its early days;
- ensuring that as far as possible those who are affected by the new system get some benefit, e.g. by smoother working, more interesting work, opportunities for personal development.

Logistic support

There are some aspects of management to which particular attention needs to be given to support PHC.

Transport

The need for an effective transport system has frequently been underestimated in planning for PHC. Transport needs to be low-cost and appropriate for each level, e.g. walking at community level; bicycles, motorcycles and donkeys at dispensaries and health centres; vehicles at district levels. Health workers may need to be encouraged to use public transport where it is available. This requires efficient local systems for reimbursing monies spent on fares. Budgets for fuel and maintenance also need to be made, based on realistic estimates of routine and non-routine journeys. Often journeys can be combined, e.g. distribution of supplies with support visits to outlying units. Full use can also be made of the natural desire of people in peripheral units to visit the centre, e.g. to settle pay queries, by encouraging training sessions, personal reporting, etc. at the centre. Transport frequently represents the most valuable resource under the direct control of a district management team, so its management should be a high priority. Scheduling, control of use, regular main-

Table 1.4.11 Transport problems and how to tackle them

Breakdown of vehicles	Ensure regular maintenance with log book for each vehicle, showing mileage and type of maintenance required
	Develop good relationships with local workshops, garages, mechanics
	Plan for temporary substitution of vehicles, bicycles, and so on
	Train users in proper upkeep and use of their vehicles
	Keep a reasonable supply of spares
	Regular vehicle replacement
Misuse of vehicles	Good supervision and training
	Good scheduling of vehicle use, so fewer opportunities for misuse
	Restrict use to named individuals
	Effective controls, log-books
	Enforceable policies on private use
High transport costs	Examine transport needs – are all journeys really necessary?
	Use low-cost transport – bicycles, by foot (a health worker, including doctors and nurses, on a bicycle or on foot gets closer to the community and becomes better known)
	Standardize vehicles, bicycles and spares
	Re-examine systems of work in the District
	Use public transport
	Work out cost per mile and transport costs for different services

Table 1.4.12 Problems and solutions in the management of drugs

Problems	Solutions
Costly drugs	
High prices	Tendering
	Procurement
	Basic list
	Review suppliers
Brand names	Use generic names
Bribery	Committee system for suppliers
Costly imports	Local production
High inventories	Control stock levels
Quality	
Poor quality	WHO certification quality assurance programme
Supplier fraud/ negligence	Bond
Deterioration	Storage
Wrong packaging	Control
No containers	Prepack
Misuse	
Wrong prescribing	Training
	Standard treatments
	Prescribe by level of use
	Overseas drug representatives
Patients' mistakes	Explain
	Community education
	Symbolic labelling

tenance, etc. should be a senior management responsibility. Where a clerical officer acts as transport officer, a clear transport policy is needed, and the transport officer given full backing to see it is carried out effectively (see Table 1.4.11).

Drugs and supplies

Although PHC emphasizes health prevention and promotion, supplies of basic drugs, vaccines, oral rehydration salts, etc. on a regular basis are essential. It is important to identify reasons for drug shortages. These can include overprescribing, overstocking, high patient demand, use of expensive brand-name drugs, poor storage, pilferage, misuse, and lack of explanation to patients. Means of dealing with such shortages include the use of standard drug lists; ordering in relation to usage, forecasted need, local health priorities, and cost; use of generic drugs, balanced programmes of prevention and cure; good storage and stock control; monitoring of drug issues; prepacking; sharing of pharmaceutical expertise and better education of prescribers and patients (see Table 1.4.12).

Standard drug lists need to be established and kept up to date. This entails reviewing existing prescribing and local disease patterns; eliminating duplications, i.e. two or more drugs serving the same purpose; removing old-fashioned and unused drugs; comparing effectiveness, convenience and cost, and choosing between alternatives. Having produced the standard drug list this needs to be followed by education in its use, the production of drug information sheets, and a review of supply and distribution systems. Such systems may be improved by the introduction of standard packs for use at health centres and dispensaries, review of ordering and storage procedures, and regular stock control to identify drug shortages and unused drugs.

Finance

It is the manager's responsibility to ensure that there is enough money to fund the activities of the organization. For a district medical officer this means making realistic estimates of expenditure, checking that adequate financial allocations are made from the central Ministry, costing new projects in good time to ensure adequate funding, and making full use of additional sources of finance from local sources, other agencies, etc. Thus, the costing of projects is a very important part of the planning process and a cost-conscious manager will always take into account the cost-effectiveness of alternative projects when deciding between them. In doing so, there must be a careful balancing of capital and recurrent costs. Capital costs are for large single items, such as buildings, vehicles and equipment. Recurrent costs are incurred on a regular basis, e.g. for salaries, drugs, fuel and main-tenance of buildings. A common problem in projects in developing countries is that the capital costs are funded through external agencies (e.g. for new health centres and vehicles) but insufficient provision is made for recurrent costs. Thus, there are insufficient funds for vehicle maintenance and fuel and there is a continual drain on resources to fund the recurrent costs of large institutions such as hospitals.

Once obtained, there must be proper budgetary control of funds to ensure their most effective use. It is a good principle of management that budgets should be held at as low a level as practicable, so as to give those who actually use resources of staff, drugs, supplies, and so on, the responsibility for controlling and using them effectively. Within a district budget, individual budgets may be based on: staff groups (e.g. a nursing budget held by the nursing officer); or programmes (e.g. an immunization or maternal and child health, MCH, programme); or facilities and catchment areas (e.g. health centres). There may be a combination of such individual 'budget centres' but it is important to identify an individual manager for each of them, e.g. head of MCH programme, health centre supervisor. These managers then have responsibility for controlling their own budgets, which may be largely expressed in terms of for example numbers of staff employed, hours worked, drugs used, miles driven, based on monthly statements and reviews. Once such budget centres are established it is then possible to make cost comparisons, for example between costs of different health centres or programmes, or between costs at different times of the year.

Day-to-day management of finance is concerned with managing petty cash, usually on an imprest system, whereby an advance of cash is given for a particular purpose and is replenished as necessary against original receipts of money spent. It is particularly important in managing such systems that workers who spend money on public transport, travel-ling allowances, etc. are recompensed quickly and efficiently.

District management and coordination

The task of district health management is complex, and much of a manager's time is spent in coordinating different activities and dealing with immediate problems that arise. To be effective, managers need to develop a range of skills and approaches which include the following:

- Taking a broad view – this entails looking at the whole needs of the district and balancing many competing priorities, clinical and non-clinical. In particular, it means listening to the needs of the community and making full use of community resources, whilst still operating within a formal bureaucratic structure. This dual responsibility is illustrated in Fig. 1.4.11.
- Personal motivation – where the manager has

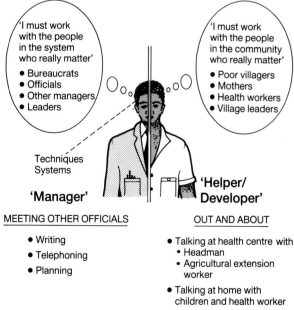

Fig. 1.4.11 The dual responsibility of a district health manager.

USING TIME WELL

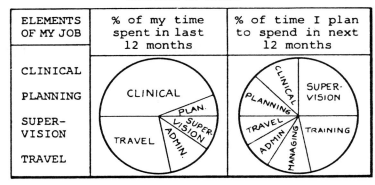

'To do' list

TODAY I MUST:

1. _____
2. _____
3. _____
4. _____
5. _____
6. _____
7. _____
8. _____
9. _____
10. _____

Review of time

ELEMENTS OF MY JOB	% of my time spent in last 12 months	% of time I plan to spend in next 12 months
CLINICAL PLANNING SUPER-VISION TRAVEL	CLINICAL / PLAN. / SUPER. / ADMIN. / TRAVEL	CLINICAL / PLANNING / SUPER-VISION / TRAINING / TRAVEL / ADMIN / MANAGING

CONSTRAINTS Things I am unable to do	DEMANDS Things I must do	CHOICES Things I can choose to do
• • • • •	• • • • •	• • • • •

BEWARE !

DO NOT BE SO PLANNED AND ORGANISED THAT YOU CANNOT MEET AND TALK TO PEOPLE

MAKE TIME ● To go out and talk to people
● Be available for people to talk to you

Fig. 1.4.12   Using time well.

positive, enthusiastic attitudes this will spread to others and enable many problems to be solved which previously appeared insurmountable.

- Building up effective working teams. Time and care spent in selecting good people will be amply repaid in the future.
- Recognizing people's potential contribution – starting with his or her own, but ensuring that every worker is able to make their best possible contribution to the work of the district.
- Using time well – this entails making good use of diaries, schedules, appointments, having daily, weekly, and monthly 'to do' lists, and reviewing time, as well as helping others to use their time effectively (see Fig. 1.4.12).
- Setting clear objectives and standards of performance which are relevant to the local situation, yet challenging enough to bring the best out of people.
- Planning the future whilst managing the present – dealing with immediate problems in ways which prevent similar problems arising in the future, and

provide a means of improving services.

- Organizing and allocating resources of money, facilities, time and supplies effectively to meet local needs.
- Decision-making – making good decisions about major issues which give other people freedom to make decisions within their own sphere of influence. Consulting others to ensure that their interests are taken into account when decisions are made.
- Delegating, motivating, and developing staff – managers who are continually concerned to train others to develop skilled, motivated and enthusiastic teams who work well together.
- Developing and maintaining systems – e.g. for drugs distribution, monitoring and evaluation, staff training, reports and reviews. Where such systems are well established and understood much of the work of the district will operate routinely and effectively.
- Monitoring and evaluating – this requires an attitude of mind which continually assesses how

programmes and work are being implemented, and makes necessary changes and adjustments at an early stage.

- Managing changes smoothly and effectively – recognizing when changes are needed, overcoming people's natural resistance to change, planning new approaches and effectively implementing them.

Management training

To be fully effective, health managers need to be well trained. This entails:

- Management training as part of basic training. Despite a crowded curriculum in medical and professional training schools, time needs to be found to give a basic appreciation of management, ideally as part of a systematic introduction to primary health care.
- Specific training and orientation when health professionals take up managerial positions, especially as members of health management teams.
- In-service training and development. Career development programmes are needed for those with an interest and potential for managerial work, in addition to regular courses, seminars, practical projects, etc.
- Team training. Management of PHC is so highly

dependent on teamwork, that it is appropriate for much management training to take place on a multidisciplinary basis, and especially for teams of managers who work together to train together.

- Personal learning. Managers need to accept responsibility for their own personal development, through systematic reading, involvement in new projects, planned visits, etc. The development of distance-learning material for managers should be a priority, with an emphasis on relating theory to work in the managers' own sphere of responsibility.

Further reading

Amonoo–Lartson R, Ebrahim GJ, Lovel HJ, Ranken JP. *District Health Care*. Basingstoke, Macmillan, 1984.

McGrath EH. *Basic Managerial Skills for All*. India, Prentice Hall, 1980.

McMahon R, Barton E, Piot M. *On Being in Charge*. Geneva, WHO, 1980.

Maneno J, Schluter P, Sjoerdsma AC *et al. Guidelines for Management of Hospital Outpatient Services*. Nairobi, AMREF, 1982.

National Council for International Health. *The Training and Support of Primary Health Care Workers*. Washington, NCIH, 1981.

O'Connor RW. *Managing Health Systems in Developing Areas*. Lexington, Massachusetts, Lexington Books, 1980.

IMMUNIZATION

J. P. Stanfield

Immunization in perspective

The most important single task in improving maternal and child health in developing countries is the prevention of infection. Immunization by the use of

vaccines is one means of achieving this – but it is important to realize that the role of vaccines varies greatly from country to country, from infection to infection and from vaccine to vaccine. Immunization is thus not a panacea in the control of infectious disease, and the strategies of an immunization programme will change as a country develops, as the disease pattern alters, and as new vaccines are produced. The vaccines will need to be defined at intervals in terms of specific needs and opportunities.

One or two examples may illustrate this. Historically, the incidence and severity of a number of infectious diseases have altered radically in the development of the so-called developed world. For instance neonatal tetanus has been eliminated in most countries of Europe and measles no longer poses a significant threat to life in childhood. This happened before the widespread availability of tetanus toxoid or measles vaccine.

In several rural villages in West Africa[1], measles mortality in children under five was found to be reduced to the same extent in villages with a regular vaccination programme against measles as in villages supervised by health care teams giving particular attention to health education and sanitation but with no measles vaccination. This study concluded that mortality had been reduced in the first case by reduction in measles incidence through vaccination, and in the second, by reduction in measles severity through improving general health and nutritional levels. Clearly a combination of inputs is needed.

In eastern Nigeria in 1968, smallpox vaccine supplies were inadequate for a mass campaign. Intensive efforts were made to identify new cases of smallpox and vaccination was confined to all individuals within a defined area surrounding each new case. Through this containment strategy smallpox was eradicated in eastern Nigeria in six months with less than half the population vaccinated.

Definitions

At the outset it is useful to be clear about the meanings of some of the terms used here.

Vaccines Vaccines are antigens derived from the naturally occurring or 'wild' infective agent against which immunity is sought. They fall into the following main categories.

Live vaccines These are infective agents developed in various ways from their wild progenitors in (a) an attenuated form in which virulence has been reduced or eliminated, or (b) as heterologous strains from animals which are very much less virulent for man and yet carry common antigens (such as vaccinia). They are usually viral, such as poliomyelitis (Sabin), measles, rubella, yellow fever, vaccinia, mumps, rabies, varicella and herpes, but can be bacterial, such as BCG.

Killed vaccines Killed suspensions of infective agent, such as pertussis, the enteric vaccines such as cholera and typhoid and the killed poliomyelitis (Salk) vaccine are used.

Toxoids These are made from purified toxins produced by the infective agent, attenuated to neutralize their toxic effect without reducing antigenicity. The diphtheria and tetanus toxoid components of the triple vaccine (DPT) are examples.

Component vaccines These are antigens originating from the infective agent. Toxoids come into this group. There has been considerable resurgence of interest recently in the field of bacterial vaccines, such as polysaccharide antigens of the capsules of pneumococci. Constituents of bacteria have been isolated and used as antigens such as ribosomal vaccines.

Immunization vs vaccination The distinction between immunization and vaccination is important, especially when an immunization programme is being evaluated and the following terms should be clearly differentiated.

The *immune status* of a community or population is the quality and quantity of immunity to a given infection or infections within that community whether through natural infection or immunization. Those who are not immune are termed *susceptible*. The *immunization status* refers to the number of people in a community or population who have been made immune through vaccination.

The *vaccination status* or *coverage* refers to the number of people in a population who have been vaccinated. In practice the immunization and vaccination statuses are used interchangeably, but it is well to remember that there may be a significant difference between the two, as for example in measles. If measles vaccine is given at six months of age, up to half of those vaccinated will not be immunized through failure of the vaccine to 'take' on account of persisting maternally transferred antibodies. If a vaccine loses its potency for any reason, i.e. through failure of the cold chain, again the percentage of those vaccinated who are subsequently immunized will progressively fall, ultimately to zero.

Thus, the success of a vaccination campaign should not only be judged by the 'coverage' though this may be important. The increase in the immune status, most simply judged by the incidence of infection, is the best measure of the success of a programme.

The present position in the developing world

Most of the commonly used vaccines of today have been available and widely adopted since the middle of this century by the developed world. The coincident improvements in socio-economic and environmental conditions have robbed immunization of a good deal of the credit for the reduction of such infections as diphtheria, tetanus and tuberculosis and of the morbidity and mortality of measles and whooping cough. In the case of poliomyelitis and smallpox the vaccines have been manifestly the main cause of the elimination of disease.

Immunization developed slowly in the Third World. Introduced into the general health services for mothers and children as a routine measure, coverage was minimal. In 1974 it was estimated that only 5 per cent of the total childhood population of the Third World had been covered by a completed schedule of primary immunization. This was despite measles causing the deaths of four million children, pertussis the deaths of half a million children, tetanus the deaths of nearly one million neonates, and poliomyelitis the crippling of up to one million children annually.

Following the success of smallpox vaccination, the World Health Organization (WHO) in 1974 launched a series of country-based initiatives entitled EPI (Expanded Programmes of Immunization). The long-term objectives were: reducing the morbidity and mortality of six major preventable infections of early childhood – diphtheria, whooping cough, tetanus (in particular neonatal tetanus), poliomyelitis, measles and tuberculosis; and immunizing all children by the year 1990. This was a vertical programme within the primary health care services of each country. It heralded a move away from the integrated approaches that were being emphasized in the wake of the Alma-Ata (1978) declaration on primary health care.

Initial progress measured on coverage (completed primary vaccination rates) is encouraging; in 1988 mean rates for countries of the developing world who had adopted EPI were BCG 63%, DPT 55%, poliomyelitis 56%, and measles 46%. The incidence of these infections has fallen in most of the countries where statistics have been considered reasonably reliable. This is especially so when due regard is paid to the counter effect due to improved reporting. The EPI programme does not yet appear to have accelerated this decline, apart from paralytic poliomyelitis. No data yet compare the incidence of non-vaccine preventable common childhood infections (such as respiratory infection and diarrhoeal disease) with the six EPI infections.

As the end of the century approached, UNICEF promoted a series of vertical programmes to support the child survival revolution. It had the twofold aim of generating more aid from the developed world and stimulating goal-orientated activities within the Third World. WHO has embarked on an accelerated programme of immunization (ACI).[2] Planning principles worked out for specific areas of activities include:

- opportunism at every contact;
- reduction of defaulting during completion of vaccination schedules;
- emphasis on the priority of controlling measles, poliomyelitis and neonatal tetanus;
- protection of large vulnerable populations exposed to high infection pressures, namely the urban poor;
- intensive publicity activities such as national immunization days, and social marketing which promotes a commercial advertising style of operation.

Primary vaccination strategies

The primary schedule for static health services is now advocated as follows.

For women of child-bearing age and pregnant women:

First contact	Tetanus toxoid
Next visit > one month later	Tetanus toxoid

For infants:

Birth	OPV (or IPV), BCG
6 weeks	OPV, DPT, BCG (if not given at birth)
10 weeks	OPV, DPT
14 weeks	OPV, DPT
9 months	Measles

For remote areas there is a mobile schedule requiring two visits:

3 to 8 months	DPT, OPV (or IPV), BCG
9 to 14 months	DPT, OPV (or IPV), Measles

In West Africa yellow fever vaccine is given on the second encounter.

Some programmes advocate 'pulse' saturation policy[3]: an immunization team stays in one area to give every child at least four doses of DPT and oral poliomyelitis vaccines (OPV), one BCG and one measles vaccination. The team moves from village to village, returning to the same village at monthly intervals until they have achieved at least 70 per cent coverage for all children. They then go to the next area. On completion of a district, after one year or so, they return to the initial villages and immunize the residual non-immunized and the new susceptibles.

Mass campaigns involve national immunization days when as many children as possible are given any or all of the six vaccines they have not completed taking. Sometimes these campaigns are in response to an outbreak of measles, poliomyelitis, meningococcal meningitis or yellow fever. In the future, new vaccines may be suitable for this activity. Follow-up at the local maternal and child health (MCH) clinic is desirable.

Current status of measles vaccine

Until recently the major problem with measles vaccine was cost. This ruled out universal use of the vaccine in the Third World. Giving less than the full dose did not work well, particularly if the cold chain was defective. The three major problems are all linked:

- the need to immunize at least 80 per cent of susceptibles to interrupt transmission;
- the percentage of susceptible infants under the age of nine months;
- the need to maintain the cold chain.

The susceptible population in the Third World is infants and children from nine months to three years. This excludes some infants under nine months, who have lost initially lower levels of maternally transferred immunity, and a small number over three years who have escaped infection. There is recent evidence that the rate of decay of maternally derived antibodies may vary with area. The reason is not known. For the time being it is reasonable to assume that inhibition of sero conversion may be present up to the age of nine months.

Below nine months of age, measles can be either as severe as that seen in older children, in babies who have received very little or no antibodies from their mothers, or so attenuated by residual maternal antibody activity as to be easily missed. The age incidence rises as over-crowding lessens, the more rural the environment and the less susceptible individuals there are in the community. The common factor in these three situations is the likelihood of meeting an infectious dose of measles virus, in other words, the infection pressure. The implication is clear. The prevention of measles below nine months of age depends on reducing the infection pressure rather than the age of vaccination.

Measles vaccination should aim to cover the age range nine months to three years. One dose of 0.1 ml (4000 plaque forming units) of current measles vaccines will infect 98 per cent or more of a susceptible population. The more effective the coverage the greater will be the 'umbrella' protection given to the remaining susceptibles. The threshold above which significant transmission is interrupted will vary, mainly with infection pressure; 80 per cent coverage is an arbitrary figure. It will be less in sparse rural populations and greater in overcrowded urban communities. In addition, in achieving adequate initial coverage it is vitally important to maintain the vaccination of fresh recruits to this age group and not allow the percentage of susceptibles to rise again. If this is not checked it will reach a critical level at which transmission re-establishes itself with an explosive outbreak of measles.

In my opinion, the maintenance of such coverage is far more important than lowering the age of vaccination, either by doses of injectable live vaccine at say six months and again at one year, or by aerosol vaccine or even killed measles vaccine at six months. First, such strategies are more expensive. Second, if they are given and fail, measles vaccine falls into disrepute. Third, concentration on effective vaccination at nine months and over will not only reduce the chances of infection for infants below nine months, but perhaps also the severity. There is a direct relationship between severity of infection and numbers of cases in each household.[4] Severity may be related to infection pressure or dosage of measles virions. Reduction in incidence of the infection will reduce infection pressure and very likely the severity of the infection. This fits with the experience of a falling mortality rate as well as a rising age incidence as the incidence of measles falls in association with a successfully maintained immunization programme.

Measles vaccination fails for two reasons: maternal antibody is present; or the cold chain is ineffective. Until recently, measles vaccine was thermolabile. Ineffective vaccine has been given, undermining confidence. There are now at least two heat stable vaccines. EPI programmes may therefore be less dependent in the future on the integrity of the cold chain.

Current status of pertussis vaccine

In combination with diphtheria and tetanus toxoid, a killed whole-cell suspension of *Bordetella pertussis* has been in use as a trivalent vaccine (DPT) for over 30 years. It is known to reduce the incidence and severity of whooping cough. The Third World was not involved in the controversy regarding post-vaccination encephalitis and subsequent brain damage. The problem of pertussis vaccine in the developed world lay in its very success. The control of whooping cough reached a point where the danger of the vaccine became more significant than the residual morbidity and mortality of whooping cough itself. This setback has had its constructive features. The reappearance of the infection in UK was caused by the fall of pertussis immunization rates. The severity of the infection was once again demonstrated beyond doubt.[5] Improved surveillance of vaccines resulted in much more realistic 'risk' estimates against which to balance their benefits.

Recently it has been estimated that the febrile convulsion risk is 0.3–9 per 100 000 doses of triple vaccine (DPT); encephalitis could be vaccine-induced in 0.1–3 per 100 000 doses; and the risk of permanent brain damage 0.2–0.6 per 100 000 doses. Compare these with the risks of whooping cough even in the apparently less severe forms in which it has reappeared in UK. Convulsions may occur in 600–8000 per 100 000 cases; encephalitis in 90–4000 per 100 000 cases; permanent brain damage in 600–2000 per 100 000 cases; and death in 100–4000 per 100 000 cases.

Death rates are highest under one year of age and especially under three months of age. In the UK, deaths per 100 000 notifications under three months were 20 in 1974/5, and 9 in 1978/9. In rural Kenya, the case fatality rate in 1984 was 2.6 per cent in the first year of life. With no maternal protection, stress has been laid on early immunization at six weeks to two months of age. In many instances a reduced dose schedule has been employed without any significant reduction in protection but with less local and generalized reactions. In Denmark, a monovalent pertussis vaccine has been given, commencing at five weeks of age, without untoward results. Since 1981 a non-cellular vaccine has been in use in Japan. Reports so far indicate less toxic side-effects and in a recent trial in Sweden whooping cough incidence has remained low. A large-scale trial in India is in progress with the intention of using the vaccine to protect infants in the first three months of life. The possibility of vaccination in pregnancy and more antigen as in tetanus toxoid, awaits a less toxic specific vaccine.

Current status of poliomyelitis vaccines

The advantages and disadvantages of killed (inactivated) and live (oral) poliomyelitis vaccines (IPV and OPV respectively) are still being compared after considerable experience of both.

The oral vaccine establishes an enteric infection with production of mucosal IgA and some circulating serum antibodies. The inactivated vaccine produces higher levels of serum antibodies, enough to interrupt invasion of 'wild' virus through the nasopharynx and intestines. An apparent disadvantage of the oral vaccine has been the very poor circulating antibody levels accompanying its use in the Third World. This may be due to a combination of the interference of effective colonization by other enteroviruses and the reduction in titre of the vaccine, through faults in the cold chain. Do circulating antibody levels correlate with the immune status? The proof of immune status is the incidence of the infection as vaccination proceeds. To overcome poor conversion rates the number of doses of the oral vaccine has been increased to four or five, the first three given with DPT vaccine at 6 weeks, 10 weeks, and 14 weeks. The current WHO schedule also advises a dose of oral vaccine as shortly after birth as possible. This should not, if possible, be given immediately before or after a breast feed because of inhibition which the high level of IgA in colostrum exerts on the establishment of vaccine colonization of the gut.

Can poliomyelitis be eradicated? A twice yearly mass national immunization day for all children under five, whether previously vaccinated or not, is advocated.[6] Community volunteers would be mobilized who could deliver the 'polio' drops. The volunteers could also notify any new cases of poliomyelitis and vaccinate all their contacts immediately. The target of reaching and maintaining 80 per cent coverage has been pledged by a number of international agencies.

Poliomyelitis has been virtually eradicated in many developed countries. The small number of cases of vaccine-associated poliomyelitis has prompted the use of inactivated polio vaccine (IPV). This can be combined with DPT in a quadruple vaccine. Given as a first dose at birth, IPV bypasses the inhibition of oral vaccine colonization produced by colostrum. A more potent IPV has been marketed recently but its cost is still too high to allow its widespread use.

Recent outbreaks of poliomyelitis in Finland and other areas have occurred in which the antigenic structure has differed slightly from the three standard serotypes. Eradication may not be as easy as smallpox though WHO has been committed to the global eradication of the infection by the year 2000.[16]

Current status of tetanus toxoid vaccine

Tetanus toxoid is one of the safest, most stable, antigenically potent vaccines in existence. Given in two doses, one month apart, it confers almost complete protection against tetanus. Subsequent booster doses given at the time of a deep and dirty wound or skin infection, at a subsequent pregnancy or at school entry, give lifelong immunity. The toxoid is an ingredient in the triple vaccine (DPT) given at 6 weeks, 10 weeks and 14 weeks of life and thereafter as a monovalent vaccine at intervals in childhood and adult life. Tetanus toxoid comes into its own in the prevention of neonatal tetanus, a far too frequent cause of neonatal mortality.

The mortality from neonatal tetanus, up to 800 000 or more annually throughout the world, is a major challenge to primary health care services.[7] Its reduction in endemic areas is as good an indicator of improved MCH services as any other single measurement, for it depends upon two crucial processes, clean deliveries and ensuring the immunity of all women in pregnancy, both of which involve supervisory contact in the antenatal period and at delivery. Antenatal tetanus immunization affects only that proportion of neonatal deaths due to tetanus, in some areas more than 50 per cent. A clean environment at delivery and immediately postpartum for mother and baby, has a greater impact on maternal and neonatal morbidity and mortality, as this eliminates not only tetanus but sepsis of all kinds.

Neonatal tetanus can be eradicated this century. Apart from the will to succeed, access to the target population appears to be the major limiting factor. Only 20 per cent of women are contacted antenatally or at delivery by the health care services. There are two main possibilities for achieving the immunity required to protect the neonate in endemic areas of tetanus. They are complementary.

One method is to immunize, either with two doses of toxoid or a single booster dose in the case of the already immunized, every woman of child-bearing age in the community. This has been attempted in a manner similar to the campaigns against measles and poliomyelitis. Mothers bringing children for immunization, as well as those attending antenatal clinics and in the process of delivering, are offered immunization.

A second approach is to maximize the contact with the pregnant population. Even a single dose of potent toxoid, given as long before delivery as possible, can produce protective levels of antitoxin in the cord blood in up to 80 per cent of deliveries. With such a single dose the percentage of babies adequately protected drops rapidly the closer to delivery it is given. A second dose at least one month after the first ensures almost 100 per cent protection, providing it is given at least a week before delivery. The key to increased contact during pregnancy is the traditional midwife. She could be trained to administer tetanus toxoid with the help of a disposable non-reusable plastic 'squeeze' injector.

The schedule recommended is a primary course of two doses of tetanus toxoid to any woman of child-bearing age, independent of whether she was immunized in infancy. The first dose should be given as early in the pregnancy as possible. A second dose can be given at least one month later and if possible more than one week before delivery is expected. Booster single doses can be given at intervals of at least one year or at the next pregnancy, whichever happens first, up to a total of five doses.

Current status of BCG vaccine

The vaccine is an attenuated *Mycobacterium bovis* strain. The many different preparations all derive from the original strain developed by Calmette and Guérin. The freeze-dried vaccine is reconstituted and given intradermally. By producing a primary focus of infection in the skin and local lymph nodes, it induces a cell-mediated immunity demonstrable by the development of tuberculin sensitivity.

The efficacy of the vaccine has been debated since its introduction. It is now thought that the vaccine protects by limiting the infection and preventing its septicaemic spread following an initial infection.[8] In Third World countries the vaccine is given shortly after birth and is usually the most widely administered. Coverage of 60 or 80 per cent is common.

In tropical environments where tuberculosis is endemic there are no contra-indications to BCG. In children with suppressed immunity, such as following measles, in the malnourished child, or in early HIV infection, it is better to have BCG than tuberculosis. In areas of high prevalence of HIV infection, infants may be exposed to tuberculosis from HIV–infected adults and should be immunized with BCG as soon after birth as possible.

With the breast-fed infant of a sputum-positive mother, INAH-resistant BCG vaccine (if available) should be used with a daily dose of INAH to the infant whilst on the breast or as long as the mother is infectious. If this vaccine is not available, the ordinary vaccine should be given and if it does not take, it should be repeated after the INAH course is finished.

The modest tuberculin skin sensitivity which follows vaccination in 90 per cent of infants persists for a variable time, depending on the degree of contact with 'wild' mycobacterial organisms. Adverse reactions in the form of large (>2 cm diameter) painful or suppurating lymph nodes have been reported more frequently with recently manufactured BCG vaccines but should not occur in more than 1 percent of vaccinations.

In very low incidence countries, the risks of complications of BCG vaccination such as local abscess formation (between 100 and 400 per 100 000 vaccinated), osteomyelitis (between 0.1 and 30 per 100 000), or septicaemia (< 0.1 per 100 000 vaccinated) are sufficient to warrant using the vaccine only to protect contacts, especially children under five, of open cases of tuberculosis.

BCG provides a useful marker for vaccination schedules now that smallpox vaccine is no longer given. BCG produces a scar in over 80 per cent of those vaccinated and if placed in a characteristic site (such as in Kenya, on the radial aspects of the forearm just below the elbow) can give an estimate of vaccination coverage especially in the first two years of life.

BCG can be used instead of tuberculin preparations to show the tuberculin reactivity of a child or a community. A reaction beginning in the first week indicates the presence of tuberculin sensitivity, which, if brisk, may indicate an active tuberculous infection unless anergy from measles or malnutrition is present. Thus, BCG can be used for protection, and also for detection, in tuberculosis control.

BCG has been used to protect against leprosy and other mycobacterial infections. The evidence is conflicting but as the vaccine appears to limit the spread of infection it is advised for contacts of infective patients.

Current status of other vaccines

Other established virus vaccines

Yellow fever vaccine is a highly antigenic and very safe vaccine. Where the infection is either endemic or epidemic it is included in EPI programmes. The schedule provides measles and yellow fever at 9–14 months. Mass vaccination campaigns have been used every few years or in response to an epidemic outbreak in South America and West Africa.

Rabies vaccine derived from human diploid cell culture (HDCV) is very effective (see p. 621). Where the animal reservoir of rabies is high, the routine immunization of children under five is recommended. This is the group particularly in danger of being bitten. Two doses given subcutaneously at a one month interval, or intradermal vaccine (0.1 ml into each limb to a total of 0.4 ml) in two doses one month apart, give a high titre of neutralizing antibodies.

Enteric vaccines

The last few years have seen very rapid advances in the isolation of pathogenic agents causing diarrhoea. These agents have been dissected into component parts and the function of each of these studied in relation to their pathogenicity. Much more is known about the genetic structure of viruses and bacteria, and methods of isolating and transferring genetic material. From this has followed the development of effective avirulent antigens as vaccines. Recent work has concentrated on typhoid, cholera, shigella and rotavirus.

Live oral vaccines have generally been found to generate the most effective gut immunity. This may be because they establish a mild invasive mucosal infection and reach the lymphocytes responsible for the production of appropriate IgA.

The simplest live enteric vaccines are either naturally avirulent strains, heterologous strains from animal hosts, or virulent strains attenuated by repeated passage.

Recombinant DNA technology has enabled a great deal of hybridization and reassortment of strains of bacteria and viruses. A virulent organism, for instance shigella, can be attenuated by introducing gene segments of an *E. coli* type. Genetic material from one pathogenic organism capable of stimulating requisite antibodies, can be inserted into another organism, either an attenuated pathogen or a non-pathogen.

By means of these exciting processes there are now vaccines against shigella and rotavirus infection. Cholera remains a problem. Most of the cholera mutants have sufficient pathogenicity to produce mild diarrhoea in field testing. This has ruled them out as vaccines. A killed cholera vaccine combined with a purified non-toxic subunit of cholera toxin has shown promise in field trials in Bangladesh.[17]

No vaccine has yet been developed for enterotoxic *E. coli* (ETEC) infection. Toxins have been isolated and their genes cloned. Work is needed to determine what should be incorporated into a live oral ETEC vaccine which will be polyvalent, stable, avirulent and protective.

Other bacterial vaccines

There is resurgent interest in bacterial vaccines. A meningococcal vaccine is a way of preventing epidemics which sweep through arid regions at regular intervals. Pneumococcal infections are as virulent as ever, particularly for children who are immune deficient, sicklers and those who have had a splenectomy. Strains are appearing which are resistant to most antibiotics.

The current vaccines are polysaccharide antigens derived from the capsules of the organisms. A problem of bacterial vaccines is the number of different antigenic types which may produce infection. Furthermore, polysaccharide antigens do not produce very effective or lasting immunity under the age of four.

There are at least three different meningococci – A,

B and C. The current vaccine provides protection against A and C, which are responsible for 90 per cent of infections. It has been used in Brazil, the Sahel area, Nepal and epidemics in other countries.

There are a number of polyvalent pneumoccocal vaccines. The most recent protects, to a varying extent, against 23 different types of pneumococci. Two doses are recommended. The first should be given at six months of age and should be repeated at two years of age, especially in high-risk children. Vaccinated groups have lower mortality.[9] There is a costly capsular vaccine against *Haemophilus influenza*.

Vaccines in vertically transmitted infections

Until recently, infections of the newborn derived from the mother have taken a low priority in the developing world. In the last few years the focus has broadened to include the intrauterine health of the fetus and the perinatal period of life. Infections transmitted from mother to child are emerging as causes of infant morbidity and mortality which demand measures of prevention. They include infections such as the coccal diseases, cytomegalovirus infection, rubella, acquired immune deficiency syndrome (AIDS) and hepatitis B.

Vaccines are available for rubella (see p. 164) and hepatitis. The incidence of rubella and rubella-negative women of child-bearing age varies from country to country. Whether to include rubella vaccination into a standard vaccine schedule in developing countries depends on the availability and cost of the vaccine. The awareness of a need for rubella vaccination will arise when the rubella syndrome emerges as a handicap. It will then be found that a considerable number of women of child-bearing age are seronegative and in need of immunizing.*

Hepatitis B infection has a variable pattern. It is common in many countries in Africa and South East Asia. As a 'hereditary' infection it is responsible for a considerable amount of chronic liver disease in adults, including hepatomas. Transmission seems to vary. In West Africa perinatal transmission is uncommon even in the presence of HBs Ag in mothers. The infection is acquired between six months and three years giving time to vaccinate the infants with HBV vaccine. In Southeast Asia transmission occurs from infected mothers to newborn infants, especially when both 's' and 'e' antigens are present. If prevention is to be undertaken, the infant should receive HB immunoglobulin within a day of delivery and, either at the same time or within a week of delivery, a dose of HBV

*Rubella vaccine is now available as a combined measles, mumps and rubella vaccine in Europe and North America (see pp. 501, 513).

vaccine. This should be repeated at one month and six months of age (see p. 183).

HIV virus infection is common in the infants of mothers with HIV virus. It may be a major cause of infant mortality if some form of prevention is not available soon (see p. 166).

Vertical transmission of malaria also occurs more frequently than was supposed; it is often veiled by a latent period of up to three months and presents a danger to infant survival. A malaria vaccine is still a long way off though it is the subject of intensive research.

Immunization technologies

The cold chain

Successful immunization coverage depends on a lot more than manufacture of effective vaccines. The environment of each vaccine has to be maintained from its exit from the factory to its entry into the person to be immunized in such a way that potency is not lost. The main problems in the environment concern temperature and light.

As the vaccines are transported and stored from manufacturer to central stores and thence to regional, district health centre, and finally local or vaccinator levels, the system through which they travel is called the 'cold chain'.[10] Each vaccine has a specified temperature range and time span between each of the links of the chain. A typical cold chain has four levels: the central store in the capital city; the regional store in the main provincial town; the health centre store and the local health post or place where the vaccinations are going to be given. The refrigerating temperature, the refrigerator capacity, the power sources and the transport refrigeration, have all been subject to intensive research in the past few years and references are available from EPI, WHO Geneva, together with a consumer's guide to all the equipment. EPI, WHO also issue a current guide to the temperature requirements and shelf life of each vaccine at each level, though the manufacturer's guide to the date of expiry at optimum temperature should also be consulted. Virus vaccines store best in deep-freeze conditions ($-20°C$) whilst toxoids and BCG should be kept just above freezing ($0-8°C$).

The major advances in refrigeration have been in solar energy as a source of power, simplified refrigerator units at health centre level and improved, less expensive cold boxes for transporting the vaccines. Using chemical colorimetric discs, monitoring of the total heat exposure from the time since manufacture and thus vaccine potency can be checked. Apart from high temperatures, vaccines can be damaged by refreezing or freezing, particularly of the killed vaccines, which can be inactivated by temperatures below 0°C.

A considerable amount of management skill is required in ensuring regular supplies of vaccines to local level through the cold chain, in estimating the correct capacity of cold chain equipment required at each level and in avoiding accumulating too much or storing too little vaccine at the various levels. Research in live vaccine production has been aimed at increasing heat stability and thus reducing the risks of loss of potency from exposure to heat due to breakdown of the cold chain. A relatively heat stable measles vaccine has been manufactured which can withstand room temperatures for a few days. The vaccines listed in decreasing order of heat stability are TT, DPT (pertussis being the least heat stable), BCG, measles and oral polio.

Delivery techniques

The site and method of vaccination bear on its effectiveness. Ease and cheapness of delivery affect the time taken to vaccinate and the recurrent cost. Oral administration is much easier, usually quicker and often less costly than injection methods.

For mass campaigns, jet injection (either intradermal or subcutaneous) is more rapid though initially more costly. A disposable non-reusable capsule injector has already been mentioned for use by midwives and traditional birth attendants in tetanus toxoid vaccination during pregnancy. It could also be used for measles and DPT vaccines.

Safety is important, especially in syringe transmitted infection. Transmission of hepatitis virus is the main problem. AIDS has not yet been shown to be transmitted in the immunization process.

The site of delivery of the antigen affects the type of antibody response. Vaccines given by mouth will stimulate the formation of surface antibodies in the mucosa of the gastro-intestinal tract, the IgA immunoglobulins, which have at least as significant protective effects as circulating antibodies. Repeated intradermal doses of antigen are very often more effective than single intramuscular doses, possibly because antigen reaches a greater number of lymph nodes. This seems to be true of rabies vaccine. Finally, delivery of vaccines by intranasal or aerosol methods may provide a more effective antibody response, as in measles. This may be as much a factor of dose as of site. Perhaps trachoma vaccine might be best delivered intraocularly.

Evaluation and surveillance

These two activities are essential accompaniments to an immunization programme. They concern 'process' and 'outcome'.

'Process' involves costs. It is estimated that the cost of vaccinating a child fully against the six EPI infections is US$5–15 per child. The study of the cost-effectiveness of vaccination programme is difficult. Two recent references are listed.[11,12] 'Process' also concerns coverage, the vaccination status of the community and the default rate. The presence and size of BCG scarring has been used to estimate initial coverage. Home-based record cards in a domiciliary survey may be helpful.

'Outcome' evaluation concerns the immune status of the population, particularly the infants and children, resulting from the programme. The best indicator of this is the incidence of the infection over a period. This needs to be compared with the incidence over a similar period before vaccination started, or in a similar unvaccinated community.

Disease surveillance has improved considerably since the strategies of prospective monitoring of 'sentinel' posts and retrospective surveys of 'cluster' homes were developed. Sentinel posts or systems consist of selected health centres or posts which regularly report disease cases. The 'cluster' method[13] of estimating certain disease incidences, such as lameness representing poliomyelitis or neonatal tetanus, entails selecting in a standard randomized way 'clusters' of homes. These are then visited and a questionnaire applied concerning livebirths, neonatal mortality, classical symptoms of, say, neonatal tetanus, lameness and immunizations given in the previous four months. Some surveys use a one-year recall, which will be less accurate but requires a smaller number of homes.

In this way several basic statistics can be obtained: including birth rates/1000 population; neonatal death rates/1000 livebirths; neonatal tetanus death rates/1000 livebirths; incidence of poliomyelitis, etc. Vaccine efficacy can be worked out on the basis of the ratio of incidence of disease per child vaccinated to the incidence of disease per child not vaccinated. The formula is as follows:

$$\text{Vaccine efficacy} = \frac{\text{Attack rate unimmunized minus attack rate immunized}}{\text{Attack rate unimmunized}} \times 100$$

Communication

In the final analysis the success of immunization stands or falls on the community response.

Methods to obtain this have varied from the extreme of coercion, through incentives, mass media appeals, nation-wide immunization days and publicity stunts, to the other extreme of creating, as time and opportunity allow, a community awareness of the importance of immunization until such time as the communities themselves want to have their children immunized (the so-called community-based approach).

The current climate favours the aggressive social marketing approach, and this indeed has shown considerable initial success. On its own it is unlikely to be sustained. Underpinning the publicity and neon lights there must be the participatory awareness and acceptance, planted in people's hearts by skilled patient communicators, that immunization is one very effective method of protecting their children. 'Child survival' may be the right phrase for collecting support for 'immunization for all by the year 1990'. It must, however, be replaced by child 'health' or 'potential' in the programmes within the Third World itself as a much more acceptable and solid motivation. For further reading two general reviews are recommended.[14, 15]

References

1. Rey M, Cantrelle P. Comparative results of two programmes: anti-measles vaccination on the one hand and health education and sanitation on the other. In: *Seminar on Immunization in Africa*, Kampala, Dec 7–10 1971. Paris, Centre Internationale de l'Enfance, 1971. pp. 63–5.
2. WHO/UNICEF. Expanded Programme on Immunization. *Planning Principles for Accelerated Immunization Activities*. Geneva, WHO, 1985.
3. Jajoo UN, Chhakra S, Jain AP. Annual cluster (pulse) immunization experience in villages near Sevagram, India. *Journal of Tropical Medicine and Hygiene*. 1985; **88**: 277–80.
4. Aaby P, Bukh J, Lisse IM *et al*. Determinants of measles mortality in a rural area of Guinea-Bissau: crowding, age and malnutrition. *Journal of Tropical Paediatrics*. 1984; **30**: 164–8.
5. Pollock TM, Miller E, Lobb J. Severity of whooping cough in England before and after the decline in pertussis immunization. *Archives of Disease in Childhood*. 1984; **59**: 162–5.
6. Sabin AB. Strategy for rapid elimination and continuing control of poliomyelitis and other vaccine preventable diseases of children in developing countries. *British Medical Journal*. 1986; **292**: 531–3.
7. Stanfield JP, Galazka A. Neonatal tetanus in the world today. *Bulletin of the World Health Organization*. 1984; **62**: 647–69.
8. Tripathy SP. The case for BCG. *Annals of the National Academy of Medical Sciences* (India). 1983; **19**: 11–21.
9. Riley ID *et al*. Pneumococcal vaccine prevents death from acute lower respiratory tract infections in Papua New Guinean children. *Lancet*. 1986; **ii**: 877–81.
10. World Health Organization Expanded Programme of Immunization. *The Cold Chain Status*. Geneva, WHO, 1984.
11. Dabis F *et al*. Measles control in Africa. *Lancet*. 1986; **ii**: 162.
12. Haaga J. Cost effectiveness and cost benefit analyses of immunization programmes in developing countries. In: Jelliffe DB, Jelliffe EFP eds *Advances in International Maternal and Child Health*, Vol. 6. Oxford University Press, 1986. pp. 195–220.
13. Henderson RH, Sundaresan T. Cluster sampling to assess immunization coverage: a review of experience with a simplified sampling method. *Bulletin of the World Health Organization*. 1982; **60**: 253–60.
14. Immunizing the World's Children. *Population Reports, Issues in World Health*. **L**(5), 1986 (Population Information Programme, Johns Hopkin University, Hampton House, 624 North Broadway, Baltimore, Maryland 21205, USA).
15. Issues in immunization in developing countries: an overview by Bruce Dick. *Evaluation and Planning Centre for Health Care Publication* 7, 1985 (Evaluation and Planning Centre, London School of Hygiene and Tropical Medicine, Keppel Street, London WC1E 7HT, UK).
16. WHO. *Expanded Programme on Immunization*. Forty-second World Health Assembly Report, 6 March 1989. Annex 2.
17. Clemens JD *et al*. Impact of B subunit killed whole-cell and killed whole-cell-only vaccines against cholera upon treated diarrhoeal illness and mortality, in an area endemic for cholera. *Lancet*. 1988 **1**: 1375–1379.

MATERNAL HEALTH

Kusum P. Shah

Maternal health in different cultures

The health and well-being of women is influenced by many factors: local and international economics; the status of women in the society; prevailing beliefs; the health service provision for women; and local customs, beliefs and practices relating to health, disease, reproduction, nutrition, etc. Women's low social status in many countries has an adverse impact on their health, nutritional status and reproductive health and use of health services. Women have many demands made on their physical and emotional energies which can leave them worn out. In addition to being wives and mothers, they may have to spend many hours in agricultural or subsistence work, fetching firewood, carrying water, leaving little time for self care or for attending health services.

Local customs and practices relating to women's health vary greatly. Some are very beneficial, others prevent women from practising adequate health and nutrition care. Examples of harmful customs are common. For example in some societies men and children eat first. Women only eat the leftovers. Muslim and Hindu women in some villages are not permitted to talk directly with any male adult of the family other than their husband, and most of them follow the 'purdah' system which further reinforces the barrier in communication. Their health and nutrition needs are often of little or no concern to their entourage and women themselves develop a reluctance to speak about these matters, even when they are given an opportunity to do so. In some communities female circumcision is widespread. Where the practice extends to infibulation (an extreme narrowing of the vagina) there are difficulties in labour, with complications such as infection, haemorrhage, prolapse and fistulae.

Child bearing

Pregnancy at a young age is a drain on a woman's strength. The risk of maternal death is higher for women under 18. Yet in some tribes and religious sects it is common practice to arrange the marriage of young girls at the onset of menarche or even earlier. Even at 16 to 17 years, girls have not yet completed their own physical growth and are at higher risk. However, having children is essential. Without children they have little status and little security for the future and their old age. In some agricultural communities an 11 year old will produce more than he eats and thus children are essential to the community. If the perinatal and child mortality rates are high, women will have large families to ensure that some survive. However, women who have many children are more likely to have complications in childbirth and die.

Poverty, environment and ill health

Socio-economic factors play a key role in maternal health and disease. Poverty leads to poor health and limited access to health care. Poor women are less likely to have formal education so they have little access to new information. They are more likely to have health problems but are less able to use health services because of the costs involved. These costs may be money for fares, medical fees, or treatment. Costs can also be in time, energy or emotion – poor women may be ashamed of their clothing.

Not only are poor women in developing countries more at risk of dying from a given pregnancy due to their own poor health and to lack of access to appropriate care, but they also undergo this risk more frequently and over a longer period of time in their lives, than do women in developed countries. Often such a woman will begin her reproductive cycle as soon as she is sexually mature but before having completed her growth. In countries where the average number of livebirths for a woman is eight, women usually experience at least 10 pregnancies. Typically, a poor woman in such a country will spend much of her adult life either pregnant or breast-feeding her children. These factors are reflected in the national variations in maternal mortality, from 2 per 100 000 in Finland to 2000 per 100 000 in Addis Abbaba in 1980.[1]

Urbanization

Rapid urbanization not only gives rise to shanty towns and urban slums but also causes disintegration of the extended family system so depriving young mothers of the vital support of the traditional rural societies. In the absence of this support, young urban mothers who have migrated from villages have to undertake work even during the later months of pregnancy and discontinue breast-feeding their babies early, which results in shorter inter-pregnancy periods.

Maternal nutrition

Malnutrition in the mother not only influences the chances of survival of her infant but also her own health. Many women in developing countries are chronically malnourished throughout their years of childbearing, both before and during pregnancy and throughout lactation. The mean weight gain during pregnancy of Indian and Sri Lankan women is as low as 5.3–6.6 kg.[2,3] Weight gains lower than this and even weight loss during pregnancy have been reported from other parts of the world, especially during hungry seasons (see pp. 254–70). In some nomadic communities dieting is practiced traditionally during pregnancy in order to allow for the easier delivery of a smaller baby. A high pregnancy wastage of 30 per cent has been observed in malnourished Indian women.[4] A major determinant of low birth weight due to intrauterine growth retardation in the Third World, is poor nutritional status of the mother both before conception and during pregnancy.[5]

According to a WHO estimate, anaemia affects 230 million women in the developing world.[6] This includes two-thirds of all pregnant women and half of all women of reproductive age. Much of the anaemia is dietary in origin but infections are also a major cause, in particular malaria and schistosomiasis. Maternal anaemia reduces resistance to infection and is associated with an increased risk of childbirth complications and mortality.

Many people argue that since women with low levels of literacy are more at risk of their children or themselves dying, teaching females to read is the key to reducing such mortality. Literacy alone is not enough. Women need status and income to improve the health of their children and themselves. Part of a health worker's role is to give women information. Then women can be empowered to make decisions for health.

Child spacing and maternal health

While the health effects of birth spacing on well-nourished mothers remain relatively unclear, the detrimental effects of too close spacing on malnourished women are well documented. Successive pregnancies deplete maternal resources and result in maternal malnutrition, anaemia and vitamin deficiencies. Better spacing of children enables mothers to recuperate from maternal depletion and rebuild their resources.

Several of the maternal health problems described earlier are associated with multiparous women with short inter-pregnancy intervals. A birth interval of less than two years is considered short in relation to a child's chances of survival; whereas a three-year interval is associated with longer survival.[7]

Women under the age of 20 years have the highest proportion of short-interval births, ranging from 39 per cent in Ghana to 69 per cent in Mexico. Urban women have a somewhat higher proportion of shorter-interval births than women living in the countryside. This finding may be related to the decline in urban breast-feeding and postpartum sexual abstinence.

Maternal mortality in developing countries can be reduced if the age at first pregnancy, birth spacing patterns and the desired size of family can be changed.

Another factor influencing the mother's health and birth interval is the survival of the preceding child. The birth interval increases from over one year, when the first of two children is stillborn or dies in the first few months, to about three years when the first child is living.

Demographic transition

Frequent breast-feeding and vigorous suckling affect birth spacing by prolonging the period of postpartum anovulation and amenorrhoea and, in some cases, by reducing the likelihood of conception once ovulation has occurred, which helps in achieving a natural birth interval of two to two-and-a-half years.[8]

In Mali, the duration of breast-feeding had a marked influence on the interval observed between two births.[9] Most of the women who breast-fed for 18 months or longer had birth intervals of more than two years and one quarter had their babies at least three years apart. On the other hand, the mean birth interval for women who breast-fed for less than a year was about two years.

An extended period of postpartum amenorrhoea of a year or longer is observed among many women in developing countries, while shorter periods of six months or less are common in women of developed countries. When mothers loose confidence in their ability to nurse their babies or have to work, they may begin to supplement breast-feeding. Lactation becomes difficult and its contraceptive effect is reduced.

The risk to the health of mother and child due to short pregnancy intervals compels consideration of pregnancy planning. To have a planned family, a number of methods of contraception are used. The ideal method of contraception should be safe, effective, aesthetically acceptable, inexpensive and reversible. It should be simple to use, easy to store and have no deleterious side-effects. It may be self-administered, should not require special skill and its application should be independent of the sexual act. There is no single method which fulfils all these criteria! Table 1.4.13 depicts the merits and pitfalls of the various methods.

Failures and successes in population control

The family planning programme in India, which was targeted to limit family size by the performance of surgical interventions, did not succeed as it lacked the important component of birth spacing. Other family planning programmes have failed in some Asian countries on account of managerial and administrative weaknesses. The programmes were unable to attract and maintain a large number of contraceptive users. Moreover, the programmes could not provide a full range of contraceptive methods.

In an attempt to meet unrealistic sterilization targets, men and women were pressurized into surgical sterilization. The impact of sterilization in developing countries is limited since in most of these countries women over 30 years of age account for no more than 30 per cent of all births, and women who obtain sterilization usually average about 32 to 33 years. Hence, the programmes achieved sterilization of couples with large families but did not help the young couples who wanted child spacing rather than limited family size. Further-

Table 1.4.13 Comparison of commonly available methods of child spacing

Methods	Characteristics						Side-effects			
	Effectiveness (%)*	For males	For females	Ease of operation	Use at coitus	Reversibility	Medical supervision needed	Menstrual	Coitus related upset	Other physical symptoms
Douche	50–60	No	Yes	Yes	Yes	Yes	Yes	No	No	No
Withdrawal coitus interruptus	60–80	Yes	No	Yes	Yes	Yes	No	No	Yes	No
Barrier methods condom	62–97	Yes	No	Yes	Yes	Yes	No	No	Yes	No
diaphragm/cap	80–97	No	Yes	Yes	Yes	Yes	Yes	No	No	No
vaginal spermicide	80–94	No	Yes	Yes	Yes	Yes	No	No	No	No
Periodic abstinence rhythm or safe period	62–89	No	Yes	Yes	Yes	Yes	No	No	No	No
Hormonal oral	81–99	No	Yes	Yes	No	Yes	Yes	Some	No	Some
injectable	96–99	No	Yes	Yes	No	Yes	Yes	Some	No	Some
implant	99–100	No	Yes	No	No	Yes	Yes	Some	No	Some
IUD	93–99	No	Yes	Yes	No	Yes	Yes	Some	No	Some
Abortion	100	No	Yes	No	No	No	Yes	Few	Yes	Some
Surgical female sterilization	99–100	No	Yes	Yes	No	Yes	Skill needed	Few	No	No
male sterilization	99–100	Yes	No	Yes	No	Yes	Skill needed	No	Few	No

* Figures are rounded off.
Adapted from Hutchings J, Lyle S. Assessing the Characteristics and Cost-effectiveness of Contraceptive Methods, PIACT paper, 1985.

more, the family planning services were not built in, or integrated with, the existing programmes of maternal and child health.

The under utilization of health services in developing countries is a distressing phenomenon. Health services have failed to provide the desired continuity of health care to women and children and have not reached those in greatest need, partly because most approaches are implemented on a vertical basis rather than on an integrated one. In some places, family planning programmes are run in isolation and do not offer ante-natal, delivery, and postnatal services. There are many needs in fertility regulation which are not met, if one considers the gap between the desire to plan a family and the practice of effective contraception. The problems faced by the health care system in extending the coverage of fertility regulation services, are further compounded by moral, religious and cultural beliefs which are often counter-promotive to the acceptance of family planning. Moreover, in some places, even though health services are available, eligible couples have no knowledge of existing contraceptive methods and their availability.

The success of a family planning programme in Singapore was based on an effective mass media campaign, as well as on group and individual moti-vational courses and the provision of family planning services, including abortions and sterilizations, in readily accessible MCH clinics and hospitals. The social changes introduced by the government encouraged female employment which influenced the age of marriage and spacing of children. Incentives were used extensively. Young educated couples have now fully accepted the two-child family and the preference for the male child has rapidly declined. The crude birth rate has declined from 42.7 in 1967 to 16.9 in 1978. Higher-order births show a persistent decline. This is accompanied by an unequivocal fall in maternal mortality.[10]

In Thailand, men typically considered family planning to be the women's responsibility and were apathetic about participating in fertility reduction efforts. Family planning was not openly discussed or publicized. Contraceptives could not be advertised in the mass media. A further barrier was the limited coverage of clinic-based family planning services. Communities were not involved in the planning and implementation of programmes. However, with the involvement of non-governmental organizations and the communities themselves, a dramatic change has occurred. Understanding of the importance of social awareness and motivation has led to the development of a wide range of culturally adapted marketing strategies

and promoted a widespread use of contraception. The number of contraceptive users increased from an average of about 47 000 new clients per year during 1965 to 1968 to almost one million by 1979. Population growth rate had a fall from 3.2–3.4 per cent annually in the early 1960s to below 2.0 per cent in 1980.[11]

The Kerala experience[12] illustrates the impact which socio-economic change has on fertility. This South Indian State is poor (per capita income US$135 compared with the Indian average of US$190) and heavily populated, yet has a high literacy rate, a falling infant mortality (55 per 1000 livebirths compared to 125 for all India) and a lower birth rate than the rest of the country (26.4 per 1000 compared with 33.3 for all India in 1978). In this socialist-leaning State there has been a major emphasis on land and income re-distribution, on female education and literacy, and on political partici-pation. These policies seem more important to implement than a specific family planning programme, if birth rates are to be affected.

Recipes for success

The acceptance of family planning by a couple depends not only on the technology available but also on other interacting factors, such as the literacy status of women, economic participation of women and the survival rate of children.

The women whose infants survive choose to stop bearing children, while those who experience infant or child deaths continue to reproduce. There is a long period between the drop in infant mortality rate and a fall in birth rates, as it takes time for awareness of better child survival to become widespread. Therefore child health care is a good basis for setting up family planning activities, as the connection between child survival and birth spacing is more easily made clear.

Use of family planning services increased further with the introduction of the home-based mother's record (see Fig. 1.4.13). By this means the health worker and traditional midwives monitor the health of the mother and her menstrual history every month during the inter-pregnancy period and educate and motivate the mother to use appropriate family planning methods for spacing of children.[13]

In order to provide the desired continuity in health care, a community-based surveillance process should include all women at grass-roots level during their reproductive age. For surveillance purposes, a compre-hensive home-based mother's record represents an appropriate technology, in its written or pictorial form, for semi-literates or non-literate mothers, traditional

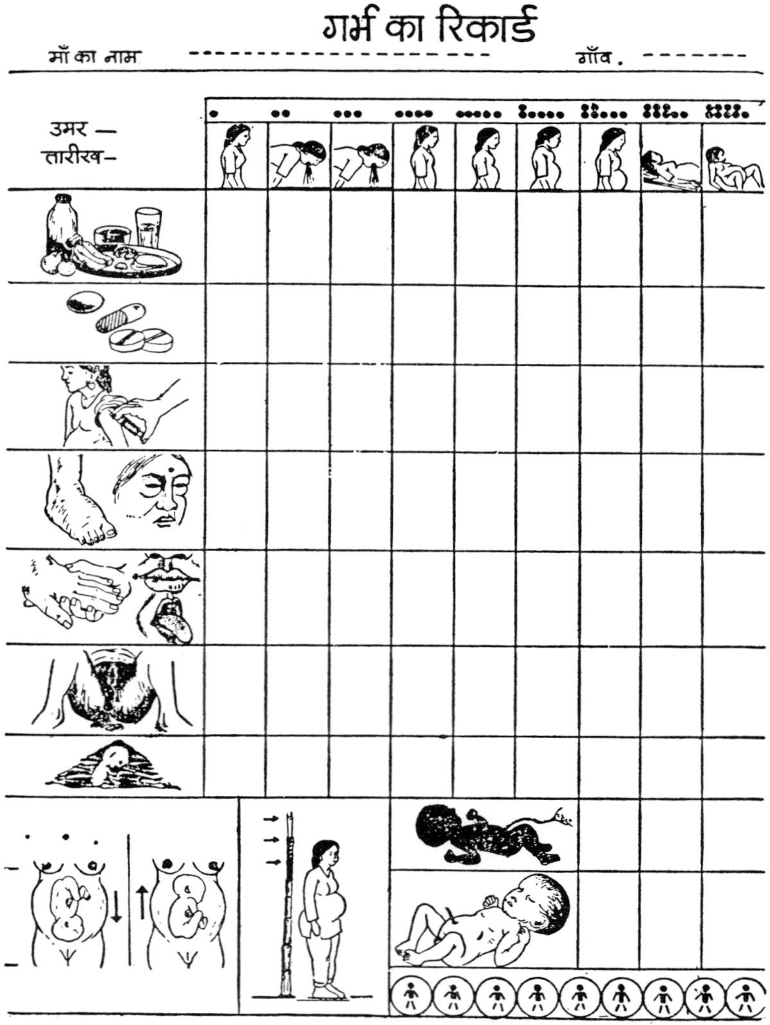

Fig. 1.4.13 Pictorial mother's record as used in India.

midwives and primary health care workers. The card could be used for the entire reproductive period of a woman (Fig. 1.4.14). Local women's associations, mother's groups or older schoolchildren, particularly girls, can play a useful role in maintaining a surveillance system using this home-based record and to identify women who are exposed to health risks associated with unfavourable reproductive patterns. Similarly they can be motivated to space their children and be provided with modern contraceptive methods.

Governments cannot hope to bring about fertility control without introducing policies which promote the status of women, raise the age of marriage and increase their job opportunities. If it falls within religious tolerance, nation-wide legislation to allow abortion on medical grounds should be introduced.

The prevention of unwanted or closely spaced pregnancies is possible. Child spacing is an alternative that should be available to everybody. Relevant sectors and health personnel should ensure the provision of information, technology and resources for families who want and need to space their children. The choice should be within the reach of all through primary health care and community organizations.

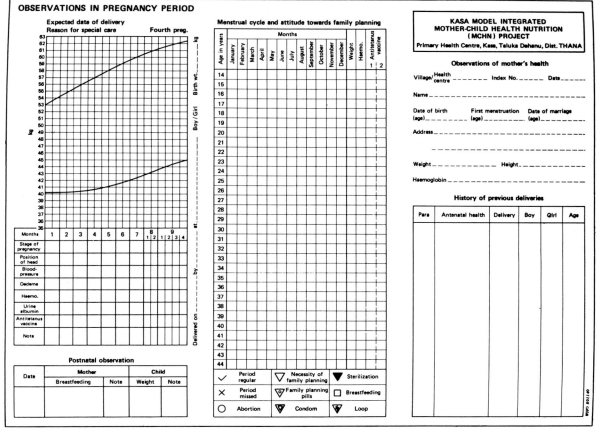

Fig. 1.4.14 Home-based mother's record. The central panel comprises of surveillance on menstrual cycle and practices of family planning. (The weights shown apply to India.)

References

1. World Health Organization. *Maternal Mortality Rates. A Tabulation of Available Information.* Second edition. FHE/86.3 Geneva WHO, 1986.
2. Shah K, Shah PM. Relationship of weight during pregnancy and low birth weight. *Indian Paediatrics* 1972; **9**: 526–31.
3. Venkatachalam PS, Shankar K, Gopalan C. Changes in body weight and body composition during pregnancy. *Indian Journal of Medical Research.* 1960; **48**: 511–17.
4. Gopalan C, Naidu AN. Nutrition and Fertility. *Lancet* 1972; **2**: 1077–9.
5. Kramer MS. Determinants of low birth weight. *Bulletin of the World Health Organization.* 1987; **65**: 663–737.
6. De Meyer E, Adiels-Tegman M. The prevalence of anaemia in the world. In: *The Health of the Family*: Some Key Issues. World Health Statistics, WHO, No. 38, 1985. pp. 302–16.
7. Wyon JB, Gordon JB. *The Khanna Study: Population Problems in the Rural Punjab.* MA, USA, Harvard University Press, 1971.
8. Huffman SL. Maternal and child nutritional status, its association with the risk of pregnancy. *Social Sciences and Medicine.* 1983; **17**: 1529–40.
9. Lews, JH, Burton N. *Breast-feeding, contraception and spacing in Mali.* Presented at the USAID Health/Population and Nutrition Conference, Gettysburg, Pennsylvania, June 19–20 1984.
10. Rataam SS, Tambiraja RL. Health benefits of appropriate timing, spacing and avoiding high parity and risks of unplanned fertility for the mother. In: Delmundo F, Ines-Cuyegkeng K, Aviado D E eds. *Primary Maternal and Neonatal Health: A Global Concern.* New York, Plenum, 1983. pp. 43–52.
11. Knodel J, Debavalya N. Thailand's continuing and

reproductive revolution. *Internal Family Planning Perspectives*. 1980; **6**: 84–97.

12. Morley DC, Rohde J, Williams G. *Practising Health for All*. Oxford University Press, 1983.

13. Hutchings J, Lyle S. *Assessing the Characteristics and Cost-effectiveness of Contraceptive Methods*. PIACT Papers Seattle, Washington, 1985.

WORKING WITH TRADITIONAL MIDWIVES

Gill Tremlett

Introduction

More than two-thirds of the world's women are delivered by traditional midwives untrained in western medicine. Many different terms are used to describe these traditional specialists. WHO uses the term traditional birth attendant (TBA), who is defined as 'a person, usually a woman, who assists the mother at childbirth and who initially acquires her skills delivering babies by herself or by working with other TBAs. This term is very narrow. People described as TBAs may provide care at puberty, pregnancy, childbirth and postnatally and advise on child care, child spacing and nutrition. Some are herbal or psychic healers.

The term 'traditional midwife' is more appropriate, 'midwife' being derived from old English 'with woman'.

Traditional midwives' skills

Traditional midwives gain skill in different ways: inheritance from relatives; apprenticeship to others with experience; experience from their own deliveries or from friends' or relatives' deliveries, or supernatural calling. In some communities women are only delivered by close relatives. In others women deliver alone, without assistance.

Traditional midwives' level of delivery skill varies greatly. Some may deliver only three to six women in a lifetime, others hundreds. Roles vary from just cutting the cord to providing psychological and physical support through pregnancy to birth and after. Some are skilled in manipulation, turning babies with abnormal lie, destructive operations, and giving herbs for controlling bleeding or increasing lactation.

Training programmes for traditional midwives

In the past, traditional midwives were unfairly blamed for much maternal and perinatal mortality or morbidity and their practice discouraged or made illegal. Now, not only are they being recognized as an essential resource in extending PHC services, but many of their non-interventionist practices are being valued and adopted by obstetric services. Common beneficial practices include: no vaginal examination, thus preventing infection; physiological management of third stage and delayed cutting of the cord so the baby gets its full complement of placental blood;[1,2] keeping mother and baby together; putting the baby immediately to the breast following delivery; and frequent demand feeding. In particular, upright positions in delivery such as squatting, kneeling or standing are beneficial to mother and child, making labour shorter, less painful and reducing fetal distress.[3]

In the 70 years since the first training programme for Sudanese traditional midwives, most programmes have provided unidirectional training with an emphasis on 'upgrading' indigenous practice.[4] Content focusses on antenatal care, high risk identification, safer home delivery, emergencies and referral. Few programmes really attempt to understand and build on traditional beliefs and practices and promote sharing of ideas and skills to upgrade the obstetric system. As a result the impact of training programmes is variable. Some report more appropriate use of services, others show decreased maternal and perinatal mortality and morbidity. However, some have found unwanted side-effects. Copying midwives' practice may result in infections from vaginal examinations, inverted uterus from inappropriate pulling on the cord, bottle-feeding or because some 'trained' traditional midwives insist that women lie on their backs in labour, the women avoid them and refuse to use the service. They go to those who follow the more traditional ways.

Therefore in training, traditional midwives must practise skills in a situation as similar as possible to their home environment. Beneficial practices must be actively promoted, harmless practices left alone. Only really harmful practices need be changed. A good starting point for a programme is to focus on what women and traditional midwives are worried about.

Four elements are essential for a successful programme:

- Learning should be two-way. Traditional midwives have very practical ideas for improving women's care and obstetric services.
- The community, traditional midwives and local women should all be involved in the selection and training process; whether it is all grandmothers as in Manicaland, Zimbabwe[5] or a few highly skilled people.
- Health professionals need to respect traditional

midwives and acknowledge their role.
- Health services must provide obstetric support and facilities for appropriate treatment of referrals, further training, follow-up and support.

References

1. Moss AJ, Monset-Couchard M. Placental transfusion: early versus late clamping of the umbilical cord. *Paediatrics.* 1967; **40** (1): 109–26.
2. Yao AC, Lind J. Placental transfusion. *American Journal of the Diseases of Childhood.* 1974; **127**: 128–41.
3. Schwartz R, Diaz AG, Fescina R, Caldeyro-Barcia R. Latin American collaborative study on maternal position in labour. Reported in *Birth and Family Journal.* 1979; **6** (1).
4. McClain C. Traditional midwives and family planning: an assessment of programmes and suggestions for the future. *Medical Anthropology.* 1981; **5** (1): 107–36.
5. Egullion C. Training traditional midwives in Manicaland, Zimbabwe, in Traditional Birth Attendants: A Resource for the Health of Women. *International Journal of Gynaecology and Obstetrics.* 1985; **23**: 247–33.

BREAST-FEEDING: PROTECTION, SUPPORT AND PROMOTION

Michael C. Latham

Advantages of breast-feeding

When the baby cries
Let him suck
From the breast.
There is no fixed time
For breastfeeding.
When the baby cries
It may be he is ill;
The first medicine for a child
Is the breast.
Give him milk
And he will stop crying.

These lines are from the epic poem *Song of Lawino* by the Ugandan poet Okot p'Bitek. The poem[1] satirizes Westernization in Africa, and these lines suggest correctly that traditional breast-feeding on demand, in sickness and in health, is best for the baby.

For most of human history nearly all infants have been breast-fed and there has usually existed good local

knowledge about breast-feeding, although practices have varied from culture to culture. Extensive studies comparing the composition and relative benefits of human milk and breast-milk substitutes have been published over the last 50 years. Although we have known for many years about the advantages of breast-feeding[2] and a good deal about human lactation, there has in the last decade been an avalanche of publications on this topic. Most of the new research has strengthened our view of the many advantages of breast-feeding over other methods of infant feeding. It is widely recommended that only breast-milk be fed to infants for the first four to six months of life.[3] Certainly in developing countries where the risks of complementary feeding usually outweigh any possible advantages, breast-feeding alone up to six months of age may be advised.

The increased interest in breast-feeding is in part due to the public controversy over the issue of bottle-feeding and the aggressive promotion of manufactured breast-milk substitutes by multinational corporations, and also because of the resurgence of breast-feeding among more educated mothers in the industrialized countries of the North. The womanly art of breast-feeding has been rediscovered in Europe and to a lesser extent in North America. Unfortunately, however, an increasing use of bottle-feeding continues to be seen in many non-industrialized countries of the South. The most serious consequences of this shift from breast to bottle are seen among poor families in Africa, Asia and Latin America.

The advantages of breast over bottle-feeding include:

- the adequacy of nutrients in human milk;
- the ready availability and convenience of breast-feeding compared with alternative feeding methods;
- the immunity conferred by anti-infective constituents in colostrum and breast-milk;
- the much enhanced risk of infections resulting from contamination with pathogenic organisms of infant formula, bottles, teats and other items used for infant feeding when compared with the relative sterility of breast-milk;
- the economic advantages for the family and the nation of breast-feeding because of the high costs of alternative methods of infant feeding;
- the good mother–child relationship fostered by breast-feeding (Fig. 1.4.15) which is more difficult with bottle-feeding;
- the apparent reduced risk of obesity, allergies and certain other health problems in breast-fed infants compared with artificially fed ones;
- the important fact that intensive breast-feeding reduces fertility by delaying postpartum ovulation and in this way assists mothers in a wider spacing of children.

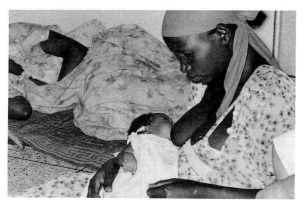

Fig. 1.4.15   Mother breast-feeding her child.

The physiological and nutritional aspects of breast-feeding are discussed in some detail (see pp. 195–208, 324–335). There is now overwhelming evidence of the health advantages of breast-feeding in terms of reduced infant morbidity and mortality when compared with artificially fed infants. These advantages accrue mainly to the two-thirds of the world's population who live in poverty, although some studies have shown lower rates of diarrhoea and other infections, and less hospitalization of breast-fed compared with formula-fed infants even in affluent communities.[4] Our knowledge of the anti-infective properties of breast-milk has increased considerably, and these are discussed elsewhere.

Problems with bottle-feeding

Whereas breast-milk is protective, alternative infant feeding methods increase the risk of infection, mainly because contamination leads to the increased intake of pathogenic organisms. Poor hygiene, particularly with bottle-feeding, is a major cause of childhood gastro-enteritis and diarrhoea. Infant formula and cows milk are good vehicles and culture media for organisms. It is incredibly difficult to provide a clean, let alone sterile, feed to an infant from the bottle under the following circumstances:

- when the family water supply is a ditch or a well contaminated with human excrement; very few households in the developing countries have their own safe supply of running water;
- when household hygiene is poor and the home environment is contaminated by flies and faeces;
- when there is no refrigerator or other safe storage space for a reconstituted formula or for cow's milk;
- when there is no turn-on stove and on each occasion someone has to gather fuel and light a fire to boil some water to sterilize a bottle;
- when there is no suitable equipment for cleaning the bottle between feeds, and where the bottle used may be of cracked plastic or an almost uncleanable soda bottle;
- when the mother is relatively uneducated and has little or no knowledge of the germ concept of disease.

There are also two ways by which artificial feeding may contribute importantly to protein–energy malnutrition (PEM), including nutritional marasmus. First, as discussed earlier, formula-fed infants are more likely to get infections including diarrhoea which then contribute importantly to poor growth and PEM in infants and young children. Second, infant formula is often overdiluted by mothers in poor families. Because of the high cost of breast-milk substitutes, the family will purchase too little, and try to stretch this by using less than the recommended amounts of powdered formula per feed. The infant may be given the correct number of feedings and the recommended volume of liquid, but each feed may be too low in its content of energy and other nutrients to sustain optimal growth. The result is first growth faltering and then perhaps the slow development of nutritional marasmus.

Economic aspects of bottle-feeding

A relatively neglected major disadvantage of bottle-feeding of infants is the serious economic consequences for poor families and nations. Manufactured breast-milk substitutes, as sold, are extremely expensive products in relation to the income of the majority of families in developing countries. The purchase of these products as substitutes for breast-milk diverts scarce family monetary resources and increases poverty.[5] In many developing countries it may cost over half the minimum or even the average wage to feed an infant adequately using an available manufactured breast-milk substitute. Table 1.4.14 illustrates the situation in three developing countries over the last two decades.

Breast-milk is produced in all countries, whereas infant formula is manufactured in only a minority of them. Therefore, for many nations, a decline in breast-feeding means an increase in the importation of manufactured breast-milk substitutes and of the paraphernalia needed for bottle-feeding. These imports may lead to a worsening of the already horrendous foreign debt problems for many developing countries. Even where formula is locally made, the manufacture is frequently controlled by a multinational corporation, and profits are exported. Therefore, the preservation of breast-feeding or a reduction in artificial feeding is in the economic interests of most Third World countries. Economists and politicians may be more inclined to support programmes to promote breast-feeding when

they appreciate that such measures will save foreign exchange. This is often of more interest to them than arguments about the health advantages of breast-feeding.

Breast-feeding and fertility

Of importance also is our increased knowledge of the relationship of breast-feeding to human fertility. For a very long time the traditional wisdom of many societies included a belief that breast-feeding reduced the likelihood of an early pregnancy. Often this belief was regarded as an old wives' tale. Scientific evidence now proves beyond question a positive relationship between on the one hand intensity, frequency and duration of breast-feeding, and on the other the length of post-partum amenorrhoea, anovulation and reduced fertility.[6,7] The physiology of the phenomenon is discussed on p. 89.

This knowledge has important implications in terms of birth spacing and population dynamics. In many developing countries, breast-feeding is now contributing more to child spacing and in prolonging intervals between births than are the combined use of the contraceptive pill, the IUD, condoms, diaphragms and other modern contraceptives. Therefore the fertility controlling benefits of breast-feeding should now be added to its other advantages. Recent data from Kenya and elsewhere suggest that women who continue to breast-feed for a long time, but who also introduce bottle-feeding in the first few months of the infant's life, may have a reduced length of postpartum amenorrhoea compared with women who do not practise early mixed breast and bottle-feeding. Therefore, the use of breast-milk substitutes in the first few months of life reduces sucking at the breast, which in turn lowers prolactin blood levels and leads to an earlier return of ovulation even for a mother who may breast-feed for a year or more. Bottle-feeding of babies is contributing to a narrower spacing between births.

Table 1.4.14   Cost of adequately formula feeding a 3–4 month old infant relative to wages or incomes

	Approx. monthly income	Cost of formula per month	Percent of wage
Tanzania (1964)	132 Shs. ($24.60)	68 Shs. ($13.60)	51%
Kenya (1976)	150 Shs. ($20.80)	88 Shs. ($12.25	58%
India (1976)	120 Rs. ($15.00)	91.5 Rs. ($11.20)	76%
Kenya (1986)	420 Shs. ($30.00)	254 Shs. ($18.15)	60%

Determinants of infant feeding

Two papers from WHO[8, 9] describe a typology of three phases and eight stages of breast-feeding situations found in countries around the world (Table 1.4.15). These show a dynamic situation, with a range from a widespread long-duration traditional breast-feeding pattern through a series of patterns of declining breast-feeding in different country subgroups, to a final pattern of widespread breast-feeding resurgence. This WHO model suggests a sequential progression through the eight stages with changes occurring within each country, first within high socio-economic status (SES) urban women, followed by their lower SES urban counterparts, and finally the rural poor. There is some value in this classification in which, for example, rural traditional India is in Stage 1, countries such as the Philippines are half way along this path and Sweden is in Stage 8.

But this kind of typology ignores the complexity of the factors that influence infant feeding and the cultural diversity of infant feeding practices. The WHO model classifies countries and communities entirely on the basis of breast-feeding prevalence and duration. But the dangerous increase in use of breast-milk substitutes in some countries such as Kenya is not at the expense either of breast-feeding prevalence or breast-feeding duration. Rather in many countries, including Kenya, mixed feeding is the common practice. Babies in the first few months of life are fed on the same day both from their mother's breasts and from the nipple of a baby bottle. This so-called 'triple nipple infant feeding'

is a common and dangerous phenomenon.[10] In a study of low-income women in Nairobi almost all women breast-fed their infants, the mean duration of breast-feeding was 16 months, and yet the majority of these same women were bottle-feeding their infants in the first few months of life. Regular use of breast-milk substitutes was reported in over 60 per cent of mothers with infants at two months and 85 per cent at three months of age (Fig. 1.4.16). Yet, using the WHO classification, these Nairobi women would be in Phase 1, Stage 1, all groups in the traditional phase.

In some developing countries (particularly in Latin America and the Caribbean) there has been a marked reduction in the prevalence and duration of breast-feeding; in others (including many in Asia) there has been a decline, particularly in the urban areas. However, the majority of rural women still breast-feed. In many parts of the world, both in whole countries and

Table 1.4.15   WHO typology of infant feeding patterns

Phases of breast-feeding prevalence and duration

Phase 1	'traditional phase' with high prevalence and duration
Phase 2	'transformation phase' prevalence of breast-feeding falling and duration becoming shorter
Phase 3	'resurgence phase' with rising prevalence and duration of breast-feeding

Typology or stages of breast-feeding prevalence and duration for national picture

Stage 1	all groups in the traditional phase (India, Zaire)
Stage 2	the lead group in Phase 2, the rest in Phase 1 (Nigeria)
Stage 3–5	prevalence and duration of breast-feeding falling (Philippines, Brazil)
Stage 6	the lead group in Phase 3, the rest in Phase 2 (Singapore, Spain)
Stage 7	the lead group in Phase 3, the other groups following close behind (USA, UK)
Stage 8	all groups in Phase 3 (Sweden)

Adapted from *WHO Statistics Quarterly*, 1982: **35(2)**:92–116 and *WHO Chronicle*, 1983;**37(1)**: 6–10.

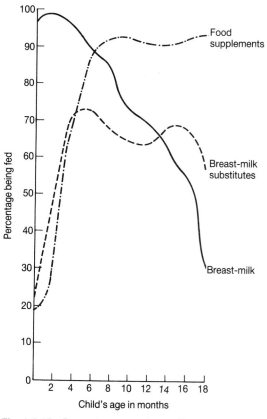

Fig. 1.4.16   Percentage current use of breast-milk, breast-milk substitutes and food supplements by age of index child adapted from data from Kenya.

in certain communities, there has been an erosion of breast-feeding in which breast-milk substitutes are increasingly used, but at the same time breast-feeding continues and is of long duration. Policies to increase breast-feeding or to reduce bottle-feeding may be different, depending on the situation in each country and on the determinants of current infant feeding practices.

It used to be assumed that a decline in breast-feeding was almost inevitable where there was industrialization and urbanization, where increasing numbers of women were entering paid employment away from home, and where modernizing influences were sweeping away traditional ways of life. Some used to say that bottle-feeding is an inevitable accompaniment of development. But this view is rightly disputed. The Scandinavian phenomenon of very prevalent breast-feeding in countries where development is advanced, where women are more liberated than elsewhere, and where female employment is high, shows that breast-feeding is possible in urban industrialized societies. Other countries, such as China, have recruited millions of women into the labour force, yet the majority of babies are still breast-fed.

Reasons most commonly given by mothers for weaning from the breast are a new pregnancy, the infant was old enough or weaned himself, the mother had insufficient milk, or illness of the mother or child. Work away from home, in most studies, has been the reason given by only a minority of women.

Reasons for decline in breast-feeding

What then are the reasons for a decline in breast-feeding or for the unnecessary use of breast-milk substitutes? These vary from country to country. The promotional practices of the manufacturers of breast-milk substitutes is one such cause. These have now been regulated in many countries, but the manufacturers continue to circumvent the accepted codes of conduct and to promote their products, even though this may contribute to infant morbidity. Another group of factors that has contributed to a reduction in breast-feeding, has been actions by the medical profession. In general, health care systems in most countries have not been adequately supportive of breast-feeding. Even in many developing countries doctors and other health care professionals have played a negative role, and have contributed to reduced levels of breast-feeding. This situation is changing, but many health professionals are relatively ignorant about breast-feeding.

Health services often do not provide adequate advice to mothers about breast-feeding prenatally, at the time of delivery, or postnatally. Too many encourage bottle-feeding and even suggest that infant formula is superior to breast-milk. Many maternity units still do not encourage mothers to breast-feed their babies in the first minutes following delivery; many do not allow mothers to breast-feed their babies on demand, nor for the babies to sleep with their mothers; and others still routinely feed newborn babies with glucose water, infant formula or both while in the maternity ward or nursery.

Many doctors wrongly believe that there are many medical contraindications to breast-feeding. They often include among these: low birth weight, Caesarean delivery, minor breast problems, and many maternal and infant health problems. None of these is very often a valid reason for not breast-feeding. A recent meeting of experts called by WHO and UNICEF[11] concluded that contra-indications to breastfeeding are very few. The situations where an infant cannot or should not receive breast-milk are very few, certainly less than one per cent of births. Yet in most hospitals around the world many infants are being denied breast-milk on the basis of wrong medical advice. Certain extremely rare congenital metabolic diseases do preclude the provision of breast-milk to an infant. For example in galacto-saemia, an infant should not receive human milk, ordinary infant formula, or cow's milk. Babies with phenylketonuria should receive a special formula low in phenylalanine only if concentrations of this in the blood reach high levels. Maple syrup disease is another contra-indication to breast-feeding.

In many studies 'insufficient milk' is cited as one of the more common reasons given by mothers for their early termination of breast-feeding or for early supplementation with infant formula. The 'insufficient milk syndrome' is not well understood either in research circles or by practising doctors and paediatricians. It is all too easy to assume simply that many women are incapable of producing enough milk to satisfy the needs of their young infants. Too often health professionals, when faced with a mother complaining of insufficient milk, simply advise her to supplement her breast-milk with bottle-feeds. Usually this is the wrong advice.[12] The maintenance of lactation is dependent on adequate nipple stimulation by the suckling infant because this encourages the release of the hormone prolactin. The cause of 'insufficient milk' may, therefore, often be that alternative feeding has replaced breast-feeding to a variable degree. Therefore, advice to provide a supplement or more supplement is almost always going to contribute to a reduction in breast-milk production. Supplementary bottle-feeds for the infant is used as a 'cure' for insufficient milk, when in fact it is the 'cause'. The most appropriate advice to a mother who wishes to breast-feed but who believes she has insufficient milk, is to help her to breast-feed more and not less, because this is likely to increase her milk production. She should try to breast-feed more frequently and for longer periods. The increased nipple stimulation will usually increase milk production. The common medical advice suggesting more supplementary bottle-feeds is likely to worsen the situation, leading to a further reduction in breast-milk production and eventual cessation of lactation.

Other reasons for the decline in breast-feeding, include a belief that it will ruin the appearance of the breasts and that a baby even in the first few months of life is healthier if formula-fed. Both these views are false but strongly adhered to, possibly as a result of media publicity about formula feeding.

Health and other actions to improve breast-feeding

Among the factors that resulted in a greater use of bottle-feeding in developing countries, two stand out as being of major importance and both include practices that lend themselves to change. These are first the promotion of breast-milk substitutes by their manufacturers, particularly the multinational corporations, and second, the failure of the health profession to advocate, protect and support breast-feeding. In the 1950s and 1960s, a small group of physicians, paediatricians and nutritionists working in developing countries, were drawing attention to the dangers of bottle-feeding and decrying the role of industry in the decline of breast-feeding.[13,14] During that time, advertising of breast-milk substitutes was widely used in newspapers and magazines, and on radio and later on television. The corporations were using 'milk nurses' to push their products in health facilities; free samples and glossy literature on their products were provided to mothers soon after delivery; and a number of other hard-sell tactics were being used.

It was not until the 1970s that public outrage in the West began to develop over these tactics, and that knowledge about the harmful effects of bottle-feeding for Third World babies became widespread. Most members of the medical profession, both in the West and in developing countries, were at best unsupportive of the growing public pressure to rein in the promotional activities of the corporations, and at worst doctors sided with the manufacturers against the critics of the corporations.

Finally, unable to resist the pressure, WHO and

UNICEF organized a meeting in Geneva in 1979 at which a handful of experts met with representatives of industry, of non-government organizations (NGOs) and of delegates from selected countries, to discuss possible regulations to control the promotion of breast-milk substitutes. This meeting probably would not have taken place had it not been for the tireless efforts of certain NGOs and their enthusiastic staff. At the 1979 Geneva conference, despite rearguard actions by the major manufacturers, a decision was made to develop a Code of Conduct and some of the main principles of a Code were agreed upon. Several meetings followed to develop wording for the Code. On 21 May 1981 the World Health Assembly overwhelmingly adopted the International Code of Marketing of Breast-milk Substitutes.[15] Only one country, the United States, voted against the Code. The Code applies to the marketing of breast-milk substitutes, and its most important article stated that 'there should be no advertising or other form of promotion to the general public of breast-milk substitutes and other items mentioned in the Code'. Other details dealt with provision of samples at sales points; contact between marketing personnel and mothers; the use of health facilities for the promotion of infant formula; and the labelling and quality of products.

The Code is not binding on member states but it suggests that goverments should take action to give effect to the principles and aims of the Code. In practice, the Code (coupled with actions such as the Nestlé boycott) has resulted in almost complete cessation of advertising of breast-milk substitutes to the public by the large manufacturers. Several countries have introduced legislation based on the international Code. The use of samples has declined but has not been halted. Many Ministries of Health are now more supportive of breast-feeding than in the past. But it is often forgotten that the Code was a compromise agreement, that it was the very minimum needed to address a small part of a large problem, that all codes have loopholes, and that industry has worked hard to circumvent the Code.

Figures are not available, but the general belief is that the major manufacturers are still spending very large sums to promote infant formula. Though advertising to the public has ceased, they are continuing to advertise to health professionals; they have worked in many countries to weaken or prevent codes from becoming law; and they are increasingly advertising to the public the use of their manufactured weaning foods for consumption by very young babies. For example, a 1984 Nestlé advertisement for Cerelac in India, claims that it 'provides a nutritionally complete feed' and that breast-milk is ideal for your baby 'but when he is four months and ready for solids consult your doctor and start him on Cerelac'. Such advertising is not forbidden by the Code, but is contrary to its spirit, and yet is practiced by a corporation which claims fully to support the Code.

The passage of the Code has led to some complacency and to a false belief that the problem has been solved. Those who worked for the Code knew that it could at best solve only a part of the problem, yet support for actions to deal with other important causes of breast-feeding decline is now more difficult to obtain. There is currently a need to strengthen and broaden the Code, by making it applicable to manufactured weaning foods as well as breast-milk substitutes, and to prevent advertising to health professionals as well as to the general public. More support is needed for NGOs involved in monitoring the Code and in their work to protect, support and promote breast-feeding.

With regard to the future role of the health profession in support of optimum infant feeding practices, there has been some progress, but much remains to be done. As stated earlier, the medical and health profession has often had a negative impact on breast-feeding. The first need then is to educate all future health workers about breast-feeding and to re-educate existing professionals. This requires improvements in training of doctors, nurses, midwives and other health professionals. In some countries major efforts are underway, using seminars and refresher courses to educate existing health workers about sound infant feeding practices.

Steps should be taken to try to ensure that in all health institutions the infant is put to the breast as soon as possible after birth, preferably within the first hour. The advantages include beneficial effects on the mother's uterus, promotion of mother–infant bonding, supply of immune substances to the newborn, and a positive influence on subsequent successful breast-feeding. In many communities in Africa, Asia and Latin America very early breast-feeding is discouraged, and in many cultures colostrum is discarded because it is not considered to be good for the baby. This is one of the few instances where traditional practices related to breast-feeding are not ideal. Efforts should be made to influence mothers about the benefits of early feeding and of colostrum fed to their infants.

The importance of rooming-in, which allows some women after delivery in hospital to remain with their infants, is now accepted but not practiced everywhere. No hospitals should remain where rooming-in is not the norm. Health professionals need to guard against influence on them by formula manufacturers, and should avoid becoming obligated to the corporations by

accepting favours, donations or even research grants from them. If the multinational corporations wish to support research or projects dealing with infant feeding they should not provide grants directly to scientists, but rather should give the funds to organizations such as WHO or UNICEF, or to national professional bodies who can then allocate the funds to scientists on a competitive basis following peer review processes.

There are three categories of activity, all allied, which need to be considered if optimum breast-feeding is to be practiced in a country or a community:[16]

- Protection of breast-feeding, which includes policies, programmes and activities which shield women, already breast-feeding or planning to breast-feed, against forces which might influence them to do otherwise.
- Support of breast-feeding through activities, both formal and informal, which may help women to have confidence in their ability to breast-feed. This is important for women who have a desire to breast-feed but have anxieties or doubts about it, or who face conditions which seem to make breast-feeding seem difficult.
- Promotion of breast-feeding through activities that are designed mainly to influence groups of women to breast-feed their infants when they are disinclined to do so or have not done so with their previous babies.

While all three categories of activity are important, the relative effort put into each should depend on the current situation in each country. Thus, where traditional breast-feeding practices are the norm but where infant formula is just beginning to make inroads, protection is the policy deserving highest priority. In contrast, in a country where the majority of women are not breast-feeding at all, the major efforts should be on promotion. To use a health analogy it can be said that protection and support are preventive measures, and promotion is a curative approach to the problem.

Protection of breast-feeding This aims to guard women who normally would successfully breast-feed, against those forces which might cause them to alter this practice. All actions which prevent or curtail promotion of breast-milk substitutes, baby bottles and teats will have this effect. A strong Code properly enforced and monitored will help protect breast-feeding. Also, measures which reduce the availability of infant formula in places where poor women shop, will be useful. Other forms of formula promotion also need to be curtailed including: that aimed at health professionals; the giving out of samples, calendars and promotional materials; and hospital visits by corporation staff. Legislative measures to curb these practices may be needed. Papua New Guinea has placed infant formula on prescription as a means to protect breast-feeding. New measures need to be adopted in some countries to reduce the promotion of manufactured weaning foods and items such as glucose for child feeding.

Support of breast-feeding In each country, this depends on those factors or problems which are making breast-feeding more difficult. In many urban areas paid employment away from home is one such factor. In this case, legislation to provide women with two to three months of maternity leave, and job security if they take unpaid leave, may be called for. Also adequate lunch-breaks to allow breast-feeding or crèches to permit babies to be fed at the work site are supportive measures. A second set of factors is related to maternal morbidity, including breast problems during lactation. Unless the health workers are supportive of breast-feeding, it is often found that mothers unnecessarily resort to breast-milk substitutes when they face such problems. A third important issue includes current health facility practices. As stated, these sometimes discourage successful breast-feeding whereas they should be supportive. Hospital regulations and practices which ensure rooming-in and on-demand breast-feeding, very early placing of the infant on the breast after delivery, and a variety of educational and other activities by health workers aimed at mothers before, during and after delivery, should all be routine practice in support of breast-feeding. Doctors need to understand that very few health conditions are absolute contra-indications for breast-feeding. In many industrialized and non-industrialized countries private voluntary agencies and non-government organizations are playing very useful roles in support of breast-feeding. La Leche League in the US and breast-feeding information groups in other countries have been important.

Promotion of breast-feeding This involves motivation or re-education of mothers (or potential mothers) who otherwise might not be inclined to breast-feed their babies. In theory, promotion is the most difficult and certainly the most costly of the three options. But in some societies, it is an essential approach if breast-feeding is to become the preferred method of infant feeding. Mass media and education campaigns to make known the disadvantages of bottle-feeding and the advantages of breast-feeding are the usual approaches. It is important to know the factors that have led to the decline in breast-feeding in an area and to understand how women regard breast and bottle-feeding. A lack of such understanding has led to failure of many promo-

tional campaigns. Social marketing techniques, properly applied, have a greater chance of success. Promotion should address not only the health benefits, but also the economic and anti-fertility advantages of breast-feeding. Often it is first necessary for politicians to be educated about these matters. Both a strong political will and an ability to implement new policies are necessary ingredients of any plan to protect, support and promote breast-feeding.

References

1. Bitek, O p'. *Song of Lawino*. London, Longman, Green and Co., 1960: 30–31.
2. Latham MC. *Human Nutrition in Tropical Africa*. Rome FAO, 1965.
3. American Academy of Pediatrics. Encouraging breast-feeding. *Pediatrics*. 1980; **65**(3): 657.
4. Cunningham AS. Breastfeeding and morbidity in industrialized communities: An update. *Advances in International Maternal and Child Health*. 1980; **1**: 128–68.
5. Greiner T, Almroth S, Latham MC. *The Economic Value of Breastfeeding*. Cornell International Nutrition Monograph Series No. 6. Ithaca, New York, Cornell University, 1979.
6. Latham MC. The relationship of breastfeeding to human fertility. In: *The Decline of the Breast*. Cornell International Nutrition Monograph Series No. 10. Ithaca, New York, Cornell University, 1982. pp. 1–21.
7. Potts M, Thapa S, Herbetson MA. Breast-feeding and fertility. *Journal of Biosocial Science* (Supplement). 1985; **9**: 1–173.
8. WHO. The prevalence and duration of breast-feeding: a critical review of available information. *WHO Statistics Quarterly*. 1982; **2**: 92–116.
9. WHO. The dynamics of breast-feeding. *WHO Chronicle*. 1983; **37**(1): 6–10.
10. Latham MC, Elliott TC, Winikoff B *et al*. Infant feeding in urban Kenya: a pattern of triple nipple feeding. *Journal of Tropical Pediatrics*. 1986; **32**: 276–80.
11. WHO. *Report on a Consultation on Infants Who Cannot be Breastfed*. Geneva, WHO, 1986.
12. Latham MC. Insufficient milk and the World Health Organization Code. *East African Medical Journal*. 1982; **58**: 87–90.
13. Latham MC. Nutritional problems of Tanganyika. In: *Proceedings of the Sixth International Congress of Nutrition*. Edinburgh, Churchill Livingstone and Co., 1964.
14. Jelliffe DB, Jelliffe EFP. *Human Milk in the Modern World*. Oxford University Press, 1978.
15. WHO. *International Code of Marketing of Breast-milk Substitutes*. Geneva, WHO, 1981.
16. Greiner T. *Infant Feeding Policy Options for Governments*. Report for Infant Feeding Consortium, Cornell University, Ithaca, New York, 1982.

Community diagnosis

Michel Pechevis

The policy of primary health care advocated since the Alma-Ata Conference in 1978 is losing its momentum in many countries despite some isolated successes. The reasons for this stagnation are numerous, and many of them are beyond the volition of health professionals. However, it may be questioned whether sufficient efforts have been made to orientate the organization and management of services and activities and the training of staff to put this policy into practice.

The concept of primary health care involves decentralization of health policies to regional and local levels, with an intersectoral approach to the problems and with participation from the population. But if it is not to remain a slogan with no concrete significance, the means must be found to develop these aspects. Community diagnosis seems to be an excellent means, indeed an essential condition, for developing primary health care.

What is community diagnosis?

The meaning of the term

'Diagnosis' is a well-known term among health professionals and the public. Before treatment is prescribed and before any decision is reached on what action should be taken, an effort is made to diagnose a patient's disease. In the same way, before health activities are developed in a particular community, an appreciation is needed of the situation in that community – its problems, needs and resources, as well as its traditions, history, etc. Only when all this is known is it possible to take appropriate measures.

The term 'diagnosis', however, may be considered too heavily weighted with medical connotations, and too static. For a community, what is needed is not only a 'snapshot' of the current situation but also to add progressively to the information obtained and to follow up the situation as it develops. Furthermore, clinical diagnosis all too often implies a passive role by the individual being 'diagnosed'. However, as we shall see, the community participates fully in its own diagnosis.

Finally, it is necessary to clarify what is meant by 'community'. The following definition was proposed at the Alma-Ata Conference on Primary Health Care:[1]

A community consists of people living together in some form of social organization and cohesion. Its members share in varying degrees political, economic, social and cultural characteristics, as well as interests and aspirations, including health. Communities vary widely in size and socio-economic profile, ranging from clusters of isolated homesteads to more organized villages, towns and city districts.

The term 'community' thus refers to a comparatively homogeneous group of individuals. By its very nature, it masks internal social differentiation, the positions of groups, and even conflicting relationships existing between them. In village communities neighbours are often rivals. It will be necessary to distinguish the groups and possibly subgroups that make up the 'community', and to determine the different problems and needs accordingly.

Furthermore, the term 'community' is more apt than 'population' or 'group of people' because what is involved is not simply a collection of individuals but the relationships that these individuals establish, and the development dynamics that such relationships make possible.

The meaning of the process

To make a community diagnosis is to identify the problems, the needs, and the resources of a community. This process is the first step in community health programme planning, as shown in Fig. 1.5.1.

This diagram is now classical, and is attractive because of its apparent logic. However, if the first step is not in the right direction it may lead health professionals to set up services and activities that have no connection with the real needs of the population. Needs that are wrongly identified may result in health programmes condemned to failure from the start because they do not coincide with the problems that the members of the community consider to be of priority. As an example: in a small town in a developing country, the health authorities had decided to set up a family

planning centre. The population was faced with a serious water supply problem, for which they had been requesting assistance from the same authorities for many months. They resented the establishment of the family planning centre, which had been imposed on them from above and which had no impact. Community diagnosis must therefore not be diagnosis *about* a given community but diagnosis *with* the community. The needs of a population may differ considerably according to whether they are defined and identified by health professionals alone or in close cooperation with the members of the community and with their participation.

As perceived by Raynald Pineault,[2] two main approaches may be used to identify health problems:

- Epidemiological. This uses various ways of measuring the health status of a population, such as indicators of mortality and morbidity.
- Psycho-sociological. This consists of identifying a population's problems and determining their importance on the basis of how they are perceived by individual members of the community. In practice, this approach is rarely used by planners, on the grounds that such information is difficult to obtain or not as accurate or as meticulously scientific as it should be.

Community diagnosis employs these two complementary approaches, and every effort is made to maintain a balance between them. This balance is essential when priorities are being established.

All health workers, whatever their responsibilities, should approach the community with the attitudes and ways of thinking of a 'general practitioner'. This means that an overall approach must be maintained, without prejudices, narrowmindedness, or a 'specialist's' preoccupation with one particular subject. As is discussed later, the methodology proposed calls for an overall approach before focussing on specific problems.

Furthermore, this approach encourages every member of the health staff responsible for a particular activity to be aware of the other health problems of the community, the complementarity of activities, and the need for integration of the various family health activities. It can only be undertaken together with the other members of the health team, the other professionals concerned, and the population, and provides an excellent opportunity for developing intersectoral cooperation and team-work.

Another essential characteristic of community diagnosis is that it is a local process. Whatever the health policy defined at central level, and the broad outline of activities planned, the activities themselves

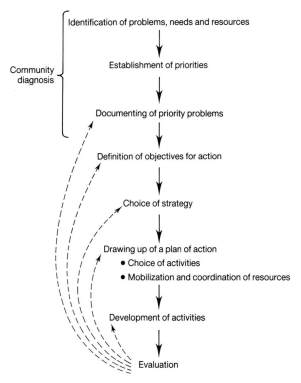

Fig. 1.5.1 Steps in the planning of a community health programme. (From Pineault R. *Union Médicale du Canada*, 1976:**105**, 1208–14 with modifications.)

are going to be carried out in the field, at local level. They will have to be adapted to local circumstances and to the real needs of the population (or communities) concerned.

If appropriate objectives for action are to be set, if activities based on the resources of a community are to be developed, and if the activities thus undertaken are to be evaluated accurately, it is necessary for local data to be available.

Information collected by the primary health care services and sent in the form of periodic reports to regional or central level is all too rarely used at local level for the planning and evaluation of activities. Community diagnosis, however, helps to restore the full value and significance of data collection, which is an essential activity of basic health services.

Community diagnosis is therefore clearly a preliminary step which is essential in order to apply a valid policy of primary health care.

'Participation' is one of the key words in the concept and definition of primary health care:[1]

Primary Health Care is essential health care made universally accessible to individuals and families in the community by means acceptable to them, through their full participation and at a cost that the community and country can afford. It forms an integral part both of the country's health system of which it is the nucleus and of the overall social and economic development of the community.

However, participation is often no more than a pious hope. One of the chief reasons for this is that the health services do not make the effort required to obtain this participation, whereas the process underlying community diagnosis, and the methods and techniques required to accomplish it, are in fact an incentive to health personnel to work *with* the community and not only *for* it. In this approach, the health professional is not simply someone 'who knows', but also someone 'who is learning' from, and with, the community. In community diagnosis, the role of health professionals is first and foremost to 'give the floor' to the community, listen attentively to what it has to say, and in this way help it to express its needs. The attitude which makes this approach possible will help to transform relationships between health personnel and the members of the community.

In a community health approach, which underlies and follows up community diagnosis, the organization of activities *starts from the community*, and this leads to a re-examination of the usual hierarchy of health services and activities, and to a reversal of the traditional pyramid, as shown in Fig. 1.5.2.

The methodology of community diagnosis

The preparatory phase

Community (and institutional) preparation

If the diagnosis is to have a truly community orientation, health professionals must involve both the community and professionals of other disciplines concerned from the preparatory phase onwards. It is essential to avoid facing the community and its representatives with a *fait accompli*, and asking them to 'participate' in a project which has already been planned without them.

Cooperation can be ensured from the start through a working group[3] or a coordinating body to bring together health professionals and members of the community. It will be for the working group to decide on the successive steps; define the objectives of the community diagnosis; determine how it is to be carried out and the methods to be used; mobilize the necessary resources; evaluate the results, and make the preliminary contacts required. In practice, however, it will often be necessary for a more limited group to start the process and extend it as and when the first contacts are made, at the same time ensuring that a satisfactory balance is maintained between professionals and representatives of the different groups in the community.

Technical preparation

This consists of:

- Briefing, and if necessary training, the people directly involved in the diagnosis, particularly the members of the working group (professionals and non-professionals). This training must of course deal with methodology, but it must also prepare those who take part in it for communication with the community, and for analysis and interpretation of the data collected.
- Planning and working out the various stages of community diagnosis.

Community diagnosis *per se*

Once the preparatory phase is completed and the working group set up, the following steps will need to be taken in succession:

- Definition of the objectives of the proposed community diagnosis.

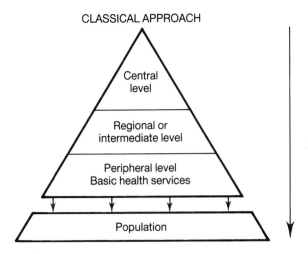

CLASSICAL APPROACH

Central level

Regional or intermediate level

Peripheral level
Basic health services

Population

Health activities are planned at central level and applied at peripheral level to the population, whose role is usually passive

APPROACH BASED ON PRIMARY HEALTH CARE

Primary health care

C O M M U N I T I E S

Peripheral level

Intermediate level (region or district)

Central level

Health activities are decided upon, planned and carried out jointly by professionals and members of the community on the basis of local identification of problems, needs and resources (community diagnosis)

The intermediate level is responsible for coordination and supervision of local activities

The central level decides on the main trends of health policy and provides the additional support needed (in human, material and financial resources) to the intermediate and peripheral levels

Fig. 1.5.2   Hierarchy of health services and activities.

- Compilation of the list of information or data to be collected.
- Identification of sources of data, choice of the most appropriate methods of data collection, and, if necessary, drawing up of instruments for data collection, taking available resources into account.
- Collection of data.
- Analysis and interpretation of the data collected.
- Identification of the problems, needs, resources, and groups at risk.
- Establishment of priorities.
- Documenting priority problems.

These steps are considered in some detail below.

Definition of objectives

Agreement must be reached from the start on what it is hoped to achieve and with what aim in view, and which community(ies) are to be included.

It may be decided that a health team should identify the priority problems and needs of children in a particular community, in order to orient or reorient the activities for which it is responsible. In other cases, a problem that has already been identified may be taken as the basis for ascertaining its true importance, or for gathering further background information to enable a suitable community programme to be established.

It may also be desirable to find out whether the establishment of a new health service in the community is justified, or to evaluate the impact of activities that have been undertaken, or simply to gain a better understanding of the community in which the health team is working.

Finally, the objective may be primarily an educational one, using community diagnosis as a practical field exercise within the basic or refresher training of health personnel.

Information or data to be collected

The information needed depends primarily on the objectives of each particular community diagnosis, but the following list may be put forward.

The characteristics of the community
General environment:

- history of the community;
- geographical characteristics of the area, and its climate;
- urban or rural nature of the area;
- distribution of population in the area; type(s) of housing;
- the main communications network;
- transportation and travel facilities.

Demography:

- population size and age structure;
- birth, death and fertility rates; age of marriage;
- migration.

Socio-economic situation:

- occupations of the community and local resources;
- employment situation; unemployment;
- socio-professional categories;
- income;
- cost of living;
- social and family organization;
- system of social protection.

Administrative and political organization:

- degree of administrative centralization;
- government policy on health;
- health and social legislation.

Cultural and religious life:

- traditions, customs, habits with regard to food, health, and reproduction;

- different ethnic groups and religions;
- leisure pursuits;
- schooling and literacy level;
- existence of cultural, political, military, religious or other associations or groups;
- modes of relationship and communication among the members of the community and between them and the outside world (mass media).

The health system:

- existing health facilities (public and private);
- current health activities (e.g. curative and preventive care, health education);
- accessibility and use of the health services by the population;
- health personnel: number, categories, training, skills;
- traditional medicine.

The classification adopted is arbitrary, and some of the items could equally well be placed under other headings. Furthermore, this list is purely indicative, and makes no claim to be exhaustive.

Data for assessing the health status of the population with special reference to children: these data cover primarily mortality and morbidity.

Relationships between the characteristics of the community and its health status   This can be done by trying to identify the factors which play a determining role (whether positive or negative) in the health status of a community and its members (particularly children). (See Fig. 1.5.3.) The negative factors are the risk factors which will need to be controlled through preventive

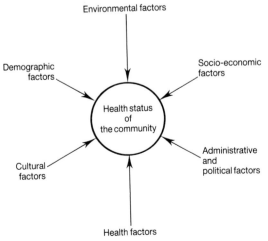

Fig. 1.5.3 Factors that may influence the health status of a community.

measures. The positive factors are the existing or potential resources which can be used, or which will need to be developed, in the programmes of activities.

The risk factors may include for example:

- difficulties of access to health services (environmental factor and health factor);
- too early or too closely spaced pregnancies (demographic factor);
- unemployment, or lack of social protection (socio-economic factor);
- certain habits such as abrupt stopping of breast-feeding as soon as another pregnancy starts (cultural factor);
- poor immunization coverage (health factor).

On the other hand the positive factors and resources which could be used for the development of community health programmes include:

- the existence of a good communications network (environmental factor);
- later age for marriage (demographic factor);
- abundant local food crop resources (socio-economic factor);
- a high literacy rate among mothers, or the existence of a dynamic women's association (cultural factor);
- health personnel skilled in primary health care (health factor).

Depending on the community some factors will play a more important role than others, and emphasis will need to be given to these when community diagnosis is undertaken.

By this method a preliminary list of information can be drawn up. Before going on to the subsequent stages, however, a number of questions should be asked, as is suggested by Brownlee:[4]

If the workers are attempting to develop a study that is truly relevant in the cultural area where they work they must also ask themselves at least four basic questions concerning each piece of information that may be sought before choosing what information they will actually gather:

1. Will this piece of information be of real use in the program we are planning? If so, just how will it be used?
2. Is the category of information meaningful in the local context?
3. If so, will the methods we are planning to use give us information that is accurate?
4. Are there any other categories of information (possibly irrelevant in our own culture) that would be important in the local culture?

Where the term 'our own culture' is used, it must be clear that this refers not only to foreign personnel taking part in community diagnosis in a country other than their own, but also to personnel who are natives of the country but are working in an area, ethnic group, socio-economic environment or socio-professional environment other than their own. For this reason, the subjects to be covered in the diagnosis must be worked out by a multidisciplinary team (part of the working group mentioned earlier for instance) which includes local personnel and members of the community.

Ways of expressing the data   Some data can be expressed quantitatively. This is the case with epidemiological data, which express the health status of the community in terms of mortality or morbidity rates or demographic data. These quantitative data will prove very useful, perhaps essential, in setting definite objectives and later on evaluating the impact of the programmes established.

The following are some examples of quantitative data:

- death rates by age; morbidity rates (e.g. incidence of measles or diarrhoeal diseases);
- birth rate;
- fertility rate;
- statistics on utilization of the health services;
- average age of marriage and average interval between births.

In addition, these indicators may be analysed by age, socio-professional category, ethnic origin, and the religion of the parents.

Other data are of a qualitative nature. They relate particularly to cultural factors and to the opinions of different population groups on health problems – their importance, their meaning, their causes, or the most effective solutions.

Every effort should be made to provide numerical data whenever possible, and to be meticulous in collection and expression of data. Health professionals must, however, beware of the magic of statistics, which can give a false impression of objectivity. The same applies to the number of subjects surveyed or interviewed. It is sometimes better to obtain more data on a small number of families than brief data on a large number.

Identification of sources of data, choice of methods, and drawing up of instruments for data collection

Once it has been decided what information should be collected, the possible sources of information will need to be identified and the most suitable methods of collection chosen.

It is necessary to determine what information is already available and what information needs to be built up. The smaller the community, the more difficult it is to obtain data which can be used or transposed directly, and the more need there will be to build up data.[5]

Information already available The working group will have to make an index of all existing information about the community or about the area in which the community is located. This may require a great deal of work and tedious searching, but it is often surprising to find how many studies, reports and documents already exist. This search also provides an opportunity to make contact with administrations and services with which it may be useful to cooperate later on.

The documents to be consulted include:

- the plan for national socio-economic development and the national health plan;
- records of births, marriages and deaths;
- health and population statistics (particularly concerning the area in which the community is located);
- reports on activities of the health services (especially those of paediatric services or MCH and family planning/birth spacing clinics);
- reports on studies or surveys already made in the area (or if none is available, in a similar area) and covering the data to be collected;
- theses and papers on the area prepared by students in medical schools or institutions for the training of health personnel or other professionals;
- the local or regional press.

Information to be built up Several complementary techniques may be used to collect specific information about the community directly.

Qualitative data. In the first place, relevant information about the life of the community should be collected. This covers primarily qualitative data, i.e. what we have termed the psycho-social approach to needs and problems.

For this purpose, it will be necessary to observe the community. Observation is one of the best ways of analysing a community's problems and needs, but it requires much more careful and meticulous work than would appear at first sight. It is also important to collect the views expressed by key persons and groups in the community, especially:

- the various professionals concerned – in the health services, the social services, education, rural development, etc;
- official community leaders – civil, religious and (if relevant) military authorities;
- traditional leaders and practitioners – tribal chiefs, medicine-men, traditional midwives;

- the various established associations and groups – women's, men's, or joint associations for sports, cultural activities, politics;
- other members of the community – school-age children, adolescents, families representing different socio-economic strata, and representatives of the various socio-professional categories.

This may be done through structured interviews. A semidirective style, or even informal conversations, often provide extremely useful information which is usually missed in systematic surveys. As Brownlee says:[4]

Every culture has ways people traditionally relax, times when they let down their defences and talk sometimes of nothing in particular, other times about what is most important to them. [This is] one of the best and most painless ways to learn about many aspects of local life.

It may also be useful to hold meetings with large or small groups, such as the community forum which is open to all members of the community. This technique can be used to complete data obtained from key persons, or to ascertain how valid and representative these data are.

Visits can also be paid to various services and public places (health services, social centres, schools, professional training centres, cultural centres, places of worship, markets, shops) and to the workshops and factories in the area.

Quantitative data Precise and quantifiable data need to be collected with the community itself, to confirm and complete the items of information shown up or surmised as a result of the non-systematic methods mentioned above, or identified through a study of existing documentation. Systematic epidemiological or sociological surveys will be required.

The choice of methodology and techniques will depend on the means (and particularly the skills) available. Some surveys can only be carried out by highly specialized personnel such as epidemiologists or sociologists. The methods chosen must therefore be those that can be planned and carried out with local personnel, even if this means some loss of precision in the information. Otherwise, community diagnosis is condemned to be a luxury activity carried out in pilot areas by a few privileged teams. An increasing number of epidemiologists now agree to take part in field activities, and this change is all to the good.

One of the roles of national and international staff responsible for establishing or developing primary health care is to work out, with the help of epidemiologists, simplified methods of data collection suitable for use in community diagnosis at local level by local staff.

This has already been done for assessment of immunization coverage under the Expanded Programme on Immunization, as well as in the Diarrhoeal Diseases Control Programme, on the initiative of WHO.[6,7] Studies are underway to adapt such methods to other fields of primary health care.

It will usually be necessary to give additional training, in the form of refresher sessions, to those who will be responsible for helping to prepare methods for data collection, draw up instruments for collection, and actually collect the data.

No single method can provide all the data needed to identify the health problems and needs of a given community and to solve them with a community health approach – that is, with the participation of the community. Only with a combination of several of the different methods that have been described, and perhaps others as well, will it be possible to achieve the objectives and at the same time remain consistent with the approach.

Data collection

The time required for data collection will depend on the objectives, the urgency of the problems to be solved, the needs to be satisfied and the resources available. It will also depend on the availability of the members of the working group. Community diagnosis should be part of the priority activities for health professionals. However, a certain amount of time will need to be set aside to prepare and put into operation some of the methods of data collection, especially surveys. The availability of members of the community may vary from one period of the year to another (according to seasonal agricultural work, for instance), and the working group should take this into account in their planning. Collection of data for community diagnosis is a more or less continuous activity, with peak periods.

Community diagnosis may be undertaken as part of a training programme. In this case, the actual collection of data will often have to be concentrated into a few days. The resulting diagnosis can only be partial and provisional and will have to be completed by the local health team. However, it is surprising how much high-quality information can be collected, within a week or even within a few days,[8,9] by a group of students who are strangers to a community.

Analysis and interpretation of data

On the basis of the data collected (whether quantitative or qualitative, statistical or non-statistical) the working group responsible for community diagnosis will try to bring out the main points. These might include:

- rates considered to be abnormal (death rates, birth rates, etc.);
- statistics that are too high or too low (e.g. data on average intervals between births, health services attendance);
- factors which have a decisive effect on the health of the community;
- the opinions of members of the community on problems or needs considered to be of priority, their perception of certain events related to health, their expectations, their willingness to change, etc.

This analysis will enable the working group to draw up a list of the chief problems and needs. In the literature as well as in professional practice, the terms 'health problem' and 'health need' are often used synonymously but a distinction should be made between them: 'A problem may be considered as objective, identifiable by an outside observer; a need is more subjective, and is connected with the individual's or the community's own characteristics'.[5]

At this point health professionals and members of the community may diverge in their perception of problems and needs, the professionals tending to give more importance to the problems highlighted by the quantitative data, and the members of the community having more feeling for the subjective and qualitative expression of the needs.

In addition, confusion frequently arises between health needs and needs for services or resources.[10] It may however be useful to distinguish clearly among these different catagories of needs, with a view to establishing priorities as well as choosing a strategy for action once the community diagnosis is completed.

Community diagnosis also consists of identifying resources. These include existing health, social or educational facilities, and the personnel available and their qualifications. The resources of the community are:

- the skills of one or another of the members or groups in the community which might be used to solve problems;
- existing community networks, both formal and informal (e.g. different associations, and also welfare networks);
- formal and informal channels of communication and meeting-places used by the community.

A great deal of imagination must be used to identify everything that can contribute to solving problems and promoting community participation.

Analysis of the data will often reveal that certain groups or individuals in the community are especially vulnerable to particular health problems, for example women with large families, adolescent girls, or weaned or bottle-fed infants. The analysis may also show a higher frequency of problems in a particular village, district of a town, or ethnic group.

Groups or individuals at risk who are identified in this way can be made the priority 'target' for health service activities. It is worth mentioning here that the concept of 'target-population', which is much used in public health, is based on an approach which may run counter to the principles of community health. It may lead health professionals to consider the community as the target and object of the activities to be undertaken, rather than as a partner and the 'subject' of these activities, in whose planning and development it is called upon to participate. That said, care must be taken not to mistake the target and give undue attention to one population group that may have been studied, to the detriment of another that is more exposed but has been missed in the diagnosis. This may happen with isolated communities that are outside the usual area of coverage or influence of the health services. One of the objectives of community diagnosis is to reveal these population groups and, together with them, identify their problems and needs.

Establishment of priorities

The priorities to be given to the problems and needs identified should be determined as far as possible with the participation of all those involved, both professionals and non-professionals, under the coordination of the original working group in which they must be represented.

At this stage, there may once more be differences in perception of the true importance and urgency of the problems and needs between the health professionals and the members of the community. It will be necessary to apply criteria which take these different perceptions into account. The criteria generally used by health professionals are as follows:

- the relative importance of the different problems, determined on the basis of statistical data (incidence or prevalence);
- the gravity of these problems (determined primarily on the basis of frequency of complications and lethality rate);
- the existence of effective control measures;
- the applicability of these control measures in the community given the resources and constraints;
- the cost of the control measures proposed.

In addition to these criteria, it is essential to take into account others of a more 'community' nature. With regard to a given problem, for example:

- whether it is recognized as frequent and/or serious by the community;
- whether the community agrees with the existing solution;
- whether the community is ready to participate in solution of the problem.

The community representatives may, without meaning to, introduce a distorted view of the priorities in the light, for instance, of the health or social facilities that they would like to see established in their area.

It may be useful to bear in mind the distinction between health needs and the need for services. The professionals may decide to undertake an information campaign among the population to give a better understanding of the importance of a specific criterion which they consider essential. The final decision (which will often be temporary) will result from dialogue or negotiation which takes the various arguments and points of view into account. The important thing is to reach decisions which the community understands, which it finds acceptable, and on which it will be willing to take action.

Documenting priority problems

Once the priority problems have been determined from the data collected and with the help of a number of criteria, it will often be necessary to complete the initial diagnosis on specific problems in order to have available all the background information required for their solution or for dealing with them.

When community diagnosis is undertaken to document a specific problem already identified by professionals or by the community, the first steps should not be left out. A global approach should be made to the characteristics of the community, while at the same time focussing on the specific problem.

Documenting a specific or priority problem means:

- defining it accurately, and if necessary reformulating it;
- establishing its causes in the community, with special reference to risk factors;
- identifying the specific or other resources which can be used to solve it.

The same process and the same methodology can be used as for the global approach to the community but in this case focussing on a single problem. Thus, identification of risk factors and resources can be based on the various factors that play a decisive role with regard to the problem concerned. Fig. 1.5.3 can be used for this purpose, placing the specific problem in the central circle.

In the same way as for the global approach to the community,¹ it is desirable to set up a working group responsible for coordination, made up of professionals and non-professionals noted for their skills or for their involvement with the problem to be documented. To illustrate this, let us take an example from among the priority health problems of children in developing countries – diarrhoeal diseases.

The problem already identified concerns a high frequency of diarrhoeal diseases and several fatal cases of dehydration in children under 5 years of age, according to the records of a health unit established in a rural community.

Identification of the community's specific features shows that it is a farming village in the tropics, located in a mountainous area, 50 km from the nearest town, and very difficult to reach during the rainy season. The dwellings are very scattered. Furthermore, the only supply of drinking water is a spring with a small flow of water located 3 km from the village (environmental factor). The health unit is in the charge of a single health worker with minimal qualifications, but who is anxious to cooperate (health factor). Finally, there is a very active women's association (cultural factor).

The problem was discovered in the records of the health unit by the supervising medical assistant, who took the initiative of setting up a working group. The government has decided to carry out a diarrhoeal diseases control programme, but its operation is more or less limited to the capital city.

The group's first task is to determine the scope of the problem, with the help of a simplified epidemiological survey. This will provide more accurate statistics on the incidence of acute diarrhoeal episodes, the lethality rate

of diarrhoea, and also the most vulnerable age-groups. The next step is to seek the possible determining factors of diarrhoea in children in the community, using epidemiological and psycho-social approaches. It will thus be possible to determine:

- the true significance of childhood diarrhoea in the community;
- the traditional practices used by the women for children with diarrhoea (some practices may be harmful, such as the systematic suppression of all fluids for a child with diarrhoea; others may be useful, such as the use of carob-bean soup or other drinks that are recognized to have antidiarrhoeal properties);
- the level of knowledge and the actual activities of the health worker with regard to prevention and/or treatment of diarrhoeal diseases and dehydration, etc.

The working group will thus have at its disposal information that will enable it to define objectives for the activities planned, to choose an appropriate strategy, and to evaluate the activities undertaken. Table 1.5.1 shows the various steps and their sequence.

Conclusion

Community diagnosis, like community health and development, is based primarily on ensuring that all health activities have their roots in the needs of the population and are carried out with their full participation. It is not a 'study' or just an observational exercise in which the observers try to remain neutral

Table 1.5.1 Steps in community diagnosis and their sequence

Steps	Duration
0. Preparation	
• Setting up of working group	
• Community preparation	
• Technical preparation	
1. Definition of objectives	
2. Drawing up of list of information	
3. Identification of sources of data. Choice of appropriate methods	
4. Collection of data (on the spot)	
5. Analysis and interpretation. Identification of problems, needs and resources	
6. Establishment of priorities	
7. Documenting of priority problems	

Key: —— Expected duration of each step.
——---- Means that this step may continue over a longer period.
---- Means that this step can or should be repeated or carried out in several stages.

and not make any changes in the running of the community (as for an anthropological study for example). The aim is not only to encourage expression of needs but also to stimulate awareness and participation in the community. It is research–action, or more precisely research–action–participation, which commits the health professionals together with the community, and leads them to share its fears as well as its hopes.

Community diagnosis is also an excellent means of doing effective field work, including work in areas far removed from big cities. It is a most exciting process according to all who have attempted it or have been involved in it, either as an actual situation or in the form of an educational exercise.

Its difficulties and its exigencies should, however, not be overlooked. It is based, as we have seen, on certain types of knowledge, skills and attitudes that by no means all health professionals possess. To participate in carrying out community diagnosis involves knowing how to make use of the various methods of data collection. It also involves knowing how to observe, how to listen, how to communicate with others, how to work as a team and how to negotiate.

Most training programmes for health professionals as yet give very little emphasis to acquiring these skills. It is urgent to review basic training, and to make up for present deficiencies with refresher training sessions. Only as health services and training programmes are reoriented in this way will it be possible to go forward in the establishment of community-based primary health care.

References

1. WHO/UNICEF. *Primary Health Care* (Report of the International Conference on Primary Health Care, Alma-Ata, USSR). Geneva, WHO, 1978. pp. 49.
2. Pineault R. Eléments et étapes d'élaboration d'un programme de santé communautaire. *Union Médicale du Canada*. 1976; **105**: 1208–14.
3. Lecorps P. *Le diagnostic communautaire*. Communication personnelle, février 1986.
4. Brownlee, AT. *Community, culture and care: a cross cultural guide for health workers*. St. Louis, C.V. Mosby Company, 1978. pp. 297.
5. Secrétariat d'Etat Chargé de la Santé, France. *Promotion de la Santé: Méthodologie. Atelier 7: Analyse des besoins d'une communauté*. Document de travail préparé par Deschamps JP. *et al*. Paris, La Documentation Française, 1986. pp. 60.
6. Henderson RH, Sundaresan T. Cluster sampling to assess immunization coverage: a review of experience with a simplified sampling method. *Bulletin of the World Health Organization*. 1982; **60**: 253–60.
7. Lemeshow S, Robinson D. Surveys to measure programme coverage and impact: a review of the methodology used by the expanded programme on immunization. *World Health Statistics Quarterly*. 1985; **38**: 65–75.
8. Amat T. *Community diagnosis in training in family planning for health personnel*. (Report on a WHO/ICC meeting, Paris 6–11 July 1981 Copenhagen, World Health Organization, Regional Office for Europe). *Public Health in Europe*. 1985; **20**: 44–50.
9. Pechevis M. Family planning training and community needs. *Children in the Tropics*. Paris, International Children's Centre, 1983; **141**: 7–46 (published both in English and French).
10. Pineault R. La planification des services de santé: une perspective épidémiologique. *Gestions Hospitalières*. 1980; **200**: 951–9.

CHAPTER 6

The doctor as teacher

Tony Waterston

Introduction

Teaching must be a central part of the work of doctors who are dedicated to the ideals of primary health care. As we near the end of the century, there is an urgent need to spread our medical knowledge far and wide. Why? Because knowledge is power; because self-reliance depends on knowledge; because the need for effective health workers is ever increasing; because children die every day due to lack of knowledge; and because doctors, in the past, have withheld knowledge and must make up for lost time. People desperately want health information but access to it is hard. All doctors must ask themselves "what am I doing to 'liberate' knowledge?"

The purpose of this chapter is to help doctors (and perhaps other health workers) to answer this question in a satisfactory way. In finding out what we can do to spread our knowledge, we need to look at the needs (and abilities) of the learner, as well as the teacher. We need to look at the ways we teach and why some of the means we have used in the past have failed. We need to recognize that doctors are not always the best teachers, and how to learn from those who may be better – sometimes non-professionals. Can we learn *with* our students? Sometimes they know more than we do, about life and the local culture. How do we balance our work in treatment and prevention with our teaching role? Which is more important? Ideally, they should always be combined, but sometimes this is a vain wish.

This chapter is aimed at the busy practising clinician rather than at the teaching hospital academic. For the former, some compromises are inevitable – it is just not possible, for instance, to teach each mother of a malnourished child about infant feeding in the course of a lengthy ward round. Nor is it desirable. But the teaching that is done can be improved, and time can be saved by teaching someone else to do what we do already. Remember though, that learning involves questioning – of accepted principles, policies and practices. We must continually question ourselves if we are to be effective teachers.

Who are we to teach?

Traditionally doctors have taught medical students, junior doctors and nurses, and our patients when we have the chance. Whom *should* we teach? Doctors are not the most effective teachers of the lay public. I shall refer a lot in this chapter to Werner and Bower's book *Helping Health Workers Learn*[1], and would encourage all doctor-teachers to read it and keep it handy. They comment that, as instructors of health workers, "Doctors have a tendency to take charge, to regard themselves as decision-makers even in areas they know little about. Feeling that even simple diagnosis and treatment are 'risky' without years of medical school, they often limit teaching of curative medicine to a few minor chores". But doctors can change their attitudes! And it is because I think they can that I put first the group for whom health 'knowledge' is most important – parents. Next come village health workers, then other professional health workers (e.g. nurses) and finally medical students and other doctors.

Parents

As child health workers, we recognize that parents take a bigger role in child-care than any professional and therefore have a great need for health information. That their intuitive approach is usually medically correct has been confirmed by research[2] and their ability to take on a more complex nursing role in hospital has also been supported by a UK study[3]. In most countries it is the mother who carries the burden of child-care; therefore it is towards her that most of our educational efforts should be dedicated. Fathers too have a great interest in children and in the past their lack of involvement may have been partly due to their exclusion from the medical process by the professionals. We should certainly do our best to include fathers in any information sharing. Opportunities for teaching in an informal situation are ever present and every consultation should include an educational encounter. Beware of long words and a patronizing manner! Remember that some parents may have had access to the same books as you and may even be more up to date, so do not disparage their view of the disease. Medical knowledge is not always based on sound science.

Formal teaching of parents (e.g. in the children's ward, out-patient clinic or antenatal clinic) is better organized by nursing or voluntary staff than by doctors, but it is up to us to ensure that time and space are given to health education. It is also important to watch and maintain the level of such teaching as well as the attitudes of the teacher to ensure that health talks are not dictatorial (see Fig. 1.1.11, p. 11).

How much should parents be taught? This can only be answered in the individual case and depends both on the parents' desire to learn and on their ability to absorb information. Some parents are so used to being treated as ignorant that they don't ask questions. We should start by demonstrating that their own knowledge and experience are valid and worthy of building upon.

Remember that parents recall little of the information that is conveyed verbally at the time of a consultation, and anything that is important should be given in writing (at the appropriate reading level). Much health education material used in the UK is too complex to be understood by parents.[4]

The field of health education and promotion for the general public is too wide to cover in this chapter but it is an extension of parent-education which many

paediatricians will wish to pursue. There is a role for child health doctors in the child to child programme,[5] in health teaching in schools, and in using the media. Most countries now have radio and television programmes on health and paediatricians are in a good position to supply accurate information through these channels. We tend to have a distrust of journalists thinking that they will misconstrue what we say, but we have to live with them and greater familiarity with their art will increase our ability to make constructive use of it.

Village health workers

It is doubtful whether doctors should ever be teachers of village health workers (VHWs) for the reasons stated below, but they should be aware of the content of the teaching programme for these workers. The doctor's teaching role will be by example rather than by precept, if we reinforce the status of the VHW. Doctors are seen as the ultimate fount of knowledge and hence if on occasion we defer to the VHW, this enhances the role of the latter in villagers' eyes (see Fig. 1.6.1).

Informal teaching of the VHW on issues as they arise is helpful. The VHW should also be consulted on ways of putting information over to the general public.

Why should doctors not teach VHWs directly?

- Doctors will find it hard to teach at the right level. Their teaching is likely to contain much science and

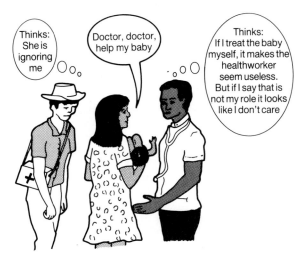

Fig. 1.6.1 A visiting health worker may weaken the position of the local health worker if he attends on his own those who come to him for treatment. The health worker should be included in the consultation. (After Werner op. cit. p10.7).

jargon and will make excessive use of the 'medical model'. It is possible to escape from this straight-jacket but once we do, it is better to concentrate on medical student and doctor teaching.

- VHWs require much more than 'medical' knowledge. They must be masters and mistresses of their culture and be familiar with basic agricultural, educational and public health principles. Most important, they must understand the political situation in their country and the political nature of their work (see 'critical awareness' below).
- Most VHW teaching will be at village level whereas most doctors work at small town or city level. It is, however, important that VHWs and doctors have contact and learn how the other works, to reduce the mystique that inevitably arises from ignorance. The same is true for the others who work with VHWs, e.g. agricultural extension workers, education extension workers, women's group leaders and local political organizers.

Nurses, medical assistants, 'paramedics'

These health workers are traditionally taught by doctors but not vice versa. Why not? (See Fig. 1.6.2.) I suggest that the reason is that doctors are supposed to be repositories of knowledge whereas nurses and 'paramedics' (in which blanket term I include speech therapists, physiotherapists and occupational therapists) are supposed to possess skills. This clearly is a gross exaggeration since doctors have skills in addition to knowledge, whereas the others have much knowledge not shared by doctors. There must therefore be a case for cross-fertilization. In addition, all these workers are expected to be part of a team in which the doctor is not necessarily the leader. Team relationships do not come easily to many teachers and must be worked at. Such work should start in the student stage with different cadres learning together. Joint project work is a better means to this end than sitting together in a classroom, though the greater number of 'paramedics' than doctors leads to an unbalanced group, particularly if nurse students are included.

Team-work aside, is it appropriate for doctors to teach nurse students? In many hospitals it will be essential to draw upon doctors but this should be done with care. On the positive side, the teaching contact should improve informal relationships between doctors and nurse teachers. However, doctors' teaching may lack relevance because of their failure to understand the level of knowledge required by nurse students. Greater guidance on nurses' learning objectives should be obtained from nurse tutors. There is a risk of the medical/nursing hierarchy (with its sexist overtones) entering the classroom (the 'oh great doctor' problem) and doctors should be aware of this.

As with all teaching, careful thought should be given to teaching methods and over-reliance on the lecture should be avoided. Bedside teaching of nurses (as of medical students) can be an effective method if properly used.

Medical students and doctors

The peripatetic nature of many medical students means that there are few readers of this book who will not encounter them either on electives or rural placements. Those meeting them in a more formal way will find guidance elsewhere.[6] What medical students relish about working in a district hospital in a developing country is the clinical experience. They see a wide variety of acute diseases and are given responsibility for patient care in a way which is rarely possible in their own medical school. The teacher should ensure that the student is not over-taxed, that a source of assistance is always available, and that a holistic attitude is engendered towards the local people and the community. There should therefore be a balance between cure and prevention, between hospital and community, and between Western and traditional medicine. The teacher should help the student to understand the 'whys' of disease seen commonly on the ward – particularly malnutrition and diarrhoeal disease (see Fig. 1.1.8).

The hospital-based doctor should also if possible consider the learning needs of doctors in the area who do not have access to 'continuing medical education'. Are TALC (Teaching Aids at Low Cost) slides in use? Is there a local medical society where problem cases can be presented? What about starting a journal club or a local newsletter? Could the scope of the national medical journal be widened? Unfortunately many such journals are heavily medical and disease-orientated, but are short of papers and may welcome an influx of fresh ideas.

Postgraduate teaching

Postgraduate teaching (or 'continuing medical education', the current in-term) will require input at national as well as at district level but the awareness of the district paediatrician of doctors' needs will be very helpful. What kind of learning facilities will attract doctors to work in rural areas? Three requirements (often all lacking) are diplomas, courses and resources.

Diplomas It is generally regarded as better for doctors to obtain a postgraduate specialist diploma in their own country than abroad. Specialist training in a developed country encourages the 'brain-drain' and is not often appropriate to the needs of the developing country. Courses or attachments which are individually chosen with the needs of the poorer country in mind, do have merit. Local postgraduate diplomas should include experience at primary care level and should emphasize the priority of primary health care (PHC); they should also place an emphasis on teaching, research and management as well as on clinical skills.[7]

It may be hard for a doctor working in a rural hospital to find time to study for a diploma, and provision of study time should be seen as a priority by the employing authority.

Courses Training requires more than simply studying for an exam and working in a busy job. Courses should be available at a national level (to cover teaching, research and management as well as the clinical areas) and time be made available to attend them – this is a financial issue which doctors might do better to campaign over than salary levels. However, there is also a case for organizing courses which can be pursued by post ('distance learning'). In either case, the trainee should be allocated to a tutor who will supervise his or her training needs.

Resources These are often in short supply. It should be the task of a Postgraduate Dean to ensure that all hospitals have appropriate learning tools which will include books (preferably appropriate reduced price editions), selected journals, tape–slide sets and the means to view them, an overhead projector, and any material produced nationally such as a newsletter. An important way in which the central hospital can support primary care is by sending specialists on teaching/consultation visits, which can include operating visits and medical out-patient clinics.

Blocks to better teaching and learning, and how to overcome them

Blocks to teaching

Perhaps the greatest block is the teacher who pays little attention to the learning needs of students, and to the eventual aims of a teaching programme. When the emphasis is on the teacher rather than on the learner, little attention is paid to the organization of teaching and to the methods used. However, owing to the failure of many medical schools to evaluate their own teaching, and the busy work pattern of most doctors, this deficiency is entirely understandable and is no reflection on the dedication of many doctor-teachers.

Blocks to learning

Lack of motivation is perhaps the greatest block to learning and this constraint should be recognized. An air of enthusiasm in a hospital for teaching sessions may take time to build up but is a necessary background factor in continuing medical education.

It is also hard for students to learn if inappropriate methods (such as lectures) are used persistently. Shortage of materials is another common block. There are students who have never been taught 'how to learn' and the knowledge they acquire is not retained. Finally, some of the subjects that students really need to learn about (how to teach, how to manage, how to solve problems) may not be taught in their locality.

How better to teach

Enthusiasm in the teacher is thought by students to be more important than the method used. The next step is to plan any formal teaching you do. Werner[1] has valuable comments on alternative teaching methods which though specially aimed at health worker training, are very relevant for doctors. He points out that 'the way they (health workers) teach can either break-down or build up people's self-confidence . . .' Doctors should examine carefully different approaches to learning – we tend automatically to adopt the lecture method because we were exposed to it ourselves, but it is a technique which discourages active thinking (see Fig. 1.6.3). The good teacher should encourage critical thinking and exploration of ideas by the students. This is much easier to do in a small group situation than a lecture theatre.

Doctors do not take easily to this form of teaching; it fits more easily into our authoritarian role to stand up at the front of a class and give a talk. Try to gain experience of other techniques by seeing them in action. Cox and Ewen[8] provide many helpful suggestions. Role play is of great value in encouraging students to question their own attitudes – this method is also particularly good for teaching multidisciplinary groups when there is an emphasis on team work. The first step in improving one's teaching is to think about the students' learning needs and how one's own style matches them. Obtain feedback from students and colleagues on your technique, and perhaps tape a lecture and listen to yourself. Is there a course on teaching methods (perhaps at a teacher's training

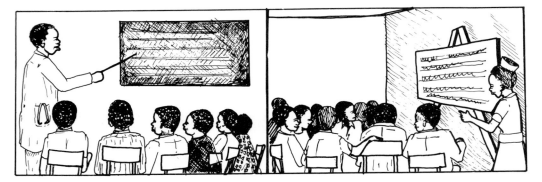

Fig. 1.6.2   All doctors should learn how to teach medical students. Nurses should also be involved in teaching medical students. (Courtesy of Taffy Naisho, AMREF, Nairobi.)

college) that you could attend? This should be obligatory for all medical school teachers.

Critical awareness

Teaching about health must also include teaching about people and their role in society. Doctors may not be much involved in this kind of teaching but should know about, and may wish to learn from, Freire's methods which are further discussed in Ref. 1. Paulo Freire was a Brazilian educator who used challenging techniques to teach literacy in the 1960s. Freire described three stages of awareness: magical awareness, when people explain the world about them in terms of myths and magic; naive awareness, when there is incomplete understanding of the social world, and an imitation of the élite but no attempt to change the social order; and critical awareness. People at this stage look more carefully at the causes of social problems and explain them through observation rather than by magic. As this awareness deepens, people develop a greater sense of self-worth and they feel able to take social action to bring about change. Awareness raising is brought about through group dialogue. The group leader's main role is to ask questions (using key words and pictures) which act as discussion starters. The group discussion aims to help the members gain confidence in themselves, to examine and later take action to change their situation, and to give them the tools to help control their lives. The method was originally used for the lay public but is also very relevant to health workers and can be incorporated into any health teaching.

Those interested in this and other teaching methods are referred to Ref. 1 and the other sources listed at the end of the chapter.

The children's doctor as a teacher in practice

Much of the foregoing theory of medical teaching may seem beyond the scope of the busy children's doctor, who is expected not only to provide curative care for the very sick children in hospital but also to organize preventive programmes in the district. Not all doctors will wish to spend time on thinking about and planning teaching, and those who are enthusiasts will feel that already their techniques are quite adequate. This may well be so but it is at least worth taking a few quiet moments from time to time to think about what one is doing. All of us are engaged in informal teaching with patients, on ward rounds, in the clinic, during time-consuming medical procedures, and in the course of visits to outlying hospitals. Maybe there is room for some improvement in how we convey our messages? In formal teaching of nurses it is worth getting together with the nurse tutors to discuss objectives. Too often a set programme of medical lectures has been maintained year after year and could do with updating. But this is better done in consultation with the nurses themselves, than by a medical imposition.

The interested teacher will find innumerable opportunities for extending the areas of teaching. Some ideas which might be discussed locally are as follows:

- a refresher course for medical assistants in the district;
- a study day for teachers;
- a local health newsletter;
- input to the local press or radio on health issues;
- a teaching/learning exchange with local traditional healers;

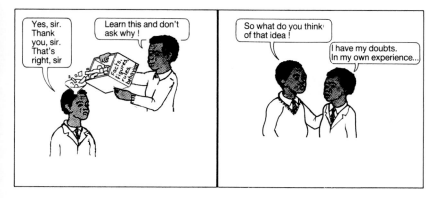

Fig. 1.6.3   A good teacher should encourage critical thinking.

- a child to child programme in local schools;
- an informal journal club or case presentation sessions, perhaps with multidisciplinary input.

There is an old Chinese saying which well expresses the good teacher's approach:

Go in search of your people: love them, learn from them, plan with them, serve them; begin with what they have, build on what they know. But of the best leaders when their task is accomplished, their work is done, the people all remark: 'We have done it ourselves'.

References

1. Werner D, Bower B. *Helping Health Workers Learn*. Palo Alto, Hesperian Foundation, 1982.
2. Spencer NJ. Parents' recognition of the ill child. In: Macfarlane A ed. *Progress in Child Health*, Vol. 1. Edinburgh, Churchill Livingstone, 1984. pp. 100–112.
3. Sainsbury CPQ, Gray OP, Cleary J. Care by parents of their children in hospital. *Archives of Disease in Childhood*. 1986; **61**: 612–15.
4. Nicoll A. Written material concerning health for parents and children. In: Macfarlane A ed. *Progress in Child Health*, Vol. 2. London, Churchill Livingstone, 1985. pp. 89–100.
5. Aaron A, Hawes H, Gayton J. *Child to Child*. Basingstoke, Macmillan, 1979.
6. Waterston T. Medical education in child health. In: Macfarlane A ed. *Progress in Child Health*, Vol. 3. London, Churchill Livingstone, 1987. pp. 199–216.
7. General Medical Council Education Committee. *Draft recommendations on the training of specialists*. London, General Medical Council, 1986.
8. Cox KR, Ewan CE. *The Medical Teacher*. London, Churchill Livingstone, 1982.

Further reading

Association for the Study of Medical Education, University of Dundee, Dundee, Scotland, publishes excellent Medical Educational Handbooks on teaching and assessment methods.

Guilbert JJ. *WHO Educational Handbook*. Geneva, WHO, 1977.

Medical Education – monthly journal published by Blackwells, UK.

Teaching Aids at Low Cost (TALC), PO Box 49, St Albans, Herts AL1 4AX, UK – excellent source of slide sets and many other teaching aids.

CHAPTER 7

Parents and children in hospital

Janet Goodall

Introduction

A five-year-old boy with scarlet fever was admitted to a British isolation hospital. Alone in a cubicle, he could see his parents call at the porters' lodge to enquire about him but there was no closer contact during his whole admission. This was in the 1940s. Forty years later, now a senior police officer, his eyes filled with tears again as he described how distressed he had been. At that age he could not understand that his parents were actually denied access. Instead, it seemed to him that they had chosen not to visit and he had felt completely rejected at a time when he needed them most.

Unhappily, this experience is not unique and neither is it now past history. There are still children all over the world whose time in hospital is one of lonely bewilderment. However excellent and caring the physical treatment of children may be, it is substandard if it overlooks their emotional well-being. Like anyone else, children not only have disorders to be corrected but feelings to be considered.

Reasons given for keeping parents out

A review of Western history may be helpful, so that those in other countries can avoid similar errors of judgment and so save their children unnecessary suffering.

Ignorance of children's needs

The first children's hospital in Britain was opened in Great Ormond Street, London, in 1852 but it was not until the early 1900s that children's wards were established in British general hospitals. Until then, children were cared for by nurses, physicians and surgeons whose major experience was with adults. Kind as most of them were, they had little insight into the personal needs of their patients. As late as 1952, only 25 per cent of British hospitals allowed daily visiting by parents and rooming-in was largely confined to normal neonatal care. Even today, ignorance remains the biggest universal problem to be overcome wherever children are cared for. Despite the increase in paediatric training and the complexities of modern paediatric care, there is still inadequate teaching on how children think and how they may see what is done for them as an abuse rather than a benefit (e.g. a child recognizes the pain but not the purpose of an injection). Physical care alone is not enough. Attention to a child's emotional well-being must include the maintenance of close family ties.

Cross-infection

In the pre-immunization and pre-antibiotic eras, there was a very real fear that illness would quickly travel round a family if one member had an infectious disease. Many old British gravestones tell us this, with their sad lists of names of young children and their parents who probably died during epidemics of measles, TB, pertussis or diphtheria – all now preventable diseases. Then, hospital care could be costly and many would die at home. As time went on access to hospital became easier. However, the fear of cross-infection meant that, however young they were, patients were admitted into solitary confinement and some would even die alone. So persistent was the fear of cross-infection that, even with the proven effectiveness of barrier nursing and despite the increasing availability of antibiotics from the 1940s onwards, the tradition of strict isolation held.

Misplaced protectiveness

In Britain, by the 1950s (thanks to pioneer work by sensitive paediatricians) children not only began to have their own wards but also free visiting or rooming-in by parents, although this was not so for those requiring more intensive care. As antibiotics multiplied, resuscitation techniques improved as well so that by the 1960s, nursing and medical care included attention to more complex life-saving machinery. It was falsely reasoned that because this could make the relatives anxious, they should be kept out as much as possible. The patient as well as the equipment became hospital property, so that visiting was strictly limited and notices were put up outside hospital wards denying access to all but two adult visitors. When special care baby units were first set up in the UK, parents were only allowed to look at their babies through a window in the unit wall. By the early 1970s, mothers (but not at first fathers!) were allowed into these units to handle and feed their babies. Only since the late 1970s have most units allowed free visiting by the whole family in turn. Even now, this is not universally true either in units for babies or on wards for older children.

Another misunderstanding often quoted was that young children were upset if visitors were allowed to come and go and were thought to settle down much better if nursed alone in hospital. It took the film *A two year-old goes to hospital*[1] and work by writers such as Bowlby[2] to understand that protest is a child's natural response to separation, to be followed by withdrawal, apathy and pining (the so-called 'settling down') if separation becomes protracted. Rejection of the returning parent or superficial sociability with hospital staff should not be treated as a joke, or an indication of staff popularity, but seen as a sign of seriously damaged emotions. This is now seen to be so important in Britain that, since 1964, the government's Department of Health and Social Security requires that any new children's wards must include accommodation for resident parents.

Overcrowding

In some parts of the world, where wards are badly overcrowded, it may be said that visitors get in the way of the ward's work and are to be discouraged. As such places often have a nursing shortage, it may be better to encourage attendants to come in to help with the child's nursing. There are already encouraging reports that this is happening and that wherever relatives help with the nursing the child is happier.[3,4]

Confidentiality

Senior doctors have been known to complain that they cannot speak privately to a child's parents if every other child has visitors who may overhear. Alternatively, the noise on a full ward may make concentration difficult, which could lead to errors of medical judgment. However, it is well documented that children are less likely to cry if their parents are there during waking hours and a private corner can usually be found for personal conversation.

Family problems

Parents sometimes find it hard to achieve either regular visiting or staying with a child in hospital because of distance, wage loss, the needs of other children, personal illness, or ignorance. Where there is an extended family, someone may well come to the rescue in a crisis if the child's needs are put first, but ignorance about such needs is the biggest reason for both professionals and parents to neglect them. Absence of visitors may be a marker of a child's social deprivation and special efforts should be made to help such a family.

Some of these arguments against parents rooming-in may sound all too familiar, as far too many of those caring for children still let them down badly by treating

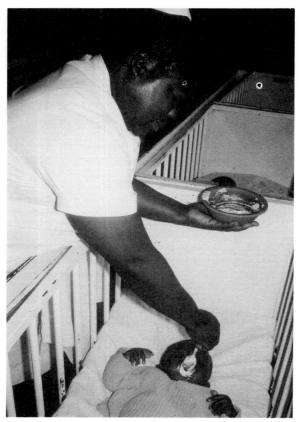

Fig. 1.7.1   Physical care alone is not enough.

their bodies well but ignoring their need for personal understanding (Fig. 1.7.1).

How children see our treatment of them

The art of all successful care-giving is to learn to see things from the patient's point of view. Perhaps the biggest single mistake we make in caring for children is to think that they see things as we do. In the great activity of our busy clinics and wards full of acutely ill or dying children, it is all too easy to overlook this aspect of care. In so doing we may save lives but leave emotional scars. Each age group is at risk.

Newborn babies

Many parents and professionals caring for babies see them almost like dolls – interesting and needing attention but mindless. Others may say, even of very young infants, that they are deliberately naughty or spiteful. Both these attitudes are wrong. Although babies are dependent on others for food and care, they also show a personal responsiveness which indicates a deep-seated interest in other people. It seems that, to them, personal relationships matter most. We now know that the sensory pathways of a newborn baby (touch, taste, smell, sound and vision) are all set at birth to respond best to human contact.[5] Breast-feeding babies can indicate at five days that they know their own mother by smell. On the first day of life, the most interesting pattern for a baby to look at is that of a face and the distance at which the child's eyes focus best is that between the parent's face and the holding arm (Fig. 1.7.2).

Because babies are born to relate, it may be very hurtful to remove them at birth to recover from the shock of being born, either alone or in a nursery with other babies in the same state. Should not each newcomer receive a loving welcome from their nearest and dearest? Instead, babies are subjected to being weighed, injected, bathed and swaddled – all extraordinary experiences after the confines of the womb and usually done by busy and sometimes impersonal hands. In many countries now, cultural traditions have been changed to allow the father into the delivery room and to allow both parents to have time with their baby right from the start, surely a fitting climax to all their expectations as well as being a comfort to the child.

Even if the baby is ill and needs special care, this early contact is to be encouraged. It has been shown that there is less cross-infection, not more, if parents are taught and allowed to handle their own children. The

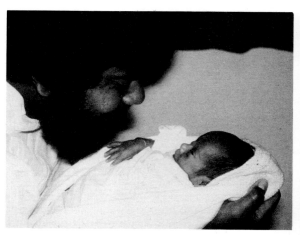

Fig. 1.7.2   The baby's focal distance.

By about ten months a child will start to search for a hidden object, so showing that what is not seen is still known to exist. This is known as the concept of permanence and until it is grasped, out of sight is out of existence. This is true of people as well as objects. If a child without this concept is admitted to hospital alone (or a mother admitted without her baby) there will be bewilderment and a sense of loss without any real knowledge of what has happened. Once the concept of permanence is achieved, however, the child will know that the parent is somewhere else and the sudden interruption of a previously close relationship (as when a child has been breast-fed but is separated from the mother) will cause acute misery and pining. In the child's eyes, this abandonment is impossible to understand (Fig. 1.7.4). In countries where the physical closeness has been the greatest, the sense of loss will be greater still, yet sadly it is in these very countries that weaning practices may include sending the child away. From riding on his mother's back, sharing her bed and having access to her breast, the child is suddenly out in the cold and has no idea that this was done with good intention. For some, the subsequent misery may be at least in part responsible for the advent of kwashiorkor (a syndrome associated with severe calorie and protein deficiency) and could be provoked by hospital admission if the mother did not come too (see pp. 335–57). We must therefore clarify the relationship of any attendant in hospital, neither assuming that she is the mother nor that she will be the permanent care-giver. Teaching about the child's needs must be given to the person who will give ongoing care and must include instruction on emotional as well as physical needs.

One to six-year-olds

As the years go by, a child's experiences will train intelligence and understanding but (although we were all children once) it surprises most adults to be shown how long it takes for a child to learn that things are not always what they seem. Imagine that you are already feeling quite ill, but are taken out of your own bed to see an alien person, three times your size and wearing strange clothes, who at once removes you from your family. You are taken into a big white room full of unfamiliar objects and the stranger holds you down on a table whilst someone else starts to torture you with sharp instruments pushed into your arm, head or back. How terrifying this would be and you might emerge scarred for life. Yet this happens all the time to small children when it is hospital practice to exclude parents whilst procedures are being performed. Everyone but the child knows that this is intended for their good and

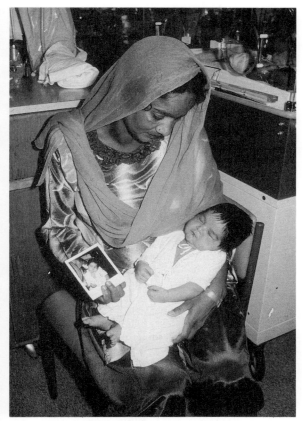

Fig. 1.7.3 A photograph for use between visits.

child becomes used to their organisms (to be met at home eventually anyway) and at the same time their relationships are all strengthened. Sadly, there are still centres where parents are kept out, even though at least one study has indicated that there is a risk of child abuse later if early attachment is interfered with in this way.[6] The roots of a relationship, present before birth, must be encouraged to grow stronger as soon as the child is born. Wealthier countries have the practice of giving a photograph of the baby to parents to keep the feelings warm (Fig. 1.7.3). Poorer countries could experiment with drawings, or giving a piece of the baby's hair as a momento.

The first year

A child in close contact with parents may indicate within weeks that their faces are familiar when seen in a group. By five months, a parent who has been away will be welcomed back with open arms and a broad smile.

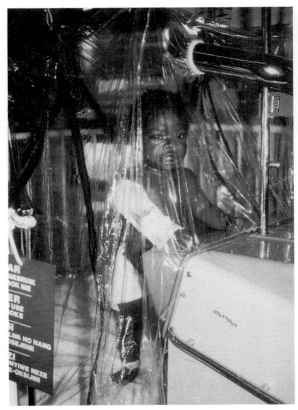

Fig. 1.7.4 Abandonment is impossible for a child to understand.

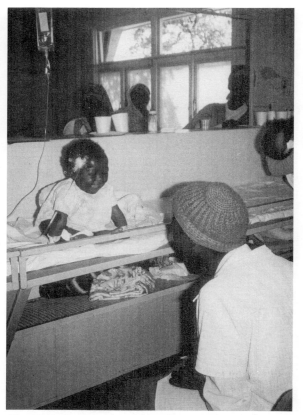

Fig. 1.7.5 Recovery is quicker with a parent present.

very few stop to think of the damage actually being done.

Children cannot be spared confusion and even distress, but to be lovingly supported through such experiences helps them to grow up instead of being permanently hurt. It is important both to offer comfort after inflicting a necessary pain and also to have on hand someone familiar and trusted to offer further reassurance. Hospitals with staff shortages may actually do their patients a good turn if they depend on parents for nursing care. Even uneducated village people can be taught simple nursing procedures (such as guarding a drip) which upset a child far less when done with care by relatives than they would if performed by a busy professional (Fig. 1.7.5).

Six to 12-year-olds

It is a sad fact that this age group may still be nursed on adult wards when paediatric beds are limited, or the special needs of children are unrecognized. Yet an adult way of thought does not emerge until adolescence and it is not in the child's best interests to be out of a paediatric environment. Even though younger children may copy adult phrases or behaviour, this is done entirely without insight. A child will still match experiences and ideas with those previously encountered and the ability to perceive differences and make correct deductions takes years to develop. It takes even longer to see things in depth and to understand double meanings.

If a family member stays with a child, or at least visits regularly, there is someone familiar to ask, but we must warn relatives (and staff) not to laugh at a child's misconceptions. To be humiliated means not to ask again and so to suffer unnecessary confusion and distress.

Over 12 years

Children now begin to understand adult behaviour and thought a little more, though inexperience and immaturity mean that such understanding is still incomplete. Also, we all become less confident in unfamiliar surroundings. Even an adult admitted to hospital can feel very overwhelmed, so that regular visiting by family and friends is important as reassurance, although a constant attendant is not as necessary at this age.

Play in hospital

Play material need not be expensive[7] but is much neglected. Play is not simply a way of keeping children occupied and out of the way, but an opportunity to offer experiences which can both educate the child and enlighten the observer. The child's understanding can grow if toys or games are available which teach about the body and about hospital procedures, making treatment less fearful for children of six years old or over. Younger children may be helped by acting out in play what they think has been happening: thus, a child seen to be violently beating a doll, or sticking sharp objects into it, may be showing how physiotherapy or an injection have been perceived as physical assault. Such insight gives an opportunity for parents or staff to demonstrate affectionate reassurance, even if the mind is too young to grasp the concept of treatment itself, so that bewilderment will then be less overwhelming. Even a very sick child can 'play with the eyes' by having interesting things to look at and will be comforted by being told a story or hearing a song. Many children have a precious object (Fig. 1.7.6) and if so this should go to hospital, too, as a comfort. Parents and others should be encouraged to meet these needs.

A visit to hospital is an opportunity for everyone to grow in understanding about the need for stimulation as an aid to development, but all too few hospitals take any trouble over this and children are still nursed in colourless and unstimulating wards with little to take their minds off their troubles.

The dying child

A child may be too ill to take much of an interest in activities but when dying, there is an even greater importance for loved members of the family to be close by. In neonatal care, after an accident, or with overwhelming infection, death may come suddenly. Parents need to be included, however intensive the care. Their voices probably reach even an unconscious child. Sudden bereavement is usually the hardest to cope with

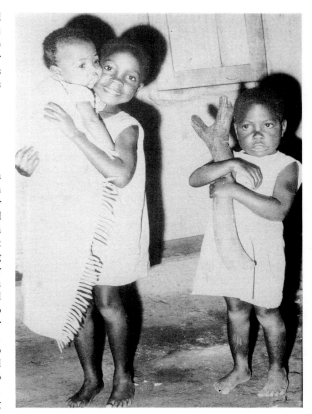

Fig. 1.7.6 Each with her 'baby'.

and parents themselves need to be prepared for what is happening.

When the process of dying is slower, the relationships established in life must be allowed to stand firm right up to the time of death. Physical comfort may be achieved by drugs and this will need to be explained to the parents who could otherwise worry about it.

Spiritual and emotional comfort cannot be prescribed but must be permitted by the hospital team, otherwise many parents will take their child away to seek this help elsewhere. Not all religions offer hope beyond death, but staff who have such hope themselves may find that parents want to hear this good news at a time when all other supports have failed. To give them quality time may be difficult in a busy schedule but is itself a recognition that child and family are more than mere physical presences. To offer personal, rather than merely professional care, may be to see life changed for the better, even at the end.

How can we change hospital attitudes?

At this stage, we may have a vision of what could be done to humanize the care of sick children and their families, but feel that we can never get policies changed in our own hospital. Space and money may be scarce, staff and government may be unsympathetic. It does take time to change attitudes but here are a few suggestions.

Teach by example Change will already have started if each of us becomes committed to seeing the emotional well-being of children as a high priority in care and by earnestly aiming to improve this in our own place of work rather than dismissing it as an optional extra.

Encourage the nurses Nurses are nurses because they have kind hearts. Many have children of their own. Tutorials on how children think are always welcomed by nursing staff. On an average ward, they may also see the benefits for themselves, as well as for the child, when a breast-feeding mother does much of the nursing herself (Fig. 1.7.7). It is only a step from this to see that older children would also be more contented and receive their treatment better when they are with someone known to them. Nurses can be relieved to know that parents may be taught basic skills (such as oral rehydration) and that to include teaching on basic hygiene may keep a child out of hospital next time. If parents are allowed to participate in care, nurses are liberated from doing everything for the children and will have more time to spend on such instruction.

Emphasis on health education Everyone working in hospital, at whatever level, should be a teacher and all should be encouraged to see this as part of their care in cooperation with the local child health demonstrators.[8]

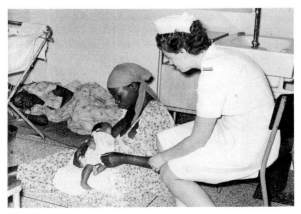

Fig. 1.7.7 Basic equipment but personal care.

Parents on the ward form a captive audience and teaching should include reference to the child's emotional needs and the use of play. Helpful guidance is available at low cost.[9]

Influence local hospital administrators This may be a harder task, as providing accommodation and possibly food for resident relatives is not immediately seen as cost-effective. The preventive aspects of such involvement could be emphasized (50 per cent of paediatric admissions are likely to be due to preventable disease) so to seize the opportunity for health education is a serious responsibility. Evidence from research indicates that the children recover more quickly (and so cost less!) if they are treated more personally.[10] Such research may be more impressive if conducted locally. It should also be emphasized that it is up-to-date to conduct paediatric care in this way so that the hospital's reputation is at stake. Support from parents, including those who may represent authority such as ministers or their wives, can be invaluable in encouraging a change of attitude both locally and in government circles. In our own hospital in the UK this has resulted in fund-raising in the local community, producing enough money to build a parents' rest-room off the ward, folding beds for parents to use on the ward at night and a play room with ample play materials for the children – all given voluntarily by concerned friends of the hospital who were made aware of our needs.

The practicalities of involving parents in the hospital care of children

Nursing and medical minds must put aside time to discuss what is needed locally and how to produce it. The experience of others will be helpful here.[11,12] For some, this will involve reorganization rather than expense. Others will have to think how to provide accommodation for resident parents, the best option from the child's viewpoint being a foldaway bed or mat close by the cot. (At home, they may share a bed, but hospitals have concrete floors as well as drips and other equipment to consider.) Toilet, laundry and eating facilities, however basic, need to be provided. Personnel trained in health education may also be nurses or even sweepers. There must be someone to act as social worker to help families work out their priorities in financial and supportive terms for the child in hospital. Depending on the size of the hospital, one person may have to supervise others or fulfil all these roles. This person must be identified as having this responsibility if plans are to develop into more than dreams and if parents are to be better informed as a result of the hospital experience.

The word 'parents' rather than 'mothers' is used deliberately here. For years we have spoken of maternal and child health as though one-parent families were the norm! Fathers have become a neglected species, yet unless the father is committed to the child's health, he will not ensure that the family income is fairly divided. Involving him in the child's care may to him be a compliment to his importance and to the mother a relief that her burden is shared (Fig. 1.7.8). In some cultures this may be hard to get across, but to encourage awareness of how the child thinks and develops provides an intellectual interest for the father which complements the mother's tender, loving care. In an extended family, other relatives may take a share in the child's care, but parents and grandmothers remain the prime targets for health education.

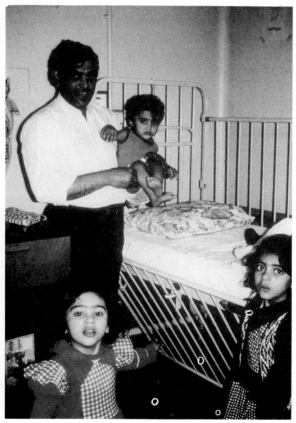

Fig. 1.7.8 Father is important too.

Including parents will save lives

One of the first things to strike me on arrival in East Africa was the sad, withdrawn expression in the eyes of many children with kwashiorkor. It became clear that many of these children had suffered a sudden, and to them inexplicable, interruption in a very close relationship, usually with the mother[13]. Some of these children died.

In contrast to these sad expressions, the radiant faces of two mothers will always stay in my memory. The first mother addressed a packed lecture theatre in her own language. It needed no interpreter to tell us of her joy in the transformation of her malnourished child to the happy little person sitting on her back and peeping over her shoulder as she spoke to us. Her message was very simple. Someone had taught her about the correct food for the child and she herself had given it. Physical nutrition and emotional nurture had gone on together, the child's life had been saved and she was taking back to the village not only the 'before and after' photographs but missionary zeal to teach others also.

The second woman was equally radiant. Her toddler had come in with diphtheria and required a tracheostomy. During this serious illness he contracted measles with pneumonia. His mother stayed at his side throughout the weeks of his illness, watching his drip, coping with nasogastric feeding, collecting his medication and guarding his tracheostomy. What sleep she had was on a small bench at his cotside and her only food was the ward's very simple diet. The combination of overcrowding with shortage of nurses almost certainly meant that he would have died without her devotion. Any other children she had could be spared this experience as she was taught about immunization during her stay, so perhaps other lives would be saved. The pride and pleasure on her face as she hitched him on to her back to take him home, was to us the most vivid testimonial that children in hospital do need to be accompanied by someone who loves them and that this can be life-saving.

References

1. Robertson J. *A Two Year-Old Goes to Hospital.* Tavistock Child Development Research Unit, London, 1953 (film).
2. Bowlby J. *Child Care and the Growth of Love.* Harmondsworth, Pelican Books, 1953 (reprinted 1980).
3. Sebikari SRK. The role of mothers in hospital. *Journal of Tropical Pediatrics and Environmental Child Health.* 1972; **18**: 96–8.
4. Sainsbury CPQ, Gray OP, Cleary J *et al.* Care by parents

of their children in hospital. *Archives of Disease in Childhood.* 1986; **61**: 612–5.

5. Klaus MH, Kennell JH. *Maternal Infant Bonding*, 2nd edn. St Louis, CV Mosby Company, 1982.

6. Lynch M. Ill-health and child abuse. *Lancet.* 1975; **2**: 317–9.

7. Aarons A, Hawes H, Gayton J. *Child to Child*, Macmillan London, 1979.

8. Mateega PH. The work of the maternal and child health demonstrators. *Journal of Tropical Pediatrics and Environmental Child Health.* 1972; **18**: 99–103.

9. Teaching Aids at Low Cost (TALC), PO Box 49, St. Albans, Herts AL1 4AX, UK.

10. Stenbak E. *Care of Children in Hospital*. Copenhagen, WHO, 1986.

11. Waterston AJR. Child health in district and rural hospitals. *Central African Journal of Medicine.* 1982; **28**: 298–303.

12. Goodall J (ed.). The hospital care of East African children (Report of a UNICEF assisted seminar). *Journal of Tropical Pediatrics and Environmental Child Health.* 1972; **18**: 46–125.

13. Goodall J. A social score for kwashiorkor: explaining the look in the child's eyes. *Developmental Medicine and Child Neurology.* 1979; **21**: 374–84.

Further reading

Beadle M. *A Child's Mind*. London, Methuen, 1972 and 1977.

Bowlby J. *Loss, Sadness and Depression*. London, Hogarth Press, 1980.

Lewis C. *Becoming a Father*. Milton Keynes, Open University Press, 1986.

Rutter M. *Maternal Deprivation Re-assessed*. Harmondsworth, Penguin, 1972.

Topics dealt with in this chapter are also illustrated by the author in tape/slide sets available from Graves Medical A–V Library, 220 New London Road, Chelmsford, Essex CM2 9BT, England.

SECTION 2

Maternal, Prenatal, Perinatal and Neonatal Care

Michael Chan

CHAPTER 1

Introduction

Michael Chan

In the past decade efforts have been made to reduce infant mortality in developing countries by primary health care interventions such as immunization programmes, the use of oral rehydration fluids for acute diarrhoea, breast-feeding, and growth monitoring. Success has been recorded in many regions including some of the poorest countries with high infant mortality rates. However, these interventions do not attack the fundamental causes of malnutrition and infection early enough to produce the needed long-term impact on health which is determined in the fetus and newborn.

It is generally accepted in most developing countries that about half the infant mortality occurs in the first four weeks of life (neonatal period) and half the neonatal deaths occur in the first week. Therefore, attention should be focussed on mothers and their newborn babies to improve survival. But in developing countries today most pregnant women do not receive health care, many births are not attended by trained people, and very little, if any, medical care is provided for newborn babies. Maternal and child health (MCH) services have been introduced as primary health care in most developing countries. Perinatal health care for the pregnant mother and her newborn baby are integral aspects of MCH and primary health care, and should be given high priority, particularly in developing countries where the majority of births in the world (estimated at 130 millions annually) take place. The perinatal period occupies less than 0.5 per cent of the average life span, yet in a number of developing countries there are more deaths within this period than during the next 30 years of life.

A healthy mother is necessary to ensure the survival and health of her children. If a mother dies, her infants and children are at great risk. Maternal health during pregnancy and safe delivery will therefore be considered in this book. Basic maternity services at primary health centres will need to be supported by good secondary and tertiary levels of care that are within the reach of women in the community, so that appropriate referrals may be made without undue delay. Facilities such as maternity villages or a mobile emergency service have been introduced in some countries with significant influence on improving maternal survival during obstetric emergencies.

Survival of the newborn baby in the first days and weeks after birth has always been hazardous, until the introduction of maternity services into industrialized countries during the twentieth century. Traditional African and Asian communities continue to delay giving the newborn baby a name until the end of the first month. This practice is a reflection of the precarious existence of the neonate because of poor care provided for pregnant women and their babies. Basic interventions during pregnancy, labour, delivery and the postnatal period could greatly improve the survival of mothers and newborn babies. Some of these measures include protection against malaria, and the administration of tetanus toxoid to pregnant mothers; the identification of high-risk pregnancies for transfer to hospital; birth to be attended by trained health workers with sterile equipment who are able to resuscitate the neonate if necessary; and supervision of breast-feeding soon after delivery, prevention of infection, and management of neonatal jaundice. Low-birth-weight infants (weighing less than 2500 g) have a higher death rate than heavier babies. More than 90 per cent of the world's 21 million low-birth-weight infants are born in developing countries. Factors contributing to this condition range from poor maternal nutrition and ill-health to premature delivery associated with short interval (less than two years) between pregnancies. Prolonging the birth interval beyond two years would reduce the infant mortality by 10 per cent and the mortality from one to four years by 16 per cent. The health of mother and infant improves if there are longer intervals between births. The survival of newborn babies has a positive effect on the acceptance of family planning by parents (Fig. 2.1.1); 60–70 per cent of women in Costa Rica, Peru, Bangladesh, Sri Lanka and Thailand with three living children wanted no further pregnancies. This influence on contraception is a strong argument in favour of maternal, prenatal, perinatal and neonatal care, and for introducing a new section to the fourth edition of this well-known book.

Perinatal mortality in developing countries

Definition

Perinatal mortality defined by the Ninth Revision of the International Classification of Diseases (ICD) comprises late fetal deaths or stillbirths and deaths in the first week of life (early neonatal deaths). The Ninth Revision recommends that babies chosen for inclusion in perinatal mortality statistics should be those above a

minimum birth weight, and if this is not available, gestation or body length should be used. The minimum values for inclusion in national and international perinatal statistics are shown in Table 2.1.1.

The duration of gestation is measured from the first day of the last normal menstrual period. Gestational age is expressed in completed days or completed weeks – events occurring from 280 to 293 days after the onset of the last normal menstrual period are considered to have occurred at 40 weeks of gestation. (See Fig. 2.1.2).

The International Classification of Diseases is revised every 10 years and the Tenth Revision is due soon. Whatever new recommendations are made for perinatal statistics, it would be difficult to improve on the proposals for international perinatal statistics in the Ninth Revision, particularly in developing countries where perinatal mortality statistics are difficult to obtain, and, those that are available are collected in hospitals. Data on perinatal deaths in the community where most babies are born, are generally not available in developing countries.

Why consider perinatal mortality?

While infant mortality rate (IMR) is a measure of socio-economic development of a country, indicators such as maternal deaths and perinatal mortality reflect the health status of women and the quality of health care received during pregnancy, labour, delivery and in the early days of life. This has been seen in the development of health care for mothers and newborn infants in the United Kingdom from the second decade of the twentieth century until now. Four phases of development have been identified:

1. 1910–30 both maternal mortality and perinatal mortality rates were high, and this led to the licensing of midwives.
2. 1931–40, maternal mortality gradually decreased but perinatal mortality remained high – sulphon-

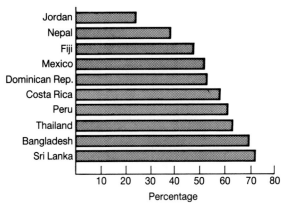

Fig. 2.1.1   Percentages of women with three living children who want no further pregnancies. (Adapted from Maine D. *Family Planning: Its Impact on the Health of Women and Children*. New York, The Centre for Population and Family Health, Columbia University, 1981.)

Table 2.1.1   Definition of babies for inclusion in national and international perinatal statistics

Minimum value	National perinatal statistics	International perinatal statistics
Birth weight	500 g	1000 g
Gestational age	22 weeks	28 weeks
Body length (crown–heel)	25 cm	35 cm

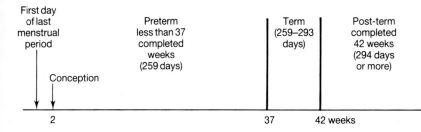

Fig. 2.1.2 Gestational age.

amides were used to treat infections during this decade.

3. 1941–70 saw a rapid decline in maternal mortality to its present low level associated with the liberal use of Caesarean section, blood transfusion and antibiotics, but the perinatal mortality rate paradoxically increased.

4. 1970–89, maternal mortality remained low and perinatal mortality declined substantially to its present low level in association with introduction of neonatal care units and technological improvements.

Experience in developed countries including the United Kingdom has confirmed the value of birth weight specific mortality, after excluding lethal malformations, as a sensitive indicator of health care quality.[1] Where health care is rudimentary, the death rate among infants weighing more than 2500 g at birth is high; this perinatal mortality rate improves when an effective system of health care for mothers and babies is provided in the community. Perinatal deaths and prevalence of low birth weight are two simple measures to monitor health care provided for women and their offspring. As the health status of a community improves, the perinatal mortality rate decreases.

A population with a higher than average proportion of low-birth-weight infants will have a higher crude perinatal mortality rate. Fifty-seven per cent of perinatal deaths occurred among babies with a birth weight of less than 2500 g although they constituted only 10.8 per cent of births in Cuba in 1973.[2] To determine how well newborn infants are being cared for, it is necessary to calculate the risks of death within different birth weight bands. Comparison of birth weight specific mortality rates indicate trends in mortality within the same population or in different populations with similar mean birth weights and birth weight distributions.

Other factors influencing perinatal mortality in developing countries are maternal age and parity. A population-based study in rural Kenya[3] showed that maternal age of 35 years or more and parity of seven or more were associated with increased perinatal mortality. A history of previous perinatal death and breech delivery were also associated with higher perinatal mortality. Studies have shown that for a given maternal weight, mothers who are taller give birth to heavier babies, whereas mothers who are fatter give birth to lighter babies. However, a study in an urban hospital in Uganda indicated that maternal weight of less than 55 kg was associated with increased perinatal deaths and low-birth-weight babies.[4] It is clear that more community-based controlled studies are needed in developing countries to identify risk factors associated with perinatal deaths, in order that interventions may be introduced for better survival.

Causes of perinatal deaths

Ideally, causes of perinatal deaths should be based on data collected in the community. But most studies on perinatal mortality have been done on deliveries in hospitals. Classification of perinatal deaths into antepartum, intrapartum, and early neonatal deaths provides a helpful framework for analysis. Intrapartum deaths occur more often among normal babies than low-birth-weight babies and are associated with inadequate supervision of labour. A survey carried out in Indian hospitals in 1977–9[5] reported a perinatal mortality rate of 66.3 per 1000 total births, an incidence of fresh stillbirths of 26.2 per 1000 total births and a ratio of fresh stillbirths to macerated stillbirths of 1.5. In a Nairobi birth survey the stillbirth rate was 23 per 1000 total births, the incidence of fresh stillbirth was 14.4 per 1000 total births and the ratio of fresh stillbirths to macerated stillbirths was 1.7.[6] In European countries where the perinatal mortality rate is around 10 per 1000, the incidence of fresh stillbirth is about 1 per 1000, and the ratio of fresh stillbirths to macerated stillbirths is around 0.2. The above figures show that improvement in care of women in pregnancy, labour and delivery produces a sharp decrease in the incidence of fresh compared to macerated stillbirth.

Clinical classification of causes of perinatal deaths

This classification assists the identification of preventable deaths where intervention is required. The Aberdeen classification[7] proposed in 1954 promoted the use of eight categories: cause unknown (premature), cause unknown (mature), trauma, pre-eclampsia, antepartum haemorrhage, congenital malformations, maternal disease, and miscellaneous. Wigglesworth, in 1980, suggested a classification based on five pathological groups analysed by birth weight.[8] This classification is simple and can be used where perinatal pathology facilities are not available (Table 2.1.2).

If deaths due to asphyxia occurring in mature infants (over 2500 g) were high, this indicates a need to improve care during labour and delivery by proper management of obstructed labour and hypertensive disorders, and preventing birth injury. In the rural Kenya study, half of all perinatal deaths were caused by either preterm delivery or birth trauma[3].

Perinatal audit

Perinatal audit should arise from the clinical classification of perinatal deaths, when health workers learn from discussion of the circumstances leading to deaths, so that future clinical management may be improved. Perinatal audit, initiated by hospital departments of obstetrics and paediatrics would involve the active participation of community-based personnel in maternal and child health services who can identify and refer high-risk mothers to appropriate levels of care.

Morbidity

In the perinatal period, morbidity may have long-term effects of mental and physical handicap. Morbidity affecting the fetus or neonate can originate at five periods of development: preconception (genetically-determined diseases), embryonic period (neural tube defects), prenatal period (intrauterine growth retardation), intrapartum period (trauma), and neonatal period (ineffective resuscitation at birth). Data collected during the perinatal period would also identify causes of morbidity.

Perinatal data collection

Perinatal mortality is the most reliable index of the quality of antenatal and obstetric care. Most deaths in the perinatal period (excluding congenital defects) are the result of complications in pregnancy and childbirth. Therefore, the following recommendations have been made on perinatal data collection in developing countries by the World Health Organization[2]:

- Maximal use should be made of available data while taking into consideration their quality.
- Linkage of data held in different locations such as hospitals, community health services and civil registers should be explored to provide a more reliable information system for routine surveillance.
- The epidemiology of perinatal mortality is required if effective policies and interventions are to be formulated and put into practice, especially outside the hospital where the majority of births take place.
- Methodologies should be developed that are simple and scientifically sound and which can be used at community level in developing countries.

Table 2.1.2 Model form for classification of perinatal deaths (after Wigglesworth, 1980)

Birth weight (g)	Normally formed macerated SB	Congenital malformation (SB/NND)	Conditions associated with immaturity (NND)	Asphyxia in labour (fresh SB/NND)	Other specific conditions	Total births	PNMR
<1000							
1001–1500							
1501–2000							
2001–2500							
over 2500							
unknown							
Total							

(SB = Stillbirth; NND = Neonatal death; PNMR = Perinatal mortality rate)

- Improved understanding of risk factors related to perinatal mortality makes possible timely antenatal interventions and referral of high-risk mothers to appropriate levels of care.

The collection of data on perinatal mortality and morbidity requires registration of births and deaths, and a system of records for pregnant women and the outcome of their pregnancies, including birth weights. Few developing countries have national statistics on perinatal and maternal deaths today. However, relevant data may be gathered from some hospitals but this will not be an accurate reflection of the situation in the community. If hospital and teaching institution staff were to extend their interest to the community, cooperation with primary health centres and village leaders would make it possible to collect meaningful information. Interest in the community must be stimulated and harnessed to ensure collection of statistics, their analysis and interpretation.

A good example of data collection of deaths in the perinatal period has come from Curacao, the largest island in the Netherland Antilles in the Caribbean.[9] This survey analysed the 223 consecutive fetal and neonatal deaths occuring in 6514 births over two years, 1984 and 1985. About 98 per cent of the deliveries took place in hospital. Full autopsies were performed on 210 deaths (94 per cent). Perinatal deaths comprised both fetal and neonatal deaths with a minimum birth weight of 500 g. Infants who died within 28 days of life were included. The crude death rate was 34.2 per 1000 total births. Death was caused by problems of preterm birth in 68 cases, 53 of whom were born before 28 weeks of gestation. Other causes of death were associated with asphyxia in 35, malformation in 28, maternal hypertension in 25, antepartum haemorrhage in 19 and miscellaneous (generalized infection, hydrops fetalis, kernicterus) in 14. No specific cause could be found in 34 deaths of whom 32 were macerated stillbirths. The authors of this study concluded that a substantial reduction of perinatal mortality could be achieved by better fetal surveillance for fetal growth retardation, improved clinical judgement and better management of fetal distress, particularly in the 58 deaths (27 per cent) at or after 28 weeks of gestation due to hypertension and asphyxia, as well as many of the macerated stillbirths. This study shows that it is possible to carry out a population-based inquiry into fetal and neonatal mortality in a region that is socially and economically disadvantaged.

References

1. Chalmers I. The search for indices. *Lancet*. 1979; **ii**: 1063–5.
2. Edouard L. The epidemiology of perinatal mortality. *World Health Statistics Quarterly*. 1985; **38**: 289–301.
3. Voorhoeve AM, Muller AS, W'oigo H. Agents affecting health of mother and child in a rural area of Kenya. XVI. The outcome of pregnancy. *Tropical and Geographical Medicine*. 1979; **31**: 607–7.
4. Holden J. *Mengo hospital maternity survey 1980*. Personal communication.
5. Mehta AC. Perinatal mortality. In: Menon MKK, Devi PK, Rao KB eds. *Postgraduate Obstetrics and Gynaecology*, 2nd Edn. Bombay, Orient Longman, 1982. pp. 195–200.
6. Mati JKG. The Nairobi birth survey – 1. The study design, the population and outline results. *Journal of Obstetrics and Gynaecology of Eastern and Central Africa*. 1982; **1**: 132–9.
7. Baird D, Walker J, Thomson AM. The causes and prevention of stillbirths and first week deaths. III. A classification of deaths by clinical cause: the effect of age, parity and length of gestation on death rates by cause. *Journal of Obstetrics and Gynaecology of the British Empire*. 1954; **61**: 433–48.
8. Wigglesworth J. Monitoring perinatal mortality: a pathophysiological approach. *Lancet* 1980; **i**: 684–6.
9. Wildschut JIJ, Nolthenius-Puylaert MCBJET, Wiedjik Y *et al*. Fetal and neonatal mortality: a matter of care? Report of a survey in Curaçao, Netherlands Antilles. *British Medical Journal*. 1987; **295**: 894–8.

CHAPTER 2

Maternal health

MATERNAL CARE
Olive Frost

Introduction

While maternal and child mortality and morbidity in some parts of the world has improved consistently over the last decades, in other areas pregnancy and child bearing continue to take their unacceptable toll. In 1984, maternal deaths per 1000 births were 6.4 in Africa, 4.2 in Asia and 2.7 in Latin America compared with 0.3 in all developed countries and less than 0.1 in northern Europe. An estimated 500,000 women, 99 per cent of whom are in developing countries, die every year from pregnancy-related causes. The 'Safe Motherhood Initiative' was launched by the WHO in 1988 to fund schemes to reduce maternal mortality in developing countries. Perinatal mortalities of more than 240 have been reported in unbooked emergency deliveries in northern Nigeria compared with 15 per 1000 births in Britain in the late 1970s. In these developing countries women very often have limited status apart from labouring in the fields and childbearing, which commences too early in life and occurs far too often. Although motherhood is so important, the mother is often ill prepared and has few resources to fulfil this role. As a result children are deprived. The health of the woman from conception to middle age is very relevant to the life of the offspring and can be represented as a cycle:

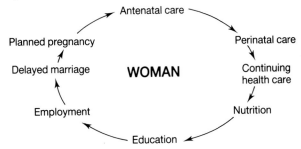

All parts of the cycle should be of interest to doctors who have contact with the child.

The choice of a mother

If the neonate could choose its mother, it should choose a woman between 20 and 35 years old with no more than three existing children, the youngest of whom should be at least two years old. When the mother was a neonate, she should have been as welcome as her brother and been given the same quality of care to ensure good nutrition and prevention of disease in childhood. When necessary, good medical and other services should have been available to her; this would usually mean a satisfactory income level in the family. She should have been educated to secondary level, and have a good basic knowledge of health. Ideally she should have had a choice as to when she married, and a choice as to when she became pregnant; acceptable contraception should have been available to her whenever she needed it. Hopefully, she would have been spared infections like rheumatic heart disease and tuberculosis which may mar future health. She should be of such a build as to make cephalo-pelvic disproportion unlikely.

Once she enters pregnancy in a stable marriage situation, a mother should receive regular antenatal care from early pregnancy, with adequate surveillance to detect abnormality and suitable medical care and treatment when necessary. The pregnancy should be free of conditions which endanger the health and life of the mother, and which prejudice the well-being of the fetus, especially those which may result in pre-term delivery, a light-for-dates infant or infection in the fetus. This would include a healthy life-style with freedom from hard physical work and from dangerous social habits such as smoking, drinking alcohol and partaking of other harmful drugs such as heroin.

Appropriate delivery should be planned with provision for dealing with any high-risk situation which may have arisen. Wherever the delivery takes place, there should be meticulous attention to cleanliness and prevention of infection. There should be clear guidelines for selection and management of high-risk labours.

Once the child is born the mother should have the time, knowledge and advice to care for him/her in sickness and in health.

For millions of neonates the choice of such a mother is impossible and it is necessary for all doctors, especially those who care for children, to do all they can to improve the quality of life of women and the care available to them wherever they are. The aim must be to plan the best use of available resources, to monitor the operation of this plan and to seek more equity in the care of different groups such as rich and poor, urban and rural.

Antenatal care

The value of antenatal care has been put beyond doubt by a detailed survey in northern Nigeria[1] Three groups of women were identified and their pregnancy outcomes compared. One group received antenatal care and remained free of complications throughout pregnancy (booked–healthy group). The next group received antenatal care but each woman had had at least one major complication during pregnancy (booked–complication group). The third group was classified as unbooked–emergencies. Maternal mortality rate per 1000 deliveries was 0.4 in the booked – healthy group, 3.7 in the booked–complication group and 29 in the unbooked–emergencies. Perinatal mortality rate per 1000 singleton births was 22 in the booked–healthy group, 74 in the booked–complication group and 243 in the unbooked–emergencies.

The principles of antenatal care are the same whether the mother is a poor, illiterate person living in a city slum or rural village, or rich and educated and living within easy reach of modern medical care.

The aim should always be that the mother is seen as early as possible in pregnancy, so that pre-existing maternal disease can be diagnosed, monitored and treated, and that pregnancy complications can be anticipated, prevented, diagnosed early and managed in the best possible way. Ideally mothers should be as healthy, if not healthier, after delivery as they were at the time of conception.

However, it is evident that though the principles of care are the same in all women, the method of delivery of care can initially be varied according to the presence of risk factors, and later according to the presence of complications (see Table 2.2.1).

The actual criteria for transfer will vary from place to place, depending on the quality and training both of primary care workers and doctors, on the equipment and facilities available and on the terrain and distances over which patients will need to be taken. An upgraded primary health centre in India could well be a suitable venue for a Caesarean section, whereas in another situation any patient in whom operative delivery may be necessary should be transferred to a maternity village a few weeks before delivery.

However, it is important that an obstetric service in a given situation should be a managed one and that all levels of workers should know when to refer or transfer a mother during the antenatal period.

Table 2.2.1 Examples of risk factors and complications where hospital booking should be considered or arranged

Maternal disease
    Malnutrition
    Anaemia
    Hepatitis
    Respiratory conditions
    Heart disease
    Diabetes
    Hypertension
    Renal disease
Past obstetric performance
    Elderly primigravida/prolonged infertility
    Multiparity (5 +)
    Bad obstetric history (e.g. stillbirth, neonatal death)
    Past Caesarean section/symphysiotomy/instrumental
        delivery/VVF repair
    Past third stage abnormality (PPH retained placenta)
Present pregnancy
    Pre-eclampsia/eclampsia
    Antepartum haemorrhage
    Malpresentation and unstable lie
    Hydramnios
    Multiple pregnancy
    Intrauterine growth retardation

PPH = post partum haemorrhage; VVF = vesico-vaginal fistula.

Risk factors

It is important that the pregnant woman is seen as early as possible in pregnancy, so that the antenatal attendant can document risk factors in the pregnancy, and classify the mother as low, middle or high risk. To do this, all mothers should have a careful history taken, and this should include details of personal and family health, a detailed history of past pregnancies and deliveries, and a history of the present pregnancy. This should be followed by a clinical examination, and whatever investigations are available and appropriate. The attendant who performs this examination should have clear guidelines about the management of each risk group, and a provisional plan for antenatal care and delivery should be made. Risk factors should be sought at each subsequent antenatal visit, and the same principles of management applied.

Maternal disease

Many mothers will enter a pregnancy without ever having had a medical examination, and the first antenatal visit is an excellent opportunity to review their state of health. This is important in order to improve the health of the mother and because many conditions deteriorate during pregnancy or contribute to pregnancy complications, which in turn adversely affect fetal outcome.

Maternal nutritional status

Ideally a woman should be well nourished at the beginning of pregnancy. In normal pregnancy there is considerable variation in weight gain with an average of 12.5 kg. This weight gain can be achieved by eating an additional 75 000 calories or 280 cal/day over the 40-week pregnancy period. Given this ideal situation, and assuming there are no other constraints on growth, the mother can support normal fetal growth while either maintaining or improving her own nutritional status.

Malnutrition, however, prevents the mother from supporting normal fetal growth and the fetus is proportionately more affected than the mother. The mechanism for this seems to be placental insufficiency. During pregnancy the placenta is the main organ for fetal nutrition, and in malnutrition placental growth is reduced and the placenta has a decreased number of villi with a reduced surface area. These changes in placental structure lead to reduced placental blood flow, which in turn leads to limitation of nutrients required for normal fetal growth. As a result, poorly nourished mothers deliver an infant of reduced mean birth weight.

It is probable that maternal malnutrition only causes growth retardation in the last trimester of pregnancy, the time when the normal growing fetus triples its weight, and rapidly accumulates body fat. If there is insufficient nutrient transfer at this stage, the fetus becomes light-for-dates or small-for-gestational dates (SFD) with a reduced weight for length and reduced skin fold thickness. In cases of more severe malnutrition, fetal skeletal growth may also be retarded and head circumference reduced. Both the duration and severity of the malnutrition affects skeletal and head growth. Severely malnourished women have at least a threefold risk of producing growth retarded babies, as compared with the general population.

As SFD infants have a significantly higher mortality and morbidity rate, it is important that the 'at risk' mother should be identified, and preventive measures applied where possible. The most specific indicator of nutritional risk is a low pre-pregnancy weight for height. A second best but more practical indicator suggested by workers in Central America, is a mid-upper arm circumference (MUAC) of less than 22.5 cm at the first antenatal visit. The ideal management for this group would be to increase their calorie–protein intake, so that they can recover their desired preweight for height, and in addition put on the 12 kg which is desirable for pregnancy. The tragedy is, that mothers in this group often do not have antenatal care, and even if they did would not have the means to change their diet in the recommended way.

Dietary supplementation of pregnant women can be an efficient and cost-effective nutritional intervention for improving fetal growth and survival in chronically undernourished populations. Studies in the Gambia, where women show marked seasonal fluctuations in energy balance, have reported encouraging results. All pregnant women were offered a dietary supplement of groundnut-based biscuits and a vitamin-fortified tea drink on six days each week and consumption was carefully supervised and measured. This resulted in a net energy increment of 431 kcal/day. In the wet season, when the women were normally in marked negative energy balance due to food shortages and a high agricultural work-load, the supplementation improved birth weight by a mean of 224 g and reduced the incidence of low-birth-weight babies (less than 2.5 kg) from 28.2 to 4.7 per cent. In the dry season, when the women were previously in positive energy balance despite an energy intake of only 60 per cent of the recommended dietary allowance, the supplement had no beneficial effect on birth outcome.[2]

In addition to protein–calorie malnutrition, mothers may have other specific deficiencies in their diet. The most common of these is iron deficiency, and this makes anaemia very common in pregnancy in many parts of the developing world. Its incidence is increased by other causes of anaemia common in the tropics.

Unless the diet of a non-pregnant healthy woman provides 40 mg of absorbed iron daily, she is likely to start pregnancy with anaemia. Even if she does absorb this amount of iron, menorrhagia e.g. due to an intrauterine device, could easily disturb the precarious iron balance. During pregnancy there is an iron gain from physiological amenorrhoea, but this is more than offset by iron loss to the fetus and placenta, and especially in the latter half of pregnancy, by blood loss at delivery and by lactation. As a result, even a healthy well-nourished woman may reach the end of pregnancy with an iron store deficit, unless she receives iron supplementation. Many tropical diets are deficient in meat and vegetables and the foods eaten may reduce the amount of iron absorbed. The likelihood that a mother in the developing world is anaemic is high. Therefore, it is important that a haemoglobin estimation is done in early pregnancy and at regular intervals. Although methods which can be used in peripheral clinics are not accurate, they do help in the selection of the mothers who need further investigation, should that be

available. If possible iron supplementation should be given to all anaemic women with appropriate dietary advice.

During pregnancy, because there is an increase in the number of rapidly dividing cells, requirement for folic acid is increased, and if this is not met folate deficiency develops. A good prophylactic measure is to prescribe 5 mg of folic acid per day.

Zinc is a current focus of interest and zinc deficiency, measured in maternal leucocytes, has been shown to be related to small-for-gestational dates (SFD) fetuses.[3] (See pp. 379–86.) Supplementation appears to be beneficial in correcting the deficiency. Pregnancy is also a time when a mother may become deficient in various minerals and vitamins. The antenatal attendant, who knows the quality of the local diet and methods used for cooking, is the best person to advise on diet and the preparation of food. Supplementation will depend on local needs and the availability of treatment.

Common medical diseases

Anaemia

Anaemia is very common in the tropics, not only because of dietary inadequacies, but because of the multiplicity of other causes contributing to it. These include conditions like chronic liver and renal disease which may cause metabolic disturbance, acute or chronic infections which may impair erythropoiesis and chronic diarrhoeal disease which impairs absorption. The investigation and treatment of these conditions should be part of the management of anaemia. Anaemia in the tropics is often severe, and a significant cause of maternal and fetal mortality and morbidity (see pp. 822–34).

Hookworm is an important cause of anaemia in many parts of the world. Each worm can extract up to 0.05 ml of blood per day. The effect of hookworm infestation will vary depending on how precarious the existing iron balance is in a particular patient. In some areas where most women are anaemic and hookworm is endemic, the best policy might be to treat all women for hookworm in early pregnancy (or when first seen); in others, a hookworm count may give the best indication as to who needs anthelmintics. Bephenium hydroxynaphthoate (Alcopar) is the treatment of choice and does not appear to have teratogenic effects. The usual dose is 2.5 g. It can be repeated in three days in heavy infestations (see pp. 633–48).

In some ethnic groups in the tropics and subtropics sickle cell disease and other haemoglobinopathies exist and appropriate investigations should be done. If homozygous sickle cell (HbSS) disease is present, the patient should be referred to hospital for all her pregnancy care, and folic acid (5 mg) prescribed throughout pregnancy. The fact that the mother has been relatively well before pregnancy does not guarantee a smooth course in pregnancy, and the complications for mother (urinary tract and chest infections, sickling crises, severe pre-eclampsia) and fetus (premature delivery, low birth weight and fetal distress) are appreciable (see pp. 822–38).

Malaria is a common cause of anaemia in endemic areas and may result in pregnancy complications, such as abortion, preterm delivery, light-for-dates fetuses and severe illness in the mother. These complications may be due to the pyrexial illness or to placental parasitization. Maternal deaths from cerebral malaria occur with acute infection during the third trimester of pregnancy in epidemic areas such as Thailand. The prevention and treatment of malaria therefore assumes great importance in endemic areas, and regular prophylaxis should be commenced with folic acid to combat anaemia. Antimalarial prophylaxis used will vary with local drug resistance and its safety in pregnancy. In the acute attack the aim is to reduce the fever as soon as possible, to eradicate the infection and to prevent relapses (see pp. 657–74).

Anaemia should be prevented or diagnosed early, but unfortunately many pregnant women are only seen when the anaemia is already severe or when it has caused complications. These patients should ideally be transferred to hospital. Severe anaemia may proceed to cardiac failure (often in the puerperium) and mild blood loss (e.g. postpartum haemorrhage) in an anaemic patient may cause severe shock or even death. Surgical and anaesthetic intervention is hazardous in anaemic patients who are less resistant to infection, which in turn may impair erythropoiesis. Anaemia is associated with late abortions, light-for-dates fetuses and preterm delivery, with resulting perinatal mortality and morbidity.

The key to reducing anaemia in pregnancy lies in dietary improvement and prophylactic therapy. The aim when treating an anaemic patient in pregnancy, is for her to have as high a haemoglobin level as possible by the time of delivery. Wherever possible, this should be achieved by oral or intramuscular therapy for the anaemia and treatment of associated medical conditions. However, there are occasions when the anaemia is severe and cardiac failure imminent or present when the anaemic patient is already in labour, or when there is infection which would prevent erythropoesis. In these situations blood transfusion may be necessary to increase the circulating cell mass, but attendants must be alert to the danger of cardiac overload and use packed cell transfusion, exchange transfusion, together with diuretics (frusemide) to reduce the danger of cardiac failure. Total dose intravenous iron infusion during pregnancy is not beneficial to maternal haemoglobin concentration. It may also increase the frequency of malaria in primigravid women.

Viral hepatitis

While viral hepatitis in pregnancy in the developed world is relatively innocuous, in the tropics it is a significant cause of maternal and fetal loss. There is evidence that its incidence is higher in the pregnant woman particularly in the third trimester, and the condition is more severe probably because of the associated protein deficiency in these women.

If the disease takes an uncomplicated course, the woman will feel better when jaundice appears and may not present at a health institution. In others the general condition does not improve, the jaundice deepens and the disease progresses and shows signs of impending hepatic failure. Coma is common, and there is evidence of clotting deficiency. Hepatic failure causes intrauterine death, and delivery may be followed by a severe postpartum haemorrhage. Once coma supervenes, the prognosis is poor and very few patients survive despite energetic treatment.

It seems that the best way to attempt to reduce the morbidity and mortality of this condition is to improve the general nutritional status of the women to avoid protein deficiency. However, when they present in an advanced state of the disease they should be given a high carbohydrate diet with vitamin supplements and low protein and salt. Hypoglycaemia should be prevented and treated and vitamin K (1 mg by intramuscular injection) given to try and improve blood clotting.

Pulmonary tuberculosis

The incidence of pulmonary tuberculosis remains high in many developing countries and it is therefore commonly associated with pregnancy. It is important that the attendant should be aware of this, and should look for a history suggestive of tuberculosis whenever the pregnant patient presents. Clinical examination of the chest should always be performed. Where there is a high incidence of tuberculosis, and chest radiography is easily available, routine screening is indicated.

If the disease is diagnosed in pregnancy the ideal management would be in-patient treatment until the disease is controlled, followed by out-patient therapy.

This would be an opportunity also for rest and advice on diet. Where this is not possible, out-patient treatment has to suffice with efficient follow-up of defaulters. Drug regimens vary with local programmes, and with cost and availability of drugs. An example would be isoniazid (300 mg) and ethambutol (15 mg/kg daily) for one year. These women are often anaemic as well and prophylactic haematinics should be prescribed.

In labour, care should be taken to maintain adequate hydration and to prevent respiratory embarrassment, and the second stage should be shortened by timely prophylactic forceps delivery or vacuum extraction which can be performed in the health centre.

Management of the neonate

In the tropics the decision as to whether to allow the infant to breast-feed has to be based on the relative dangers of tuberculous infection from the mother, and disease and death from unhygienic bottle-feeding.

If the mother has been effectively treated the child should breast-feed but should also receive BCG vaccination in the neonatal period. This should be repeated at about six weeks if tuberculin testing is negative. Should the mother still be infectious at the time of delivery she must be given antituberculous therapy immediately. If INAH-resistant BCG is available it should be given to the infant at birth; the infant breast-fed and protected from tuberculosis by prophylactic INAH. This should be continued until Mantoux conversion occurs. Should INAH-resistant BCG not be available, the child can be given ordinary BCG at birth, followed by temporary segregation from the mother (while the breasts are manually expressed) and the commencement of INAH prophylaxis and breast-feeding. This should be continued until the mother is non-infectious, or the child has achieved Mantoux conversion.

Heart disease

Physiological changes in pregnancy and labour

Pregnancy is a time of added strain to the cardio-vascular system. Cardiac output rises in the first trimester, continues to rise until about 32 weeks, and remains at this high level until term. Heart rate increases 10 to 15 beats per minute, reaching its peak near term, while stroke volume is highest in early to mid pregnancy. Blood volume increases variably in different women most rapidly during the first 20–30 weeks of gestation, and continuing gradually to term.

Plasma volume often increases more than red cells, causing a lowering of haemoglobin values if iron supplies are insufficient. Labour and delivery impose a further burden on the heart, and this is compounded by pain and anxiety.

The problem of heart disease in pregnancy

In developed parts of the world, the incidence of heart disease in pregnancy has lessened and changed in pattern; less rheumatic heart disease is seen, and more congenital heart disease, often post-surgery. However, in poorer countries, rheumatic heart disease is still common, and pregnant patients with heart disease are a significant risk group. Pregnancy may be the first opportunity for diagnosis, and antenatal clinic staff should be alert to this.

Clinical classification of physical disability in the non-pregnant state, and the nature of the lesion are the best guide to prognosis when sophisticated investigation is not available.

The aim of medical care throughout pregnancy and delivery is the prevention of cardiac failure and the other complications of heart disease. The patient must therefore be seen more often and by the most experienced personnel available. She must rest more than her healthy sister, and may need to be admitted to hospital for prolonged periods. Anaemia should be prevented, or energetically treated when diagnosed. Dental extractions should be covered with antibiotics and infections, e.g. in the chest, regarded as potentially dangerous. Antibiotics should be given in labour also. Tachycardia, cardia arrhythmias, pulmonary oedema and cardiac failure should be looked for, diagnosed early and treated. If anticoagulants are needed heparin is safe in pregnancy.

Ideally the patient should be resting in hospital when she goes into labour (digoxin causes earlier and shorter labour) and this should be as pain- and anxiety-free as possible. Conduction anaesthesia is ideal if available, and if Caesarean section is necessary for obstetric reasons, it can be done under epidural anaesthesia. The condition of the mother should be very closely monitored, and the second stage shortened by forceps delivery. Intravenous oxytocics should usually be avoided, and particular vigilance taken during the hours following delivery, as complications are more likely at this time. Return to normal activity should be gradual and contraceptive advice should be given in the hope that birth intervals will be prolonged and family size limited. Sterilization may be indicated in some cases.

Diabetes

Diabetes and pregnancy are an unhappy partnership. Pregnancy is a diabetogenic state and therefore makes diabetes worse, and diabetes is associated with many complications in pregnancy, from preconception to puerperium. Diabetic pregnancy outcome will only be successful when the diabetes is controlled meticulously from preconception through delivery, and this requires, if possible, the supervision of an experienced physician and obstetrician, the availability of drugs and equipment for monitoring and a motivated, cooperative patient. All this emphasizes the difficulty of achieving good results in diabetic pregnancy in much of the developing world.

Principles, however, remain. If a woman is known to be a diabetic, she should be counselled about the importance of preconception diabetic control and advised about antenatal and delivery care. An estimation of glycosylated HbA if available, reflects the degree of metabolic control in a patient over the previous months. During pregnancy, the ideal management is to maintain a blood glucose below 120 mg/100 ml (approx. 7 mmol/l), and this often needs a controlled diet and changing combinations of soluble and isophane insulin, which in turn requires an efficient monitoring system. This is often very difficult to achieve in the Third World, but every effort should be made to see the pregnant diabetic regularly and adjust treatment according to blood glucose levels. Prolonged hospitalization may be the only way to achieve this, and patients and their families need to be convinced that one or two well-supervised pregnancies with successful outcome are far better than several resulting in perinatal death. The severity of the diabetes is a guide to the outcome of pregnancy, but all need close surveillance.

Diabetes may be diagnosed for the first time in pregnancy. The attendant should look for factors such as unexplained stillbirth or neonatal death, or a history of a baby weighing more than 4000 g in a previous pregnancy, and investigate these patients as early as possible.

Routine screening by urine examination for glucose and further investigation of those with glycosuria, remains sound practice. However, the availability of resources and the prevalence of diabetes in the population, will determine the extent of screening. It is far better to screen potential diabetics routinely than to screen all patients while reagents last and then screen nobody.

The obstetric management should look for complications in the fetus caused by the diabetes, monitor growth and well-being of the fetus by whatever methods are available and decide on the optimum time and method of delivery. In early pregnancy it is important to assess the gestation as accurately as possible from menstrual history, uterine size and ultrasound examination if available. Ultrasound examination will also assist in the diagnosis of fetal abnormalities. This early contact with the mother is an opportunity for convincing her of the importance of good diabetic control and for teaching her any home monitoring methods that are available. As the pregnancy progresses, the obstetrician should look for signs of hydramnios and excessive fetal growth, which are evidence of poor control and fetal compromise, as well as for pregnancy complications such as hypertension and pyelonephritis, which may have more sinister effects in the diabetic than the normal pregnancy. Preterm labour, intrauterine deaths and neonatal morbidity are also more common in diabetic pregnancy.

Fetal well-being has to be assessed by whatever methods are possible. Clinical assessment of fetal size and the presence of hydramnios remain important, even if regular antenatal fetal heart monitoring and ultrasound examinations are available.

If insulin-treated diabetic control is satisfactory and there is no evidence of fetal compromise, macrosomia, hydramnios or pre-eclampsia, then labour can be induced at 37 to 38 weeks. If diet alone has achieved good control, and providing there is no evidence of placental insufficiency, induction can be left to 39 to 40 weeks, allowing more possibility of spontaneous labour. Intravenous infusion of 5 per cent glucose is commenced one hour before and continued at 80 ml per hour. A simple regimen would be to give 14 units isophane insulin subcutaneously; others prefer to give half the normal morning dose of soluble insulin. Rupture of the forewaters is performed and intravenous syntocinon infusion in normal saline commenced. Progress should be good and the labour complete within 12 hours. Close monitoring of the fetal heart is essential, with maternal blood sugar estimation done every two hours and the infusion adjusted to keep this between 4 and 8 mmol/l. Failure to progress will justify intervention and delivery by Caesarean section. Mothers with a previous bad obstetric history will need delivery by elective Caesarean section at 37 weeks. Care should be taken in the 24 hours after delivery, as hypoglycaemia may result from postpartum increased sensitivity to insulin. The mother's insulin requirements will then usually return to prepregnancy levels.

Following delivery, contraceptive advice should be

given and the parents reminded again of the advisability of limiting family size.

Hypertension

The older the childbearing population, the more common is hypertension and its complications. This will usually be due to essential hypertension, but may also be due to renal disease and to rare causes like phaeochromocytoma, coarctation of the aorta and Cushing's syndrome. The importance of chronic hypertension in pregnancy is that it is one of the major predisposing factors of pre-eclampsia and also intra-uterine growth retardation.

Chronic hypertension can only be diagnosed with confidence in pregnancy if it is known to be present outside pregnancy, or if a blood pressure of 140/90 or over is found on two occasions before 20 weeks. If a pregnant patient is first seen in the middle trimester, the usual physiological decrease in blood pressure may mask such hypertension, and if she is seen later in pregnancy it is difficult to distinguish between this and pre-eclampsia. Treatment is only necessary in pregnancy for maternal reasons, and a maximum blood pressure of 160/100 would be an acceptable level of control. The drug methyldopa (dosage 250–500 mg three times a day) is preferred, as it has proved not to have teratogenic or other adverse effects on the fetus. However, more recently labetalol, a combined α – and β – adrenoceptor blocking drug (dosage 100–200 mg three times a day) is becoming more widely used. Diuretics would only rarely be needed for control of hypertension; it should be noted that they have disadvantages in superimposed pre-eclampsia. It is important to remember that a raised blood pressure, whenever it is found, implies a significant risk and the patient must be seen more often and referred to hospital if necessary. These patients will often need varying periods of hospitalization.

Renal disease

The most common renal complication of pregnancy is acute pyelonephritis which presents with pyrexia, pain, frequency, and vomiting. It may cause abortion, preterm labour and intrauterine death. Antibiotic therapy should be aggressive (commenced while waiting for bacterial culture sensitivities) and continued for about three weeks. After cessation of treatment, regular urine cultures should be taken. Seventy per cent of these patients will have had asymptomatic bacteriuria, and if tests are available it is worth screening for bacteriuria early in pregnancy. The 2 to 5 per cent of patients who

have bacteriuria should be treated prophylactically with antibiotics and then followed up.

Chronic renal disease may coincide with pregnancy and the course of pregnancy varies with the severity of disease. Deterioration in renal function may occur in patients with reflex nephropathy. Good antenatal care is mandatory, with close cooperation between obstetrician and physician. The particular problems to look for are:

- hypertension, its effects and treatment;
- a deterioration in renal function and the possibility of superimposed pre-eclampsia;
- early diagnosis and treatment of latent or acute urinary tract infection;
- problems with fetal growth and well-being.

When complications occur, hospital admission should be arranged and appropriate advice should be given for contraception and planned future pregnancies.

Drugs and pregnancy

Many drugs have an adverse effect if taken during pregnancy. Therefore advice against taking any drug in pregnancy unless they are absolutely essential is wise. The main adverse effect in early pregnancy is the production of congenital malformations, and in late pregnancy the growth and functional development of the fetus may be affected. Unfortunately, animal trials do not always detect human teratogenicity and a drug has to be used for a long time before its safety is assured. Despite its capacity to produce such dramatic congenital malformations, thalidomide was prescribed for four years before the association was confirmed, and this experience should remind all to prescribe very cautiously in early pregnancy. Where a mother is already on treatment, the drug should only be continued if essential for the preservation of maternal health. The doctor should always prescribe the least toxic drug available with the same therapeutic effect.

The second important group of drugs in pregnancy are those which the mother 'prescribes' for herself: smoking, which causes a reduction in birth weight and increased perinatal mortality; alcohol, which in sufficient dosage causes the fetal alcohol syndrome and opiate addiction, with its effects on pregnancy, the fetus and the neonate. Every effort should be made to obtain a clear history of these addictions, so that appropriate advice can be given to stop their use, and the pregnancy managed in the best possible way.

Past obstetric performance and menstrual history

A mother's performance in previous pregnancies is extremely important, and time spent taking a detailed history is time well spent. It is imperative that all health workers are taught to take accurate histories, and that their history-taking is monitored continually. If staff are taught to fill in high-risk factors with a red pen, their understanding can also be monitored.

A primigravid will have no past to reveal her obstetric behaviour, but age and general health will be indicators of risk. A teenage pregnancy brings many problems, e.g. educational deprivation, late booking, increased incidence of pre-eclampsia and problems of child management. It is tragic when a girl becomes a mother with responsibility for another child before she herself has completed her childhood. Older age brings its problems too, even when not associated with multiparity, and the age when a woman becomes an elderly primigravida needs to be defined in a given population. It is important to establish the date of the last menstrual period as accurately as possible, difficult as this is when women often become pregnant while still breast-feeding, or when menses are not established after stopping the contraceptive pill. Ultrasound examination is the most accurate means of assessing gestational age when this is uncertain. Even in women with reliable dates, measurement of the biparietal diameter on ultrasound between 12 and 18 weeks predicts the date of delivery more accurately than calculations based on the date of the last menstrual period.

Pregnancies after the fifth child become progressively more hazardous (e.g. from anaemia, hypertensive disease, unstable lies, precipitate labour, ruptured uterus and postpartum haemorrhage). It is important to ensure that the mother mentions stillbirths, as well as livebirths, in the history. The historian should search for problems in previous pregnancies like anaemia, urinary tract infection, antepartum haemorrhage, hypertension, intrauterine death before labour, and obtain a detailed history of the duration and outcome of labour. Instrumental delivery may be for non-recurrent causes, but may also be due to mild disproportion. Caesarean section and symphysiotomy are indications for hospital delivery, though the latter may have ensured a large enough pelvis for subsequent vaginal delivery.

A history of a retained placenta and postpartum haemorrhage is also important. If possible the duration of gestation, birth weight, occurrence of congenital malformation and neonatal morbidity should be noted, and a history of stillbirth or neonatal death sensitively handled.

This aspect of the history is very useful for determining risk factors, and should be confirmed where possible by perusing notes of the previous pregnancy. Decisions should then be made as to where and by whom antenatal care should be performed, and where the patient should deliver. Minimally trained staff need very clear referral criteria, e.g. short stature, weight loss, and continuing supervision to ensure that referrals are timely and for appropriate reasons. The criteria need to be worked out in the local situation and to take distance, transport facilities, etc. into consideration.

The present pregnancy

Another aspect of antenatal care is the identification of problems in the present pregnancy, both by history and clinical examination. Symptoms of nausea, abdominal pain, vaginal discharge or bleeding should be elicited, and further investigations done where necessary. It would be impossible in a chapter like this to detail abnormalities to be sought, but some important ones will be mentioned.

Pre-eclampsia

This condition has many names, but pre-eclampsia does at least give one characteristic of the disease – the fact that it may lead to convulsions. Traditionally, pre-eclampsia was defined as the presence of two signs from the triad of oedema, hypertension and proteinuria, but is now realized that oedema is very common in normal pregnancy and hypertension with significant proteinuria are more reliable signs. The disease has widespread effects (cardiovascular, renal, hepatic, cerebral, haematological, uterine and placental), but aetiology is unresolved. It is usually a disease of the primigravid pregnancy, and has serious complications both for mother and fetus.

The aim of antenatal care is early diagnosis and appropriate management of the pregnancy, to prevent eclampsia and other maternal complications, and intra-uterine death or morbidity of the fetus. Increased rest reduces the progress of pre-eclampsia and so it is important to detect hypertension early and to advise rest and more frequent visits to the antenatal clinic for review. Such mothers could also be referred for specialist care. The mother may need to be admitted to a maternity village, a health centre or a hospital for rest.

Unfortunately, many women do not present to the

health service until pre-eclampsia is already severe i.e. a blood pressure of 160/110 or over, heavy proteinuria, oliguria, cerebral or visual disturbances and pulmonary oedema or cyanosis. The principles of management of severe pre-eclampsia are the same, and it is imperative that all levels of staff should treat the condition as an emergency and admit the patient to hospital as soon as possible.

The steps in management are:

- maintenance of an airway;
- treatment of convulsions;
- control of blood pressure;
- stabilization of mother;
- delivery of infant.

The treatment of convulsions should commence at the point when the patient meets the health service. Maternity assistants can start treatment with either magnesium sulphate or diazepam (choice depending on local policy) intravenously or intramuscularly, while they accompany the patient to hospital. Treatment should then be continued and monitored carefully in hospital. These drugs may reduce the blood pressure to some degree, but hypotensives are usually needed as well. The most commonly used drug is hydrallazine, either in intermittent or continuous intravenous dosage. As it may cause a rapid fall in blood pressure, close monitoring is essential. When the mother is fairly stable (usually 2–4 hours after admission) delivery should be expedited either by induction of labour or Caesarean section where necessary. These patients need the most experienced personnel to give the anaesthetic and intensive care should be continued for some days.

Antepartum haemorrhage

The three common causes for bleeding from the genital tract after the 28th week of pregnancy are placenta praevia, abruptio placentae and bleeding of undetermined origin. Fetal mortality is high in all.

The most common mode of presentation is slight bleeding without pain or shock. These patients have to be regarded as cases of placenta praevia until proved otherwise, and need hospital admission because of the danger of further bleeding. Following admission the pregnancy should be assessed carefully, a haemoglobin estimation should be performed, prophylactic or therapeutic haematinics given, and every effort made to obtain compatible blood in case transfusion is necessary. Vaginal examination should not be performed. Two or three days after cessation of bleeding a speculum examination should be performed to exclude any incidental cause of bleeding like carcinoma of the cervix. The next step is to localize the placenta by whatever method is available. Ultrasound is the most effective and least invasive method, but care should be taken in interpretation of reports. If placenta praevia can be excluded, the patient can usually be discharged, but she must still be considered a high-risk patient. If a placenta praevia is present, the woman must stay in hospital until 38 weeks, when a vaginal examination is performed under anaesthesia, followed by surgical induction or Caesarean section. If no method of placental localization is available, the patient should ideally stay in hospital until 38 weeks, when she can be examined under anaesthesia and the placenta located digitally. There will be a few cases of placenta praevia who cannot be managed conservatively because of the quantity of bleeding, and these need to be delivered urgently by Caesarean section.

Some women will be seen with clinical signs of abruptio placentae, i.e. bleeding from separation of a normally situated placenta. This bleeding may be completely revealed when the degree of shock corresponds to the amount of bleeding, concealed when the patient may be very shocked with no apparent blood loss, or commonly a mixed pattern may occur. Typically, in abruptio placentae the dominant symptom is pain, and the patient may be pale and shocked when she arrives. A normal blood pressure may be deceptive as the pre-abruptio blood pressure may have been raised. The abdomen will be tender, the uterus woody hard, the fetal parts not palpable and the fetal heart usually not heard. Active management is imperative, and should include sedation (with morphine), rapid assessment of general condition, review of haematological state (including haemoglobin, fibrinogen titre, presence of fibrinolysis) liberal transfusion with central venous pressure monitoring in severe cases, and induction of labour. In the rare case where the baby is alive and not too preterm, a Caesarean section may be indicated. During labour, progress must be assessed by regular vaginal examination, as monitoring uterine contractions is usually impossible. Oxytocin infusion may be necessary, and if there is no progress Caesarean section may be the best management, even with a dead baby. Whatever the method, postpartum haemorrhage is a real hazard, and everything possible should be done to prevent it and minimize its effects. Transfusion is often inadequate even when there is no scarcity of blood, and patients need haematinics for varying periods of time to restore iron stores. It is important too, that they do not embark upon another pregnancy too soon.

Hydramnios, malpresentation, unstable lie and multiple pregnancy

Antenatal clinic visits give the opportunity for regular abdominal palpation and the diagnosis of hydramnios, malpresentations, and multiple pregnancy.

The official definition of hydramnios is over 1500 ml liquor, and if it is diagnosed, associated abnormalities of the fetus, such as multiple pregnancy, fetal abnormality and hydrops should be sought and confirmed by X-ray or sonar. Maternal diabetes or chorioangioma of the placenta may be associated too. Occasionally the mother may need to be admitted for rest because of severe hydramnios, and if discomfort is marked, liquor may have to be removed by amniocentesis. The labour is high risk, and the attendant may have to deal with malpresentation, prolapsed cord, multiple pregnancy and postpartum haemorrhage. Oesophageal atresia or oesophageotracheal fistula may be present in the neonate, and should be excluded soon after birth by passing an endotracheal tube.

Breech presentation

The incidence of breech presentation is 2–3 per cent and the two common aetiological factors are prematurity or any factor that prevents the spontaneous version which has normally occurred by about the 34th week of pregnancy. Because of the hazards of breech delivery, there is a natural desire to avoid it if at all possible, and this has led to the practice of external cephalic version. This is usually done around 34 weeks if there are no contra-indications such as hypertension, antepartum haemorrhage and previous Caesarean section. Despite the satisfaction of doing a successful external cephalic version, it is not a procedure without complications and there is no evidence that it reduces the frequency of breech presentation at the beginning of labour.

Breech delivery

If perinatal mortality and morbidity are to be avoided, breech deliveries must be conducted by experienced personnel and Caesarean section should be performed if breech presentation is accompanied by any other complications, e.g. contracted pelvis, a large baby, footling presentation or a bad obstetric history. It is therefore imperative that breech presentation is diagnosed antenatally so that the decision to deliver vaginally or by Caesarean section can be taken before the onset of labour. Prolapse of the cord is more common in breech presentation and vaginal examina-tion performed when the membranes rupture. Delay in the first stage may be a sign of disproportion and abdominal delivery should be done sooner rather than later. It is often difficult to establish when the second stage commences because parts of the breech can pass through an undilated cervix and give the mother a desire to push. Therefore, the mother should be discouraged from pushing until the anterior buttock is fully visible, or until vaginal examination has verified full dilatation with the presenting part below the ischial spines. Ideally an epidural anaesthetic should be administered during the first stage and if possible an anaesthetic should be available in the delivery room during the second stage in case one is required. If there is non-descent of the breech in the second stage, the only management is Caesarean section. A pudendal block should be performed for breech delivery if there is no epidural anaesthesia, and this facilitates timely episiotomy. Delivery as far as the umbilicus should be spontaneous, the legs can then be flexed and delivered and a loop of cord brought down. When the anterior scapula is visible, the arms can be flipped out, the back gently rotated uppermost and the baby allowed to hang by its own weight. The head will flex and descend slowly and when the nape of the neck is showing the attendant should extend the infant upwards by its ankles and deliver the head slowly and carefully. Many prefer to use Wrigley's forceps to control the delivery of the head, especially where there is no epidural anaesthesia, and this allows an assistant to suck out the upper respiratory tract before the baby breathes. A problem may be extended arms, and these should be delivered by the well-documented Lovset's manoeuvre. The worst difficulty is failure of the head to descend and this can be due to an incompletely dilated cervix, poor flexion of the head, previously unrecognized disproportion, or hydrocephalus. Flexion of the head, and downward traction using the Mauriceau–Smellie–Veit manoeuvre may succeed. Occasionally there is a place for cervical incision or emergency symphysiotomy but this should only be performed by experienced people. Hydrocephalus will often necessitate craniotomy to effect delivery.

Unstable lie and other malpresentation

Another finding in the antenatal period which is likely to end in malpresentation is a transverse or an unstable lie, and these are more common in grand multiparous patients. If repeated attempts at external cephalic version do not result in stabilization, it is wise to admit the patient at about 38 weeks to a maternity village or hospital where medical care is quickly available should she go into labour with uncorrected malpresentation. External cephalic version in very early labour, when the uterus has developed some degree of tone, may be effective and result in an uncomplicated labour. Should the membranes rupture in a case like this, vaginal examination should be done immediately to exclude a prolapsed cord. If a prolapsed cord is found, or if a shoulder presentation persists, Caesarean section is the only safe course. Some centres use stabilizing induction in the management of these cases, i.e. uterine activity is induced with syntocinon after 38 weeks and the membranes are ruptured after the onset of regular contractions to release enough liquor to stabilize the presenting part; following this labour should progress normally. It is essential that such a procedure is monitored very closely by experienced staff. Should a woman arrive in labour with an arm or shoulder presentation, she should be transferred to hospital and a Caesarean section be performed if the baby is alive. If the baby is dead, decapitation with an instrument like the Blond–Heidler saw or large scissors is preferred. The risk of ruptured uterus must always be considered in these cases.

Face and brow presentation are only rarely diagnosed in the antenatal clinic, so these presentations are usually encountered for the first time in labour. When diagnosed, the mothers should be transferred to a centre where Caesarean section is possible, as this is the only management in brow presentation, and is often needed in a persistent mento-posterior face presentation. Mento-anterior presentations may deliver spontaneously, but may also need forceps delivery.

Multiple pregnancy

The average incidence of multiple pregnancy is about 1:80, but it varies in different communities and racial groups. The diagnosis is suspected when the uterus is large for dates, or when three fetal poles are palpated, but it is imperative to confirm the suspicion with either X-ray or sonar. Multiple pregnancy is associated with many complications of pregnancy, e.g. exaggerated symptoms like tiredness, vomiting or oedema, anaemia (including folic acid deficiency) and other nutritional deficiencies, pre-eclampsia, hydramnios, malpresentations and preterm labour. Increased rest should be advised during pregnancy and the mother may have to be admitted for this. The labour, too, is high risk and wherever possible should be in hospital.

There is no reason why the management of the delivery of the first twin should differ from the singleton, but methodical steps should be taken to ensure the safe delivery of the second. The comments

about anaesthetic requirements for breech delivery apply also in multiple pregnancy. Once the first twin is delivered, and the cord clamped in the usual way, the abdomen should be palpated to ascertain the lie and the presentation of the second twin, and an external cephalic version done if necessary. Artificial rupture of the membranes should follow, and sometimes syntocinon infusion is needed to initiate contractions. If delivery is at all delayed in a vertex presentation, forceps delivery or vacuum extraction should be performed. In a second twin, internal podalic version and/or breech extraction are not dangerous because of the amount of room available in the uterus, and because the membranes are only recently ruptured. However, a second twin, larger than the first, could cause unexpected trouble. As postpartum haemorrhage is a very real hazard in twin delivery, intravenous ergometrine should be given prophylactically. When a patient is admitted with a retained second twin, an experienced person should make the necessary decisions regarding delivery, taking into consideration the mother's general condition, the lie and presentation of the fetus and whether it is alive, the duration of ruptured membranes and the dilation of the cervix.

Intrauterine growth retardation

Intrauterine growth retardation is never an easy diagnosis in the antenatal period, and it becomes even more difficult when mothers are unsure of their dates and facilities, e.g. sonar for establishing gestational maturity, are not available. The most widely used definition is a weight below the third centile and this is one of the three main causes of perinatal mortality. Though intrauterine growth retardation has many known causes e.g. socio-economic circumstance of mother, malnutrition, pre-eclampsia, hypertension, abruptio placentae, smoking and infections, the aetiology in the majority is unknown.

Clinical suspicion of intrauterine growth retardation may occur when a mother loses weight or fails to gain weight, when a uterus appears small for dates or when there is oligohydramnios. Symphysis-fundus measurements are helpful, especially if serial and carried out by the same person. Failure in growth may be confirmed by serial ultrasonography and this may also identify a fetal abnormality. Once suspicion is aroused the fetus is in the high-risk category, and every effort should be made to establish whether it is likely to die *in utero* if there is no intervention. Available methods in hospital will vary from fetal movement counts to antenatal cardiotocography to oestriol assays and other estimates of placental function, but without these one has to rely on clinical estimate of growth and size.

Management is not easy, especially where facilities are limited. Every effort should be made to treat any identifiable underlying maternal condition and to increase blood flow to the uterus by bed rest. If possible, management is then conservative until about 37 weeks, when delivery can be induced. A reduction in fetal movements or serial oestriols will point towards early delivery, as will a critical fetal reserve pattern (reduced baseline variability, absence of accelerations and repeated late decelerations in response to Braxton–Hicks contractions) on cardiotocography. In this group continuous observation in labour is the ideal, and the best technology available should be used. The quality of neonatal intensive care available will be a guide as to how early in pregnancy a fetus can be delivered and survive.

Labour

The development of care in labour seems to have been somewhat similar in many different parts of the world. Initially birth is usually an entirely female event and the men of a community are totally excluded. Generally speaking certain females, e.g. grandmothers, experienced friends or an individual from the community are recognized as expert and they conduct deliveries. There is no formal training and birth is regarded as a dirty event. There is therefore no comprehension of the importance of cleanliness and sterility, and dirty aprons rather than sterile gowns are donned. These traditional birth assistants are independent, and there is no control of their activities.

At some stage there is the establishment of a 'rival' group of trained professional midwives, and there is an attempt to train the traditional midwife. The two groups may then work together with the traditional midwives usually supervised by the professional group. A parallel development is the realization that at some stage intervention is necessary for the good of the mother and child, and doctors (who are often male) enter the scene as the performers of intervention. Sometimes this can go on to the excessive medicalization of labour with, at some point, a cry from women that the process has gone too far.

But in most of the developing world this is not likely to happen, and the need to use traditional midwives and other lowly trained workers will continue.

The pattern of labour

The uterus, while accommodating and nurturing a growing conceptus, is also preparing to expel it at the appropriate time. Throughout pregnancy, but with increasing frequency as pregnancy progresses, contractions occur. In early pregnancy they tend to be irregular in pattern, of low amplitude and of short duration, but as term approaches they become more regular, larger and stronger. They imperceptibly change into the efficient contractions of labour which dilate the cervix and cause fetal descent. At this stage the contractions are painful and recognized by the mother as the onset of labour.

Clinically labour is divided into two stages, the first stage from the perceived onset of contractions to full dilatation of the cervix, and the second from full dilatation to the delivery of the baby. The first stage is further divided into a latent phase which seems to be a preparatory phase when little dilatation or descent occurs, and an active phase when full dilatation is achieved, and, in addition, an appreciable amount of descent. Descent continues and the fetus is delivered in the second stage. The relationships and effects of the different phases are illustrated in Fig. 2.2.1.

It is not possible to monitor labour merely by feeling abdominal contractions or by designating time limits. However, measuring the process of dilatation of the cervix and descent of the head gives an indication of normality and assists in the early diagnosis of delayed labour. The representation of this dilatation and descent in a graphical form greatly clarifies the progress of labour and this 'partogram' can accommodate many other observations too.

Delay in labour

A simple classification of delay in labour is:

- delay in the latent phase of labour;
- protracted dilatation and descent throughout the active phase of labour;
- an arrest of dilatation and descent following initial satisfactory progress.

Delay in latent phase

The latent phase commences when the mother is aware of regular painful contractions and continues until the cervix is about 3 cm dilated, when the active phase with its accelerated dilatation usually commences. It is not possible to distinguish between false labour and the latent phase of labour except by hindsight. So if

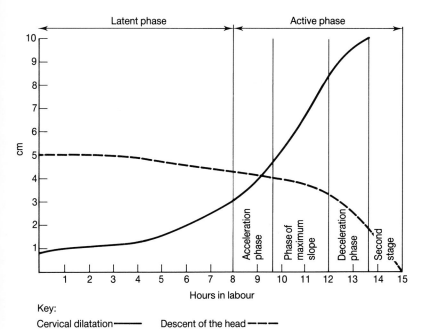

Fig. 2.2.1 Progress of normal labour.

Key:

Cervical dilatation——— Descent of the head – – –

contractions continue without interruption for more than about 12 hours in primigravid mothers, and 6 hours in multiparous ones without cervical dilatation, a prolonged latent phase can be diagnosed. The most common cause for a prolonged latent phase appears to be too early administered sedation, or heavy medication for pain relief, but some causes are idiopathic. Fortunately a delayed latent phase does not necessarily lead to delay in active labour, and the best management is sedation to allow the mother to rest. Following the resultant sleep, about 85 per cent will be in active labour, 5 per cent will continue with ineffectual contractions, and contractions will have stopped in the 10 per cent or so who were in false labour. The only patients who need to have labour stimulated in the latent phase, are those who have a good reason for induction, e.g. evidence of intra-amniotic infection or hypertensive disease.

Protracted dilatation and descent

A slow rate of dilatation and descent in the active phase of labour is much more serious than a delay in the latent phase. The cause of this pattern is unknown, but it is associated with cephalo-pelvic disproportion, mal-positions and deflexion attitudes. These reasons do not

necessarily cause the inefficient uterine action; the latter may fail to resolve the malposition. Careful vaginal examination at regular intervals should reveal any specific cause, such as brow presentation, and the decision can be taken to perform Caesarean section. Contractions can be improved in strength and frequency by using syntocinon stimulation and the subsequent progress of labour carefully assessed. Meticulous monitoring of maternal and fetal condition is essential in these difficult cases. Given time, many will deliver vaginally but others will need Caesarean section, especially those associated with disproportion. Fig. 2.2.2 illustrates the progress in a protracted labour.

Arrest of dilatation and descent

Arrest disorders differ from the last group in that the delay in dilatation and descent occurs after a period of satisfactory dilatation. Many of these, too, occur in association with disproportion and if evidence of this is confirmed it will be safest to deliver by Caesarean section. If disproportion or malposition are excluded, then most will probably respond well to syntocinon and deliver vaginally, but needless to say careful maternal and fetal monitoring remains essential. Fig. 2.2.3

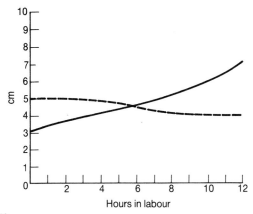

Key:

Cervical dilatation ——————   Descent of the head —— —— ——

Fig. 2.2.2   Protracted dilatation and descent.

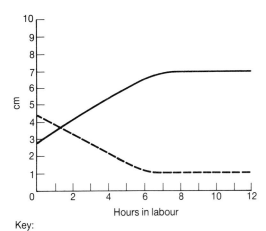

Key:

Cervical dilatation ——————   Descent of the head —— —— ——

Fig. 2.2.3   Arrest of dilatation and descent.

illustrates an arrested labour. Early recognition of delay is the key to good management and graphic representation of labour offers the best method of doing this.

Recording observations in labour

The secret of good care in labour is regular observations, so that abnormalities are detected, and appropriate steps taken in management.

Observations in labour can conveniently be divided into fetal, maternal and those which indicate the progress of the labour. Most observations should be taken half-hourly, but a few (like maternal temperature) need only be done routinely every four hours.

The fetus

In an ideal labour the fetus should remain well and show no signs of distress. However, if a fetus is particularly vulnerable (e.g. a small-for-dates fetus) or if a labour is unusually problematical or prolonged, there will be distress and this should be identified as early as possible. The clinical methods of assessing the condition of the fetus are: observing the colour of the liquor, listening to the fetal heart rate and assessment of moulding of the fetal head. The last is especially significant when there is disproportion.

Meconium staining of the liquor has long been recognized as ominous, and even when it is not accompanied by an abnormal heart rate, there is the ever present danger of meconium aspiration.

The optimal time to listen to the fetal heart is before and throughout a uterine contraction, as this gives the opportunity to note changes in rate associated with the contraction. Decelerations occurring in the early part of the contraction may only be a result of pressure on the fetal head, but late decelerations may indicate anoxia, and a full assessment of the patient by the most competent person available is needed. Persistent bradycardia is also sinister (the normal fetal heart rate is a regular rate of 120–160/min throughout contractions). If electronic or ultrasound monitoring and biochemical evaluation of the fetal blood pH are available, they should be used in the cases of heart rate abnormality and the most competent person available should make a considered judgement on the management of the patient.

In the cases of disproportion, four-hourly assessment of fetal skull moulding is an aid to diagnosis and management. This should be done in an objective way, so that the observations of different examiners can be compared.

The mother

Unfortunately childbirth is often regarded as a 'natural' event in a mother's life, so much so that it is considered that no special care is required, and if the woman is damaged or dies in the process it cannot be avoided. But what greater tragedy is there than a 16-year-old primigravid dying of sepsis after a five-day labour, or a 35-year-old mother of six children dying of haemorrhage because her relatives would not donate blood?

The mother also deserves careful, continual monitoring of her general condition in labour, and in addition the experience should be made as pleasant as possible for her. Her pulse rate should be recorded half-hourly and the blood pressure and temperature four-hourly. The urine should be examined and measured whenever passed and notice taken if the bladder is not empty.

Reassurance and explanation should be given throughout labour and sedation and analgesia when needed. When abnormalities are detected their cause should be diagnosed and the appropriate management initiated, e.g. antibiotics if there is any evidence of infection, or intravenous fluids if the mother is dehydrated.

The progress of labour

A short efficient labour resulting in the delivery of a live healthy infant is pleasing to all, but unfortunately many labours are abnormal and because they are not adequately managed they end in tragedy. The more high risk the population, the greater the proportion of abnormal labours.

There are three essential components to the monitoring of labour:

1. The recording of the quality and frequency of uterine contractions.
2. Measuring the dilatation of the cervix.
3. Measuring the rate of descent of the fetal head.

Recording uterine contractions Contractions should be monitored and the observations recorded half-hourly. It is important to be objective, both with the frequency of contractions, e.g. 1:10, 2:10, and with their length, e.g. 20 s, 40 s. Terms like medium/strong contractions can be misleading, and may mean different things to different people. The quality of contractions taken with the rate of progress is a guide to the cause of delay.

Measuring the dilatation of the cervix Ideally also the dilatation of the cervix in centimetres (not in fingers or fractions) should be measured four-hourly, and the rate of dilatation calculated so that it can be compared with normality. It is of course essential that vaginal examinations should be performed with full aseptic technique; indeed labour attendants often need to be taught the basics of the importance of cleanliness and asepsis in labour, both in a traditional midwife hut and so-called modern hospitals.

Measuring the rate of descent of the fetal head The position of the head needs to be recorded four-hourly too, and the best method is to record the amount of head above the pelvic brim, as well as distance from the ischial spines, as caput formation and moulding can confuse all but the very experienced.

Once attendants are disciplined to keep an accurate record of the progress of labour they can be taught the specific signs which cause concern, what action to take, and to whom to refer the mother should this be necessary. It is imperative that delay should be diagnosed early, the cause ascertained and the appropriate management instituted. This may be continuing observation, uterine stimulation with oxytocics (in the primigravid patient) or Caesarean section.

The second and third stages of labour

The same vigilance is necessary in the second stage of labour, so that appropriate action can be taken in cases of distress or delay. Usually this means instrumental delivery (either forceps or vacuum extraction), but sometimes Caesarean section is essential even at this time. Symphysiotomy may need to be considered too.

It is extremely important that those who attempt instrumental delivery should be adequately trained; knowing when instrumental delivery is appropriate is more important than knowing how to do it.

The third stage also is potentially hazardous, and attendants should know how to manage both normal and abnormal third stages.

The composite partogram

The recording of all these observations on one graph greatly assists in providing a comprehensive picture of the progress of labour, and the early diagnosis of delay. Methods of alerting lowly trained staff to danger can be included on it. An example of a partogram is shown in Fig. 2.2.4.

Provision of community care

In the developed world, care in labour can be thought of at a personal level. Should the woman be delivered at home or in hospital? Should care be by a community midwife and a general practitioner, or a hospital midwife and a consultant obstetrician? Sophisticated and technological care is available to all.

However, in much of the developing world facilities are very limited, and the aim should be for hospital and health centre facilities to be reserved for the high-risk patients while low-risk patients are delivered at home, the midwife hut, or a village clinic by minimally trained staff.

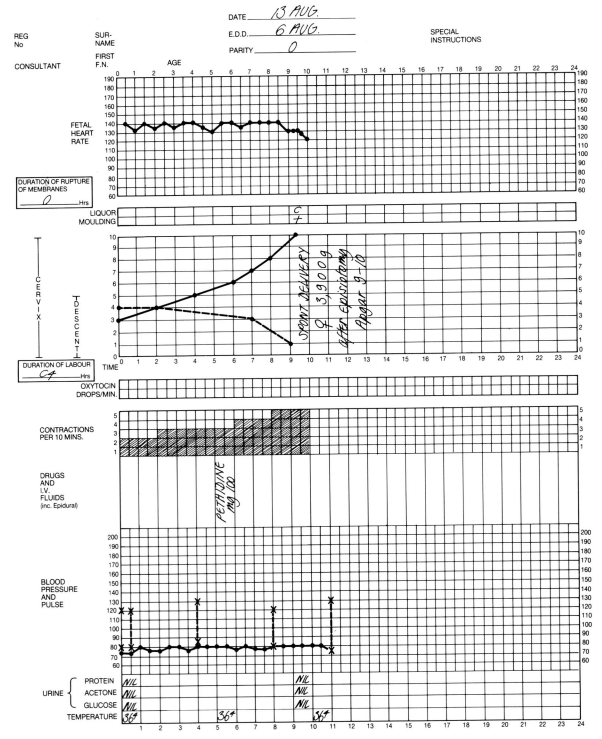

Fig. 2.2.4 An example of a partogram.

In each region there is a need for an organizational plan for obstetric services (the region will vary in size according to local population and terrain) and specialist obstetricians and midwives should take responsibility not only for the patients who attend the hospital or health centre, but also those who deliver in the community.

For a system like this to work, staff need to be adequately trained and continually monitored, both on their clinical performance, the importance of clean delivery and on their adherence to the plans laid down at regional level. The duties of each grade of staff should be clearly defined, and each should know when and where to refer the patients. Where climate and/or geography make referral impractical, certain groups of staff may need to be equipped to do tasks normally performed by higher grade staff. Operational procedures should cover antenatal care, labour and the postnatal period, and there should be close liaison with maternal and child health services in other regions.

Such services if adequately resourced, and if provided by caring men and women of vision, vigour and discipline, can revolutionize obstetric care for a population, significantly reduce maternal and perinatal mortality, and complications like vesico-vaginal fistula and ruptured uterus can disappear. The women of this world deserve this sort of care.

References

1. Harrison KA. Child bearing, health and social priorities: a survey of 22 774 consecutive hospital births in Zaria, Northern Nigeria. *British Journal of Obstetrics and Gynaecology*. 1985; **92** (Suppl. 5): 1–119.
2. Prentice AW, Watkinson M, Whitehead RG *et al.* Prenatal dietary supplementation of African women and birth weight. *Lancet*. 1983; **i**: 489–92.
3. Simmer K, Thompson RPH. Maternal zinc and intrauterine growth retardation. *Clinical Science*. 1985; 395–9.
4. Lawson JB, Stewart DB. *Obstetrics and Gynaecology in the Tropics and Developing Countries*. London, Edward Arnold, 1974.

MATERNAL LACTATION
Dorothy A. Jackson, M. W. Woolridge, Stella Imong, J. D. Baum

There is no doubt that breast-milk is the most suitable food in early infancy, and breast-feeding is particularly advantageous in poor communities. Despite this the growth of breast-fed babies in many developing countries shows signs of 'faltering' from as early as three months of age[1] This is particularly evident when children of poor families are compared with children of privileged families[2], raising the possibility that disadvantaged mothers may not be able to produce breast-milk of adequate quantity and quality to meet the nutritional requirements of the growing infant, and protect against infection.

Quantity of breast-milk

The quantity of milk produced by mothers in developing countries is difficult to measure, especially in traditional societies, where infants are fed 'on demand', frequently and at irregular intervals.

The most widely used method of estimating breast-milk production is by weighing the infant before and after feeding (test-weighing). An accurate balance is essential, especially when infants feed frequently and so take small amounts of milk at each feed, yet research centres in developing countries have often had to make do with spring balances, which are inexpensive but inaccurate.

Bringing mothers to a hospital or research institute and changing nursing patterns from demand-feeding to feeding at scheduled times for convenience of measurement, may have the effect of depressing milk yield.[3] The relationship between daytime and night-time milk intake can be variable[4], but because night-time breast-feeding is difficult to measure, some earlier studies simply measured daytime intakes or multiplied 12-hour day intakes by a constant, giving inaccurate estimates of the total milk intake. Recent studies have recognized the importance of avoiding disturbance to natural feeding patterns, and new techniques of measurement have been developed with this objective in mind.[5, 6]

Taking account of the methodological problems involved, the typical milk output in the first six months of lactation of mothers from developing countries is about 600–700 ml/day, but some earlier studies have reported values as low as 400 to 500 ml in India and Papua New Guinea.[3] The adequacy of lactation in developing countries has been assessed against the milk yields of well-nourished Western women. For many years, a value of 850 ml/day was taken as the Western 'norm', even though this was only the mean value from a study which reported milk outputs ranging from 250 to 1500 ml/day.[3]

Recent studies and re-evaluation of earlier data now suggest that typical breast-milk production by Western mothers is around 700–800 ml/day.[3, 7] The milk yields in developing countries are about 100 ml/day less than those in industrialized countries, but one should also bear in mind that the range in milk production in both developing and industrialized countries is very great: some disadvantaged women have high milk yields, some privileged women have low yields. Factors which may contribute to such individual variation are discussed later.

Quality of breast-milk

As with milk yields, the assessment of milk quality depends on the methods used to collect the data, in particular, the procedures for obtaining milk samples and the biochemical techniques used to analyse composition.

Fat, the breast-fed infant's main energy source, is the most variable component of breast-milk, increasing as much as fivefold from the start to the end of a feed and also varying diurnally in a predictable manner.[8] There are marked differences in composition between colostrum and mature milk, with fat and protein concentration decreasing over the course of lactation while lactose concentration increases. Estimates of milk composition therefore depend on the proportions of fore and hind milk sampled, the time of day at which samples are taken and the stage of lactation.

Bearing these sources of variation in mind, the concentrations of fat, protein and lactose in breast-milk produced by women from developing countries are broadly similar to values obtained in Western countries, despite differences in the dietary intakes of the two groups. However, lower fat and protein concentrations and lower whey protein:casein ratios have been reported from some developing countries.[7] Table 2.2.2 shows the ranges of constituents reported in breast-milk

Table 2.2.2 Constituents in breast-milk taken by infants aged 1–12 months

	Industrialized countries	Developing countries
Lactose (mm/l)	18–223	181–227
Protein (excluding non-protein nitrogen) (g/100 ml)	0.7–1.41	0.82–1.31
Fat (g/100 ml)	2.85–4.99	2.73–4.57

taken by infants between 1 and 12 months of age, obtained using a variety of methods.[9]

The amount of fat consumed by lactating women does not greatly affect the total fat concentration of breast-milk, since women on the low-fat, high-carbohydrate diets characteristic of developing countries can synthesize fatty acids from glucose in the breast. This results in a greater proportion of medium-chain fatty acids, (e.g. lauristic and myristic acids) compared with women on high-fat diets, in whom the fatty acid composition of breast-milk resembles that of the diet. In women with very low energy intakes, breast-milk fatty acid composition is similar to that of the body fat stores, indicating mobilization of body fat for breast-milk synthesis.

Water-soluble vitamins (thiamine, riboflavin, vitamin C, folic acid, B_6, pantothenic acid, B_{12}) and to a lesser extent, fat-soluble vitamins (A and D), tend to occur in lower concentration in breast-milk from mothers in developing countries, reflecting low maternal dietary intake. Little is known of mineral and trace element composition of breast-milk, but calcium concentrations may be lower in mothers from developing countries.

Factors influencing breast-milk quantity and quality

Maternal nutrition

The gross composition of breast-milk from women in developing countries is comparable with that of Western mothers, although the amount of milk produced appears to be slightly less. The similarity in breast-milk production and the ability of mothers from poorer nations to undergo repeated, prolonged lactation is perhaps surprising considering that women in many developing countries apparently subsist on diets providing only 40 to 70 per cent of the energy intakes of well-nourished lactating western women (an average of 1600 cal/day compared with 2300 cal/day).[10]

Nevertheless, comparison of well-nourished and deprived groups in the same country and observations on lactational output during seasonal decreases in food availability, suggest that poor maternal nutrition may be the cause of smaller breast-milk yields; and where nutritional intake is very low, milk composition may also be affected.

Numerous studies have sought to test this hypothesis experimentally by supplementing the mother's nutritional intake during lactation. Such intervention studies have yielded contradictory results which are difficult to interpret due to differences in study design, type and quantity of supplements and duration of supplementation. The evidence for 'feed the nursing mother, thereby the infant' is weak, since although two-thirds of the studies reported some improvement, the increase in milk yields was small and in two studies accompanied by a decrease in nutrient content. Vitamin supplementation did appear to increase vitamin concentrations in breast-milk, but improvement of the maternal diet generally had little positive effect on energy, protein, fat and lactose concentrations in breast-milk. As a practical intervention to improve milk output and gross composition, supplementation of lactating mothers does not therefore seem to be cost-effective.[7]

The lack of success of such interventions may have been because the amounts of supplements provided were not sufficient to increase dietary intake significantly, or because supplements were provided over too short a time. However, even in a long-term study carried out in the Gambia in which net energy intakes of lactating mothers were increased by 46 per cent (over 700 cal/day), and protein raised to well above the daily WHO recommended allowance (thus eradicating the energy and protein deficit during the 'hungry season'), the effect of supplementation on milk volume was negligible. The effects on composition were also small: milk protein increased by 7 per cent but total energy showed no change (an 8 per cent increase in fat was offset by an 8 per cent decrease in lactose).[11] Mothers did, however, derive some benefit from the supplementation programme in that they reported fewer ailments and greater 'well-being'.

The extra energy and protein provided in the form of supplements during the Gambian study did not appear to be used to increase milk production or substantially increase fat stores, since the average net weight gain of supplemented mothers was 1.8 kg, which if weight gain was due to deposition of adipose tissue, would account for only 7 per cent of the extra energy consumed.

It has been suggested that the ability of mothers on very low calorie diets to produce milk volumes only slightly less than those of well-nourished mothers, may be due to raised maternal metabolic efficiency[12] and preferential channelling of nutrients to the breast through elevated prolactin levels, and that when extra energy is provided, much is wasted through relaxation of metabolic efficiency. A reduction in physical activity is also likely to be an effective method of adjusting to low energy intakes, but this did not appear to be the case in the Gambia, where lactating women were as active as non-pregnant, non-lactating women except during the traditional postpartum month of confinement.

The poor diets of women in many parts of the world are cause for concern, since there clearly are costs to functioning at such an extreme level of efficiency. Low energy intakes during pregnancy, for example, result in small babies, with all the attendant problems associated with low birth weight. However, since milk production does not seem to be strongly limited by maternal nutrition during the period of lactation, attention to mechanisms which control the infant's 'demand' for milk may offer an alternative approach to improving lactational output.

Infant demand

Frequency of breast-feeding

Very large milk volumes, averaging 1000 ml/day (after adjustments have been made for the test-weighing method used) have been reported for Australian mothers who belong to breast-feeding support groups. Wet nurses and mothers suckling twins also produce large quantities of breast-milk. It has been argued that such outputs are potentially achievable by any woman, provided that true 'demand-feeding' is practiced, i.e. the infant feeds frequently and the breast is emptied at each feed.[9] Frequent feeding has been found to increase breast-milk output up to the first month of life and in populations where there is a wide range in the number of breast-feeds, infants who feed more frequently or suckle for longer consume more milk. The physiological basis for this effect appears to be that sucking stimulates secretion of prolactin, which in turn increases milk yield.[13]

It is generally thought that limits to feeding do not occur in traditional 'demand-feeding' societies, where the timing and duration of feeding are supposedly dictated by the infant's demand rather than the mother's schedule. In reality, the baby's access to the breast may be limited by the mother's need to resume her usual work as the baby grows older, or by seasonal increases in farming activities. Thus, even in traditional societies, opportunities for breast-feeding during the daytime may be controlled by the mother. This may provide an alternative explanation for the decrease in milk outputs observed in some countries during the 'hungry' season; this is the time of heaviest farm work, when the mother is forced to spend much of the day away from her child.

In many traditional societies the infant has free access to the breast at night since mother and infant sleep side-by-side. Night-time feeding is then more under the control of the infant, and as the amount of milk taken during the daytime decreases, night-time feeding makes an increasingly important contribution to total breast-milk intake as the infant grows older.[18] In industrialized countries, however, night-time milk intake decreases with increasing age due to the practice of cutting out night-feeds to ensure an uninterrupted night's sleep for the mother.[2]

Supplementary food

A further major influence on lactation is supplementary feeding. The timing of first introduction of supplements is very variable; in a study of nine countries, supplementary foods were commonly given well before the age of six months.[2] Traditionally, supplements may be introduced at a particular age for cultural or religious reasons. In general, this would be part of the process of weaning the infant from breast-milk on to solid foods, during which a gradual decline in the number of breast-feeds is paralleled by an increase in the number of supplementary feeds. However, mothers may start to introduce supplements unusually early, or give breast-milk substitutes, if they feel that their infant is not growing well or that their milk supply is no longer sufficient to supply the baby's needs, for example, if the baby appears to be hungry after breast-feeding.

In this case, supplementary foods should ideally contribute extra nutrients to those received from breast-milk. However, some studies have shown that young infants receiving supplements consume less breast-milk than exclusively breast-fed infants of the same age, and that when the number of supplementary feeds is increased, the number of breast-feeds decreases. Rather than truly supplementing breast-feeding, early feeding of supplements may only substitute for breast-feeds, perhaps a deliberate policy by the mother to release her from breast-feeding, and so permit her to resume work activities. If supplementary foods are of poor nutrient quality and low energy density, there is a danger that total nutrient intake will fail to meet the needs of the growing infant, leading to malnutrition.

The early replacement of breast-feeds by bottle-feeds

or supplements may decrease milk intake and eventually reduce milk production, since the suckling stimulus which maintains milk synthesis will be diminished. A downward spiral of reduced milk production encouraging greater use of supplements and consequently even further reduction in milk output may result.

Infant size

If the baby has free access to the breast, and maternal milk production is not limited, intake will depend on the infant's appetite. Correlational studies have shown that larger (heavier) infants consume more milk than smaller infants of the same age, and that among young infants, those who were heavier at birth consume more than infants of lower birth weight. However, the direction of such associations is not clear: larger infants may have bigger appetites and be better at withdrawing milk from the breast; alternatively, consumption of more milk may result in a heavier infant. A second possibility is that the association between milk intake and infant weight is due to maternal nutrition during pregnancy, which influences birth weight and might also affect subsequent lactation performance.

Morbidity

Providing that the mother does not deliberately reduce breast-feeding when the baby is ill, infections do not usually affect breast-milk intake, although intake of solid foods is often reduced.[14] Some infants may not be able to suck effectively if they are too weak and tire easily (e.g. due to malnutrition or cardiac disease) or if they are neurologically impaired. Such infants consume little milk, which is likely to result in decreased maternal milk production due both to inadequate stimulation of the nipple and inadequate removal of milk from the breast. Maternal anxiety about the health and well-being of the infant may also interfere with milk production by inhibiting the oxytocin-mediated milk ejection reflex.

Hormonal contraception

While breast-feeding confers a degree of protection against conception, the effect appears to be less pronounced in well-nourished mothers and cannot be guaranteed for the individual.[13] Breast-feeding mothers therefore still require advice on contraceptive methods, especially after the first two months of lactation.

High dosages of combined oestrogen–progesterone oral contraceptives have been found to depress milk yield and also decrease protein, fat, lactose, and mineral content of breast-milk while low-dose progesterone-only pills do not appear to adversely affect lactation. Depot-medroxyprogesterone acetate (DMPA) is a long-acting injectable contraceptive widely used in developing countries. Doses of 300 mg given at six-month intervals appear to increase milk volume while decreasing fat, protein and calcium concentrations.[15] DMPA is also secreted into the breast-milk at concentrations approaching maternal plasma levels, but so far no adverse effects on infants have been reported. These results suggest caution in recommending hormonal contraceptives. Where there is no alternative to birth control by pharmacological means, low-dose progesterone-only pills are least risky, since concentrations in breast-milk are very low, and there are no apparent effects on lactation.

Conclusions

The World Health Organization recommends that infants should be exclusively breast-fed for the first four months of life. Present information suggests that the quantity and quality of milk produced are not greatly limited by maternal nutrition during lactation, except in the most severe circumstances; however, the maternal diet does influence the vitamin content of breast-milk. Milk intake can be maintained by allowing the infant maximum access to the breast, and encouraging frequent feeding, especially at night. Supplementary foods should be introduced to augment nutritional intake rather than replace breast-feeds, at least in the first few months of life, to avoid reducing milk intake and impairing milk production. If hormonal contraceptives are prescribed they should be low dose, and preferably progesterone only. Changes in hospital routine, national breast-feeding promotion programmes, legislation to protect women's rights, facilities for breast-feeding in places of work, and local information, counselling and support schemes are all methods by which the prevalence and duration of breast-feeding can be increased.[15,16,17]

References

1. WHO. *The Quantity and Quality of Breastmilk.* Geneva, WHO, 1985.
2. WHO. *Contemporary Patterns of Breastfeeding.* Geneva, WHO, 1981.
3. Ashworth A, Feachem RG. Interventions for the control of diarrhoeal diseases among young children: improving lactation. *Bulletin of the World Health Organization.* 1985; **63**: 165–84.
4. Imong SM, Jackson DA, Woolridge MW *et al.* Indirect test-weighing: a new method for measuring overnight breastmilk intakes in the field. *Journal of Pediatric Gastro-enterology.* 1988; **7**:699–706.
5. Coward WA, Cole TJ, Sawyer MB, Prentice AM. Breast-milk intake measurement in mixed-fed infants by administration of deuterium oxide to their mothers. *Human Nutrition, Clinical Nutrition.* 1982; **36C**: 141–8.
6. Woolridge MW, Jackson DA, Imong SM *et al.* Indirect test-weighing: a non-intrusive technique for estimating night-time breastmilk intake. *Human Nutrition, Clinical Nutrition.* 1987; **41C**: 347–61.
7. Whitehead RG. Effect of diet on maternal health and lactational performance. In: Whitehead RG ed. *Maternal Diet, Breastfeeding Capacity and Lactational Infertility.* United Nations University, 1983. pp. 24–53.
8. Jackson DA, Imong SM, Ruckphaopunt S *et al.* Circadian variation in fat concentration of breast milk in a rural Northern Thai population. *British Journal of Nutrition.* 1988; **59**: 349–63.
9. Hartmann PE, Rattigan S, Saint L, Supriyana O. Variation in the yield and composition of human milk. *Oxford Review of Reproductive Biology.* 1985; **7**: 118–67.
10. Whitehead RG. Measured dietary intakes of lactating women in different parts of the world. In: Whitehead RG ed. *Maternal Diet, Breastfeeding Capacity and Lactational Infertility.* United Nations University. 1983. pp. 12–23.
11. Prentice AM, Roberts SB, Prentice A *et al.* Dietary supplementation of lactating Gambian women. I. Effect on breastmilk volume and quality. *Human Nutrition, Clinical Nutrition.* 1983; **37C**: 53–64.
12. Illingworth PJ, Jung RT, Howie PW *et al.* Diminution in energy expenditure during lactation. *British Medical Journal.* 1986; **292**: 437–41.
13. McNeilly AS, Lunn PG, Delgado H. The role of prolactin on the contraceptive effect of lactation and the influence of breastfeeding practices and of maternal dietary status. In: Whitehead RG ed. *Maternal Diet, Breastfeeding Capacity and Lactational Infertility.* United Nations University, 1983. pp. 72–81.
14. Martorell C, Yarbrough C, Yarbrough S, Klein RE. The impact of ordinary illness on the dietary intakes of malnourished children. *American Journal of Clinical Nutrition.* 1980; **33**: 345–50.
15. Laukaran VH. Breastfeeding and the use of contraceptives. *Outlook.* 1985; **3**: 2–5.
16. Feachem RG, Koblinsky MA. Interventions for the control of diarrhoeal diseases among young children: promotion of breastfeeding. *Bulletin of the World Health Organization.* 1984; **62**: 271–91.
17. Lechtig A, Jelliffe DB, Jelliffe EF. The first workshop on national breastfeeding programmes in Latin America. *Journal of Tropical Paediatrics.* 1986; **32**: 274–5.
18. Imong SM, Jackson DA, Wongsawasdii L, *et al. Journal of Pediatric Gastroenterology and Nutrition.* 1989; **8**:359–70.

CHAPTER 3

Prenatal health

Michael Chan

Fetal growth

The birth weight at term of a baby of an elite well-nourished mother anywhere in the world is more than 3 kg. Any newborn baby whose birth weight is less than 2.5 kg is classified as being of low birth weight. Delivery before full-term or 37 completed weeks of gestation is one cause of a neonate being of low birth weight; such an infant is a preterm baby. A term infant of low birth weight is one who is small-for-gestational dates (SFD). Preterm low-birth-weight babies are usually appropriate for gestational dates but some are both preterm and small-for-gestational dates. Any newborn infant weighing 1.5 kg or less is called a very-low-birth-weight baby (VLBW), and one weighing 1 kg or less is an extremely-low-birth-weight baby (ELBW).

Factors affecting growth

Most normal fetuses have similar rates of growth during the first two trimesters of pregnancy. Slowing of fetal growth usually occurs in the last trimester when one-third of the birth weight is acquired. Factors affecting fetal growth are to be found in the fetus, the mother or the environment.

Environmental factors

Women living at high altitude, such as the Andes in Colombia, are shorter and lighter than their sisters at sea-level, and tend to give birth to low-birth-weight babies. Low social class women have the highest frequency of small-for-gestational dates babies related to a number of adverse maternal factors.

Maternal factors

Nutrition A baby's birth weight is influenced by the size of the mother. Small women tend to give birth to low-birth-weight babies. Maternal size is an indicator of the quality of nutrition the mother had as a girl. Improving the nutrition of girls leads to increase in birth weights of their babies, as observed in emigrant Japanese in America.

Birth weight shows a greater relationship to the weight of the mother before pregnancy than to weight gained during pregnancy. In a study in Uganda, maternal weight of less than 55 kg was associated with an increase in the number of low-birth-weight infants compared with heavier women.[1] For a given maternal weight, mothers who are taller give birth to heavier babies than shorter women. Thin mothers who give birth to small-for-dates babies are less able to mobilize their fat stores than mothers of normal weight babies. Energy intake during pregnancy influences fetal growth in thin women, as demonstrated in Birmingham Asian mothers receiving food supplements in the last trimester of pregnancy. Heavier babies were born to thin mothers who had shown poor weight gain and little increase in triceps skin fold thickness earlier in pregnancy. Well-nourished mothers of similar height did not benefit.[2]

Maternal undernutrition must be severe before fetal growth is affected. Observations during the acute famine in Holland in 1944–5, showed that fetal growth was affected when maternal food intake was under 1500 calories a day during the last trimester of pregnancy. There was a decrease of 300 to 400 g in birth weight and these infants had a significant increase in mortality during their first three months but with no long-term effects in the survivors. Women who were in their first trimester of pregnancy during the famine had more stillbirths or premature deliveries with increased death rate.

Chronic undernutrition of mothers is common in developing countries. Fetal tissues take priority over the mother's body when there is an energy deficit. Supplementing the diet of malnourished mothers who are protein or energy deficient can increase the baby's weight at birth. In a study in Guatemala, dietary supplementation of malnourished mothers in the latter half of pregnancy reduced the incidence of low-birth-weight babies by 40 per cent.[3] The greatest gains were associated with increased calorie intake. The effects on birth weight may be more marked if a food supplement is given at an earlier stage of pregnancy and if it is sustained throughout gestation as shown by the studies in the Gambia[4]. (See pp. 324–35). High-protein food supplements alone have proved harmful in some pregnancies, increasing the risk of deliveries before 30 weeks of gestation and of neonatal death.[5] But a supplement enriched with protein will not be harmful if recommended dietary allowances are followed within the framework of a regular diet.

Some mothers of small-for-gestational dates babies have an eightfold increased risk of another SFD infant in subsequent pregnancies.

Age Young teenage mothers and women over 35 years of age tend to have low-birth-weight babies.

Parity First babies usually weigh less than their siblings.

Chronic disease Impaired transfer of nutrients through the placenta occurs in mothers with hypertension, pre-eclampsia, renal disease and poorly controlled diabetes mellitus.

Alcohol and smoking The adverse effects of cigarette smoking on the placenta are probably mediated through nicotine and carbon monoxide and lead to chronic fetal deficiency of oxygen and retardation of intrauterine growth. These result in a decrease in birth weight and an SFD baby.

The daily consumption of 45 ml of absolute alcohol by a pregnant woman will lead to slow fetal growth, increase in preterm delivery and fetal malformations. Alcoholic mothers who drink 90 ml of absolute alcohol daily tend to produce babies with features of the fetal-alcohol syndrome – severe stunting, microcephaly, mental retardation and typical facies of maxillary hypoplasia, short palpebral fissures, ptosis, squint and hairy face.

Fetal factors

Boys are born heavier than girls by about 140 g at full-term, because of their faster growth after 36 weeks of gestation.

In multiple pregnancies such as twins, fetal growth is slower after 32 weeks gestation compared with singletons. Abnormal fetuses with genetic defects or intrauterine infections suffer growth retardation by the middle of the second trimester. Congenital defects are found in 3–5 per cent of SFD infants. Hormones, particularly thyroxine and insulin, influence growth in the latter half of pregnancy. Thyroxine deficiency results in a reduction in body length, delayed ossification of bones and impaired brain maturation. Insulin excess increases the laying down of fat in the fetus, as seen in the infant of a poorly controlled diabetic mother. Infants of women with gestational diabetes (prediabetic women) tend to be large and have macrosomia. Lack of insulin production causes severe growth retardation.

Intrauterine growth retardation

Intrauterine growth retarded newborn infants are usually defined as those whose birth weights are less than the 3rd centile for gestational age. Body weight and gestational age distribution curves are available for boys and girls of most European populations. In the absence of growth charts for race-specific populations in developing countries, standards such as Fig. 2.3.1 may be used in the subtropics and tropics.

Growth retardation experiments in animals suggest that for tissue such as brain with only a limited period when cell multiplication can occur, growth restriction at this sensitive time would result in permanent stunting. If growth restriction occurs throughout the period of brain growth, there is also permanent stunting of body growth. No satisfactory explanation has so far been found to explain the stunting of body growth in association with restricted growth during the period of brain growth.

In a large series of postmortem studies on intra-uterine growth retarded newborns (birth weight more than two standard deviations below the mean), Gruenwald[6] found all organs of these babies were lighter than expected, but the brain was least affected and the liver and thymus most affected. These infants had relatively large heads, a moderate reduction in length and the greatest reduction in weight. Recent studies show that they have thinner than normal skin folds. They account for the majority of SFD infants in developed countries, are described as asymmetrically growth retarded and are the result of growth failure during the last trimester of pregnancy. Growth retarded infants with equal reduction in brain and body size, and

normal skin fold thickness are described as symmetrically growth retarded; they are the product of chronic placental insufficiency and growth failure before the last trimester.

Intrauterine growth retardation contributes to a substantial proportion of infants of low birth weight (<2500 g) in some developing countries in Asia and Latin America. Fetal malnutrition is the cause of intrauterine growth retardation in these developing countries. The incidence of intrauterine growth retardation was reported as 24 per cent in a poor urban population of Guatemala city.[7] Many studies underestimate the incidence of intrauterine growth retardation because they do not include infants whose birth weights fall below the 3rd centile but who weigh more than 2500 g.

Asymmetrically and symmetrically growth retarded infants can be distinguished at birth using the formula weight/length $^3 \times 100$, described by Rohrer[8] as the ponderal index. Data from Guatemala City on 848 intrauterine growth retarded newborns analysed by the ponderal index (PI) showed 177 (20.8 per cent) had PI below the 10th percentile (indicating subacute fetal malnutrition) and 671 (79.1 per cent) had PI values above the 10th percentile (indicating chronic fetal malnutrition).[7] The same PI analysis applied to a rural Guatemala population of 143 intrauterine growth

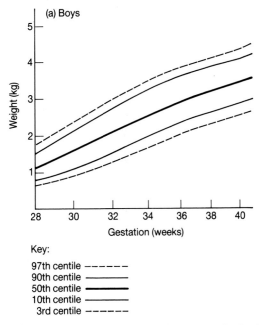

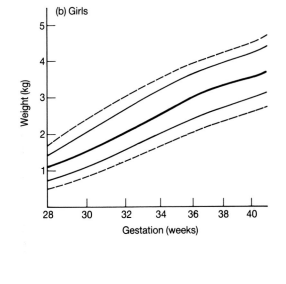

Key:

97th centile – – – – –
90th centile ————
50th centile ▬▬▬▬
10th centile ————
3rd centile – – – – –

Fig. 2.3.1   Body weight and gestational age distribution curve for British boys and girls. (After Gairdner D and Pearson J 1985, *Archives of Diseases in Childhood*; **60**. © Castlemead Publications).

retarded newborns, found 68.5 per cent to have chronic fetal malnutrition, and among 188 rural South African infants, 67.5 per cent were chronically malnourished *in utero*. Infants with chronic fetal malnutrition remain lighter, shorter, and with smaller head circumference till at least three years of age. They also score the lowest in tests of mental development from three years to school age. Villar and his colleagues make the gloomy prediction that in Latin America at least 2 million infants born every year are, already destined at birth, to remain undergrown and underdeveloped[7]. Similar studies are required in other developing countries to monitor and prevent chronic fetal malnutrition.

Antenatal detection of fetal growth retardation

Poor weight gain during pregnancy is common in developing countries; mothers may put on no more than 6 kg instead of the 12 kg gained by their counterpart in industrialized countries. The result of this insufficient weight gain during pregnancy is a greater risk of growth retarded babies of low birth weight. Accurate assessment of intrauterine growth depends on the ability to measure fetal maturity and fetal size accurately. If a pregnant woman is sure of her menstrual dates, prediction of the expected date of delivery is correct to within 14 days in 90 per cent of cases. Many women in developing countries are not sure of their dates because of irregular periods or frequent pregnancies. The measurement of symphysis – fundal height plotted on a graph can detect intrauterine growth retardation as early as 28 weeks. Symphysis – fundal graphs are simple to use and indicate when to refer a patient for an ultrasound check.[9] Ultrasonography is the most accurate method of assessing fetal maturity in these circumstances. In the first trimester, crown–rump length is measured and in the second trimester, before 20 weeks, biparietal diameter gives accurate assessment of fetal maturity by ultrasound.

Fetal loss

There is a paucity of information on the epidemiology and pathology of fetal loss in developing countries. However, it is generally accepted that fetal death or stillbirths occur in late gestation (from 28 weeks onwards) or intrapartum during labour and delivery. Stillborn fetuses in late gestation are usually macerated with no specific lesions found in many of them. Congenital malformations and lesions corresponding to asphyxia are found in a minority of these macerated fetuses. About 5 per cent of stillbirths and perinatal deaths have abnormal chromosomes and an equal number have malformations.

Deaths of normal fetuses occur in late gestation because of failure of placental function. Tests of placental function measuring placental hormone levels are not feasible in developing countries. However, failure of fetal growth may be detected with ultrasonography and the fetus delivered before term by surgery to prevent fetal loss. Haematological disorders associated with isoimmune haemolysis from incompatible blood groups or of a non-isoimmune basis (homozygous α-thalassaemia) lead to hydrops fetalis and fetal deaths.

Intrapartum fetal deaths are mainly a result of asphyxia due to prolonged labour. In developing countries, where the majority of births take place unsupervised by a trained attendant at home, intrapartum fetal deaths from asphyxia account for a disproportionately large number of stillbirths. These fetal losses are eminently preventable by primary health care of pregnant women in the antenatal period, during labour and timely intervention by assisted delivery, details of which are given on pp. 136–53. Congenital defects and isoimmune disorders are found in a minority of intrapartum fetal deaths.

Congenital defects

Major malformations are found in 2 per cent of infants at birth and the incidence rises to about 5 per cent with congenital defects detected later in childhood. A major malformation has serious medical, surgical or cosmetic consequences. A recognized pattern of malformations with a known cause is called a syndrome. About half the major congenital defects found in newborn infants have a genetic basis attributable to chromosome abnormalities (Down's syndrome, etc.), single mutant genes (achondroplasia) and multifactorial inheritance (cleft lip and palate, cardiac defects).

There are certain congenital defects that are particularly common amongst people in the tropics and subtropics. Polydactyly is common in African infants. Cleft lip with or without cleft palate has ethnic differences in its frequency: it is high (3 or 4 in 1000 livebirths) in Orientals (Chinese, Japanese), intermediate (1 in 1000) in Europeans and low in Africans. These frequencies persist after migration from their homelands, suggesting that the defect is genetic in origin. Consanguinity is practised in several ethnic groups in the Indian subcontinent and in the Middle East with unions between first cousins or uncles and nieces accounting for more than half of their marriages. Uncle–niece marriages are unique to Southern India. There is evidence in Britain that consanguinity increases perinatal mortality due to congenital malformations in the Pakistani communities of Bradford[10] and Birmingham.[11] Consanguinity increases the incidence of rare recessive conditions, and to a lesser extent, of multifactorial or polygenic disorders.

Teratogens

Agents that injure the developing fetus and induce congenital defects are teratogens. They include drugs, hormones, vitamins, poisons, radiation and alcohol. Information on teratogenic agents has come from animal experiments, some observations made as long ago as 1930, when pigs born to sows on a diet deficient in vitamin A were found to lack eyeballs. Before 1962, when the effects of thalidomide on the human fetus became evident, teratogens were discovered accidentally. Since the thalidomide disaster when affected babies were born with limb abnormalities, all drugs prescribed during pregnancy have been kept to a minimum and their teratogenic potential monitored. Antimetabolic and antineoplastic agents are potent teratogens. Vitamin A is a unique teratogen because both excess and deficiency of the vitamin produce deformities of the central nervous system (CNS) in animals.

Factors that determine teratogenesis are the age of the fetus when the agent acts on it and the dosage. The vulnerable period for producing malformations in the human fetus is between the 21st and 36th days of pregnancy, when the neural tube is open and limbs and organs are in a critical phase of development. The timing of malformations is exact, with only a day separating the formation of defects of the heart from those of the kidney. The dosage effect may be seen with alcohol where the equivalent of 45 ml consumed daily by the pregnant mother slows fetal growth and 90 ml daily may result in a baby with microcephaly, mental retardation and typical facies.

Pathogens that infect the fetus, particularly rubella virus, *Toxoplasma gondii*, *Treponema pallidum*, cytomegalovirus and herpesvirus, produce congenital defects of major consequence (see pp. 163–74). Many young women in the tropics do not have antibodies against rubella and would benefit from vaccination to prevent their future babies being affected with congenital deafness, cardiac defects, cataracts, and microcephaly. Maternal diabetes mellitus predisposes to congenital malformations. Amniotic constrictive bands cause limb defects and oligohydramnios leads to compression and postural congenital defects such as club feet

and torticollis. Neural tube defects are now thought to be related to folic acid deficiency and trials are in progress in Britain where women are being given folic acid supplements during pregnancy and compared with a control group. No cause is detectable in about 40 per cent of congenital malformations such as intestinal atresias, exomphalos and diaphragmatic hernia.

Management

Every infant with a major congenital defect should have a diagnostic evaluation to detect genetic causes and environmental factors. Some malformations of the heart, limbs and intestines are amenable to surgical correction, and usually require transfer to a specialist unit with a paediatric surgeon. Complicated congenital malformations, however, will continue to contribute to perinatal and neonatal mortality, as they do in developed countries. Prenatal diagnosis of severe malformation of the CNS, such as anencephalus and myelomeningocele with measurement of serum α-fetoproteins and ultrasound diagnosis in the fourth month of pregnancy, followed by abortion of the affected fetus, has been a factor in the reduction of the number of babies born with neural tube defects in the UK. However, even before these measures were introduced, a decline in neural tube defects had begun.

Prenatal diagnosis

Prenatal diagnosis to detect an affected fetus in order to terminate the pregnancy is practised in most industrialized and some developing countries. The steps in prenatal diagnosis are to visualize the fetus, usually by ultrasonography, and to obtain fetal tissue, blood or fluid for biochemical or cytogenetic analysis, using amniocentesis, chorionic villus sampling, or fetoscopy and fetal blood sampling. Chorionic villus sampling was pioneered in China in the 1960s and is now the preferred method of prenatal diagnosis because it is done at seven to nine weeks of gestation through the cervix, either by aspiration through a cannula under ultrasound control or under direct vision using an endoscope. Once an adequate sample is obtained, the maternal decidua is carefully removed to leave chorionic villi derived from the zygote. Chromosome preparations can be made rapidly for identification, e.g. of Down's syndrome, and DNA samples for the diagnosis of autosomal dominant disorders (tuberous sclerosis, neurofibromatosis), autosomal recessive conditions (thalassaemia, sickle cell disease), and X-linked diseases (haemophilia, Duchenne muscular dystrophy).

The application of prenatal diagnosis in developing countries depends not only on the level of cytogenetic technology but also on the national population control policies and the religious beliefs of the people.

PRENATAL INFECTIONS

Many infections occurring in pregnancy may be sub-clinical and their adverse effects limited to the fetus and newborn infant. The agents known to cause fetal infection are listed in Table 2.3.1. (See also pp. 600–23.)

Clinical and pathological findings in newborn infants who have experienced intrauterine infection in early gestation include:

- prematurity or low birth weight at term;
- developmental anomalies in the cardiovascular system, central nervous system, and skeleton;
- florid peri- and postnatal infection with inflammation such as adenitis, encephalitis, hepatitis, pneumonia;
- IgM antibodies in umbilical cord blood;
- prolonged virus shedding in secretions and excretions;
- late onset diseases such as juvenile diabetes and possibly malignant tumours.

There is an overlap in the clinical features of congenital toxoplasmosis, rubella, cytomegalovirus, herpes, and syphilis (the TORCHES group) in the neonatal period. These infections all cause congenital disease with defects of varying degree. They may present with the following features in common: skin rash, jaundice, hepatosplenomegaly, central nervous system involvement, and radiological changes in the growing ends of bones. The frequency of these infections is high in children and adults in the tropics.

Table 2.3.1 Agents causing fetal infection

Viruses	Bacteria
Rubella virus	*Listeria monocytogenes*
Cytomegalovirus	*Mycobacterium tuberculosis*
Hepatitis B virus	*Treponema pallidum*
Ebstein–Barr virus	
Herpesvirus hominis	**Parasites**
Human immunodeficiency	Filaria
virus (HIV)	Malaria
Vaccinia virus	*Toxoplasma gondii*
Variola virus	Trypanosomes
Varicella-zoster virus	
Poliovirus	
Parvovirus B19	

The diagnosis of fetal infections depends upon the recovery of the infecting agent and/or the detection of raised immunoglobulin M (IgM) which does not cross the placenta from mother to fetus. Although produced in small amounts by the normal fetus, IgM is the first immunoglobulin to be produced after infection and is found in high concentrations in the fetus subject to intrauterine infection.

Congenital rubella

The teratogenic effects of the rubella virus were first reported in 1940 by Gregg[12] who described the association between neonatal cataracts and first trimester maternal rubella infection. These infants were often deaf and had congenital heart disease.

Pathogenesis

When a pregnant woman is infected, the rubella virus passes through the placenta to affect the fetus. The virus disseminates in the fetus and persists in tissues until some time after delivery. The earlier the infection occurs in pregnancy, the more likely the risk of fetal damage. Stigmata of congenital rubella in the neonate decreases from 75 per cent of seropositive infants whose mother was infected in the first two months of pregnancy, to 52 per cent in the third month and 17 per cent in the fourth month. Congenital rubella is rare after 20 weeks of gestation.

The extent of fetal damage is also related to the stage of pregnancy when infection occurs. Multiple defects are more likely to be seen in a fetus infected in the first 12 weeks. Deafness may be the only defect associated with infection beyond 16 weeks.

Neonatal signs and symptoms

Jaundice, thrombocytopaenic purpura and hepato-splenomegaly are usually present in the newborn infant, together with eye abnormalities, heart murmur and CNS signs. Intrauterine growth retardation is present in one-third of these infants. The full spectrum of congenital rubella defects is shown in Fig. 2.3.2. Eye defects include cataracts and microphthalmos, with glaucoma developing in a small proportion. Cardio-vascular defects are a result of endothelial damage of large blood vessels and produce a high incidence of patent ductus arteriosus and peripheral pulmonary artery stenosis. Central nervous system effects include microcephaly, cerebral palsy and mental retardation. Deafness may be the only defect and is usually

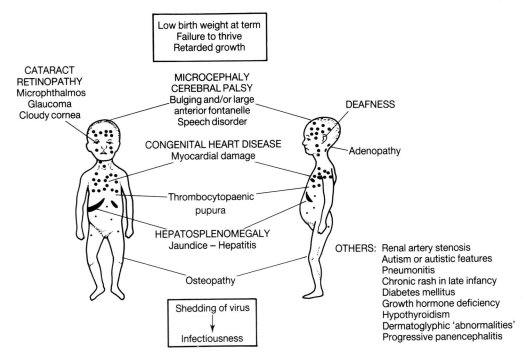

Fig. 2.3.2   Manifestations of congenital rubella.

sensorineural and bilateral. Hepatitis with prolonged jaundice may be seen in some cases. Thrombocytopaenic purpura is found in most cases at birth but does not persist after the neonatal period. Radiographic examination of the long bones shows irregular translucencies and an irregular trabecular pattern ('celery stalk').

Late presentation

Congenital rubella is a potentially progressive condition and damage may not become apparent until infancy and childhood, e.g. hearing impairment may develop or deteriorate after birth. Many affected infants present beyond the neonatal period, particularly in developing countries. Therefore, infants with neurological and eye defects, deafness and congenital heart disease should be investigated for congenital rubella. Other forms of 'late onset' disease include rubelliform rash, interstitial pneumonitis, hypogammaglobulinaemia, thymic hypoplasia, encephalitis and diabetes mellitus, but these manifestations are infrequent.

Diagnosis

The diagnosis of congenital rubella can only be made by virus isolation from throat swab and urine (for up to 12 months of age) or by serology. The presence of raised levels of IgM in cord blood or in neonatal blood is suggestive of congenital infection by a number of agents. The presence of IgM rubella antibody indicates rubella infection and positive tests may be found up to six months of age. Rubella haemagglutination inhibition (HI) antibody persisting beyond six months of age when passively acquired maternal antibodies would have disappeared, is another useful method of diagnosis. The presence of antibody in a single serum sample between six months and three years of age can be useful retrospective evidence of congenital infection, as natural infection is uncommon during this period.

Prevention

Congenital rubella can be prevented by active rubella immunization of all susceptible school-age girls and women of childbearing age who are shown to have no rubella antibodies. Pregnancy should be avoided for three months after vaccination. Vaccination during pregnancy should be avoided because vaccine virus has been isolated from some fetuses. There is little or no evidence that the vaccine virus is teratogenic. Pregnant women suspected of having rubella should be investigated. The first sample of serum should be taken as soon as possible after exposure (within 10 days) and if there is detectable antibody the person may be considered immune as a result of past infection or immunization. If antibody is not detected a second specimen should be tested 14 to 21 days later. A fourfold rise in antibody titre denotes a recent rubella infection and therapeutic termination of pregnancy may be offered after the risk of an affected handicapped infant is explained. Administering immunoglobulin to such women is of no value.

Congenital cytomegalovirus (CMV)

Cytomegalovirus (CMV) is one of the herpes viruses, human (β) herpesvirus 5. Most healthy adults and children with CMV infection experience no symptoms or a mild illness of fever with or without respiratory symptoms. In Western countries such as the UK, Europe and North America the prevalence of CMV antibodies in adults is 30–50 per cent. However, in many tropical and subtropical countries almost all adults have CMV antibodies. Studies of children in developing countries indicate that all are infected by two to five years of age. Reactivation of latent CMV infection may occur during pregnancy in immune women and about 10 per cent may excrete virus from the cervix. In West Africa more than one per cent of women known to be seropositive before conception gave birth to infants with congenitally acquired CMV infection. This indicates that the presence of maternal antibody does not prevent congenital infection which has also been reported in consecutive pregnancies. However, analysis of fetal infections resulting from reactivation of latent CMV shows that damage is highly unlikely to occur in these infants.

Fetal damage is most likely to occur with primary maternal infection during the first half of pregnancy.[13] During primary CMV infection the virus will infect the fetus in 25–50 per cent of cases. In industrialized countries the rate of congenitally acquired CMV infections is between 0.5 and 1 per cent and the proportion of infants with clinical disease is between 0.05 and 0.1 per cent. Women with primary CMV infection in pregnancy infect their offspring through the placenta if they have depressed cell-mediated immunity to CMV. In contrast, the proportion of congenitally acquired infections in developing countries is well above 1 per cent but there is no evidence so far that these infections contribute towards the development of congenital anomalies.

Neonatal signs and symptoms

Of the 0.5 per cent of British neonates with congenital CMV infection the majority (90 per cent) are asymptomatic. In later childhood about 10 per cent of asymptomatic neonates become deaf. Severe disease is rare, but those affected have a high (20–30 per cent) infant mortality and those who survive are severely handicapped with microcephaly, blindness, deafness and mental retardation. Clinical features of congenital CMV disease are shown in Table 2.3.2.

There is no easy way to prevent the birth of babies damaged by CMV either by reliable prenatal diagnosis or an acceptable vaccine.

Herpesvirus hominis

Primary infections with Type I strains in adults are rare because of high prevalence of infection in childhood. Genital infections, mainly caused by Type 2 strains, present the greatest hazard to the neonate in lower socio-economic groups. Infection may occur from ascending infection following rupture of membranes or during the passage through an infected birth canal. Infants whose mothers acquire primary genital herpes in the third trimester are most at risk of low birth weight, preterm delivery, and neonatal infection.[14]

Neonatal clinical features

Three forms of perinatal disease have been recognized: localized superficial herpes, localized central nervous system disease, and disseminated herpes. In localized herpes, the infant presents towards the end of the first week with a vesicular skin rash, kerato-conjunctivitis, and vesicles in the mouth. There is no evidence of other systems being involved. Localized CNS disease presents with the above features together with

Table 2.3.2 Clinical features of congenital CMV disease

Low birth weight	Hepatosplenomegaly
Microcephaly	Hepatitis
Cerebral calcification	Jaundice
Chorioretinitis	Haemolytic anaemia
Encephalitis	Thrombocytopaenia
Hypotonia	Pneumonitis
Mental retardation	

non-specific signs of meningitis. Disseminated disease presents earlier in the first week, and half have neurological disease as well. Infants with disseminated disease are critically ill with hypotension, peripheral vasoconstriction, renal failure, jaundice with hepatosplenomegaly, respiratory symptoms (e.g. apnoea) because of underlying pneumonitis, and generalized bleeding associated with disseminated intravascular clotting.

Diagnosis

Vesicle fluid, CSF or conjunctival scrapings should be examined microscopically after Giemsa staining, for intranuclear inclusions. If possible, viral cultures should be done on vesicle fluid, CSF, urine and stool samples. The CSF may show typical changes of viral meningitis with up to 200 lymphocytes/mm^3 and minimal alteration of glucose and proteins.

Management

The antiviral agent acyclovir, given for at least 14 days, has been successful in reducing mortality and morbidity. Other antiherpetic agents such as adenine arabinoside, cytosine arabinoside and idoxuridine are all very toxic and are not recommended.

Avoidance of vaginal delivery reduces the frequency of herpesvirus hominis infection in the newborn, provided that when the membranes have already ruptured, Caesarean section is performed within four hours.

Medical and nursing staff with labial herpes or herpetic skin lesions should apply acyclovir cream to their lesions. They should probably not handle babies.

Human immunodeficiency virus (HIV)

Since 1981, there has been a dramatic increase in reports of human immunodeficiency virus (HIV) infection and acquired immuno-deficiency syndrome (AIDS) in men and women in subsaharan Africa. Some of the highest incidence rates of AIDS in the world have been reported from countries in central and East Africa. The World Health Organization's mid-1988 rates for AIDS reported on 1 August 1989, identified Zaire as the African country with the highest rate of 99 per 100 000 people, followed by Malawi with 51, Uganda 42, Burundi 38.5, Central African Republic 23, Rwanda 18.9, Kenya 18.8, Zambia 17.6 and Tanzania 17.3. The USA with a rate of 36.6 per 100 000 has the highest incidence of AIDS in the

Western world; France with 11.1 is the highest in Europe, and the UK has a rate of 3.55. The Health Minister of Kenya reported that seven new cases of AIDS were diagnosed each day of 1989 in his country, and an estimated 200 000 Kenyans were infected with HIV out of a population of 23 million. The survival of AIDS patients in Africa is very poor compared with that of North Americans, e.g. only 7.5 per cent of AIDS patients in Tanzania survived more than three months after diagnosis, compared with more than two years for most patients in the USA.

African women have a higher risk (about twice the rate) of HIV infection than men. In Kenya, for example, 25 per cent of prostitutes in three towns were infected but only 8 per cent of promiscuous men were seropositive in a survey in 1988. HIV infection is a sexually transmitted disease and, therefore, in most of Africa prostitutes are at highest risk. In Dar-es-Salam, capital of Tanzania, 42 per cent of women working in bars were infected in 1988, and this was double the infection rate in 1986.

Pregnant women in some African countries have a high incidence of HIV infection. In Kinshasa, Zaire, 8 per cent of pregnant women attending antenatal clinic were seropositive for HIV antibodies in 1984–5, and 8 per cent of infants in the first nine months of life were also seropositive.[4] Of more than a thousand women attending antenatal clinic in Kampala, Uganda, 13.4 per cent were HIV-positive in 1986, but the proportion had risen to 24 per cent by 1988. All babies of seropositive women received HIV antibodies transplacentally transferred, and one in three of these infants had died at the end of one year.

Pregnancy does not appear to make HIV-infected women more likely to develop full-blown AIDS.

Most cases of AIDS in children have been reported in offspring of mothers infected with HIV. Transplacental passage of the virus occurs in early (16 weeks) and late (36 weeks) gestation, and Caesarean section does not seem to protect the fetus from infection. The prevalence of HIV infection and AIDS in newborn babies of mothers with HIV antibodies has been increasing with longer follow-up studies. HIV-carrier mothers with symptoms have a higher chance of transmitting perinatal infection than asymptomatic mothers. Half of the babies aged six months born to intravenous drug-addicted mothers with HIV antibodies were seropositive in an Italian study. Not all infants born to intravenous heroin-addicted mothers with HIV infection are likely to be infected, unless maternal infection occurred during pregnancy. About 10 per cent of these infected infants develop AIDS during the first year with persistently enlarged lymph nodes, diarrhoea, failure to thrive and *Pneumocystis carinii* pneumonia. The prognosis for children with perinatal HIV infection must be assumed to be poor until suitable drug therapy is available. Meanwhile, perinatal HIV infection will increasingly become a major public health problem, particularly in Africa where an estimated 6000 babies infected with HIV were born in Zambia in 1987.[15]

Management

All the babies of HIV-carrier mothers should be breast-fed in developing countries. There is no convincing evidence that HIV infection occurs through breast-milk. Zidovudine, azidothymidine or AZT (3-azido-3-deoxythymidine) was licensed in 1987 for use in the management of serious manifestations of HIV infections in patients with AIDS or AIDS-related complex (ARC). The drug inhibits HIV replication by insertion of azidothymidine triphosphate into the developing chain of viral DNA. Zidovudine has so far been used only in adults and has been found to significantly reduce the death rate from AIDS. But serious toxic effects have been observed during the treatment of HIV-infected patients with zidovudine. Anaemia requiring blood transfusion, leucopaenia and neutropaenia have frequently led to reduction and discontinuation of the drug. These haematological complications are the result of bone marrow toxicity. Until the safety of zidovudine has been more extensively evaluated, its use is unlikely in asymptomatic infected children.

Acquired immunodeficiency syndrome, AIDS, is the disease attracting greatest attention in the world in the late 1980s. However, in spite of coordinated international research, little is known about this disease in developing countries. Efforts to develop a vaccine are unlikely to be rewarded for another decade. Therefore, prevention of this sexually transmitted disease in adults is the only means of controlling and reducing the incidence of perinatal HIV infection.

Varicella zoster virus

Congenital varicella

Mothers who develop chickenpox before the 20th week of pregnancy have given birth to infants with congenital varicella infection. Affected babies are small-for-dates, have cutaneous scars, limb and digit hypoplasia or atrophy, eye defects, convulsions, cortical atrophy and mental deficiency. Prognosis is poor with many dying in the perinatal period, and most survivors are handicapped. Direct damage to fetal tissue or its nerve supply by a varicella vesicle probably produces the congenital defects. Congenital varicella is probably extremely rare as most women with first trimester varicella either abort spontaneously or have a normal baby.

Perinatal varicella

Women who develop chickenpox within two or three weeks of delivery may infect their infants, and 20 per cent show signs of neonatal varicella. Babies born five or more days after the mother developed varicella will often be born with a chickenpox rash but have some transplacental immunity and so survive. Infants born within five days of the appearance of the maternal rash usually develop chickenpox 5–10 days after delivery and have a high death rate. Therefore, these infants should all receive a dose of zoster immune globulin (ZIG) 1.25 ml by intramuscular injection as soon after delivery as possible. This is followed by a course of acyclovir intravenously for at least 10 days.

Occasionally, newborn infants acquire varicella by contact with an infected child or adult. This form of neonatal chickenpox is mild and requires no treatment.

Syphilis

Fetal infection occurs in 40–50 per cent of women with primary syphilis. Infection in the mother may lead to spontaneous abortion, stillbirth, an infected infant without signs of disease at birth but developing later in life, or to the birth of a normal uninfected infant.

Clinical features

Many infants with congenital syphilis appear normal at birth and may only develop signs of the disease weeks, months, or occasionally, years later. Early features of congenital syphilis resemble the lesions of secondary syphilis in adults (see also pp. 590–1).

Early-onset congenital syphilis is a serious life-threatening disease and may present with anaemia, oedema, jaundice, failure to thrive and pyrexia, in the absence of typical mucocutaneous lesions and other local signs of the disease. Conversely, the infant may show florid mucocutaneous lesions without significant constitutional disturbance. Hepatomegaly is usual, and may be accompanied by splenomegaly and lymphadenopathy.

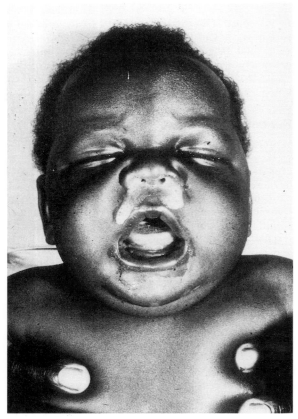

Fig. 2.3.3 Newborn infant with profuse nasal discharge 'snuffles' of congenital syphilis.

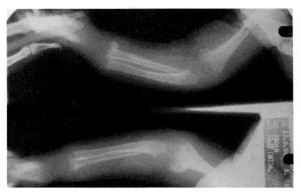

Fig. 2.3.4 Widespread periostitis of the radius and ulna in an infant with congenital syphilis.

Skin lesions are common but vary both in character and distribution. The rash is usually maculo-papular, but circinate lesions are the most characteristic eruptions seen. Involvement of the skin of palms and soles is usual and provides one of the most typical localizing features of the rash of congenital syphilis. The palms and soles become red, mottled, and swollen with superficial desquamation.

Rhinitis or 'snuffles' is a characteristic early sign (Fig. 2.3.3). Ulceration of nasal mucosa produces a profuse mucopurulent discharge which may be blood-stained, and produces excoriation around the nose and on the upper lip. Destruction of the nasal cartilage and bone will in time produce a flattened nasal bridge and the 'saddle-nose' of congenital syphilis.

Lesions at the mucocutaneous junctions of the mouth, nose, anus and vulva are common and produce moist fissuring and bleeding. Healing of deep fissures leads to radiating scars or rhagades, typical stigmata of congenital syphilis. Condylomata which are plaques with moist surfaces may occur around the anus and female genitals.

Osteochondritis, a frequent and typical sign may present as dactylitis, fracture, or pseudoparalysis. Radiological examinations of the bones around elbows, wrists and knees show multiple and widespread changes that help in the diagnosis of congenital syphilis (Fig. 2.3.4). Osteochondritis is evident by widening and alteration in density of the epiphyseal line, and by irregular destructive lesions in the epiphyseal end of the metaphyses. Widespread periostitis in bones of the limbs may also involve the skull. Radiological signs of congenital syphilis may not be evident in the neonatal period but become obvious during the early months of life. They may show spontaneous regression after the sixth month.

Meningitis and hydrocephalus may occur with congenital syphilis. Even when there is no clinical evidence of CNS involvement the CSF may be abnormal with a moderate increase in lymphocytes, increased protein, normal glucose and positive serological tests for syphilis.

Diagnosis

A high index of suspicion is required for clinical diagnosis. Radiological examination for typical bone changes is usually helpful. Fluid from skin lesions should be examined for *Treponema pallidum* on dark-ground microscopy. Serological tests for *Treponema pallidum* in developing countries may produce false-positive results in people who have been infected with *Treponema pertenue* or yaws. Infection with yaws provides some protection against syphilis. Diagnosis of congenital syphilis may be difficult in partially treated women. Seropositivity for syphilis in the young infant does not prove active disease because of transplacental transfer of maternal immunoglobulins. Conversely, negative serology in the newborn does not preclude the diagnosis of syphilis.

Management The following are indications for treatment:[16]

- Clinical and/or radiological signs of syphilis.
- Mother with syphilis:
  (a) untreated
  (b) inadequately treated
  (c) treatment status unknown
  (d) treatment with drugs other than penicillin.
- Infant apparently normal but serological titre rising or persistently high.
- Syphilis suspected but follow-up of infant cannot be ensured.

Penicillin is the drug of choice in treatment. Aqueous procaine penicillin 30 mg (50 000 units per kg body weight daily by intramuscular injection for 10 days) is the recommended regimen. Long-acting benzathine penicillin 60 mg (100 000 units per kg body weight) may be given in a single intramuscular dose if follow-up is not possible.

Tuberculosis

Tuberculosis is prevalent in almost all tropical developing countries and constitutes a special risk during pregnancy and lactation to mothers and babies (see also pp. 519–52). The management of an infant of an infected mother poses special problems. Isolation of the baby from the infected mother is usually not feasible and is, in any case, undesirable because it would inevitably signal the end of breast-feeding and expose the infant to all the hazards of artificial feeding. The policy advocated here for infants of tuberculous mothers has been proved effective, and is as follows:

- Maintain breast-feeding (except where this is precluded by the gravity of maternal illness).
- Treat the mother for tuberculosis.
- Give the infant prophylactic isoniazid in a single dose of 10 mg/kg daily. This prophylactic medication to continue until the mother is confirmed to be sputum-negative by repeated sputum examination.
- Carry out BCG immunization in the infant using isoniazid (INH) resistant BCG.

Results are best where infected mothers have been detected by antenatal screening and antituberculous treatment instituted during pregnancy.

Congenital tuberculosis

Criteria for the diagnosis of congenital tuberculosis were described by Beitzke in 1935.[17] There must be proof that the lesion is tuberculous, and in this regard a primary complex in the liver is usually of intrauterine origin. If the liver primary complex is absent, the infection should be obvious in the fetus or in the neonate at birth or during the first week. Neonatal tuberculosis is the result either of intrauterine infection or of inhalation of tubercle bacilli during or soon after birth through intimate contact with an adult with active pulmonary tuberculosis.

Transplacental infection occurs when the pregnant mother has clinical tuberculosis or a recent primary infection. In the former, miliary lesions are present in the placenta but not in the latter.

There is an absence of cellular response in the host, the primary focus and lymph nodes are caseous with abundant tubercle bacilli. The peripheries of the lesions contain few lymphocytes and no giant cells.

Clinical features

The neonate with congenital infection may present with hepatomegaly and jaundice due to obstruction of bile drainage by enlarged lymph nodes at the porta hepatis. The primary focus is in the liver but sometimes a primary complex is found in the lung due to dissemination through the ductus venosus.

The infant may also present with pneumonia (tachypnoea, cyanosis, moist sounds), anaemia and hepatosplenomegaly, with radiological evidence of widespread pulmonary infection involving both lungs, mediastinal and hilar lymph nodes. There is no liver lesion in this clinical syndrome, the source of infection probably being the amniotic fluid, maternal genital tract or mouth-to-mouth resuscitation by an adult with active pulmonary tuberculosis. Examination of the gastric aspirate for acid-fast bacilli is the best diagnostic test. The infected neonate is not sensitive to tuberculin.

Treatment

Isoniazid (20 mg/kg daily) combined with streptomycin (20 mg/kg daily) or rifampicin (10–20 mg/kg daily) together with a third drug is recommended. Rifampicin should not be given continuously for more than three months because of its effects on liver function, while streptomycin should be withdrawn after eight weeks as it is an ototoxic drug. Steroids have no place in treatment because of the lack of a host reaction. The infant with congenital tuberculosis should be vaccinated with isoniazid-resistant BCG to encourage active immunity. Breast-feeding should be encouraged and, if infected, mother must be treated with antituberculous drugs.

Toxoplasmosis

Toxoplasma gondii is a protozoal parasite whose whole life-cycle can be completed only in the intestine of the cat. Cats excrete millions of oocysts that become infective after maturation. These oocysts are ingested by cattle, sheep, pigs or other animals in whom spread and multiplication occurs in the same way in body tissues as in humans. Human infection is usually through eating infected pork or mutton that is raw or undercooked. Infection by contact with cats may play a role in rural regions and under conditions of poor hygiene (see also p. 934).

Infection with *T. gondii* during pregnancy may be asymptomatic or present as an influenza or glandular fever type of illness. The developing fetus may be infected at any stage of gestation but the risk is highest (70 per cent) in the third trimester. Infections in early pregnancy may cause abortions. Most damaged infants are infected in the first and second trimester. Severe congenital toxoplasmosis in the newborn presents as low birth weight at term, jaundice, hepatosplenomegaly, anaemia, thrombocytopaenia, meningoencephalitis and hydrocephalus. Extensive necrosis of the brain cortex leads to intracranial calcification, while periventricular damage around the aqueduct results in hydrocephalus. One-third of congenitally infected infants have neonatal symptoms and about one-quarter die. A baby with congenital toxoplasmosis may have the triad of hydrocephalus, intracranial calcification and chorioretinitis. Asymptomatic infants with congenital infection may show abnormalities in the CSF (raised protein and increased cells). On follow-up these infants may have damage involving the brain, eyes or ears.[18]

Serology to detect toxoplasma IgM antibodies by ELISA confirms the diagnosis.

Treatment

The antibiotic, spiramycin, is used by the French to treat pregnant women known to have been infected. Three-week courses, repeated after two-week inter-vals free of treatment from the time of diagnosis until delivery were beneficial (23 per cent of 388 treated women had infants with congenital toxoplasmosis compared with 61 per cent of those who were untreated). The majority of congenital infections in both groups were subclinical and severe cases were uncommon in both the treated (2 per cent) and the untreated (5 per cent). For the neonate, alternating courses of spiramycin (100 mg/kg daily) for four to six weeks with pyrimethamine (1 mg/kg daily) and sulphadiazine (50 mg/kg daily) for three weeks have been recommended for the first year, although no clear evidence of clinical benefit has been found.

The prognosis for seropositive infants who are normal in the neonatal period with no intracranial calcification is good. For those with neurological problems or systemic disease in the neonatal period the outlook is bleak and most survivors are handicapped. However, congenital toxoplasmosis is a rare cause of mental handicap compared with Down's syndrome.

Prevention

All pregnant women should eat well-cooked meat and stay clear of cats and their faeces.

Trypanosomiasis

Trypanosomes are protozoa that produce two distinct diseases in man. African sleeping sickness is caused by *Trypanosoma (brucei) gambiense* and *T. (brucei) rhodesiense* and transmitted by *Glossina* (tsetse) flies. Chagas disease found in Latin America is caused by *Trypanosoma cruzi* and transmitted by large Triatomidae bugs (see pp. 675–82).

Congenital African trypanosomiasis

Classical sleeping sickness is uncommon in the indigenous population of West Africa where *T. brucei gambiense* is endemic, except during epidemics. The disease frequently is mild in contrast to that associated with *T. rhodesiense* found in East Africa which is serious and fatal.

Congenital African trypanosomiasis has been reported with both varieties although most cases involve *Trypanosoma gambiense*. Fever and anaemia with trypanosomes in the blood and/or cerebrospinal fluid of the infant in the first weeks of life is the usual presentation of congenital infection. Lymphadenopathy is not a feature of the congenital disease although it is characteristic of infection acquired after birth. Traub *et al.*[19] described a case of congenital trypanosomiasis due to

T. rhodesiense in a Zambian infant delivered at 36 weeks of gestation by Caesarean section for fetal distress. Her mother was in coma, had numerous trypanosomes in her blood and died three days after the delivery. A year earlier, she had started on a course of treatment for trypanosomiasis but after three doses of suramin she felt better and absconded. The baby girl weighed 2.46 kg at birth and remained asymptomatic until the ninth day when she became febrile with an eye discharge and oral candidiasis. She was clinically anaemic and on the 19th day her Hb was 10.5 g/dl, falling to 7.7 g/dl by the 13th day. A thin blood film showed increased rouleaux formation and trypanosomes. Parasitaemia was high at 490/μl. Examination of the CSF showed 40 WBC/μl with 90 per cent lymphocytes, increased protein of 92 mg/dl and trypanosomes. Serum IgM was 165.4 mg/dl on the 32nd day before treatment but fell to 18 mg/dl on the 99th day. Suramin was given by intramuscular injection on alternate days starting with 10 mg, increasing to 20 mg and ending with 37.5 mg. Melarsoprol (Mel B) to clear the CNS infection was started after the course of suramin. The first course comprising 0.1 ml of a 3.6 per cent solution of melarsoprol was injected intravenously on three consecutive days. The second and third courses totalled 0.6 ml and 0.9 ml, respectively, with a week's interval between courses.

Congenital African trypanosomiasis has also been reported in infants born outside endemic regions to infected mothers. Lingam *et al.* (1985) described an African child born and raised in London, who was healthy but attracted medical attention because of signs of retardation in psychomotor development at 18 months of age. Conception had occurred in Kinshasa, Zaire, and his mother had remained in Africa until the last trimester of pregnancy when she travelled to London. When examined at 18 months, the child had evidence of meningoencephalitis with raised levels of IgM in the CSF. *T. gambiense* was demonstrated in both blood and CSF. Treatment with suramin and melarsoprol was followed by some improvement.

In congenital infection in endemic areas, trypanosomes are found very early in the CSF and even before they are detected in the blood. Increased rouleaux formation in the blood should raise the suspicion of trypanosomiasis. IgM is usually high in the blood and low in the CSF during the neonatal period in infected infants.

Trypanosomiasis during pregnancy usually leads to abortion, hydramnios and shortened gestation with preterm delivery.

Pentamidine and suramin are effective in trypanosomiasis without CNS involvement. Melarsoprol and nitrofurazone are active drugs in all stages of trypanosomiasis. Congenital trypanosomiasis is treated with a combination of suramin and melarsoprol irrespective of the infecting species. Suramin is given first in three injections (5, 10 and 20 mg/kg respectively) on alternate days. This is followed by intravenous melarsoprol (3.6 percent solution) in three courses of three days each: 0.1 ml (0.36 mg) given on three consecutive days, 0.2 ml (0.72 mg) daily on three consecutive days, and finally 0.4 ml (1.44 mg) daily on three consecutive days.

Congenital Chagas disease

Chagas disease is a major public health problem in South America where more than 65 million people living in rural areas are exposed to infection by *Trypanosoma cruzi*. The first case of congenital Chagas disease was described in Venezuela. Since then reports have emerged from Argentina, Brazil and Chile. The frequency of congenital Chagas disease is higher than suggested by the number of cases reported. Studies in Chile, Argentina, and Brazil have shown that 0.5–2 per cent of low-birth-weight infants weighing less than 2000 g had congenital Chagas disease.

Trypanosoma cruzi enters the fetal circulation through the placental trophoblast in acute, latent or chronic maternal disease. In most cases of transplacental infection the mother is asymptomatic. The diseased placenta is large, and in cases when the fetus is hydropic, it is indistinguishable from the placentitis of syphilis or toxoplasmosis. Abortions occur when the placenta is massively diseased. Congenital Chagas disease has been observed to recur in subsequent pregnancies.[20]

Clinical features

Most newborn infants with Chagas diseases are of low birth weight and may be either preterm or small-for-dates. Manifestations of congenital infection may be obvious at birth or occur after a few months. Anaemia, jaundice, oedema, petechiae, hepatosplenomegaly, tremor and convulsions are common features. Anaemia may be so severe as to require blood transfusion. Dysphagia with inflammatory infiltration of the oesophagus and absence of nerve cells of the myenteric plexus, interferes with feeding and has been described in a few cases. Prognosis of congenital infection depends upon the intensity of parasitaemia. Several organs including heart, oesophagus, brain, skin and skeletal muscle show pathological changes with inflammation, giant cells (a distinctive feature) and granulomas. Parasites have been found either in the muscle fibres or in the reticuloendothelial system with giant cells.

Diagnosis of congenital Chagas disease in the newborn is made on the presence of *Trypanosoma cruzi* amastigotes in the blood using a fresh thin blood smear or a thick drop preparation. An indirect immuno-fluorescence reaction using anti-IgM detects IgM of fetal origin specific for *T. cruzi*. High levels of fetal IgM and IgA have been observed on the first and fifteenth day after birth. A direct agglutination test using sera treated with 2-mercaptoethanol has also been introduced as a simple method of diagnosing congenital Chagas disease.

No satisfactory treatment for Chagas disease is currently available. Nifurtimox, a nitrofuran derivative, may be used in the treatment of congenital Chagas' disease (25 mg/kg daily for at least three months). Nifurtimox is usually administered with phenobarbitone (5 mg/kg daily) to prevent neurological side-effects of tremors and irritability. Benznidazole, a derivative of 2-nitro-imidazole, has been used on a limited scale in congenital Chagas' disease (5 mg/kg daily for 60 days).

Malaria

Pregnancy and malaria

Pregnancy is associated with an increased susceptibility to clinical malaria and severe infection in semi-immune women in areas of high malarial endemicity (see pp. 657–74). The prevalence of malaria is highest during the second trimester of pregnancy and primigravidae are at greatest risk.[21] There is evidence of suppression of antibody formation and depression of cell-mediated immunity to explain this increase in malaria infection in pregnant women. Severe anaemia results from the destruction of sensitized red cells and the depression of erythropoiesis. Malaria in pregnancy may cause abortions and an increase in premature labour. Heavy infections of the placenta with *Plasmodium falciparum* occur in immune mothers, particularly primiparous women. Microscopic examination of the infected placentae show large intervillous accumulations of parasitized erythrocytes together with monocytes containing ingested pigment. In addition, the trophoblastic basement membrane shows irregular thickening with protrusion of syncytio-trophoblast into the basement membrane. These pathological changes prove that *P. falciparum* damages the placenta and interferes with the blood supply to the fetus. Therefore, malaria in pregnancy leads to intra-uterine growth retardation and a high frequency of small-for-gestational-dates infants; mean singleton birth weights being depressed by about 170 g.

The incidence of congenital malaria is low in infants of immune mothers but is more frequent in babies born to non-immune women. The factors protecting the neonate against malaria include the placenta which acts as an effective filter of parasites, passively acquired maternal antimalarial IgG antibodies, fetal haemoglobin and a diet of milk. A cross-sectional survey in the Gambia showed that there was a seasonal fluctuation in antimalarial IgG in cord blood but this did not follow the pattern in pregnant women. During the wet season when parasitaemia and antibody levels rose steeply in pregnant women, antibody levels in cord blood fell. The authors suggested that the placenta infected with malaria acted paradoxically as a barrier to the passage of antimalarial IgG from mother to fetus.

Malarial parasites experience retardation of growth in erythrocytes containing fetal haemoglobin. These findings suggest an explanation for high gene frequencies of thalassaemias in malaria-endemic areas because of the protection against malarial parasitaemia offered by fetal haemoglobin. An exclusive milk diet has been shown to suppress malarial infection in infants and experimental animals by depriving the parasite of para-aminobenzoic acid required for its growth in the erythrocyte.

Congenital malaria

Congenital malaria may occur with infections of *P. falciparum*, *P. vivax* and *P. malariae*. Keitel *et al.*[22] described a case of congenital quartan malaria which presented with the nephrotic syndrome at 21 months of age. The drug-addicted mother had acquired her infection by syringe inoculation in a non-malarious area. Complete remission of the nephrotic syndrome occurred following antimalarial treatment.

Factors responsible for the transplacental transmission of malaria are not fully understood but placental damage, either overt or occult, has been suggested as a probable route. The role of placental damage was probably crucial in the transmission of *P. vivax* malaria to one non-identical twin born in Birmingham. The first twin of a primigravid woman from India, delivered as a vertex presentation assisted by Wrigley's forceps, showed no evidence of malaria on repeated blood film examination. The second twin was a transverse lie who was delivered by breech extraction after an internal version under general anaesthesia. This infant became febrile when 42 days old, developed splenomegaly, anaemia (Hb 6g/dl) and had *P. vivax* in the blood.

Clinical features

Infants with congenital malaria are usually well at birth but develop symptoms of fever, jaundice, abdominal distension and pallor from 5 to 20 days of age. Severe anaemia and massive splenomegaly are found in most infants. Clinical presentation is similar irrespective of the type of malarial infection. Women living in areas of unstable malaria may transmit the infection to their fetuses in spite of treatment. In South East Asia, a region of unstable malaria, untreated *P. falciparum* infection in a teenage primigravid Malay mother during the last trimester of pregnancy resulted in a neonate developing congenital malaria on the third day of life presenting with jaundice and parasitaemia. Serological tests showed specific IgM antibodies against *P. falciparum* at titre 1:64 in maternal blood, cord blood and in the baby during the first fortnight of life. Since maternal IgM antibodies do not cross the placental barrier, *P. falciparum*-specific IgM antibody in the neonate was probably a primary antibody response and confirmed intrauterine infection.

Treatment

Chloroquine is the drug of choice in the treatment of congenital malaria. An initial dose of chloroquine (10 mg/kg) is followed by a similar dose six hours later. Two further doses of chloroquine (5 mg/kg) are given on the second and third day of treatment.

The widespread development of chloroquine-resistant *P. falciparum* infection has led to the use of quinine as the drug of choice in regions of unstable malaria; in Papua New Guinea, East Africa and parts of Central and West Africa. Quinine in a dose of 10 mg/kg every eight hours for seven days, may be given by mouth; intravenous infusion in 30 ml of 5 percent dextrose per dose of quinine over eight hours, may also be used. Cardiac arrhythmias (prolonged QT and T-wave flattening), hypotension and hypoglycaemia may follow rapid intravenous infusion.

To ensure eradication of exoerythrocytic forms of *P. vivax*, a 14 day course of primaquine (0.5 mg/kg daily) is given after the chloroquine. Primaquine should *not* be given to infants with glucose-6-phosphate dehydrogenase (G6PD) deficiency.

Protection of pregnant women

Pregnant women are at risk of severe malaria during the second and third trimester. Semi-immune women become anaemic with malaria and their offspring are subject to intrauterine growth retardation because of placental damage by *Plasmodia*. Non-immune mothers are likely to transmit the malarial parasite to their infants. Therefore, it is prudent to protect all pregnant women living in endemic areas against malaria by chemoprophylaxis using pyrimethamine (25 mg weekly), proguanil (100 mg daily) or chloroquine (200 mg weekly). Visitors who leave a malarious country must remember to continue chemoprophylaxis for at least four weeks. In chloroquine-sensitive regions of stable *P. falciparum* malaria I recommend 200 mg of chloroquine once a week; in regions of unstable malaria where the *P. falciparum* is resistant to chloroquine, a combination of chloroquine (200 mg weekly) and proguanil (100 mg daily) is currently recommended by the World Health Organization.

Chloroquine-resistant *P. falciparum* malaria in South East Asia has spread to Latin America and East Africa and necessitated the use of combinations of pyrimethamine with dapsone (Maloprim) or pyrimethamine with sulphadoxine (Fansidar). But the use of these drugs in pregnant women is controversial because of the alleged embryopathic action of pyrimethamine or possible effects of long-acting sulphonamides on the haemopoietic organ of the fetus, and the reports of agranulocytosis associated with Maloprim. The search for new antimalarials has identified Mefloquine, a drug structurally related to quinine and Qinghaosu, a compound extracted from the herb *Artemisia annua* and used in China for 2000 years. Both compounds are being developed and evaluated under the auspices of the WHO.

Neonates who require blood transfusions or exchange transfusion in malaria endemic areas might be at risk of transfusion-acquired malaria. It is recommended that these infants receive a curative course of chloroquine following their transfusion. In areas now known to have chloroquine-resistant malaria, the new antimalarial compounds should be used.

References

1. Holden J. *Mengo hospital maternity survey 1980*. Personal communication.
2. Wharton B. Food growth and the Asian fetus. In: Wharton B ed. *Topics in Perinatal Medicine 2*. London, Pitman, 1982. pp. 7–16.
3. Lechtig A, Delgado H, Martorell R *et al*. Effects of maternal nutrition on infants growth and mortality in a

developing country. In: *5th European Congress of Perinatal Medicine, Uppsala, Sweden.* 1976. pp. 208–20.

4. Prentice AM, Watkinson M, Whitehead RG *et al.* Prenatal dietary supplementation of African women and birth weight. *Lancet.* 1983; **i:** 489–92.

5. Stein Z, Susser M, Rush D. Prenatal nutrition and birth weight: experiments and quasi-experiments in the past decade. *Journal of Reproductive Medicine.* 1978; **21:** 287–99.

6. Gruenwald P. Pathology of the deprived fetus and its supply line. In: Elliott K, Knight J, eds. *Size at Birth.* Ciba Foundation Symposium No. 27. Amsterdam, Associated Scientific Publishers, 1974. pp. 3–9.

7. Villar J, Altobelli L, Kestler E, Belizan J. A health priority for developing countries: the prevention of chronic fetal malnutrition. *Bulletin of the World Health Organization.* 1986; **64** (6): 847–51.

8. Rohrer F. (Index of state of nutrition). *Munschener Medizinische Wochenschrift.* 1921; **68:** 580.

9. Westin B. Gravidogram and fetal growth. *Acta Obstetrica et Gynaecologica Scandinavica.* 1977; **56:** 273–82.

10. Barnes R. Perinatal mortality and morbidity in Bradford. In: Macfadyen IR, Mac Vicar J, eds. *Obstetric Problems of the Asian Community in Britain,* London. Royal College of Obstetricians and Gynaecologists, 1982. pp. 81–7.

11. Terry PB, Bissenden JG, Condie RG, Mathew PM. Ethnic differences in congenital malformations. *Archives of Disease in Childhood.* 1985; **60:** 866–79.

12. Gregg NM, Beavis WR, Heseltine M *et al.* Occurrence of congenital defects in children following maternal rubella during pregnancy. *Medical Journal of Australia.* 1945; **ii:** 122–6.

13. Stagno S, Pass RF, Cloud G *et al.* Primary cytomegalovirus infection: predisposing maternal factors. *Journal of the American Medical Association.* 1986; **256:** 1904–5.

14. Brown ZA, Vontver LA, Benedetti J *et al.* Effects on infants of a first episode of genital herpes during pregnancy. *New England Journal of Medicine.* 1987; **317:** 1246–51.

15. Panos Dossier 1. *AIDS and the Third World,* 2nd Edn. The Panos Institute, 1987. pp. 37–43.

16. Wilcox RR. Treatment of syphilis. *Bulletin of the World Health Organization.* 1981; **59:** 655–63.

17. Beitzke H. Uber die angeborne tuberculose infektion Ergebnisse der Gesamten. *Tuberkulose-Forschung.* 1935; **7:** 1–30.

18. Remington JS, Desmonts G. Toxoplasmosis. In: Remington JS, Klein JO, eds. *Infectious Diseases of the Fetus and the Newborn Infant.* Philadelphia, WB Saunders, 1983. pp. 143–263.

19. Traub N, Hira PR, Chintu C, Mhango C. Congenital trypanosomiasis: report of a case due to *Trypanosoma brucei rhodesiense. East Africa Medical Journal.* 1978; **55:** 477–81.

20. Bittencourt AL. Congenital Chagas disease. *American Journal of Diseases of Children.* 1976; **130:** 97–103.

21. McGregor IA, Wilson ME, Billewicz WZ. Malaria infection of the placenta in the Gambia, West Africa: its incidence and relationship to stillbirth, birthweight and placental weight. *Transactions of the Royal Society of Tropical Medicine and Hygiene.* 1983; **77:** 232–44.

22. Keitel HG, Goodman HC, Havel RJ *et al.* Nephrotic syndrome in congenital quartan malaria. *Journal of the American Medical Association.* 1956; **161:** 520–3.

23. Lingam S, Marshall WC, Wilson J. Congenital trypanosomiasis in a child born in London. *Developmental Medicine and Child Neurology.* 1985; **27:** 670–4.

CHAPTER 4

Perinatal health

OBSTETRIC PROBLEMS AND PERINATAL MORTALITY

David Goodall

Management
Preterm labour
  Causes

Prevention
Management
Stillbirths

Perinatal mortality rates have declined in all developing countries over the past two decades, but this fall has been more dramatic in some countries than in others. In countries such as Singapore, perinatal mortality rates now compare favourably with western countries. However, other countries, such as India, still have a wide variation in perinatal mortality rates between rural and urban centres, indicating that many problems remain (Table 2.4.1). As perinatal mortality rates usually refer to the outcome of deliveries in health facilities, it must be realized that in situations where over 90 per cent of women may be delivering at home, perinatal mortality rates quoted from centres are of little value. Recently, measurement of neonatal mortality rates (in particular neonatal tetanus mortality rates) within the community in India has been attempted with some success through retrospective questionnaires delivered by community health workers at home visits. This has so far not been extended to stillbirths and thus perinatal mortality rates.

Table 2.4.1 Perinatal mortality rates (PMR: mean per 1000 births) in India, 1980

Institution	Mean PMR
Rural health centre	85.1
Teaching hospital	71.3
General hospital	62.8
Private trust hospital	43.5
Private clinics	34.5

Data from Mehta A. Perinatal mortality survey in India. *Third International Seminar on Maternal Mortality*, Delhi, 1982. © Federation of Obstetric and Gynaecological Societies of India.

One of the main reasons for the decline in perinatal mortality rates in hospital centres is the utilization of antenatal care facilities by an increasing number of patients. Many studies have clearly shown the dramatic impact of antenatal care in reducing stillbirth and early neonatal mortality rates. Without such antenatal care these rates remain unacceptably high. Increased acceptance of antenatal care by mothers is dependent on many factors, chief among which are the educational and socio-economic status that influence the desire and ability to obtain antenatal care. Age and high parity continue to be associated with high mortality.

Antenatal care allows the development of the strategy of 'high risk' and 'low risk' in obstetric management. The higher the risk, the greater the need for more experienced medical and nursing supervision with better and more sophisticated facilities to deal with obstetric problems. In most Third World situations highly technical care can be provided to a mere fraction of all pregnancies and deliveries. Thus the need for assessment of perinatal risk and referral of obstetric problems to more central and better equipped units becomes a necessity. The accessibility of such units to women living remotely becomes a crucial issue in the reduction of perinatal and indeed maternal mortality and morbidity.

As outlined on pp. 136–53, the identification of maternal problems allows a strategy for improving maternal health through the antenatal care system. Such conditions as anaemia in pregnancy, hookworm infestation, tuberculosis, malaria, tetanus, and poor nutrition can be managed in the antenatal clinic in primary health centres with resulting reduction in perinatal mortality and morbidity. Antenatal care provides the opportunity to identify obstetric problems which may give rise to stillbirth and perinatal death. This will include recognition of the following conditions: toxaemia in pregnancy, antepartum haemorrhage due to placenta praevia or abruptio placentae, diabetes mellitus, preterm labour, multiple pregnancy, breech or other fetal malpresentations, prolapsed cord, intrauterine growth retardation, cephalo-pelvic disproportion. Early recognition and diagnosis of these conditions enables steps to be taken to minimize the risks to mother and baby, such as a decision to refer the pregnant woman for appropriate care and management. Antepartum haemorrhage and difficulties during labour are two of the major obstetrical problems causing perinatal mortality followed by toxaemia of pregnancy and medical conditions such as diabetes mellitus.

Management

The management of the common obstetric problems that contribute to perinatal mortality is outlined on pp. 136–53. The optimum management of these conditions is best done by obstetricians with the support of hospital staff and facilities. However, good management can be provided at primary health care level on condition that basic and sound guidelines are followed. This is typified by the management of pre-eclamptic toxaemia. Hypertension with diastolic blood pressure of 110 mmHg or more is an indication for the use of intravenous hydrallazine (40 mg in 500 ml of isotonic saline) together with diazepam (40 mg in 500 ml of 5 per cent dextrose). Artificial rupture of the membranes should be performed if the cervix is favourable, and syntocinon infusion commenced to establish labour. Urine output should be monitored carefully. Once full cervical dilatation is reached, delivery should be expedited in the second stage either by forceps or vacuum extractor. Syntocinon (5 or 10 units) should be given intravenously in the third stage instead of ergometrine or syntometrine. If eclampsia with convulsions occurs, management is even more urgent. Immediate sedation with intravenous diazepam is followed by the regimen as outlined above. Artificial rupture of the membranes should be done without delay as the cervix is usually favourable in this condition. Management of antepartum haemorrhage and intrapartum problems is outlined on pp. 136–53.

Preterm labour

Preterm labour has been defined by the World Health Organization as labour where infants are delivered before 37 completed weeks of pregnancy. It may occur spontaneously and place the newborn infant at considerable risk. Sometimes preterm labour may be intentionally induced in order to avoid other risks which the fetus may face, such as severe pre-eclampsia or rhesus isoimmunization. In either case survival will depend on the degree of support and the quality of facilities provided by the neonatologist. If there is a well-equipped full-time specialist unit, then neonatal survival after 30 weeks of gestation may be about 80 per cent. Where there is no such care available, neonatal mortality may be high for gestations between 30 and 36 weeks. Since neonatal intensive care units are rare in most parts of the developing world, the first responsibility of the obstetrician is to prevent preterm labour occurring wherever possible; to prevent preterm delivery if labour has started, and when preterm labour is inevitable to make it as safe for the baby as possible.

Causes

Attempts have been made to identify women 'at risk' of preterm labour, but this has not been easy because its aetiology is complex and poorly understood. Some occur for no apparent reason, sometimes following a previous preterm delivery. Others may be associated with causal factors such as antepartum haemorrhage, twins, hydramnios, ruptured membranes, urinary tract infection, and other conditions such as malaria, torsion of an ovarian cyst, or a laparotomy.

Prevention

Women who have evidence of the risk factors listed above can be seen frequently in the antenatal clinic, perhaps admitted to hospital for rest and observation, and may sometimes be given β-sympathomimetic drugs (orciprenaline, isoxisuprine, salbutamol, or ritodrine) to reduce uterine activity. Urinary tract infections and malaria should be diagnosed and treated promptly.

If there has been a history of a preterm labour the details should be carefully elicited, in particular, if associated with rupture of membranes. This may suggest the possibility of cervical incompetence for which a Shirodkar suture or similar method of cervical circlage, such as a Macdonald or Wurm stitch, can be inserted at about 14 weeks gestation, often with the delivery of a healthy baby near term.

Management

To confirm preterm labour the patient must be examined to check if there is any effacement and/or dilatation of the cervix. Preterm labour should not be confused with other causes of abdominal pain such as urinary tract infection. If the diagnosis is confirmed the first decision must be whether it is right to try to prevent delivery. Accuracy of estimation of gestational age and maturity is extremely helpful in this regard and is not difficult if facilities for routine antenatal ultrasound scanning are available. Menstrual period dates are often unreliable because of the absence of antenatal care and supervision. If neonatal care is of a high standard, nature can be allowed to take its course. If there is evidence of placental insufficiency, often associated with hypertension, or a suspicion of infection with maternal pyrexia and tachycardia, it will be better to allow labour to proceed. Otherwise, in most circumstances it is worthwhile attempting to prevent labour. Even if the membranes have ruptured, as long as there is no infection and no other unfavourable factors, β-sympathomimetic drugs can be given. If labour is in the latent phase it may be stopped for days and even weeks, but in the active phase drugs are unlikely to be effective. The drugs are usually given as an intravenous infusion (ritodrine 50 mg or salbutamol 5 mg in 500 ml dextrose 5 per cent solution) and the rate adjusted and increased until uterine contractions cease or the maternal pulse rate exceeds 120 beats per minute. If the pulse rate rises above this the patient usually complains of feeling unwell, experiences palpitations and is unable to tolerate the drug. The infusion should be continued for at least six hours after the last contraction at a reduced rate and some obstetricians will give it for 24 hours. Thereafter the drug may be given orally for two or three days. If the patient has any history of cardiac disease, these drugs are contra-indicated.

In many situations the first line management of preterm labour will take place at the peripheral clinics or health centres; it may, therefore, be appropriate to administer the drug, if available, as an aerosol inhalant allowing the nurse midwife to initiate treatment before transfer. With prompt intervention before 3 cm dilatation of the cervix, labour can be delayed up to 10 to 14 days.

Often labour continues in spite of various efforts, and then care has to be taken at the delivery itself. A generous episiotomy will reduce pressure on the rather soft neonatal skull. A prophylactic forceps delivery has been advocated but this must be done with extreme care and is best with Wrigley's forceps. Epidural anaesthesia will minimize some of the risks. Fetal malpresentation (particularly breech) carries the frequent risks of cord compression and of partial delivery through a not-fully-dilated cervix, thereby trapping the baby's head. It was thought, therefore, that delivery in such cases by Caesarean section would increase neonatal survival and decrease morbidity. Some reports have shown that there is no significant difference in outcome between breech babies born vaginally under epidural anaesthesia in controlled situations and Caesarean section, although the latter is still considered by many the best and safest method of delivery.

Stillbirths

Stillbirths or fetal deaths are discussed on p. 161. The total number of perinatal deaths in countries such as India, can be divided approximately into 65 per cent stillbirths and 35 per cent first week deaths (of the latter, 75 per cent occur within 48 hours). Of the stillbirths, 25 per cent occur before labour due to intrauterine death of the fetus, and 40 per cent occur intrapartum. Undoubtedly some are inevitable, such as those due to severe fetal abnormality (like renal agenesis or anencephaly), but many are preventable. Early recognition and control of maternal conditions such as diabetes and hypertension can lead to a more favourable outcome. In many cases fetal loss is associated with failure of placental function which may be evident by fetal growth retardation. If this is detected a decision can be made to induce labour early or even deliver by Caesarean section and thereby avoid the risk.

Intrapartum fetal deaths are usually the result of intrauterine asphyxia. This is frequently associated with hypertension or pre-eclamptic toxaemia, antepartum haemorrhage due to abruptio placentae or placenta praevia, or prolonged labour because of cephalo-pelvic disproportion or fetal malpresentation. Sometimes it may be due to cord compression. Many mothers may present themselves when the problems are far advanced and it is too late because stillbirth has already occurred, and saving the mother's life becomes paramount. However, stillbirth is still too often a result of a failure to recognize that labour is not progressing normally and thereby missing the opportunity to take appropriate action which can lead to a livebirth.

The use of the partogram is the best method of ensuring early recognition of a delay in the progress of labour at primary health centre level as well as in hospital units. Its role in the routine management of labour has been discussed (see pp. 136–53) and we remain convinced that the widest possible introduction of the partogram at primary health care level will

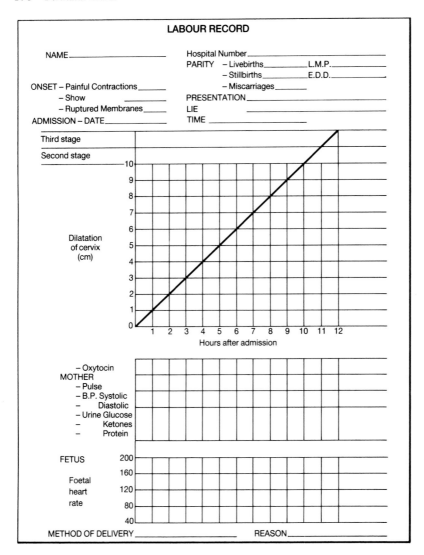

LABOUR RECORD

NAME_____   Hospital Number_____
                         PARITY   – Livebirths_____L.M.P._____
                                  – Stillbirths_____E.D.D._____
ONSET – Painful Contractions_____   – Miscarriages_____
      – Show   _____   PRESENTATION_____
      – Ruptured Membranes_____   LIE   _____
ADMISSION – DATE_____   TIME _____

Third stage

Second stage

Dilatation of cervix (cm)

10
9
8
7
6
5
4
3
2
1
0

1 2 3 4 5 6 7 8 9 10 11 12
Hours after admission

MOTHER
 – Oxytocin
 – Pulse
 – B.P. Systolic
 –   Diastolic
 – Urine Glucose
 –   Ketones
 –   Protein

FETUS

Foetal heart rate

200
160
120
80
40

METHOD OF DELIVERY_____   REASON_____

V.E. date_____ Time_____   REMARKS

Cervix_____	Effaced/Not Effaced thick/thin
Application_____	close/loose
Dilatation_____	cms
MEMBRANES_____	intact/ruptured
LIQUOR_____	clear/meconium
PRESENTING PART____	Vertex/Breech/
Station_____	−2/−1/0/+1/+2

A
R   L
P

Fig. 2.4.1   One of the simplest forms of partogram used for ensuring early recognition of a delay in the progress of labour.

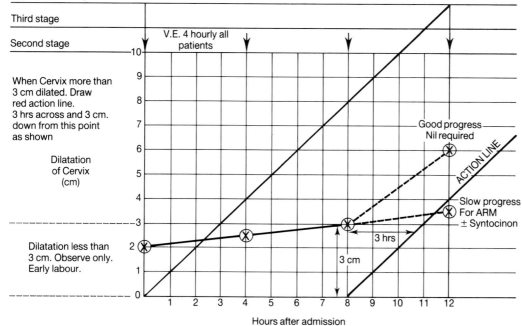

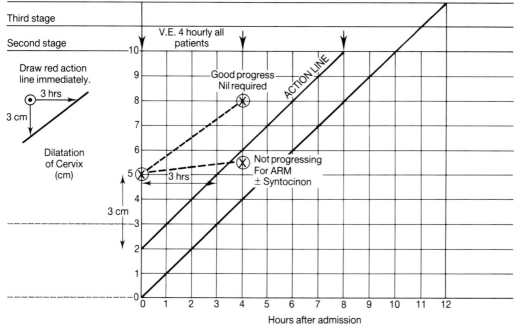

Fig. 2.4.2 Partogram filled in for (a) admission in early labour, and (b) admission in established labour. VE = vaginal examination.

reduce substantially the complications of labour that lead to stillbirths and perinatal death.

One of the simplest forms of partogram which can be used is shown in Fig. 2.4.1. As illustrated in Fig. 2.4.2 when labour is established and the cervix is more that 3 cm dilated, an action line is drawn at 3 hours across and 3 cm down. Subsequent vaginal examination in 4 hours will indicate whether progress is normal or action such as performing ARM (artificial rupture of the membranes) or commencing syntocinon infusion is necessary. Trained staff will subsequently be alerted as to the need for medical intervention.

Finally, it is most essential that all staff involved in the provision of maternity services and obstetric care should be encouraged to keep a careful record of both maternal and perinatal deaths. Regular meetings at different levels must be held to discuss the problems which have led to fetal loss and an attempt made to separate avoidable from unavoidable factors. Such an enquiry must not be with the purpose of apportioning blame, but rather with the intent of establishing more informed and better routine practices which will ensure greater success for the team in its aim of safe delivery for mother and child.

PERINATAL INFECTIONS

Michael Chan

Neonatal tetanus	*Chlamydia trachomatis*
Hepatitis B	Amoebiasis
Ophthalmia neonatorum	Listeriosis
Gonococci	References

The fetus grows in a sterile environment protected from infection by the placenta and the amniotic sac. Rupture of the membranes exposes the infant to infectious agents present in the birth canal. At delivery, the newborn infant comes into contact with a contaminated environment, particularly with the organisms derived from his mother's rectum. However, these organisms are of limited pathogenicity and are antibiotic-sensitive bacteria. If breast-fed the neonate's gut flora is much less likely to contain pathogenic coliforms than if bottle-fed.

The umbilical cord is an important site of infection. Poor hygiene when cutting and dressing the umbilical cord causes neonatal tetanus, one of the major causes of death in newborn infants in developing countries. Bacterial colonization of the umbilicus is common and can lead to septicaemia, another important cause of neonatal deaths.

Neonatal tetanus

Epidemiology

Tetanus is an important cause of avoidable morbidity and mortality in the newborn baby. It is a disease related to unhygienic local conditions and customs at birth, rather than to climate. Neonatal tetanus is more prevalent in rural than in urban areas.

Results of community-based surveys on neonatal tetanus in developing countries, reviewed in 1984, showed that mortality rates ranged from less than 5 to more than 60 per 1000 livebirths[1]: these deaths represented between 23 and 72 per cent of all neonatal deaths. From these results it is estimated that tetanus claims the lives of over half a million newborn infants every year. Neonatal tetanus is a substantially under-reported disease in many developing countries. Routine reporting systems identify only about 2 to 5 per cent of the estimated number of all tetanus cases. More reliable and accurate estimates of the incidence and mortality from tetanus are therefore required.

Neonatal tetanus mortality rates should serve as an index of the quality and the extent of utilization of the maternal health services and of the impact of immunization programmes. As with other aspects of primary health care, the elimination of neonatal tetanus calls for full commitment by government and other bodies with responsibility for the care of women and children.

Prevention

Tetanus in newborn infants can be prevented by aseptic management of the umbilical cord at birth. The persistence of neonatal tetanus in many developing countries reflects the lack of rudimentary obstetric services for large sections of the population, particularly in rural communities. Education of traditional birth attendants in hygienic handling of the umbilical cord at birth – washing hands with soap before assisting in childbirth, cutting the cord with sterile instruments, using sterile ligatures for the cord, avoiding harmful umbilical cord dressings and applying antiseptics to the cord – has resulted in a sharp decline in the prevalence of neonatal tetanus in a number of communities in developing countries.

Active immunization of pregnant women with tetanus toxoid prevents the disease but, unfortunately, those in greatest need of protection are not likely to attend antenatal clinics. At least two doses of tetanus toxoid 0.5 ml each (i.m.) separated by two months give effective immunity against tetanus.

Passive immunization of neonates at risk is the most frequently employed preventive measure in paediatric practice. The administration of 750 units of antitetanus serum to infants born in high-risk circumstances will provide protection.

Pathogenesis

Clostridium tetani is a Gram-positive rod, 2.5 μm by 0.5 μm with spherical terminal spores, found in animal faeces and contaminated soil. Spores of *Cl. tetani* are highly resistant to heat, chemicals and antibiotics, but can be destroyed if autoclaved. They can survive for many years in dry dust or earth. A strict anaerobe, *Cl. tetani* produces two toxins, tetanospasmin and tetanolysin. Tetanospasmin is a potent exotoxin with high affinity to nervous tissue. Within the CNS the toxin is bound to gangliosides; its action on motor neurones is similar to that of strychnine, inducing hypertonicity, spasms and seizures. The toxin also produces overactivity of the sympathetic nervous system resulting in tachycardia, arrhythmias, labile hypertension, peripheral vasoconstriction and sweating.

Controversy surrounds the mechanism and route of absorption of tetanus toxin, but evidence tends to favour a neural rather than a vascular route. Once bound to tissue, tetanus toxin cannot be dissociated or neutralized.

Clinical features

The incubation period of neonatal tetanus varies from 3 to 14 days. The severity of the disease is greater with a shorter incubation period. Rigidity and spasm of muscles are typical of tetanus. Muscle rigidity involves the masseters, abdominal muscles and erector muscles of the spine; it persists throughout the illness. Muscle spasm is intermittent, varying with severity of the disease.

Trismus due to spasm of the masseter muscles, occurring a few days after birth is the presenting symptom in more than half the patients. It is followed by stiffness of the neck muscles and difficulty in swallowing. The infant is irritable, restless and unable to feed. Spasms of spinal muscles occur next and result in opisthotonus. This is accompanied by flexion and adduction of the arms and clenching of the fists. Spasms become prolonged from seconds to minutes. The patient is conscious and crying because of the intense pain as muscle spasms become more powerful and are easily precipitated by any stimulus. Fever is common, probably due to overactivity of muscles. Spasms of laryngeal and respiratory muscles may lead to asphyxia and cyanosis.

The natural history is one of increasing severity during the first seven days, followed by a plateau in the second week, and gradual abatement over the next two to six weeks. The majority of neonates who die from tetanus have bronchopneumonia or aspiration pneumonia. In spite of the high fatality rate of neonatal tetanus, assisted ventilation and intensive care, when available, can reduce the death rate substantially.

Management

There is no agreed standard regimen of management for neonatal tetanus. Efficacy of treatment will be influenced by the incubation period, interval between the first symptom and the first spasm, frequency and duration of spasms, fever and respiratory complications.

Skilful nursing care is life-saving: it prevents aspiration pneumonia and atelectasis, and reduces stimuli that precipitate spasms and seizures. Patients are best cared for in open wards where they are in easy view of nurses with access to resuscitation equipment. Mothers should observe and care for their babies. Feeding is by naso-gastric tube with expressed breast-milk. Drugs are given by intravenous infusion with 5 per cent glucose solution.

- *Penicillin* (100 000 units or 30 mg per/kg per day) is given for five days to eliminate *Cl. tetani*. Concomitant infections should be treated with broad-spectrum antibiotics, e.g. ampicillin (50–100 mg/kg per day).
- *Tetanus antitoxin* can only neutralize unbound circulating toxin and has no effect on toxin-fixed nerve cells. Although the CNS is usually damaged by toxin before symptoms appear, patients given antitoxin have usually fared better than those not given any. Specific antitetanus human immuno-

globulin is the preparation of choice (3000–5000 units i.m.). Equine antitetanus serum (ATS) is the most widely used antitoxin and should be given as early as possible, either as a single i.m. dose of 5000 units or 750–1500 units daily for three doses. There may be benefit in giving 50–100 units ATS intrathecally early in the disease. There is no convincing evidence that periumbilical infiltration of ATS has a significant effect on outcome.

The following schedule of sedation is recommended for general use in tetanus neonatorum:

1. *Immediate control of spasms*
   Paraldehyde   0.3 ml/kg i.m., and/or
   Diazepam   1–2 mg/kg i.m. or i.v. (i.v. dose has to be given slowly to avoid respiratory arrest).
                   The higher dose of diazepam is recommended for the more severe cases.

2. *Continued sedation* (via naso-gastric tube)
   Phenobarbitone   5 mg/kg   × 6 hourly
   Chlorpromazine   2 mg/kg   × 6 hourly
   Diazepam   1–2 mg/kg × 6 hourly

Total respiratory paralysis using curare combined with intermittent positive-pressure ventilation with intravenous nutrition has greatly reduced mortality from neonatal tetanus. However, this intensive care management raises questions about the reasons for the disparity in health services that on the one hand are insufficiently developed to prevent this dreadful disease, but on the other hand can employ expensive modern technology to treat it.

The value of corticosteroids in the management of neonatal tetanus remains unproven and any possible benefit must be balanced against the risk of infection.

Hepatitis B

Epidemiology

There are about 300 million asymptomatic carriers of hepatitis B virus (HBV) world-wide and the majority are in developing countries. The prevalence of hepatitis B surface antigen (HB$_s$Ag), the marker for the carrier of HBV in apparently healthy adults, varies from 0.1 per cent in Western Europe and North America, to 6–12 per cent in China, and 15–20 per cent in some parts of West Africa and the Far East.

Transmission of the virus from carrier mother to her newborn infant during the perinatal period is an important route of infection. Carrier mothers who are 'e' antigen-positive transmit HBV to their neonates in about 70 per cent of cases. The expression of 'e' antigen seems to be determined genetically; most Chinese carrier women are 'e'-positive (40%) compared with African carrier women (15%). Of children born to Chinese carrier mothers between 40 and 70 per cent become carriers; to African mothers about 30 per cent; to Indian mothers 6–8 per cent; and to European mothers almost none.[2] Perinatal transmission of HBV among Arab women is low.

Most infants who are infected acquire HBV during birth. Virus probably gets squeezed across the placenta during delivery and may be detected in cord blood by a sensitive test, such as radioimmunoassay. Antenatal infection with a high titre of HB$_s$Ag in cord blood is rare. Apart from infection through chronic carrier mothers, there is also a substantial risk of infection in the newborn baby if the mother has acute HBV infection in the second or third trimester of pregnancy or within two months after delivery.

Clinical features

Infected neonates do not usually develop jaundice and remain asymptomatic. HB$_s$Ag appears in their blood between six weeks and four months after birth and persists so that most of these infected infants become chronic carriers of the virus. A small number of infants with HBV develop jaundice, have a fulminant illness and die with massive liver necrosis for reasons that are not clear. Although the clinical course for perinatally infected infants is usually mild, their long-term prognosis is hazardous because of the increased risk of chronic liver disease and primary hepatic carcinoma in adulthood. Prospective studies in Taiwan showed that 40 of 41 cases of hepatocellular carcinoma detected in a five-year study had HB$_s$Ag in their blood. A Chinese boy who became a carrier with 'e' antigen in his blood after birth, died of hepatoma seven years after his perinatal infection.

Management

Breast-feeding should not be discouraged because transmission of HBV through breast-milk or by ingestion of blood from excoriated nipples is negligible compared with the infant's exposure to contaminated maternal blood at delivery. Furthermore, the dangers of not breast-feeding in developing countries, such as bacterial infections and hypoglycaemia, are more important than the very small chance of the neonate becoming infected through breast-milk of a carrier mother. These neonates, if given hepatitis B vaccine at birth, will not even be exposed to this small risk from breast-milk. Specific hepatitis B immunoglobulin given soon after birth and repeated at intervals will prevent persistent carriage of most exposed infants by modifying the infection. A 75 per cent protection rate was reported from Taiwan in a controlled trial of hepatitis B immunoglobulin given at birth and repeated twice at intervals of three months.

Once the carrier state has developed it cannot be terminated by any therapeutic agent currently available. Active immunization against hepatitis B virus should therefore have priority in communities with high carrier rates. Vaccines currently available in Western countries are expensive but centres in a number of Asian and African countries are setting up production of a cheap and effective vaccine. Trials with smaller doses of vaccine administered by intradermal injection have reported that $4\,\mu g$ (about half the intramuscular dose) give good HBV surface antibody response in excess of 100 MIU/ml of serum.

The scheme of passive–active immunization of high-risk neonates of mothers with surface antigen in the UK and USA consists of: hepatitis B immunoglobulin 200 mg (200 IU) by intramuscular injection within 48 hours of delivery; hepatitis B vaccine $10\,\mu g$ (0.5 ml) by intramuscular injection at birth, one month later, and a third dose six months after the first. The dose of hepatitis B vaccine produced by recombinant DNA technologies e.g. recombinant yeast vaccine, should be $20\,\mu g$ (1 ml). This schedule may be difficult to implement in developing countries. In mothers carrying HB_sAg without the 'e' antigen, it is suggested that HBV vaccine can be given at one and six months without the immunoglobulin within a day or two of birth, and vaccine immediately thereafter.

A successful clinical trial of hepatitis B vaccine in Senegal reported a schedule which may be more appropriate. The scheme consisted of hepatitis B vaccine $5\,\mu g$ (of HB_sAg) administered by subcutaneous injection into the upper arm at birth, repeated at 6 months and 12 months. Anti-HB_s antibodies were detected in 90 per cent of infants just before the third dose and in 95 per cent two months after.[3]

Ophthalmia neonatorum

Eye infections in the neonate reflect the prevalence of venereal disease in many urban populations of the developing world. Recent studies in Africa have found ophthalmia neonatorum in 5–15 per cent of all newborn infants. Both *Chlamydia trachomatis* and *Neisseria gonorrhoeae* have been isolated from infected neonates.[4]

Gonococci

Gonococcal infection is prevalent in many parts of Africa and Asia, with up to 15 per cent of antenatal clinic attenders infected in Africa.

Gonorrhoea is usually an asymptomatic disease in women who transmit the infection to their infants during passage through the birth canal. The infant's eyes become red and inflamed with swollen lids and purulent discharge one to five days after birth. Both eyes are usually infected with pus oozing from tightly closed lids that are severely congested and oedematous. Keratitis, corneal ulceration and panophthalmitis are serious complications of untreated gonococcal ophthalmia. It is rare for the infant to have systemic illness.

Diagnosis is made by microscopic examination of the pus for Gram-negative intracellular diplococci and confirmed by culture if possible. Gonococci are delicate organisms requiring inoculation on to prewarmed agar and incubation in 10 per cent carbon dioxide.

Treatment consists of local and systemic antibiotic therapy. Crystalline penicillin eye drops (20 000 units/ml) are instilled hourly for the first 24 hours (after swabbing the eyes clean), then at gradually lengthening intervals for three to five days. Four doses of crystalline penicillin (200 000 units) are given by intramuscular injection at six-hourly intervals. Penicillinase-producing strains of gonococci have been reported in developing countries. A report from Singapore of ophthalmia neonatorum caused by β-lactamase-producing *Neisseria gonorrhoeae*, responded to kanamycin therapy. The parents of infected babies should also receive treatment.

An effective method of preventing gonococcal ophthalmia is the instillation of 1 per cent silver nitrate eye drops at birth, a practice unfortunately now abandoned in many countries. Application of tetracycline eye ointment is also an effective prophylactic and it also prevents *Chlamydia* infection.

Chlamydia trachomatis

This intracellular organism is responsible for hyperendemic trachoma, the world's most common eye disease, causing blindness in some two million people in Africa, the Middle East and the Far East. *C. trachomatis* has recently been reported to be the most common cause of ophthalmia neonatorum in West Africa.[4]

Clinical features

C. trachomatis is the cause of ophthalmia neonatorum that develops 4–10 days after birth and can present either as severe conjunctivitis, similar to gonococcal infection, or as mild 'sticky' eyes. Sometimes the eye infection may be obvious in the first five days of life. There may be acute mucopurulent discharge, conjunctival injection and oedema of the eyelids. One or occasionally both eyes may be infected, the palpebral conjunctiva being hyperaemic with mild to moderate chemosis of the bulbar conjunctiva. Chlamydial follicles appear on the conjunctivae within two weeks. The disease may become chronic with the development of pseudomembranes, corneal micropannus and scarring.

Newborn infants develop respiratory tract complications (rhinitis, pharyngitis, otitis media and pneumonia) if the infection is not treated for more than three weeks, the spread occurring via the tear duct. These complications may also occur before three weeks.

A swab of the eye discharge should be examined with Gram-stain to exclude gonococcal infection. A scraping should be taken from the conjunctiva as chlamydia are to be found inside epithelial cells and their inclusion bodies may be identified by Giemsa, iodine, or fluorescent-antibody staining. Culture in irradiated McCoy cells treated with idoxuridine provide highly sensitive methods for isolation of *C. trachomatis* but is usually not available in developing countries.

Treatment

Treatment consists of topical 1 per cent chlortetracycline eye (ointment applied four times daily) together with oral administration of erythromycin stearate (at 50 mg/kg daily in four divided doses for two weeks). Chloramphenicol is partially effective but aminoglycosides are ineffective. Laboratory examination of conjunctival scrapings should be repeated after two weeks. The parents should also be treated with oral erythromycin (250 mg four times daily for two weeks).

C. trachomatis infection is now recognized as a sexually transmitted disease and occurs in many countries where trachoma has never been a prevalent endemic disease.

Other causes

Conjunctivitis may be caused by other pathogens, particularly *Staphylococcus aureus*, and will usually respond to topical neomycin or chloramphenicol eye drops.

Amoebiasis

Entamoeba histolytica, a unicellular protozoal parasite, has a global distribution and frequently causes intestinal disease in communities with poor sanitation in warm climates. Patients present with chronic diarrhoea and passage of loose stools with excess of mucus. Pregnant women may transmit the parasite to their newborn infants through faecal contamination at birth.

Clinical features

Infants born by vaginal delivery are well until the second week when they become fretful and pass loose stools with blood streaks. Their mothers develop diarrhoea with mucus before delivery and have not received treatment or have been inadequately treated. The infant's stools examined under the microscope are positive for *Entamoeba histolytica*. This presentation may sometimes be mistaken for necrotizing enterocolitis.

Amoebic proctocolitis and liver abscess have been reported in a 21-day-old African female infant with a week's history of diarrhoea streaked with blood.[5] The infant was febrile, dyspnoeic and fed poorly. She had a distended abdomen with an enlarged liver 5 cm below the costal margin and an ulcer extending from the anus into the rectum. Amoebae were recovered from the ulcer. The infant made a good recovery on treatment with metronidazole.

Treatment

Metronidazole (50 mg/kg daily in three divided doses for 5 to 7 days) is the treatment of choice for amoebiasis.

Listeriosis

Listeria monocytogenes is a Gram-positive, non-sporing motile rod that is an anaerobe. Of the four antigenic serotypes, types 1 and 4 are the main causes of infection in man. Listeria may be a normal resident of the intestinal tract with potentially pathogenic properties. Rectal carriage by pregnant women is higher during an epidemic, and symptomless carriage of *L. monocytogenes* in the genital tract may be associated with a history of recurrent abortion.

Infection of the fetus is often associated with a non-specific, flu-like, pyrexial illness in the pregnant mother. Fetal infection in early pregnancy results in abortion; in later pregnancy it causes stillbirth or preterm labour associated with meconium-stained liquor and an infected baby.[6] Severe chorioamnionitis found with perinatal listeriosis suggests that infection is by the ascending pathway of the birth canal.

Clinical features

Congenital listeria infection presents soon after birth as pneumonia and septicaemia, with *L. monocytogenes* isolated from the vagina of more than one in three mothers of such infants. Most infected infants are preterm and have a high mortality of 35–55 per cent. Microabscesses and granulomas containing *L. monocytogenes* are found at autopsy, particularly in the lungs, liver and spleen.

Neonatal infection acquired during birth from the mother's genital tract, or later by cross-infection, presents as septicaemia and meningitis days or weeks after a normal delivery. Granulomatous inflammation of the meninges may lead to microabscesses in the brain, but neonatal listeriosis has a lower mortality and survivors are unlikely to have neurological sequelae compared with congenital infection.

Treatment

Suspected neonatal infection should be treated before firm bacteriological confirmation. Penicillin or ampicillin with gentamicin or kanamycin are more effective against listeria than other agents alone or in combination. Maternal infection during pregnancy, presenting as septicaemia, may be successfully treated with ampicillin and such treatment prevents perinatal disease. The prognosis of perinatal listeriosis depends on the extent of fetal or neonatal infection at diagnosis.

References

1. Stanfield JP, Galazka A. Neonatal tetanus in the world today. *Bulletin of the World Health Organization*. 1984; **62**: 647–69.
2. Flewett TH. Can we eradicate hepatitis B? *British Medical Journal*. 1986; **293**: 404–5.
3. Coursaget P, Yvonnet B, Sarr M *et al*. Clinical trial of hepatitis B vaccine in a simplified immunization programme. *Bulletin of the World Health Organization*. 1986; **64**: 867–71.
4. Mabey D, Hanlon P, Hanlon V *et al*. Chlamydial and gonococcal ophthalmia neonatorum in the Gambia. *Annals of Tropical Paediatrics*. 1986; **7**: 177–80.
5. Axton JHM. Amoebic proctocolitis and liver abscess in a neonate. *South African Medical Journal*. 1972; **46**: 258–9.
6. Evans JR, Allen AC, Stinson DA *et al*. Perinatal listeriosis: report of an outbreak. *Pediatric Infectious Diseases*. 1985; **4**: 237–41.

CHAPTER 5

Neonatal health

NEONATAL CARE
Michael Chan

Neonatal care has to be provided both in the community, based at the primary health centre, and at the district hospital. Staff at the primary health centre and the hospital can give optimum care if they cooperate and integrate their services for mothers and newborn babies.

The health of the newborn infant is closely related to factors present during pregnancy, labour and birth. Care should be provided using the 'at risk' approach by detecting mothers and babies who are likely to have problems that may be life-threatening and refering them, preferably before delivery, to trained persons based in hospitals with the facilities to treat and prevent these complications. Good neonatal care, therefore, begins before birth in the antenatal period and during labour, as described on pp. 136–53.

Delivery

Most deliveries are normal, with the baby presenting by its head. A trained birth attendant will ensure that the baby's head is delivered gradually, to avoid sudden decompression and tearing of the tentorium that will produce a potentially fatal subdural haematoma. When the head is born, the baby's nose and pharynx are cleared of mucus by suction, using a catheter with a hand or mouth-operated mucus trap. The baby's eyes may also be wiped with a sterile swab. The baby's body is usually delivered soon after the shoulders have emerged from the birth canal and the baby takes the first breath. Immediately after the infant is born the mother is shown her baby. The newborn infant is covered in a clean dry towel until the umbilical cord stops pulsating or the placenta is expelled. This delay in clamping and cutting the umbilical cord gives time for blood to flow into the infant and prevent anaemia. The umbilical cord must be tied with sterile material and cut with a clean blade or knife. The occasional case of haemorrhage from the umbilical cord because of loose cord ties, makes it necessary for inexpensive disposable cord clamps to be made for developing countries. After the skin is dried, the baby is wrapped in clean linen before being presented to the mother to be suckled at her breast and to be kept warm beside her in the security of her arms. Putting the newborn to the breast immediately after birth should be encouraged because it has the following beneficial effects:

- it stimulates the release of oxytocin which induces uterine contraction and helps prevent postpartum bleeding;
- it promotes mother–child bonding;
- it helps to improve the performance of breast-feeding;
- it prevents heat loss from the baby;
- it keeps the birth attendant occupied and prevents unwarranted interference during the third stage of labour.

Routine care of the normal newborn

The newborn should be weighed after delivery because the birth weight is an indicator of risk, particularly if this is below 2.5 kg. This measurement is the beginning of growth monitoring and should be continued in infancy and childhood. The recording and charting of birth weight on a health card is currently not practiced in the majority of deliveries that take place at home, but it is strongly recommended. Suitable weighing scales that are portable, inexpensive and easy to use are being developed and tested for use by birth attendants. Newborn babies weighing 2 kg or less would require the attention of a doctor.

Keeping babies warm

It is customary to bathe newborn babies for physical and ritual cleanliness. This practice at night has caused hypothermia, particularly in low-birth-weight infants. Bathing should, therefore, be delayed until the sun is shining, unless warm water is available. Blood may be wiped off the baby's skin with a clean cloth without bathing, and vernix should be left overnight to reduce heat loss. However, if there are strong objections to it, vernix may be removed by applying oil to the baby's skin. Newborn infants lose heat rapidly if not kept in a warm environment and adequately clothed. Babies whose body temperature falls below 35°C have a higher death rate than those kept warm. This is of great importance in the low-birth-weight infant. Breast-feeding is essential to the survival and health of newborn infants in developing countries, where mother's milk is the best source of nutrients and protection against infection. The baby should be fed on demand and mothers may lie down when breast-feeding. Ten minutes of suckling on one breast gives sufficient milk. No prelacteal feeds of water, glucose, honey, powdered milk or animal milk should be given because they may be contaminated, be of the wrong concentration, and most importantly, discourage the baby from feeding adequately at mother's breast.

Prevention of infection

In most traditional communities, umbilical cord dressings are applied and this is a common cause of neonatal tetanus. It is, therefore, prudent to apply antiseptic dressings such as gentian violet (1 per cent solution) or triple dye to the umbilical cord to discourage parents from using contaminated dressings.

Newborn infants are more susceptible to infection than children. They pick up gut and respiratory tract flora from their mothers and others who have close contact with them. Fortunately, these microbes are largely non-pathogenic and sensitive to antibiotics, so there is no point in trying to protect full-term neonates from colonization by these sources. Breast-milk contains antibodies to common pathogens in the home environment and so newborn infants should be breast-fed. In hot climates, daily baths with clean warm water and soap will reduce bacterial colonization of the neonate's skin.

Babies born in hospital should be protected from the pathogenic, antibiotic-resistant flora that colonize medical staff. This is effectively done by hospital staff paying rigorous attention to hand washing before handling any newborn infant.

Examination of the newborn

The purpose of a full physical examination of a newborn infant in the first days of life is to:

- identify conditions that require immediate treatment, such as congenital dislocation of the hip;
- detect abnormalities that require long-term supervision and treatment, such as congenital heart defect;
- identify conditions with genetic implications, such as Down's syndrome, other chromosome abnormalities, and neural tube defects;
- detect conditions that are a variation from normal and might worry mothers;
- assess the gestational age, particularly of low-birth-weight infants.

A systematic approach will save time and abnormalities will not be missed. First, a record should be made of the name, sex, birth date, birth weight, head circumference (the maximum occipito-frontal measurement which is 33–37 cm for a term infant), and length of the newborn. The last three measurements in metric units should be plotted on a centile chart.

General examination will show obvious external defects that have been detected by the birth attendant and parents, such as cleft lip and palate, and extra digits.

Head

Caput succedaneum is the oedematous thickening of the scalp in the presenting part (usually the parietal region), which is obvious after prolonged labour and disappears within two days. The anterior *fontanelle* is in the shape of a diamond measuring 1–5 cm across; it is concave and may be seen to pulsate. The posterior fontanelle is triangular and smaller than the anterior fontanelle, with the sagittal sutures connecting the fontanelles. *Craniotabes* (softening of the skull bones) is often a normal finding over the posterior parietal bones near suture lines. When more generalized, it may be a sign of early rickets or osteogenesis imperfecta. *Cephalhaematoma*, a collection of blood between the periosteum and skull bone, is the result of trauma at delivery, and appears as a soft bump over the posterior parietal region, restricted to one side of the head by the skull sutures. It usually takes about six weeks to resolve. Sometimes cephalhaematomas may be large and bilateral, producing significant anaemia and jaundice during the neonatal period. When organization of the blood and calcification start at the edges of a large cephalhaematoma, the clinical findings may simulate a depressed fracture. Parents are always worried about large cephalhaematomas and need firm, repeated reassurance so as to prevent them from interfering and introducing infection.

Examination of the mouth would include palpation with a finger to detect a *submucous cleft* of the soft palate, which would cause regurgitation of milk through the nose and inhalation pneumonia. *Oesophageal atresia* should be suspected if the infant has frothy mucus dribbling persistently from the mouth. A radio-opaque feeding tube should be inserted into the stomach and contents aspirated for testing with blue litmus (there should be no acid if there is atresia) and a lateral chest X-ray taken to locate the position of the tube. A tracheo-oesphageal fistula may be present in oesophageal atresia. Surgery is the only treatment. An infant with *Pierre-Robin syndrome* has a receding chin, a cleft palate and glossoptosis with occlusion of the airway when lying supine. The infant should be nursed prone to prevent the tongue falling backwards.

Skin

Irrespective of pigmentation, almost all newborn infants look pink at birth. *Pallor* may be a sign of severe anaemia due to bleeding (internal or external), transfer of blood from one twin into the other, or pooling of blood in the placenta as in birth asphyxia. Blood transfusion may be necessary. *Milia* are white pin-head sized spots of tiny sebaceous retention cysts found on or around the nose which disappear after a few weeks. *Erythema toxicum* (urticaria neonatorum) is a blotchy red rash associated with pin-head spots containing eosinophils. They occur in the first week of life and may persist for one or two days but are of no clinical significance. *Purpura* presenting only on the face and head is usually due to stasis from pressure on the neck during delivery. Subconjunctival haemorrhages may also be associated with this localized purpura. Generalized purpura associated with a deficiency of platelets requires investigation to exclude intrauterine infection or immune thrombocytopaenia.

Vascular naevi can be divided into two types. *Capillary haemangiomas* may present as *portwine stains* that are flat, may be extensive and do not resolve. Portwine naevi situated in the distribution of the trigeminal nerve may be associated with intracranial vascular anomaly (Sturge–Weber syndrome). Diffuse capillary naevi appearing as pinto patelus or 'stork marks' on the face, eyelids or occiput are common and resolve after a few months. *Cavernous haemangiomas* (strawberry marks) start as a red spot, grow larger over several weeks, and become raised. They are common in preterm babies, affecting girls more than boys. These naevi resolve spontaneously in 90 per cent but the process which begins after six months of age takes years to complete. A *dermal sinus* is a midline pit anywhere along the spine but mainly in the neck and coccyx. The sinus may connect with the spinal cord, in which case it requires surgical excision to prevent bacterial infection and meningitis.

Spine

A neural tube defect may occur along the length of the vertebral column and involve skin and spine (spina bifida). Extensive defects are associated with paralysis of the lower limbs with club feet, the anal sphincter, and the bladder. The surgical management of open extensive neural tube defects in the lower thoracic and upper lumbar region has a poor outcome. In developing countries where specialist surgery is not available, treatment is not an option and these babies usually die from meningitis and hydrocephalus.

Cardiovascular system

The infant should be pink. Both brachial and femoral pulses should be easy to feel. If *femoral pulses* are difficult to feel, coarctation of the aorta should be suspected.

A *systolic murmur* is usually due to a patent ductus arteriosus (PDA), and this murmur disappears after the first week. A long murmur appearing after the first week is usually the result of a ventricular septal defect *(VSD)* or mild pulmonary stenosis with no symptoms. Most VSDs close spontaneously before the infant reaches the age of five years.

If there is a murmur and the infant is feeding poorly or has a respiratory rate faster than 60/min at rest, multiple heart defects should be suspected. A chest radiograph and ECG should be done to confirm the diagnosis.

Respiratory system

Examination of the respiratory system includes the respiratory rate, chest expansion and auscultation. A normal newborn has a regular respiratory rate of less than 60 breaths per minute. The preterm infant usually has a periodic breathing pattern. Indrawing or recession of the chest on inspiration is a sign of respiratory disease.

Abdomen

The liver edge is palpable up to 2 cm in many normal infants. The tip of the spleen is normally palpable. Isolated splenomegaly may be normal, but if associated with other features, fetal infection should be suspected; it may also be found in haemolytic jaundice. The kidneys and bladder should also be located and enlargement detected. Any palpable mass in the abdomen, though rare, should be investigated with ultrasonography.

Genitalia

A complete set of normal external genitalia should be present. A hooded prepuce suggests *hypospadias* with the uretheral orifice at the base of the glans penis. If the urethral meatus is adequate and there is no curvature of the penis (chordee), no immediate treatment is needed. The infant must not be circumcised.

If the urethral orifice is nearer the perineum, the *adrenogenital syndrome* should be considered. In the adrenogenital syndrome, cortisol secretion fails and the adrenals produce excessive androgen. Girls become virilized, with enlargement of the clitoris and fusion of the labia. Vomiting and dehydration with low serum sodium (hyponatraemia) may occur in the salt-losing type of adrenogenital syndrome, requiring intravenous fluid replacement and cortisol treatment.

Small hydrocoeles usually disappear spontaneously during the first month. Undescended testis is common in preterm infants; the testes usually descend during the first three months after birth.

In girls a small amount of *vaginal bleeding* is common five to seven days after birth, and follows excretion of maternal or placental oestrogens transmitted to the fetus before birth. White vaginal discharge or prolapse of the vaginal mucosa are normal.

Breasts

In either sex physiological enlargement of the breasts may occur towards the end of the first week. This enlargement, sometimes unilateral, resolves within a few weeks. A watery discharge may be expressed but parents and birth attendants should be discouraged from squeezing the baby's breasts.

Central nervous system

Alertness of the infant and symmetry of spontaneous movements should be noted. The normal posture of the limbs of a term infant is in flexion. If one limb is not flexed then injury to nerve roots, e.g. brachial plexus, or fracture of clavicle, humerus or femur should be excluded.

The tension of the anterior fontanelle and the width of the fontanelle should be palpated while the infant is at rest.

A more detailed neurological examination is not required unless there is a special indication.

Congenital dislocated hip and dislocatable hip

This is the most important asymptomatic congenital abnormality to detect as treatment is extremely effective. The frequency of this abnormality is about 1 in 200 livebirths. Girls are more likely to have dislocated hips, especially after breech delivery, and there is a high incidence in some families. Recognition requires adequate training and practice, and the following method is recommended. (See also pp. 912–3.)

With the infant on her back, the degree of abduction of the femora at rest is noted. The knees and hips are flexed to a right angle (90°) and the greater trochanter is grasped between the examiner's thumb anteriorly and the fingers posteriorly. In the Ortolani manoeuvre the examiner gently attempts to abduct the hip fully. Failure to achieve this indicates that the hip is dislocated. Gentle traction on the leg together with continued abduction will return the head of the femur into the acetabulum. If the Ortolani test is normal, the Barlow manoeuvre should be applied to detect the dislocatable hip (Fig. 2.5.1).

In the Barlow manoeuvre, each leg is held in slight abduction. Holding the knees must be avoided as this produces dangerous leverage. An attempt is then made to move each femoral head gently forwards into or backwards out of the acetabulum. Results fall into one of three groups:

1. No movement of femoral head – normal hip.
2. Femoral head moves forwards – dislocated hip.
3. Femoral head moves backwards – dislocatable hip.

Movement of the femoral head in and out of the acetabulum is the only reliable sign. It may be accompanied by a 'clunking' sensation, but this must be distinguished from a ligamentous click which has no pathological significance.

Dislocated and dislocatable hips require similar treatment. As soon as the diagnosis is made clinically, a Von Rosen, Barlow or similar padded malleable splint is applied to keep the hips abducted and flexed. The splint remains in place for three months and during this time the infant should be bathed and washed without removing the splint. It is essential that the splint is periodically adjusted to allow for the infant's growth and to ensure that the hips are not being over-abducted.

Radiographs of the hips are generally not of value in diagnosis in the neonatal period. Ultrasound examination has significantly improved the detection of congenitally dislocated hips.

The management should be carried out in conjunction with an orthopaedic surgeon. When the splint is removed almost all treated infants have normal hips. Late diagnosis leads to permanent secondary damage to the hips that often need several orthopaedic operations.

Club foot

Muscular imbalance due to the posture of the infant's feet *in utero* is the most common cause of club foot. In postural club foot it should be possible to dorsiflex the foot fully and to obtain inversion to 90°. The mother can be taught to manipulate the foot through the whole range of movements after each feed, although the shape usually reverts to normal within a few weeks, even without treatment. In contrast, in structural club foot the range of passive movements is restricted, and orthopaedic advice on strapping, manipulation, or serial plasters is needed within 24 hours of birth. Club feet may be associated with neural tube defects.

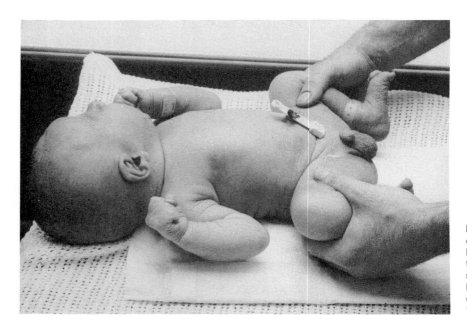

Fig. 2.5.1 Barlow's manoeuvre for examining the newborn for congenital dislocation of the hip. (With permission from SJ Steele and NRC Roberton, *Gynaecology, Obstetrics and the Neonate*, 1984, Edward Arnold.)

Extra digits

Digits should be counted with the infant's palm open, or an extra thumb may be missed. Polydactyly or extra fingers and toes are often familial and vary from an apparently normal digit to a skin tag. The latter can be tied off with a sterile silk thread and will separate by aseptic necrosis.

Resuscitation of the newborn

All babies at increased risk should be delivered in a unit with full respiratory support facilities and trained staff. High-risk deliveries include multiple pregnancy, preterm, fetal distress, abnormal presentation, prolapsed umbilical cord, antepartum haemorrhage, meconium staining, diabetic mother, difficult instrumental delivery (high forceps), and a heavily sedated mother. The resuscitation trolley should be fully equipped for endotracheal intubation and intermittent positive-pressure ventilation with oxygen. A model, assembled locally at a fraction of the cost of a commercial trolley, is illustrated in Fig. 2.5.2. To this should be added a clock with a secondhand, stethoscope, and face mask system. Endotracheal tubes should be provided in three sizes: 2.0, 2.5 and 3.0 mm (FG10, 12 and 14). After washing, endotracheal tubes can be sterilized by autoclaving. An umbilical vein catheter set and syringes of 1, 10 and 20 ml should be readily available.

Assessment of the infant

Most babies start breathing within 10 seconds of the pharynx being sucked out. Routine suction is usually unnecessary unless the amniotic fluid is meconium or blood-stained. Aggressive pharyngeal suction is a powerful vagal stimulus provoking reflex bradycardia and can delay the onset of spontaneous respiration. If the baby breathes promptly everything will probably be alright. If necessary, the baby can be encouraged to breath by skin stimulation such as flicking the baby's feet. Any baby who does not respond must be transferred immediately to the resuscitation trolley.

Start the clock as soon as the baby is free from the mother. As soon as the baby is on the resuscitation trolley assess the five components of the Apgar score (Table 2.5.1) which should be completed by one minute. The heart rate is counted by listening with a stethoscope. Action is taken according to Table 2.5.2.

Alternatively, respiratory efforts should be checked first. If they are present and regular but producing no tidal exchange, the baby is blue because the airway is obstructed. This can be overcome by extending the baby's neck. An airway should be inserted if the baby has choanal atresia (with blockage of both nostrils) or Pierre-Robin syndrome, to overcome the obstruction. If respiratory efforts are feeble or absent, count the heart rate over 10–15 seconds using the stethoscope. When the heart rate is more than 80 per minute, repeat skin stimulation, and if this fails proceed to face mask resuscitation. Mouth-to-mouth (including baby's nose) resuscitation is satisfactory in an emergency. Put in an oral airway and extend the baby's neck. Blow very gently with puffed cheeks, just enough to inflate the baby's chest.

Face mask resuscitation

Effective ventilation can only be achieved if there is a tight seal between the mask and the baby's face. Therefore, face masks must have a soft continuous ring (Fig. 2.5.3) with a 500 ml reservoir. Slightly extend the baby's neck, hold the jaw forward, then introduce an oropharygeal airway before applying the mask. Make sure that the chest is moving and the lungs are being inflated. Better tidal exchange can be achieved by introducing oxygen into the face mask at 4–6 litres per minute. Make sure that the oxygen flows through a pressure valve and does not exceed 30 cm of water. The baby's lungs should be inflated at a rate of 30 times per minute. Listen to the baby's chest within the first 10 inflations to check that there is air entry into both lungs

Table 2.5.1 The Apgar score

Sign	Score		
	0	1	2
Appearance (colour)	Blue/pale	Body pink; extremities blue	Completely pink
Pulse (heart rate)	Absent	<100	>100
Grimace (reflex activity)	No response	Grimace	Cry
Activity (muscle tone)	Limp	Some flexion of limbs	Active motion
Respiration (respiratory effort)	Absent	Slow, irregular	Regular: strong cry

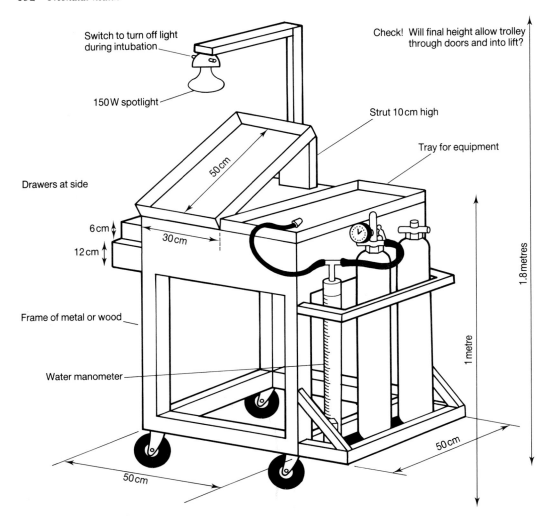

Fig. 2.5.2 Isfahan infant resuscitation trolley (with minor modifications). Equipment includes: General – stethoscope, oxygen supply, spotlight bulb, endotracheal tube connector, manometer, suction motor; Shallow drawer – neonatal airway(s) size(s) 00 (000), laryngoscope (Seward, other), spare bulbs and batteries, scissors, naloxone (Narcan-Neonatal) – 5 ampoules, sodium bicarbonate – 2 ampoules, dextrose 20 per cent – 2 ampoules, Vitamin K₁ (Konakion) – 5 ampoules, (5FG suction catheters); Deep drawer – endotracheal tubes (L, M, S sizes), cord clamps or ties, mucus extractors, aluminium foil, sterile swabs, syringes, needles. (With permission from Fawdry RDF, *Tropical Doctor*, 1983: April; 66.)

and that the heart rate is above 100 per minute. If the heart rate falls below 80 per minute, proceed immediately to endotracheal intubation.

Endotracheal intubation

A straight bladed laryngoscope is best for performing intubation. It must be held in the left hand and the baby's neck slightly extended, if necessary, by an assistant. Pass the laryngoscope down in the midline until the epiglottis comes into view. The tip of the blade is passed immediately over the epiglottis so that the vocal cords are brought into view. Press lightly on the cricoid cartilage with the fifth finger of the hand holding the laryngoscope and the view of the larynx is improved. As the airway tends to be filled with fluid, a suction catheter is introduced with the right hand to clear the upper airway. Once the vocal cords are visible insert the endotracheal tube, using the right hand, and remove the laryngoscope blade, taking care that this does not displace the tube out of the larynx. Attach the endotracheal tube either to a T-piece system,

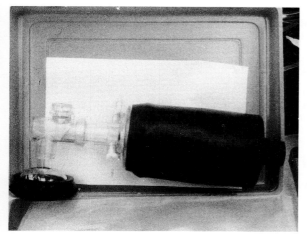

Fig. 2.5.3 Face mask with reservoir.

Table 2.5.2 Action to be taken after the Apgar score

Apgar score at 1 min	Action
8 to 10	None – normal infant
4 to 7	Oxygen by face mask and observe
0 to 3	Laryngoscopy, suction, endotracheal intubation or mouth-to-mouth resuscitation

incorporating a 30 cm water blow-off valve in the inspiratory line, or to a neonatal manual resuscitation device. Maintain the initial inflation pressure for two or three seconds to help the lung expand. The baby can be ventilated at a rate of 30 per minute allowing one second for each inflation.

Inspect the chest wall for movement and confirm by auscultation that both lungs are being inflated. If there is no air entry the endotracheal tube is in the oesophagus; and if this happens remove the tube immediately and reintubate. If only one lung, usually the right, is being inflated, try withdrawing the endotracheal tube by 1 cm while auscultating the left chest; and left lung should have air entry by this manoeuvre. Should there be no improvement, the possible causes include pneumothorax, diaphragmatic hernia, or pleural effusion.

External cardiac massage

If the heart rate falls below 30 per minute, external cardiac massage must be started. Place both hands round the chest and press on the sternum with both thumbs at a rate of 100 to 120 compressions per minute. This will achieve about three compressions for every ventilation. If there is no dramatic improvement within 10 to 15 seconds, the umbilical vein should be catheterized using a 5 French gauge catheter. The umbilical cord is cut 2 or 3 cm from the abdominal skin and the catheter inserted into the vein until there is free flow of blood up the catheter. The baby should be given 3 mmol of sodium bicarbonate per kg body weight over 2 or 3 minutes. This is given by mixing 8.4 per cent sodium bicarbonate solution (1 ml contains 1 mmol) with an equal volume of 10 per cent dextrose. A term baby will receive 20 ml and a low-birth-weight baby

10 ml, while continuing external cardiac massage and intermittent positive-pressure ventilation. A baby who fails to respond at the end of the injection requires 1 ml of 1 in 1000 adrenaline intravenously or injected directly down the endotracheal tube. This method of resuscitation should be continued for 20 minutes. If the baby does not make at least intermittent respiratory efforts, resuscitation should be stopped.

Meconium aspiration

If there has been meconium staining during labour, direct laryngoscopy should be carried out immediately after birth to prevent aspiration leading to respiratory distress, complicated by pneumothorax and infection. If meconium is seen in the pharynx or around the vocal cords, intubate the baby immediately (even if the baby is vigorous at birth). Place a piece of gauze over the open end of the endotracheal tube and apply mouth suction to the tube while removing the endotracheal tube, and then reintubate with a new tube. Provided the baby's heart rate is above 60 per minute this procedure can be repeated until meconium is no longer recovered. It is important that the baby does not gasp during the suctioning, and an assistant can hold the chest with two hands to prevent this happening. Speed is essential in this procedure. Intravenous naloxone (40 μg) is recommended for all babies who become pink, have a satisfactory circulation on resuscitation but fail to start adequate respiratory efforts. Their mothers have usually been given opiate sedation.

Preterm infants

Babies who are less than 32 weeks gestation may have a lower morbidity and mortality if a policy of active resuscitation is adopted. However, there is no firm evidence that a rigid policy of routine intubation of all babies less than 28 or 30 weeks leads to improved outcome. Unless the operator is very skillful, intervention may produce severe hypoxia in a previously lively baby. All babies under 32 weeks gestation should be given face mask resuscitation at 15 to 30 seconds unless there are adequate respiratory efforts. Endotracheal intubation should be started if satisfactory respiratory efforts are not achieved by 60 seconds.

In all infants, start the clock on the resuscitation trolley when the baby is out of the vagina; as soon as the baby is on the trolley dry him, and wrap him in warm towels; assess the features of the Apgar score at about 60 seconds of age. Most neonates will be pink, vigorous and breathing satisfactorily by this stage. If they are not, follow the flow diagram.

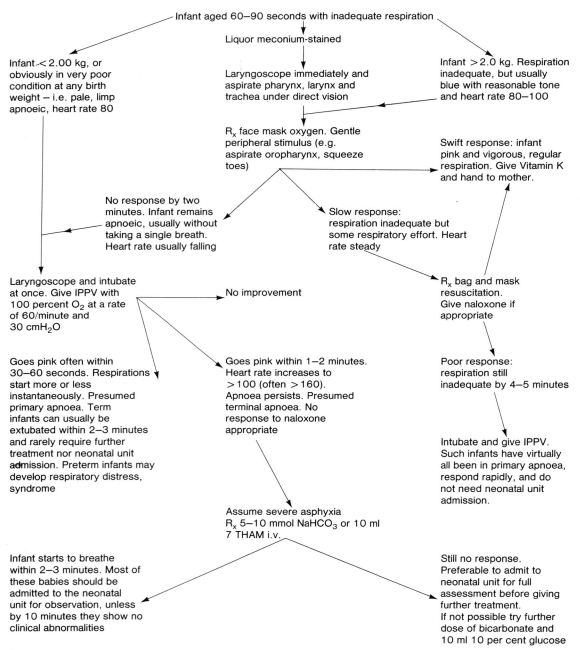

Fig. 2.5.4   Resuscitation of the newborn. (Reproduced with permission from NRC Roberton, *A Manual of Neonatal Intensive Care*, 1986, Edward Arnold.)

Pneumothorax and diaphragmatic hernia

The baby that is vigorous with a normal heart rate, marked respiratory distress and remains very cyanosed in oxygen, probably has an anatomical problem. A diaphragmatic hernia is suggested by mediastinal shift, poor air entry in the left chest, and a scaphoid abdomen. The baby should be intubated, given intermittent positive-pressure ventilation and have a chest X-ray. If possible, a surgeon should be summoned.

A pneumothorax may be spontaneous or the result of over-vigorous positive-pressure ventilation, particularly if a small endotracheal tube has been passed into a segmental bronchus. The signs suggesting a pneumothorax are:

- shift of the trachea and mediastinum;
- hyper-resonant hemithorax;
- distended abdomen;
- vascular changes such as cyanosis of the thorax and pallor of the abdomen.

If the infant is deteriorating rapidly, there will be no time to confirm the diagnosis by X-ray. Insert a wide-bore needle (No. 19 or 21) attached to a 10 or 20 ml syringe, into the second intercostal space in the mid-clavicular line. It there is a pneumothorax the air will rush into the syringe and push up the plunger, the infant's condition will improve, and a chest drain should be inserted. If you are wrong, no harm will have been done to the baby.

Other lung malformations, such as pulmonary hypoplasia of Potter's syndrome, and major defects in the heart, make resuscitation impossible and are usually fatal.

A practical scheme for resuscitation of the newborn baby has been recommended by Roberton and is shown in Fig. 2.5.4

FEEDING THE NEONATE
Indira Narayanan

Initiation of breast-feeding

Breast-feeding of the newborn infant may be influenced by a number of factors, e.g. social, economic and educational differences, variations in health status of mothers, the degree of their emancipation, the need to work, knowledge and involvement of health professionals and administrators, and policies and priorities of clinics, institutions, governments, etc.

The international collaborative study of the WHO indicated that there were three main feeding patterns (see p. 98). In Category I, breast-feeding was less frequent and was rarely continued for six months. Countries such as Hungary and Sweden and women of higher social classes in other countries, were in this category. In some of these countries, over 30 per cent of women did not even initiate breast-feeding. In Category III, breast-feeding was prolonged and almost universal and less than 2 per cent failed to initiate breast-feeding. This group was comprised of primarily rural mothers and the urban poor from developing countries and, interestingly, the higher social class in Zaire. Category II included most of the other mothers who fell between Category I and III.

Another interesting change that has been noted in the past decade or two, is that the practice of breast-feeding has actually increased in privileged women in advanced industrialized countries. This has not been the case in the Third World, where the higher social classes, in spite of commencing breast-feeding in large numbers, tend to supplement breast-milk very early with other milks and then rapidly discontinue breast-feeding. While these women are a relative minority in the Third World, their behaviour is important not only for their own infants but for the population at large, as they are often the trend-setters faithfully copied by less privileged women who can ill afford to do so.

As many factors influence infant feeding, it is essential for all health professionals to be familiar with various aspects of the subject so that they can provide appropriate active support to mothers, in order to avoid and even reverse some harmful practices.

This section deals only with initiation of breast-feeding of the neonate and lays stress on practical aspects.

Advantages of breast-feeding

Although universally applicable, the benefits of breast-feeding can best be appreciated in developing countries where the risks of bottle-feeding are very high. The nutritive advantages of breast-milk are low protein content, appropriate casein–whey ratio (40:60 in contrast to 80:20 as in cow's milk), presence of essential polyunsaturated fatty acids and medium-chain triglycerides, low solute load and high calcium–phosphorus ratio (2:1). The high lactose content supports the growth of *Lactobacillus bifidus*, which prevents excessive colonization of the gut with pathogenic organisms. The nutritive value of human milk is far superior to bovine milks and many of the formulas available in some Third World countries. Even in the specially adapted, so-called 'humanized' milk formulas available in other countries, certain nutrients present in human milk are either absent or in low concentrations. These include milk lipases which aid in the digestion of fat, and amino acids such as taurine.

Table 2.5.3   Anti-infective factors demonstrated in human milk

Secretory IgA
Lactobacillus bifidus growth factors
Lactoferrin
Lactoperoxidase
Complements (C1–9)
Lipids (unsaturated fatty acids)
Interferon
Milk cells – T and B lymphocytes and macrophages

(Reproduced by kind permission of Barker Publications, from Narayanan I, *Postgraduate Doctor*, 1986; **9**: 148–54.)

Another unique feature of human milk is the presence of anti-infective factors listed in Table 2.5.3. There is now objective evidence that breast-milk does indeed afford active protection against some infections.

Other practical advantages are that it is more economical, requires no preparation, is less time-consuming than bottle-feeding, and is associated with a lower incidence of colic and constipation. It is the natural way of feeding and is very supportive of mother–infant bonding. The latter benefit, however, needs to be cautiously stated, especially in developing countries where the other advantages are more glaringly obvious. If for any genuine reason a mother is unable to breast-feed, she should not be made to feel guilty.

Another advantage of breast-feeding which has received much publicity is the contraceptive effect. Studies have indicated that women who suckle their babies frequently on demand have longer birth intervals between siblings than in women whose infants are bottle-fed. This benefit of 'frequent suckling' is vitiated when supplementary feeding with semisolids or other milks is started. In any case, it is an unreliable contraceptive method in individual cases. In the Third World where increasing population is a major problem, recommendation of other appropriate methods of birth control at the relevant time must continue. In certain underprivileged areas, however, breast-feeding may be the only method of birth control being practiced, even if unknowingly. In such instances, health professionals should encourage frequent suckling, avoid other milks, and institute intense health education for acceptance of other appropriate contraceptives before supplementary feeding is initiated.

The let-down reflex

In this physiological reflex, milk is ejected as drops or a thin spray from the nipple due to contraction of the myoepithelial cells within the breast. This can occur before or during feeds and may be noted in the contralateral breast when the infant is sucking on one side. It is controlled by the hypothalamic–pituitary axis and is therefore also governed by the psychological status of the woman. Milk may drip from the breasts when the mother is emotionally stimulated by, say, the cry of the baby or near feed times when the breasts are heavy. Anxiety and depression may have inhibitory influences.

This reflex has received increasing attention over the last two decades. However, although it may help to introduce some milk into the infant's mouth, the bulk is actively sucked by the baby. It is in fact tempting to speculate as to whether it is a vestigeal reflex. In sea-living mammals, such as whales and dolphins, this draught or let-down reflex may be far more important as large quantities of milk can be 'pumped' into the infant's mouth during the short feeding periods.

This reflex may, at times, have an element of nuisance value in certain classes of women, especially when they are out of the home. Leakage of milk and unsightly staining of clothes may be an embarrassment; a clean cotton wad or cloth placed inside the brassiere will help. It should be changed frequently, as prolonged soaking can predispose to nipple cracking and infection.

The first feed

There are many traditional practices related to the feeding of the newborn infant in developing countries, particularly relevant to the first feed. For example, there is a tendency to delay initiation of breast-feeding even up to the third day. Many Indian women do this because it is a family custom or because certain ceremonies need to be carried out before feeding, such as washing of the breast by an older sister or mother-in-law, and some traditionally wait for night fall. A number of women actually believe that they have no milk at this stage and hence do not attempt to initiate feeding. Some state that the early milk looks 'different' and may be 'unclean'. During this interim period other items such as glucose, sugar, jagaree ('gur'), honey, herbs or spices ('ghuttis') are dissolved in water and given to the infant. Animal milks may also be offered during the first few days until the breast-milk flow increases. These have been termed 'inaugural' or 'prelacteal' feeds. There is some risk in these practices of contamination, aspiration from forced feeding and even adverse toxic effects on the infant. For example, infants have been brought in to hospital with features of opium toxicity after reportedly ingesting some of these feeds. Mothers need to be motivated to initiate breast-

feeding as soon as possible after the delivery. They need to be told that the colostrum in the breast is adequate for the baby during the first few days and that it has certain constituents which the baby should not be denied. Delayed feeding may also predispose to painful engorged breasts.

In some extended or joint families with elderly women such as the mother-in-law, traditions are deep-rooted and it may be extremely difficult to change such harmful practices completely. In some cases it has been considered by some to be more sensible to compromise and to permit administration of relatively safer solutions, such as a small amount of sugar or glucose mixed with boiled water, given in as clean a manner as possible for the ceremony. Soon after this the mother should be urged to start breast-feeding. It should be stressed to her that her milk is adequate and that early initiation and frequent suckling on demand will promote milk formation and avoid breast engorgement. While honey may be satisfactory for these inaugural feeds, some cases of botulism have been attributed to it. Some authorities, on the other hand, are of the opinion that making compromises over these early feeds may actually augment their use.

The practice of underprivileged mothers 'discarding colostrum' has perhaps been over-publicized and even misunderstood. Many of these mothers actually only express extremely small volumes and what is really of practical importance to the baby, is to encourage early suckling after this brief expression.

Much has been written in Western literature on the importance of early skin-to-skin contact between a naked baby and the mother, not only in supporting mother–infant bonding but also in promotion of breast-feeding. Reports from the Third World are very few. Recently carefully controlled studies from Thailand indicate that there is no significant difference between early and late contact in breast-milk intake. In traditional societies there is frequent close contact between the mother and infant, even if clothed. Further controlled prospective studies are needed from various parts of the world and different social classes, to identify the important influencing factors before radical changes are made to traditional community practices.

The technique of feeding

Position during feeding

In traditional societies, women frequently feed their babies lying down during the night. This position is also convenient soon after delivery, especially if the mother has had an episiotomy. There is, in practice, nothing wrong in feeding the infant in any comfortable position. It may, however, be sensible to raise the head of the baby, possibly to avoid otitis media and ensure that the nostrils are clear. The latter can be achieved by the mother turning over onto one side and feeding from the breast which is upper-most. Placing the baby prone, after burping, on a firm surface without a pillow is also beneficial and avoids inhalation of vomitus.

Frequency of feeding

It is universally acknowledged that demand feeding is more physiological than time-scheduled feeding every three or four hours. It is important for health professionals and mothers alike to realize that the frequency of demand shows considerable variation. At times, the baby may want a feed after one hour or even earlier, and at other times sleep for three to five hours. With a little experience and commonsense, a mother can learn to distinguish the various reasons for her baby's crying. Frequent suckling in the first few days is particularly beneficial in promoting milk formation, in preventing breast engorgement and in avoiding the temptation to introduce a bottle-feed. At this sensitive time of bonding between mother and baby, the mistaken notion on the part of the new mother that the breast-milk is 'inadequate' should be strongly resisted by reassurance and health education.

Night feeds

Infants differ greatly in their behaviour at night. Babies of some lucky mothers sleep soundly through the night. Others, however, wake up regularly in the early stages, even more frequently than in the daytime. This is distressing to some mothers. Initially, it is convenient to explain to the mother that the infant has not yet learnt the social differences between day and night. Many babies settle down by one or two months, but some may demand night feeds longer. This is not uncommon in less privileged communities where mothers seem to accept this, and, as noted above, sleep with their babies. Problems are more frequent in the middle and upper social classes. Some women need emotional support and guidance on planning their household work and to enable them to rest during the day. Joint or extended families may be supportive at such times.

Administration of water

There is now evidence to suggest that exclusive breast-feeding in the early months is of great benefit both to the infant and mother. Because of the low solute load, extra water between feeds is not required. In fact, many infants do not even accept water. It has been argued in a lighter vein, that had nature intended a newborn infant to have water, an extra breast would have been provided for this purpose. Administration of water is particularly hazardous in developing countries, as it is frequently a source of contamination.

Hygiene related to breast-feeding

The importance of personal hygiene cannot be over-emphasized particularly in underprivileged women in the tropics, as it is not uncommon to have thrush even in exclusively breast-fed babies. Mothers must be advised to wash their breasts with soap and water once or twice a day and to bath daily. In some communities it is traditional not to permit a mother to take a bath for some days after the delivery. In such cases, she should be advised to wash at least her breasts, under-arms and genitalia daily with soap and water. Daily changes of undergarments and blouses are also advisable. However, repeated cleaning of the breast with soap and water before each feed is not only unnecessary but may actually result in drying of the skin and promote sore nipples.

Stool characteristics of the breast-fed infant

The black sticky meconium is replaced within a few days by greenish stools, which then turn yellow. Between the third and fifth day, breast-fed babies pass stools frequently, at times with a greenish tinge and at times bright yellow with separate curdy and watery portions. They also tend to move their bowels soon after a feed and this requires no treatment. The baby passes up to twenty or more stools a day, if the small volumes of stool or watery portions evacuated at the time of passing wind are counted as separate motions. Whether this stool frequency is related to the increased milk secretion, coupled with a transient physiological deficiency of intestinal lactase in the infant, is not clear. It certainly is not infective in origin and is self-limiting. The baby continues to be normal, active and readily accepts feeds. Mothers only need reassurance and emotional support during this period when 'masterly inactivity' is the only acceptable remedy.

After this phase the stool pattern varies considerably. Many babies tend to pass five to eight stools a day in addition to evacuating small watery portions in between, especially when passing wind. Some pass stools less frequently, and a few, once every day or two. The stools, however, remain relatively soft in spite of the fact that babies tend to squirm and strain excessively during bowel movement. This is in contrast to the harder stools typical of bottle-fed babies who may be frequently constipated.

Maternal diet during lactation

Here too, dietary practices are governed by tradition and mothers are often given special foods for the express purpose of producing adequate breast-milk and also of ensuring that the mother does not eat anything which will upset the infant's digestion. Some diets tend to contain an excess of fat and result in unnecessary weight gain, especially in the higher social classes. Mothers should be advised to eat a balanced diet (about a fourth more than in the prepregnancy period), and in general be guided by their appetite. They also need adequate fluids.

Common problems: prevention and management

Flat or retracted nipples

Ideally, these should be detected and managed in the early antenatal period. Mothers should be instructed to stretch the skin near the nipple and to gently pull out the nipple several times a day after applying oil or cream. While this helps in some cases, it is difficult to manage the truly retracted nipple which, fortunately, is less common. Some larger, vigorous babies may still manage to grip the areola and suckle, especially if the breasts are soft. However, where there is difficulty a nipple shield (Figure 2.5.5), sterilized by boiling or with sodium hypochlorite, may be used. This type of nipple shield is different to the shell used in some advanced industrialized countries for collecting milk dripping from the breast. Use of the nipple shield is easier than repeated expression of milk and feeding by bottle or spoon. It may further have a therapeutic effect as it helps to draw out the nipple. It is important to detect and manage this problem early before painful breast

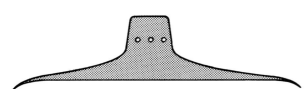

Fig. 2.5.5 The nipple shield which can be tried as an alternative to direct breast-feeding or feeding of expressed milk in suitable cases of flat, retracted or sore nipples.

engorgement discourages the mother from breast-feeding her baby.

Sore nipples

Cracked or sore nipples appear to be more common in primiparous mothers, particularly in higher social classes. Prevention is definitely better than cure. Mothers should be instructed to introduce as much of the areola as will comfortably go into the baby's mouth and not let the infant 'bite' on the nipple. Again, if the baby goes off to sleep at the breast the nipple should be gently eased out after depressing the baby's chin if necessary. Application of an emollient (oil, cream or lanolin) after feeds may help. Antiseptic sprays have not been found to be beneficial. Bloody discharge is not a contra-indication to feeding. If the nipple is very painful, use of a nipple shield or expression of milk for feeding may be helpful.

Engorged breasts

Some mothers do not put the baby to the breast on the first day or two if the breast feels soft and 'empty', only to end up with painful engorgement of the breast on the third or fourth day. Prevention again is far better than cure. Once engorgement has set in, the areola is stretched and the infant finds it difficult to grip on it and suck. Expression of the milk will soften this area and the baby can suck out much of the milk. Any further excess of milk or hard lumpy areas must be relieved by gentle local massage and expression, following, if necessary, hot or cold fomentation. Women in developing countries seem to prefer a hot water bottle to ice packs. On the whole, manual expression is better than the use of a pump in the Third World, but some may prefer the pump. Care must be taken to ensure that the skin is not abraded during expression, either by rubbing with the thumb or by pressure with the edge of the pump's funnel.

Mastitis/breast abscess

Prevention and early management of engorged breasts and good personal hygiene can avoid these problems. Early use of suitable antibiotics in suspected infection can prevent abscess formation. Although mastitis is now not considered a true contra-indication for breast-feeding, in practice, babies may refuse to suck on the affected side as the taste of the milk may be altered. In such cases, mothers can continue to feed on the normal side, and express and discard milk from the infected breast. Once an abscess develops, it has to be incised.

Again, although attempts should be made to support breast-feeding, in practice it becomes very difficult because of local pain, pus discharge, and the need for a dressing. Hence, avoidance of such a problem is of paramount importance.

Refusal of the breast

At times an infant may actually refuse the breast and scream vehemently. Trying to squeeze some milk into the mouth is generally unsuccessful. To make matters worse the baby is quite willing to suck from a bottle. The best method is to place the infant on the shoulder, quieten him and then try to breast-feed again. After a few attempts suckling may be re-established. If all attempts are unsuccessful, expressed breast-milk or boiled water may be taken in a sterilized bottle and offered to the baby. As soon as the baby starts suckling, the bottle should be gently removed and the breast nipple slipped in. Whether this problem is really a temper tantrum or is due to discomfort is not clear. A calm but firm attitude is essential on the part of the health professional to support breast-feeding. In the long run this is better than commencing bottle-feeds in a hurry.

Breast-feeding and neonatal jaundice

There are a number of reports indicating that jaundice, both in the early and later neonatal periods, is more significant in breast-fed infants. In practice, it is seldom severe enough to worry about brain damage. It is also effectively treated by phototherapy. Thus, there is no justification for stopping breast-feeding in cases of neonatal jaundice. This dictum is particularly important in the Third World. There is some evidence to suggest that frequent suckling may result in lower bilirubin levels.

Breast-feeding and haemorrhagic disease of the newborn

The relation between haemorrhagic disease due to vitamin K deficiency and breast-feeding is well documented. The American Academy of Pediatrics recommends the use of prophylactic parenteral vitamin K_1 (0.5–1 mg) soon after birth. More recently, oral vitamin K_1 (1–2 mg) has also been shown to be beneficial and may be an acceptable alternative in situations where intramuscular injections are difficult to administer.

Maintenance of the 'figure'

Cosmetic aspects related to breast-feeding may, at first glance, seem superfluous in a developing country. However, the high social classes seem to have very similar stresses and requirements all over the world. Hence, where relevant, mothers must be told that breast-feeding, if properly done, will not spoil the figure. There is even evidence to suggest that the maternal fat deposited during pregnancy is actually utilized during lactation. In addition, the shape and size of the breast is also influenced by the genetic profile, the woman's posture, the support given to the breasts during pregnancy and lactation, and the diet. Even women who have never breast-fed can have sagging breasts. As noted above, excess of fat in traditional diets may lead to inappropriate weight gain. A sensible balanced diet, exercise, care in maintaining a proper posture and adequate support for the breasts, will aid in maintaining the figure.

Adequacy of milk and lactational failure

Hospital and community-based studies in developing countries have indicated that the most common reason for early administration of other milks is 'inadequacy' of breast-milk and the age of supplementation is progressively earlier in urban slums and among the elite. It is not likely that the urban woman is biologically different to her rural counterpart. The higher prevalence of lactational inadequacy in privileged groups excludes major nutritional deficiencies as a cause. Hence, social stresses and in some cases the need to go to work may be contributory factors. Another detrimental practice is the introduction of a bottle-feed in early infancy, even when there is adequate milk, just 'to get the baby used to it'.

Mothers themselves frequently begin to have doubts about the adequacy of their milk, not realizing that demand feeding really implies frequent feeding. Test weighing of the baby before and after every feed, while being a well-known research tool, is not of practical importance in the assessment of lactational failure in daily clinical practice. It may even be fallacious if not properly carried out. One of the best guides is the weight gain monitored on standard growth cards at acceptable periodic but not too frequent intervals.

True biological lactational failure must be extremely rare but inadequacy, secondary to predisposing factors noted in Table 2.5.4, is well known. The single common denominator appears to be inadequate suckling and all attempts must be made to avoid or minimize the factors stated in the table as a preventive

Table 2.5.4   Factors predisposing to 'lactational failure'

Factors in the baby
Prematurity/low birth weight
Birth asphyxia
Illness
Defects, e.g. cleft palate

Maternal factors
Poor motivation or ignorance leading to discontinuation of
    feeds for minor ailments, administration of infrequent, strict
    time-scheduled feeds, etc.
Inappropriate management of local problems in the breast,
    e.g. flat and sore nipples, engorgements
Sedation (also influences the baby)
Over-anxiety
Excessive fatigue
Heavy smoking
Drugs, e.g. oral contraceptives

Environmental factors and hospital practices
Separation of the baby from the mother
Painful interventions, e.g. episiotomy, Caesarean sections
Early introduction of bottle-feeds
Use of pacifiers
Inadequate support and guidance from health professionals
High-pressure advertisement of baby foods

(Reproduced with permission from Narayanan I, *Indian Journal of Paediatrics*, 1985; **52**: 167.)

measure. Management includes advice of a balanced nutritious diet, plenty of fluids, nipple stimulation or exercises and frequent suckling. Where another milk has already been started, mothers should be advised to offer the breast before every 'top' feed to increase the sucking stimulus. If there are simple harmless dietary home remedies suggested by older women in the family, these too can be followed. Certain drugs have been utilized for purposes of lactation. These include oxytocin (2–4 units placed in contact with buccal mucosa or given as a nasal spray) before every feed or alternate ones, and metoclopramide (commonly 10 mg t.i.d.). These have been tried with some success. Their use, however, should be supervised by informed medical personnel, as in theory at least, there may be side-effects in the mother or infant.

Lact-aid consists of a fine siliconized rubber tube one end of which is attached to a sterile polythene bag or a feeding bottle filled with milk and the other end taped to the breast nipple. It has also been used to promote milk flow as the infant's effort to draw out milk from the bag or bottle serves to provide sucking stimulus to the breast, but care has to be taken to avoid contamination and infection.

Mothers should be advised to continue breast-feeding as long as possible but supplementation with

appropriate semisolids is essential between four and six months of age.

Contra-indications to breast-feeding

In developing countries, especially in the underprivileged group where the risks of bottle-feeding are high, there are very few contra-indications to breast-feeding and the conventional recommendations in standard textbooks are not in general applicable. Each mother and baby should be evaluated on an individual basis and the risks of introducing other milks carefully weighed against those of continuing breast-feeding. When the mother is seriously ill (too ill to be with the baby) feeding can be discontinued temporarily or on a permanent basis, depending on the nature of the illness. In the former case, repeated expression of milk is needed to avoid engorgement of the breast and to maintain flow of milk.

Maternal tuberculosis, hepatitis B, HIV-AIDS and malaria which are common in the Third World are not contra-indications. Guidelines for babies of tuberculous mothers are given in Figure 2.5.6. (See also pp. 169, 519–552.)

As far as maternal drugs and breast-feeding is concerned, it is expedient to evaluate and balance the

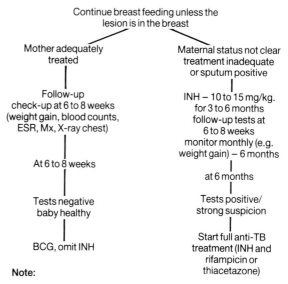

Continue breast feeding unless the
lesion is in the breast

Mother adequately
treated

Maternal status not clear
treatment inadequate
or sputum positive

Follow-up
check-up at 6 to 8 weeks
(weight gain, blood counts,
ESR, Mx, X-ray chest)

INH – 10 to 15 mg/kg.
for 3 to 6 months
follow-up tests at
6 to 8 weeks
monitor monthly (e.g.
weight gain) – 6 months

At 6 to 8 weeks

at 6 months

Tests negative
baby healthy

Tests positive/
strong suspicion

BCG, omit INH

Start full anti-TB
treatment (INH and
rifampicin or
thiacetazone)

Note:

If the mother is not likely to come for follow-up, give BCG at birth
INH = isoniazid, Mx = Mantoux test

Fig. 2.5.6 Suggested guidelines for the management of babies born to tuberculous mothers. (Reproduced with kind permission of Barker Publications from Narayan I, *Postgraduate Doctor*; **9**: 148–54.)

dangers of drugs secreted in the breast-milk and the risk of introducing bottle-feeds. It is not within the scope of this chapter to review this subject. However, the most frequently used drugs, such as common antibiotics and occasional analgesics, are not contra-indicated. Long-acting sulphonamides are not recommended, especially in the first postnatal week, because of the risk of neonatal jaundice. Later, if their use is unavoidable as in some peripheral centres, breast-feeding can be continued. Tetracyclines tend to stain the teeth and bones and should not be used. Theoretically, chloramphenicol has some risks, but in practice the amount excreted in the milk is small and not likely to cause the 'grey baby syndrome'. However, better alternatives should be used when available. Oral contraceptives are also better avoided until two months after birth (see p. 156).

On the whole, a practical approach to the administration of drugs to pregnant and lactating women is to use them only when absolutely necessary and then to choose the relatively safer alternatives. If a definitely harmful drug is unavoidable, breast-feeding will have to be discontinued. Since discontinuation of breast-feeding has serious implications in the Third World, the decision must be taken by a competent informed person after careful deliberation.

Use of expressed breast-milk

Where the infant cannot suck directly from the breast, milk should be expressed and given to the infant. Practical guidelines appropriate for developing countries are indicated in Table 2.5.5. Manual expression appears to be the best and most economical. Electrical pumps are expensive and those with narrow tubes difficult to sterilize. Cylindrical pumps such as the Kaneson's variety and those with wide mouths and 'necks' may be suitable alternatives as they can easily be cleaned and sterilized, either by boiling or with sodium hypochlorite. However, the commonly available cheap pumps consisting only of a funnel and a rubber bulb should not be used, as they are associated with gross contamination.

The few controversies associated with the use of human milk, especially banked milk, for small preterm babies in advanced industrialized countries are not applicable to the Third World. In fact, human milk has been shown to decrease the occurrence of infections and actually improve the outcome of these high-risk low-birth-weight infants in developing countries.

Promotion of breast-feeding

Education of health professionals is essential and stress

Table 2.5.5 Practical guidelines for the use of human milk in developing countries (for infants who cannot accept direct breast-feeding)

1. Give clear instructions to the mother and supervise the collection where possible. Hence, in hospitals, it is better to collect milk in the nursery than in the maternity wards.
2. Hands and breasts should be washed with soap and water. If the skin tends to get dry apply cream, oil or lanolin after expression.
3. Milk can be collected directly into sterilized, wide-mouthed cups.
4. Manual expression is best. Sterilized Kaneson's pumps and others with wide mouths and necks may be good alternatives. Electric pumps are expensive and need careful sterilization – especially the tubing. The conventional old-fashioned pumps consisting of just a funnel and a rubber bulb should not be used.
5. Utilize the milk rapidly. Milk for later feeds can be stored in the refrigerator in the first shelf under the freezer but not for more than 24 hours.
6. In hospital send samples for bacteriological analysis periodically.
7. Human milk is useful both in hospital and domicilliary care of low-birth-weight infants.
8. As the infant gets stronger allow intermittent suckling on the breast for short periods to promote milk flow, and commence direct breast-feeding as soon as possible.

(Reproduced with kind permission of Barker Publications from Narayanan I, *Postgraduate Doctor*, 1986; **9**: 148–54.)

should be laid on practical aspects and provision of answers to questions commonly raised by mothers, rather than on theoretical aspects, if they are to provide any meaningful support to mothers. The staff should gain expertise in giving advice not only on medical problems but also social ones some of which are described in this chapter. Continued support to mothers is essential, particularly in urban communities, to avoid unnecessary supplementation with other milks. Use of mass media may also be beneficial. Table 2.5.6 suggests some guidelines for promotion of breast-feeding in hospitals. In a situation with limited resources and staff and a large population, it is important to define priorities. For example, time needs to be spent on advising urban mothers of the middle and higher social classes on the techniques of feeding, its advantages, prevention and management of problems such as sore nipples, engorged breasts, etc. This may be unnecessary for the urban poor and rural mothers. Hence, it is essential to identify the major local problems and act accordingly.

The problem of the working woman is ever on the increase. A few practical guidelines include advice on taking more of the leave due after the delivery, unless there are medical reasons for rest during pregnancy or

Table 2.5.6 Guidelines for promotion of breast-feeding in hospital and health centres

1. Do not ask mothers to purchase feeding bottles and formulas in advance, at or before the delivery. Prescribe them only when unavoidable.
2. Avoid separation of the mother and baby, even for short periods.
3. Motivate for early initiation of breast-feeding.
4. Promote frequent suckling on demand.
5. Resist the temptation to introduce formula feeds in the first few days after birth.
6. Do not stop breast-feeding unnecessarily.
7. If separation of the infant is unavoidable, minimize the period and advise frequent expression of milk. Call mother to the nursery. Mothers may also stay in the neonatal special care units.
8. Advise a nourishing balanced diet, adequate fluids and rest. Give encouraging emotional support to the mother.
9. Do not prescribe oral contraceptives.
10. Ensure prevention, early detection and treatment or appropriate advice for problems such as engorged breasts and sore, flat or retracted nipples.

(Reproduced with kind permission of Barker Publications from Narayanan I, *Postgraduate Doctor*, 1986; **9**: 148–54.)

the employment is stressful and involves heavy physical work. Exclusive breast-feeding should be continued until the milk flow is well established and preferably up to two to three weeks before the mother is due to restart work. At this time, supplementation with another milk by bottle or a cup and spoon and continued breast-feeding when the mother is at home is advisable. Breast-feeding at night can provide essential nutrition to the baby in a poor agricultural community where women must work in the fields.

Expression of milk at work during the lunch break will aid in preventing engorgement and excessive leakage. In the Third World it is difficult in most situations to utilize this milk, as facilities for continued refrigeration are inadequate.

Provision of more part-time jobs, creches at the place of work, and safer methods of transport will be beneficial. Uniform provision of maternity leave in governmental and non-governmental sectors and, where possible, longer leave would also be helpful. However, a reasonable balance between the infant's and mother's requirements and family's economic needs must be maintained. The problem is not a simple one and mothers cannot always resolve matters on their own. Society too has a responsibility in this issue; it is an investment for the future.

Further reading

Helsing E, Savage King F. *Breast-Feeding in Practice: A Manual for Health Workers.* Delhi, India, Oxford University Press, 1982.

La Leche League International. *The Womenly Art of Breast-Feeding.* Illinois, USA, Franklin Park, 1981.

Narayanan I. Human milk in the developing world: to bank or not to bank? *Indian Journal of Pediatrics.* 1982; **19**: 395–9.

Narayanan I. Nutrition for the low birth weight and preterm infant: developing country concerns. *Journal of Human Nutrition* 1985; **39A**: 242–54.

Narayanan I. Breast feeding and infection. *Postgraduate Doctor.* 1986; **9**: 148–54.

World Health Organization. *Collaborative Study on Breast-Feeding Practices.* Geneva, WHO, 1980.

Bottle-feeding and other methods of oral feeding

While there is no doubt about the superiority of breast-feeding there will on occasion be very genuine indications for resorting to other methods of feeding and the use of other milks. The decision is not easy and should never be taken lightly, especially when dealing with underprivileged women. Although a mother has the right to choose the type of feeding for her infant, only educated well-informed mothers are able to appreciate the benefits of breast-milk and the potential risks of other methods of feeding. The underprivileged have no real choice and none should be offered.

Indications for bottle-feeding

The following are indications for bottle-feeding:

- the death of the mother and where a suitable wet nurse is not available or not acceptable;
- genuine insufficiency of breast-milk where appropriate methods to improve the milk supply have failed or have been inadequate;
- genuine contra-indication to breast-feeding;
- working women where it is not feasible or safe to express and preserve breast-milk for the working period;
- where the infant is premature or sick and is unable to suck from the breast; attempts must be made

to procure expressed breast milk where possible and safe before resorting to other milks.

Types of bottles

A variety of bottles are available (Fig. 2.5.7). The wide-mouthed bottle which can be cleaned easily is ideal. Glass bottles are cheaper but breakable. Non-breakable plastic containers are more expensive and only good-quality ones can withstand boiling. The boat-shaped bottle has two ends: the front is covered by the teat for sucking and the back with a rubber cap or teat which can be lifted up during feeding to allow entry of air, thus avoiding a vacuum and ensuring a free flow of milk. The narrow ends, however, make cleaning more difficult, especially for underprivileged women and this often outweighs the above advantage. Unfortunately, the most common types of bottle used by many underprivileged women are small 'medicine' bottles on to which are slipped rubber teats. The extremely narrow necks and broad 'shoulder' make adequate cleaning virtually impossible and, where such bottles are coloured, it is difficult to see the dirt.

Even poor mothers are likely to have an appropriate wide-mouthed bottle at home and can buy a 'slip on' wide nipple without a screw-cap ring. This is cheaper than the conventional feeding bottle. Alternatively, the mother can be advised to use one of the other methods of feeding, e.g. cup and spoon.

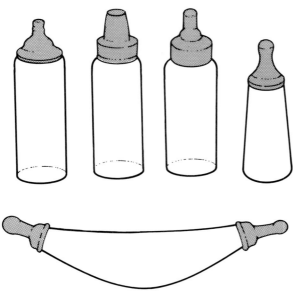

Fig. 2.5.7 Various types of bottle used for feeding infants.

Cleaning and sterilization of bottles

Underprivileged mothers have problems of lack of resources for procuring items and fuel, and a scarcity of water – a lethal combination for maintenance of adequate hygiene. Methods of cleaning and sterilization should be as simple as possible and if the infant is thriving there may not always be a need to be rigid in the procedures in difficult situations. However, if there are recurrent episodes of diarrhoea then great care should be taken to adhere to the instructions noted in this section and in Appendix 1.

Bottles should be cleaned with a detergent. Very poor mothers can use any available soap. Although some health workers permit the use of salt or ash, it appears better to motivate mothers to spend money on soap than on treatment of the repeated infections acquired in a poor environment.

Chemical sterilization

In developing countries, bottles are frequently sterilized by boiling. Use of sodium hypochlorite is not common in the Third World, except in private clinics and hospitals and higher social classes. However, this might be a good method for underprivileged women who could afford to buy only one bottle and light the fire only once a day for cooking purposes. Only a little of the concentrate need be diluted with a larger quantity of water and the solution only has to be changed once every 24 hours. Controlled trials in field situations in different social classes are required but the chemical method does seem to have great potential. It is also very useful during travel.

Practical guidelines for the cleaning and sterilization of bottles and technical aspects of feeding are noted in Appendix 1 and 2. Some mothers, especially from the lower social classes tend to make the hole in the teat too large. In contrast other mothers, often from the more educated group, tend to have such a small hole in the teat that the infant's intake becomes inadequate because of prolonged sucking and tiring.

Types of milk

Where expressed breast-milk is not available from the mother or a safe suitable donor, an alternative milk is required. The milks commonly used include:

- cow milk;
- buffalo milk;
- cooperative diary milk – a partially defatted milk consisting of cow or buffalo milk or a combination of both;

- full-cream formulas;
- adapted formulas.

Although, in some instances, milk from other animals (such as goat or camel) may be used, the most common source is bovine. The salient features of more commonly used milks are given in Tables 2.5.7 and 2.5.8.

As far as the nutritional features are concerned, where breast-milk is not available one of the adapted formulas would be best for the neonate, or at least partially adapted formulas where attempts have been made to alter the casein–whey ratio nearer to that of human milk (40:60) and lower the protein and salt load. However, these formulas are very expensive and because of this may be overdiluted. Further, in some areas only fresh bovine milks may be available. Some dilution is required because of the high content of protein with an inappropriate casein–whey ratio of 80:20 and a high solute load. It has been estimated that

a dilution of 2:1 of cow milk with water and addition of 5 per cent sucrose (about 1 teaspoon full per 100 ml etc) has the following composition:protein 2.2 g/dl, carbohydrate 8.1 g/dl, fat 2.5 g/dl, and an energy content of 63 kcal/dl (265 kJ/dl).[1] At the same time, addition of water carries a considerable risk of

Table 2.5.7 Composition of human and some animal milks

Milk	Energy kcal/dl (kJ/dl)	Protein (g/dl)	Carbo-hydrate (g/dl)	Fat (g/dl)
Human	67–75(281–315)	0.9	7	2.7–4.5
Cow	66 (277)	3.5	5.0	3.5
Buffalo	103 (433)	4.3	4.5	7.5
Goat	76 (319)	3.7	4.5	4.8

(Data from Hambreus L. *Pediatric Clinics of North America*, 1977; **24**:17–36 and Passmore R, and Eastwood MA, *Human Nutrition and Dietetics*, 1986, Churchill Livingstone. p. 211.)

Table 2.5.8 Major characteristics of common types of milk

Type	Protein	Carbohydrates	Fats	Miscellaneous
Human milk	0.9 g/dl Homologous protein Casein–whey ratio = 40:60 Amino acids suitable	7 g/dl High lactose content Energy content = 67–75 kcal/dl (281–315 kJ/dl)	2.7–4.5 g/dl Contains MCT, PUFA and lipases	Anti-infective factors Low renal solute load = 80 mOsm/l Ca:P ratio = 2.3 Iron low but utilization high Vitamins variable – dependent on mother's diet
Starting formulas	1.5–1.6 g/dl Heterologous protein Total protein variable Casein–whey ratio = 80:20 Phenylalanine high Taurine and cystine low	6.9–7.4 g/dl Lactose and maltodextrins Energy content = 65–7 kcal/dl (273–81 kJ/dl)	3.4–3.8 g/dl Low in MCT and PUFA	Renal solute load = 105–110 mOsm/l Ca:P ratio = 1.2–1.3 Vitamins and minerals supplemented
Adapted formulas	1.5–2.3 g/dl Heterologous protein Based on cow milk or soy protein Casein–whey ratio = 40:60 Taurine and cystine added in some formulas	7.2–10.6 g/dl Lactose and glucose/ polymers Energy content = 69–80 kcal/dl (269–336 kJ/dl)	3.5–5.3 g/dl MCT and PUFA added	Renal solute load = 95–100 mOsm/l Ca:P ratio = 1.4–2.0 Vitamins and minerals supplemented
Cow milk	3.5 g/dl Heterologous protein Total protein high Casein–whey ratio = 80:20 Phenylalanine high Taurine and cystine low	5.0 g/dl Lactose Energy content = 67 kcal/dl (281 kJ/dl)	3.5 g/dl Low in MCT and PUFA	Renal solute load = 220 mOsm/l Ca:P ratio = 1.3 Vitamins and minerals mostly inadequate

MCT = medium chain triglycerides; PUFA = polyunsaturated fatty acids. (Reproduced with permission of Blackwell Scientific Publications from Narayanan I, *Journal of Human Nutrition*, 1985; **39**: 242–54.)

contamination and reduces the concentration of other essential nutrients. Further, mothers in the Third World already tend to dilute milk excessively, actually adding 2–4 parts water to one part milk. In some situations the milk may be adulterated with water at the place of purchase. Thus, in practice, the need for dilution has to be underplayed and in some instances mothers actually need to be told not to add any water.

Infants on animal milks and most formulas require boiled water in between feeds. When the infant is constipated, as frequently happens with artificial milk, adding some sugar in the water may help. Fruit juices in practice are unsafe, particularly in the hands of uneducated mothers. They are usually given in too small quantities, excessively diluted and the fruit is often not fresh enough to provide adequate vitamin C. In the manner given (strained) it is not of much use in preventing constipation. Further, poor hygiene in preparation and administration may actually result in recurrent diarrhoeas. Babies may be better off with multivitamin supplements (with iron after three months) procured where possible from a nearby health centre.

Where buffalo milk is being used for older infants, part of the fat can be reduced by removing the cream from the top of the milk after boiling and cooling to room temperature. However, removal of cream from the milk after prolonged or overnight storage in the refrigerator is not good, as most of the fat is lost. Skimmed milk and condensed milk are not suitable, as the growing infant needs fat and the latter is too sweet.

Fresh milks tend to spoil quickly in the tropics without refrigeration. It may help to keep the container cool in water in earthen pots and reboil the milk in between feeds after adding a little water to prevent it from getting excessively concentrated. In situations where a mother cannot buy milk twice a day from a refrigerated source, a powdered formula may need to be prescribed for the late night and early morning feeds.

Thus, where breast-milk is not available the alternative should be chosen after careful consideration of local availability, climatic conditions, and socio-economic and educational status of the parents, especially the mother.

Volume of feeds

Although in theory normal infants require 110 cals/kg (462 J/kg) and 150–200 ml/kg, it is better not to specify the volume for mothers of normal babies. Otherwise excessive anxiety and even forced feeding may occur, if infants do not consume the 'prescribed' volumes. Periodic weighing at appropriate intervals will check if growth is normal.

Other methods of oral feeding

A cup and spoon is the most common alternative method of feeding. The salient features and comparison with bottle-feeding noted in Table 2.5.9 are based on a preliminary controlled evaluation by I. Narayanan. Further studies are required in this area and also on the use of traditional feeding devices. Figure 2.5.8 shows the two main prototypes based on the structures of most utensils. The small cup-like device which is filled from a larger cup, is like a modified 'spoon' and produces less spillage than a spoon as the projecting portion is placed inside the mouth. The rest of the features are similar to those of spoon feeding (Table 2.5.9) but there is a greater risk of 'forced feeding'. The teapot like utensil with a spout is not suitable, as the narrow spout is very difficult to clean. For the same reason, a dropper is not suitable. Some underprivileged women soak a piece of cloth or cotton in milk and squeeze it into the infant's mouth – a method so full of risks, especially of contamination, that it obviously cannot be recommended.

In conclusion, as methods of feeding other than suckling on the breast are associated with a number of potential risks, the decision for their use should be taken only after great deliberation. The responsibility should ideally rest with a knowledgeable, experienced health professional in conjunction with a well-informed mother. Furthermore, it is the duty of the health staff concerned to ensure that the mother is given clear instructions on the practical aspects appropriate to her socio-economic and educational background, to avoid or minimize complications such as diarrhoea and malnutrition.

Table 2.5.9   Features of alternative methods of oral feeding

Advantages	Disadvantages
Bottle-feeding	
Provides emotional satisfaction of sucking	More costly
Faster than spoon feeding	Relatively high risk of contamination
	Permits mother to see how much the baby sucks but risk of 'over-feeding'
Use of cup and spoon	
More economical	Time-consuming
Readily available in all households	More difficult
Easier to clean	More spillage
	Risk of choking
	More problematic in infants under four months of age; easier in older babies

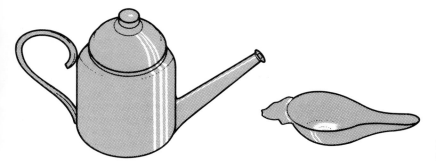

Fig. 2.5.8 Traditional feeding devices.

References

1. Brostrom K. Human milk and infant formulas: Nutritional and immunological characteristics. In: R.M. Suskind ed. *Textbook of Paediatric Nutrition*. New York, Raven Press, 1981. pp. 41–64.
2. Hambreus L. Proprietary milk and human breast milk. *Pediatric Clinics of North America*. 1977; **24**: 17–36.
3. Passmore R, Eastwood MA. *Human Nutrition and Dietetics*. Hong Kong, ELBS/Churchill Livingstone, 1986. pp. 211.
4. Narayanan I. Nutrition for the low birth weight and preterm infant: developing country concerns. *Journal of Human Nutrition*. 1985; **39A**: 242–54.
5. Committee on Nutrition, A.A.P. Nutritional needs of the low birth weight infants. *Pediatrics*. 1977; **60**: 519–30.

Appendix 1

Instructions for cleaning and sterilization of feeding bottles

- Check the hole in the teat by putting milk in the bottle and inverting it. For a normal healthy newborn infant the milk should come out as a stream and then as drops. If there is no hole or if it is too small, make a proper hole by plunging a red-hot sewing needle through the tip of the teat. Mothers should be told not to use hair pins or scissors to make the hole.
- Separate the rubber teat and the supporting plastic ring. Clean the items with a detergent which does not leave a powdery residue after rinsing. Take care to check the grooves and hole in the teat.
- Sterilization by boiling
  Place the washed bottles erect in container of cold water, taking care to completely immerse them. Cover, bring to the boil and boil for 10 min. Drain off a portion of the water so that the tops of the bottles are clear, to facilitate easy removal of individual bottles when required.
  Slot the rubber teats into the supporting rings and place them upside down along with their top covers when required. Pour boiling hot water over them, cover, and boil for 3–5 min. Drain off the water totally, as rubber spoils more quickly with prolonged soaking in hot water.
  Having several bottles and boiling them all together once or twice a day, saves time and fuel and provides a sterile bottle for each feed.
- Chemical sterilization
  Use sodium hypochlorite (0.5 per cent), following the instructions of the manufacturer carefully.
  Use a plastic or glass container to prepare the solution and ensure that the bottles and teats with the rings and top covers are totally immersed with the air expelled. If any items tend to float, submerge them with the aid of a plastic sieve or spoon.
  Items washed with soap and water must be soaked for 45 min. It is more practical to keep them in the solution until the next feed. At that time remove the bottle and nipple, draining off the fluid into the same container. Rinsing, if carried out, should be done only with boiled water.
  Make up a fresh solution after 24 hours.
- Do not touch the inside of a sterilized bottle or the portion of the teat that goes into the infant's mouth.
- When the bottle is taken out for travel, fix the nipple upright and cover it with an additional sterilized plastic cover. Do not invert the nipple into the ring and the bottle because the tip of the teat is likely to become contaminated when it is refixed in the upright position for feeding later on.
- Rinse the bottle as soon as possible after a feed to make subsequent cleaning easier.

Appendix 2

Practical guidelines for bottle-feeding

- Hold the infant in the lap with the head and shoulders raised in a comfortable position. Never leave the baby unattended with the bottle propped-up on a pillow.
- Check the hole by inverting the bottle. If the hole is blocked, hold the bottle firmly in one hand in the horizontal position and tap sharply on the other end. Do not squeeze the nipple with the fingers.
- The average infant takes 10–20 min to finish a feed. If the baby sucks vigorously but takes excessively long to finish the feed and becomes hungry quickly, the nipple hole is probably too small. If the baby tends to choke and splutter during the feed the hole may be too large.

- During the feed tilt the bottle so that the tip of the teat is filled with milk, to avoid excessive aerophagy.
- Burp the infant after the feed by placing him on the shoulder or sitting him up on the lap and gently stroking or patting his back.
- Feed the baby on demand, giving him as much as he will take at a time. Prepare sufficient volumes so that in some feeds at least a small amount of the milk is left, indicating that the baby has had his fill.
- If an infant leaves much of the feed unfinished, it can be consumed by another sibling or the mother. If this is not feasible, the milk can be kept in the refrigerator with a nipple cover and given again after changing the teat, and, if required, after rewarming in a bowl of warm water. If there is no refrigerator, the milk can be kept in a covered container, placed in a dish of water to keep cool and if necessary boiled again before use.

LOW-BIRTH-WEIGHT INFANTS
Michael Chan

Definition	Management
Incidence	Special care for preterm infants
Aetiology	Prevention of low birth weight
Types of low-birth-weight infant	Anticipation of the birth of low-birth-weight infants
Clinical complications	References and further reading

Definition

The 29th World Health Assembly in 1976 defined low-birth-weight (LBW) infants as those less than 2500 g (up to and including 2499 g) at birth[1]. In practice most weighing machines for babies in developing countries are not constructed to be accurate below 20 g.

Paediatricians in developing countries take into special care nurseries, babies with a birth weight of 2000 g or less. As a result, data on babies between 2000 g and 2500 g are often not available. For the sake of international comparison, data should be collected on the above basis as defined by the World Health Assembly.

Incidence

Of the 21 million LBW babies born world-wide in 1979, 90 per cent (more than 18.9 million) were in developing countries. The Indian subcontinent had the highest proportion of LBW babies (31 per cent) compared with Asia (excluding India) 20 per cent, Africa 15 per cent, Latin America 11–13 per cent, Europe and North America 7–8 per cent. An estimated 20 million LBW babies were born in 1982, about 16 per cent of the total global births.[2] More than 7 million LBW infants are born every year in India.

Low-birth-weight infants suffer increased mortality rates during the perinatal, neonatal and postneonatal periods. One study from India typifies the hazards facing LBW newborn infants in developing countries. Ghosh *et al*[3] surveyed 27 394 consecutive singleton births in Safdarjung Hospital, a district hospital in New Delhi, of whom 2072 died (986 fetal and 1096 neonatal deaths), giving a perinatal mortality of 75.6 per 1000 births. The lowest perinatal mortality rate (PNMR) was 16.7 for babies of 3001–3500 g birth weight. The PNMR of those weighing between 1501–200 g and 2001–2500 g was 340.5 and 46.7 respectively. Perinatal mortality was lowest (27 per 1000 births) in full-term infants; this increased to 137 per 1000 in the 34–36 weeks of gestation group and was more than 500 per 1000 in those under 33 weeks of gestation.

A population-based study in Brazil found that LBW babies were 17 times more likely to die in the perinatal period than babies weighing 2500 g or more. Perinatal mortality was very high among preterm babies, being five times more than in the general population.[4] LBW babies comprised 71 per cent of babies who died in the neonatal period and were 24 times more likely to die in the first month than babies with birth weight of 2500 g or more.[5]

Postneonatal mortality is also increased in LBW infants, particularly in the early months of life. This is associated with respiratory infections, diarrhoeal disease and other infections.

Ideally, all LBW babies merit neonatal care because of their high perinatal mortality rate.

Aetiology

There are numerous factors contributing to low birth weight, many of which have been discussed on pp. 158–74.

Maternal factors

Literacy and income, if low, increase the risk of delivering LBW offspring. Other factors include:

- Pregravid weight of less than 45 kg
- Loss of weight during pregnancy
- Short stature <150 cm
- Teenage pregnancy
- Short birth interval
- Malnutrition
- Anaemia
- Smoking and tobacco chewing
- Hard work during the third trimester
- Maternal infections: malaria, TORCH group, tuberculosis and chronic infections

- Pregnancy complications: toxaemia, antepartum haemorrhage

Fetal factors

- Preterm delivery
- Multiple pregnancy
- Intrauterine infections
- Congenital abnormalities

Types of low-birth-weight infant

The two main types of LBW infant are *preterm* and *small-for-dates* (SFD) term infants. Preterm infants may be appropriate-for-gestational-age (AGA) or SFD. SFD term infants may be divided into asymmetrical infants with low birth weight but head circumference and length not decreased for gestation, and symmetrical infants in whom birth weight, length and head circumference are all decreased. Symmetrical LBW babies have been subjected to severe chronic placental insufficiency. Asymmetrical LBW infants are the result of acute nutritional deficiency during the third trimester. In developed countries, the majority of LBW babies are preterm.

What is the frequency of these types of LBW infant in developing countries? This question can be answered by examining epidemiological data. In India where a number of studies have been done, the statistics from Ahmedabad (Mehta, personal communication) are fairly typical. The vast majority (82 per cent) of LBW infants are SFD and their survival is better than preterm infants of the same weight (Table 2.5.10). Bhargava et al.[6] reported that in the birth weight group 1501–2000 g, 30–45 per cent are preterm, the rest being term or post-term infants. In the birth weight group 2001–2500 g, 85 per cent or more are term infants and only 13–15 per cent are preterm. Similar differences are seen in the same birth weight groups between hospital and community based studies.

Table 2.5.10   Birth weight, gestation and deaths in the Civil Hospital, Ahmedabad

Weight (kg)	Preterm			Term		
	Number born	Fetal deaths	Perinatal deaths	Number born	Fetal deaths	Perinatal deaths
<1.0	91	33(36%)	90(99%)	0	0	0
1.0–1.5	139	54(38.8%)	129(92.8%)	9	4(44.4%)	8(88.8%)
1.5–2.0	101	25(24.7%)	69(68.3%)	247	8(3.2%)	30(12.1%)
2.0–2.5	66	6(9%)	11(16.6%)	1564	44(1.8%)	67 (4.3%)
2.5–3.0	0	0	0	2006	40(2%)	78 (3.9%)

(Data courtesy of D.K. Mehta, 1985.)

Dawodu and Laditan[7] studied LBW infants in Ibadan, Nigeria. These infants comprised 8.2 per cent of 6135 live births in six health centres in the city. Of the LBW 236 (62 per cent) were SFD and most of them (87 per cent) were term infants; 146 (38 per cent) of LBW were AGA and of this group 79 per cent were preterm.

Similar trends have been reported in Latin America with 42 per cent of LBW babies being preterm and 58 per cent having a gestational age of 37 weeks or more and probably growth-retarded.[4]

Identification of SFD and preterm infants

Small-for-dates (SFD) term infants and preterm, appropriate-for-gestation (AGA) LBW infants can be identified either by using maternal dates of the last menstrual period, or by clinical methods of gestational assessment. As maternal dates may not be remembered, assessment of gestational age in the first days of life will have to be employed.

Gestational assessment depends upon signs of neurological development and changes in skin, subcutaneous tissues, joints and external genitalia.

The Dubowitz[8] method of gestational assessment uses both neurological and non-neurological criteria with a system of scoring; the total score being plotted against a regression line graph to obtain the gestation in weeks (Fig. 2.5.9a–d). The Dubowitz assessment should normally be done by doctors.

The Farr score is a rapid assessment scheme devised in Newcastle upon Tyne and subsequently modified.[9] It relies solely on non-neurological physical signs, details of which are given in Table 2.5.11.

A simple method of assessing gestational age at birth has been devised and used in India (Table 2.5.12).[10] (See also pp. 296–7.) Simple means of assessing gestational age should also be taught to birth attendants and nurse-midwives so that they may identify the preterm infant for referral to hospital for special care.

Clinical complications

The complications of LBW infants may be divided into those that mainly affect preterms and those that are commonly encountered amongst SFD infants suffering from intrauterine growth retardation (see Table 2.5.13).

Preterm babies are likely to suffer from hypothermia, inability to suck feeds, respiratory distress syndrome due to lack of surfactant in the lungs, infections, jaundice and bleeding.

Small-for-dates babies are prone to develop

Table 2.5.11   Rapid assessment of gestational age at birth. (Devised by Farr *et al.*, 1966 and modified by Parkin, Key and Clowes, 1976, *Archives of Disease in Childhood*; **51**:259–63.)

Skin texture
Pick up fold of abdominal skin
0 = very thin, gelatinous
1 = thin and smooth
2 = smooth, medium thickness, rash, superficial peeling
3 = slight thickening, superficial
4 = thick, parchment-like, superficial or deep cracking

Skin colour
Inspect when baby is quiet
0 = dark red
1 = uniformly pink
2 = pale pink, variable over body
3 = pale, only pink over ears, lips, palms and soles

Breast size
Measured by picking up breast tissue
0 = no breast tissue palpable
1 = breast tissue on one or both sides <0.5 cm
2 = breast tissue both sides, one or both 0.5–1.0 cm
3 = breast tissue both sides, one or both >1 cm

Ear firmness
Palpate and fold the upper pinna
0 = pinna soft, easily folded, no recoil
1 = pinna soft, easily folded, slow recoil
2 = cartilage to edge of pinna, soft in places, ready recoil
3 = pinna firm, cartilage to edge, instant recoil

Gestational ages (mean) and Newcastle score

1 = 27 weeks	5 = 36 weeks	9 = 40 weeks
2 = 30 weeks	6 = 37 weeks	10 = 41 weeks
3 = 33 weeks	7 = 38.5 weeks	11 = 41.5 weeks
4 = 34.5 weeks	8 = 39.5 weeks	12 = 42 weeks

hypoglycaemia and hypocalcaemia (if fed on cow milk) and suffer from infection. They are also likely to have congenital defects from intrauterine infections such as rubella, cytomegalovirus (CMV), toxoplasmosis and, syphilis.

Management

Routine care of low-birth-weight infants

Identification   Identification of LBW babies depends upon weight being recorded at birth.

Birth weight All babies should be weighed at birth and therefore, all birth attendants should be equipped with a Salter spring weight scale with a plastic hammock in which the baby is placed. This instrument is accurate to the nearest 50 g. The weight should be recorded on an infant health care chart.

Gestational assessment Preterm AGA and SFD babies

Neurological sign	Score					
	0	1	2	3	4	5
Posture						
Square window	90°	60°	45°	30°	0°	
Ankle dorsiflexion	90°	75°	45°	20°	0°	
Arm recoil	180°	90–180°	<90°			
Leg recoil	180°	90–180°	<90°			
Popliteal angle	180°	160°	130°	110°	90°	<90°
Heel to ear						
Scarf sign						
Head lag						
Ventral suspension						

Fig. 2.5.9 (a) The Dubowitz method of gestational assessment. Neurological criteria. (Reproduced by permission of *Journal of Pediatrics*; **77**:1–10 © 1970.)

External sign	Score				
	0	1	2	3	4
Oedema	Obvious oedema hands and feet; pitting over tibia	No obvious oedema hands and feet; pitting over tibia	No oedema		
Skin texture	Very thin, gelatinous	Thin and smooth	Smooth; medium thickness Rash or superficial peeling	Slight thickening; superficial cracking and peeling, esp. hands and feet	Thick and parchmentlike; superficial or deep cracking
Skin colour (infant not crying)	Dark red	Uniformly pink	Pale pink; variable over body	Pale; only pink over ears, lips, palms or soles	
Skin opacity (trunk)	Numerous veins and venules clearly seen, especially over abdomen	Veins and tributaries seen	A few large vessels clearly seen over abdomen	A few large vessels seen indistinctly over abdomen	No blood vessels seen
Lanugo hair (over back)	No lanugo	Abundant; long and thick over whole back	Hair thinning, especially over lower back	Small amount of lanugo and bald areas	At least half of back devoid of lanugo
Plantar creases	No skin creases	Faint red marks over anterior half of sole	Definite red marks over more than anterior half; indentations over less than anterior third	Indentations over more than anterior third	Definite deep indentations over more than anterior third
Nipple formation	Nipple barely visible; no areola	Nipple well defined; areola smooth and flat; diameter <0.75 cm	Areola stippled, edge not raised; diameter <0.75 cm	Areola stippled, edge raised; diameter >0.75 cm	
Breast size	No breast tissue palpable	Breast tissue on one or both sides; 0.5 cm diameter	Breast tissue both sides; one or both 0.5–1.0 cm	Breast tissue both sides; one or both 1 cm	
Ear form	Pinna flat and shapeless, little or no incurving of edge	Incurving of part of edge of pinna	Partial incurving whole of upper pinna	Well-defined incurving whole of upper pinna	
Ear firmness	Pinna soft, easily folded, no recoil	Pinna soft, easily folded, slow recoil	Cartilage to edge of pinna, but soft in places, ready recoil	Pinna firm, cartilage to edge, instant recoil	
Genitalia Males	Neither testis in scrotum	At least one testis high in scrotum	At least one testis right down		
Females (with hips half abducted)	Labia majora widely separated, labia minora protruding	Labia majora almost cover labia minora	Labia majora completely cover labia minora		

(Adapted from Farr *et al*, *Developments in Medicine and Child Neurology*, 1966; **8**:507.)

Fig. 2.5.9   (b) Non-neurological criteria

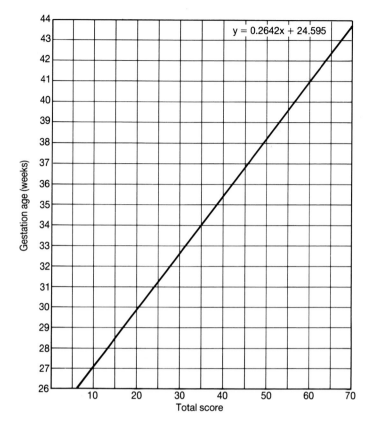

Fig. 2.5.9 (c) Total score plotted against regression line graph to obtain gestation in weeks. (Reproduced by permission of *Pediatrics*; **45**:937; © 1970.)

born at term may be distinguished by clinical methods of gestational assessment. A simplified method using only three characteristics – plantar creases, breast nodule and ear cartilage firmness – is applicable to all newborns within two days of birth, and it has a 95 per cent confidence limit of 11 days.

Breast-feeding Early breast-feeding for all LBW babies especially SFD infants will prevent hypoglycaemia. Babies unable to suck should be fed through a stomach tube. Breast-milk contains anti-infective factors and prevents infection in LBW infants. Feeding should be started before two hours of age. If possible, blood glucose should be monitored using Dextrostix. Glucose should not be used for feeding LBW babies after birth because it stimulates insulin secretion and results in hypoglycaemia.

Temperature LBW babies carried in a sling next to the mother's breast under her clothes, have survived well in the Colombian highlands. Simple means of keeping babies warm include wrapping in aluminium foil or in cotton wool held in place by a thin cloth, taking care to cover the head, and using well-covered hot water bottles and radiant heat from electric lamps. In hospital, LBW babies may be covered with plastic sheets below the neck, and warmed in a room with heaters to maintain the air temperature at 28–30°C.

Vitamin K₁ Vitamin K₁ (Konakion) administered by injection (1 mg) or by oral preparation will prevent haemorrhagic disease of the newborn.

Infections Infections may be prevented by exclusive breast-feeding, washing hands before and after touching newborn babies and by judicious use of antibiotics. Group B streptococcal infections may mimic respiratory distress syndrome but respond to a course of

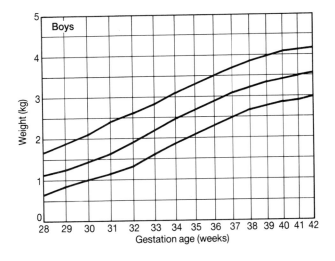

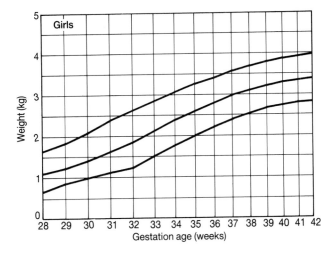

Fig. 2.5.9 (d) Weight charts for newborn Caucasian babies (with 10th, 50th and 90th centiles). (Reproduced by permission of *Pediatrics*; **45**:937 © 1970.)

benzylpenicillin injections (60–90 mg/kg in four divided doses). *E. coli* infections may be followed by septicaemia and meningitis.

Septicaemia A baby with septicaemia is unwell and does not feed well. The heart rate may be disproportionately high for body temperature. There may be jaundice, purpura and episodes of apnoea. If septicaemia is suspected and the cerebrospinal fluid (CSF) is normal, intramuscular ampicillin (100 mg/kg in three divided doses) together with gentamicin (5 mg/kg in two divided doses) is given for 7–10 days. The blood levels of gentamicin before and after a dose should be monitored, if possible, to prevent ototoxicity from high levels. This is a vital part of the effective and proper use of antibiotics in neonates in special care nurseries.

Meningitis Early symptoms of meningitis are similar to those of septicaemia. Late features are vomiting, a high-pitched cry, convulsions and raised anterior fontanelle tension. Neck stiffness is rare. If there is an increased number of pus cells in the CSF and the smear shows Gram-negative rods or no bacteria, treatment is given (see pp. 234–5, 238).

Urinary tract infection In early life urinary tract infection can cause kidney damage. Detection and prompt

Table 2.5.12 A simple method of assessment of gestational age at birth (scores given in parenthesis)

Characteristics	≤27 wks	28 wks	29 wks	30 wks	31 wks	32 wks	33 wks	34 wks	35 wks	36 wks	37 wks	38 wks	39 wks	≥40 wks
1. LENS Vessels in the pupillary membrane seen with an ophthalmoscope set at + 20 D. (For objectiveness note diameter of clear area and relation to total diameter of lens visualised)	Vessels all over the lens (Score 0)		Clearing < ½ lens diameter (Score 1)		Clearing – ½ lens diameter (Score 2)		Small loops at edge clearing > ½ lens diameter (Score 3)			Lens completely clear or with occasional strand or a faint loop (Score 4)				
2. BREAST NODULE Size of the breast nodule (not nipple) noted by picking up between index finger an thumb.	No breast tissue (Score 0)							Breast nodule < 0.5 cm (Score 1)		Breast nodule 0.5 cm– 1.0 cm (Score 2)			Breast nodule > 1.0 cm (Score 3)	
3. EAR FIRMNESS Noted by palpation. Test recoil after folding of upper pinns.	Folds into bizarre shapes; no recoil (Score 0)		Very soft; slow recoil on folding (Score 1)				Some cartilage; ready recoil after folding (Score 2)				Firm with cartilage; instant recoil after folding (Score 3)			
4 PLANTAR CREASES Note grooves on the soles. (Fine superficial lines not so significant as they also occur with drying and intrauterine growth retardation)	No creases (Score 0)	Very faint lines anterior ½ (Score 1)			Red marks over anterior ½ and grooves over anterior ⅓ (Score 2)				Grooves over more than anterior ⅓ (Score 3)			anterior ⅓	Extensive creases; deep grooves over anterior ⅓ (Score 4)	

RELATION OF THE TOTAL SCORE WITH THE GESTATIONAL AGE

0–<27 wks.	2–29 wks.	4–30 wks.	6–32 wks.	8–34 wks.	12–38 wks	14–>40 wks.
1–28 wks.	3–29½ wks	5–31 wks.	7–33 wks	11–37 wks.	13–39 wks.	

Note: First feel for the breast nodule. If it is not palpable the infant is likely to be less than 34 wks. Assessment can be made by the lens alone. If the lens is clear or if the breast nodule is well felt, evaluate the breast tissue, ear firmness, and plantar creases and add 4 for the lens. An alternative in the latter cases (i.e. over 34 wks.), is to assess the gestational age by the breast nodule, ear firmness, and plantar creases and take the average. *Assessment by the total score decreases the effect of intrauterine growth retardation.* (Reproduced by permission of *Pediatrics*; **69**:27 © 1982)

Table 2.5.13 Clinical complications of low-birth-weight infants

Complications	Preterm	Term
Failure to suck	+ +	0
Hypothermia	+ +	+
Hypoglycaemia	+	+ +
Infections	+ +	+ +
Respiratory distress syndrome	+ + +	0
Meconium aspiration	0	+
Jaundice	+ +	+
Congenital defects	+	+ +
Bleeding (IVH, Pulmonary haem)	+ +	±
Polycythemia	0	+ +
Prenatal asphyxia	±	+

IVH = intraventricular haemorrhage

treatment in the neonate is very important. Boys are affected more commonly than girls in contrast to later childhood and adult life when the converse is true. *E. coli* is responsible for nearly 80 per cent of cases. The collection of uncontaminated urine specimens from the newborn requires patience and attention to detail. The perineum should be washed with soap and water, rinsed, and dried with sterile swabs before a collecting bag is applied, or the infant is held or placed over a sterile collecting dish. Freshly collected uncentrifuged urine is examined for bacteria by microscopy. If bacteria are present, treatment should be given using a combination of ampicillin and gentamicin as for septicaemia.

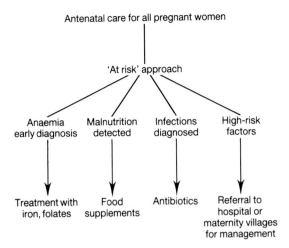

Antenatal care for all pregnant women

'At risk' approach

| Anaemia early diagnosis | Malnutrition detected | Infections diagnosed | High-risk factors |

| Treatment with iron, folates | Food supplements | Antibiotics | Referral to hospital or maternity villages for management |

Fig. 2.5.10   Intervention to prevent low birth weight.

Special care for preterm infants

Feeding

Preterm infants should be fed with mother's milk because its composition is appropriate for the gestational age of the baby. Infants born before 34 weeks of gestation are unlikely to suck at the breast and they should be fed by a polythene tube inserted into the stomach. Expressed breast-milk from the baby's mother is collected into sterilized containers and used as soon as possible. Raw milk from the infant's mother is easily digested, particularly the fat which provides valuable calories. Breast-milk is also crucial for the preterm neonate in developing countries because of its anti-infective properties. This benefit has been demonstrated in India amongst mothers from lower social groups.[11] The milk is fed in measured amounts using a syringe with the milk flowing by gravity. Babies may also be fed expressed breast-milk by spoon, the milk having been collected into a sterile cup. Feeding of all preterm infants should be supervised by nursing staff who encourage mothers to administer the feeds.

The infant is weighed daily for a gain in weight. This should be of the order of 18 g/kg daily. When this occurs, the baby is being fed adequately. Feeds should be given every two or three hours. The infant should be encouraged to suck at the breast as soon as possible.

Problems of artificial feeding   Artificial milks have a number of differences in composition that may be harmful to LBW preterm infants. If these milks are not

properly prepared, they have a high osmolality which will increase the solute (e.g. sodium) load on the immature kidneys and also lead to necrotizing enterocolitis. The volume of milk fed is initially 60 ml/kg body weight and this is increased by 20 ml/kg daily upto 200 ml/kg; an SFD baby would require daily increments of 30 ml/kg. If the infant is under a radiant heater or a phototherapy unit, fluid volume should be increased by 40 per cent. Casein is much higher in cow milk than human milk, and the essential amino acids (taurine, alanine, arginine) for preterm infants are usually inadequate in milk formulas, particularly taurine in milk. Preterm infants fed on artificial milk tend to pass hard stools because of the fat content and composition. The absorption of calcium from artificial milks is also poor because of the inappropriate calcium to phosphorus ratio; this may lead to rickets. Because of all these problems it is best to feed preterm babies in developing countries on breast-milk.

Oral multivitamin supplements including iron are recommended for all preterm infants.

Warmth

Preterm babies in warm climates are at risk of heat loss because adults assume that the environmental temperature is sufficient to maintain a normal body temperature. This assumption is incorrect because the LBW preterm infant has a large body surface area relative to its weight. Heat loss is also increased because of a high cerebral blood circulation, high skin blood flow with limited peripheral vasoconstriction and poor subcutaneous tissue insulation, a hypotonic posture at rest, and a smaller mass of brown fat than the term baby. Heat production in the neonate, particularly the LBW preterm infant, is mainly through non-shivering thermogenesis of brown fat; shivering occurs only when the environmental temperature is 15°C or less. Brown fat is found superficially (between the scapulae) and along the aorta. In response to cold, catecholamines are released which act directly on brown fat generating heat (2.5 calories/g brown fat per minute) by hydrolysis of triglycerides to free fatty acids and glycerol. Oxygen is consumed in this process.

There is a zone of environmental temperature in which heat production and oxygen consumption are at a minimum – the thermoneutral range. For a 2 kg baby lying naked in an incubator, it is 32–34°C, and for a swaddled infant 24–29°C in the first week.

Survival of the neonate is related to body temperature. The environmental temperature of a closed room may be raised by heaters. A baby may be warmed by radiant heat from an electric heater made with two 60 W light bulbs in a metal casing placed 40 cm above the baby.

Respiratory distress syndrome (RDS)

Preterm infants are prone to suffer respiratory distress due to a deficiency of surfactant in the lungs. Surfactant consists of lipoproteins, mainly phosphatidyl choline (lecithin) synthesized in the Type II or granular pneumocytes of the alveolar epithelium during the third trimester of gestation. Therefore, the more immature the infant, the more likely is he to suffer from respiratory distress syndrome. Not all preterm infants develop RDS, particularly if their lecithin to sphingomyelin (L:S) ratio is more than 2:1. The shake test or foam stability test is a fairly good predictor of lung maturity but it is much less effective in predicting lung immaturity. However, it is a simple test that can be done without the help of a laboratory. Gastric or pharyngeal aspirate to be tested (0.5 ml) is shaken with 0.5 ml of 95 per cent ethanol (alcohol) in a small glass tube. After 15 minutes the persistence of bubbles at the surface indicates lung maturity.

The preterm infant subjected to perinatal hypoxia, acidaemia and cold is at high risk of developing RDS. Infants born to inadequately controlled diabetics have an increased incidence of RDS. Preterm infants greater than 32 weeks of gestation and delivered by Caesarean section before the onset of labour, are also at greater risk of developing RDS.

Clinical features RDS presents within four hours of birth in an infant with: tachypnoea (above 60 breaths per minute); sternal retraction, intercostal and sub-costal recession, and an expiratory grunt. Chest radiograph shows a reticulogranular pattern due to atelectasis, and radiolucent air-filled major airways or 'air bronchogram'. In severe cases the lungs are as opaque as the cardiac shadow. It is essential to X-ray the chest as soon as possible after any infant develops signs of respiratory distress. This prevents any delay in starting appropriate therapy for the respiratory illness.

Signs should be present before four hours of age, should still be there at four hours of age, and should persist for some period beyond four hours of age. Without added inspired oxygen the infant is cyanosed. Ausculation of the lungs shows reduced air entry, with a few crepitations. The heart rate tends to be fixed at 120–130 per minute, and the blood pressure is 20–25 per cent lower than normal (44–60 mmHg) for gestation. The infant is inactive, lies in a 'frog' position,

and has moderate generalized subcutaneous oedema owing to increased capillary leakiness. Only small amounts of urine are passed and meconium may not be passed until the third or fourth day of life.

In uncomplicated RDS, surfactant reappears in the lungs at about 36–48 hours of age. The illness gradually gets worse over the first 36 hours, it then stabilizes for 24 hours, and improves from 60 to 72 hours. Recovery is usually complete by the end of the first week.

Pathophysiology The alveoli collapse when the lungs are depleted of surfactant and the lungs become very stiff. There is exudation of plasma into the alveoli and airways.

The proteins in this exudate clot and form the characteristic hyaline membranes that line the bronchioles and alveolar ducts. Because the lungs are stiff, lung compliance falls to 25 per cent of normal, the work of breathing is increased, there is increased intrapulmonary shunting of arterial blood leading to severe hypoxaemia and hypoventilation, causing respiratory acidosis. Other clinical features of RDS are secondary to hypoxia, e.g. hypotension, vascular damage, severe metabolic acidaemia, and decreased perfusion of other tissues such as kidneys, intestines and brain.

Treatment The aim is to keep the baby alive until he starts to synthesize his own surfactant 36 to 48 hours after birth. This is done by avoiding hypoxaemia, acidaemia and hypothermia which inhibit surfactant synthesis, and having complete control of the baby's cardiorespiratory, electrolyte and renal homoeostasis. In developing countries, this can be difficult to achieve because it requires trained nursing staff, equipment and doctors specialized in intensive care.

As far as possible the following should be monitored: heart rate, arterial oxygen (PaO_2), concentration of oxygen delivered to the baby, respiratory pattern and activity, body temperature and blood pressure. The following outline of management should be instituted:

1. The baby's body temperature must be maintained at 37°C by increasing the environmental temperature and covering him with a clear plastic sheet.
2. Acid–base homoeostasis should be achieved so that the arterial blood pH is above 7.25 (H^+ below 65 mmol/l) so that surfactant synthesis is not inhibited. A base deficit in excess of 5 mmol/l indicates metabolic acidaemia and every effort should be made to discover its cause (e.g. hypotension, hypoxaemia, sepsis, anaemia or a

metabolic error) and to correct it by appropriate means. Solutions of sodium bicarbonate or THAM should be used with care; THAM should only be used if the infant is being ventilated. Sodium bicarbonate should usually be used and the rate of infusion should not exceed 0.5 mmol/min. The dose used may be calculated from the formula: dose in mmol of sodium bicarbonate = base deficit (mmol/l) × body weight (kg) × 0.4 (sodium bicarbonate 8.4 per cent solution contains 1 mmol of bicarbonate per ml). This calculated dose will always undercorrect the acidaemia and the blood gases should be checked within an hour.

Respiratory acidaemia ($PaCO_2$ raised) is found in all cases of RDS and may reach 13.3 KPa (100 mmHg) or more if untreated. As $PaCO_2$ increases cerebral blood flow and causes intraventricular haemorrhage (IVH), it should not be allowed to rise above 9.3 KPa (70 mmHg). A rise in $PaCO_2$ indicates the following: (i) steady rise means mechanical ventilation is likely to be needed; (ii) sudden rise may be due to a pneumothorax, collapsed lung lobes, misplaced endotracheal tube; (iii) gradual rise at the end of the first week in a ventilated, previously stable LBW infant, may be due to a patent ductus arteriosus (PDA). Respiratory stimulants (vandid, nikethamide) have no role in the management of the hypercapnoea of RDS.

3. Oral feeding should be omitted for the first two or three days of life, because most cases have paralytic ileus. Glucose electrolyte infusions given via an umbilical artery catheter or through a peripheral vein, will maintain hydration and blood glucose. Expressed breast-milk (1 ml every hour) may be started on the third day through an oro-gastric tube.

4. Sick neonates are poor at excreting water so great care should be taken to prevent excessive fluids by infusion. In RDS, fluid overload leads to complications such as a PDA, necrotizing enterocolitis and chronic lung disease. Therefore, fluid intake should be kept at 60 ml per kg over 24 hours in the first few days.

5. Infants with severe RDS are often hypotensive in the first few hours. Blood should be given if the haematocrit is less than 40 per cent and albumin or plasma given if the haematocrit is above 45 per cent. Initially, 15 to 20 ml/kg of blood or plasma is given. Chronic iatrogenic hypovolaemia and anaemia are caused by frequent sampling during intensive care, so top-up blood transfusions of 10–15 ml/kg should be given when the haematocrit falls below 40 per cent.

6. Oxygen therapy is needed to keep the PaO_2 in blood in the range 8–12 KPa (60–90 mmHg). The lower limit is chosen to avoid acidaemia with PDA and decrease surfactant synthesis, and the upper limit to minimize development of retinopathy of prematurity and possible blindness. The retinopathy (retrolental fibroplasia) is a disease of prematurity with the death of retinal capillaries when perfused with blood of high PaO_2. The disease is rare in infants over 30 weeks of gestation and above 1.5 kg birth weight. The problems of monitoring oxygen therapy are not discussed here but may be found in textbooks devoted to neonatology (e.g. Roberton NRC. *A Manual of Neonatal Intensive Care*, 2nd Edn, Edward Arnold, 1986). Oxygen may be administered by headbox and this is usually satisfactory for most infants with RDS in the first two or three days. The oxygen should be warmed and humidified. Other methods of delivering oxygen above 60 per cent concentration include continuous positive airways pressure (CPAP) and mechanical ventilation. These techniques are not without complications and should be done only by specialists trained in intensive care.

7. Drug therapy includes diuretics, e.g. frusemide (1.5 mg/kg once, and repeated if necessary after six hours) for cardiac failure or pulmonary haemorrhage, and antibiotics (penicillin and gentamicin).

Prevention   Corticosteroid therapy has been shown to reduce the incidence of RDS in preterm deliveries at 32–34 weeks of gestation. It should be avoided in women with hypertension and or proteinuria (preeclampsia). Betamethasone sodium phosphate or dexamethasone sodium phosphate (12 mg daily) are convenient since they need to be given only once daily for two days. To be effective the steroid must be given to the mother at least 12 and preferably 24 hours before delivery.

Prevention of low birth weight

The majority (80 per cent) of births occur in the community or at home where deliveries are conducted by traditional birth attendants (trained or untrained) or relatives. It is not possible to provide care for such infants in special care baby units because of the constraints of economy, trained personnel and availability of suitable inexpensive equipment. The logical step in the management of LBW infants appears to be a concerted effort aimed at its prevention rather than care after birth. The following strategies, consistent with national health policies, utilize the infrastructure for health delivery in a cost-effective manner (Fig. 2.5.10).

Health education

The highest priority should be accorded to health education for the masses because of its long-term benefits. Health education programmes should emphasize the importance of child spacing, the avoidance of smoking and alcohol during pregnancy, antenatal care, nutritious diet during pregnancy, treatment of anaemia and maternal protection against malaria, tetanus and rubella. Programmes involving increasing community participation are essential to successful mass education and utilization of existing health care facilities.

Population awareness of low birth weight

The effects of low birth weight on survival and morbidity, the risks of neurological sequelae and failure to thrive should be publicized by mass media to the population, particularly amongst high-risk communities such as primigravida. It should be clearly stated that while it may be possible with timely intervention and appropriate care of the pregnant woman to prevent the occurrence of LBW infants, it will be difficult to prevent an adverse outcome after birth. The slogan 'prevention is better than cure' will have to be adopted.

Antenatal care

The role of antenatal care in improving the outcome of pregnancy is well documented; in southern India the mean birth weight of infants whose mothers had antenatal care was 2964 g compared with 2710 g for those who did not. Initial educational campaigns should seek to highlight the necessity of early registration of pregnancy and regular antenatal checks. The exact number, frequency and timing of antenatal visits remains a matter for debate. However, the importance of periodic antenatal checks must be repeatedly emphasized. Pregnancy weight gain may be monitored by weighing and by mid-upper arm circumference measurement.

Maternal nutrition

The need for extra nutrition for the pregnant woman is a fact well accepted by most communities. Education is needed on the use of inexpensive and readily available foods in adequate quantities by the pregnant woman. Customs and beliefs may act as constraints on adequate utilization of existing food resources, e.g. while pregnant women accept food supplements, they do not always use these for themselves. The family, therefore, must be made to appreciate that the pregnant woman needs to be accorded the highest priority for adequate nutrition.

Rest and conservation of energy

Customs which benefit the outcome of pregnancy should be encouraged. The practice of delivering the first born at the parental home is to be commended because the burden of daily household chores tend to diminish when the expectant woman is looked after by her mother. It offers the expectant woman an opportunity for adequate rest and nutritional intake to improve the outcome of pregnancy. Another benefit from this practice would be the decrease in cohabitation in later months of pregnancy and thus a decrease in the risks, if any, of early spontaneous rupture of membranes or premature labour. Further studies are indicated in this field.

Utilization of MCH facilities

Basic primary health care is usually provided but most services remain grossly under-utilized. Reasons for non-utilization include distance, non-availability of drugs, facilities and health workers, or the community's lack of trust in the system.

Anticipation of the birth of low-birth-weight infants

'At risk' approach

Several factors contributing to the causation of low birth weight are identifiable through careful clinical history, examination and simple laboratory tests. Early identification and appropriate care of pregnant women at risk of delivering a low-birth-weight infant would be the aim of this 'at risk' approach. The success of this approach would depend upon selection of risk factors or a scoring system which can be used by a basic health worker (see Table 2.5.14).

Fetal monitoring

Biophysical monitoring in early diagnosis of fetal growth failure has been established in recent reports. Ultrasonography, although ideal for this purpose may not be freely available. It would be more appropriate to

Table 2.5.14 Simplified scoring system

Factor	Score
1. Maternal age <20 or >35 years	1
2. Parity 0 or >4	1
3. Previous Caesarean section	2
4. Previous perinatal death	2
5. Acute maternal illness (fever, diarrhoea, etc.)	2
6. Fetal malpresentation	2
7. Antepartum haemorrhage	2
8. Maternal height <140 cm	2
9. Maternal Hb >7 g/dl	2
10. Gestation <9 months	3

A score of 3 or more indicates high risk of perinatal mortality. (Reproduced with permission from Bhargava *et al*, *Indian Pediatrics*, 1982; **19**:209–15.)

use gravidograms which are a record of fundal height and abdominal girth at different gestational periods. Such graphs are now available and should be incorporated in antenatal records. A weight gain in pregnancy of <0.5 kg per month especially in already malnourished women, (initial mid-upper arm circumference of <22.5 cm) is also a high risk indicator for LBW (see p. 138).

Prolonging birth interval – contraception

Temporary methods of contraception are necessary to prolong the birth interval beyond 24 months. This will reduce the delivery of preterm LBW infants. Intrauterine devices, barrier methods and oral contraceptives are effective methods.

Delaying marriage age

This method, effective in China, is being applied in India to prevent teenage pregnancies.

References

1. World Health Organization. *International Classification of Diseases 1975 Revision*. Vol. 1. Geneva, WHO, 1977.
2. World Health Organization. The incidence of low birth weight: an update. *Weekly Epidemiological Record*. 1984; **59**: 205–12.
3. Ghosh S, Bhargava SK, Saxena HMK, Sagreiya K. Perinatal mortality: report of a hospital based study. *Annals of Tropical Paediatrics*. 1983; **3**: 115–19.
4. Barros FC, Victoria CG, Vaughan JP, Estanislau HJ. Perinatal mortality in southern Brazil: a population-based study of 7392 births. *Bulletin of the World Health Organization*. 1987; **65**: 95–104.
5. Barros FC, Victoria CG, Vaughan JP *et al*. Infant mortality in southern Brazil: a population based study of causes of death. *Archives of Disease in Childhood*. 1987; **62**: 487–90.
6. Bhargava SL, Sachdev HPS, Ramji S, Iyer PU. Low birth weight: aetiology and prevention in India. *Annals of Tropical Paediatrics*. 1987; **7**: 59–65.
7. Dawodu AH, Laditan AA. Low birth weight in an urban community in Nigeria. *Annals of Tropical Paediatrics*. 1985; **5**: 61–6.
8. Dubowitz LMS, Dubowitz V, Goldberg C. Clinical assessment of gestational age in the newborn infant. *Journal of Pediatrics*. 1970; **77**: 1–10.
9. Parkin JM, Key EN, Clowes JS. Rapid assessment of gestational age at birth. *Archives of Disease in Childhood*. 1976; **51**: 259–63.
10. Narayanan I, Dua K, Prabhakar AK *et al*. A simple method of assessment of gestational age at birth. *Pediatrics*. 1982; **69**: 27–32.
11. Narayanan I, Prakash K, Bala S *et al*. Partial supplementation with expressed breast-milk for prevention of infection in low birth weight infants. *Lancet*. 1980; **ii**: 561–3.
12. Bhargava SK, Srinivasan S, Kishan J. A simplified scoring system for identification of high risk births. *Indian Pediatrics*. 1982; **19**: 209–15.

Further reading

Kramer MS. Determinants of low birth weight: methodological assessment and meta-analysis. *Bulletin of the World Health Organization*. 1987; **65**: 663–737.
Roberton NRC. *A Manual of Neonatal Intensive Care*, 2nd Edn, London, Edward Arnold, 1986.

NEONATAL JAUNDICE
Michael Chan

Jaundice is commonly found in newborn infants in Africa, South-east Asia, the Pacific, the Mediterranean and Latin America. Neonatal jaundice received high priority in 1984 at a Geneva consultation of senior paediatricians from these regions with World Health Organization officials, when they identified serious diseases affecting child health not covered by WHO programmes in developing countries.[1]

There are geographical and racial differences in the pattern of severe neonatal jaundice which reflect the interaction of genetic and environmental factors. When compared with European babies, normal full-term infants of Chinese, Greek and Japanese origin tend to have higher maximum bilirubin levels that reach their peak at four or five days of life.

Neonatal jaundice is almost always due to a rise of unconjugated bilirubin in the blood. It is difficult to detect in dark-skinned babies, and may become severe in the presence of pathological causes (Table 2.5.15) before medical attention is sought. When this happens, the newborn baby may show evidence of brain damage because of the deposition of unconjugated bilirubin in the basal ganglia producing kernicterus. Kernicterus may be fatal but most babies survive with deafness, and varying degrees of athetoid cerebral palsy and mental retardation. The primary dentition is also stained yellow-brown in survivors of kernicterus.

Pathophysiology

Bilirubin is produced by the degradation of haemoglobin; one gram forming 600 μmol (35 mg) of bilirubin. Bilirubin production in the normal newborn infant is 8–10 mg/kg body weight per day – more than double that of adults. This is the result of a larger relative red cell mass (at birth the newborn has a haemoglobin concentration of about 20 g/100 ml), a shorter red cell life span, ineffective erythropoiesis from perinatal stress, and intestinal reabsorption of bilirubin from the duodenum and proximal small intestine. The enterohepatic recirculation of bilirubin in the newborn results from the action of the intestinal enzyme β-glucuronidase, reserves of bilirubin in meconium, and the absence of appropriate intestinal flora to degrade bilirubin to urobilinogen.

In the European term infant, serum bilirubin concentration increases from 35 μmol/l (2 mg/100 ml or dl) to a peak of 85–100 μmol/l (5–6 mg/100 ml or dl) on the third day, after which it declines to the level at birth by the end of the first week. Premature infants have a higher maximum bilirubin reached on day five or six and a slower decline. On the other hand, postmature infants and some small-for-dates infants have a minimal postnatal rise in serum bilirubin. In general, any newborn infant whose serum bilirubin concentration exceeds 175–210μmol/l (10–12 mg/dl) by the third day of life should be considered to have a pathological cause for the jaundice. Bilirubin in the blood is bound to serum albumin during its transport to the liver where it is conjugated to glucuronic acid in a process catalysed by the microsomal enzyme, uridyl diphosphate (UDP) glucuronyl transferase. Glucuronyl transferase activity is low at birth and increases gradually to attain adult levels by 14 weeks.

Table 2.5.15 Causes of severe neonatal jaundice in the tropics

Glucose-6-phosphate dehydrogenase (G6PD) deficiency
ABO blood group and other minor blood group
  incompatibilities
Bacterial sepsis
Extravasated blood – cephalohaematomas
             – extensive bruising (breech delivery)
Prematurity
Dehydration and starvation
Drugs that bind albumin (kanamycin, sodium salicylate,
  sulphonamides)
Rhesus haemolytic disease (uncommon)

As the concentration of serum bilirubin rises, the capacity of albumin to bind unconjugated pigment is used up so that unbound or free bilirubin increases. Free bilirubin is toxic to the brain. As its concentration in the brain increases, the infant becomes irritable or lethargic, sucks poorly and vomits its feeds. With the establishment of kernicterus, abnormal neurological signs appear such as hypertonia, paralysis of upward gaze, opisthotonus, high-pitched cry, fever, apnoea and convulsions. When the total unconjugated serum bilirubin level reaches 350μmol/l (20 mg/dl), toxic levels of free bilirubin are probably achieved in the brain of full-term infants. Preterm infants who are ill, may develop kernicterus at total unconjugated serum bilirubin levels as low as 210μmol/l (12 mg/dl).

Clinical presentations

Infection

Jaundice which develops suddenly in any newborn infant in the first week of life should alert the doctor to the diagnosis of infection and appropriate investigations and treatment should be instituted.

Glucose-6-phosphate dehydrogenase (G6PD) deficiency

Severe jaundice presents on days three to five and may be noticed for the first time in the second week of life. Some infants may present before the third day but significant jaundice in the first 24 hours is rare. As this red cell enzyme deficiency is inherited in a sex-linked recessive manner, the majority of infants affected are boys. Haemolysis occurs rapidly in G6PD-deficient neonates exposed to potent haemolytic agents such as naphthalene.

More than 400 million people in Africa, the Mediterranean and South-east Asia are G6PD deficient. The gene for this condition is said to have been perpetuated because heterozygous carriers suffer less severely from *P. falciparum* malaria. The G6PD molecule comprises 515 amino acids in two identical chains. Therefore, mutations resulting in amino acid substitutions easily occur and more than 300 variants of G6PD enzymes have so far been identified.[11] They have been classified into five groups.[2]

- Class 1: severe enzyme deficiency associated with chronic non-spherocytic haemolytic anaemia
- Class 2: severe enzyme deficiency (<10% of normal)

- Class 3: moderate to mild deficiency (10–60% of normal)
- Class 4: very mild or no deficiency (60–100% of normal)
- Class 5: increased enzyme activity (more than twice normal)

Individuals with normal G6PD enzyme activity possess the B^+ variant which has a half-life of about 62 days. Enzyme variants belonging to classes 2 and 3 are commonly associated with severe neonatal jaundice. The Mediterranean variant found in Greece and the Canton variant in China have a half-life of a few days and are examples of class 2 enzyme variants. The A^- variant found in west Africa is a class 3 variant.

Glucose-6-phosphate dehydrogenase (G6PD) is the enzyme which catalyses the conversion of glucose 6-phosphate to 6-phosphogluconate in the first reaction of the pentose–phosphate pathway of aerobic glycolysis (Fig. 2.5.11). It participates in the reduction of nicotinamide adenine dinucleotide phosphate (NADP) to NADPH. Glutathione (GSSG) is converted to its reduced form (GSH) by the transfer of H^+ ions from NADPH in the presence of glutathione reductase. Reduced glutathione is an intracellular buffer that protects red cells from damage by oxygen-derived free radicals, produced in excessive amounts during the metabolism of some drugs and chemicals. The sulphydryl (SH) radical of reduced glutathione neutralizes such radicals as hydrogen peroxide (H_2O_2) and superoxide (O_2-) in the presence of glutathione peroxidase. G6PD-deficient red cells lack reduced glutathione (GSH) and are, therefore, susceptible to damage leading to haemolysis by these radicals.

The association of neonatal jaundice and G6PD deficiency was first recognized in 1960 by Smith and

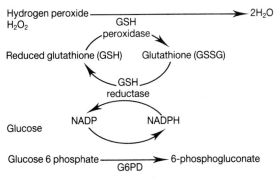

Fig. 2.5.11 The pentose-phosphate pathway of aerobic glycolysis.

Vella who reported 13 newborn infants in Singapore with kernicterus.[3] Similar reports followed from Greece, Sardinia, Turkey, Hong Kong, Taiwan and Thailand in the 1960s, and from Africa and the West Indies and in black Americans in the 1970s and 1980s. Common features were apparent in these reports. Although the frequency of G6PD deficiency in these at-risk populations varied between 2 and 20 per cent, it was found more commonly in neonates with severe jaundice and those presenting with kernicterus. Most of those affected were boys.

Neonates with G6PD deficiency invariably have a reduced red cell life span. Although haemolysis is the main cause, jaundice rarely presents on the first day of life. Preterm infants with G6PD deficiency and those with serious infections such as pneumonia and septicaemia are at high risk of developing kernicterus.

Low birth weight

The *preterm* infant born before 37 weeks of gestation is at risk of developing jaundice because of immaturity of the glucuronyl transferase enzyme system. When associated with birth asphyxia, respiratory distress or sepsis, kernicterus may occur at serum bilirubin levels of 200 μmol/l (12 mg/dl).

The *small-for-dates* infant may be polycythaemic or suffer from hypoglycaemia, both conditions that lead to jaundice.

Infants of diabetic mothers are usually born preterm although they may be of normal weight or large. They become jaundiced because of prematurity associated hypoglycaemia and bruising due to birth trauma.

Blood group incompatibility

ABO blood group incompatibility is numerically much more important in developing countries than rhesus incompatibility. In ABO incompatibility, the mother usually has blood group O and the baby either group A or B.

Infants with rhesus isoimmunization are usually rhesus (D) positive born to rhesus (D) negative mother. Such infants of primigravid mothers may have mild jaundice only unless the mother has been previously immunized by an incompatible rhesus (D) positive blood transfusion. With successive pregnancies, the fetus will be affected with increasing severity. The severely affected infant with rhesus isoimmunization may be very anaemic at birth with severe heart failure, and peripheral oedema (hydrops fetalis), hepatospleno-megaly and rapid onset of jaundice.

Prolonged jaundice

The many causes of jaundice persisting beyond ten days is listed in Table 2.5.16. Of these, hypothyroidism and galactosaemia should be sought for by investigations because they are two treatable causes of mental retardation.

In the 1970s breast-milk was reported to be associated with persisting jaundice in Western countries. Recent studies have shown that breast-feeding on demand is not associated with jaundice, in contrast to less frequent feeding. This is due to the rapid clearance of meconium from the bowel in demand feeding, which reduces the enterohepatic recirculation of bilirubin. Breast-feeding on demand is normal practice in traditional communities in developing countries, and, therefore, explains its infrequent association with neonatal jaundice.

Diagnosis

Jaundice in the newborn infant is best detected by blanching the skin on the nasal bridge or the tip of the nose. The severity of neonatal jaundice is associated with its spread from the face to the trunk and extremities of the limbs (Fig. 2.5.12).

The day of appearance of jaundice may help in the diagnosis of the underlying cause. Jaundice appearing in the first day of life is probably due to haemolytic disease associated with rhesus isoimmunization or with ABO incompatibility. Transplacental infections with rubella, cytomegalovirus, herpes simplex, syphilis and toxoplasmosis may also present with jaundice, and other associated signs on the first day. Jaundice

Table 2.5.16   Causes of prolonged neonatal jaundice

Unconjugated bilirubin
G6PD deficiency
Hereditary red cell membrane disorders – spherocytosis, elliptocytosis, stomatocytosis
Infection – chronic or low-grade bacterial or viral, congenital malaria
Hypothyroidism
Galactosaemia

Obstructive jaundice (mixed bilirubin)
Hepatitis – rubella, hepatitis B, cytomegalovirus
Galactosaemia
Biliary atresia
Inspissated bile syndrome
Biliary obstruction (choledochal cyst, band, tumour)
Inherited defects (α_1-antitrypsin deficiency, Dubin–Johnson, Rotor)

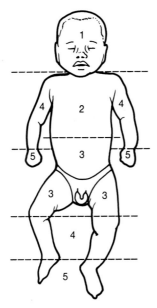

Fig. 2.5.12 Spread of skin jaundice in the newborn. Skin zones: 1 = 4–8 mg/100 ml; 2 = 8–12 mg/100 ml; 3 = 12–16 mg/100 ml; 4 = 14–18 mg/100 ml; 5 = 16–20 mg/100 ml. (Reproduced from Kramer LI, *American Journal of Diseases of Children*, 1969; **18**:454–58. © 1969, American Medical Association.)

occurring after the first day of life is associated with other causes listed in Table 2.5.15.

Severity of jaundice

Management of neonatal jaundice is dependent on the severity of jaundice based upon the level of total serum bilirubin. Mild neonatal jaundice is diagnosed when the total serum bilirubin is less than 175 μmol/l (10 mg/dl). Moderate cases of jaundice have a bilirubin level of between 175 and 210μmol/l (10 to 12 mg/dl) in preterm infants and up to 260 μmol/l (15 mg/dl) in full term infants. Severe jaundice is present when the total serum bilirubin level is above 12 mg/dl in preterm infants or above 15 mg/dl in term neonates. All infants with severe jaundice should be examined for evidence of kernicterus, the earliest features of which are disturbance with feeding such as poor sucking, vomiting, drowsiness, hypotonia and sluggish reflexes. When kernicterus is established, abnormal neurological signs appear with hypertonia replacing hypotonia, paralysis of upward gaze giving the 'sun-setting' sign in the eyes, opisthotonus (retracted neck and arched back), high-pitched cry, involuntary movements or twitching of the limbs, high fever and convulsions.

Investigations

Serum bilirubin   A serum bilirubin estimation should be done to determine the severity of the jaundice in all infants with jaundice on the first day or with jaundice in skin zones 2 to 5 (Fig. 2.5.12). (See also p. 982.) In hospitals where neonatal jaundice is a common problem, direct reading of serum bilirubin can be obtained using a photometric instrument. Although expensive, it will be cost-effective in personnel, reagents and time. Both unconjugated and conjugated bilirubin should be estimated.

If a serum biliburin determination is not available, a perspex icterometer (Fig. 2.5.13) can be equally useful to estimate the severity of the jaundice. The icterometer, first devised by Gosset in 1960, identifies the degree of jaundice of the blanched nose matched with yellow strips from grades 1 to 5; grade 4 being equivalent to a total serum bilirubin of 15 mg/dl.[5] In black infants, better correlation is obtained by blanching the gum instead of the nose in direct sunlight. The correlation between serum bilirubin concentrations and icterometer grading in black neonates is shown in Table 2.5.17.

Full-term infants with an icterometer grading below 4 and preterm infants with grading below 3 may be followed up with the icterometer. Jaundice during the first day of life and infants with icterometer grades above 3 or 4, should be referred to a centre with laboratory facilities to do further investigations, such as serum bilirubin estimation and blood grouping. Sick neonates and very-low-birth-weight infants (under 1500 g) should be referred with lower icterometer readings. Despite the availability of more complex and expensive devices for transcutaneous bilirubinometry, the icterometer continues to serve as a cost-effective screening device for neonatal hyperbilirubinaemia.

Blood tests   Haemoglobin concentration, blood film examination and reticulocyte count are three simple

Table 2.5.17   Mean and +2 SD bilirubin levels for each icterometer grading

Icterometer grading	Total bilirubin (mg/dl)	
	Mean	+2 SD
2	5.50	7.54
2½	7.39	10.67
3	8.66	13.14
3½	12.18	14.79
4	15.10	18.40
4½	19.65	22.09

(Reproduced with permission from Hamel BCJ, *Tropical Doctor*, 1982; **12**:213–4.)

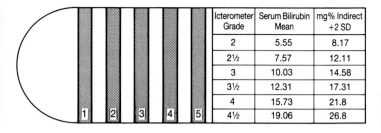

Icterometer Grade	Serum Bilirubin Mean	mg% Indirect +2 SD
2	5.55	8.17
2½	7.57	12.11
3	10.03	14.58
3½	12.31	17.31
4	15.73	21.8
4½	19.06	26.8

Fig. 2.5.13 The icterometer. (Sole makers: Thomas A. Ingram & Co., PO Box 305, Birmingham B19 1BB, UK.)

tests that can be done at primary health level to detect haemolysis.

Blood groups and direct Coomb's test If the mother is group O rhesus positive, the baby group A or B rhesus positive, and the direct Coomb's test on the baby's blood is positive or weakly positive, then ABO incompatibility may be the cause of the jaundice. Maternal serum should be examined for anti-A and anti-B haemolysins. Spherocytes are found in the baby's blood film. In communities where rhesus isoimmunizations occurs, the diagnosis is made when the baby is rhesus positive, the mother rhesus negative and the direct Coomb's is positive. If the baby is rhesus negative and the direct Coomb's test positive, other antibodies of the rhesus system (C or E) should be looked for as well as Kell and Duffy groups.

Erythrocyte G6PD enzyme screening tests These tests should be done in populations where G6PD deficiency is common. They depend on the presence of the G6PD enzyme which induces the formation of NADPH (reduced nicotinamide adenine dinucleotide phosphate). The NADPH is responsible for the reduction of dyes such as brilliant cresyl blue or methylene blue with colour change from blue to pink. G6PD-deficient red cells are unable to reduce methylene blue or brilliant cresyl blue. During the past 15 years, a fluorescent screening spot test has been widely used because it is more sensitive than other tests. NADPH produced by normal red cells fluoresces under ultraviolet radiation. With G6PD deficiency, NADPH is not produced in sufficient quantities to cause fluorescence. This method requires only a spot of blood 1 cm in diameter on blotting paper for accurate screening of G6PD enzyme. Specimens of blood may be sent through the post to a central laboratory for the fluorescence test.

Screening tests for infection These should be done where appropriate (see pp. 233–40).

Management of neonatal jaundice

Management depends on the severity of jaundice. Neonates with mild to moderate jaundice may be underfed and have an element of dehydration. These infants should have an increase in the frequency of breast-feeding. Mothers with an inadequate flow of milk may need more fluids to drink and even a galactogogue such as metoclopramide hydrochloride (10 mg three times a day). The level of serum bilirubin should be monitored daily to detect severe neonatal jaundice.

Treatment of severe jaundice

Adequate hydration

Dehydration is a significant cause of jaundice in some breast-fed babies who are not given feeding on demand. Sick, low-birth-weight, preterm neonates may also be dehydrated. If there are no contra-indications, such infants should have their fluid intake increased to 150 ml per kg per 24 hours by tube feeding or by intravenous infusion of 5 per cent dextrose solution.

Pharmacological agents

Phenobarbitone can induce the enzymes of bilirubin glucuronidation but it takes about 48 hours for the drug to take effect. It also makes the neonate sleepy and feed poorly, and may cause respiratory depression in preterm infants. Therefore, phenobarbitone cannot be recommended for the treatment of neonatal jaundice.

It has been noted that jaundice in preterm infants starts to clear once they have opened their bowels. However, the use of laxatives to lower serum bilirubin in the neonate is not justified.

Phototherapy

Phototherapy is the most commonly used treatment for

severe neonatal jaundice in the world. The routine use of phototherapy has significantly reduced the need to resort to exchange blood transfusion. The indications for phototherapy are jaundice in the first 24 hours, and severe neonatal jaundice without clinical evidence of kernicterus.

Phototherapy (with light of wave length 450–460 nm) reduces the amount of unconjugated bilirubin in plasma by isomerization of the bilirubin to produce water-soluble isomers which are slowly excreted, by intramolecular photoconversion between pyrrole rings to produce lumirubin which is rapidly excreted, and photo-oxidation of bilirubin to colourless mono- and di-pyrrols. All these compounds are not toxic to the brain. Isomers including lumirubin are formed immediately phototherapy starts. They are yellow and cannot be distinguished by the bilirubinometer but they are non-toxic.

Effective phototherapy should deliver to the infant a minimum irradiance of 1 mW/cm² in the 420–480 nm range (blue light). This level of irradiance may be obtained by using a phototherapy unit comprising at least seven 20 W white daylight fluorescent tubes placed 40 cm above the naked infant. A time record should be kept of the duration that phototherapy units are switched on because fluorescent tubes in phototherapy units have a useful life of 200 hours only. Therefore, fluorescent tubes in phototherapy units should be replaced regularly.

Neonates undertaking phototherapy should be nursed naked for maximum benefit from the breakdown of bilirubin in the skin. It is wise to shield the eyes with a gauze mask, although retinal damage observed in experimental animals has never been reported in human babies. Phototherapy in preterm infants is generally used when the serum bilirubin rises to 200 μ mol/l (12 mg/dl) or earlier in the very immature. In the full-term infant, phototherapy is used when the bilirubin has risen to 300 μ mol/l (17.5 mg/dl). The age of the infant and the rate of rise of serum bilirubin are important factors when considering the start of phototherapy – the younger infant and the infant with a rapid rise of bilirubin require phototherapy at lower levels of serum bilirubin.

Side-effects of phototherapy include increased water loss associated with absorbed photon energies, skin rashes associated with histamine release, and diarrhoea from increased excretion of bilirubin products. Neonates under phototherapy require additional fluid – about 10 to 15 per cent extra daily. Skin rashes and diarrhoea are transient. Body temperature should be recorded to avoid the risks of hypo- or hyperthermia. Phototherapy should not be given to infants with conju-gated bilirubin because their skin turns a deep brown colour due to photodegradation of porphyrins.

Exchange transfusion

Exchange transfusion is the only method of reducing the level of bilirubin rapidly when it has reached potentially toxic concentrations or when the infant is showing early clinical evidence of kernicterus. The first exchange transfusion ever performed was on an infant with severe haemolytic disease due to rhesus isoimmunization.[7] It not only removed the bilirubin, but it also removed haemolytic antibody and corrected anaemia. Exchange transfusion has also been used for the following: severe non-haemolytic anaemia; neonatal septicaemia with bleeding from disseminated intravascular coagulopathy (DIC); hypoxaemia in hyaline membrane disease; and to remove drugs in depressed neonates.

Feeding should be withheld for three hours before the exchange transfusion to prevent aspiration of vomited gastric contents; if time does not allow this, the stomach contents should be aspirated.

Blood used for exchange transfusion should be free of infective agents such as malarial parasites, hepatitis and HIV viruses, and should preferably be less than 48 hours old. Older blood will have more potassium in the plasma and may lead to hyperkalaemia in the baby. The ABO group of the donor blood may be that of the baby, if baby and mother are ABO compatible. In cases of ABO incompatibility, it is best to use blood group O reconstituted with ABO plasma. Group O whole blood is an alternative if it has been screened and found to be free of haemolysins. Rhesus-negative blood of the same group as the infant is preferred in cases of rhesus isoimmunization. If this is not available, group O rhesus-negative blood can be used. In all cases of exchange transfusion, cross-matching against mother or baby's blood should be performed before the procedure. If more than one exchange transfusion is required, the donor blood should be of the same ABO group as that used for the first transfusion.

Although heparinized blood is advocated by some, there are disadvantages to the use of heparin. The blood must be used promptly, and heparin may interfere with albumin binding of bilirubin due to the increase in plasma non-esterified fatty acid levels. Therefore, blood drawn into citrate phosphate dextrose (CPD) or CPD adenine is recommended for exchange transfusion. CPD anticoagulated blood has a higher pH than blood drawn into ACD (acid citrate dextrose) anticoagulant, and it also retains its 2.3 DPG enzyme levels (regulating the release of oxygen to the tissues) better during storage. A minor degree of acidosis occurs with the use of CPD blood but most infants are able to correct this without difficulty. The blood for exchange transfusion should preferably be warmed to body temperature with care to avoid haemolysis.

The standard technique for exchange transfusion is to introduce a polyvinyl end-hole catheter under strict aseptic conditions up to 7 cm into the umbilical vein in a full-term infant (see p. 1004). This will ensure that the catheter tip is in the hepatic vein or inferior vena cava, and a free flow of blood is obtained. The aim is to exchange twice the infant's blood volume (2 × 85 ml/kg body weight) in two hours using 20 ml aliquots of blood. Smaller volumes of 10 ml may be indicated in sick or preterm infants. Each cycle of withdrawing 5, 10 or 20 ml of baby's blood and injecting 5, 10 or 20 ml of donor's blood should take 4 or 5 minutes, taking at least 2 or 3 minutes for the infusion. Throughout the exchange the infant should have continuous ECG monitoring, or at least the heart rate should be counted every 10 minutes and recorded. The baby must be closely observed for skin colour, respiratory rate, and body temperature. The whole procedure must be timed and recorded.

The citrate in ACD blood combines with calcium to form calcium citrate and may give rise to hypocalcaemia. Therefore, 1 ml of a 10 per cent calcium gluconate solution is administered after each 100 ml of citrated blood exchanged. In sick infants with acidosis, sodium bicarbonate should be given in appropriate dosage to maintain arterial pH at 7.3. Prophylactic antibiotics are not indicated as a routine. Serum bilirubin should be measured before and at the end of the transfusion. After exchange transfusion, the baby should be given phototherapy. Bilirubin concentration is usually monitored at regular intervals four hourly after transfusion, and exchange transfusion repeated if indicated.

Albumin priming to increase bilirubin removal has been advocated. One gram of 25 per cent serum albumin per kilogram of body weight may be given intravenously to the infant one or two hours before exchange transfusion. Albumin (6.25 g) may be added to the unit of blood immediately before exchange transfusion by removing 90–100 ml of supernatant plasma. Administration of albumin in donor blood increases the amount of indirect bilirubin removed by 35 or 40 per cent.

If at any stage during exchange transfusion there are signs of respiratory failure, the procedure must be discontinued immediately, and the infant resuscitated with suction and oxygen. Hyperkalaemia may develop if the blood preserved in ACD or CPD is more than two

or three days old. It causes ventricular dysrrhythmias but can be corrected by giving 1 or 2 ml of 10 per cent calcium gluconate intravenously under ECG monitoring. Acidaemia should be corrected and resonium (0.5 g/kg) given by mouth or per rectum. Resonium can be repeated four-hourly until the potassium is below 7.0 mmol/l.

Prevention of severe jaundice

In populations at-risk of severe neonatal jaundice in the subtropics and tropics, the screening of neonates for the G6PD enzyme is warranted. A simple fluorescence test using blood collected on blotting paper is adequate for screening. Infants with G6PD deficiency should be protected from exposure to haemolytic agents such as naphthalene and oxidant drugs that produce free radicals (Table 2.5.18). Naphthalene has been reported to be a potent haemolytic agent in G6PD-deficient neonates in Greece[8] and Singapore.[9] It can be inhaled and absorbed through the skin to induce haemolysis and fragmentation of red blood cells by the oxidizing properties of α-naphthol. Even normal red cells may be haemolysed by naphthalene. Therefore, all G6PD-deficient babies should not be exposed to naphthalene, e.g. clothes stored in mothballs, balms and lotions containing naphthalene.

G6PD-deficient neonates should be observed for jaundice, and parents informed about haemolytic agents and given a list of drugs and chemicals which are to be avoided (Table 2.5.18).

G6PD deficiency is genetically heterogeneous;

Table 2.5.18 Drugs and chemicals to be avoided in G6PD deficiency

Antimalarials: primaquine, pamaquine, pentaquine
Sulphonamides: sulphanilamide, sulphapyridine, sulphadimidine, sulphacetamide, salicylazosulphapyridine (Salazopyrin)
Sulphones: *diphenylsulphone (Dapsone), *sulphoxone, glucosulphone sodium (Promin), sulphamethoxazole (in co-trimoxazole)
Antibacterial agents: nitrofurans (nitrofurantoin, furazolidone, nitrofurazone), nalidixic acid
Anthelmintics: niridazole, stibophan
Analgesics: acetophenetidin (Phenacetin), acetylsalicylic acid (Aspirin) in large doses
Miscellaneous: Dimercaprol (BAL), *phenylhydrazine, *Arsine, *acetylphenylhydrazine, probenecid, vitamin K water-soluble analogues
Chemicals: *naphthalene (mothballs), methylene blue, toluidine blue
Faba bean (*Vicia faba*)

* These drugs and chemicals may cause haemolysis in normal individuals if given in large doses.

different genetic variants have different susceptibilities to haemolytic risk from drugs. A drug found to be safe in some G6PD deficient subjects may not be as safe in others.

Mothers who are breast-feeding their babies with G6PD deficiency should abstain from eating fava beans and avoid contact with mothballs. Herbal medicines may also have haemolytic properties.

Early detection of G6PD deficiency and appropriate education of parents not only prevents severe neonatal jaundice but also brain damage and death from kernicterus.

Environmental illumination of obstetric wards in the tropics may have effects on the incidence of neonatal jaundice. Architectural modifications to an obstetric ward in Papua New Guinea involved extension of the roof overhangs to a width of several metres.[10] These extensions excluded most of the daylight from the ward. An alarming increase in the incidence of severe neonatal jaundice from 0.5 to 17 per cent occurred after the modifications. Other causes for the increase in neonatal jaundice were excluded. This observation has important implications for the design of obstetric wards and nurseries in the tropics. They should be built with windows facing north–south for coolness, and roof overhangs should be limited to one metre to allow entry of adequate indirect sunlight and illumination to help prevent neonatal jaundice. The use of natural illumination from indirect sunlight has been found to be of therapeutic value during the day in the tropics; if used with care it can reduce the need to use phototherapy units during daylight hours.

References

1. World Health Organization. Serious childhood diseases: priority issues and possible actions at family, community and health centre levels. Report of an informal consultation. Geneva 9–11 July 1984, WHO MCH/85.3.
2. Yoshida A, Beutler E, Motulsky AG. Human glucose-6-phosphate dehydrogenase variants. *Bulletin of the World Health Organization*. 1971; **45**: 243–53.
3. Smith GD, Vella F. Erythrocyte enzyme deficiency in unexplained kernicterus. *Lancet*. 1960; **1**: 1133–4.
4. Kramer LI. Advancement of dermal icterus in the jaundiced newborn. *American Journal of Diseases in Childhood*. 1969; **18**: 454–58.
5. Gosset IH. *Lancet*. 1960; **i**: 87–8.
6. Hamel BCJ. *Tropical Doctor*. 1982; **12**: 213–14.
7. Diamond LK. Erythroblastosis fetalis or haemolytic disease of the newborn. *Proceedings of the Royal Society of Medicine*. 1947; **40**: 546.
8. Valaes T, Doxiadis SA, Fessas P. Acute haemolysis due to naphthalene inhalation. *Journal of Pediatrics*. 1963; **63**: 904–15.
9. Wong HB. Singapore kernicterus: a review and the present situation. *Bulletin Kandang Kerbau Hospital Singapore*. 1966; **5**: 1–8.
10. Barss P, Comfort K. *British Medical Journal*. 1985; **291**: 400–1.
11. Luzzatto L, Mehta A. Glucose-6-phosphate dehydrogenase deficiency. In: *The Metabolic Basis of Inherited Disease*, 6th Edn. New York, McGraw Hill, 1989.

CONVULSIONS IN THE NEWBORN
Michael Chan

Presentation and diagnosis	Further reading
Management	

Presentation and diagnosis

Convulsions in the neonate are difficult to detect with the untrained eye. They are usually subtle (minor eye movements) and involve transient changes in breathing pattern. Full-term infants also have tonic or clonic convulsions which may be focal or generalized. Preterm infants may have brief tonic seizures and adopt a decerebrate posture with ophisthotonus, extended and internally rotated limbs, eyes diverging outwards and downwards, apnoea, cyanosis and bradycardia.

The major causes of neonatal convulsions are hypoxia with cerebral oedema, intracranial haemorrhage, meningitis, metabolic disturbances, kernicterus, narcotic drug withdrawal and congenital defects of the brain such as microcephaly and hydrocephaly. Intrapartum asphyxia produces hypoxia and ischaemia of the brain due to hypotension; in preterm infants this can give rise to periventricular leucomalacia in the region of the pyramidal tracts leading to spastic diplegia in survivors. Intracranial bleeding may occur as subdural, subarachnoid, intracerebral, or periventricular haemorrhage (or intraventricular, occurring mainly in infants of birth weight below 1500 g). The common metabolic causes of neonatal convulsions are hypoglycaemia, hypocalcaemia, hyponatraemia and hypernatraemia. Hypoglycaemia is most likely to occur in the small-for-dates baby. Pyridoxine deficiency is a rare cause of recurrent convulsions in the neonate. Kernicterus has been described in the previous section and is eminently preventable. Drug withdrawal only occurs in babies of mothers who are narcotic drug addicts. After 24 hours of age, the neonate may be irritable, tremulous, hyperactive, hypersensitive to sound and have a high-pitched cry, tachypnoea, respiratory distress, apnoea, rhinorrhoea or a blocked nose, sneezing, wakefulness, lacrimation, with weight loss or failure to gain weight. Friction marks on the skin are the result of restlessness.

The convulsing neonate should be investigated with the following tests wherever possible: blood glucose, white blood count with differential, electrolytes, blood urea, calcium, lumbar puncture and ultrasound brain scan. If the fontanelle is tense and bulging, a subdural tap may help to diagnose a haematoma and relieve the pressure on the brain (see p. 1012). Cranial transillumination is helpful in the rare cases of hydranencephalus where the cerebral hemispheres are replaced by bags of fluid, and the head glows like a Chinese lantern.

Management

- Place the baby on his side and clear the airways by suction of the pharynx.
- Oxygen is given in high concentration with a funnel until convulsions cease.
- A blood glucose test (dextrostix) is done and if the result is below 1.4 mmol/l (25 mg/dl) hypoglycaemia is presumed, and treatment given. A feeding tube is passed into the stomach and expressed breast-milk is given, if the baby cannot suck, at 60 ml/kg in 24 hours. One hour after starting the milk drip, blood glucose is checked again by dextrostix. If hypoglycaemia is still present, 10 per cent dextrose solution is given by intravenous drip.
- The infant is nursed prone to prevent aspiration pneumonia.
- If birth asphyxia is the cause, phenobarbitone (10–20 mg/kg) is given as a bolus intravenous injection to control convulsions. If it does not have any effect, paraldehyde (1 ml) is given by deep intramuscular injection or per rectum; diazepam (1 or 2 mg) intravenously, or phenytoin (10 to 20 mg/kg) intravenously may also be used. When the convulsions are under control, phenobarbitone (5 mg/kg) is given for maintenance. It is important to measure the blood level of phenobarbitone for optimum management.

Most asphyxiated neonates who are neurologically abnormal soon after birth recover completely even if they have suffered convulsions, and begin to suck their feeds. Prolonged delay in the ability to suck is an indication of future sequelae such as developmental retardation, cerebral palsy, hemiplegia and microcephaly.

Further reading

Roberton NRC. Neurological problems. In: *A Manual of Neonatal Intensive Care*, 2nd Edn. London, Edward Arnold, 1986.

BLEEDING IN THE NEWBORN
Michael Chan

Physiology of haemostasis	Haemorrhagic disease of the newborn
Screening tests	Late haemorrhagic disease
The role of vitamin K	Other types of bleeding
Causes of neonatal bleeding	References

Newborn infants are at risk of bleeding because of a combination of physiological and pathological factors. Blood vessels in the neonate are fragile and easily traumatized. Blood clotting factors are present in low concentrations at birth, there being no transplacental transfer of clotting factors from mother to fetus. Therefore, factors II (prothrombin), VII, IX and X, which are dependent on vitamin K, achieve half the adult levels in full-term infants, and are even lower in the preterm. Factors XI and XIII are also low. These clotting factors reach concentrations found in adults only in the third postpartum month.

Risk factors for bleeding in the neonate include trauma and asphyxia at birth, the transplacental transfer of anticoagulants and anticonvulsants in mothers taking these drugs, and sepsis with associated disseminated intravascular coagulation (DIC). These conditions have effects on blood vessel walls, clotting factors, platelets and the fibrinolytic system.

Physiology of haemostasis

The process that leads to the arrest of bleeding involves platelets, clotting factors, red cells and the vascular endothelium. A complex series of biochemical reactions is set in motion whenever the vascular endothelium is injured. Platelets are attracted to the exposed subendothelium and they are induced to aggregate. Thrombin is formed on the surface of these platelet masses and it then generates insoluble cross-linked fibrin which causes the platelets to aggregate irreversibly into a platelet–fibrin meshwork forming an effective barrier to further bleeding (Fig. 2.5.14).

Under normal circumstances when fibrin is deposited on blood vessel walls or in tissues, it is slowly broken down into soluble fibrin split products (FSP) by plasmin. Plasmin is a proteolytic enzyme that splits arginine and lysine bonds; it can also attack fibrinogen and factors V and VIII. Plasminogen is the inactive precursor of plasmin normally present in plasma, urine and tissue. The fibrinolytic system, like the coagulation system, is normally held in check by a series of inhibitors, and is in a state of dynamic equilibrium with the coagulation system.

Screening tests

Whole blood clotting time   This measures the time taken for whole blood to clot in a glass tube under standard conditions of obtaining the sample and conducting the test. It may be prolonged in severe haemophilia, afibrinogenaemia, clotting factor deficiency, thrombocytopaenia, and haemorrhagic disease of the newborn. The whole blood clotting time is often normal in these disorders if the defect is not severe. The test is non-specific, requires careful techniques of blood drawing and laboratory methodology, and a large volume (5 ml) of blood (see p. 978). It cannot be recommended in the initial diagnostic evaluation of a bleeding infant.

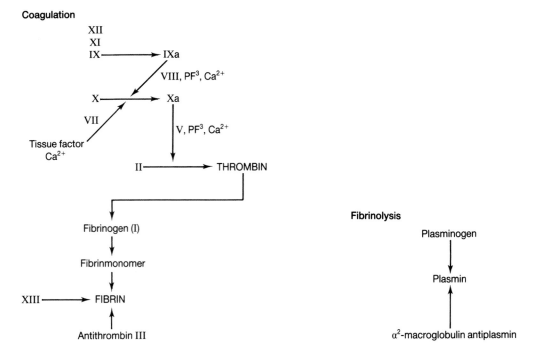

Fig. 2.5.14   The process of clotting and fibrinolysis in the blood. (PF^3 = platelet factor 3; Ca^{2+} = calcium.)

Bleeding time   This measures the time required for a wound of standardized size to stop bleeding and is a measure of platelet number and function. It is generally prolonged in thrombocytopaenia, thrombasthaenia, von Willebrand's disease and disseminated intravascular coagulation (DIC). In the Ivy method, the puncture is performed on the dorsal surface of the forearm and in the Duke method, the puncture is in the earlobe. The Duke method should never be done in infants and children because of the difficulty in applying pressure to the wound in case bleeding should persist.

Platelet count   This should be done if platelets are not seen in an ordinary blood film.

Prothrombin time (PT)   The one-stage PT or Quick Test is done by adding tissue factor (complete thromboplastin) to citrated plasma, followed by recalcification. The PT measures factors VII, X, V, II and fibrinogen. It is a little affected by heparin.

Activated partial thromboplastin time (APTT)   This is the most sensitive screening test of plasma clotting factors available. Citrated plasma is incubated with an inert surface-activating agent (kaolin, celite, bentonite) and a partial thromboplastin (cephalin, inosithin) as a platelet substitute, followed by the addition of calcium. The APTT is designed to detect deficiencies of all clotting factors except VII and XIII. It will be prolonged in the presence of heparin or other anticoagulants.

Fibrin degradation products (FDP)   Intravascular fibrin is broken down by plasmin and degradation products appear in the blood. The presence of increased quantities of FDPs in serum indicates fibrinolysis which is usually secondary to disseminated intravascular coagulation.

The role of vitamin K

Vitamin K is not required for the synthesis of factors II, VII, IX and X; it activates precursor proteins into proteins with clotting activity. These precursor proteins (PIVKA or proteins induced in vitamin K absence) are clotting factor precursors that require carboxylation to become functional. They are synthesized in the liver and are carboxylated into active proteins in hepatic microsomes. Marked increases may be observed in the concentration of factors II, VII, IX and X in plasma often within one hour of vitamin K administration.

Hypoprothrombinaemia observed at the time of birth, is usually the result of reduced production of the precursor protein and not of vitamin K deficiency. Some full-term infants who have experienced complications of labour and delivery, are born with ratios of precursor protein to coagulant protein that are indicative of vitamin K deficiency. Reduced concentrations of factor IX commonly observed in normal full-term infants are a result of inadequate synthesis of the precursor protein, and not a sign of vitamin K deficiency.

Administration of vitamin K to the healthy full-term infant prevents the decrease in prothrombin activity, factors VII and X which is consistently found by the prothrombin time test and the activated partial thromboplastin time. The results of these tests are invariably prolonged if vitamin K is not administered.

Coumarin and its analogues block the action of vitamin K on the precursor proteins, so that the concentration of precursor proteins is increased in the plasma.

Large doses of water-soluble synthetic analogue, vitamin K_3 (Synkavit) causes haemolysis in neonates and result in hyperbilirubinaemia and kernicterus. Vitamin K_1 (phytomenadione; fat soluble and occurring in green vegetables) is safe and effective in doses as small as 0.5–1.0 mg by intramuscular injection. Vitamin K can also be given orally. An oral dose of 1 mg vitamin K_1 gives peak plasma concentrations 300 times the normal adult concentrations (which in turn exceed cord blood concentrations by a factor of 10^3) but only 5 per cent of those achieved after intramuscular injection of the same dose. Therefore, oral vitamin K_1 is entirely adequate for preventing haemorrhagic disease of the newborn.

Causes of neonatal bleeding

Although there are many possible causes of bleeding in newborn infants, most cases in developing countries are related to trauma, asphyxia with acidosis, sepsis with disseminated intravascular coagulation, vitamin K-associated haemorrhagic disease, and umbilical cord bleeding because of inadequate ligatures. Rare causes of neonatal bleeding include inherited factor deficiencies such as haemophilia (VIII), hypofibrinogenaemia (I), V, VII, IX, X, XI, and XIII, thrombocytopaenia and platelet function disorders.

A common problem in diagnosis is that of spurious melaena in the newborn who swallows maternal blood, for example, in the case of a mother with antepartum haemorrhage. Apart from an accurate history, spurious melaena is best diagnosed by using an alkali-denaturation test for fetal haemoglobin in the melaena passed by the affected neonate. This test is the Apt Test – sodium hydroxide 1 per cent solution mixed with haemolysate in the ratio 1:4; if there is no colour change, the blood contains fetal haemoglobin; if the solution turns pink to yellow-brown, adult haemoglobin is present.

Haemorrhagic disease of the newborn

This term was first used in 1894 by Townsend[1] who described 50 infants (31 of whom died) with bleeding on the second or third day of life from the gastro-intestinal tract, umbilicus, nose, skin, and internal organs.

Haemorrhagic disease of the newborn usually affects healthy full-term infants. Bleeding occurs spontaneously during the first week usually on the second and third days but sometimes after the seventh day. Bleeding is usually from multiple sites such as the gut, umbilicus and nose, as described by Townsend, including venepuncture sites; if the bleeding is severe, anaemia and hypovolaemia are obvious.

The majority of these babies in developing countries are born of multigravid mothers, are almost always breast-fed, and have not been given vitamin K. The vitamin K content of breast-milk is low and lower than that of cow's milk. Infants of epileptic mothers who have taken phenobarbitone and phenytoin in pregnancy are prone to develop haemorrhagic disease of the newborn.

Investigations show that the bleeding time is normal, the clotting time is prolonged (9 to 30 minutes), prothrombin time is very prolonged (30 to 720 seconds with control of 14 seconds) and PTT prolonged. Factors II, VII, IX, and X are 5 per cent or less of normal values.

Management consists of giving 1 or 2 mg of vitamin K_1 by intravenous injection; this corrects the clotting defects within one or two hours by activating the precursor proteins. Intramuscular injection may produce muscle haematomas and oral administration is slow to cancel the bleeding. Synthetic water-soluble vitamin K analogues (Synkavit) which induce haemolysis and hyperbilirubinaemia must not be used.

Prevention of bleeding in newborn infants

An oral dose of 1 to 2 mg of vitamin K_1 or 0.5 to 1 mg by intramuscular injection should be given to all newborn infants to prevent haemorrhagic disease of the newborn.[2]

Late haemorrhagic disease

Vitamin K deficiency presenting with bleeding after the second week of life, usually between 4 and 8 weeks, has been described mainly in South-east Asia in the 1960s[3,4] and 1970s[5], but reports also appeared in Britain[6], Japan[7], and North America[8] in the late 1970s and 1980s. The characteristic presentation is severe intracranial haemorrhage of sudden onset which leads to death or severe central nervous system dysfunction. The affected infants described have all not received vitamin K at birth. In Japan, this late neonatal vitamin K-dependent intracranial haemorrhage occurs in one in 4500 infants and in one in every 1700 breast-fed infants who have not been given vitamin K prophylaxis.

The early South-east Asian reports of this late haemorrhagic disease described intracranial haemorrhage only or in combination with purpura and gastro-intestinal bleeding in infants between 4 and 8 weeks of age. All had low levels of factors II, VII, IX and X which responded to vitamin K therapy. The overall mortality rate was high (37 per cent) in infants with intracranial haemorrhage. The aetiology of this syndrome, named late haemorrhagic disease or acquired prothrombin complex deficiency (APCD) of infants, remains unclear. In Singaporean and Thai patients hepatomegaly was common and there was slight impairment of liver chemistry but with no specific histological changes on autopsy examination. Herbal remedies administered to the breast-feeding mother or to the neonate before the onset of haemmorhage have been reported and suspected to be of aetiological significance. Vitamin K administration or blood transfusion produced clinical improvement and corrected the haemostatic defects.

Other types of bleeding

Intracranial haemorrhage occurring after traumatic delivery, such as in breech presentation, instrumental delivery and prolonged labour associated with cephalopelvic disproportion, usually results in subdural haematoma or subarachnoid haemorrhage. Preterm low-birth-weight babies who develop surfactant-deficient respiratory distress syndrome (hyaline membrane disease) often become anoxic and may develop intraventricular bleeding even if given vitamin K. Drugs that protect the integrity of capillaries in the brain, such as ethamsylate, reduce the likelihood of intraventricular haemorrhage. Pulmonary haemorrhage is also associated with anoxic damage to fragile capillaries.

Vitamin K is administered for these types of bleeding in the hope of raising the levels of prothrombin, factors VII, IX and X to reduce the extent of haemorrhage. Blood (fresh, if possible) transfusions are necessary in the management of these serious forms of neonatal bleeding.

References

1. Townsend CW. The haemorrhagic disease of the newborn. *Archives of Paediatrics*. 1894; **11**: 595–65.
2. American Academy of Pediatrics.*Pediatrics*. 1961; **28**: 501–7.
3. Chan MCK, Wong HB. Late haemorrhagic disease of Singapore infants. *Journal of Singapore Paediatric Society*. 1967; **9**: 72–81.
4. Tan KH. Severe hypoprothrombinaemic bleeding in breastfed young infants. *Singapore Medical Journal*. 1969; **10**: 43–9.
5. Bhanchet P, Tuchinda S, Hathirat P *et al.* A bleeding syndrome in infants to acquired prothrombin complex deficiency – a survey of 93 affected infants. *Clinical Pediatrics*. 1977; **16**: 922–8.
6. Cooper NA, Lynch MA. Delayed haemorrhagic disease of the newborn with extradural haematoma. *British Medical Journal*. 1979; **i**: 164–5.
7. Motohara K, Matsukura M, Matsuda I *et al.* Severe vitamin K deficiency in breast fed infants. *Journal of Pediatrics*. 1984; **105**: 943–5.
8. Lane PA, Hathaway WE, Githens JH, Rosenberg DA. Fatal intracranial haemorrhage in a normal infant secondary to vitamin K deficency. *Pediatrics*. 1983; **72**: 562–4.

NEONATAL INFECTIONS
Michael Chan

Immune system	Buffy coat examination
Practical approach to infection	Counterimmunoelectrophoresis
Clinical features	Swabs and cultures
Neonatal septicaemia	Lumbar puncture
Neonatal meningitis	Radiological examination
Neonatal pneumonia	Treatment
Osteomyelitis	Antibiotics
Necrotizing enterocolitis	Supportive therapy
Diagnosis	Prevention
White blood cell count	References
Platelet count	

Newborn babies are prone to infections because of the many risk factors to which they are exposed, and with which their immune systems are unable to cope. Some of the factors that increase the risk of infection are maternal in origin, such as urinary tract infection and prolonged rupture of membranes (>24 h). Other factors include preterm delivery, birth trauma, intrapartum hypoxia, low birth weight, male sex, unhygienic handling at birth, and invasive procedures such as intravenous infusions. Studies in Liverpool showed that babies of birth weight below 1500 g had three times more infection than heavier babies admitted for intensive care.

Immune system

Functions of cell-mediated immunity such as the delayed hypersensitivity response are not apparent until some weeks after birth. However, the thymus, the source of T cells associated with cell-mediated immunity, is large and well developed. Preterm infants have a reduced number of T cells; active T cells are reduced even in term infants. Non-specific defence mechanisms are not optimal, e.g. complement, fibronectin and opsonin concentrations are low in serum, and phagocytosis is inefficient.

The only immunoglobulin to cross the placenta is immunoglobulin G (IgG) which is acquired during the last weeks of pregnancy. Preterm infants, therefore, may have very low levels of IgG and be at risk of severe infection. Synthesis of IgG is not efficient until six months after birth. The level of IgM is low at birth unless there has been intrauterine infection. In term infants the level of IgM reaches half the adult level by six months. Synthesis of IgA occurs after birth. Secretory IgA is abundant in colostrum and breastmilk. Secretory IgA consists of two molecules of IgA joined together by a J-chain and a secretory component; this appears in the infant's intestine at four weeks of age. Maternal secretory IgA in breast-milk protects the suckling infant against *Escherichia coli* and infection by Gram-negative bacteria commonly found in hospital nurseries. Secretory immunity is measured by concentrations of IgM, IgA and IgA antibodies to *E. coli* which are higher in the saliva and nasal secretions of breast-fed babies in the first six weeks of life compared with bottle-fed infants.[1]

Practical approach to infection

Neonatal infections can be prevented by simple measures such as routine hand-washing of all attendants, including mothers and family members, before they touch newborn babies. The consequences of neonatal infections are serious: for example, neurological handicap after meningitis, and a high death rate with septicaemia.

Neonatal infections should be treated with effective antibiotics used in combination, and before bacterial culture results are known. If bacterial cultures are negative, antibiotics may be stopped without completing a course of five or seven days. This practice has not been found to be detrimental to the well-being of neonates in developed countries. A major obstacle to the effective management of neonatal infections in developing countries is the lack of information about the common bacteria that infect newborn infants. Every effort should, therefore, be made to identify the microorganisms that infect sick newborns. This may be done by routine cultures of blood, cerebrospinal fluid, urine and skin swabs. Reliable culture results depend upon a good-quality microbiological laboratory with adequately trained staff and regular supplies. Changing patterns of micro-organisms have been reported in neonatal nurseries in developed countries; similar trends are also being monitored in some hospitals in developing countries. These changes in the type of infecting microorganism depend on the type of antibiotics used and the development of resistant strains of bacteria. Therefore, bacterial surveillance in neonatal nurseries is essential to good practice.

Clinical features

Neonatal septicaemia

Septicaemia is a major cause of death in neonates with infection. Clinical features of septicaemia vary according to the type of onset. In early onset septicaemia, presenting in the first 72 hours of life, there is peripheral circulatory failure and respiratory distress with a fulminating course. Later onset septicaemia usually occurs after the fifth postnatal day and manifests with non-specific signs such as lethargy, poor feeding, jaundice, apnoeic attacks, abdominal distension and low body temperature (below 36°C). Preterm babies are at high risk of septicaemia, but those born at term are not spared. Sclerema, a diffuse, non-oedematous, hardening of the subcutaneous tissues is an ominous sign associated with a mortality rate approaching 100 per cent.

Early onset infection is acquired from the maternal birth canal just before, or during, delivery. Septicaemia presenting later is usually a nosocomial infection acquired from the hands of attendants or from neonatal care equipment such as unsterile needles, resuscitation masks and contaminated incubators. The infecting microorganisms that cause septicaemia in developing countries are mainly Gram-negative bacteria, the most common being *E. coli, Klebsiella pneumoniae* and *Pseudomonas aeruginosa*, as well as *Staphylococcus aureus* and *S. epidermidis*. Group B streptococci are a significant cause of septicaemia in Britain and N. America. More research into the aetiology of neonatal septicaemia is required in developing countries.

In industrialized countries, deaths from septicaemia range from 20 to 70 per cent, the higher rate occurring with fulminating early onset group B streptococcal infection with meningitis. Late onset infection has a lower mortality rate of 10 to 20 per cent. The prognosis of neonatal septicaemia in developing countries is, in general, poorer than in industrialized countries because of delayed diagnosis and the lack of trained nurses and doctors to provide specialized care for these gravely ill babies. The incidence of neonatal septicaemia was 5.6 per 1000 livebirths and the mortality rate was 31 per cent in a special care nursery in Nigeria.[2] Neurodevelopmental sequelae have been reported in about 20 per cent of survivors of septicaemia, in spite of new antibiotics and improvements in intensive neonatal care.

Neonatal meningitis

Meningitis occurs as a consequence of bacteraemia; bacteria entering the neonatal bloodstream through the immature gastro-intestinal or respiratory tracts or as a complication of arterial or venous catheterization. The disease is more common in the first week than at any time in the neonatal period. There is often a history of late pregnancy complications such as urinary infection or prolonged rupture of membranes, and the incidence of birth asphyxia is high.

Early clinical signs are vague, non-specific and may not appear to be related directly to the central nervous system. The following features have been found in newborn infants with meningitis (in descending order of frequency): raised temperature, lethargy, anorexia or vomiting, respiratory distress, convulsions, irritability, jaundice, a bulging or full fontanelle, diarrhoea, and neck stiffness.

The cry of the affected infant may be abnormal and high-pitched. Skin rashes – erythematous, maculopapular or purpuric – may sometimes be found on clinical examination. Sclerema is a late sign. Hepatosplenomegaly and easily palpable kidneys are frequent findings. Central nervous system malformations predispose to meningitis; these defects range from large myelomeningoceles to midline congenital dermal sinuses that are easily missed unless actively sought.

Gram-negative bacteria that inhabit the intestine are often the infecting organisms, although the group B (β-haemolytic) streptococcus is an important cause of neonatal meningitis in N. America. *E. coli* is the most common cause of meningitis in Britain with 80 per cent of strains carrying the invasive K1 capsular antigen. *Listeria monocytogenes* may be a cause of septicaemia and meningitis. It is acquired during birth from the maternal genital tract, or later by nosocomial transmission and cross-infection.

Neurological complications, particularly hydrocephalus, may occur during the acute illness, often in the second week while the infant has ventriculitis. Hydrocephalus may also present with increasing head size at any stage after bacteriological cure of the meningitis. In most cases a permanent shunt for CSF has to be inserted between the cerebral ventricles and the heart, when the CSF is sterile and the protein is below 1–2 g/l. This will prevent damage to the brain from increasing intraventricular pressure which may eventually lead to cortical blindness. Cerebral abscess is a rare complication, except in neonatal meningitis due to *Citrobacter*. It presents with signs of increased intracranial pressure in a neonate who is not responding to treatment.

The mortality rate from meningitis varies with the causative organism and the gestational age of the neonate. It is higher in preterm than term infants. The mortality rate for *E. coli* meningitis is about 30 per cent, group B streptococcus 20 per cent and listeria 15 per cent. Permanent CNS damage occurs in 20–30 per cent of survivors in Europe and America. This includes cerebral palsy, mental subnormality, convulsions, cortical blindness and deafness.

Neonatal pneumonia

Pneumonia may occur as a feature of severe early onset septicaemia, commonly due to microorganisms acquired from the maternal birth canal, in particular group B streptococci. Septicaemia, pneumonia with septicaemia, and meningitis are the main presentations of newborn infants infected with group B streptococci. Pneumonia may also be an isolated infection developing after the first six hours of life, or it may be a complication of infants receiving endotracheal intubation and ventilation for respiratory distress syndrome (hyaline membrane disease).

The newborn with pneumonia presents with respiratory distress – tachypnoea, dyspnoea, grunting, intercostal and subcostal recession (indrawing), and cyanosis in air. Preterm infants may have apnoea. A raised temperature is usual in term infants, and hypothermia in preterm ones. Cough is rare, but if present, is an important symptom. Other signs of systemic infection may be detected. Percussion and auscultation of the neonatal chest may not be rewarding. In some cases, localized crepitations may be heard. Tachypnoea and radiological changes are a common combination of findings in neonatal pneumonia. Causative organisms are similar to those of septicaemia.

Osteomyelitis

Neonatal septic arthritis and osteomyelitis are rare infections usually associated with group B streptococci and *Staphylococcus aureus*, and to a lesser extent, Gram-negative bacteria, in Britain. Isolated arthritis and osteomyelitis of the hip joint may occur as a complication of femoral venepuncture, when coliform infection is common. In view of this complication, femoral venepuncture has been abandoned in all progressive neonatal units. Blood should only be sampled from peripheral veins of hands and feet using sterile disposable needles.

Septic arthritis and osteomyelitis often coexist in the neonate, because the infected metaphysis of the bone lies within the capsule of the adjacent joint. The disease may present in one of three ways:

- pseudoparalysis of a limb because of pain, often with swelling but little inflammation over the infected joint or bone;
- on investigation of a neonate with non-specific signs of infection;
- incidentally on radiological examination of an ill infant.

Necrotizing enterocolitis

Necrotizing enterocolitis (NEC) is primarily a disease of the preterm low-birth-weight baby, particularly those weighing less than 1500 g. Term infants may also suffer from NEC during an outbreak in the neonatal nursery, and they become ill in the first week of life; they account for 10 per cent of NEC cases.

The onset of NEC may be gradual or sudden. The preterm baby has non-specific signs of infection with lethargy, low body temperature, and apnoeic spells followed by abdominal distension, bile-stained vomitus, and passage of blood in the stools. Tests show a low platelet count, and on X-ray, dilated loops of bowel with thickening of the gut wall and pathogno-monic bubbles of intramural gas (pneumatosis intestinalis) or intrahepatic venous gas, may be visualized. Peritonitis and bowel perforation may occur in the terminal ileum and ascending colon. The mortality from NEC is between 20 and 40 per cent in industrialized countries.

NEC is associated with hypotension and hypoxia which reduce the oxygenation and perfusion of the neonate's bowel, resulting in ischaemic damage. Other factors of aetiological significance are the use of umbilical arterial catheters, fluid overload, feeding of artificial milk to sick preterm infants, and bowel infection.

Diagnosis

Positive microbiological culture from body fluids is the most definite diagnostic test of infection in the neonate (see p. 979). However, microbiological services are not readily available in most developing countries. Where there are facilities for bacterial cultures, results take 24 hours or longer to be available. A plethora of haematological and serological methods have been tested in the search for rapid and simple means for diagnosing infection in neonates, but without success. Even where a combination of tests have been found to have a high sensitivity (being positive in cases confirmed by blood cultures), they often have poor predictive accuracy because many uninfected babies are also positive.

Therefore, the following investigations should always be carried out in an infant suspected on clinical grounds of being infected:

- full blood count, differential WBC, platelet count;
- stain and culture swabs of nose, throat, umbilicus, external ear, and skin or eye lesions;
- rectal swab/stool culture;
- blood culture;
- lumbar puncture with stain, microscopy, chemical analysis, and culture;
- urine collected in a sterile bag for microscopy and culture;
- chest X-ray.

A clinical decision about treatment must then be made on the basis of clinical findings and the results of tests that are immediately available. If in doubt, treatment with antibiotics should be started without delay.

White blood cell count

The white blood cell (WBC) count is the most useful rapid test when evaluating infection in the neonate. Total WBC counts are not helpful in the diagnosis of infection, particularly in the first 48 hours, because the normal range is so wide; it also varies with gestational age and postnatal age. Absolute neutrophil counts are more helpful and normal values for term and preterm infants are documented. Normal absolute neutrophil counts have been found in about 20 per cent of infected infants. In the first 48 hours of life, neutropaenia (below $2.0–2.5 \times 10^9/l$ or 2000–2500/mm^3) is an indicator of bacterial infection. After the second day, both neutropaenia and neutrophilia (above $7.5–8.0 \times 10^9/l$ or 7500–8000/mm^3) are suggestive of bacterial infection.

Another useful indicator of infection can be detected on blood film examination for immature cells of the neutrophil series (band cells, myelocytes, metamyelo-cytes) to obtain the ratio of immature cells to total neutrophils by dividing the number of immature cells by the total number of neutrophils. The maximum normal ratio is 0.16 in the first 24 hours, 0.14 by 48 hours, and 0.13 by 60 hours where it remains until the fifth day. Thereafter the maximum normal ratio is 0.12 until the end of the first month. In most reports, a high ratio above the maximum normal value accurately predicted sepsis in 80 per cent of infected babies, and it was normal in 90 per cent of infants without infection. An abnormal ratio together with a low absolute neutrophil count is very suggestive of infection.

These tests of WBC counts may also be abnormal in infants with birth asphyxia, convulsions, periventric-ular haemorrhage, and pneumothorax.

The presence of toxic granulations in neutrophils may also indicate infection.

Platelet count

Thrombocytopaenia at birth is associated with many intrauterine infections such as rubella, cytomegalovirus

(CMV), herpes and toxoplasmosis. It may also be a non-specific and late indicator of bacterial infection. About half the neonates with proven bacterial infection will have platelet counts below $100 \times 10^9/1$ or $100\,000/mm^3$ but they may be obviously septicaemic.

Buffy coat examination

The buffy coat is a thin layer seen between the plasma and the red cells when a blood sample is centrifuged or allowed to settle. It contains most of the white cells and may also contain bacteria if a bacteraemia is present. Microscopic examination of the buffy coat stained with Gram, methylene blue, or acridine orange is a useful method for rapid diagnosis of bacteraemia in neonates suspected of infection.

Counter immunoelectrophoresis

Counter immunoelectrophoresis (CIE) is a sensitive method of detecting bacterial antigens in blood, CSF or urine. Commercial kits for CIE using latex particle agglutination give a result within a few minutes and are a rapid and reliable way of detecting group B streptococci. The use of CIE may be limited in developing countries because of its cost.

Swabs and cultures

These should be taken as soon as possible because in the first 24 hours of life, the microorganisms that have colonized the baby in these superficial sites are likely to be those responsible for systemic infection. The swabs should always be moistened initially (if the site is dry) with sterile water or transport medium but not with saline.

In early onset septicaemia, the infant's gastric aspirate should be sent for bacterial examination, and a high vaginal swab taken from the mother since she is the likely source of the infection. Infants receiving intensive care with assisted ventilation should have secretions sucked out of the endotracheal tube and sent for microscopy and culture. The tips of all tubes removed from ill babies – umbilical cannulae, thoracentesis tubes, and central vascular lines used for total parenteral nutrition – should be placed in a sterile universal container and sent for culture.

Secretions likely to contain a large number of organisms should be examined under the microscope, after Gram-staining or acridine orange, for immediate identification to assist with the choice of antibiotics.

Blood for culture should be obtained from a peripheral vein after thoroughly cleaning the overlying skin with an iodine-containing solution, which is allowed to dry before the venepuncture is done. After 1.0 ml of blood has been collected in a sterile syringe, the needle is withdrawn and changed for a new one to inject the sample into the blood culture bottle. The bottle cap and top should be thoroughly disinfected before the blood is injected. Blood should not be sampled from an indwelling arterial or venous cannula, unless it has only just been inserted under sterile precautions. If venous blood is allowed to drip into the culture bottle through a needle from which the hub has been removed, it is likely to give false-positive blood culture results. The iodine solution should be washed off the baby's skin to prevent burns after the blood has been obtained.

Lumbar puncture

Lumbar puncture should be done on all sick babies, particularly those in whom meningitis is suspected (see p. 1011). The only exception may be infants with known respiratory infection whose condition may be made worse by a lumbar puncture. The procedure must be performed with strict sterile precautions. CSF should be collected in three bottles: the first bottle is sent for microscopy and culture, the second for biochemical tests and the third sample collected into a fluoride bottle for glucose estimation.

CSF glucose levels must be estimated with simultaneous measurement of blood glucose; the mean CSF glucose is 75–80 per cent of the blood glucose in normal neonates. A low CSF glucose of <1.0 mmol/l (18 mg/100 ml) strongly suggests meningitis. Any white cell count in CSF $>30/mm^3$ is indicative of meningitis. When blood-stained CSF is obtained, the ratio of red to white blood cells should be calculated and compared with the ratio in peripheral blood. In uninfected CSF this ratio is 500:1 or more. The upper limit of protein in normal CSF is 1.5–2.0 g/l in term neonates and up to 3.0 g/l in preterm infants. In meningitis, CSF protein levels are above normal; very high levels (>6.0 g/l) are associated with a poor prognosis and a high incidence of postmeningitic hydrocephalus.

Microscopy of CSF after Gram- or acridine orange-staining is a most important investigation in the diagnosis of meningitis. It can detect bacteria and even determine the antibiotics to be used.

Radiological examination

An X-ray of the chest should be part of the investigation of any neonate suspected of infection, irrespective of the presence of respiratory symptoms. Any infant with abdominal distension, vomiting, diarrhoea or bloody stools should have an X-ray of the abdomen in two positions: antero-posterior AP, and a left lateral film.

Treatment

Antibiotics

Antibiotics should be given to the neonate suspected of infection immediately after specimens for culture have been obtained. The choice of antibiotics depends on the suspected infecting bacteria and their sensitivity, and any cultures already available from the baby or mother. It is customary to use a combination of a penicillin with an aminoglycoside such as penicillin G with gentamicin or netilmicin. Ampicillin and gentamicin are preferred if listeria is suspected. The majority of Gram-negative bacteria are sensitive to gentamicin or netilmicin. This combination is usually effective when used for babies born in hospital and admitted within the first 72 hours. For infants admitted from outside the hospital after the third day, flucloxacillin would be the penicillin of choice because of the likelihood of staphylococcal infection. If pseudomonas infection is prevalent, a third antibiotic, piperacillin or ceftazidime (a third-generation cephalosporin) should be added. Metronidazole is added to the penicillin and aminoglycoside combination if necrotizing enterocolitis is diagnosed. Coagulase-negative staphylococci such as *S. epidermidis* tend to be resistant to antibiotics in common neonatal use, and vancomycin may have to be used.

All antibiotics for treating infected neonates should be given intravenously. Oral antibiotics are inefficiently absorbed and intramuscular injections are hazardous because they may damage nerves and produce abscesses due to the small muscle bulk of neonates. Recommended dosages of antibiotics are given in Table 2.5.19.

Table 2.5.19 Dosages of antibiotics

Drug	Dose	Age/Birth weight	Dosages in 24 hours
Ampicillin	30 mg/kg/dose	<7 days	2
		7–14 days	3
		<7 days with meningitis	4
	50 mg/kg/dose	>7 days with meningitis	4
Cefotaxime	30 mg/kg/dose	<7 days	2
		>7 days	3
Ceftazidime	30 mg/kg/dose	<7 days	2
		>7 days	3
Cefuroxime	30 mg/kg/dose	<2 kg and <7 days	2
		>2 kg or >7 days	3
Chloramphenicol	12.5 mg/kg/dose	<7 days	2
	(for meningitis)	7–14 days	3
Flucloxacillin	30 mg/kg/dose	<2 kg and < 7 days	2
		7–14 days	3
		>14 days	4
		>2 kg at all ages	4
Gentamicin	2.5 mg/kg/dose	<7 days	2
		>7 days	3
(infuse over 20 min at least do not combine with carbenicillin in same infusion)			
Metronidazole	7.5 mg/kg/dose	All ages and gestations	3
Netilmicin	3 mg/kg/dose	<7 days	2
		>7 days	3
Penicillin	25 000 units/kg/dose with meningitis	<2 kg and <7 days	2
		>7 days	3
		<7 days	3
		>7 days	4
	50 000 units/kg/dose with meningitis	>2 kg and <7 days	2
		>7 days	3
		<7 days	3
		>7 days	4
Piperacillin	100 mg/kg/dose	All ages	2
Vancomycin	15 mg/kg/dose	All weights and <7 days	2
		>7 days	3

(Adapted from Roberton NRC. *A Manual of Neonatal Intensive Care*, 2nd Edn. Edward Arnold, 1986.)

The antibiotics prescribed should be reviewed after 48 hours when the culture results are available. If the cultures are negative and the baby is well and does not appear to be infected, antibiotics should be stopped. If the baby is not well, the antibiotics should be continued for seven days even though the cultures are negative.

Monitoring antibiotic therapy by measuring drug concentrations in plasma is an essential part of good management in neonates. It is essential to know if adequate therapeutic levels are being achieved in babies with severe infection such as septicaemia and meningitis.

The antibiotic treatment of neonatal meningitis is difficult and contentious. Meningitis caused by group B streptococcus, listeria, haemophilus, pneumococcus and meningococcus is not usually associated with ventriculitis, and so intravenous high doses of antibiotics such as penicillin and gentamicin are effective. Chloramphenicol, in the dose 50 mg/kg daily, is safe and effective without complications of the grey-baby syndrome of circulatory collapse. Treatment should be continued for at least 14 days with these antibiotics.

Meningitis caused by *E. coli* and other Gram-negative bacteria is often accompanied by ventriculitis which requires the use of third-generation cephalosporins, such as ceftazidime or cefotaxime, that penetrate the meninges in the absence of inflammation. Roberton[3] has summarized the treatment of meningitis as follows:

- An aminoglycoside in conventional doses should always be included in antibiotic treatment because it penetrates the inflamed meninges in useful quantities, and is important in treating the coexisting septicaemia.
- Parenteral antibiotic treatment should be maintained for three weeks.
- Intrathecal treatment by the lumbar route is of no value.
- The appropriate therapy for Gram-negative meningitis should be intravenous gentamicin, cefotaxime or latamoxef for 21 days. Appropriate changes can be made when culture and sensitivity results are available.
- If the organism is unknown, triple therapy is started with penicillin, gentamicin and ceftazidime.

Intraventricular therapy should be considered when there is failure to improve within 24 to 48 hours of commencing the above treatment, or in the presence of ventricular dilatation or periventricular enhancement on ultrasound. Ventricular puncture to examine the CSF should precede treatment. To avoid repeated punctures, an Ommaya or Rickham reservoir should be inserted into the ventricle. Therapy should be for at least two weeks after the CSF in the ventricles is clear.

Other measures in the treatment of neonatal meningitis include fluid restriction to 30 or 40 ml/kg during the first few days (to prevent cerebral oedema), and anticonvulsants to control seizures, e.g. phenobarbitone with a loading dose of 20 mg/kg.

Supportive therapy

Regular monitoring of neonates with infection should include frequent blood pressure measurements and a meticulous fluid balance chart. The infant must be weighed regularly to assess the state of hydration. Daily blood counts and plasma electrolytes should be done as a routine.

Intravenous infusion and sampling of arterial blood should be done through peripheral cannulae because indwelling central lines may act as foci of infection (see pp. 1002–7).

Neonates with severe infection become hypothermic and require warmth which is best supplied by servo-controlled incubators.

In Gram-negative septicaemia, shock may be a feature and it should be treated with plasma or blood transfusion, depending on the haemoglobin level. If the blood pressure is low (<40 mmHg systolic) an immediate infusion of plasma in a dose of 10 ml/kg should be given over 15 to 30 minutes and the response noted. Another plasma infusion or an infusion of dopamine should be given if the blood pressure does not rise.

Acid–base status must be checked because metabolic acidosis is frequent in severe infections. Metabolic acidosis (pH <7.20, base excess < –10 mmol/l) should be half corrected. Blood gases should be measured on arterial samples only.

Plasma electrolytes may be abnormal such as excessive losses of sodium and potassium, particularly in NEC, and gastroenteritis. These losses should be replaced, and electrolytes monitored daily.

Calories are required but they cannot be given by mouth because of concomitant ileus. Intravenous infusion of 5 per cent dextrose provides calories but blood glucose must be monitored regularly and hypoglycaemia corrected. Vamin, which is a solution of amino acids and vitamins, may be given with the dextrose.

Respiratory support may be needed for some ill babies who develop apnoea. Intermittent positive airways pressure may be necessary.

Exchange transfusion with fresh whole blood is of value in the management of severe neonatal infection. Antibiotics should be added to the blood before the exchange transfusion in babies with septicaemia. The exchange transfusion should be performed through an umbilical venous catheter as for severe neonatal jaundice, but only one-volume is changed (see p. 1004).

Prevention

The single most important measure used for the prevention of neonatal infections in hospital nurseries is the scrupulous washing of hands of all attendants – nurses, doctors and parents, before they handle babies. Almost everybody carries *Staphylococcus epidermidis*, micrococci and diphtheroids as resident flora on their skin. Transient organisms are also carried on the hands and these are likely to be Gram-negative bacteria in a hospital environment. The transient flora can largely be removed by washing with soap and clean running water. Antiseptic solutions are necessary to remove resident flora. Studies have shown that right hands tended to be washed less effectively than left hands by right-handed people.[4] Even the most careful hand wash may be totally negated by those who turn off contaminated taps with their washed hands. Hospital washbasins should have taps with long handles that can be turned off with the elbows. Bars of soap should not stand in wet dishes; soap should be kept dry. Squamous particles carrying bacteria are dispersed into the air as hands are washed with soap, and bacterial dissemination is reduced only when antiseptics are used. A hand lotion containing alcohol, glycerol, and chlorhexidine, used instead of handwashing, prevents bacterial dissemination and skin damage owing to frequent washing.

The wearing of gowns, overshoes and masks routinely in hospital nurseries has not been found to be important in the prevention of infection and has been abandoned in progressive units in developed countries.

References

1. Stephens S. Development of secretory immunity in breastfed and bottlefed infants. *Archives of Disease in Childhood*. 1986; **61**: 263–9.
2. Okolo AA, Omene JA. Changing pattern of neonatal septicaemia in an African city. *Annals of Tropical Paediatrics*. 1985; **5**: 123–6.
3. Roberton NRC. Infection in the newborn. In: Roberton NRC ed. *Textbook of Neonatology*. Edinburgh, Churchill Livingstone, 1986. pp. 725–81.
4. Taylor LJ. Evaluation of hand washing techniques. *Nursing Times*. 1978; **74**: 54–5.

CHAPTER 6

Organization of perinatal care

S. K. Bhargava, S. Ramji and I. Bhargava

Perinatal and neonatal care in the past two decades have been revolutionized in developed countries, resulting in a dramatic fall in maternal, perinatal and neonatal morbidity and mortality. This has largely been possible due to provision of well-organized and quality care-oriented perinatal services. However, in most developing countries this care has remained static or neglected for decades.[1] Several factors have contributed to this. They include limited resources in terms of finances and health, limited personnel with adequate training, absence of facilities or poor management and scanty utilization of maternal and child-care facilities. In addition, inhibitions due to deep-rooted social customs, beliefs and taboos, and logistic problems in supply and maintenance of services have contributed significantly to the present situation. The gap between what is done and what could be done is increasing and underlines the problem of organization and delivery of good quality perinatal services.

Ideally, a perinatal care programme should be one which ensures provision of essential components of perinatal care (Fig. 2.6.1) and utilizes maximally, the existing infrastructure of health delivery. It should be culturally acceptable to the community, technologically appropriate, manageable within the existing resources and cost-effective to meet the national or regional goals.

It should primarily fulfil the 'felt needs' of the community and provide primary to tertiary levels of care, closely linked to each other and supported by a good referral system. It should be able to deliver good quality medical care and have an outreach training and education programme for providers and users of this care system. It should have the capability to initiate or participate in research programmes relevant to local or national needs.

Delivery of perinatal care

Regionalization of perinatal care and its delivery through a well-linked three-tier system is being increasingly accepted as a method of health delivery to pregnant women and their newborns. This system helps to define areas of activity, levels of care, quality control, logistic supplies and phases of development and/or delivery of services. While several developed countries have already initiated this kind of programme, in the countries of the Third World it still remains an experimental measure, but recent reports of its use are encouraging.

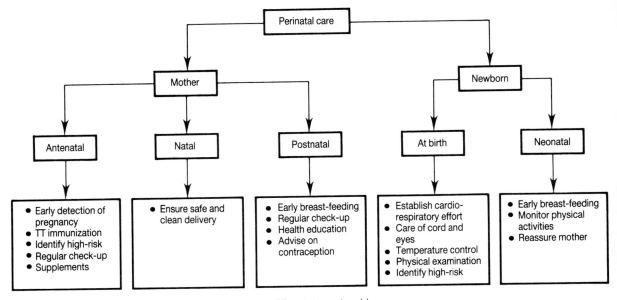

Fig. 2.6.1   The essential components of perinatal care. TT = tetanus toxoid.

Regionalization of perinatal care

This concept implies providing perinatal care to a defined population or a geographically delineated area. The scope of coverage and area of activity are determined by the size of population, birth rate, and maternal, perinatal and infant mortality rates. This requires a referral system and organized communication and transport facilities from periphery to centre.

Three-tier system of perinatal care

The three-tier system envisages provision of services at primary or level I, secondary or level II and tertiary or level III, to be provided for all pregnant women and their offspring during the antenatal, natal, postnatal and neonatal periods. (See Table 2.6.1.) Secondary care units are recommended for centres with 2000–5000 births and tertiary care units for those with 5000 births or more. This is expected to provide adequate patient load and will therefore be cost-effective.

Primary care

Primary care has to be accorded the highest priority and needs a major share of resources for its successful delivery. It is intended for all parturient mothers and their newborns at grass-roots level, irrespective of rural

Table 2.6.1   Indications for appropriate level of care for newborn infants

Level I (primary)	Level II (secondary)	Level III (tertiary)
Term or post-term neonates: normal weight, clinically normal, Apgar score ⩾8, uncomplicated course in early neonatal period	Weight 1301–2000 g or >4000 g Mid-arm circumference <7.5 cm at birth Gestation 33–36 weeks Moderate birth anoxia (Apgar 3–7) Respiratory distress (Silverman score ⩽5) Infants with abnormal behaviour or weight patterns Infants with metabolic, haematologic or any other problem Moderate to severe jaundice	Weight ⩽1300 g Gestation <33 weeks Severe birth asphyxia (Apgar score <3) Respiratory distress (Silverman score >5) Critically sick neonates needing life-support systems Infants with life-threatening problems or congenital malformations

(After Bhargava *et al.*, *Annals of Tropical Paediatrics*, 1986; **6**:225–31.)

Table 2.6.2   Primary perinatal care

Care	Place	Delivered by	Task expected	Supplies	Logistic support	Community support and awareness
Antenatal	Home	Dai/TBA	Detect pregnancy Confirm pregnancy Risk assessment Referral, if high-risk	Measuring tape		Health education – use MCH services – antenatal checks – immunization
	Home/ health centre	Nurse midwife	Confirm pregnancy High-risk identification Complication recognition e.g. toxaemia, PPH, IUGR and treatment TT immunization Nutrition supplementation Appropriate referral, when needed	Weighing scale, height measure, measuring tape, BP apparatus, haemoglobino- meter, urine analysis kit	Antenatal cards for recording, TT vaccine, iron and folic acid supply, first line antimalarials	– nutrition – rest – breast-feeding – family welfare – risks of bottle-feeding Voluntary support for MCH services
Intranatal	Home	TBA	Clean, safe delivery	Delivery kit		
	Home/ health centre	Nurse midwife	Management of at-risk mother and infant Referral and transportation when needed	Ambu bag and mask	Transportation	
Postnatal	Home	TBA	Examination of mother and baby during first week Initiation and establishment of early breast-feeding and lactation		Family welfare, nutrition	
	Home/ health centre	Nurse midwife	Identify complications e.g. PPH, infection and referral if needed Advise on contraception			
Neonatal	Home	TBA	Care of normal newborn i.e. feeding, temperature Risk detection	Measuring tape, spring balance		
	Home/ health centre	Nurse midwife	Examination for risk identification and malformation Recognition of sick newborn Treatment and referral of sick newborn	Weighing scale		

TBA = traditional birth attendant; TT = tetanus toxoid; PPH = postpartum haemorrhage; IUGR = intrauterine growth retardation; BP = blood pressure.

or urban community, and hospital or home delivery. Such services are to be accessible to all to ensure optimum utilization, the main goal of providing the care. Table 2.6.2 outlines the actual delivery of perinatal care, expected tasks of health staff, supply needs and some aspects of community education and community participation.

Antenatal care

The most crucial period for a successful outcome of pregnancy is the antenatal period, when both the expectant mother and the developing fetus may either be at unrecognized risk or become at-risk if not cared for appropriately. However, in countries where the outcome of the pregnancy (maternal or fetal) has been generally unfavourable, poor antenatal care due to inadequate provision of care, lack of awareness about the facility or a careless attitude of the family, has been identified as a major contributory factor. While providing antenatal care, it is important to identify the users and ensure that it is made available and sufficiently accessible for them to utilize it optimally.

Figure 2.6.2 provides a plan for antenatal care which is linked to objectives for determining risk and ensuring appropriate medical care. These requirements are often compromised in traditional rural communities where it may be difficult to obtain compliance due to family or social factors. The exact number of visits and frequency of timing of antenatal visits should be kept flexible but not compromised to ensure at least the minimum of perinatal care (Fig. 2.6.2).

At-risk approach

The use of the 'at risk' approach in maternal and child-care is increasingly advocated. This approach recommends essential care for all and maximum care for those who are at risk of morbidity and mortality.

This will mean making them more accessible to maternity facilities or making maternal facilities more accessible to them. It can be used at all levels of care, particularly at primary level, during the antenatal period, where the visits of an expectant mother for antenatal checks are few and limited. Several risk-scoring methods have been described in the literature for use during antenatal, intranatal and postnatal periods.[2] These vary in their detail. It is often necessary to adopt a realistic and practical view in the choice of a risk-scoring method. For community use it has to be simple and comprise factors which can be identified by a primary health care worker in a primary care setting. Table 2.5.14 on p. 220 suggests a modified simplified scoring system for use at primary level. It is based largely on factors which can be identified antenatally by any level of primary care worker.

Intranatal care

Safe and clean delivery remains the main objective of intranatal care. Table 2.6.3 provides essential components of a delivery and newborn care kit. Mucus suction trap for oropharyngeal suction, infant weighing

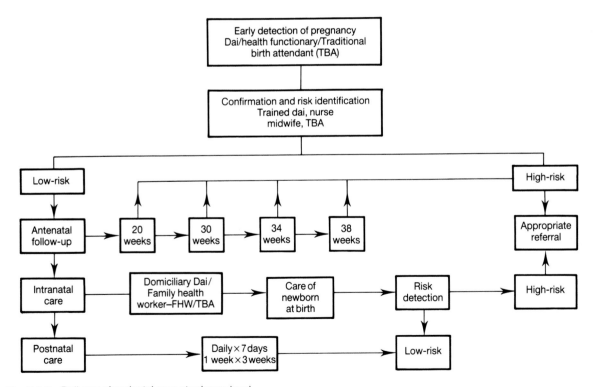

Fig. 2.6.2   Delivery of perinatal care at primary level.

Table 2.6.3 Traditional birth attendant's kit for safe delivery and newborn care

1. Soap
2. Plastic sheet
3. Cotton and gauze pads
4. Thread or ligature
5. Razor blade
6. Mucus suction trap (may be disposable)
7. Spring balance (reusable)
8. Measuring tape (reusable, fibreglass)

(After Bhargava *et al.*, *Annals of Tropical Pediatrics*, 1986; **6**:225–31.)

scales (spring or beam balance), a measuring tape, and provision of extra warmth if necessary, ensure safe delivery. A physical examination of the newborn for timely identification of risk and congenital malformations should be an integral part of intranatal care.

Postnatal care

A postnatal mother needs to be looked after for postdelivery complications, such as bleeding and infection. She requires advice on adequate rest, nutritious diet, establishing early and successful lactation and breast-feeding and has to be warned against introduction of early bottle-feeding.

Secondary and tertiary care

Secondary and tertiary perinatal care have to be delivered through specialized obstetric and paediatric neonatal services. These would include provision of biomedical, biophysical and biochemical investigations and monitoring facilities. Such care requires an obstetrician and a neonatologist and has to be largely organized in a hospital setting.

Neonatal care

All newborns, irrespective of their place of birth, weight or gestation, need to be looked after at birth and in the immediate neonatal period. The initial care is aimed at successful establishment of cardiorespiratory effort, prevention of aspiration, hypothermia and infections. A physical examination has to be performed for recording body measurements, gestational age assessment and detection of fetal growth retardation and malformations.

The indications for different levels of care for the newborn are given in Table 2.6.1. It is estimated that 80–85 per cent of all births need only primary care, 10–15 per cent secondary care and 1–5 per cent tertiary care.[3]

Primary care

Primary or level I care should be provided to all newborns, irrespective of whether they are at low or high risk. In developing countries, where the majority of births occur at home, care has to be organized at home or at a primary health centre.

Primary neonatal care, whether at a primary centre or at home, must include the basic features outlined earlier in care at birth. The early neonatal care should concentrate on observations for physiological events (i.e. passage of urine and meconium), early onset of pathological jaundice and promotion and maintenance of successful breast-feeding. A constant vigil for deviations from normal will help identify the 'at-risk' newborn and ensure early transfer to an appropriate higher level of care.

It is better to transfer a baby *in utero* than '*ex utero*'.

Secondary care

Secondary or level II care is required for infants who are 'at risk' (Table 2.6.1) and need continuous and close clinical monitoring. A number of these 'at-risk' infants will be delivered by 'at-risk' mothers who will already be at level II/III care. They may need support for maintenance of body temperature, fluid and nutritional requirements or intervention by specific therapeutic modalities. Such care is, therefore, totally nurse-based and requires a paediatrician trained in neonatalogy. The infant is monitored by a nurse for body temperature, weight, respiratory and heart rate, feeding, intake and output record, respiratory distress, jaundice, hypoglycaemia, oxygenation, drugs, etc. It is preferable to record these events on a nursing chart for close supervision and prompt and appropriate action.

Tertiary care

Tertiary or level III care is indicated for infant survival of high-risk infants with one or more life-threatening problems or diseases which may cause permanent sequelae later in life (Table 2.6.1). The infants in this type of care need continuous clinical, biochemical and biophysical monitoring. The care is delivered through highly trained nursing personnel and neonatologists. It further requires support of several disciplines such as anaesthesiology, haematology, nephrology, surgery and supportive laboratory and radiodiagnosis and imaging services.

All vital signs, such as body temperature, respiratory effort, heart rate and blood pressure are monitored through electronic monitoring. The ambient oxygen and the arterial oxygen tension and acid–base status are monitored continuously or intermittently. This is supported by the presence of a well-equipped laboratory within the neonatal care complex.

Equipment for newborn care

The need to support physiological functions and treat pathological states is most acutely felt in the newborn period. There has been a tremendous upsurge in the availability of a wide variety of equipment for newborn care, but the actual choice of equipment depends on the level of care and availability of resources for purchase and maintenance. Most of the equipment is expensive and needs to be imported from developed countries. It, therefore, becomes necessary to list the activity and level of care in order of priority and organize different levels of care in a phased manner. Table 2.6.4 provides a list of essential equipment for different levels of care and the approximate costs.

Delivery room and care at birth

It is ironical that inspite of the awareness that birth asphyxia is the most common preventable neonatal disorder, and the need for its prompt and immediate management at birth, provision of suitable space and equipment often remains neglected. All places where deliveries occur (except home deliveries) should be equipped with resuscitation equipment. In its simplest form, this comprises a table with provision to keep the baby at an angle, a light source, radiant warmer, Ambu bag, infant laryngoscope, endotracheal tube and intravenous infusion, oxygen and suction facility. Several models of neonatal resuscitation tables or trolleys are available and the choice will depend on financial resources (see p. 192).

Primary care

The basic need at this level is to keep the baby warm. Warmth can be provided by hot water bottles in pockets on the sides of the crib (where electricity is not available), a lamp with a 100 W bulb or radiant warmers. Low-birth-weight infants may be wrapped in aluminium foil or strapped to the mother's body between her breasts. Adequate oxygenation can be provided by a head box with added oxygen. Phototherapy units may be required to avoid unnecessary referrals in countries where neonatal jaundice is a common problem.

Secondary care

In addition to equipment for primary care, incubators, temperature, cardiac and respiratory monitors, apnoea alarm, intravenous infusion pumps and facilities for exchange transfusion are mandatory for this level of care.

Several kinds of incubator are available, including ambient temperature control, servo-control and open intensive care bassinets. A combination of an ambient temperature control incubator and open intensive care bassinet with servo-temperature controlled facilities is recommended for minimizing expenses without compromising the quality of care. An open infant care system has been found to be particularly useful owing to ease of maintenance and sterilization for reuse.

Tertiary care

Continuous monitoring of vital signs, acid–base status, maintenance of body temperature and cardio-respiratory effort, necessitates availability of bio-physical, biochemical and biomedical services for this kind of care. It is necessary to equip such levels of care with baby cardiac, respiratory, and non-invasive blood pressure monitoring. For maintenance of adequate oxygenation, oxygen analyser, blood gas and trans-cutaneous pH, O_2 and CO_2 monitors are recommended. Respiratory effort often needs to be supported by ventilators. It is ideal to have volume and pressure-limited ventilators, though these are extremely expensive and difficult to obtain and maintain. In the initial state of development, therefore, a pressure-limited ventilator may be used, as it meets most requirements. It may be necessary to provide a compact, multiple point, noiseless air compressor where piped compressed air facilities are not available.

While providing for tertiary care, it is necessary to have supportive biochemical, radiodiagnostic and imaging facilities for prompt diagnosis.

Design for neonatal units

The necessity for and functional size of newborn units depends on community or regional needs. It is generally accepted that a community or hospital with an annual birth rate exceeding 2000, needs a neonatal special care unit. Accepting that about 20 per cent of livebirths need special care, a 15–20 bed unit would probably be ideal. The unit should be located adjacent to the delivery rooms to facilitate early and rapid transportation of high-risk newborns.

The space in a neonatal special care unit may be

Table 2.6.4 Equipment needs for newborn care

Equipment	Level I	Level II	Level III	Approx. (US$)
Delivery room and resuscitation				
Resuscitation bag and mask	+	+	+	50–100
Neonatal laryngoscope with straight blade (No. 0)	+	+	+	20–50
Endotracheal tubes (size 2, 2.5, 3 mm) with adaptors	+	+	+	
Warmer				
Radiant warmer	+	+	+	1000
Lamp with 100 W bulb	+	−	−	20
Suction facility				
Mucus trap	+	+	−	1
Pedal-operated	+	+	+	100–200
Electric-operated	*	*	+	400
Resuscitation trolley (O_2, suction facility, radiant warmer, Apgar timer)	−	*	+	5000
Neonatal care				
Warming devices				
Lamp with bulb (100 W)	+	*	−	
Radiant warmer	*	+	+	
Incubators				
Ambient temperature control	−	+	+	4000
Servo-control	−	*	+	10 000
Open intensive care bassinet	−	*	+	8000
Cardiac monitors	−	*	+	8000
Respiration/apnoea monitor	−	*	+	500
Blood pressure monitor	−	*	+	
Invasive				8000
Non-invasive (Doppler)				2000
Oxygenation				
Oxygen hoods	+	+	+	50–200
Oxygen analyser	−	*	+	1000
Transcutaneous O_2 and CO_2 monitors	−	−	+	10 000
Ventilators				
Pressure limited	−	−	+	10 000
Volume limited	−	−	+	15 000
Phototherapy units	+	+	+	700–20
Blue lamps				
White fluorescent tubes (200 W)				
Exchange transfusion sets	−	+	+	
Infusion units				
Measured volume burette	+	+	+	3
Infusion pumps	−	*	+	500
Weighing scales	+	+	+	20–50
Spring balance				
Beam balance				
Laboratory equipment				
Microscope	−	+	+	500–1000
Neubauer chamber and pipettes	−	+	+	50
Haemoglobinometer	−	+	+	20
Microcentrifuge	−	*	+	200
Bilirubinometer	−	+	+	1500
Blood gas analyser	−	*	+	15 000
Micro method facility for sugar, calcium, electrolytes, urea	−	*	+	2500

− Not needed, * optional, + essential.

considered to be made up of areas for patient and non-patient care activities.

Area for patient care activities

This should preferably be large and open to facilitate mobility of equipment and personnel, rather than partitioned cubicles. It is recommended that about 4–5 m² be provided for each level II bed and about 7–9 m² for each level III bed; particular care must be taken to provide adequate conveniently placed wash basins and electrical outlets (4–12 per bed depending on level of care) in a patient care area.

Areas for non-patient care activities

These areas may include a scrub-and-gown area at entry, nurse's station, storage room, formula room, mother's room (where mothers can feed babies and foster maternal-infant bonding), laboratory, nurses' and duty doctors' room, soiled utility room (must be separate but contiguous, with dual access).

Staff and training needs

In the community where perinatal care has to be delivered at home or in a health centre, a trained birth attendant for a population of 500–800 is recommended. An auxiliary nurse midwife with specifically defined tasks for providing maternal and child-care is required for a population of 2500–3000. Two medical officers with training in perinatal and newborn care are

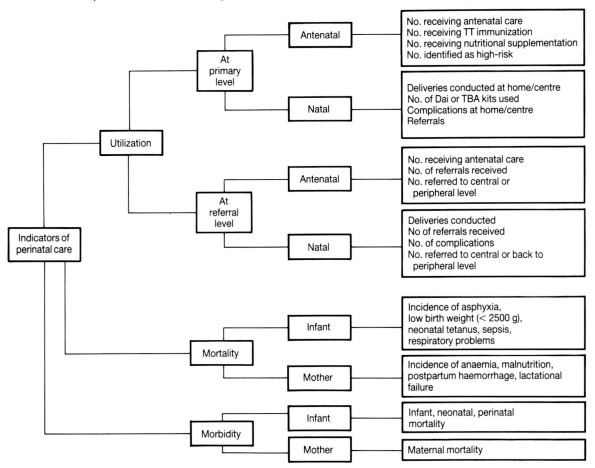

Fig. 2.6.3 Monitoring of perinatal care services. TT = tetanus toxoid.

recommended for a primary health centre covering a population of 100 000.

At the hospital, nurse–patient ratios of 1:10 for level I, 1:4 for level II and 1:1 for level III are recommended. Full-time paediatricians caring mainly for newborn babies are required for the organization and delivery of secondary and tertiary neonatal care.

The training needs for each category of health personnel, namely birth attendants, nurse midwives, in-service nurses and doctors, medical and nursing students, have to be very clearly defined. All training should be related to tasks expected to be performed by a health worker who should undergo training or reorientation periodically.

Monitoring perinatal care

It is essential to devise a system which monitors or audits delivery of perinatal care. These indicators are likely to vary from unit to unit and should essentially be based on objectives for which these services are provided. Figure 2.6.3 gives in a flow diagram a monitoring system based on utilization of services and maternal and neonatal morbidity and mortality. Such a system is particularly likely to be useful in situations where perinatal services are being developed and are linked to cost-effectiveness. Wherever possible death rates in mothers and babies should be collected, although such information may be difficult to obtain in the community. One of the simplest methods of monitoring would be to weigh all babies born and to calculate the proportion below 2.5 kg. This information could be collected by trained birth attendants and recorded on health cards analysed at health centres.

References

1. Bhargava SK. Perinatal care (Editorial). *Indian Pediatrics*. 1983; **20**: 547–8.
2. Bhargava SK, Srinivasan S, Jaikishen P. Simplified scoring system for identification of high risk birth. *Indian Pediatrics*. 1982; **19**: 209–15.
3. Jhamb U. A prospective study of morbidity and mortality of high risk infants. Thesis submitted to University of Delhi, in part fulfilment of Doctor of Medicine (Paediatrics), 1984.
4. Bhargava SK, Ramji S, Sachdeva HPS, Iyer PU. Delivery of perinatal care in India: priorities and policies. *Annals of Tropical Paediatrics*. 1986; **6**: 225–31.

SECTION 3

Growth and development

Michael Parkin and Paget Stanfield

CHAPTER 1

Introduction

Michael Parkin

The Child increased in wisdom and stature and in favour with God and Man

St Luke, New Testament.

Growth and development, in physical, intellectual, emotional and social terms, are the essential biological characteristics of childhood. A child is not a small adult but is a developing human being who changes from a newborn baby, through infancy, toddlerhood and the early school years into an adolescent and finally, a mature adult. The corollary of development is dependence, particularly upon the mother. Initially this is complete but as development progresses so should independence.

Recognition of the child as a developing and a dependent person places certain responsibilities upon all concerned with children, parents, professional people and politicians. They must ensure that children receive what is needed, whether as food, protection, stimulation and teaching, sleep, play or love, to enable them to grow, to develop and to gain in independence.

There are special and important implications for medicine. Paediatrics is not a subspeciality of adult medicine like the organ specialities but is the medical care of children who have special characteristics and needs.

Disease in childhood affects growth and development. Measurement of growth and development is therefore an essential skill for paediatricians, as these are indications of health in individual children and in communities. The pattern of disease and the clinical picture and long-term consequences of diseases in children are affected by the stage of development at which they occur. Finally, the care of sick children should be appropriate for their stage of development and dependence and should never be considered without the mother, who has an essential role as observer and nurse.

CHAPTER 2

Physical growth

GROWTH IN CHILDHOOD
A. S. Paynter and Michael Parkin

Introduction

Physical growth is the increase in size of the body that occurs as a result of the multiplication and increase in size of cells. The process begins with fertilization of the ovum and continues until adult life. Within tissues it occurs in three phases. The first is cell division, a very rapid increase in the number of cells without increase in their cytoplasmic content. This phase occupies the first 22 weeks of intrauterine life. In the second phase, cell division continues but more slowly; however, the rate of protein synthesis is as rapid and there is an increase in the size and complexity of the cells. In the third phase, cell division has stopped and cells grow only in size. The age at which one phase changes to the next varies in different tissues. Neurones cease cell division as early as 18 weeks after fertilization. The total number of muscle cells also is fixed early in intrauterine life. Neuroglia continue cell division for two years after birth, while the cartilage at the growing ends of bone continues mitosis until the epiphyses close. Regenerative tissue including bone marrow and epithelia continue mitosis throughout life, though this constitutes replenishment rather than growth. In general, most of the growth in late intrauterine life and childhood consists of phase three and this process of increase in cell size may continue into adult life, for example in the muscles of a weight lifter.

Because physical growth varies in rate and pattern in different tissues and different regions of the body, measurement of growth is not simple. In principle it involves repeated assessment of the size of some part of the individual. In practice, several measures may be used. Total body weight is a measure of all body tissues. Height, or in the younger child, length, indicates skeletal size. Skin fold thickness, which may be assessed by Harpenden callipers, either just over the triceps muscle or just below the scapula, is a measure of fat. Skull circumference reflects a combination of skeletal and brain size. Mid-upper arm circumference, a very easy measurement to make and one requiring very simple equipment, is affected by bone, muscle, skin and fat. No single index can truly reflect the intricate process of growth, and so indices are best used in combination. Usually the single most useful measure is height or length as it measures only one tissue – bone.

The growth curve, growth standards and centiles

Growth is most easily understood when represented graphically, and a growth chart is a very valuable tool in monitoring the health of children. A growth chart incorporates two concepts; the pattern of longitudinal growth and normal variation or distribution. Serial measurements of the size (e.g. height) of a child from birth to adulthood plotted against age on a graph give a longitudinal representation of the growth of that child, as shown in Fig. 3.2.1. Figure 3.2.2, in contrast, shows the distribution of the heights of 100 boys at the age of five years. Fifty boys (50 per cent) have heights below, and 50 per cent above 108 cm. This is therefore referred to as the 50th centile or median. Three per cent have heights less than 99 cm and this is therefore referred to as the third centile. Similarly, the 97th, 90th, 75th, 25th, and 10th centile points are identified, the given centile being defined as that value below which a given percentage of observations occur. If measurements of these 100 boys were repeated throughout their childhood and the corresponding centile points joined, a longitudinally produced centile chart would be formed. To make meaningful charts, however, large samples of children need to be studied throughout childhood. In practice, the data used for charts often come from

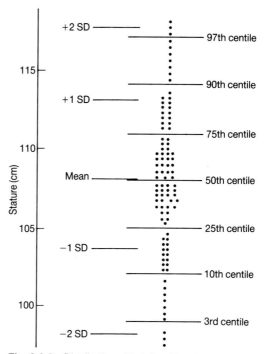

Fig. 3.2.2 Distribution of height of 100 boys aged five years.

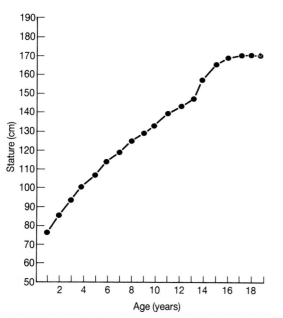

Fig. 3.2.1 Longitudinal representation of the growth of a boy from birth to 18 years.

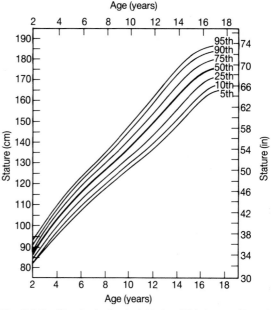

Fig. 3.2.3 Standards for height for USA boys. (Data from National Center for Health Statistics; cross-sectional charts.)

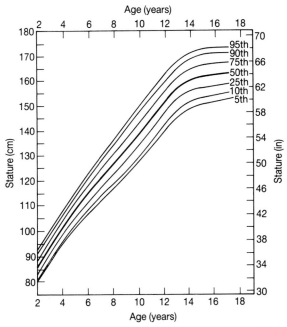

Fig. 3.2.4 Standards for height for USA girls. (Data from National Center for Health Statistics; cross-sectional charts.)

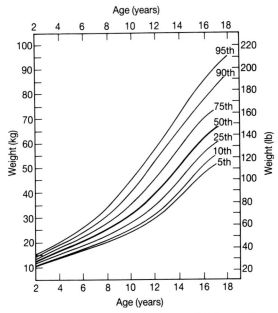

Fig. 3.2.5 Standards for weight for USA boys. (Data from National Center for Health Statistics; cross-sectional charts.)

mixed cross-sectional and longitudinal studies in which several short-term overlapping longitudinal groups are linked. For example, Figs 3.2.3–3.2.6 are examples of height and weight charts for boys and girls drawn up by the National Centre for Health Statistics, USA.

As the distribution of heights is normal or Gaussian, the median or 50th centile height is the same as the mean. Of the observations in Fig. 3.2.2, 68 per cent fall within the range of +1 and −1 standard deviations (SD) or 4.5 cm from the mean, and 95 per cent fall within the range of +2 and −2 SD. The relationships between centile points and standard deviation are also shown in Fig. 3.2.2. It can be seen that the +2 and −2 SD points are approximately the 97th and 3rd centile points respectively.

Growth velocity

Growth velocity or growth rate is growth per unit time. The height curve represents distance travelled, while a growth velocity curve represents speed. It is clear from a standard height chart, e.g. Fig. 3.2.7a, that velocity of growth varies through childhood. The lines are steep in the first two years, become less steep thereafter until the pubertal growth spurt, when they become steep before they finally flatten. This phenomenon is represented

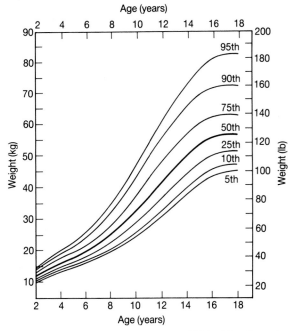

Fig. 3.2.6 Standards for weight for USA girls. (Data from National Center for Health Statistics; cross-sectional charts.)

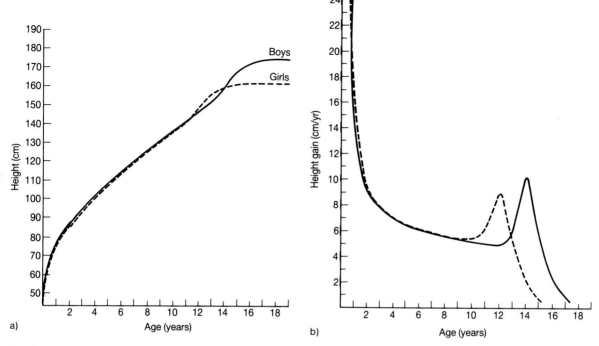

Fig. 3.2.7   (a) Typical individual height-attained curves for boys and girls (supine length to the age of two years; integrated curves of Fig. 3.2.5). (b) Typical individual velocity curves for supine length or height in boys and girls. These curves represent the velocity of the typical boy and girl at any given instant. (From Tanner JM, *Foetus into Man*, 1978, © Castlemead Publications.)

better in the growth velocity curve (Fig. 3.2.7b) which plots growth as centimetres per year against age.

The pattern of growth

Intrauterine growth

Intrauterine growth is very rapid, as is shown in Fig. 3.2.8a, a prenatal growth curve continuing into postnatal life, and Fig. 3.2.8b, the velocity curve for the same data. The most rapid stage of intrauterine growth is between 18 and 22 weeks and represents a phase of rapid mitosis, the first phase of growth. After this, cell division is slower, phase one giving way to phases two and three. Growth in late fetal life and postnatal life consists of an increase in the cytoplasmic content of cells rather than cell multiplication.

Growth in childhood

The pattern of growth in childhood is demonstrated by the distance charts and velocity charts for height

(Fig. 3.2.7a and b). Though body mass is a far less precise measurement of growth than height (as it represents a mixture of all tissues) the general pattern of weight gain is similar to that of linear growth, and this pattern is followed by most organs and tissues of the body such as the liver, kidney and spleen. However, there are some important exceptions, particularly the brain, the reproductive organs, the lymphatic tissues and fat. Figure 3.2.9 shows the different growth patterns for these organs compared with the general curve. The brain continues to grow rapidly after birth, reaching 90 per cent of its adult size by the age of five and 95 per cent by age eight. The reproductive organs on the other hand remain infantile throughout childhood and grow rapidly at puberty. The lymphatic tissue has an interesting pattern of growth, growing rapidly and reaching twice its adult mass before puberty and then regressing. The subcutaneous fat layer (measured by skin fold thickness) has a curve of its own, reaching its peak at the end of the first year and then decreasing in content (i.e. having a negative growth velocity) until the age of six to eight when it begins to increase once more. Girls have less initial loss and more

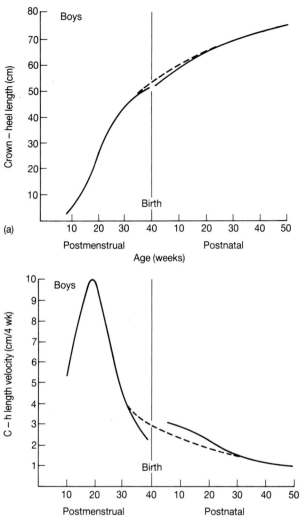

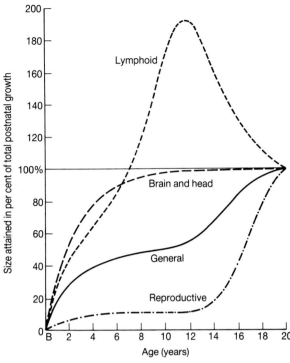

Fig. 3.2.9 Growth curves of different parts and tissues of the body, showing the four chief types. All the curves are of size attained, and plotted as percentage of total gain from birth to 20 years, so that size at age 20 is 100 on the vertical scale. *Lymphoid type*: thymus, lymph nodes, intestinal lymph masses. *Brain and head type*: brain and its parts, dura, spinal cord, optic apparatus, cranial dimensions. *General type*: body as a whole, external dimensions (except head), respiratory and digestive organs, kidneys, aortic and pulmonary trunks, musculature, blood volume. *Reproductive type*: testis, ovary, epididymis, prostate, seminal vesicles, fallopian tubes. (From Tanner JM, *Foetus into Man*, 1978. © Castlemead Publications.)

Fig. 3.2.8 Distance (a) and velocity (b) curves for growth in body length in prenatal and early postnatal periods. Diagrammatic, based on several sources of data. The continuous lines represent actual length and length velocity; the interrupted line the theoretical curve if no uterine restriction took place. (Tanner JM, *Foetus into Man*, 1978, © Castlemead Publications.)

subsequent increase than boys (Fig. 3.2.10). The decrease in fat content after the first year has an interesting practical application. The mid-upper arm circumference remains almost static between the ages of one and five years as muscle and bone mass increase while fat decreases (Fig. 3.2.11). In areas where mal-nutrition is rife, the precise age of children is often not known. Measurement of the mid-upper arm circumference in children between the estimated ages of one and five years is a useful tool in evaluating the nutritional status of these children.

Growth in puberty

Throughout childhood, boys are slightly taller than girls and this difference originates in late fetal life. The difference is marginal, being only about a centimetre until the age of 11. Boys and girls both have a growth spurt at puberty. In girls this growth spurt occurs

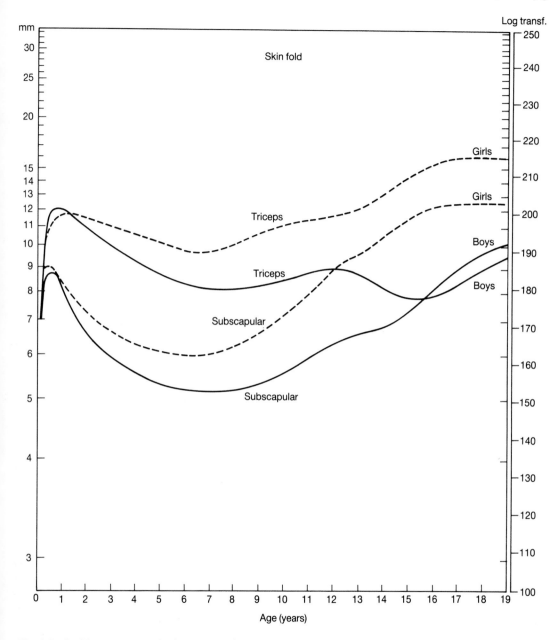

Fig. 3.2.10 Distance curve of subcutaneous tissue measured by Harpenden skin fold callipers over triceps (back of upper arm) and under scapula (shoulder blade). Scale is mm on the left and logarithmic transformation units on the right. British children, 50th centiles. (From Tanner JM, *Foetus into Man*, 1978, © Castlemead Publications.)

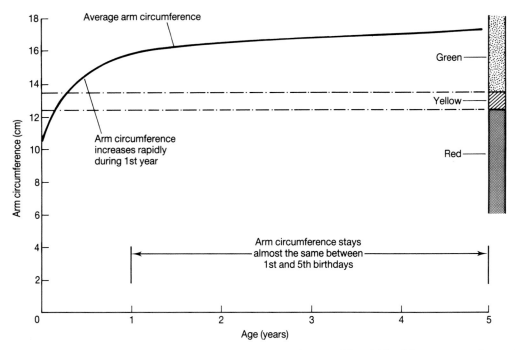

Fig. 3.2.11   An arm-circumference-for-age graph. The circumference of the middle of the upper arm changes little from ages one to five years. (Reproduced with permission from Morley D and Woodland M, *See How They Grow*, 1978, Macmillan.)

earlier – preceding the growth spurt of boys by two years. The peak growth velocity in girls (9 cm/year) occurs at a mean age of 12. Boys have a greater peak velocity of 10.3 cm/year at a mean age of 14. As girls achieve their pubertal growth spurt earlier, they overtake boys and remain on average taller until the age of 13.5 when the boys overtake again to attain an adult height 8 cm taller than their female peers. Most body tissues are involved in this growth spurt, but the most marked growth is in bone and muscle.

Variation

The growth patterns described so far are based on observations made in Western countries. This does not imply that these are the only normal patterns, or that growth of children elsewhere should conform to them. They have been used to illustrate growth patterns. They are nothing but an aggregate of certain observations made on growing children at a certain time and place, and reflect the genetic and environmental influences on those children. There is considerable variation in human growth world-wide, and it is not always easy to disentangle genetic from environmental influences in this variation.

In any population there is a wide range of normal growth, influenced by genetic and environmental factors. There is also wide variation in average adult height between different peoples, which has been assumed to result from genetic differences. For example, the Japanese, South Indians, New Guinea Highlanders and the pygmies of central Africa are small. On the other hand, Polynesians are big and tall, as are some American Indians. How much of this variation is genetic and how much environmental?

There is probably little variation in growth rate in early fetal life but differences in growth rate occur in late fetal life. A slowing down of fetal growth may occur as a result of poor placental circulation due to maternal disease, or as a result of poor maternal nutrition. The wide variation in mean birth weights in different countries is predominantly a reflection of the widely differing standards of maternal health and nutrition in these countries.

The difference in postnatal growth patterns throughout the world is also largely due to differing standards of health and nutrition in different populations. Careful and extensive growth studies have been done in people of different ethnic origins both in their original homelands and in different parts of the world to which they have migrated. These studies have demonstrated that some of the variation in the growth patterns of different ethnic groups is attributable to genetic factors, but that environment is by far the more important factor influencing final adult height.[3]

All European populations grow in a very similar manner, although in all countries children in well-off homes grow faster than those in poor homes. On average, the tallest populations are those in the north-west of Europe, i.e. Norway, Sweden, North Germany and Holland. The heaviest Europeans, both absolutely, and relative to heights, are those of north-central Europe, Czechoslovakia and Poland.[3]

People in the Indian subcontinent and in Mediterranean countries resemble Europeans in growth and body proportions, although in many areas undernutrition and disease undermine optimal growth. There is a marked difference in growth between the well-off and the poor, the well-off approximating European growth rates.[3]

The growth of many Africans in Africa is also limited by poor nutrition and disease, but well-off Africans grow in height and weight very much as do Europeans (Fig. 3.2.12). In the United States, children of African descent, on average, are taller and heavier at all ages than children of European descent.[3]

Though optimally growing Africans do not differ significantly in size from optimally growing Caucasians, they differ in their body proportions. They have longer limbs and correspondingly shorter trunks, broader shoulders and narrower hips, and less subcutaneous fat.[3]

The Chinese and Japanese differ from Europeans and Africans in their pattern of growth. Even those growing up under conditions of optimal growth are shorter than their European or African counterparts. There are two reasons for this: first, their legs grow slowly so that, as adults, they have relatively shorter legs; second, they attain skeletal maturity and therefore stop growing, a little earlier than Europeans or Africans.[3]

In summary, although there are minor genetic differences in growth patterns in people of different ethnic groups, there is a much wider difference in size and growth velocity between the rich and the poor within the same group. This difference between rich and poor is apparent in all communities throughout the world. The main reason for people in many parts of the world being small and growing slowly is their poverty, and not their genes.

Growth standards

Any attempt to measure growth involves comparing the growth of an individual or population with some standards. Which standards should be used? Should each country have its own national standard, and each community its own community standard, or should there be a single internationally accepted standard? Drawing up standards is an extremely time-consuming and expensive exercise and would prove an insurmountable task in many areas. Separate standards would make comparisons difficult and create a Tower of Babel. There are, however, valid objections to any one country or population having to subscribe to the standards of another.

While the major factors responsible for variation in growth are environmental, there are minor differences in growth patterns of people of different races. If standards are to be acceptable internationally, then they must be drawn up from a truly internationally representative population. Two sets of standards have been widely used in the past and neither has fulfilled this requirement. The first set of standards were the Harvard standards. These were drawn up by the Harvard School of Public Health and based on data collected from children of North European stock in Boston in the 1960s. The samples were small and unrepresentative but the standards were used all over the world for nutritional surveys because they were the only ones available at the time. The other widely used set of standards were the London standards. The sample population for these standards was taken at random from London schools in the 1960s and was very extensive. The preschool sample was derived from births in central London at the same time. In spite of the sample being extensive, it was not internationally representative. Recently, a new set of standards has been issued by the National Centre for Health Statistics (NCHS) in the USA. The data were collected between 1971 and 1974 from surveys mounted specially to sample the whole childhood population in a proportionate way with multiethnic representation. These standards therefore come closer than the previous standards to fulfilling the requirements of the international community and have been accepted for international use by the WHO (Figs 3.2.3–3.2.6).[4]

Influences upon growth

Several factors influence human growth. Some of the genetic factors that influence it have been described and others, including inherited or chromosomal

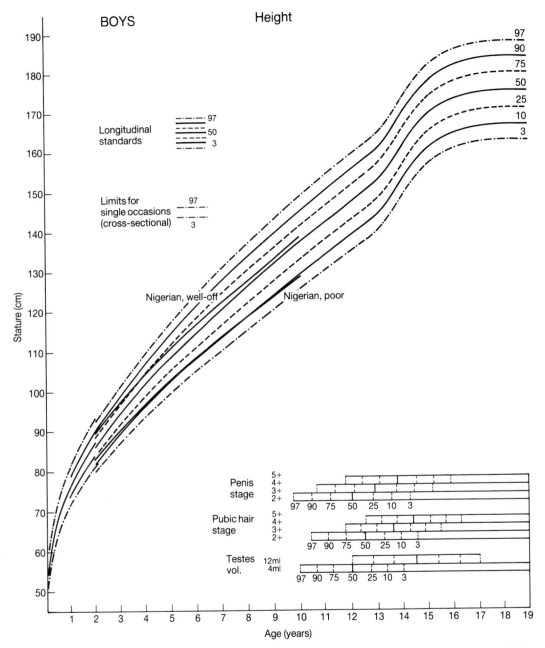

Fig. 3.2.12   Average growth in height of two groups of boys in Ibadan, Nigeria, plotted on British Standards for a well-off group and an indigent group. (Data from Janes, 1975, as quoted in Eveleth and Tanner, *Worldwide Variation in Human Growth*, 1976, Cambridge University Press, p. 216.)

abnormalities, are discussed on pp. 275–80. Here, some important environmental influences on growth are considered.

Intrauterine environment

Any noxious influence that can cause the death of a fetus can, in a smaller dose, cause growth retardation. The final outcome of the effect of the intrauterine environment on growth can be assessed by measuring the size of the full-term baby. If one excludes those babies who are born too soon, birth weight reflects fetal growth, and is a good (though retrospective) indicator of maternal health and nutrition. There is considerable variation world-wide in mean birth weight (Table 3.2.1) which is largely a reflection of differing standards of maternal nutrition. In Tanzania, for example, the mean birth weight of African children of low income groups was 2.9 kg, whereas the mean birth weight of children of the same ethnic group but of higher income groups was 3.3 kg, which compares favourably with the mean birth weight of European babies.[1]

Average weight gain during pregnancy varies with nutritional status of mothers (see Table 3.2.2) in some areas mothers gain relatively little weight in pregnancy, and in very deprived groups at times of food shortage, some mothers actually lose weight in pregnancy.[2]

Table 3.2.1 Mean birth weight of some groups of people in different countries

Group	Country	Weight (kg)
Lumi	New Guinea	2.4
Indian	India	2.74
Indian	Malaysia	2.73
Tanzanian	Tanzania	2.95
West African	Senegal	2.97
Chinese	Malaysia	3.01
West African	USA	3.11
Caucasian	UK	3.35
Caucasian	USA	3.32

(From Meridith HV, *Human Biology*, 1970; **42**: 215, by permission of Wayne State University Press.)

Table 3.2.2 Average weight gain during pregnancy in some different countries

Country	Weight gain (kg)
USA	17.0
UK	11.7
Tanzania	9.1
Uganda	8.4
South India	6.0

The birth weight of the baby is in part a reflection of the mother's health and nutritional status in pregnancy. Growth failure, due to poor maternal nutrition, occurs in the last few weeks of pregnancy and results in poor fat and energy storage in the fetus in those weeks. The outcomes of pregnancies during the wartime famine in Holland from October 1944 to May 1945 were studied extensively. Mothers exposed to a very low calorie intake (less than 1500 cal per day) during the third trimester of pregnancy had low-birth-weight babies (birth weight diminished by 9 per cent). However, mothers exposed to very low calorie intake during the first and second trimesters of pregnancy and whose calorie intake was restored during the third trimester had no significant reduction in the birth weights of their babies.

In some poor agricultural communities there is a seasonal variation in weight gain during pregnancy, and corresponding variation in birth weights of babies. It has been demonstrated in the Gambia that pregnant women had a weight gain of 1200 g per month if pregnant during the dry season, but a gain of only 500 g per month if pregnant during the wet season. This difference in maternal weight gain was reflected in the birth weight of babies. Babies born after a wet season pregnancy were 200 g lighter than those born after a pregnancy of relative plenty. Nutritional supplements to these women had an effect when given during the lean wet season, increasing the weight gain in pregnancy and birth weights of the babies, and had no such effect during the dry and more plentiful season.[6]

Anaemia is a common antenatal problem in many developing countries and is associated with an increased risk of low birth weight and perinatal mortality. One study in East Africa showed that 42 per cent of mothers with a haemoglobin of less than 7.4 g/100 ml had babies weighing less than 2500 g.[2]

There is considerable overlap between the influence of maternal infection and nutrition on the growth of the fetus. Malarial infection of the placenta is an important contributory factor to low-birth-weight babies in areas where malaria is endemic. Urinary infection is estimated to affect about 4.5 per cent of pregnant women and birth weights of infants of such mothers are lower than those of mothers without bacteruria.[2] Lepromatous leprosy in the mother is associated with low birth weight and is discussed further on pp. 561–5. During pregnancy the viral infection rubella, in addition to causing multiple congenital abnormalities in the fetus, also causes intrauterine growth retardation.

Toxaemia of pregnancy through poor placental circulation causes intrauterine growth retardation, as does any condition that causes hypertension during pregnancy.

Smoking in pregnancy has an adverse effect on the growth of the fetus. Babies of mothers who smoke tend to be lighter and shorter than babies of non-smokers. There is also an increased risk of prematurity in babies of smoking mothers. Excessive alcohol consumption during pregnancy can result in intrauterine growth retardation as part of the fetal alcohol syndrome.

Factors influencing the growth of the infant and young child

The two most important factors that influence growth of the infant and young child are nutrition and infection. It is often difficult to disentangle the one from the other; where malnutrition is rife, infections are common and together they lead a macabre dance which causes devastation to child life, growth and health. During starvation or illness the child's growth slows down and may even stop. However, if after this period there is

adequate or compensatory nutrition, then this is followed by a catch-up period in growth and the child will regain the previous centile line. This may occur in two ways. In complete catch-up growth the growth velocity increases so rapidly that the original curve is attained and thereafter growth proceeds normally. In some instances the growth velocity is not rapid enough for this but maturity is delayed, the child continues to grow at a normal velocity below the centile lines, and because of a prolonged period of growth, ultimately reaches the original centile line. Children have an astonishing capacity to return to their normal growth centile and usually do so completely, provided they are well-fed and looked after during the period of rehabilitation. However, if the insult or period of poor nutrition occurs in early fetal life, during the phase of rapid cell multiplication, then potential for growth is limited and catch-up is incomplete. Figure 3.2.13 shows the growth, in weight, of an actual child in a poor central American community. For the first six months of life, breast-feeding kept the child growing well.

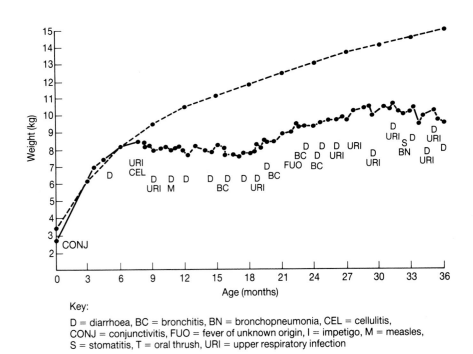

Key:

D = diarrhoea, BC = bronchitis, BN = bronchopneumonia, CEL = cellulitis,
CONJ = conjunctivitis, FUO = fever of unknown origin, I = impetigo, M = measles,
S = stomatitis, T = oral thrush, URI = upper respiratory infection

Fig. 3.2.13 This chart plots the growth of an actual child in a poor Central American community and tells a story typical of the childhood of millions in the developing world. Based on studies by L. J. Mata, J. J. Urrutia and A. Lechtig for the Institute of Nutrition of Central America and Panama (INCAP). (From *State of the World's Children*, 1982, by permission of Oxford University Press.)

Thereafter, with weaning, the baby received less high-energy food than required. While this degree of malnutrition is not severe enough to be manifest in any clinically obvious form, it results in suboptimal growth with an increase in the risk of infection. This in turn exacerbates malnutrition, and so the cycle continues and severely compromises the growth of the child. Any one of these infections in a poorly nourished child could prove fatal or tip the child into clinically obvious malnutrition in the form of kwashiorkor or marasmus. Sadly, this pattern of poor nutrition, illness and poor growth is the lot of many millions of children in many less materially advanced countries of the world and is an indictment to what we are pleased to call twentieth century industrial civilization. Such children fail to reach their growth potential, not as a result of a single insult of malnutrition or severe infection, but as a result of constant suboptimal nutrition and infection which result in the initial growth failure and prevents the opportunity of convalescence and catch-up.

Methods of measuring growth and nutritional status

The best method of assessing the health and nutrition of the individual child is by longitudinal monitoring of growth. Weight monitoring and the use of the growth charts is central to the concept of child care in developing countries. It is also important, for epidemiological reasons, to survey children in a community to make an objective assessment of their nutritional status. This is done by measuring one or more parameters of growth on a sample population and comparing them with a standard. The methods used will depend on the tools and personnel available to do the survey and the information available on the children measured, particularly their ages.

Weight-for-age and height-for-age

It is simple to measure the weight or height of a child and compare this with an accepted standard if the age is known. Many surveys done world-wide in the 1960s and 1970s used the Harvard Standards. Arbitrary cut-off points were taken as criteria for malnutrition. Children who weighed less than 80 per cent of the Harvard mean were considered malnourished and those less than 60 per cent of this mean, severely malnourished; 80 per cent of the mean for weight is approximately the third centile, or -2 SD. Using height for age, children less than 90 per cent of the Harvard mean were considered 'stunted' and children below 80 per

cent of the mean severely stunted; 90 per cent of the mean for height is approximately the third centile or -2 SD, while 80 per cent is approximately -3 SD.

Waterlow[7] described a classification of malnutrition using both weight and height for age as shown in Table 3.2.3. This classification is useful in that it distinguishes those children with acute malnutrition who will be in group II (wasted) from those with chronic under-nutrition who are stunted (group III). The disadvantage in the method is that, although height is a far more accurate reflection of growth in the long term, it is often difficult to measure accurately in community surveys. There is a tendency to place the genetic or constitutionally small child into the category of undernutrition. This may also occur with the premature infant during the first year of life.

Using a weight chart for community surveys

Many community health programmes in developing countries use growth charts as a means of health surveillance of children. These charts can be used for quick cross-sectional surveys by taking one chart for boys and another for girls and plotting on them the weights against age for all children measured that day (Fig. 3.2.14a). Plastic overlay sheets can be superimposed on these charts to enable the scatter of weights to be analysed according to centile lines[5] (Fig. 3.2.14b). Kits for this simple method are available from Teaching Aids at Low Cost, PO Box 49, St Albans, Herts, AL1 4AX, UK. They are a useful method of auditing the work of a community clinic with little extra effort.

Mid-upper arm circumference

In many communities with suboptimal nutrition it is difficult to ascertain the exact age of children, and therefore impossible to apply growth standards. As has been pointed out earlier, the mid-upper arm

Table 3.2.3 Waterlow's classification

| | | Weight for age | |
		>80%	<80%
Height for age	>90%	Normal I	Wasted II
	<90%	Stunted III	Stunted and wasted IV

(With permission from the *British Medical Journal*, 1974; **4**: 89.)

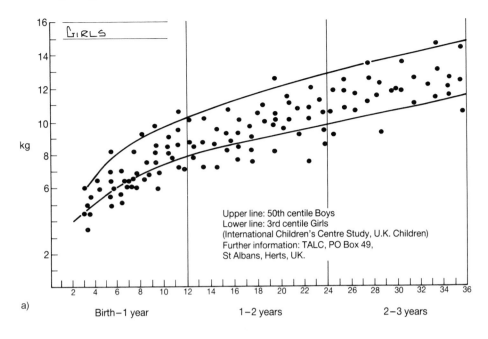

Upper line: 50th centile Boys
Lower line: 3rd centile Girls
(International Children's Centre Study, U.K. Children)
Further information: TALC, PO Box 49,
St Albans, Herts, UK.

a)

Birth–1 year   1–2 years   2–3 years

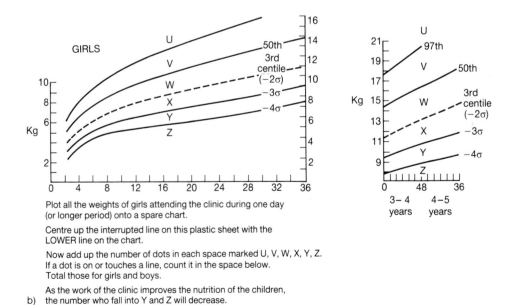

Plot all the weights of girls attending the clinic during one day
(or longer period) onto a spare chart.

Centre up the interrupted line on this plastic sheet with the
LOWER line on the chart.

Now add up the number of dots in each space marked U, V, W, X, Y, Z.
If a dot is on or touches a line, count it in the space below.
Total those for girls and boys.

As the work of the clinic improves the nutrition of the children,
b)   the number who fall into Y and Z will decrease.

3–4 years   4–5 years

Fig. 3.2.14   (a) A chart on which are plotted weights of the girls attending a clinic over a period of a week. Over this can be placed a plastic sheet as shown in (b), and the number of dots falling into each area counted. The lines suggested are those arising from a 1972 WHO consultation group (WHO 1977). (With permission from Morley D and Woodland M, *See How They Grow*, 1979, Macmillan.)

circumference changes little between the ages of one and five (Fig. 3.2.11). At one year of age there is a good deal of fat under the skin, while at five years there is more muscle and less fat, but the total circumference remains almost the same. Measurement of the mid-upper arm circumference of children between these ages is a simple way of identifying malnourished children and of estimating the size of the problem in a community. The Shakir strip is a simplification of this method. A strip of plastic which may be obtained by removing the emulsion from an old X-ray film, has the various cut-off points colour coded as shown in

Fig. 3.2.15. This may be used instead of a measuring tape. Though this is a very simple method of assessing nutritional status, and is not very accurate, it is a useful tool to help sensitize communities to the problem of poor nutrition in their areas. A more sophisticated mid upper arm circumference (MUAC) metre (Fig. 3.2.16) can be used for measuring arm circumferences at different ages (from 1 to 12 years). It is more accurate, but is more difficult to make and a little more difficult to use. As a method of growth monitoring it is probably less effective than weight for age and the growth chart.

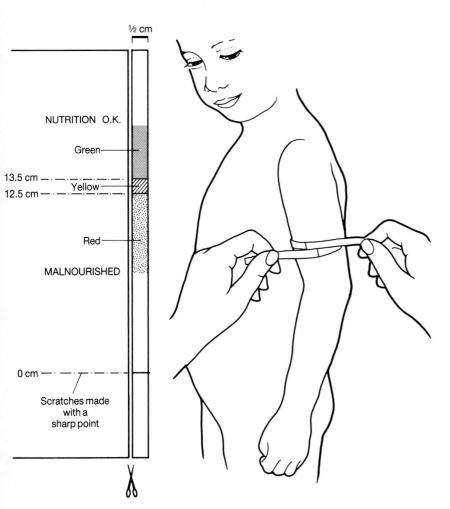

Fig. 3.2.15 Most hospitals and clinics have old X-ray films which can be used to make the Shakir strip. To do this the film emulsion is soaked in strong soda or bleach and then scrubbed off. When all the emulsion is off the plastic should be clear. The plastic is then scratched with a sharp point in three places, at 0, 12.5 and 13.5 cm. A sharp point is used to make one single line. Both sides of the film are coloured using the spirit type of felt pen, which smells. To use, the strip is placed round the arm so that it lies on the skin (it should not be pulled so tight that the skin wrinkles). (With permission from Morley D and Woodland M, *See How They Grow*, Macmillan, 1979.)

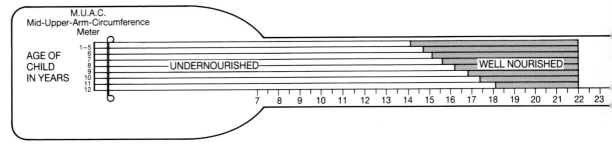

Fig. 3.2.16   The MUAC meter can be used for measuring arm circumference at different ages.

Weight-for-height

Another method of assessing the nutritional status of children of uncertain age is to compare their weight with their height. Save The Children Fund have produced a simple 'life size' weight for height chart with height on the 'Y' and weight on the 'X' axis. Cut-off areas are colour coded as shown in Fig. 3.2.17. The child is weighed and then measured at the point on the chart appropriate for this weight. The poorly nourished child, being thin, is comparatively tall for weight and falls within the red section. This method has its limitations as it identifies only those children with acute malnutrition; those with chronic malnutrition who are stunted are missed as being both short and light for their age, although they are the appropriate height for their weight.

Measuring techniques

Height

Height needs to be measured accurately, as an error of one or two centimetres may make a significant difference when interpreting growth data, particularly velocities. Accurate measurement of height does not need sophisticated equipment, provided attention is paid to detail in measurement. Height can be perfectly adequately measured against a perpendicular wall with a triangular or book-shaped object brought down on the child's head. It takes at least two people to do this, as one has to position the child and the other, at the right moment, bring the book down on the child's head. The longer side of the book, the spine, should be in contact with the wall and the shorter side of the book in contact with the top of the child's head. Contact of the book with the head must extend well out, at least to a point above the forehead. The child stands with his heels against the bottom of the wall, his shoulders, buttocks and head touching the wall while he looks straight forward, so that his earholes are in the same horizontal plane as the lower border of his eye sockets. He is asked to stretch up as much as he can, to make himself as tall as he can, take a deep breath and relax his shoulders, while the observer applies gentle pressure upwards to the bony prominences just behind the ears. When this position has been reached, the other observer brings the book down with the spine against the wall to touch the top of the child's head. The position on the corner of the book is marked on the wall and this is then measured exactly.

Much more sophisticated and expensive equipment is available with a counterbalanced headboard and a digital readout. This eliminates the need for two observers and though ideal is not available in the situations in which most children need to be measured. It must be emphasized that accuracy in measuring the height is dependent on the technique rather than the equipment used. However, various aids may be used to make this procedure simple, including the Oxford Life Size Height Chart and the Save The Children Weight-for-Height Chart used in developing countries (Fig. 3.2.17). Attention must be paid to ensuring that these charts are pinned up so that the heights they measure are exact.

In children of less than two years it is almost impossible to measure height accurately and so the measurement loses its meaning. Length is the appropriate measure but is much more difficult, and in addition, it is more difficult to find a home-made substitute for the supine length machine. The best that can be advised is a right-angled board such as a bed with a low headboard and a plank put along it. The infant's head must be held with the ear/eye plane vertical. The ankles are gently pulled to stretch the child and the legs are straightened, the feet turned up vertically; a triangle is then brought against the feet and its position on the

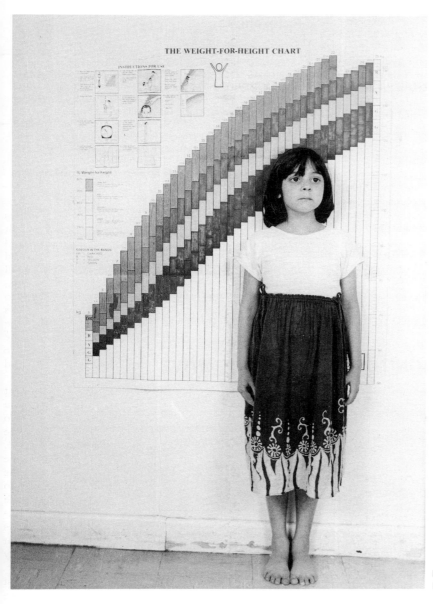

Fig. 3.2.17 The Save the Children Fund Weight-for-Height Chart.

bed marked. Because measuring length is more prone to errors than measuring height, it is a less valuable tool for use in the community.

Weight

Though weight is theoretically less suitable for monitoring growth than is height, it is so much easier to do, particularly in young infants, that it is a much more practical clinical tool. Ideally a frequently calibrated beam balance should be used but this is not available in many clinics. For older children, bathroom scales, provided they are frequently calibrated, may suffice. For younger children a spring balance has been found to be very effective. The child is suspended by a sling with holes for his legs. Two varieties of scale are in use, one which weighs to an accuracy of 0.5 kg and the other which weighs to an accuracy of 100 g. This is a useful tool and central to well-baby clinics the world over. It is perfectly adequate for growth monitoring in the under-fives' clinic. The intervals on the commonly used growth charts are 500 g, as finer divisions tend to confuse health workers and are of no great significance for children weighed less frequently than monthly.

Skin fold thickness

The skin is pinched up between finger and thumb and measured by Harpenden callipers, which exert a gentle standard grip and measure the skin fold thickness in millimetres. The measurement is made at two sites, half way down the back of the arm, the triceps skin fold thickness and, just below the angle of the scapula, the subscapular skin fold thickness.

References

1. Ebrahim GJ. *Practical Mother and Child Care in Developing Countries*. Basingstoke, Macmillan Press, 1978.
2. Ebrahim GJ. *Care of the Newborn in Developing Countries*. Basingstoke, Macmillan Press, 1979.
3. Eveleth PB, Tanner JM. *Worldwide Variation in Human Growth*. London, Cambridge University Press, 1976.
4. Hamill PVV, Drizd TA, Johnson CL *et al*. Physical growth: National Center for Health. Statistics as percentiles. *American Journal of Clinical Nutrition*. 1979; **32**, 607–29.
5. Morley D, Woodland M. *See How They Grow*. Macmillan Press, 1979.
6. Prentice AM, Whitehead RG, Watkinson M *et al*. Prenatal dietary supplementation of African women and birth-weight. *Lancet*. 1983; **i**, 489–92.
7. Waterlow JC. Some aspects of childhood malnutrition as a public health problem. *British Medical Journal*. 1974; **4**: 88–90.

Meredith HV. Body weight at birth. *Human Biology*. 1970; **42**: 215.

Morley D. *Paediatric Priorities in the Developing World*. Butterworths, 1974.

Tanner JM. *Foetus Into Man*. Open Books Publishing Ltd, 1978.

MAKING GROWTH MONITORING MORE EFFECTIVE
Gill Tremlett

Parents and other relatives are usually aware of a child's growth, i.e. whether the child is developing well or failing to thrive. They may judge a child's weight when lifting or carrying the child on their back, and observe not only these physical changes but also developmental milestones, the child's mood and emotional maturation. Although health workers have only been interested in observing children's growth and development in communities in developing countries since the 1950s, they have been able to add precision to observations and to use them in health surveillance.

Growth is a sensitive indicator of health. The aim of growth monitoring is to give information about a child's health and to detect problems at a stage when action can be taken relatively easily. For example, observations of weight-for-age charts show that the growth curve is usually abnormal 6 or even 12 months before a child presents with kwashiorkor or marasmus.[1] Regular growth monitoring may also be of value in assessing the results of rehabilitation programmes.

However, monitoring of growth is useful only if some action, such as nutrition advice, treatment or referral, can be taken when problems are identified. When food is very scarce, mothers and health workers may see no benefit in simply weighing children and growth monitoring may actually become a barrier to mothers' seeking advice or treatment. In addition, health workers have reported that mothers may avoid the clinic when their children are failing to thrive, if they feel that staff or relatives blame them for not feeding their children properly.

Methods of growth monitoring

Growth may be assessed by repeated measurements of weight, height or arm circumference; each method has particular advantages.

Weight-for-age

This method involves the regular weighing of a child and plotting the observations on a suitable chart. It encourages the provision of comprehensive health care, linked with regular supervision. The child's medical history and the use of preventive services such as immunization as well as the weight, may be recorded on the chart. If the chart is kept by the mother it helps to provide continuity of care and to stimulate collaboration between family and health services.

Weight-for-height: thinness chart

A child's height can be related to weight; a child who is comparatively tall for weight is likely to be thin or undernourished. This measurement is appropriate when decisions have to be made about services to children who are not being seen on a regular basis or whose ages are not known. It may be useful for monitoring the progress of acutely malnourished children in intervention programmes to a community.[2]

Arm circumference

Measurement of arm circumference is usually done with a measuring strip or tape and provides another useful indicator of severe current malnutrition in under-fives, whether or not stunting is present.[3, 4] This technique is cheap and relatively easy to perform. The measurement does not require knowledge of a child's age and simple strips may be designed for use by non-literate workers.[5]

Features of a successful programme

Growth monitoring programmes[6] have been found to be most successful if they include the following:

- A community-based approach. This requires support from community workers.
- Reliance on paramedical personnel who have been

effectively trained. Training programmes should be developed by professionals familiar with local problems. They should be carried out on-the-job and close to trainees' homes, with continued education and supervision through frequent meetings of health workers and supervisors.
- Adequate supplies and manpower.

It has also been shown to be helpful to build on[7]:

- Local customs, such as neighbourhood meetings and fathers' clubs.
- Traditional knowledge about feeding. Mothers may advise each other about ways of making food more palatable, how to coax a sick child to eat, preparing small snacks from leftovers or stealing a little extra from the family pot without the father noticing!
- Traditional forms of growth measurement such as rings or strings around a child's wrist or leg.[7]
- Traditional beliefs in the need for preventive action.

Problems with growth monitoring programmes

Attitudes and understanding of clinicians, health workers and families

Hospital clinicians may not be committed to growth monitoring[8] and may fail to pay attention to the growth charts completed by field staff. Such lack of commitment can be overcome when the benefits are seen.[9]

Health workers may not understand their role in growth monitoring. They may not have been adequately trained or know what action is needed if the growth pattern is abnormal. Their commitment may be eroded if much of their day is spent in completing forms or filing,[6] a problem avoided if records are held by the mother.

Many primary health workers have problems in all aspects of using growth charts: weighing the child, completing the chart, interpreting the growth pattern or identifying the action to be taken. These arise if teaching is not geared to solving individual mother's problems but consists of blanket answers with a didactic approach. Publications such as the WHO *Guidelines for Training Health Workers in Nutrition* and those produced by TAPS (Technologia alternative na Promoçao da Saude, Brazil), VHAI (Voluntary Health Association of India) and TALC (Teaching Aids at Low Cost)[1] are suitable for practical training of health workers. However, manuals and exercises related to the use of growth charts cannot replace apprenticeship to a senior health worker. Less experienced health workers need to practise techniques of decision-making, counselling and communication under supervision. Without this they can easily fall into the trap of giving standard advice which is not really related to the problem the mother is experiencing.[7]

There is a great need for health workers to recognize and understand the significance of different growth patterns. Firstly, the position of one recording on the growth chart at first visit gives no indication of growth. If the recording is below the lower centile line on the growth chart it may be that this is a normal small child, or one who has had an infection or was of very low birth weight. 'Growth' can only be assessed when there are two, three or more recordings through time.

Secondly, growth curves that follow the shape of the centile lines on the growth chart are normal. Even if the child's age is not accurately known, a few weighings will show if a child is growing well with a growth curve that follows the shape of the centile curves. The term 'Road to Health' used to describe the area between specific centile curves is counterproductive and dangerous. It may cause anxiety if single weights or growth curves are outside this area. Also, health workers may fail to act when growth failure occurs but the weight is still inside the 'Road to Health' area.

Thirdly, one of the most significant indicators of adequate rehabilitation after an episode of growth retardation, due either to dietary inadequacy or to infection or to both, is the 'catch-up growth'. This occurs when the slope of the child's growth curve is steeper than the centile curves. The child's growth is adequate when the growth curve begins to follow the shape of the centile curve which the child should have been following before the infection or nutritional problem. If the child is not getting enough food, or the infection is not dealt with adequately, or both, the child will not catch up and the child's growth curve will not follow the shape of the previous centile curve. With repeated episodes of infection and/or malnutrition, the growth curve may become a series of steps downwards, never regaining a growth curve that follows the original centile.

In addition to basic training in the use and interpretation of growth charts, health workers need guidelines[8] for action. These include:

- Clear and simple checklists, such as the things to be done before each clinic.
- Protocols for action about nutritional advice and screening for common diseases if a child has faltering weight.

- A referral policy which is essential to give credibility to a service.
- The use of at-risk registers of children in need of special care. Keeping a duplicate of their records will enable staff to monitor and evaluate their efforts for individual children.[9]
- Simple methods of evaluation.

Mothers may lack understanding of the purpose of growth monitoring. Understanding does not depend so much upon a mother's literacy as the health worker's interest in sharing information.[10, 11] Sadly mothers are often not given an explanation of the results of monitoring.

Some mothers are so occupied with surviving that regular clinic attendance is difficult, while others do not attend unless weighing is tied to other benefits, such as treatment, immunization or food supplements.[12, 13] Many mothers find the costs of using services outweigh the benefits. These costs include time, money, energy, embarrassment and even the fear of the complications of immunization. Ways that have been found to help include:

- Giving the growth chart to the family as their child's passport to the health service. This emphasizes the family's key role in the child's care. Do not use duplicate records except in unusual circumstances: they take time to find and when they are used mothers do not see the point of bringing their own card.
- Sharing the meaning of the chart with the family and other local people, for example school teachers who can include it in the curriculum.
- Having respect for local people and using them to monitor children's weights for example, by starting weighing circles.
- Minimizing waiting by holding clinics at convenient times and places and by improving 'lines of flow' in the clinic.[14] Use essential waiting time constructively for group discussions.
- Opening small clinics in poor areas so that the poor are not shamed away from clinics held in richer areas.

Growth monitoring linked with culturally appropriate education can assist families to learn more about the relationship between diet and health. This in itself may lead to reduced morbidity and mortality.[15-17] Usually, however, the impact of growth monitoring is less direct and it is up to the health worker to use the growth chart when discussing with the mother the action needed for her child.

Equipment

Charts may be too complex, take too long to complete and the social details on them may cause embarrassment. Scales may be difficult to read, frightening for children or not robust enough for prolonged use.

When choosing equipment it is important to consider who will use it, where will they work and what will be done with the results.[2, 18] The advantages of high-cost, accurate equipment in a relatively centralized clinic must be compared with those of low-cost, less accurate equipment which can be used anywhere. It may be better, if resources are limited, to use arm circumference and focus on wide coverage rather than insist on accurate assessment with scales kept in a small number of inaccessible centres.

Ideally, equipment for assessing growth should be accurate, easy to use, cheap, easily transportable and durable. Locally made scales have advantages as they are often familiar to workers, cheap and can be repaired easily. Their disadvantage is that they may be less accurate than more sophisticated scales but in field practice it is not normally necessary to have an accuracy of greater than 100 g. If a spring balance is used, rapid needle movement may be a problem and this can be overcome by using 90 cm of bicycle inner tube between the scale and the child as a damper[19] (Fig. 3.2.18).

It is important to decide if the growth chart is for health workers or local people and whether it is to focus on growth alone and identify children at risk or to help health workers to provide comprehensive care. Many developments in growth charts increase their complexity and this is usually a disadvantage, particularly if they are primarily for mothers.[20-22] It is necessary to assess mothers' understanding of different designs. For example, in Nigeria, mothers understood more easily charts with a straight base-line and bars (Fig. 3.2.19) rather than a stepped base-line and dots representing the weight (Fig. 3.2.20).

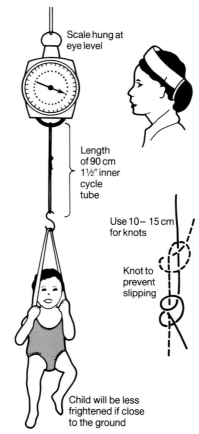

Scale hung at eye level

Length of 90 cm 1½″ inner cycle tube

Use 10–15 cm for knots

Knot to prevent slipping

Child will be less frightened if close to the ground

Fig. 3.2.18 Using a bicycle inner tube to damp needle movement.

importance of the family's own observations. The understanding, energy, will and commitment of the health worker is more important than any assessment technique. Techniques are simply tools to allow the committed health worker to be more effective.

Focus for the future

In the past, growth monitoring has often been carried out as an isolated activity or as one of several vertical programmes eg. immunization, FP, oral rehydration. Such vertical programmes can avoid a real political commitment to childrens' well-being. The challenge is to link all the key aspects of child health surveillance to promote normal growth and development. The focus for the future, therefore, is to help health workers to look at all aspects of the child and to recognize the

References

1. Morley DC, Woodland M. *See How They Grow*. London, Macmillan, 1979.
2. Nabarro D, Verney J, Wijga A. *The Weight-for-Height Chart Project*. Save the Children Fund. Evaluation Report No. 3, 1982–84.
3. Anderson M. Comparison of anthropometric measures of nutritional status in preschool children in five developing countries. *American Journal of Clinical Nutrition*. 1979; **32**: 2339
4. Velzeboer MI, Selwyn BJ, Sargent F *et al*. The use of arm

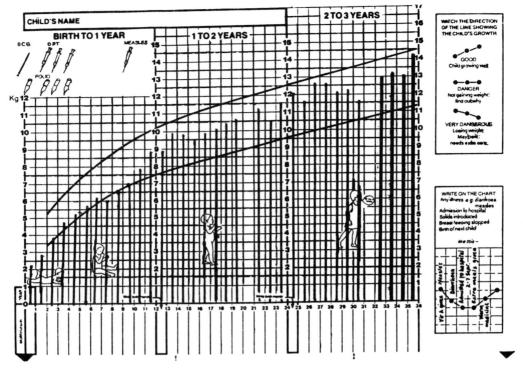

Fig. 3.2.19 A growth chart with a straight base-line and weights represented by bars.

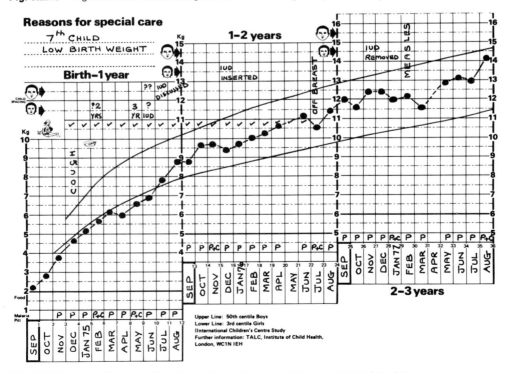

Fig. 3.2.20 A growth chart with a stepped base-line and weights represented by dots.

circumference in simplified screening for acute mal-nutrition by minimally trained health workers. *Journal of Tropical Pediatrics*. 1983; **29**: 159–66.

5. Ramachandran K, Parmar B, Jain J *et al.* Limitations on film strip and bangle test for identification of mal-nourished children. *American Journal of Clinical Nutrition*. 1978; **31**: 1469.
6. Gwatkin D, Wilcox J, Wray J. *Can Health and Nutrition Interventions make a Difference*. (Washington DC Overseas Development Council Monograph 13, 1980).
7. Rohde JE, Ismail D, Sutrisno R. Mothers as weight watchers: the road to child health in the village. *Journal of Tropical Pediatrics and Environmental Child Health*. 1975; **21**: 295–7.
8. WHO, *Guidelines for Training Community Health Workers in Nutrition* (WHO Offset Publication No. 59, Geneva, 1981).
9. King M. Clinics for under fives in Zambia and Malawi. *Tropical Doctor*. 1971; **1**: 36–8.
10. APHA. *Primary Health Care Issues: Growth Monitoring*. (1981; Series 1, No. 3: 70).
11. UNICEF. *How are Children Growing?* (Collection and analysis of weight-for-age data about groups of children, 1982).
12. Kimmance KJ. Evaluation of the work of a mobile out-patient unit in Swaziland. *Journal of Tropical Pediatrics*. 1970; **16**: 62–7.
13. Stephens AJH. The impact of health care and nutritional education on an urban community in Zambia through the under five clinics. *Journal of Tropical Medicine and Hygiene*. 1975; **78**: 97–105.
14. Morley DC. A medical service for children under five years of age in West Africa. *Transactions of the Royal Society for Tropical Medicine and Hygiene*. 1963; **57** (1): 79–94.
15. Growth monitoring: intermediate technology or expensive luxury? *Lancet*. 1985; 1337–8.
16. Scrimshaw NS. Myths and realities in international health planning. *American Journal of Public Health*. 1974; **64**: 792–8.
17. Alderman M, Wise P, Ferguson R *et al.* Reduction of young child malnutrition in rural Jamaica. *Journal of Tropical Pediatrics and Environmental Child Health*. 1978; **24**: 7.
18. Shakir A. The surveillance of protein–calorie mal-nutrition by simple and economic means (a report to UNICEF). *Journal of Tropical Pediatrics and Environmental Health*. 1975; **21**: 69.
19. Wilkinson KN. A damping system for under fives weighing scales. *Transactions of the Royal Society for Tropical Medicine and Hygiene*. 1982; **76** (1): 77–8.
20. Tremlett G, Lovel H, Morley D. Guidelines for the design of national weight-for-age growth charts. *Assignment Children*, No. 61/62, UNICEF, 1983.
21. Wit JM, Davies C, Moltof J. Introduction of a home and clinic-based growth chart in Dominica. *Tropical Doctor*. 1984; **14** (1): 34–40.
22. WHO. *A Growth Chart for International Use in Maternal and Child Health Care: Guidelines for Primary Health Care Personnel*. Geneva, WHO, 1978.

SHORT STATURE
Michael Parkin

Definition
Identification of patients with treatable disorders
  Differential diagnosis
  Strategy for identification

Reassurance of those with good prognosis
Practical help for those who cannot be treated
Further reading

Short stature may be a sign of disease but it also may be a disability or source of anxiety in itself. A doctor therefore has three responsibilities in relation to short children:

- to identify as early as possible those who may benefit from treatment;
- to give an informed prognosis in order to reassure those who do not need treatment;
- to help and give practical advice to those who will always be very short and who cannot be treated.

Definition

As there is no demarcation between normal and abnormal stature the definition of the short child is arbitrary. The usual rule is that any child whose height falls below the third centile for his community is considered to be short. The mean heights of children of most racial groups living in a satisfactory environment are remarkably similar and so internationally accepted growth charts such as those produced by Tanner in the

UK or the National Center for Health Statistics in USA, are suitable for most countries.

Identification of patients with treatable disorders

To identify patients with treatable disorders it is essential to be clear about the main causes of short stature.

Differential diagnosis

Genetic

There are two groups of genes, acquired from both parents, that affect the height of a child; those that determine final height and those that affect rate of growth.

Children who, for genetic reasons, will be short adults are likely to be short throughout childhood. They will otherwise be normal, their heights are unlikely to be far below the third centile and their growth velocity will be within the normal range. If investigated, their bone age will usually be within one year of their chronological age, while endocrine and other tests will be normal. Their predicted height, calculated on the basis of present height, age and bone age, will be within the expected range for their family. This expected range may be determined from 'target height' which is the mid-parental centile, the mid-point between the mother's and the father's height centiles. Under normal circumstances, 95 per cent of children will have a final height within 10 cm of this target height. This method of identifying genetically short children assumes that the parents are healthy and that, if short, they do not themselves have a pathological cause for growth failure.

Children who are late developers will also be short throughout childhood. They will otherwise be healthy but will have a rather slow growth velocity, particularly when other children are beginning their puberty growth spurt. They will have a delayed but otherwise normal puberty and reach a final height within the normal range for the family. Their bone ages will be significantly retarded but other investigations normal. Usually, there will be a history of similar delay in a close relative.

It is possible for a child to be both genetically short and genetically delayed. This combination may result in the child's height being well below the third centile, especially at the age when other children have begun their puberty growth spurt.

Low birth weight

Short children of low birth weight are an heterogeneous group, including some with a pathological cause of shortness beginning before birth, e.g. children with chromosomal abnormalities, congenital infection or some syndromes. However, others are basically normal babies whose intrauterine growth has been restrained because of some abnormality of the pregnancy. Such children, light for dates at birth, often will have an increased growth velocity and catch up to their appropriate centile by six months. However, if the intrauterine failure to thrive began early in pregnancy, i.e. before 34 weeks, growth may be impaired.

Nutrition

Restraint of growth is part of the adaptation of a child to an inadequate calorie intake, whatever the cause. Growth failure therefore is an invariable feature of chronic undernutrition and is evident in children with kwashiorkor and marasmus. In communities in which chronic undernutrition is common, a high proportion of young children are stunted, i.e. short in stature rather than wasted or thin. The reason for this is not fully understood but may be related to the hormonal response to undernutrition, which includes a low level of plasma somatomedin.

Under-nutrition may be caused by disease, particularly of the intestinal tract; the presence of such disease should be considered in short children with intestinal symptoms or other evidence of malabsorption.

Chronic disease

Any disease that affects the internal environment over a long period of time will impair growth. Short stature, therefore, is seen in children with cyanotic congenital heart disease, chronic renal failure, chronic respiratory disease and poorly controlled diabetes. However, it is not usual for a child with chronic systemic disease to present with growth failure; it is more commonly found incidentally in children who present with symptoms relevant to the condition. Nevertheless, chronic disease, including renal disease, sickle cell disease and chronic infections, including malaria and kala azar should be considered in any short child who is vaguely unwell or has other symptoms.

Bone dysplasias

There are many such conditions. The most severe are

evident at birth, while some cause growth failure only later in childhood. The basic underlying cause is known in only a few, such as the mucopolysaccharidoses and familial vitamin D-resistant rickets. All are inherited, those by autosomal recessive genes being relatively common in countries where cousin marriage is frequent. However, they have different modes of inheritance and it therefore is essential for a precise diagnosis to be made before genetic advice is offered. This involves at least a full radiological skeletal survey. There is no specific treatment for most of these conditions but very occasionally orthopaedic surgical intervention is necessary to correct gross limb deformities.

Syndromes

Short stature forms part of many dysmorphic syndromes, most of which are rare. However, some are recessively inherited and should be considered, especially in families in which there are consanguinous marriages (Table 3.2.4).

The most common syndrome is Turner's syndrome which occurs once in about 3000 girls and should be considered in any very short girl. Recognition before puberty will enable replacement oestrogen and progestogen to be offered at the appropriate age, i.e. when other girls are entering puberty. The heights of these girls may be increased slightly by treatment with low-dose oestrogen, anabolic steroids or growth hormone but the benefits do not yet seem enough to justify the wide use of such expensive or risky treatments.

Endocrine disorders

Cortisol excess Growth failure always occurs in children with Cushing's syndrome and therefore this diagnosis

Table 3.2.4 Syndromes involving short stature

Name	Clinical features			
	Mental retardation	Inheritance	Birth weight	Other
Aaskog syndrome	−	X-linked dominant	Normal	Hypertelorism and ptosis. Minor abnormalities of hands and genitalia
Bloom syndrome	−	Autosomal recessive	Low	Predominantly occurs in Jews. Facial telangiectasia. May develop malignant disease
Cockayne syndrome	+	Autosomal recessive	Normal	Onset of poor growth and development with tremor and unsteady gait, deafness and retinal abnormalities at about two years
De Lange syndrome	+	Usually sporadic	Low	Hirsutism. Beaked upper lip
Hallerman–Streiff syndrome	−	? Autosomal dominant	Normal	Cataracts. Hypoplasia of nose, jaws and teeth. Atrophy of skin
MMM syndrome	−	Autosomal recessive	Low	Similar to Russell–Silver but with small head and no asymmetry
Noonan syndrome	Mild	Usually sporadic but occasionally dominant	Low–normal	Pulmonary stenosis. Cryptorchidism. Webbed neck
Progeria syndrome	Mild	Usually sporadic	Low–normal	Alopecia, loss of subcutaneous fat, periarticular fibrosis, arteriosclerosis and premature death
Robinow syndrome	−	? Autosomal dominant	Normal	Macrocephaly. Hypertelorism. Short forearms and hypogonadism
Rubinstein–Taybi syndrome	+	Usually sporadic	Low–normal	Broad thumb and toes. Maxillary hypoplasia. Cryptorchidism
Russell–Silver syndrome	−	Sporadic	Low	Head circumference less stunted than height. Usually slim. Often asymmetry of limbs
Seckel syndrome (bird-headed dwarfs)	+	Autosomal recessive	Low	Microcephaly. Hypoplastic face and prominent nose. May be other skeletal abnormalities, e.g. scoliosis
Smith–Lemli–Opitz syndrome	+	Autosomal recessive	Low–normal	Hypogonadism, abnormal facies and brain defects

need be considered only in those fat children who also are short. Its effect on growth is the main contra-indication to prolong steroid therapy in childhood.

Thyroid deficiency Thyroxine is necessary for the normal growth of cartilage and bone and so short stature associated with marked delay in bone age occurs in children with hypothyroidism, both congenital or acquired. Hypothyroidism as a cause of growth failure is particularly common in areas of iodine deficiency and endemic goitre.

Growth hormone deficiency Children with severe growth hormone deficiency usually grow slowly from an early age, are plump and have an immature facial appearance. However, there are many common causes of growth hormone deficiency. It may be hereditary, idiopathic or associated with developmental abnormalities of the brain or pituitary, while acquired deficiency may follow cranial irradiation or head injury or result from tumours affecting the hypothalamus, e.g. craniopharyngioma, pinealoma or optic nerve glioma. Many children with these disorders will also have deficiency of other pituitary hormones, particularly the gonadotrophins. Some children, while producing growth hormone in response to pharmacological stimuli, may not produce normal amounts physiologically. This group, which has been given a number of labels, e.g. neuro-secretory dysfunction, normal variant short stature or physiological deficiency, may be difficult to distinguish from genetically short children with growth delay. However, at present, the role of growth hormone in this group of children is not certain and treatment should not be considered unless there is marked growth failure.

Deprivation

In all countries of the world the growth of children from poor families is less good than that of advantaged children. Although in many cases the predominant reason is nutritional deficiency, this is not the only explanation. In developed countries, in temperate regions, the food intake of poor children who are growing slowly has been shown on average to be greater than that of children from advantaged homes who are growing well. It is probable that the calorie requirements of some deprived children are increased, while emotional deprivation in itself may impair growth. Deprivation, nutritional, physical or emotional, undoubtedly is the most common cause of growth failure throughout the world.

Strategy for identification

Although only a small minority of short children will benefit from specific treatment, it clearly is important to identify these. In addition, poor growth may draw attention to many children who need special help to compensate for environmental disadvantage. A proposed strategy follows.

School entry assessment

All children should be measured at school entry and their heights compared with an appropriate standard on a centile chart. Although it may be optimal for growth failure to be identified before this age, it is not usually practical.

- Children whose heights are well below the third centile and those who are less short but who are unwell should be referred at that stage for paediatric assessment.
- Children who are short and in whom the cause seems environmental, should be given appropriate extra help in terms of food, stimulation or care and be reviewed.
- All children whose heights are under the tenth centile should be remeasured a year later and those who are growing slowly, i.e. less than 5 cm a year, should have a paediatric assessment.

Hospital assessment

The initial objective of hospital assessment is to identify those children with a pathological cause of growth failure and separate them from those with familial short stature or growth delay. To do this the main information needed is:

- as accurate an age of the child as possible;
- the heights of parents and, if possible, their ages at puberty;
- body proportions and, if abnormal, a radiological skeletal survey;
- weight for height;
- physical examination;
- bone age and skull X-ray;
- haemoglobin and haemoglobin electophoresis, i.e. sickle cell disease, thalassaemia;
- serum creatinine or urea;
- chromosomes or buccal smear for Barr bodies in girls;
- thyroid function tests.

Children who are very short but remain without a

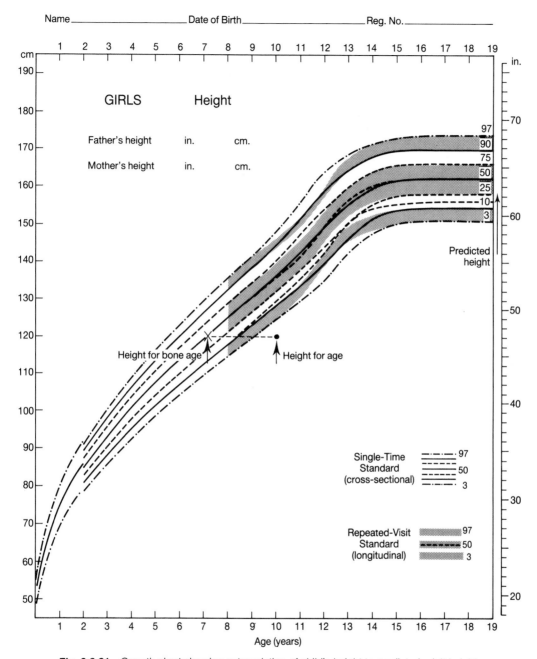

Fig. 3.2.21 Growth chart showing extrapolation of child's height to predicted adult height.

diagnosis after interpretation of this information, are likely to be those with delayed development or growth hormone deficiency. If they are growing slowly, further assessment should probably be made by a paediatrician with an interest in endocrinology and will include measurement of growth hormone levels after pharmacological or physiological stimuli.

This strategy should result in those children who need treatment or other intervention because of their growth failure, receiving it before the age of six or seven years.

Reassurance of those with good prognosis

The majority of short children will have a final adult height that is within the normal range without treatment, i.e. they have a good prognosis. It is clearly important to reassure anxious children and their parents about this. To do so involves making as accurate a prediction of final height as possible. This may be calculated by using the child's present height and age and bone age by the following methods:

- A Greulich–Pyle bone age estimation and the Bayley–Pinneau prediction tables.
- A Tanner–Whitehouse bone age with the prediction equation produced by Professor Tanner and his colleagues.
- Plotting the child's height for age and height for bone age on a growth chart and extrapolating to adult age the mid-point of the line joining these. Generally this is the most practical method and has the advantage of being easily understood by parents and even children (see Fig. 3.2.21).

None of these methods is completely accurate but any is good enough to enable informed reassurance to be given.

Practical help for those who cannot be treated

Children with bone dysplasias and some syndromes,

including Turner's syndrome, are likely always to be very short. Bone lengthening procedures are occasionally carried out but it is unlikely that these will ever be done commonly. Paediatricians, therefore, have a responsibility to try to give practical advice to these patients. If intellectually normal, they should be encouraged to go to ordinary schools and to look forward to employment. Interestingly, very short adults have more difficulty in getting a job than doing a job. They are likely to need help with clothing, with practical aspects of living at home and at school, and with mobility, and advice about future pregnancy. Most important of all, paediatricians should help all to remember that a person's worth is not related to his size but to the way he uses his talents, his love and his life.

Further reading

Bayley N, Pinneau SR. Tables for predicting adult height from skeletal age: revised for use with the Greulich–Pyle hand standards. *Journal of Pediatrics*. 1952; **40**: 423–41.

Brook CGD, Hindmarsh PC, Smith PJ, Stanhope R. Clinical features and investigation of growth hormone deficiency. *Clinics in Endocrinology and Metabolism*. 1986; **50**: 479–93.

Greulich WW, Pyle SI. *Radiographic Atlas of Skeletal Development of the Hand and Wrist*, 2nd Edn. Stanford University Press, 1959.

Parkin JM. The short child. In: Brook CGD ed. *Clinical Paediatric Endocrinology*. Oxford, Blackwell Scientific Publications, 1981; 113–33.

Preece MA, Law CM, Davies PSW. The growth of children with chronic paediatric disease. *Clinics in Endocrinology and Metabolism*. 1986; **15**: 453–77.

Smith DW. *Recognizable Patterns of Human Malformation*, 3rd Edn. Philadelphia, WB Saunders, 1982.

Tanner JM, Whitehouse RH. Clinical longitudinal standards for height, weight, height velocity, weight velocity and stages of puberty. *Archives of Disease in Childhood* 1976; **51**: 170–9.

Tanner JM, Whitehouse RH, Marshall WA *et al. Assessment of Skeletal Maturity and Prediction of Adult Height (TW2 Method)*. London, Academic Press, 1975.

Wynne-Davies R, Hall CM, Apley AG. *Atlas of Skeletal Dysplasias*. Edinburgh, Churchill Livingstone, 1985.

CHAPTER 3

Puberty and its disorders

Michael Parkin

Puberty refers to the physical changes of adolescence, the period of life between childhood and adulthood.

Endocrine basis of puberty

In fetal life the gonads are stimulated by placental hormones, and when the level of these fall after birth, the baby's own gonadotrophins are temporarily activated. During the first year gonadotrophin activity becomes relatively quiescent but even at this stage the gonads, at least in girls, are not completely inactive and cycles of follicular development of low amplitude and long periodicity occur. Between the ages of five and eight years in boys and girls there is an increase in adrenal androgen production and at this stage, for reasons as yet unclear, the hypothalamus begins to produce pulses of gonadotrophin-releasing hormone of increasing amplitude and frequency. This leads to a gradual increase in the blood levels of the gonado-trophins, luteinizing hormone (LH) and follicle stimulating hormone (FSH) which stimulate gonadal development. The physiological changes of puberty are dependent upon the resulting gonadal steroid hormones.

Physical changes of puberty

The first sign of puberty in boys is enlargement of the testes. The prepubertal testes are usually about 2 ml in volume and as a result of the stimulating effect of gonadotrophins they increase in size. As this growth of the testis consists mainly of development of the seminiferous tubules under FSH control rather than the testosterone-producing Leydig cells which are under LH control, there is not a close relationship between the size of the testes and the development of other signs of puberty. However, usually when the testes are 6–8 ml in volume increase in size of the penis, pubic hair development and the growth spurt begin.

In girls, the development of the ovaries is not evident clinically though it may sometimes be demonstrated through ultra-sound examination. The first clinical signs of female puberty, therefore, are in the target organs, enlargement of the breasts and pubic hair development. The growth spurt in girls, which is probably caused by low levels of oestrogens, begins two years earlier than in boys. The menarche usually does not occur until a late stage of puberty. The clinical signs of puberty in girls are caused by oestrogens and androgens, the latter derived by metabolism of adrenal and ovarian androsterone.

In clinical practice it is helpful to define the stages of development of the main manifestations of puberty, the criteria usually used being based on the scoring system of Tanner (see Tables 3.3.1–3.3.3).

Timing of puberty

The age of onset of puberty is variable and seems to be under both genetic and environmental control. In the

Table 3.3.1   Stages of development of the genitalia in boys

Stage 1	Preadolescent. Testes, scrotum and penis are about same size and shape as in early childhood
Stage 2	Scrotum slightly enlarged, with skin reddened and changed in texture. Little or no enlargement of penis at this stage
Stage 3	Penis slightly enlarged, at first mainly in length. Scrotum further enlarged than in Stage 2
Stage 4	Penis further enlarged, with growth in breadth and development of glans. Scrotum further enlarged than in Stage 3; scrotal skin darker than in earlier stages
Stage 5	Genitalia adult in size and shape

Table 3.3.2   Stages of pubic hair development for boys and girls

Stage 1	Preadolescent. The vellus over the pubes is not further developed than that over the abdominal wall, i.e. no pubic hair
Stage 2	Sparse growth of long, slightly pigmented downy hair, straight or slightly curled, chiefly at the base of the penis or along the labia
Stage 3	Considerably darker, coarser and more curled. The hair spreads sparsely over the junction of the pubes
Stage 4	Hair now adult in type but area covered is still considerably smaller than in the adult. No spread to the medial surface of thighs
Stage 5	Adult in quantity and type with distribution of the horizontal (or classically 'feminine') pattern. Spread to medial surface of thighs but not up linea alba or elsewhere above the base of the inverse triangle (spread up linea alba occurs late and is rated Stage 6)

Table 3.3.3   Stages of breast development

Stage 1	Preadolescent: elevation of papilla only
Stage 2	Breast bud stage: elevation of breast and papilla as small mound. Areola diameter enlarged over Stage 1
Stage 3	Breast and areola both enlarged and elevated more than in Stage 2 but with no separation of their contours
Stage 4	The areola and papilla form a secondary mound projecting above the contour of the breast
Stage 5	Mature stage: papilla only projects, with the areola recessed to the general contour of the breast

Table 3.2.1–3 from Tanner JM and Whitehouse RH, *Archives of Disease in Childhood*, 1976; **51**: 170–9.

UK, the first signs of puberty begin by age 11 years in 50 per cent of girls and by 11.5 years in 50 per cent of boys. However, as it is not easy to ascertain the first signs of puberty in large numbers of children, data on the age of puberty in most countries is based on the age of menarche. This is delayed by chronic undernutrition and amongst almost all populations, girls in well-off families reach the menarche earlier than those from disadvantaged families, while girls from an urban environment tend to mature earlier than those from rural areas (Fig. 3.3.1). The median age of menarche in different countries of the world is shown in Table 3.3.4.

Once puberty has begun, the sequence of changes varies little though the time taken for them to develop does. Fifty per cent of girls take four years to go through all the stages of puberty, while some take only 18 months and a few more than five years.

Table 3.3.4   Age of menarche in various populations.

Country	Year	Mean ± SE	
Australia (Sydney)	1970	13.0	
Canada (Montreal)	1969	13.1	± 0.04
Chile (Santiago – middle class)	1970	12.6	± 0.12
Cuba (Havana)	1973	12.8	
(Rural)	1973	13.3	
Egypt (Nubians)	1966	15.2	± 0.3
England (London)	1966	13.0	± 0.03
Finland	1969	13.2	± 0.02
Holland	1965	13.4	± 0.03
Hungary (West)	1965	13.1	± 0.01
India (Lucknow)	1967	14.5	± 0.17
Iraq (Baghdad – well-off)	1969	13.6	± 0.06
(Baghdad – poorly-off)	1969	14.0	± 0.05
Italy (Cararra)	1968	12.6	± 0.04
(Rural – near Naples)	1969	12.5	± 0.02
Japan	1966–7	12.9	± 0.01
Mexico (Xochimilco)	1966	12.8	± 0.18
New Guinea (Bundi – highlands)	1967	18.0	± 0.19
(Kaipit – lowlands)	1967	15.6	± 0.25
New Zealand (Maori)	1969	12.7	± 0.07
(non-Maori)	1969	13.0	± 0.02
Norway (Oslo)	1970	13.2	± 0.01
Poland (Warsaw)	1965	13.0	± 0.04
(Rural)	1967	14.0	± 0.02
Senegal (Dakar)	1970	14.6	± 0.08
Singapore (rich)	1968	12.4	± 0.09
(average)	1968	12.7	± 0.09
(poor)	1968	13.0	± 0.04
Turkey (Istanbul)	1967–9	12.36	± 0.01
USA (European origin)	1968	12.5	± 0.11
(African origin)	1968	12.8	± 0.04
USSR (Moscow)	1970	13.0	± 0.08

(From W. A. Marshall, *Human Growth*, 1978, Balliere Tindall, pp. 141–82.)

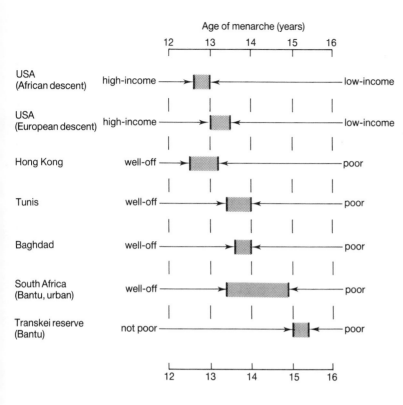

Fig. 3.3.1 Median ages of menarche in well-off and poor population samples. (From Eveleth PB and Tanner JM, *Worldwide Variation in Human Growth*, 1976 Cambridge University Press.)

Disorders of puberty

There are two broad disorders of puberty: failure of puberty to develop at the usual time, that is delayed puberty, and early development of puberty or some of its manifestations, that is precocious puberty or pseudo-puberty.

Delayed puberty

Any definition of delayed puberty is arbitrary and is affected by the usual age of puberty in the country concerned. Delayed puberty is a clinical problem when a child feels different from his or her peers. However, in most societies, if there are no signs of puberty by age 15 years in a girl or 16 in a boy, puberty should be considered to be delayed. There are three possible causes for this:

Genetic or constitutional delay

Twin studies have shown that the age of onset of puberty is under genetic control and so delay in puberty often affects several members of a family.

Impaired general health

Puberty is frequently delayed in chronically sick children, particularly those who are malnourished. The main reason for the secular trend towards earlier puberty in some developed countries is thought to have been improved nutrition and living conditions over the last century. Nutritional differences are probably the reason for the different mean ages of menarche in children from advantaged and disadvantaged groups within a country.

Children with delayed puberty for familial reasons or as a result of impaired nutrition will have endocrine test results, especially the luteinizing releasing hormone (LRH) test, which are characteristic of younger but normal children. Clinically they are usually short and on radiological examination have delayed bone age.

Specific endocrine disorders

Disorders of the hypothalamus, pituitary or gonads may lead to failure of puberty. Children with these disorders, with the exception of Turner's syndrome, are usually of normal stature for their age. Investigations to clarify the diagnosis include measurement of sex hormones before and after an injection of human chorionic gonadotrophin and estimation of gonadotrophins before and after LRH.

Precocious puberty

Evidence of secondary sexual characteristics before the age of eight years in a girl or nine in a boy is usually considered as precocious puberty.

True precocious puberty

True precocious puberty is when all the features of puberty (including the growth spurt) develop early and is more common in girls than in boys. It is occasionally caused by an intracranial tumour or other organic disorder such as the McCune Albright syndrome. However, usually there is no obvious cause, although a small anatomically insignificant hamartoma of the hypothalamus may be responsible.

The main disadvantage of precocious puberty is that final height is often stunted as a result of early epiphyseal closure. In addition, the appearance of maturity in a young child may cause psychological stress. Active treatment is usually unnecessary but if it is thought appropriate, the LRH analogue, Buserelin, given intranasally, is probably the most logical though very costly agent.

Pseudoprecocious puberty

Pseudoprecocious puberty means that only some signs of puberty develop early. In boys these may be androgen signs, e.g. pubic hair and penile development without enlargement of the testes. In girls, they may be isolated androgen signs, such as pubic and axillary hair, or oestrogen signs such as breast or labial development. If these signs are advancing rapidly, a pathological source of the relevant hormones must be considered, e.g. congenital adrenal hyperplasia or adrenal, testicular or ovarian tumours. However, the most common conditions, premature thelarche and premature pubarche are usually innocent and require no treatment.

Premature thelarche, the early development of breast tissue with no other sign of puberty, may be the first manifestation of early or true precocious puberty. In children under the age of two or three years, however, it is likely simply to indicate delay in the quiescent phase of gonadotrophin production and to disappear spontaneously. It has been suggested that it sometimes is the result of the ingestion of food containing drugs with oestrogen effects, resulting from these chemicals being fed to animals, but there is little evidence to support this.

Precocious pubarche, the early development of pubic hair, is usually associated with slightly advanced growth and bone age and an increased level of adrenal androgens in blood and urine. It is probably an exaggeration of normal prepubertal adrenal action.

Disorders of puberty may cause much anxiety to children and parents. Most are self-limiting and benign and the probable basic abnormality can often be deduced from the clinical picture. However, full investigation, which requires sophisticated laboratory facilities, is indicated in the occasional child with marked delay or rapid development of signs of puberty.

Further reading

Normal puberty

Brook CGD. Endocrinological control of growth at puberty. *British Medical Bulletin.* 1981; **37**: 281–6.

Brook CGD. Puberty. In: *Growth Assessment in Childhood and Adolescence.* Oxford, Blackwell Scientific, 1982.

Brook CGD, Stanhope R, Hindmarsh P, Adams J. The control of the onset of puberty. *Acta Endocrinologica Suppl. 279.* 1986; **113**: 202–6.

Eveleth PB, Tanner JM. *Worldwide Variation in Human Growth.* Cambridge, Cambridge University Press, 1976. pp. 213–9.

Marshall WA. Puberty. In: Falkner F, Tanner JM eds. *Human Growth*, Vol. 2. London, Bailliere Tindall, 1978. pp. 141–82.

Marshall WA. Normal puberty. In: Brook CGD ed. *Clinical Paediatric Endocrinology.* Oxford, Blackwell Scientific, 1981. pp. 193–206.

Marshall WA, Tanner JM. Variation in pattern of pubertal change in girls. *Archives of Disease in Childhood.* 1969; **44**: 291–303.

Marshall WA, Tanner JM. Variation in pattern of pubertal change in boys. *Archives of Disease in Childhood.* 1970; **45**: 13–23.

Tanner JM. Endocrinology of puberty. In: Brook CGD ed. *Clinical Paediatric Endocrinology.* Oxford, Blackwell Scientific, 1981. pp. 207–23.

Disorders of puberty

Brook, CGD. Early puberty and late puberty. In: *Growth Assessment in Childhood and Adolescence.* Oxford, Blackwell Scientific, 1982.

Chaussain, JL. Late puberty. In: Brook CGD ed. *Clinical Paediatric Endocrinology*. Oxford, Blackwell Scientific, 1981. pp. 240-7.

Lancet (Leading Article). Precocious development in Puerto Rican children. *Lancet*. 1986; **i**: 721-2.

Pasquino AM, Tebaldi L, Cioschi L, *et al*. Premature thelarche: a follow-up study of 40 girls. *Archives of Disease in Childhood*. 1985; **60**: 1180-2.

Pescovitz OH, Comite F, Hench K, *et al*. The NIH experience with precocious puberty. *Journal of Pediatrics*. 1986; **108**: 47-54.

Rayner PHW. Early puberty. In: Brook, CGD ed. *Clinical Paediatric Endocrinology*. Oxford, Blackwell Scientific, 1981. pp. 224-39.

CHAPTER 4

Development

CHILD DEVELOPMENT
P. Morrell

The normal pattern of development

Pathways of development

The development of the infant and young child proceeds along various interrelated pathways in a relatively predictable fashion (see Table 3.4.1). It is convenient to look at these pathways separately for the purpose of clarity although it is recognized that none occurs in isolation. These pathways can be defined as follows.

Gross motor development

The development of posture and independent mobility is usually observed in three positions (Figs 3.4.1–3.4.10):

- Ventral suspension – the child is held under the abdomen and the position of the head and limbs observed in relation to the trunk.
- Prone position – the child is laid on the abdomen and the ability to lift the head and eventually the body on to hands and knees observed.
- Upright posture – this progresses from observing head control when the baby is sitting, to sitting alone and thence to standing, walking and running.

Manipulation

The ability of the child to reach for, grasp and manipulate objects, follows the loss of the primitive grasp reflex and becomes more sophisticated through infancy and childhood (Fig. 3.4.11). As with gross motor function, the sequence of fine motor development does not vary.

Comprehension and social skills

This area is the most difficult to define and to examine. Various milestones can be described such as the social smile, watching a mirror and waving goodbye, but the experience of the examiner in observing the baby's general alertness and curiosity about her surroundings is probably a better guide.

Age (months)	Ventral suspension	Prone position	Upright position
0			
3			
4			
6			
7			
9			
13			

Fig. 3.4.1 Sequence of gross motor development.

Language

The development of speech is probably the most variable of all the aspects of development and is closely linked with general understanding. The newborn baby can already imitate some of the mother's sounds and gradually develops vowel sounds over the first few months, consonants by six months and the first words with meaning by about one year. Over the next two or three years the child begins putting words into phrases and then into sentences with increasing intelligibility.

General principles

The work of such pioneers as Arnold Gesell[1] has elucidated certain principles that may be stated as follows:

- The sequence of each pathway of development does not vary, although the rate of development is variable. Thus, a child must sit before standing and walking, even though the age at which the child walks varies from 8 to 18 months in the normal population.
- The rate of development along different pathways is variable. Thus, a child may be precocious in motor development but delayed in language development.

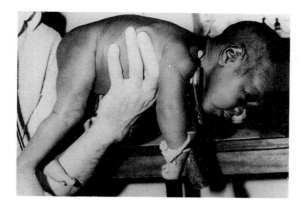

Fig. 3.4.2 Ventral suspension: neonate.

- Infant development is dependent upon neurological maturation. A skill cannot be achieved until there is maturation of all the neuromuscular components involved.
- Generalized mass activity is replaced by individual responses. Thus, the general agitation of the neonate presented with a toy is replaced by the fine index finger approach at the end of the first year.
- Motor development proceeds in a cephalo-caudal direction. Thus, head control develops before truncal control which precedes upright posture.
- Some primitive reflexes must be lost before voluntary movement occurs, e.g. the primitive grasp reflex must disappear before a voluntary grasp can develop.

Variations in the normal pattern of development

Whilst obeying the general principles of development, a child may exhibit certain variations which must be appreciated to avoid labelling a normal child as deviant.

These variations have been well described in gross motor development where it is seen that some children attain mobility in different ways. The most common variant is that of the bottom shuffler, when the child is able to shuffle around the floor on its bottom, often very rapidly. Children with this variant of development rarely crawl before they walk and walk later than average, usually at about 18 months but sometimes not until 28 months. It is interesting that this form of progression seems to have a familial tendency.

Table 3.4.1 The major points of development along various pathways of development at certain key ages

	6 weeks	3 months	6 months	9 months
Gross motor	Pull-to-sit: head lags behind body Held sitting: holds head erect momentarily Prone: head turned to side Ventral suspension: head held in line seconds	Pull-to-sit: minimal head lag Held sitting: head steady, back straight Prone: lifts head on forearms Ventral suspension: head above line of body, hips and shoulders extend	Pull-to-sit: arms up to be lifted Held sitting: sits erect few seconds Prone: lifts head and chest on hands, rolls prone to supine	Sits steadily with forward lateral and backward protective reflexes Starts to crawl on stomach or hands and knees Starts to stand holding on to furniture
Fine motor	Still shows grasp reflex	Holds object placed in hand few seconds	Palmar grasp of object Mouthing objects May transfer objects Drops first object for second	Grasps small objects between thumb and 2nd and 3rd finger Index finger approach to objects Holds objects in both hands
Vision	Follows object 23 cm from face to midline Turns to light	Follows through 180° Hand regard Defensive blink		Visually very attentive Watches dropped objects
Communication and comprehension	Activity lessens to spoken voice Smiles to friendly face Startles to loud sound	Longer vowel sounds in response to mother (coos) Quietens to soft bell May search for sound source Recognizes breast or bottle Pleasure at bathing and handling	Vowels and consonants – da, ma, ba Laughs Stretches arms to be lifted Smiles at mirror image	Two syllable consonant sounds – baba, mama, dada Imitates sounds Recognizes strangers Chews food – holds and eats biscuit Enjoys interactive games Locates sounds accurately Shouts to attract attention Understands 'no' Holds bell and rings it

12 months	15 months	18 months	2 years	3 years	4 years
Crawls on hands and knees Walks around furniture May take 1–2 steps alone May crawl upstairs	Walks several steps alone with legs apart and arms raised Often falls Creeps upstairs	Walks steadily with arms down; starts to run Kneels on floor Walks upstairs with help, creeps back downstairs Climbs on to chair	Runs steadily Walks backwards Stoops to pick object from floor Walks upstairs holding rail	Up stairs one foot per step Down stairs 2 feet per step Jumps off step Stands on one foot for few seconds	Down stairs one foot per step Skips on one foot Climbs trees
Neat pincer grip of small object (finger and thumb) Mouthing stops Grasps two cubes in one hand	Casts objects to ground wanting them to be retrieved Builds 2-block tower Puts bricks into container Holds pencil with palmar grasp – to and fro scribble Helps turn pages of book Throws ball overhand	Builds tower of 3–4 bricks Turns few pages of book	Builds tower of 6 or 7 bricks Makes train of 2 or more bricks Unscrews lids of jars Holds pencil between thumb and 2 fingers Imitates vertical and circular scribble Hand laterality established Turns pages singly Throws ball well	Builds tower of 8 or 9 bricks Copies circle, imitates cross, draws simple man Cuts with scissors May do buttons	Copies gate of bricks Copies cross, draws man (head, face, trunk, may include arms and legs)
First words with meaning Jargons persistently Understands few single words and simple commands 'give it to mummy' Looks at books Begins to show interest in pictures Points to desired object Claps bricks together Knows own name Holds spoon but not yet able to use it Plays 'pat-a-cake' and waves 'bye-bye'	3–6 words with meaning Understands many single words Points to needs Follows simple commands Drinks from cup Using spoon to feed Helps with dressing	5 to 20 words A lot of jargon Responds to simple commands Identifies pictures by pointing Knows 1 or 2 body parts Takes off shoes and socks Starting to indicate toilet needs Enjoys nursery rhymes	Over 50 clear words Starting to use 2–3 word phrases Starts to use pronouns Identifies pictures Knows 3–4 body parts Obeys complex commands Takes off most clothes Tries to put on shoes and socks Indicates toilet needs May be dry by day Feeds well with spoon and cup Demands mother's attention Tantrums if frustrated	Normal speech Asks questions Repeats 3 digits Understands numbers Follows prepositions (under, behind, upon) Knows colours Gives full name, age and sex Plays with other children	Listens to and tells stories Counts up to 10 More independent Has sense of humour Dramatic play

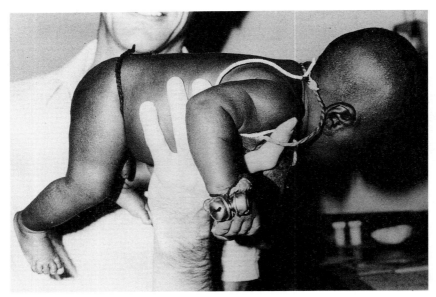

Fig. 3.4.3 Ventral suspension: two to three months.

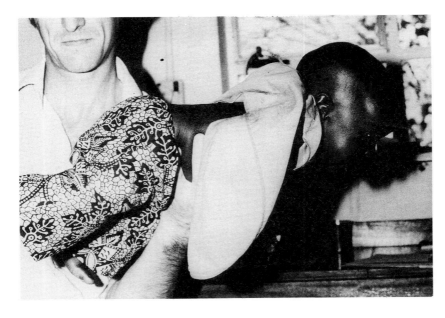

Fig. 3.4.4 Ventral suspension: over four months.

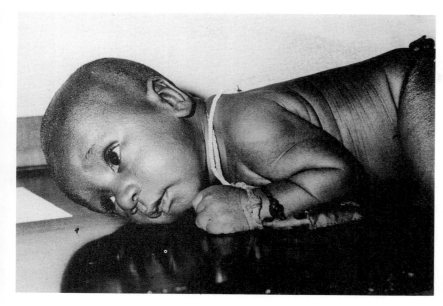

Fig. 3.4.5 Prone position: neonate.

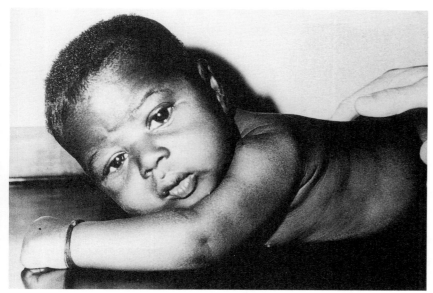

Fig. 3.4.6 Prone position: two months.

Influences on development

Nutrition

The classic studies of Dobbing[2] show a period of rapid brain growth in man from about 10 weeks post-conception to about two years postnatal life (Fig. 3.4.12). This work has led to the 'vulnerable period' hypothesis, which postulates that during this period the brain is susceptible to various insults including nutritional deprivation. There is a vast literature devoted to the effect of malnutrition upon neurological development. Studies have looked at the

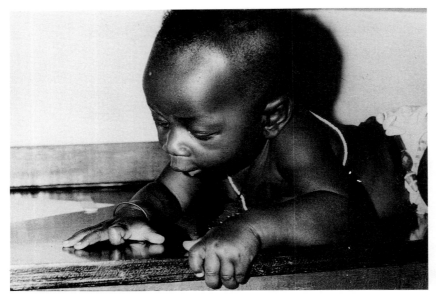

Fig. 3.4.7   Prone position: three to four months.

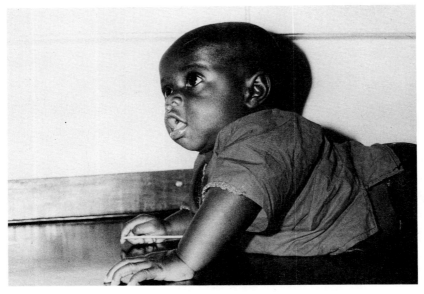

Fig. 3.4.8   Prone position: six months.

pathology of the brain in malnourished animals and humans, the growth of the brain inferred from head growth in malnourished children, and the neurological development of children under conditions of severe or moderate malnutrition. There are, however, many methodological problems in all these studies.

Pathological studies are usually limited by small numbers of subjects. Nevertheless, most of these have shown some adverse effect in terms of reduction in brain size, total cell number, disturbance in brain cell architecture and neuronal myelination.

An alternative approach has been to look at the effect

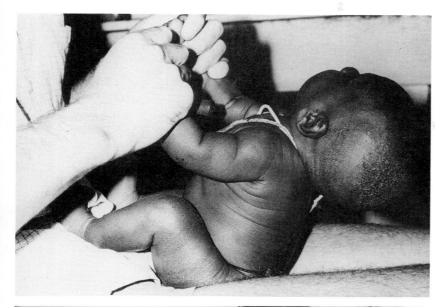

Fig. 3.4.9   Pull-to-sit: neonate.

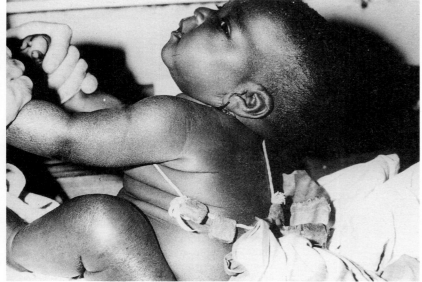

Fig. 3.4.10   Pull-to-sit: three months.

of prenatal malnutrition upon future development. At birth these babies fall below the tenth percentile birth weight for gestational age, corrected for any racial differences. Babies in this group are at particular risk of brain damage due to hypoglycaemia, asphyxia and polycythaemia occurring soon after birth. Congenital malformations, infections *in utero* such as rubella and maternal drugs such as alcohol, may cause abnormal brain development and also result in intrauterine growth retardation. If such babies are excluded, there remains a group who are small primarily because of poor placental function. When this occurs late in

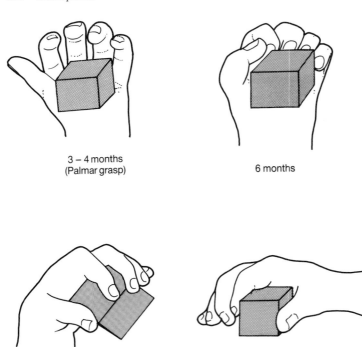

3 – 4 months
(Palmar grasp)

6 months

8 months

10 – 12 months
(Pincer grasp)

Fig. 3.4.11   The development of manipulation.

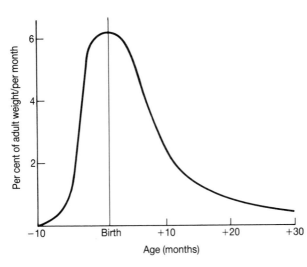

Fig. 3.4.12   Human brain growth spurt expressed as velocity curve of increase in weight with age. (Reproduced with permission of Elsevier Scientific Publishers Ireland, from Dobbing J and Sands J, *Early Human Development*; 1979; **3**: 79–83.)

gestation then there are probably no major adverse effects on brain development. However, if growth retardation occurs before 26 weeks then affected babies show significant differences in test scores at five years.

Clinical studies that measure the developmental progress of malnourished children are fraught with problems and most are subject to criticism. Many rely on developmental tests that have not been validated for that population and provide a 'developmental quotient' that is often meaningless in that context. This may be acceptable if comparisons are made within the population but, nevertheless, most tests used measure abilities that are as much a function of rearing practices as of neurological maturation. Very few published surveys take account of such important variables as perinatal events, gestation and intercurrent infections. Only recently has the effect of mothering skills and stimulation been acknowledged as having a central role upon development, while other factors such as genetic potential and recurrent or chronic illness also play an important part.

Examination of evidence from these studies indicates the following:

- Severe protein–energy malnutrition in infancy combined with an environment providing little stimulation probably results in permanent intellectual harm.
- The adverse intellectual consequences of severe malnutrition may be modified by a stimulating environment if this is introduced before three years of age.
- If improved nutrition and better stimulation are given to a group of children at risk, then the intellectual outcome of these children is significantly improved. This improvement is related to the age of the child, the younger infants showing the greatest effect.

Environment

There is little doubt that the environment plays a major part in the development of the infant, although the permanence of this effect is more controversial. Studies of children raised in institutions with little or no stimulation, e.g. 'The Creche' in Beirut, show marked retardation in development which appears to catch up when they are placed in a normal environment.[3] However, it seems that severe deprivation for longer than three years may have permanent effects, particularly in intellectual, language and personality development.

Culture and race

The French worker, Geber first suggested that the African Negro infant displayed precocious gross motor development.[4] Many workers have since agreed that African babies seem to sit, crawl and walk earlier than Western Caucasian babies.[5] These differences also persist in American Negro infants compared with their Caucasian counterparts. Some people, however, argue that these classical studies depend on data which has not been rigorously formulated and that the apparent motor advancement can be explained by other factors. A study of Ugandan babies showed that their mothers employed specific training techniques and developed an expectation that the infant would achieve a milestone at a particular time.[5]

It seems likely that the gross motor precocity, if present, is most marked in the first six months and declines thereafter, although it may never disappear. It has also been shown, somewhat surprisingly, that infants from poorer homes develop motor skills more rapidly than those from a more advantageous environment.[6]

Other aspects of development have been studied and language development also has been described as

Table 3.4.2 Comparison of development in Gambian, other African and European infants

Developmental milestone	Age milestone reached (months)		
	Gambian infants	Other African studies	European infants
Sitting	5	5	8–9
Crawling	8	6	9–10
Standing with support	9	6	8–9
Walking	14	10	13
Mature grasp	7–8	9	9–10
Speech (3 words)	12–15	10–11	10–12

(Reproduced with permission from Illingworth RS. *The Development of the Infant and Young Child: Normal and Abnormal*, Churchill Livingstone, 1975.)

occurring earlier in African infants.

Table 3.4.2 shows the mean age of attainment of various milestones of a group of Gambian infants (personal data) compared with a composite estimate from other African studies and an accepted European standard.[7] It must be remembered that great variability exists between different populations even of similar race and often between subpopulations such as children from adjacent villages in the same country. The data in Table 3.4.2 confirm the early precocity of African infants.

Gestational age at birth

The infant born before term differs in development both qualitatively and quantitatively from the term baby. Notwithstanding the fact that preterm birth may put the baby at increased risk of brain damage, the gestation of the baby must always be allowed for when observing a baby's development.

It is unclear how far one should adjust the chronological age when assessing a preterm baby. Some authors have suggested that the child should be assessed as reaching term only at the expected date of delivery, e.g. a 32-week gestation baby will be expected to sit at a chronological age of 10 months compared with 8 months in a full-term baby. Other workers, however, have suggested that the preterm baby catches up to a certain extent and it may be more sensible to assess the development as midway between the chronological age and the estimated post-term age.

Gross motor development may be unusual in that the preterm infant may show an unusual form of muscular development with hypertonus and brisk reflexes together with an odd upright posture reminiscent of early spastic diplegia. Such infants eventually may turn out to be perfectly normal, so this transient dystonia should be recognized and the parents reassured.

Genetic factors

To accept that inheritance plays a part in the development of the child implies that a child has an innate 'intelligence' and this is sometimes disputed. Various authors have studied the effect of different rearing patterns on the abilities of twins, the development of infants placed in foster homes compared with the intelligence of their parents and the abilities of infants of parents known to be mentally handicapped. Obviously other factors such as metabolic defects and chromosomal anomalies must be excluded before conclusions are reached. It is also important to realize that, in general, parents of greater intelligence provide more opportunities for intellectual stimulation for their children. Taking these factors into account, it seems that the intelligence of the parents does play a small but significant role, even when allowance is made for differences in stimulation.

Other factors

Chronic illnesses, such as tuberculosis and cyanotic heart disease, are associated with delayed development, although this may not be permanent and may improve when the child recovers. Many factors play a part, such as undernutrition and prolonged periods in hospital, during which the child may be denied the advantage of play.

The place of the child in the family is significant with, on average, first-born infants developing faster and subsequent children achieving progressively less irrespective of social class. It is also recognized that girls generally develop faster than boys, although their eventual ability is probably similar.

Examination

Gestational assessment

The clinical assessment of gestational age is important in assisting management of the infant as well as for epidemiological purposes. Clinical assessment must be used in conjunction with and as confirmation of the obstetric assessment of gestation.

The assessment of gestation may be made by applying scores to various physical and neurological signs which change in character as the baby matures (e.g. Dubowitz and Goldberg[8]). Thus, the hypotonia of the preterm baby may be assessed by various techniques, e.g. the scarf sign, the heel to ear test. The predominant extensor tone of the preterm baby can be demonstrated by the square window sign. The physical characteristics examined include the skin colour and thickness, the size of the breast nodule, the flexibility of the ear and the appearance of the genitals. A simple and rapid method of clinically assessing gestation has been described by Parkin using just four physical characteristics to derive a score which is accurate to within two weeks.[9] This may be combined with the neurological criteria described by Robinson for greater accuracy[10] (Fig. 3.4.13).

These methods have been standardized on British babies and certain characteristics such as skin colour and lanugo hair are obviously difficult to compare in African or Asian babies.[11] It has been suggested, however, that these objections may be overcome if the baby is examined very soon after birth before skin pigmentation has developed.

The primitive responses

'It is as if Nature had put them there so that we could test if the circuits are properly laid and expect that things would work satisfactorily when the current is switched on' (Mary Sheridan).

The immature brain displays certain reflexes that disappear as the central nervous system matures but provide a valuable insight on the integrity of neural function. Some of the important ones are described below. Persistence of primitive responses for longer than usual may indicate cerebral dysfunction.

Moro reflex

This is stimulated by sudden extension of the neck usually performed by holding the baby supported in one hand and allowing the head to drop back a short distance. The baby responds by abduction and extension of both arms with opening of both hands followed by the arms coming together in an embrace and the hands closing. This reflex is present at birth and disappears by three months. An abnormal response, such as extreme sensitivity or sluggishness of response, may indicate a cerebral lesion. Asymmetry of response may indicate paralysis of the affected arm due to nerve damage to the brachial plexus or to a fractured humerus (see Figs 3.4.14 and 3.4.15).

Grasp reflex

An object, usually a finger, is placed into the palm from the ulnar side. The baby responds by grasping the object. When the baby's hand is raised the baby responds by flexing the muscles of the forearm so that it can be lifted from the cot. A similar response, the

This simple scoring system can be performed even in an ill baby without manipulation or movement at *any* time in the first two days of life; more complex techniques only marginally improve the accuracy (J. M. Parkin *et al.*, 1976, *Arch. Dis. Child.*, **51**, 259–263). It is permissible to award 'half' scores where a characteristic appears to fall between the scored definitions. The technique is accurate to within ± 15 days in 95 per cent of babies when the score is more than 2. In very immature babies repeated examination at about weekly intervals in order to determine the age at which some critical primitive reflexes appear will eventually enable a more accurate assessment to be made of gestational age at birth (R. J. Robinson, 1966, *Arch. Dis. Child.*, **41**, 437–447).

Mean gestational ages derived from total scores of skin colour, skin texture, breast size and ear firmness

Score	Gestational Age (d)	(w)
1	190	27
2	210	30
3	230	33
4	240	34½
5	250	36
6	260	37
7	270	38½
8	276	39½
9	281	40
10	285	41
11	290	41½
12	295	42

Appearance of certain critical primitive reflexes

Criterion	Gestation in weeks if:− Present	Absent
Pupil reaction* to light (using pen torch)	>29	<31
Eyelids blink when glabella is tapped. (A generalized grimace does not count)	>32	<34
Neck and/or elbows flex when baby is pulled up by the wrists from prone	>33	<36

* The reaction of the pupils is not easy to see in very small babies, and this test should only be attempted gently and briefly on a healthy thriving baby by an experienced person.

Definitions

SKIN COLOUR   Estimated by inspection when the baby is quiet.
0 dark red
1 uniformly pink
2 pale pink, though the colour may vary over different parts of the body, some parts may be very pale
3 pale; nowhere really pink except on the ears, lips, palms and soles

SKIN TEXTURE   Tested by picking up a fold of abdominal skin between finger and thumb, and by inspection.
0 very thin with a gelatinous feel
1 thin and smooth
2 smooth and of medium thickness; irritation rash and superficial peeling may be present
3 slight thickening and stiff feeling with superficial cracking and peeling especially evident on the hands and feet
4 thick and parchment-like with superficial or deep cracking

BREAST SIZE   Measured by picking up the breast tissue between finger and thumb.
0 no breast tissue palpable
1 breast tissue palpable on one or both sides, neither being more than 0.5 cm diameter
2 breast tissue palpable on both sides, one or both being 0.5–1 cm in diameter
3 breast tissue palpable on both sides, one or both being more than 1 cm in diameter

EAR FIRMNESS   Tested by palpation and folding of the upper pinna.
0 pinna feels soft and is easily folded into bizarre positions without springing back into position spontaneously
1 pinna feels soft along the edge and is easily folded but returns slowly to the correct position spontaneously
2 cartilage can be felt to the edge of the pinna though it is thin in places and the pinna springs back readily after being folded.
3 pinna firm with definite cartilage extending to the periphery, and springs back immediately into position after being folded.

Fig. 3.4.13   Assessment of gestational age by external characteristics at 0–48 hours.

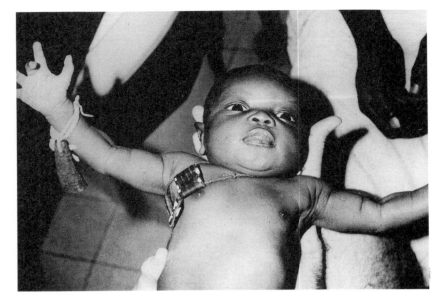

Fig. 3.4.14 The Moro reflex: stage one.

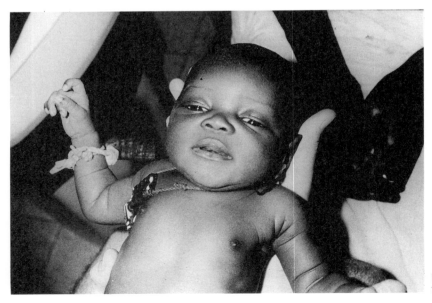

Fig. 3.4.15 The Moro reflex: stage two.

plantar grasp, can also be elicited by stimulating the sole of the foot, which causes flexion of the toes. The palmar grasp is present at birth and disappears by two to three months before the development of voluntary grasping.

Rooting reflex

The corner of the mouth is stimulated by gentle stroking with the finger. The baby responds by opening the mouth, turning the head towards the stroked side and protruding the tongue towards that side. This reflex is present at birth and disappears over the first few months.

Sucking reflex

A finger is placed into the baby's mouth and the hard palate gently stroked. The baby responds by closing the mouth and making sucking movements with the tongue. This reflex is present at birth and never really disappears but becomes submerged in voluntary sucking.

Stepping reflex

The baby is held upright so that the soles of the feet touch a hard surface. When tilted forwards the baby takes alternate stepping movements with the legs. This reflex is present at birth and disappears by three months (see Figs 3.4.16 and 3.4.17).

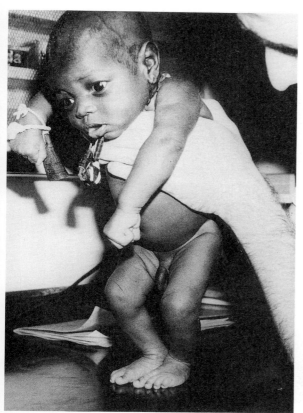

Fig. 3.4.16 The stepping reflex: stage one.

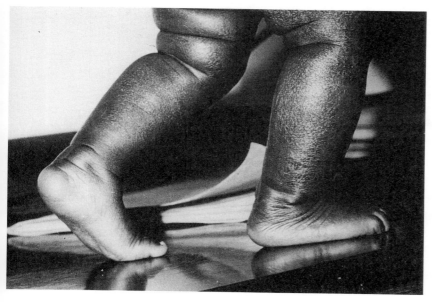

Fig. 3.4.17 The stepping reflex: stage two.

Placing reflex

The baby is held upright with the dorsum of the foot touching the edge of a table and responds by lifting the leg up on to the surface of the table. This reflex is present at birth and probably does not disappear but becomes submerged in voluntary action at about nine months (see Figs 3.4.18 and 3.4.19).

Asymmetric tonic neck reflex

With the baby lying flat the head is rotated to the side. The baby responds by extending the arm and flexing the leg on the side towards which the head is turned and flexing the arm and extending the leg of the other side. This reflex usually appears after birth, often not until two months of age and seems to prepare the baby for

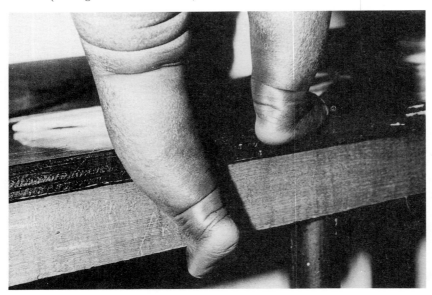

Fig. 3.4.18 The placing reflex: stage one.

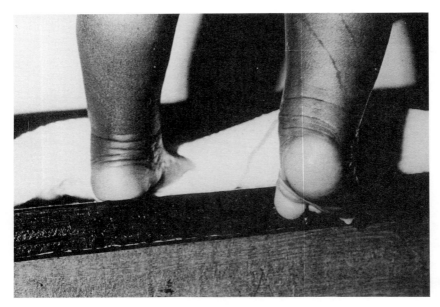

Fig. 3.4.19 The placing reflex: stage two.

visually directed reaching. It disappears at around four months but persistence of this reflex is found in infants developing cerebral palsy.

Landau response

The baby is held in a position of ventral suspension with a hand under the abdomen. At about four months the head lifts and the limbs flex. A positive response indicates neurological integrity.

The protective responses

To maintain a stable sitting position the baby must develop the ability to support itself with its arms if it falls forwards, sideways or backwards. The forward and lateral protective responses develop at about six to seven months and the backward responses at about nine months (see Fig. 3.4.20).

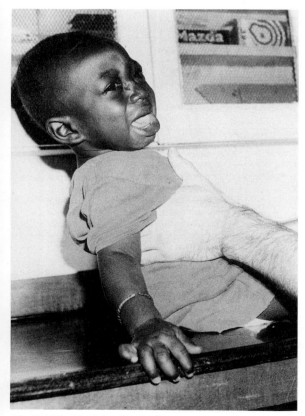

Fig. 3.4.20 The lateral protective response.

Parachute response

The baby is lifted under the arms and then tilted head down as though the examiner is going to throw it to the ground. At about nine months the baby will outstretch its hands towards the ground as though to protect from a fall.

Examination of muscle tone

Assessment of muscle tone is a valuable guide to the neurological integrity and maturity of the baby. This may be examined in three basic positions:

- Pull-to-sit. The baby is grasped by the forearms whilst lying supine and pulled to a sitting position. The attitude of the head in relation to the trunk is observed. The normal full-term infant will hold the head in line with the trunk for a few seconds although it may then droop. If the head lags behind the trunk this may indicate neurological depression or prematurity.
- Ventral suspension. The baby is suspended by a hand of the examiner beneath the abdomen and the position of the head and limbs assessed. The normal full-term infant will hold the head in line with the trunk with the limbs partially flexed. Marked drooping of the head and limbs indicates central nervous system depression or prematurity (Fig. 3.4.21).
- Prone position. The baby is placed face down on a firm surface. A normal full-term baby will lift the head to one side. The body remains flat on the surface.

Several workers have described various standardized techniques for the neurological examination of the newborn, the most valuable of which are probably those of Prechtl[12], Brazelton[13] and Dubowitz and Dubowitz.[14]

Developmental screening

This may be defined as an examination to identify those children who are failing to achieve developmental milestones for various reasons. It should be appreciated that children with developmental delay may catch up and therefore failure of a screening test does not necessarily indicate abnormality. This is different from normal children identified by the screening test as false positives.

When formulating a screening test it is valuable to use initial, median and limit ages. The initial age is the age at which a few children first show that particular

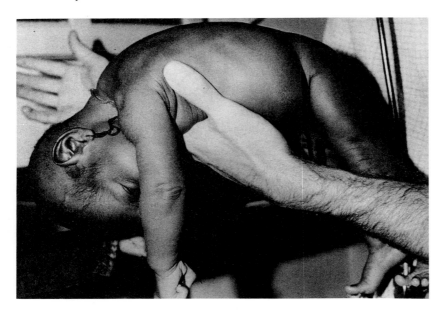

Fig. 3.4.21   Hypotonia in ventral suspension.

ability. The median age is when half the children show that ability and the limit age when most children show the ability. The initial age is used when assessing handicapped children: if they can perform that ability they may be considered to have reached at least that developmental age. The limit age provides a useful guide when screening a population of those children who need to be referred for more detailed assessment; if the milestone abilities are not reached by the stated ages then further investigations are indicated (Table 3.4.3).

If screening enables handicapped children to be identified then there should also be a mechanism for further management. There is little evidence that early diagnosis of physical or mental handicaps affects final outcome, although early physiotherapy may enable children with cerebral palsy to make the best use of unaffected muscles. It is logical also to assume that early education of children with mental handicap may be of some benefit. Early diagnosis of a developmental problem enables the best support to be given to a family in terms of an explanation of the diagnosis, a prognosis for the future and genetic counselling.

A screening test for developmental delay should be rapid and simple to apply. There must be little observer-to-observer variability, the tests used should not be affected greatly by the child's mood and should be able to be performed with as little special equipment as possible and in any environment. An ideal test would have 100 per cent sensitivity (sensitivity is the ability of a test to identify correctly those who have the disorder)

Table 3.4.3   Limit ages for various milestones

Age (months)	Milestone
2	Attention to objects
3	No head lag when pulled to sitting position
5	Reaches out for objects
6	Asymmetric tonic neck reflex disappeared
10	Sits steadily
	Bears weight on legs when held standing (unless bottom shuffler)
	Chews lumpy food
18	Walks independently
	Has stopped casting or mouthing objects
20	Says single words with meaning
28	Puts 2 or 3 words together to make phrases
36	Talks in sentences

and 100 per cent specificity (specificity is the ability of a test to identify correctly those who do not have the disorder). However, in practice, often an improvement in one of these is associated with a deterioration in the other.

The predictive value of a screening test of any condition depends upon its prevalence. With a rare condition, even a test with high specificity gives rise to a large number of false positives because of the high number of normals. It is not surprising, therefore, that studies of the predictive value of screening for developmental delay show that they are very good at predicting normal children but poor at identifying abnormalities. A failed screening test often only confirms parental suspicions, while those at greatest risk of developmental problems are least likely to attend clinics and to have parents least likely to express concern.

One of the most widely used screening tests is the Denver Developmental Screening Test (Fig. 3.4.22a) first validated in Denver by Frankenburg and Dodds.[15] Since then it has been used extensively in many countries. With training, this test may be used satisfactorily by a wide range of health personnel with a minimum of equipment and cost. It is important that its use in different cultures should follow careful standardization for that country. This has already been accomplished in several countries.[16] A screening test used by the Forth Valley health board enables a progressive graphic display of a child's development which can indicate faltering or catch-up growth similar to a growth chart (Fig. 3.4.22b).

Developmental assessment

Developmental screening tests identify children with developmental delay who require further examination. Developmental assessment involves an expert opinion which may provide a diagnosis of normality or confirm abnormality. There are many facets to assessing a child's abilities which are difficult for one person to provide. A paediatrician with training in developmental medicine and child neurology has probably the widest experience and is able to coordinate the assessment and provide the parents with a diagnosis and discussion of future plans. Other specialists examine a particular aspect of the child's development and may include a child psychologist (educational or clinical) who can administer appropriate psychological tests, a physiotherapist to assess muscular development and a speech therapist to assess language development.

The assessment will usually consist of a detailed history, including the pregnancy and birth: e.g. gestational age, asphyxia, jaundice, convulsions. There will usually be an assessment of the child's development using a diagnostic, as opposed to screening, test such as the Griffiths[17,18] or Bayley scales.[19] It must be remembered that this provides a measurement of development at that moment and makes no allowance for any later catch up. Much has been written about the predictive value of such tests and many feel that these tests have little to offer in terms of future attainment. There is some evidence that the predictive value of infant intelligence tests is better for children with mental handicap than for children of higher intelligence.

Much of the physical examination is performed by observation of the child at play. Gross motor abilities can be judged as the child walks from toy to toy and any abnormalities of gait observed. The ability of the child to climb steps and jump can be observed with the aid of a small wooden slide. Attention should be centred upon the ability to stoop to the ground and recover, which may reveal proximal muscle weakness of muscular dystrophy (the child 'climbs' up its legs to stand – Gowers sign).

The child's manipulative ability should be assessed by observing the way it handles toys when the maturity of grasp is witnessed. A child with mild cerebral palsy maintains a very clumsy grasp using the palm as support, rather than a fine finger–thumb grasp, when asked to build a tower of bricks or draw with a pencil. A tremor or athetoid movements can be noted as the child reaches for a toy. Mirror movements may be seen in the contralateral limb, indicating poor coordination. Hand–eye coordination may be observed when the child is asked to complete a jigsaw puzzle.

The concentration powers of the child may be seen by whether the child completes tasks. The child's reaction to sounds and the spoken word should be observed as a clue to deafness.

The special senses

Testing hearing in infancy

Clinical testing of an infant's hearing can start shortly after birth and thereafter should be repeated at about seven months, 18 months, three years and four and a half years. These repeat tests will detect those infants whose hearing has been affected by chronic infection. A few cases of congenital infection may worsen with age and not be apparent on the earlier testing.

Profound deafness may be detected shortly after birth using the 'blink reflex' or 'aural palpebral reflex'. This test can be used at any age and is also useful in older children with mental handicap who cannot respond to conventional testing. It is dependent upon the baby blinking in response to loud noises. The examiner stands behind the baby at arms length from either ear, makes a loud 'Ba' noise and observes whether the baby blinks. Failure to respond does not confirm deafness but indicates the need for further testing.

Testing should take place in a room with about 6 m clear space. The room obviously should be in a quiet location if not completely sound-proof.

The history preceding the examination should include any perinatal risk factors such as severe

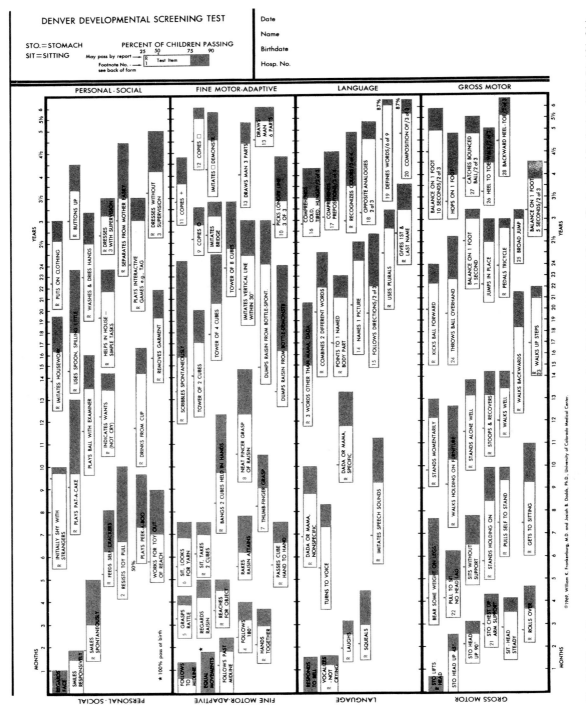

Fig. 3.4.22 (a) Denver developmental screening test. (With permission from Frankenberg WK and Dodds JB, *Journal of Pediatrics*, 1967; **71**: 181–91.)

Gross motor

Social

Vision and fine motor

Hearing and language

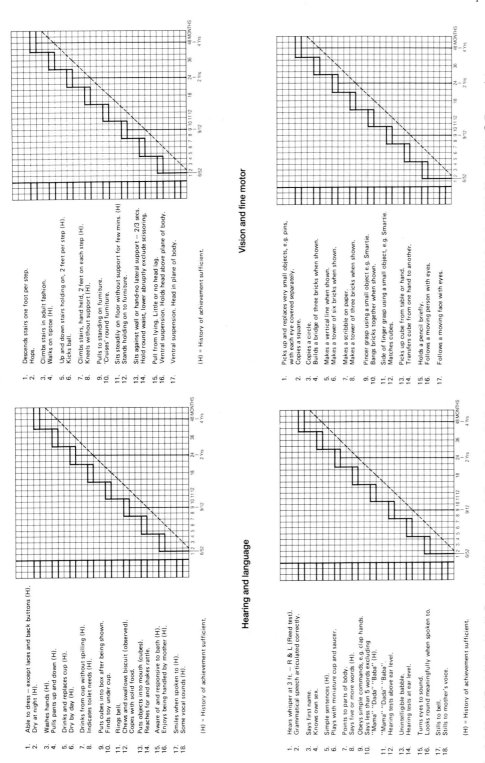

Gross motor

1. Descends stairs one foot per step.
2. Hops.
3. Climbs stairs in adult fashion.
4. Walks on tiptoe (H).
5. Up and down stairs holding on, 2 feet per step (H).
6. Kicks ball.
7. Climbs stairs, hand held, 2 feet on each step (H).
8. Kneels without support (H).
9. Pulls to standing on furniture.
10. 'Cruises' round furniture.
11. Sits steadily on floor without support for few mins. (H)
12. Stands holding on to furniture.
13. Sits against wall or hand-no lateral support — 2/3 secs.
14. Hold round waist, lower abruptly exclude scissoring.
15. Pull from lying. Little or no head lag.
16. Ventral suspension. Holds head above plane of body.
17. Ventral suspension. Head in plane of body.

(H) = History of achievement sufficient.

Social

1. Able to dress — except laces and back buttons (H).
2. Dry at night (H).
3. Washes hands (H).
4. Pulls pants up and down (H).
5. Drinks and replaces cup (H).
6. Dry by day (H).
7. Drinks from cup without spilling (H).
8. Indicates toilet needs (H).
9. Puts cubes into box after being shown.
10. Finds toy under cup.
11. Rings bell.
12. Chews and swallows biscuit (observed).
13. Copies with solid food.
14. Puts objects into mouth (cubes).
15. Reaches for and shakes rattle.
16. Aware of and responsive to bath (H).
17. Enjoys being handled by mother (H).
17. Smiles when spoken to (H).
18. Some vocal sounds (H).

(H) = History of achievement sufficient.

Vision and fine motor

1. Picks up and replaces very small objects, e.g. pins, with each eye covered separately.
2. Copies a square.
3. Copies a circle.
4. Builds a bridge of three bricks when shown.
5. Makes a vertical line when shown.
6. Makes a tower of six bricks when shown.
7. Makes a scribble on paper.
8. Makes a tower of three bricks when shown.
9. Pincer grasp using a small object e.g. Smartie.
10. Bangs bricks together when shown.
11. Side of finger grasp using a small object, e.g. Smartie.
12. Matches cubes.
13. Picks up cube from table or hand.
14. Transfers cube from one hand to another.
15. Holds a pencil briefly.
16. Follows a moving person with eyes.
17. Follows a moving face with eyes.

Hearing and language

1. Hears whisper at 3 ft. — R & L (Reed test).
2. Grammatical speech articulated correctly.
3. Says first name.
4. Knows own sex.
5. Simple sentences (H).
6. Plays with miniature cup and saucer.
7. Points to parts of body.
8. Says five or more words (H).
9. Obeys simple commands, e.g. clap hands.
10. Says less than 5 words excluding "Mama" "Dada" "Baba" (H).
11. "Mama" "Dada" "Baba".
12. Hearing tests above ear level.
13. Unintelligible babble.
14. Hearing tests at ear level.
15. Turns eyes to sound.
16. Looks round meaningfully when spoken to.
17. Stills to bell.
18. Stills to mother's voice.

(H) = History of achievement sufficient.

Fig. 3.4.22 (b) Forth Valley Health Board child health record. (From Barber JH, Boothman R and Stanfield JP. *Health Bulletin*. 1976; **May**: 80–91. © Econoprint Ltd., UK.) The top level of each step represents the 'initial' to the 'limit' ages at which normal children achieve the two abilities indicated at that level in all four major areas of development. If the child achieves both these tests a mark is placed on the top step in line with her age. If she achieves only one, then the mark is placed on the lower level. If she fails to achieve either test, then the two below are applied and the mark is placed appropriately on the top or lower level of the step. Failure to achieve these entails progressively lower pairs of tests. An arbitrary dotted line indicates the threshold below which referral is advisable.

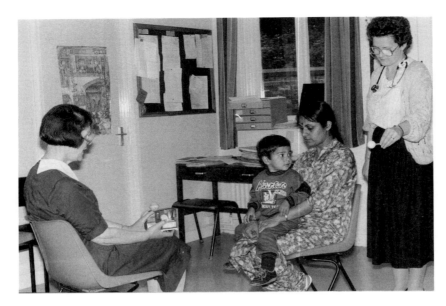

Fig. 3.4.23   Testing hearing by distraction tests.

neonatal jaundice, antenatal rubella or other viral infection and a family history. The mother should be asked about a baby's response to quiet and loud noises. The extent of vocalization should be ascertained. At seven months, the infant should have extensive vowel-based babble with the emergence of some consonant sounds. The deaf baby is either very quiet or has vocalization with little intonation and no consonants. With the older child, the extent of language development, especially comprehension, should be assessed. It is useful to assess the content of the child's play, which in a deaf child of average intelligence should be normal.

At seven months, hearing is assessed using distraction tests (Fig. 3.4.23). The equipment required is an ordinary china cup and teaspoon, a Nuffield or Manchester rattle and the examiner's voice. The infant is seated on the mother's lap facing the first examiner who sits a few metres away holding a toy to attract the infant's attention. The second examiner stands behind the infant, out of vision, and makes the appropriate sounds at either side of the infant. The infant will then turn to the source of the sound. The bowl of the cup is gently stroked to produce a quiet noise (about 35–40 dB). This is done 1 m from each ear at the level of the ear for a seven-month-old. The Nuffield rattle is moved with a stirring motion (producing a sound level of 35–40 dB) held 30 cm from the ear. The examiner then uses his/her voice to produce sounds of varying frequencies at low intensity. The aim should be to talk

very softly without whispering. A high-frequency sound is ss-ss-ss and low frequency, oo-oo-oo. It is important to include simple conversation to ensure a response to speech. The examiner speaks at about 1 m from each ear. The positive response is a definite turn of the head to the appropriate side. A failure at seven months is an indication for repeat testing in one month and referral to specialist services if the infant fails again. It is possible to obtain a sound-level meter to check the examiner's ability to produce sounds at an appropriate level.

The distraction tests are only useful for babies under 18 months. Over this age a normal infant may fail to turn to the stimulus. At this age, however, the infant may respond to appropriate toys and pictures and certainly by two years, tests using these may be attempted. These obviously have to be modified for different languages to ensure a selection of high- and low-frequency sounds. The child is shown five small toys, a cup, spoon, car, doll and brush. The toys are placed on a table with the mother and child sitting on one side and the examiner on the other. The examiner then names each toy in turn and asks the child for each of them. When happy that the child understands the test, the examiner retreats a short distance, covers his/her mouth to avoid lip reading and asks the child in a low voice to hand each toy on request to the mother. This test can be repeated with the older child (three years and above) using seven toys, a doll, ship, plane, car, knife, fork and spoon. At this age, picture tests can evaluate high-frequency hearing. The child is presented with a card showing six pictures, a ship, seat, feet, chick, pig and fish and the test administered as for the toy test. All the above tests are described in detail by Dr Mary Sheridan in the Stycar Hearing Test Manual.[20]

If the child has no speech, then it is possible to test hearing by conditioning responses. The usual method is to ask the child to place a brick in a container in response to a sound produced by the examiner. These tests can usually be performed by children with a mental age of two-and-a-half years. The child is presented with a pile of bricks and a suitable container and every time the examiner makes a sound the child is encouraged to place a brick in the container with praise for a successful attempt. As soon as the child understands the game the examiner withdraws to about 3 m, covers his/her mouth with the hand and continues the test starting with a fairly loud sound, gradually lowering the voice until the response ceases. A convenient low-frequency noise is 'go' and a high frequency 'ss'.

The conditioning test can also be performed using an audiometer. This may be a free-field audiometer or a pure-tone audiometer with headphones. The free-field audiometer produces pure tones at varying frequencies and varying loudness. This can be used for distraction tests as well as the conditioning tests but is no use below the age of one year, as small infants often do not respond to pure tone sounds. In older infants, it should be held 1 m from the ear for distraction tests. Conditioning tests are performed as described above with the free-field audiometer, but it is essential that the child receives no clues that the audiometer is being operated, i.e. the control knob must be out of sight. A pure-tone audiometer also produces sounds of differing frequencies and intensities but this is done through headphones and so each ear may be tested much more accurately. However, it does require the cooperation of the child and therefore is usually unsuccessful below the age of three years.

Neonatal hearing testing can be undertaken using brainstem-evoked response testing. An electrode on the scalp detects electrical activity produced in the brainstem by the stimulus of applied sound. A typical wave-form is produced and analysed by computer. This is a very sensitive and objective test but limited by its cost and also the time required.

Chronic secretory otitis media

The Eustachian tube of a child is poorly supported by cartilage and may be obstructed by enlarged adenoids.

Infants and young children often develop upper respiratory infections which spread along the short Eustachian tube to the middle ear, giving rise to acute otitis media with effusion. When the acute infection has subsided the effusion may persist, exacerbated by the partially obstructed Eustachian tube. This condition is described as chronic secretory otitis media or 'glue ear'. Clinically, the tympanic membrane appears retracted with a loss of the normal landmarks and the light reflex. Not surprisingly, the presence of fluid in the middle ear often affects hearing and some studies estimate that 5–10 per cent of children of school age may be affected. The hearing loss tends to be worse in the low frequencies and because of its recurrent nature may be difficult to detect. It may lead to behavioural and learning difficulties in the school child. Apart from the clinical appearance and the hearing loss, the diagnosis can be confirmed using an acoustic impedance bridge to measure tympanometry. This measures mobility of the tympanic membrane fairly simply and painlessly. Fig. 3.4.24 shows results obtained from a normal ear and from a child with glue ear.

The treatment of glue ear is to give an adequate course of an appropriate antibiotic. If this is not successful then myringotomy to drain the mucoid material and the insertion of grommets to help aerate the middle ear may be necessary.

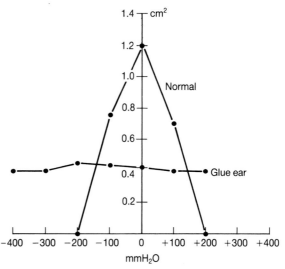

Fig. 3.4.24 Impedance from normal ear and from a child with glue ear.

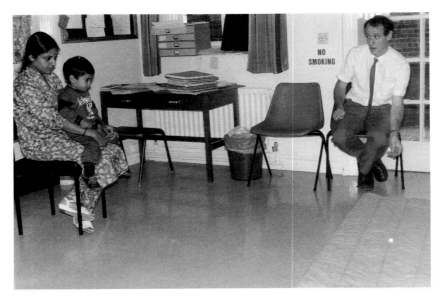

Fig. 3.4.25   Testing vision with Stycar rolling balls.

Development of vision

The retinal response to light and moving objects as shown by reflex responses of blinking, pupillary contraction and eye movements, occurs even in preterm infants.[21] During the first few weeks of life the infant starts to gaze around and may fix on objects. Body activity and respiration rate change in response to this. The ability to retain information is short and each appearance of a stimulus is perceived as a new event.

Awareness of an object involves discrimination between it and its surroundings. At first this is mainly on the basis of brightness gradients with possible colour discrimination. Development of accommodation begins during the second month and is comparable to that of adults by four months.

At five months, interest in familiar patterns declines with habituation. Thereafter, a novel object arouses more interest. Before three months the infant is unaware of the association between visual and tactile sensory patterns. At three months, the infant stretches out a hand towards an object and glances repeatedly to and fro between hand and object. At four months, the infant grasps the object and ceases to look at the hand. The infant learns by visual and tactile exploration to discriminate between objects and towards the end of the first year, realizes that objects have a permanent identity. Until then it is not possible for the infant to gain any real understanding of environment, for each object has to be explored anew as it appears.

Considerable development is required before the child can perceive with the same efficiency and rapidity as the adult. Complex shapes are not perceived accurately until five or six years of age which is particularly important with the printed word. The exact nature of environmental spatial relationships is not understood until seven years of age. (See Table 3.4.4.)

Testing vision in infancy

Clinical testing of vision can start at birth and should probably be examined again at six weeks, six months, one, two, three and four-and-a-half years. Testing should ideally include fundoscopy, examination of eye movements, testing of acuity, peripheral field testing and colour vision tests.

Testing of visual acuity under six months is mainly a qualitative examination which basically tests the

Table 3.4.4   Summary of visual development

Pupillary reaction	30 weeks gestation
Lid closure to bright light	30 weeks gestation
Visual fixation present	Birth
Fixation well developed	2 months
Visual-following well developed	3 months
Binocular vision well developed	6 months
Optic nerve myelination complete	7 months to 2 years
Normal adult acuity	2 years

infant's ability to see. A red ring or white ball on a string or the observer's face is passed in front of the infant's face and any following movements of the eyes are observed. Conjugate eye movements and the presence of a squint can be examined. Nystagmus raises the possibility of severe visual loss. At birth, the depth of vision is about 30 cm and therefore testing should start at that distance with a gradual withdrawal as the child grows.

From six months, the Stycar tests are most suitable for testing infants and young children.[20] (See Fig. 3.4.25.) The graded ball test is used from six months to two years and employs 10 white balls (0.3–0.6 cm diameter). Distant vision is tested in very young infants by rolling the balls across the floor at a distance of 3 m and watching the infant's eye following. In the older infant, the balls are mounted on sticks and with the examiner hidden behind a screen, presented at either side of the screen, with the examiner watching the child's response through a slit in the screen. Peripheral vision can also be tested with the balls mounted on sticks. Near vision is tested with tiny sweets, currants or balls of paper.

From two to three years the miniature toys test can be used. A set of seven small toys is given to the child and with the examiner standing 3 m away the child is asked to match a toy presented by the examiner. The ability to discriminate between the bowl of a tiny spoon and the prongs of a similar fork at 3 m is a good test of visual discrimination.

From about two-and-a-half years the Stycar letter tests can be used. The child is given a card portraying from five to nine letters (A O U C H L T V X). The younger child is given fewer letters or non-alphabet test cards. The examiner stands at 3 or 6 m (the distance used obviously affects the interpretation of the results) and shows the child one letter using a small flip-over book. These letters are accurately graded from large to small. The child must then point to the appropriate letter on the chart to show recognition. The smallest letter accurately matched gives a measure of the child's visual acuity, and this can be done for each eye in turn. Near-vision can be tested using a card providing graded letters from which the older child can read.

Diagnosis of squint

A squint occurs when the visual axis of one eye is not directed at the same point of fixation as the other. Stereoscopic vision develops in the first six months of life and is dependent upon an appropriate sensory input. Presentation of two different images causes suppression of the less-clear image and then amblyopia.

Squints may be associated with refractive errors, neurological disease (congenital cranial nerve palsy, cerebral tumours) or disease of the eye (cataracts, optic atrophy).

Two types of squint can be distinguished:

- Non-paralytic: there is no defect in the extra-ocular muscles or specific nerve palsy. The squint may be convergent or divergent.
- Paralytic: caused by a third nerve palsy (divergent squint, downward deviation of the eye, ptosis of the upper lid), a fourth nerve palsy (vertical deviation of the eye often with the head tilted to the opposite shoulder) or a sixth nerve palsy (limited abduction of the eye).

Methods for detection of squint are:

- Corneal reflection: a light is shone in the infant's eyes and the reflections on each cornea compared. They should be central in each pupil.
- Cover test: each eye is encouraged to fix on an object whilst the other eye is covered. If a squint is present then the eye takes up fixation when uncovered and returns to the deviated position when occluded.

Development and assessment of the blind child

About one half of blind children will have additional handicaps but, notwithstanding this, the development of a blind child progresses along different pathways from that of the sighted child.

The sighted child relies upon many visual stimuli to initiate gross motor function. Hand regard and playing with feet whilst supine encourages head lifting and eventually sitting. The blind child does not have these stimuli. Because of lack of early stimulation the blind child tends to be hypotonic and this exacerbates motor delay. Lack of visual stimulation will discourage the infant from crawling. The blind child receives no visual clues to aid language development, e.g. the change in expression accompanying 'yes' or 'no'. Speech, therefore tends to be echolalic. Therefore, the usual assessment techniques are inappropriate for blind children and special scales have been developed.[22]

Developmental surveillance

Developmental surveillance means all the activities related to the detection of developmental problems at the level of primary care. Developmental screening checks the development of children thought to be normal and is part of developmental surveillance, which also includes preventive measures such as immunization and education of parents.

The first aim of developmental surveillance is to prevent handicap through the early detection of correctable abnormalities such as hypothyroidism and phenylketonuria, by screening tests in the neonatal period eg. dislocated hips, cataracts, visual problems including squint and hearing problems.

The second aim is to detect the following handicaps early so that therapeutic services may become involved: cerebral palsy; mental handicap; visual handicap; deafness; language disorders; behaviour disorders; malnutrition; short stature.

Developmental surveillance should be supported by effective diagnostic and therapeutic services. Table 3.4.5 suggests a few key ages when simple screening tests can be applied and is largely derived from the report on child health services in England 'Fit for the Future'.[23] It is essential that surveillance is adapted to the needs of the community and that screening tests are simple to apply and clearly distinguish normal from abnormal.

Table 3.4.5.   A model for developmental surveillance

Age	Examination
Birth	The need for resuscitation should be recognized, the Apgar score being a reasonable tool for training workers
	The initial examination should include testing of the hips for stability, the eyes for cataracts and the testes for descent
	The mother and baby interaction should be observed and any anxieties discussed; this principle applies to all future examinations
6–10 days	This is a useful time to re-examine the hips and possibly the heart but more importantly to reassure the mother about the normality of her baby
6 weeks	Visual function can be assessed
	The stability of the hips should be checked again
	Feeding difficulties may be discussed
7–8 months	This age is most useful for review of the motor development as most babies will be sitting, rolling and bearing weight by now
	All babies should be reaching out with both hands although the mature grasp will not have developed
	Cerebral palsy should be detectable at this stage
	This is the ideal age to test hearing and most babies will also respond to vision testing
	The growth of the head should be assessed
18 months	Most infants should be walking by now and further evaluation should be made if not
	Manipulation can be assessed using small bricks
	Vision and hearing should be reassessed
	Most babies will be saying their first words by this age
2–3 years	The overall development can be assessed using standard guidelines
	Language is an important component at this age
	Behaviour difficulties are common at this age and can be discussed
4–5 years	It is important just before the child enters school to assess language development, vision and hearing, behaviour disorders and problems with fine motor coordination which may lead to specific learning difficulties

References

1. Gesell A. *The First Five Years of Life*. London, Methuen, 1978.
2. Dobbing J, Sands J. The quantitative growth and development of the human brain. *Archives of Disease in Childhood*. 1973; **48**: 757–67.
3. Dennis W. *Children of the Creche*. Englewood Cliffs, NJ, Prentice-Hall, 1973.
4. Geber M, Dean RFA. The state of development of newborn African children. *Lancet*. 1957; **1**: 1216–18.
5. Ainsworth MDS. *Infancy in Uganda: Infant Care and the Growth of Love*. Baltimore, Johns Hopkins Press, 1967.
6. Warren N. African infant precocity. *Psychological Bulletin*. 1972; **78**: 353–67.
7. Illingworth RS. *The Development of the Infant and Young Child: Normal and Abnormal*. Edinburgh, Churchill Livingstone, 1975.
8. Dubowitz LMS, Goldberg C. Clinical assessment of gestational age. *Journal of Pediatrics*. 1970; **77**: 1–10.
9. Parkin JM, Hey EN, Clowes JS. Rapid assessment of gestational age at birth. *Archives of Disease in Childhood*. 1976; **51**: 259–63.
10. Robinson RJ. Assessment of gestational age by neurological examination. *Archives of Disease in Childhood*. 1966; **41**: 437–47.
11. Parkin JM. The assessment of gestational age in Ugandan and British newborn babies. *Developmental Medicine and Child Neurology*. 1971; **13**: 784.
12. Prechtl HFR. *The Neurological Examination of the Full Term Newborn Infant*. London, Heinemann, 1977.
13. Brazelton TB. *The neonatal behavioural assessment scale*. London, Spastics International Medical Publication, 1984.
14. Dubowitz L, Dubowitz V. *The Neurological Assessment of the Preterm and Full Term Newborn Infant*. London, Spastics International Medical Publications, 1981.
15. Frankenburg WK, Dodds JB. The Denver Develop-

mental Screening Test. *Journal of Pediatrics.* 1967; **71**: 181–91.

16. Bryant G, Davies K, Newcombe R. The Denver Developmental Screening Test: achievement of test items in the first year of life by Denver and Cardiff Infants. *Developmental Medicine and Child Neurology.* 1974; **16**: 484–93.

17. Griffiths R. *The Abilities of Babies.* London, University of London Press, 1967.

18. Griffiths R. *The Abilities of Young Children.* Chard, Somerset, Young & Son, 1970.

19. Bayley N. Comparisons of mental and motor test scores for ages 1–15 months by sex, birth order and race, geographical location and education of parents. *Child Development.* 1965; **36**: 379.

20. Sheridan MD. *Manuals of Instruction for Stycar Tests of Vision, Hearing and Language.* Windsor, UK, NFER Publishing Co Ltd, 1968 and 1975.

21. Vernon MD. Development of visual perception. In: Gardiner PA, McKeith RC, Smith V eds. *Aspects of Developmental and Paediatric Ophthalmology Clinics in Developmental Medicine*, No. 32. London, SIMP with Heinemann Medical, 1969. pp. 1–4.

22. Reynell J, Zinkin P. New procedures for the developmental assessment of young children with severe visual handicaps. *Child: Care, Health and Development.* 1975; **1**: 61–9.

23. Department of Health and Social Security. *Fit for the future. Report of the Committee on Child Health Services. (Chairman: SDM Court)* London, HMSO, 1976.

DISABILITY IN CHILDHOOD
P. Zinkin

In all countries there is rightly great emphasis on saving children's lives through the prevention and management of acute conditions. However, when prevention and treatment fail, or are inadequate, little attention is paid to those children who become disabled as a result.

It is often said by doctors and those concerned with health planning and management, that disabled children are not a priority. But when the duration and depth of physical, social and economic hardship are considered, it is evident that disability *is* a priority for those families affected by it. Social justice alone should determine that there is access to rehabilitation for all children in the world who have a lifetime of disability ahead of them. However, children in developing countries not only are more likely to be affected by disability, but they and their families are least likely to receive help and understanding. It is sad when doctors and nurses are included in those that do not perceive the needs and rights of disabled children.

Social inequality and disability

All children are not at equal risk of impairment leading to disability, just as they are not at equal risk of disease and death. Children in poor families, in poor communities, in poor countries have the highest risk.

Not only is this inequity manifested in the causes of

impairment leading to disability, but it is compounded by the poorer children being less likely to receive help and care when they are disabled.

In a household and agency study[1] in Bangladesh, 24 858 families in rural areas and 15 350 families in urban areas were surveyed. Disabled children were found in 2.01 per cent of rural families and 1.80 per cent of urban families. In the rural areas the highest proportion of families with a disabled child were the landless day-labourers, and in the urban areas, day-labourers engaged in 'petty business' had a high proportion of affected children.

The proportion of children who were not receiving any 'treatment' at the time of the survey was 93.65 per cent in the rural areas and 86.21 per cent in the urban areas; 29.42 per cent of rural children and 22.76 per cent of urban children had *never* received any 'treatment', and this included traditional treatment.

This picture is probably fairly typical of many developing countries. Although it is likely that the children were being helped by their families, and some promising initiatives are under way, rehabilitation and stimulation of development are being denied to the majority of disabled children in the world.

Definitions

The World Health Organization[2] recommended the following definitions in relation to childhood disability:

- *Impairment* Any loss or abnormality of psychological, physiological or anatomical structure or function.
- *Disability* Any restriction or lack of ability to perform an activity in the manner or within the range considered normal for a human being, resulting from an impairment.
- *Handicap* A disadvantage for a given individual, resulting from an impairment or disability, that prevents or limits the fulfilment of a role that is normal depending on age, sex, social and cultural factors for that individual.
- *Rehabilitation* This includes all measures to reduce the impact of the disabling conditions and enables the disabled to achieve social integration.
- *Community-based rehabilitation* Involves measures taken at community level to use and build on the resources of the community, including disabled people themselves, their families and the whole community.
- *Aim of rehabilitation* The main aim of rehabilitation is to enable disabled children to pursue their lives with maximum dignity and self-reliance as members of their own families and communities.

In line with current international usage the term 'impairment' will be used for a loss or abnormality and the term 'disability' for its effect. The terms 'children with impairments', 'children with disabilities' or 'disabled children' will be used rather than the term 'handicapped children' perhaps more familiar to British paediatricians. This last term is often used as if an impairment was implied and can be confusing, especially in international circles. However, the term 'mental retardation' is in such common usage that it will be used together with the term preferred by WHO which is 'children with difficulties in learning'.

Problems with definitions

Criticism of these definitions used by doctors and health workers has been made by disabled people's organizations, because of their medical orientation, emphasizing the deficiencies of the individual, rather than those of society. It is not made clear that the major disadvantages to a child with an impairment come predominantly from the physical, social and cultural environment. In other words, it is the environment that is handicapping (or disabling).

Medical definitions are useful when establishing the cause of an abnormality or loss and enables a 'diagnosis' to be made which might lead to cure or prevention. Sometimes, a specific diagnosis is required for research purposes. However, labelling children by their diagnosis, such as Down's syndrome or 'spastic', has rarely benefited the individual child in everyday living.

It is important to recognize that it is possible to offer effective developmental help and rehabilitation to a child without establishing a definitive diagnosis.

Categories of definitions

There are reasons other than medical ones for categorizing disabled children. For example, if a benefit is to be made available to certain disabled children, there is an administrative need to define disability so that the benefit goes to those for whom it was intended.

Different categories may be used by educational authorities, which effectively include or exclude children in a school system. Similarly, registration of disabled people may be made for legal reasons, for example, if there is a legal requirement to employ a percentage of disabled people within an institution.

An example of a different way of looking at a disability which focuses on society, is the definition of 'mental retardation' proposed by Gold of the Institute for Child Behavior and Development, Illinois. This states that 'mental retardation refers to a level of function that requires from society significantly above average training procedures . . .' and that, 'the height of a level of functioning is determined by the availability of training, technology and the amount of resources a society is willing to allocate and not by significant limitations in biological potential'. This is an example of the removal of barriers that the disabled person faces.

Definitions and prevalence

It is apparent that the definition used may affect the apparent prevalence of a disability. A high prevalence of developmental disorders and disability is more likely to be found when a paediatrician interested in child development is in the area. When facilities for hearing-impaired children are provided for the first time, the problem is recognized more frequently, and parents may bring children to be seen about whom they have been concerned for some time. Depending on the definition of hearing loss, the prevalence can vary 30 fold.

There may be many reasons for using definitions that include or exclude certain groups of people, which are not always totally objective. For example, definitions which give high prevalences might be preferred for propaganda reasons to draw attention to disabled children and the lack of resources available for them. A limiting definition might be preferred by government to show that adequate services are being provided for most of the children with disabilities.

The size of the problem

Estimates of the percentage of children with disabilities vary. Prevalence rates depend on the age group being considered as well as the definition. WHO and UNICEF have commonly used the figure of one in ten as a guide but WHO now adopts the figure of 7 per cent for developing countries. This figure has been criticized[3] as being too high. Although some studies have shown a higher prevalence than this, it is a daunting figure to cope with for practical purposes. By initially including only 'severe disability' or 'disability that could easily be helped by rehabilitation' prevalence rates of around 2–3 per cent are produced. However, even when the lower figure is used, it has been found that 15–18 per cent of families have a disabled member.

There are many reasons why accurate data are not easily found. Good surveys are expensive; WHO[2] estimated in 1984 that the cost of a household sample survey is in the region of $50 000–$100 000. The cost might be justified, if it resulted in the development of adequate rehabilitation services for disabled children. Unfortunately, in many countries this is not the case and much scientific and epidemiological work goes simply into defining a problem that is already only too well understood by those who are experiencing it.

Age also has to be taken into account. Some disabilities, although present and visible at birth, may not be notified until a later age. Other impairments are visible, but only disable the child later. Some 'invisible' impairments, existing but not visible, may only present later as disabilities whilst others are acquired during childhood. Some disabilities are present at birth but their effects are so severe that the child dies in the early years of life.

Another complicating factor in estimating the prevalence of disability is that where attitudes are negative, services sparse or not understood and trusted, disabled children are hidden. In addition, a child defined by health professionals as disabled may not be perceived as such by parents or local health workers. In rural and poor urban areas other problems, not seen as important by the medical profession, may seem far more important to the family. It would appear sensible to take the families' own definition of need for rehabilitation as a criterion. However, there may be many reasons for a family not to seek help. The main reasons are poverty, especially where medical care has to be paid for, and lack of knowledge about what can be done.

Causes of impairment

In developing countries most of the primary causes of impairment, which underly disability, are preventable. The causes are similar to those that result in death and disease, although there are some differences.

The most important causes of impairment in children are those related to poverty and include:

- infectious and parasitic diseases;
- malnutrition;
- trauma, including war and armed conflict, accidents and burns;
- conditions associated with inadequate care during pregnancy, delivery and the neonatal period;
- congenital and hereditary conditions;
- chemicals, drugs and radiation.

Primary prevention

Given the basic causes, much disability could be prevented through measures taken against malnutrition, adequate supplies of clean water (a prerequisite to improved hygiene), adequate prenatal and postnatal care, care at delivery, immunization programmes, genetic counselling and the prevention of accidents and war. Most, but not all of these measures are included in primary health care programmes. As stated by the United Nations when launching the World Programme of Action concerning Disabled Persons for the decade of disabled persons in 1983, 'In most countries the prerequisites for achieving the purposes of the Programme are economic and social development, extended services to the whole population in the humanitarian area, the redistribution of resources and income and an improvement in the living standards of the population. It is necessary to use every effort to prevent wars leading to devastation, catastrophe and poverty, hunger, suffering, diseases and mass disability of people and therefore to adopt measures at all levels to strengthen international peace and security, to settle all international disputes by peaceful means and to eliminate all forms of racism and racial discrimination in countries where they still exist. Without effective remedial action the consequences of disability will add to the obstacles to development. Hence, it is essential that all nations should include in their general development plans immediate measures for the prevention of disability, for the rehabilitation of disabled persons and for the equalization of opportunities'.[4]

Early detection and secondary prevention

Once a child has a 'permanent' impairment it is important that measures are taken to mitigate the effect of the impairment and the disability.

Most of these measures are more effective if carried out early in a child's life, or soon after an accident or illness, depending on the cause of the condition. Secondary prevention is one of the main reasons for advocating early detection of impairment.

Secondary problems directly related to the impairment may be physical, developmental, social, psychological and educational.

Some examples are listed of the important consequences of physical impairments that can be prevented.

Physical

Prevention of deformity and contractures

Contractures frequently occur in conditions such as burns, poliomyelitis, cerebral palsy, spinal cord lesions such as in meningomyelocoele. They occur near joints which are not fully moved through their range due to general weakness, weak muscles or pain. Appropriate prevention is through techniques such as positioning, passive movements, stretching exercises, splinting and by encouraging active movements that counteract the deforming tendency. It is much better if these measures are incorporated into play. Specific details of these and other measures may be found in appropriate reference material (e.g. Ref. 5).

Prevention of pressure sores

Pressure sores occur over bony protuberances when a child spends many hours without moving. The local circulation of blood in the area is impeded and necrosis and infection occur. They can be very dangerous as infection may lead to septicaemia.

They occur in children who spend long periods without moving, or without moving that specific part of the body, such as those who are severely ill, malnourished, have a spinal lesion, muscular dystrophy or incorrectly adjusted plaster casts or splints.

Preventive measures are improvement of general nutrition, movement and exercise, frequent change of position, skin care and keeping the surface under the part clean, dry and smooth.

Prevention of urinary infections and serious constipation

Repeated urinary infections leading to renal failure may be a cause of death in children with spinal lesions. Prevention is through good high-fibre diet, regular bladder emptying (which may require catheterization). Automatic bowel and flaccid bowel need different programmes, and manual emptying may be necessary.

Developmental

Although development traditionally is assessed in different areas, they are linked to one another. For example, a child who is not mobile is not able to learn by exploring the environment. Once those caring for a child are aware of this, as a development need, the child can be taken to different parts of the room or compound, so that the child has the opportunity to examine things outside usual unaided reach. Similarly, a child with a hearing impairment can be helped at an early age through other methods of total communication, including speech, reading and signing, so that social development is less retarded.

Social

Almost all disabled children are additionally disabled by lack of appropriate social learning experiences. It is important that they have a chance to interact with the same range of people as other children. This does not only mean other children but adults in all of the situations that are part of the everyday social life of children of the same age.

Psychological

This is a complex area, but an important aspect is that in addition to the impairment, the disabled child almost always has a lowered self-esteem. This may be so low that motivation is affected, thus further impeding the child's development. Lowered self-esteem may come about from the attitudes of society and peers but doctors and parents often inadvertently play a negative role. Faced with a child who, for example, cannot walk, parents and doctor become concerned for the child to be as 'normal' as possible. Although this is generally positive, if the whole emphasis is on the inability to walk and all possible measures are undertaken to help the child do so, then when this predictably fails after many years, the child may consider it to be a personal failure. The child may also feel that she/he has failed the parents (and therapists) and self-esteem is lowered. At what point it is better to accept the child's limitations depends on many factors but at no stage should the focus be on the child's defects.

Classification of disability

For a detailed classification of disabilities the WHO *International Classification of Impairments, Disabilities and Handicaps* can be consulted.[6] This system is useful for medical classification but, for helping disabled children a functional system has been advocated by WHO. It includes both children and adults, and forms the basis of a suggested rehabilitation programme. The classification covers individuals with the following:

- fits;
- difficulty in learning;
- difficulty with hearing and/or speech;
- difficulty in seeing;
- strange behaviour;
- no feeling in the hands and/or feet (leprosy);
- difficulty with moving.

This very simple system is not likely to be used by doctors but can be used by lay people in the community for identifying disabled children. Belmont[7] has devised a scheme which has been proved useful internationally for identifying developmentally retarded children.

Assessment

Definition and purpose

Assessment has been defined as the 'systematic collection, organization and interpretation of information about a person and his situation'.[8] This is not of itself a useful activity for a disabled child and the family, unless the purpose is clear.

The purpose of assessment is to analyse the disabled child's present situation in order to find ways of helping the child reach optimal potential. This may seem idealistic, since very few able-bodied children in developing countries have such an opportunity. However, whereas helping resolve economic problems would contribute more than medical help to most families, this is not entirely true where disabled children are concerned. In all societies and economic groups, disabled children (and adults) are disadvantaged first by their impairment and then by society. Assessing the present situation of a disabled child in a problem-solving way can be helpful.

Method

Assessment involves the family, the community and services, as well as the child. Although the objective of assessment is to help solve problems, the emphasis should always be on the positive qualities of the child and family. This is not only a kindness or to encourage the parents psychologically but for the practical reasons. Developmental help begins with what the child can do, not with what the child is unable to do. Even the most retarded child can do something, perhaps smile or protest, and this achievement can be the starting point of a programme for that child. The method of assessment depends on the problems presented but generally includes information from the parents and an assessment of the child's functioning in different areas of development. A carefully taken history and observation of the child with the parents, preferably at home, during play or daily activities such as feeding and bathing, often gives more useful information than formal psychological or other tests.

There are many different ways of looking at areas of development and it is difficult to suggest a scheme that can work satisfactorily for all children in all cultures. For assessing the developmental needs of young children in order to offer help in specific areas, a developmental framework that includes the following may be useful:

- locomotion and posture;
- fine movements (especially of the hands);
- communication, both non-verbal and verbal (hearing, comprehension of language and speech);
- vision;
- social behaviour, including play and understanding;
- cognitive function;
- the child's feeling.

The last is extremely important and is surprisingly commonly left out of paediatricians' assessments.

The child's achievements in each area of development are noted. There is no real need to relate these to the child's actual age or compare the child with other children, except perhaps for diagnostic purposes. It is more important to see how the child is functioning in each area of development in order to help the child to the next stage. So-called developmental quotients are misleading and have no place in the assessment of a child with an impairment, since the area of function affected by the impairment cannot be averaged with other areas. In any case, the wide range of normality in different groups of children from different backgrounds makes a nonsense of such quotients.

Examining different areas may be helpful in understanding the child's strengths and in deciding if general progress is being held up by lack of progress in one area. If so, the decision has to be made as to whether to try to stimulate the child in that specific area of development or to compensate for it in other ways. For example, a child who is totally blind needs special help in other areas of development. The child will learn to use touch and hearing to find out about objects which other children can see. A child who is well advanced in all areas of development except locomotion may be helped to walk, or, if this seems to be impossible, then some sort of walking aid could allow the child to explore the environment (Fig. 3.4.26).

The next stage of assessment could include psychological and sensory tests and investigations, but it is often more appropriate to listen very carefully to the parents as they present their concerns and problems.

Assessment also has a diagnostic function. For example, with a child of three years who is not speaking at all, assessing the development in different areas may show that the child functions within the range of activity expected for 95 per cent of children of that chronological age in all areas except understanding and speech. This would indicate that the child had a hearing impairment until proved otherwise. On the other hand, a three-year old child functioning in all areas of development like a one-year-old except motor development, would most likely have mental retardation.

Rehabilitation

General needs

Children with disabilities have the same health, emotional and educational needs as those without disabilities. They are much less likely to have these needs attended to unless each is treated primarily as a child who happens to have an impairment.

For example, in countries where malnutrition is a problem, disabled children are more likely to be affected than able-bodied children. This is true for all types of disability but obviously children with feeding difficulties, such as those with cerebral palsy, are most at risk. Cerebral palsy should always be considered in a young child with malnutrition, especially when the siblings are well-nourished and if the mother says that the child is difficult to feed. This is too easily assumed to be a lack of competence or even care on the mother's part. The satisfactory nutritional status of the older siblings indicate that the mother is perfectly competent and careful in feeding her children. A neurological examination of such a child will clarify the reasons for her failure to thrive and may reveal that the feeding difficulty is due to a bulbar palsy associated with cerebral palsy.

Immunization is also much more likely to be ommitted for a disabled child; health workers forget or think that the child has such serious problems that immunization is not important. In addition, there are mistaken ideas amongst doctors about contraindications.

Special needs

If a child with a severe impairment is to reach an optimum level of development, there are several special needs:

- The reduction of the effects of the impairment. For example, the provision of a hearing aid may reduce the effects of impaired hearing in a deaf child, although alone it will not help the child to communicate better. Another example is positioning a child with cerebral palsy in such a way that the effects of spasticity are minimized.
- The prevention of direct secondary effects, for example contractures in cerebral palsy.
- The child's experience should be enlarged to correspond to, but not necessarily mimic that of an able-bodied child.
- In every society the barriers to a child's adjustment and development are only partly determined by impairment. Social attitudes play an equal, and

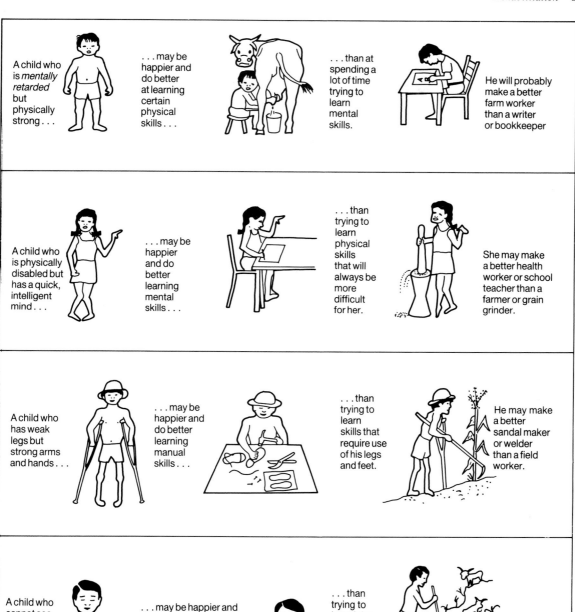

A child who is *mentally retarded* but physically strong . . .

. . . may be happier and do better at learning certain physical skills . . .

. . . than at spending a lot of time trying to learn mental skills.

He will probably make a better farm worker than a writer or bookkeeper

A child who is physically disabled but has a quick, intelligent mind . . .

. . . may be happier and do better learning mental skills . . .

. . . than trying to learn physical skills that will always be more difficult for her.

She may make a better health worker or school teacher than a farmer or grain grinder.

A child who has weak legs but strong arms and hands . . .

. . . may be happier and do better learning manual skills . . .

. . . than trying to learn skills that require use of his legs and feet.

He may make a better sandal maker or welder than a field worker.

A child who cannot see but has a good sense of hearing, touch, and rhythm . . .

. . . may be happier and do better learning skills that depend mainly on hearing and touch . . .

. . . than trying to learn jobs that are much more difficult without eyesight.

He will probably make a better village musician than a goat herder or hunter.

Fig. 3.4.26 Children with certain areas of weakness or disability often also have other areas of strength or ability. When deciding what work skills a child should be helped to develop, it is generally wise to pick those in areas where the child is strongest. (From Werner D, *Disabled Village Children*, 1987. Hesperian Foundation.)

often dominating, role. Changes in society's attitudes to disability in general are an important part of the child's needs.

Practical rehabilitation

When a health worker can offer no cure a feeling of inadequacy is common. The health worker may feel irritated when the parents do not seem to accept advice and may subconsciously find fault with the mother to justify these feelings. This may lead to the mother not being given the vital help she needs with the problems she faces in her everyday handling of the child.

The time and frustration that a mother may experience in feeding a child with cerebral palsy, or toileting a child with learning difficulties, or trying to let a child with severe visual impairments dress itself have to be lived with to be really understood. Many health workers, including doctors, do not themselves know, and regrettably some are not interested in finding out, how to help in these everyday problems. Where therapists are available they may be able to offer help but in most areas there are insufficient paediatrically trained therapists.

There are fortunately now some excellent sources of help. Details of many useful techniques for helping parents with these problems may be found in the WHO Manual *Training Disabled People in the Community*[9] and, for more detail, in David Werner's excellent book, *Disabled Village Children*.[5] Although intended for non-professionals this book is strongly recommended for doctors. Further help in specific areas are Refs 10 and 11 on cerebral palsy and Ref. 12 for blind children.

Basic problem solving

Many problems can be helped by the following basic approach:

- Analyse with the mother exactly what the problem is.
- Help with her priorities, not your own.
- Establish the short-term goals to overcome this problem to enable the child to progress to the next stage of development in that area.
- Break down the process necessary to achieve the short-term goal into very small steps.
- Take these steps one at a time.
- Usually the specific difficulty is part of a general problem in, say, dressing and the particular step is best tackled during the normal process of dressing and not isolated from it. Do the whole task in the normal way. Say what is being done in simple

language, encouraging the child to do the parts of the task the child finds easiest, extending these gradually to include more difficult steps and finally the whole task.
- Reward the child with praise for effort, not necessarily for succeeding. Although other rewards may be used, the best reward is the child's feeling of accomplishment. This is facilitated when the task consists of small achievable steps. Every effort should be made to enable the child to experience some control over the environment.
- Support the mother, concentrating on her emotional and practical needs.

The main areas of daily living in which problems occur are feeding, toileting, dressing and washing and examples of these are discussed below.

Feeding

Problems in feeding may occur with sucking and swallowing, regurgitating, vomiting, refusing food, refusing anything other than liquids or inability to chew. Solutions depend on the cause of the problem. For example, in cerebral palsy, positioning the child and finger feeding (normal in most cultures) may help.

Toileting

Problems include incontinence, inability of the child to move outside to the latrine, and danger in use of the latrine because the child has to crawl over the hole, becoming dirty and infected. Solutions might include a bladder programme (explaining that this may take a long time, but should include an explanation that the child is not deliberately incontinent to annoy the carer), mobility aid to encourage independence, adjustment of the latrine, preferably cementing around it, and adapting a support.

Dressing

Problems in dressing might be that the child is stiff, and arches the back, or throws off anything the mother puts on. Types of solution could include positioning, as in a child with cerebral palsy.

The family

The birth of a child with an impairment leading to disability has traumatic emotional and psychological implications for the family. It can also be an economic

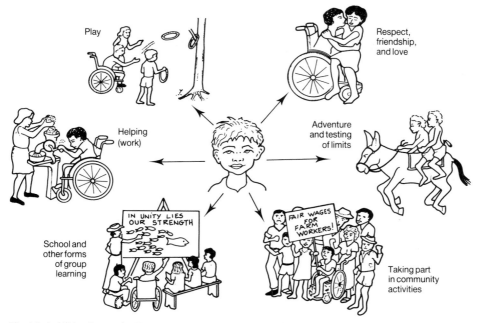

A disabled child growing up has the same needs as other children, for ...

Play

Respect, friendship, and love

Helping (work)

Adventure and testing of limits

School and other forms of group learning

IN UNITY LIES OUR STRENGTH

FAIR WAGES FOR FARM WORKERS!

Taking part in community activities

Fig. 3.4.27 Disabled children's needs. From Werner D, *Disabed Village Children*, 1987. Hesperian Foundation.

burden, especially in poor countries. Not only are there medical bills to pay, perhaps throughout the child's life, but there are adaptations to the home, equipment, and the loss of the expected economic contribution from the affected child and, in part, from the carer.

The birth of a child with an impairment is usually traumatic for the parents. They go through a period akin to mourning, as if the able-bodied child they were expecting had died. They must not be labelled as rejecting or uncooperative but treated with respect and understanding. With patience and the demonstration of genuine concern through practical measures, most parents will themselves come to respect and enjoy their child. It is also important that the medical personnel attending the child show through their actions and attitudes that they believe that disabled people should have equal rights and opportunities (Fig. 3.4.27).

Probably parents are less rejecting of disabled children than many doctors. For example, in a group of 206 disabled children seen in the Muhimbili hospital in Tanzania, Okeahialam[13] reported that 'All parents showed great concern for their children and were willing to discuss their condition at length. Many of them, particularly the mothers, expressed a feeling of guilt and shame. It became obvious from these interviews that the effect of the handicapped child on the social harmony of the family is tremendous. In six cases, the mother had been divorced because of the child and had to bear the burden alone. On the whole it was impressive to find the emotional involvement of the parents in the care that could be provided for their children'.

The concern that parents show was manifested in the fact that in searching for help for their child, one third of the children came from outside the town and some had travelled more than 100 km to the hospital. In addition, in relation to 76 per cent of the children, their parents had consulted traditional healers on three or four occasions.

Other parents or parents organizations and groups may give great support. If no parent group exists, the doctor may help parents to meet. The doctor's role should be that of facilitator, simply putting parents in touch, and any temptation to take over the group if it is not going the way the doctor wants, must be resisted. Parents' groups become increasingly important as the extended family system breaks down, through urbanization, migrant labour and other economic pressures.

The community

It has been emphasized that children with impairments are handicapped by society's attitudes and organization. Attitudes to handicapped people may range from hostility and mocking, through indifference and pity, to love and recognition of them as people with equal rights and faults. What determines societies' attitudes to disabled children and adults is complex, and includes social and spiritual values, economic and health policies, and community education. Above all, the economic conditions of the community may be so poor as to leave no resources for those that might need more than average help.

It is important to remember that within any given community there are different attitudes just as there may be within the same family. Communities are not homogenous and identifying those with positive attitudes may provide one of the foci for change.

The influences that change the attitudes of a society are also complex but include the following:

- Providing good community rehabilitation services. These show the family and community that a lot can be done to enable disabled children do more than they thought possible. This can give hope to the immediate family and interest the community.
- Integration. If a community is used to seeing disabled children, particularly knowing them as they develop, it is more likely to accept their presence than if the children appear from an institution at the age of 16.
- Access. Integration is difficult without access. Doctors should set a good example by ensuring that their premises, and all new buildings with which they are associated have access for disabled people.
- Parent group campaigns.
- Community education. This can be done through radio programmes, posters, leaflets, puppet shows and television where appropriate.
- Disabled adults organizations. By demanding equal opportunities, rights and responsibilities, and showing that we are all dependent on each other, a new approach is possible.
- By helping disabled people themselves to get suitable training and employment in different fields, particularly the health sector. Disabled people often make very good village health workers.[5]

Health workers have a special role in changing attitudes. The only attitudes we can really change are our own. We can support parents' organizations and self-help groups. We must not exclude any disabled child from care or services.

The services

Services for disabled children have been mainly based on institutions. These tend to be in urban areas and reach only a small percentage of a developing countries' disabled children. Many are associated with hospitals, and provide 'outpatient treatment'. These tend to treat the child as a patient and not as a developing individual within a family and community.

Other institutions provide day or residential care. They are expensive to run and often most of a country's professionals work in them. A serious problem of an institution-based approach is that of integration.

The ultimate aim of rehabilitation is the integration of the disabled child into the family and community, so that the child is able to pursue life with maximum dignity and self-reliance. Given this aim, it does not make sense to separate a child from family and community and hope to be able to integrate the child later. In many developing countries disabled children are already part of their families, although they are less often truly integrated into the life of their community with equal access to education, play, and meaningful employment and civic responsibilities in later life.

In Britain, historical events led to children with disabilities becoming separated even from their families. This happened mainly through the residential special schools. The argument in favour of these was that as children with special needs were scattered geographically, scarce resources would be better used if they were brought together, but it was also felt that parents were incapable of looking after children with specific impairments (especially visual and hearing impairments). It is significant that, unlike most of Europe, there is a tradition of boarding schools in certain sections of British society, and this has had an influence on special education.

The arguments against residential schools are several. First, only a part of the money spent on the school goes on education. The rest is spent on the upkeep of the institution, the building, the gardens, kitchen, laundry, and all the costs that a family usually expects to pay for its members.

Second, although the child may make some educational gains, if not too unhappy to learn, a young child is liable to lose the inner emotional strength that continued care by the same loving family gives. This inner confidence helps through the difficult times in life. Disabled children have a harder practical and psychological future than average, and so they need this inner security and family support more, not less, than other children. Residential institutions take away decision-making, responsibilities, variability in daily events and experiences of family life.

Third, the family also needs to understand the special education their child is receiving in order to be able to continue it. For example, if a hearing-impaired child is being taught to communicate using a signing system, the parents and family, and preferably the local community as well, need to know it.

The arguments against residential schools are not necessarily valid for all special schools, but an analysis of resources allocated for such schools might show that an integrated school or class is a better use of them. In this case, resources could be used, for example, for a special teacher supporting class teachers, teacher training, small groups of children with similar disabilities in ordinary schools or care persons to attend to children's special needs in the classroom. In India, blind children have been accepted into ordinary classrooms, sitting next to a helpful friend, and with the teacher, advised by a specialist teacher, remembering to say everything she writes on the board. Nevertheless, integrated education is not without problems, especially for hearing impaired children.

Institution-based outreach services

Many professionals have realised the limitations of both day and residential institutions and some are developing outreach services. This is based on the recognition that assessment of a child in a specialist centre is incomplete since it does not allow assessment of the daily living conditions of the child and family, including their assets and difficulties. The following observations may be made at home visits:

- children usually perform better in their own homes;
- the implications of the recommendations made by doctor and therapist on the mother's workload;
- the role, both positive and negative, of other family members;
- the economic and functional implications for the family;
- the inappropriateness and sometimes unnecessary complexity of some recommendations;
- the ease with which mothers are able to express their opinions in the familiarity of their own homes;
- above all, the creativity of the family in finding their own solutions to the disabled child's problems.

However, when professionals undertake home visits this can be even more expensive, since even fewer children can be seen and transport has to be paid for. The same considerations apply to mobile clinics, but in addition, these do not have the advantage of home visits.

Community rehabilitation

Experience in the assessment and rehabilitation of children with disabilities from countries with vastly different resources has shown that the emphasis should be on the child in the community. The role of professionals and institutions is to support parents, local volunteers, teachers, play groups and other community structures, rather than to take over the child's care from them. This is not as a second best for developing countries but should be the basis of rehabilitation for all. This is a changing area and different community-based rehabilitation programmes are underway in many countries. There is no rigid correct programme and each country and locality should produce its own locally appropriate programme.

The reasons for advocating a community-based approach are:

- integration is facilitated;
- the home is emphasized;
- community and family resources are mobilized;
- when professional resources are few, some help can be made available to all disabled children; this is done by demystifying the components of rehabilitation so that non-professionals can carry out most of the steps.

Community resources

The resources in the community may include:

- a few motivated people, disabled people themselves and their relatives and friends;
- an interested school teacher who could use the child-to-child programme or support integrated education;
- playgroups;
- parents;
- voluntary agencies.

Parents' organizations

Over the past few years disabled people in many countries of the world have formed their own organizations so that the voice of disabled people themselves is heard. Basically the organizations are pressing for equal rights, which though rarely denied in nations' constitutions are often denied by attitudes and practices.

Parents of children with disabilities have also formed

support, self-help and pressure groups in many countries of the world. Often these are organized round specific disabilities. They have had different functions. Some groups have raised money for research and care, some have organized their own care and support, most have been active and effective in improving public attitudes. Professionals must listen to and learn from parents' organizations. They have shown us a vast potential resource of great understanding and creativity which forms one of the essential foundations of rehabilitation.

Practical advice and technology

The World Health Organization's manual, *Training the Disabled Person in the Community*, consists of 'packages' which are simple problem-based training instructions on how to help the disabled person in his or her own home. All disabilities are included and there is advice on making simple equipment, working with teachers and community leaders and guidelines for translating and adapting the manual. Local workers may be trained to select and use appropriate packages. It has been suggested that this approach places too big a burden on already over-burdened families whilst the better-off continue to be served by the limited number of institution-based professionals. This is not the intention and all projects have received support from professionals. Some have suggested that a 'top down' approach is not the best way of approaching a community programme. Nevertheless, it is important that community programmes have international and government support in order to reach the world's disabled people who at present have no access to rehabilitation.

As well as the WHO schemes there are other approaches. A project in Mexico bases the work on a village rehabilitation centre run by disabled people with the guidance of David Werner. These young disabled people advise mothers of disabled children who come for the day, or stay in the village, for a short period of time.

The book mentioned earlier, Disabled Village Children, developed from the experiences of this project.

There are many other examples of community rehabilitation from India, Zimbabwe, Jamaica, Pakistan, Nepal, Guyana and many other countries. They all involve disabled people and the families of disabled children to different extents. The focus is on the different ways of support given to a child with a disability by a locally appropriate rehabilitation worker. This person might be a family member, a community volunteer, an existing health worker, a teacher, or in countries with sufficient professional personnel, a therapist or a special education teacher.

Community rights

Parents and the community have a right to government resources and although self-help is desirable, government has a responsibility to all its citizens, including disabled children. An important role for paediatricians is sometimes to remind government of this responsibility and to promote equal opportunities for children with disabilities.

Community strengthening

It may be difficult economically for poor communities, living in stressful conditions, to focus, even briefly, on their disabled members. Community rehabilitation is more likely to have a place where there is already a community-based programme in primary health care in the spirit of the Alma-Ata declaration. In countries where social justice is not often mentioned, it is not likely that any but the better-off disabled will be helped, except through local initiatives, which can be quite inspiring. A good time to introduce rehabilitation and help for the disabled child is when community development, education, health care and mother-and-child health plans are being made. When nobody is left out of these plans, all members of the community may benefit, including disabled children.

Conclusions

This chapter has explained that the focus should be on the child with a disability and the family, supported by a locally appropriate rehabilitation worker. This person might be a family member, a community volunteer, a primary health care worker, or, in countries with sufficient personnel resources, a therapist or special teacher. The community worker, appropriate for each country and locality, must in his or her turn receive support from committed professionals. These will share some of their skills, learn new ones, becoming teachers and helping to resolve complicated problems.

Community rehabilitation workers with professional support could make essential services available to many disabled children who are at present neglected. At the same time specialized services should be made available through proper referral systems and the professional gain a new role, not just to provide for those who are fortunate enough to live near them, but to those whose need is greatest.

Home-based services are an important part of the picture but community-orientated local rehabilitation centres, such as described by Werner and Miles, are needed to support already over-burdened families. Both community and institutions are necessary for rehabilitation services and together with voluntary groups can form a sure foundation on which to build services for disabled children.

References

1. Mia A, Islam MH, Ali MS. Situation of handicapped children in Bangladesh. *Assignment Children, UNICEF.* 1981; **3/54**, 199.
2. WHO. *World Health – Rehabilitation for All.* Geneva, WHO, 1984.
3. Miles M. *Where there is no Rehabilitation Plan.* Peshawar, Pakistan, Mental Health Center, 1985.
4. WHO. *World Program of Action Concerning Disabled Persons.* 1984.
5. Werner D. *Disabled Village Children.* Palo Alto, USA, Hesperian Foundation, 1987.
6. WHO. *International Classification of Impairments, Disabilities and Handicaps (ICIDH).* Geneva, WHO, 1980.
7. Belmont L. *Screening for Severe Mental Retardation in Developing Countries.* Bishop Bekkers Institute for the Promotion of Research into Mental Retardation (PO Box 415, 3500 AK Utrecht, The Netherlands), 1984.
8. Hall DMB. *The Child with a Handicap.* Oxford, Blackwell Scientific Publications, 1984.
9. Helander E, Mendis P, Nelson G. *Training Disabled People in the Community.* Geneva, WHO, 1983.
10. Levitt, S. *Treatment of Cerebral Palsy and Motor Delay.* London, Blackwell Scientific Publications, 1977.
11. Finnie, N. *Handling the Young Cerebral Palsied Child at Home.* Dutton-Sunrise (2 Park Avenue, New York, NY 10016, USA), 1975.
12. Fichtner, D. *How to Raise a Blind Child.* Christoffel Blindenmission (Nibelungenstr. 124, D-6140 Bensheim 4, GDR), 1979.
13. Okeahialam TC. The handicapped child in the African environment. In: *The Child in the African Environment.* East African Literature Bureau, 1975. pp. 371–9.

CHAPTER 5

Nutrition

NUTRITIONAL NEEDS OF HEALTHY INFANTS

R. G. Whitehead and A. A. Paul

Infancy and the early preschool period of life represent a particularly dynamic phase of growth and development. The velocity of growth attained in terms of g/kg body weight/day exceeds that found during puberty and is equalled only by the rate of a child's intrauterine growth during the last trimester of pregnancy. It is also a time of major physiological and metabolic changes, influencing not only the ability of children to digest and absorb nutrients but also their subsequent capacity to assimilate these nutrients for new tissue synthesis, body maintenance, activity and other essential processes.

Human milk as a nutritional standard

To take account of these rapid developmental changes, it is usual to list nutrient needs during infancy in three-monthly increments. During the earliest of these there is, in theory at least, an almost perfect model of what the child requires. Recommended daily allowances (RDAs) at this age, for most nutrients, are based on the amounts the baby would receive during an average day of breast-feeding.

It has become customary to assume that the volume of milk consumed by the average child each day is about 850 ml and when this is coupled with the average concentration of a particular nutrient within breast-milk, a basic guide-line value is obtained for the daily needs of that nutrient. It is frequently forgotten, however, that even in the case of healthy mothers feeding healthy babies, there is a substantial day-to-day variation in the volume of milk consumed not only between mother-child pairs but also within the same mother-child pair. The data in Fig. 3.5.1, for example, summarize this variation in two-month-old babies from Cambridge, UK, all of whom were being exclusively breast-fed. The total variance is about 50 per cent of the mean. To what extent this variation in intake is a direct reflection of the variation in needs of different children and in the same child, is not so clear. Whilst for dietary energy it is known that the hunger reflex does link these two processes, for virtually all of the specific nutrients there is little or no evidence for a feed-back control mechanism.

It is not just variation in milk volume which needs to be considered. Whilst the total energy, carbohydrate, fat and protein concentrations in breast-milk are relatively stable and little influenced by anything other than the most extreme dietary deficiencies or excesses, this is not so true of the other nutrients, particularly the vitamins. Thus, breast-milk vitamin concentrations tend to be substantially higher in the USA than in the UK because of the more widespread use of fortified foods and commercial vitamin preparations in the USA. What concentrations are 'biologically normal' is not certain.

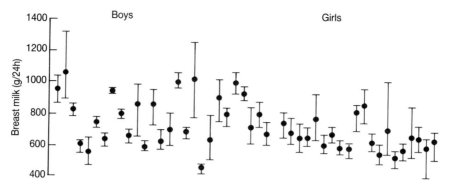

Fig. 3.5.1 Variations in the volumes of breast-milk consumed by Cambridge (UK) babies at two months. The daily mean values for each child over the four-day measurement period are indicated by •; the vertical line shows the day-to-day range for each child over the same period.

Breast-milk does not provide the simple and absolute 'gold standard' for defining the nutritional needs of young babies.

Nutritional complexities of weaning

After about three months, depending on individual needs and interaction with the mother, infants begin to need more food than the mother can provide because of physiological and/or sociological constraints. When this time is reached, most of the world's babies are given food in a totally different physical and chemical form than they have met before; not only is it semisolid, the chemical composition of the constituent nutrients is also quite different.

Ideally, and as recommended in the British DHSS standard guide-lines on the subject,[1] the earlier additional foods are provided, the more like human milk these should be. If, for any reason, additional foods have to be introduced at a particularly early age, the best option is probably a carefully formulated and prepared infant milk. However, this is expensive and so most of the world's children are given foods little better than the most basic of cereal gruels. These do not supply the range or the amounts of the different nutrients required, and many of the nutrients present may be biologically unavailable. Furthermore, the infant's gut may not be sufficiently well developed to make optimal use of nutritional components that are readily digestible in the older individual.

Under the unhygienic conditions in which most mothers and babies in the Third World have to live, it is difficult to make up foods which are not contaminated with potentially pathogenic microorganisms. Although in the Third World emphasis on infant feeding is rightly being placed on breast-feeding, the need for safer weaning foods must also receive attention. Studies in The Gambia have shown that traditional weaning foods used for young infants can be just as hazardous, in a bacteriological sense, as commercial milk products.[2] Providing a breast-fed child with supplements under the conditions which prevail in much of the developing world is potentially dangerous, whatever the source of the raw materials and however good they might theoretically be in nutritional terms. In The Gambia, for example, it is common practice in rural areas to prepare infant foods from cereal sources in quantities which are sufficient to meet the needs of the whole day, rather than just one meal. These are then stored at ambient temperatures for up to 12 hours and fed to the child when hungry. Even in the first hour after preparation the contamination is dangerously high, particularly during the wet season when the incidence of diarrhoeal disease related to faltering of growth is at its greatest. Foods not consumed fresh become progressively more seriously contaminated and are almost inevitably so after eight hours. There is little point in designing diets to meet the precise nutritional needs of the infant and toddler if these efforts are only to be wasted via nutrient losses arising from diarrhoea and vomiting.

Requirements for energy and protein

Throughout the world the principal guide-lines used by doctors and nutritionists when considering needs for dietary energy (calories) and protein are the recommendations of the UN agencies. These are revised approximately every 10 years or as new information becomes available; towards the end of 1985, FAO/WHO/UNU published their latest joint report.[3] The method of approach in this new report, and consequently the contents, differ in a number of important ways from the previous report.[4]

The primary yard-stick for estimates during early infancy remains the amount of milk the 0–3-month-old healthy child receives during a typical day of breast-feeding from a well-nourished mother, who is dedicated to this mode of feeding as the sole source of sustenance for her child. This latter proviso is very important because the amount of milk taken by the young baby at each feed is dependent on his degree of hunger and clearly this will be modified if other foods have been made available however small in amount.

Energy requirements up to three months

FAO/WHO/UNU[3] reviewed measured volumes of breast-milk intake from a number of parts of the world. These had all been measured by test-weighing, a procedure which requires the accurate weighing of the baby before and after each and every feed. All the studies indicated a similar pattern of change with age: the volume of milk being consumed by the baby rising rapidly during the first month of lactation but, in most children, reaching a virtual plateau of 750–850 ml/day by one or two months. Milk intakes then tended to remain more or less at this level until the mother began to introduce supplementary feeding, after which values fell again. This basic pattern of change with age has been reported from all over the world on numerous occasions, and typical examples from the literature for both Western and Third World countries[5] are shown in Fig. 3.5.2. From these data, it was apparent that even in exclusively breast-fed babies, during the first three months of life, the volume of milk being consumed was not keeping pace with the increasing size of the baby and thus it had to be concluded that the volume of milk/kg body weight which the child receives falls off as the baby grows older.

The mean value for the energy concentration in breast-milk adopted by the FAO/WHO/UNU consultancy was 70 kcal/100 ml (290 kJ). A similar value has been adopted by most national and international expert committees, from analysis of the protein, fat and carbohydrate of expressed breast-milk. As there was little evidence to suggest that major changes in total energy concentration occur, certainly during the first three months of lactation, the same factor was used throughout. Because of this, not only did the calculated volume of milk ingested per kg body weight fall quickly during early infancy, so did the intake of dietary energy

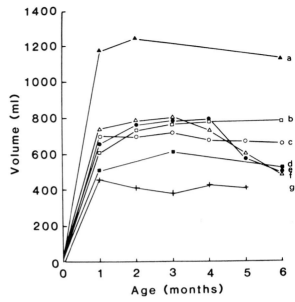

Fig. 3.5.2 Pattern of change in infant breast-milk intakes with age from studies carried out in different parts of the world: (a) Australia; (b) Sweden; (c) Gambia; (d) Zaire; (e) Sweden; (f) United Kingdom; (g) Zaire. (Reproduced by permission of *Pediatrics*, **75**: 189 © 1985.)

expressed on the same basis, presumably reflecting the pattern of requirements.

In considering the conclusions of the FAO/WHO/UNU consultancy it should be noted, however, that in practice the milk consumed at progressive stages within a given feed has a variable energy content. Because the fat content at the beginning of a feed (the fore milk) from each breast is low, the initial energy content is also low, but rises as the feed proceeds. There has been speculation[6] that energy estimates on milk obtained by complete manual expression might over-estimate the true energy intake obtained during normal lactation, particularly during the early ages of infancy when breast-milk is produced by the mother in considerable abundance. At this time the baby never needs to 'work' for the more energy-rich hind milk but might have to do so later when needs are greater. Whether or not corrections will need to be introduced in the future remains to be seen.

Energy requirements after three months

For their re-examination of energy requirements in infants beyond three months, the FAO/WHO/UNU committee carried out a detailed literature search on the

FAO = Food and Agricultural Organization, UNU = United Nations University food intakes of healthy young infants from a range of Western countries. The study was confined to such children to ensure that family food constraints or illness were unlikely to influence the data.[7] The ranges of mean dietary energy intakes at progressive stages during infancy from this survey are shown in Fig. 3.5.3. Although there is considerable variation, it will be immediately apparent that the great majority of the mean intake values at virtually all of the different ages were lower than the corresponding WHO/FAO (1973)[4] estimates which assumed that energy requirements fall only slowly from around 500 kJ/kg (120 kcal/kg) at 0–3 months to 440 kJ/kg (106 kcal/kg) at one year, in an essentially linear manner. Subjecting the literature data to mathematical analysis to determine the statistical best fit (Fig. 3.5.4) again confirmed that food energy intake, and hence presumably needs, did initially fall more steeply than had previously been

assumed, and the consultancy reasoned that by six months it would be safe to conclude that the average requirement for dietary energy was probably not more than 400 kJ/kg. Prompted by the results shown in Fig. 3.5.4, the consultancy concluded that energy needs might well rise again in the second half of infancy (on a per kg body weight basis) to accommodate the increased activity of children once they start to crawl and then walk. To account for this, the estimated needs per kg body weight were gradually raised again by a total of some 5 per cent from six months to one year.

Protein needs

The concentration of protein in the breast-milk consumed by the baby was also assumed to be a fixed value during the first three to four months of life and the value adopted was 1.15 g protein/ 100 ml. After

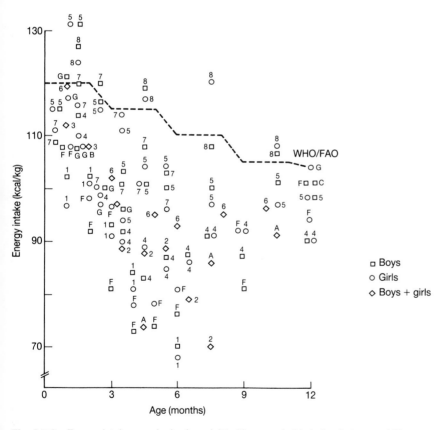

Fig. 3.5.3 Energy intakes per kg body weight of boys and girls in the first year of life compared with WHO/FAO (1973)[4] recommendations. The numbers and letters relate to the original reference. (Reproduced with permission from *Journal of Human Nutrition*, 1981; **35**: 339–48.)

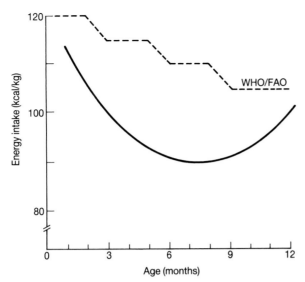

Fig. 3.5.4 The statistical best-fit line of the data in Fig. 3.5.3 expressed as the quadratic regression of energy intake per kg body weight on age. Energy $= 123 - 8.9$ (months) $+ 0.5$ (months)^2.

combining this factor with the corresponding volume of milk estimated to be consumed at each age, the resultant estimate of protein intake formed the basis of the recommendation up to four months. Essentially, therefore, the basic principle in setting protein needs up to three months was the same as for energy.

After this age, however, rather than calculating protein needs on observed intake, as energy needs had been estimated, protein requirements were derived from nitrogen balance data from studies carried out on healthy young children from various parts of the world. From the raw nitrogen balances, maintenance requirement values for zero growth and nitrogen equilibrium on milk and egg protein were calculated by regression analysis, although sweat and other miscellaneous losses had to be accounted for by the re-addition of small nitrogen increments. Maintenance values at subsequent stages during childhood were determined by linear interpolation between the infancy estimates, and those concluded to be appropriate for the average adult were obtained by nitrogen balance.

A second series of values, calculated to be the egg or milk protein increment needed to support a velocity of growth which would follow the international 50th centile reference curve, were added to all the resultant estimated maintenance protein requirements. In making these growth allowances it was necessary, however, to incorporate a safety margin allowance of 50 per

cent into the calculations. To correct for the efficiency of protein utilization during growth, a further 70 per cent was incorporated. The validity of these two increments was justified by the closeness of fit of the resultant value for maintenance plus growth with the protein intakes of young breast-fed babies, when the same assumptions were applied to these ages.

Thus, information on the protein composition of human milk drunk by young babies not only forms the direct basis for recommendations in early infancy, it also has an important if more indirect bearing on the derivation of estimated needs in older babies and toddlers. As with dietary energy, it is important that paediatricians and nutritionists have an appreciation of any scientific 'loose ends' which could have a bearing on the application of the recommendations. The key value of 1.15 g protein/100 ml was calculated after an analysis of the nitrogen content in breast-milk samples from various countries. The protein content was derived by multiplying the total nitrogen content by the basic factor of 6.25. Such a calculation is only valid if one can assume that all the nitrogen in breast-milk is in the form of proteins, peptides or amino acids or can readily be converted into such substances for protein anabolic purposes. A significant proportion of milk nitrogen is known, however, to consist of urea and other low molecular weight nitrogenous components. There are important gaps in our knowledge as to the extent to which these can be reutilized for protein synthesis or whether they might have some other protein sparing effect.

A further complication is that part of the protein in breast-milk is present as 'protective factors', substances believed to be important for protecting the child against intestinal disorders such as the diarrhoeal diseases. If the protective factors are to play their supposed role in the small intestine they must, at least in part, avoid digestion in the small gut as occurs with the other dietary proteins.[8] It is possible, however, that nitrogenous degradation products from the safety factors might still become available to the body as a result of subsequent bacterial action in the large gut. At present this is only speculation and nutritionists must admit that they do not know precisely how much of the non-protein nitrogen and the immunoproteins in breast-milk is available for tissue building. We need more exact data on the dietary availability of the different nitrogenous compounds in human breast-milk if we are to have a completely satisfactory estimate of dietary protein needs, not only during early infancy, but also in the older toddler, because of the importance attached to breast-milk as the primary indicator of what nature considers to be an adequate supply of protein for the rapidly growing child.

FAO/WHO/UNU (1985) recommended allowances

Energy

The latest set of estimated metabolizable energy needs and requirements for high-quality protein, such as that from milk or eggs, are summarized in Table 3.5.1: the corresponding WHO/FAO (1973) values are given for comparison. The changes introduced for energy have already been discussed. Essentially, they indicate that previous estimates for most stages during infancy may have been too high. Between three and six months, for example, it was calculated that the average child should be able to grow satisfactorily on up to 20 per cent less dietary energy than was previously considered necessary.

One practical consequence of this is that calculations designed to determine the length of time for which exclusive breast-feeding should be able to satisfy all the calorific needs of the average baby, suggest that this period is greater than previously thought.[9] The same calculation also has an important bearing on when to start weaning and on the quantitative extent to which breast-feeding needs to be supported by supplementary or complementary feeding as the baby grows older. For example, instead of the average requirements for a boy being 900 ml of milk at two months, 1100 ml at four months and 1250 ml at six months (values found in practice only at the upper limit of the intake distribution), recalculation suggests that only 775, 875 and 1000 ml (values much closer to the measured mean) are needed.

However, the new recommendations were based on data from healthy babies brought up in the Western style: that is fed and then encouraged to sleep for substantial portions of the day so that the mother can resume her activities. In countries where the baby is carried on the mother's back and thus tends to be awake more, the energy needs may be somewhat higher. This needs additional investigation.

Protein

The new protein recommendations are also given in Table 3.5.1 and at first sight seem similar to those of WHO/FAO (1973). This is misleading, however, as the data are expressed in terms of milk or egg protein, and the biological value of the proteins in most solid and semisolid foods given to infants, particularly in the Third World, is unlikely to be as high. Protein quality must be taken into account and the suggested way this should be achieved has now changed. The new recommendations, unlike the older ones, advise that when adjusting for protein quality, corrections for both digestibility and amino acid content should be considered.

Whilst, in general, in the adult and older child, only a digestibility correction may be necessary, in the younger child and particularly the infant and toddler, because of enhanced amino acid requirements relating to rapid growth, an amino acid composition correction factor as well as a digestibility correction, frequently become obligatory, especially for protein sources of poorer quality. The FAO/WHO/UNU 1985 report[3] provides detailed information on how this can be achieved and Table 3.5.2 shows the effect of the newer considerations on protein requirements from practical diets in selected parts of the world. The analysis indicates, for example, that children being weaned onto typical food stuffs consumed in Tunisia or India would, according to the FAO/WHO/UNU (1985) recommendations, need some 20–30 per cent more protein than would have been judged adequate on the basic calculations carried out using guide-lines suggested by the earlier committee. This, coupled with the tendency for

Table 3.5.1 A comparison of the daily energy and protein needs of infants estimated by the two United Nations Agency Consultancy Committees. Protein recommendations expressed as milk or egg protein. Reproduced with permission from *Energy and protein requirements*: report of a Joint FAO/WHO Ad hoc Expert Committee, no. 522, WHO, 1973, and *Energy and protein requirements*: report of a Joint FAO/WHO/UNU Expert consultation, no. 724. WHO, 1985.

Age (months)	Energy (kJ/kg)		Protein (g/kg)	
	1971	1981	1971	1981
0–3	500	485	—	—
3–6	480	415	—	1.86
6–9	460	400	1.62	1.65
9–12	440	420	1.44	1.48

Table 3.5.2 A comparison of the daily protein requirements of young children aged 1–1.5 years after correcting typical traditional family diets for both protein quality and digestibility according to FAO/WHO/UNU (1985) or just protein quality as in FAO/WHO (1973). (Source as for Table 3.5.1)

	Protein requirement (g/kg)				
	1971		1981		
Country	Egg	Traditional diet	Egg	Traditional diet	% change between reports
Tunisia*	1.23	2.05	1.26	2.60	+24%
India†	1.23	1.76	1.26	2.13	+21%
United States‡	1.23	1.54	1.26	1.30	−16%

* Assumed 1971 protein score: 60; 1981 digestibility: 85 amino-acid score: 57.

† Assumed 1971 protein score: 70; 1981 digestibility: 81 amino-acid score: 73.

‡ Assumed 1971 protein score: 80; 1981 digestibility: 100 amino-acid score: 97.

lower recommended energy needs, has clear implications for desirable protein concentrations in local weaning foods.

Individual variation

In infants and young children, as well as in adults, there is a fundamental interpretational difference between the estimates we give for energy needs on the one hand, and for protein and other nutrients on the other. With energy, the tabulated requirement value is always for the average individual within the community at a given age. With nutrients, it is the amount calculated to be necessary to cover the needs of the great majority of persons, the value nominally stated being the mean plus 2 SD, or about the 97th centile requirement of the population as a whole. In other words, the recommendation is substantially above the estimated needs of the average individual. This statistical difference between RDAs for dietary energy and the nutrients is of fundamental importance but often ignored, perhaps because of a lack of understanding of the theories behind it.

There are a number of reasons. First, whilst there is a natural hunger and dietary feed-back system operative for energy, it is debatable whether similarly effective mechanisms exist for the other nutrients. Thus, with energy it is reasonable to assume that if one makes available, to a large enough group, sufficient to cover average energy needs then each individual will, over a period of days, automatically have available sufficient of the community food to select his/her specific needs. Clearly with the nutrients, however, in the absence of any biological control mechanism, there would be no reason why the group nutrient supply should be distributed according to each individuals physiological needs. The only safe thing to do under such circumstances is to set the individual recommendation at a value where the needs of virtually all the people in a group would be met. A further practical consideration is that any slight excess intake of nutrients is unlikely to give cause for concern because within the ranges under consideration, no physiological harm should result if the majority of individuals do over-consume nutrients beyond their specific needs, but of course the same assumption cannot be made with energy: even a moderate excess intake would gradually lead to obesity, in this case infantile obesity.

In interpreting the adequacy of the diet of a community, we should thus not expect the average nutrient intake to equal the recommended value, as one would with energy. Rather, under conditions in which intakes happen to equate exactly with RDAs, one would expect the 97th centile intake value to equal the recommended value. Failure to recognize this has led to incorrect use of tables of Recommended Daily Allowances.

RDA tables should never be used, by themselves, to define the extent of nutritional deficiency within a community, nor to diagnose malnutrition of an individual. The only valid conclusion one can make from RDA tables, is that the greater the deficit between the measured intake and the recommended allowance, the greater is the statistical risk that a given intake might be health limiting. The correct way to diagnose a state of dietary deficiency is by direct examination of the people concerned. This point is discussed again later.

Requirements for vitamins and trace elements

Although vitamins and trace elements are required in only relatively small amounts, the young child requires a whole host of these microconstituents for satisfactory growth and development (see also pp. 367–86). The most complete list of vitamin and trace element allowances for infancy, as indeed for people of all ages, is produced by the United States Food and Nutrition Board of the National Academy Sciences, National Research Council (NRC).[10] Although Americans tend to be generous in their recommended allowances, particularly for the vitamins, their conclusions do not vary too dramatically from those of other national and international committees. In the latest NRC (1989)[10] tables, 13 vitamins and 15 minerals are listed. The currently available recommendations of the British Department of Health[24] for infancy and for children aged 1–12 years are summarized in Table 3.5.3. These recommendations are under review, and a wider selection of minerals and vitamins will be included in the new publication.

Safe ranges of intake

For some of the trace elements and the electrolytes (sodium, potassium and chloride), safe ranges are given rather than single figures. This is partly because the information on which the suggested intakes are based is less complete than that used to determine the other RDAs, and the values are more tentative. The NRC also emphasized, however, that it would be unwise to

Table 3.5.3 Recommended daily amounts of micronutrients for the UK during infancy and the early pre-school child period. Reproduced from DHSS, *Recommended Daily Amounts of Food, Energy and Nutrients for Groups of People in the United Kingdom. Report on Health and Social Subjects no. 15.* London, HMSO, 1979, with permission of the Controller of HMSO.

Nutrient	Under 1 year	1 year	2 years
Vitamin A (μg retinol equivalents[a])	450	300	300
Vitamin D (μg cholecal-ciferol)	7.5	10	10
Vitamin C (mg)	20	20	20
Thiamin (mg)	0.3	0.5	0.6
Riboflavin (mg)	0.4	0.6	0.7
Nicotinic acid equivalents[b] (mg)	5	7	8
Calcium (mg)	600	600	600
Iron (mg)	6	7	7

[a] Retinol equivalent = 1 μg retinol or 6 μg β carotene or 12 μg other biologically active carotenoids.
[b] 1 mg nicotinic acid equivalent = 1 mg available nicotinic acid or 60 mg tryptophan.

habitually exceed the upper level of intake of some of the trace elements and so a recommended range is more appropriate.

There is growing recognition that some of the trace elements, e.g. fluoride or selenium, although known to be essential nutrients in small amounts, are also potentially toxic above a critical level. The custom of providing safe ranges rather than single safe amounts is likely to be extended to most of the other nutrients in the deliberations of future expert committees, as similar considerations relating to both deficiency and excess apply. Such an approach should also lead to a better appreciation of the practical purpose behind dietary recommendations.

Nutrient availability from the gastro-intestinal tract

Deficiences of trace elements can arise for a number of reasons, in addition to poor chemical dietary content. The complex problem of reduced nutrient availability is now recognized to be of considerable importance, particularly in the Third World (see pp. 867–8).

Where children or their mothers depend on cereal sources for the majority of their mineral intake, there is the possibility that chelation with phytate or 'dietary fibre' might limit the amount of each mineral available for assimilation. Zinc has been particularly implicated

in this respect, but all of the divalent cations are equally prone to this effect.

Another complicating factor involving the gastro-intestinal tract is that absorption can also be influenced either by metabolic syndromes such as steatorrhea or, alternatively, clinical disorders such as intestinal parasitism.

Metabolic interactions between different nutrients represent a yet further complication.[11] Such interactions tend to occur between minerals of similar atomic make-up. For example, high intakes of elements such as copper or manganese can depress iron absorption because of competition at the intestinal binding sites. Nutrient interactions can, however, be both positive or negative in their effects.

Nutrient interactions involving trace elements also occur with other types of nutrient and not just at an intestinal level. Zinc, for example, is necessary for the mobilization of vitamin A from the liver into plasma and hence to vitamin A status (just one example of many where zinc and vitamin A interact). The amount of iron potentially available from the diet also depends on the overall chemical make-up of diet. While haem iron from animal sources tends to be readily available, the non-haem iron, such as that present in vegetable foods, is much more poorly absorbed. Dietary ascorbic acid can markedly improve the absorption of non-haem iron and meat has a similar potentiating effect.[11]

Thus, it is important to think about dietary requirements, infant feeding and nutritional status, within a broad physiological perspective and not just in terms of simple food composition and dietary intake. As a reasonable generalization, it can be concluded that for as long as the young infant is fed a well-balanced diet, such as breast-milk, the risks of nutrient deficiences are not great. It is usually only when the weaning process is introduced that this becomes a potential problem, especially in the Third World where mothers have a limited variety of local food-stuffs available to them and cannot afford to buy the carefully formulated commercial foods so commonly consumed in the West. Under such circumstances, it is crucial for breast-feeding to continue for as long as possible during weaning as this will remain, for most children, the only chance to 'supplement' their intake of nutritionally inadequate, basic cereal foods and other staples with essential trace elements. In the absence of a high-quality food like milk, either human or cow's, it is very difficult to meet the exacting nutritional recommendations made by expert committees for the infant and young toddler, particularly with respect to minerals such as calcium or zinc.

The importance of nutritious mixes of different types

of food for the older toddler and preschool child is well appreciated in the Third World and a number of valuable community development programmes have been set up to achieve this end, such as the *kitobero* mixtures designed by the Mwanamugimu unit in Uganda.[12] Strictly speaking, however, these have mainly been formulated to ensure a balanced supply of the different amino acids from the various vegetable protein sources: designers have rarely attempted to come to terms with the true complexity of infant dietary needs in the same way as the manufacturers of diets of the more fortunate western babies.

Vitamin and mineral supplements

The scientific basis for setting allowances of the micronutrients is not as well-developed as it is for protein and energy. As a result, expert committees set recommendations which tend to err on the side of safety and set margins which are unnecessarily large. When these recommendations are used for interpretational purposes, measured intakes are frequently found to be substantially lower.

This leads to much controversy and confusion about whether or not to introduce 'therapeutic' supplements of the relevant vitamins and minerals. The answer varies from nutrient to nutrient and from environment to environment. Children brought up in the customary western way will rarely need supplementary vitamin A, for example, as cow's milk, infant formulas, commercial infant cereals and human milk, all contain adequate amounts of retinol and related compounds. In such children a bigger danger is that the supplementary administration of vitamin A may lead to toxicity. This is a good example of where it would be wiser to give a safe range rather than just a safe level of intake in RDA tables. The United States Committees on Drugs and on Nutrition[13] advise against giving more than 10 000 IU per day.

Whilst with vitamin A there is little likelihood of deficiency in the West, routine vitamin D medication is frequently recommended for exclusively breast-fed children because of the small amount present in human milk. Again, the extent to which this really is necessary is debatable. It has been postulated that vitamin D status in early infancy is determined by the vitamin D supplied *in utero* across the placenta, rather than via the diet after birth.[14] Certainly in the rat, newborns have sufficient vitamin D to maintain them throughout lactation.[15] However, no extra vitamin D is necessary for infants fed evaporated milk, whole milk and infant formulas. As with vitamin A, there is a potential risk of toxicity and an upper limit of 400 IU/day has been set in the United States.[16]

In the Third World, however, the quality of a mother's milk depends on her nutritional status, in so far as the vitamins are concerned, and mothers living on diets typical of the deprived sectors within the developing countries may produce milk low in specific vitamin content such as of vitamin A, thiamin, riboflavin, vitamin C and vitamin B_{12}.[17] In such circumstances it is better to supplement the mother, but the attention of paediatricians needs to be drawn to the possibility of such deficiencies in babies breast-fed for extended periods by undernourished mothers.

Assessment of nutritional adequacy of breast-feeding and weaning

There are many gaps in our knowledge concerning the nutritional needs of babies and young toddlers. There is no reason to conclude that a nutritional deficiency state necessarily exists if the measured dietary intake of the wide range of different nutrients does not match the recommended allowance. Where this is suspected it can only be confirmed with any degree of certainty by direct investigation of the children.

Unfortunately detection or diagnosis on clinical grounds, even of advanced deficiency, can be difficult because of the frequent absence of specific diagnostic signs. Equally, biochemical measurements on body fluids and other tissues can be difficult to interpret because of inadequate base-line data on normal tissue values. Additionally, imbalances such as of the trace elements can complicate the interpretation of clinical and biochemical data because of the interactions described above. For example, anaemia can be a manifestation of iron, copper, nickel or cobalt deficiency, or of selenium, zinc or molybdenum excess. Furthermore, in the types of countries where such problems are prevalent, it is least likely that the necessary laboratory sophistication will be available.

Most deficiency states are, however, associated with faltering of growth and for most paediatric investigators anthropometry will remain the most appropriate investigative tool, at least in terms of detecting that something is wrong even if it is not always clear what is the problem. Even with basic anthropometry, however, one is not free from problems relating to adequate interpretational reference data. Paul and colleagues[18,19] have recently pointed out that the current international reference growth curves for infancy, based on the growth of Western children measured a number of years ago, may now be unrepresentative of the type of growth patterns seen in children brought up in accordance with more modern dietary recommendations.

Public health advice on infant feeding and on weaning practices has altered markedly over the past 10 years in the West and, at least among the more educated and well-off sectors of the community, there are signs that this advice is being acted upon. Progressively more babies are being breast-fed and the introduction of solids is now occurring much later. The probable effect that this has had in lowering total energy intake has already been referred to and there is evidence that this has had subtle but important effects on the pattern of growth. These are important for the interpretation of corresponding Third World data.

The basic principle behind using growth curves for assessing the adequacy of breast-feeding and weaning practices, is that a given child or community of children should grow parallel to one of the centile lines of a set of reference data. The size of the individual child, and even of the population mean of the community under investigation, might be greater or smaller than the 50th reference centile but the basic assumption is that the centile lines represent the ideal pattern of change with age. The guide-lines most frequently used for this purpose are the WHO reference centiles,[20] based in turn on the NCHS standards of the United States.[21] What is not always appreciated, however, is that the basic data for these standards were collected between 1929 and 1975 and the great majority of the children aged 0–3 years used were bottle-fed from an early age and weaning solids were given early, even from one month or less. A number of studies of growth among healthy babies in Europe, America and Australia have indicated that patterns of both weight, height and skin fold growth and development have changed now that breast-feeding is becoming popular again and solids are not being commenced until three to six months. The importance of these new findings has been reviewed by Whitehead and Paul.[18] Arguably, if growth standards based on over-fed babies are used to judge the growth of babies who are initially breast-fed and not introduced to weaning foods until after four months, there is a danger that the onset of diet-induced poor growth might be suspected when it should not be.

As might have been anticipated with the lower dietary energy intake, skin fold thicknesses and measures of adiposity are affected the most. Fig. 3.5.5 provides an idea of how the distribution of the values for triceps and subscapular skin fold thickness in Cambridge, UK, children[19] who were studied in the 1980s, compared with the Tanner values[22] for the same measurements collected earlier; there are substantial differences. The Cambridge data are essentially the same as those in studies published from Germany and Australia.[18]

Not only is adiposity affected but so is growth in weight and height. Fig. 3.5.6 shows the corresponding Cambridge, UK, data for boys' weights compared with the NCHS references but divided into those who were given solids before and after four months. This analysis of contemporary data illustrates well the marked influence of weaning practices on infant growth. The

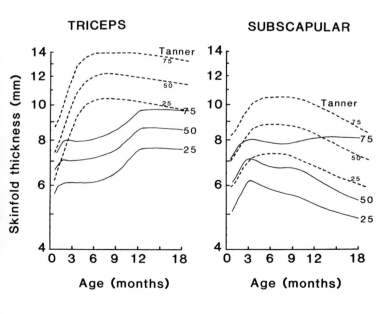

Fig. 3.5.5 The range (25–75th centiles) of triceps and subscapular skin fold thicknesses among Cambridge (UK) infant boys in comparison with the standards for British children produced by Tanner and Whitehouse. (Data reproduced from *Acta Paediatrica Scandanavica*, 1986; **233**: 14–23 and *American Journal of Clinical Nutrition*, 1985; **41**: 459–63 © American Society for Clinical Nutrition.)

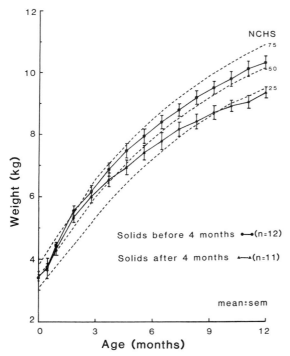

Fig. 3.5.6 Growth in weight of Cambridge (UK) boys, initially breast-fed who started weaning before and after four months. (Reproduced from *Acta Pediatrica Scandanavica*, 1986; **233**: 14–23.) Reference curves are from *NCHS*, 1977, pp. 78–1650.

children weaned after four months were essentially being fed in accordance with current dietary recommendations, and if larger amounts of data on similarly fed children could be collected, it would surely represent a more rational reference for the pattern of change in growth. A similar slippage across growth centile lines to that seen in Fig. 3.5.6 has been demonstrated for length as well as for weight for length.[19]

These data were derived from relatively small-scale studies, the aim having been merely to test various hypotheses relating to diet and growth, not to produce new growth standards. The results do caution paediatricians and paediatric investigators not to interpret their clinic and community growth data, particularly on Third World infants and toddlers, in an uncritical manner.

Whilst the Cambridge, UK, growth data cannot be looked upon as providing an adequate new reference for infant growth, it is salutary to see what would happen if existing young child growth data in the literature were interpreted on the basis of NCHS reference centiles, on the one hand, and the Cambridge data on the other. In such a comparison it would be assumed that the onset of a distinct and persistent downward trend in growth relative to the standard, represented the time when the

'mixture' of breast-milk and weaning foods begin to become nutritionally inadequate.[18] In a set of data from a relatively well-off urban community in The Gambia,[23] this would have been two months on the basis of NCHS, but four months with Cambridge babies as a reference. A similar re-interpretation, indicating a later age when public health action might be merited, was demonstrated for a number of countries including Papua New Guinea and Kenya.[18]

Conclusions

Knowledge of what is nutritionally the best for the infant and young preschool child is by no means as well-defined scientifically as it should be. Hence, it is not possible to provide the type of cast-iron advice that many would wish. However, this early period of growth is particularly dynamic and in the past its true complexity has tended to be over-simplified. This situation would appear to be changing and the reader is encouraged to keep abreast of new nutritional and anthropometric data being produced in this crucially important area of human biology and public health.

References

1. DHSS. Present day practice in infant feeding, 1980. *Report on Health and Social Subjects No. 20.* London, HM Stationery Office, 1983.
2. Barrell RAE, Rowland MGM. Commercial milk products and indigenous weaning foods in a rural West African environment: a bacteriological perspective. *Journal of Hygiene* (Cambridge). 1980; **84**: 191–202.
3. FAO/WHO/UNU. Energy and protein requirements. *World Health Organization Technical Report Series No. 724.* Geneva, WHO, 1985.
4. FAO/WHO. Energy and protein requirements. *World Health Organization Technical Report Series No. 522.* Geneva, WHO, 1973.
5. Whitehead, RG. The human weaning process. *Pediatrics.* 1985; **75** (suppl.): 189–93.
6. Lucas A, Gibbs JAH, Baum JD. The biology of drip breast milk. *Early Human Development.* 1978; **2/4**: 351–61.
7. Whitehead RG, Paul AA, Cole TJ. A critical analysis of measured food energy intakes during infancy and early childhood in comparison with current international recommendations. *Journal of Human Nutrition.* 1981; **35**: 339–48.
8. Raiha NCR. Protein in the nutrition of the preterm infant: biochemical and nutritional considerations. *Advances in Nutritional Research.* 1980; **3**: 173–206.
9. Whitehead RG. Infant physiology, nutritional requirements and lactational adequacy. *American Journal of Clinical Nutrition.* 1985; **41**: 447–58.
10. Food and Nutrition Board. *Recommended Dietary Allowances*, 10th Edn. Washington DC, National Academy of Sciences, National Research Council, 1989.

11. Levander OA, Cheng L (Eds). Micronutrient interactions: vitamins, minerals and hazardous elements. *Annals of the New York Academy of Sciences.* 1980; **72**: 355.

12. Alleyne GAO, Hay RW, Picou DI, Stanfield JP, Whitehead RG. In: Whitehead RG ed. *Protein–Energy Malnutrition.* London, Edward Arnold, 1977.

13. American Academy of Pediatrics. Joint committee statement of committees on drugs and on nutrition. *Pediatrics.* 1971; **48**: 655.

14. Fraser DR. The physiological economy of vitamin D. *Lancet.* 1983; **i**: 969–72.

15. Clements MR, Fraser DR. Quantitative aspects of vitamin D supply to the rat fetus and neonate. *Calcified Tissue International.* 1984; **36** (suppl. 2): S31 (abstract).

16. American Academy of Pediatrics. Committee on Nutrition: The prophylactic requirement and the toxicity of Vitamin D. *Pediatrics.* 1963; **31**: 512–25.

17. Fomon SJ, Strauss RG. Nutrient deficiencies in breast-fed infants. *New England Journal of Medicine.* 1978; **299**: 355–7.

18. Whitehead RG, Paul AA. Growth charts and the assessment of infant feeding practices in the Western World and in developing countries. *Early Human Development.* 1984; **9**: 187–207.

19. Whitehead RG, Paul AA, Ahmed EA. Weaning practices in the United Kingdom and variations in anthropometric development. In: Wharton BA ed. Food for the Weanling. *Acta Paediatrica Scandinavica.* 1986; Suppl. 233: 14–23.

20. WHO. *A Growth Chart for International Use in Maternal and Child Health Care.* Geneva, WHO, 1978.

21. Hamill PVV. *NCHS Growth Curves for Children, Birth to 18 Years.* US Department of Health, Education and Welfare Publication PHS, 1977. pp. 78–165.

22. Tanner JM, Whitehouse RM. Revised standards for triceps and subscapular skinfolds in British children. *Archives of Disease in Childhood.* 1975; **50**: 142–5.

23. Rowland MGM. The 'why' and the 'when' of introducing food to infants: growth in young breast-fed infants and some nutritional implications. *American Journal of Clinical Nutrition.* 1985; **41**: 459–63.

24. DHSS. *Recommended Daily Amounts of food Energy and Nutrients for Groups of People in the United Kingdom. Report on Health and Social Subjects No. 5.* London, HM Stationary Office, 1979.

PROTEIN-ENERGY MALNUTRITION
V. Reddy

Nutritional deficiencies constitute major public health problems in the tropical and subtropical regions of the world. Though the deficiency diseases are primarily due to inadequate diets, they are closely related to the poor socio-economic and environmental conditions prevailing in these areas. Among these, protein–energy malnutrition (PEM) is the most widespread. It affects mostly children under five years of age, as their nutritional requirements are relatively greater than those of adults.

PEM is particularly serious postweaning and is often associated with infection. Respiratory infection and diarrhoea are the most common diseases that precipitate severe PEM and death.

The high prevalence of malnutrition not only takes a heavy toll on life but can also impose severe handicap on survivors. There is evidence to suggest that PEM has lasting effects on growth and development of children, learning ability, social adjustment, work efficiency and productivity of labour. Thus, malnutrition has serious repercussions for human development and national productivity (see pp. 867-8).

Terminology

As the name suggests, protein–energy malnutrition results from deficiency of protein and energy as calories in the diet. Strictly speaking it is not one disease but a range of pathological conditions arising from inadequate diet. A number of terms have been used in the past, and some are still in use, to describe the various clinical syndromes that are now recognized to be only variants of PEM.

The term kwashiorkor was first introduced by Dr Cicely Williams in 1935. This is a local term used by the Ga tribe in Accra, West Africa, meaning sickness of the weanling. The other terms used in those early years, when the aetiology of the condition was not fully understood, include 'infantile pellagra', 'nutritional oedema' and 'nutritional dystrophy'. Later, the term 'protein malnutrition' was introduced when it became widely accepted that kwashiorkor was due to a deficiency of protein in the diet. More recently, recognizing the importance of calorie deficiency in the aetiology of this condition, the term has been changed to protein–calorie malnutrition or protein–energy malnutrition.[1] This expression reflects the current concept that both protein and energy deficiencies are the causative factors.

PEM covers a wide spectrum of clinical stages, the extreme forms being kwashiorkor and marasmus, while the milder forms express themselves as varying degrees of growth retardation. The manifestations vary, depending upon the severity and duration of the deficiency and the age of the child. Superimposed infection and other concomitant nutritional deficiencies further complicate the picture. This explains why no complete agreement exists among clinicians with regard to the terminology and classification of PEM. The more typical syndromes seen in advanced stages of the disease are, however, easy to identify. These include kwashiorkor, marasmus and marasmic kwashiorkor.

Kwashiorkor

Kwashiorkor is characterized by oedema, apathy and low body weight. In addition, there may be dermatosis, hair changes, hepatomegaly, diarrhoea and mental changes.

Marasmus

This condition is characterized by very low body weight, loss of subcutaneous fat, muscle wasting and absence of oedema. When an infant below one year of age develops this condition, often as a result of early weaning, it is described as 'infantile marasmus'. The same condition seen in an older child, which is mainly due to insufficient food, is termed 'late marasmus'.

Marasmic kwashiorkor

Combined forms with clinical signs of both marasmus and kwashiorkor are included here. They show gross wasting as well as oedema.

Classification

Several methods have been suggested for the classification of PEM (see pp. 254-80). The choice of classification depends on the purpose for which it is used, for example in clinical studies or community surveys.

Classification for clinical purposes

On the basis of the clinical picture, patients with severe PEM are classified into three groups: kwashiorkor, marasmus and marasmic kwashiorkor.[2] McLaren and co-workers proposed a scoring system in which points were given for various clinical signs such as oedema, dermatosis and hair changes. However, this classification has been criticized since equal weighting was given to clinical signs which do not have the same importance.[3] A simple-classification is that proposed by the Wellcome Working Party. In this, reduction in body weight below 80 per cent of the Harvard standard (50th centile) is considered as malnutrition. This corresponds approximately to the Harvard third centile. Only two criteria are used to classify the malnourished children — the presence or absence of oedema and the deficit in body weight. This gives rise to four groups as shown in Table 3.5.4.

Children with oedema who weigh between 60 and 80 per cent of the expected weight for age are classified as kwashiorkor. It was recognized, however, that children

Table 3.5.4 Wellcome classification of malnutrition

Malnutrition	Body weight (% of standard*)	Oedema
Underweight	80–60	–
Marasmus	<60	–
Kwashiorkor	80–60	+
Marasmic kwashiorkor	<60	+

*50th centile of Harvard Standard. (Reproduced from Wellcome Trust Working Party. *Lancet*, 1970; **ii**: 302.)

with oedema and other signs of kwashiorkor should be so classified even if their body weight is more than 80 per cent of the standard.

Those without oedema and weighing less than 60 per cent of the standard are considered to have marasmus. Children with oedema and a body weight less than 60 per cent of the standard are diagnosed as marasmic kwashiorkor. Children without oedema weighing 60–80 per cent of the standard are simply classified as underweight.

Classification for community surveys

The most widely used classification of PEM is that suggested by Gomez. It is based on the deficit in weight for age, and 90 per cent of the Harvard Standard is taken as the cut-off point for separating normal from the malnourished children. Malnutrition is subdivided into three degrees as shown in Table 3.5.5.

First, second and third-degree malnutrition are defined as 75–90 per cent, 60–75 per cent and < 60 per cent respectively, of expected weight for age. Jelliffe proposed a modification of this classification with four groups at intervals of 10 per cent of body weight deficit.[26] Bengoa included all cases with oedema in third-degree malnutrition, regardless of body weight.[5]

Classification on the basis of weight for age is useful to assess the magnitude of the problem in a community. However, it does not indicate the duration or type of malnutrition. Moreover, difficulties may be encountered in some communities where the precise ages of the children are not known.

The Joint FAO/WHO Expert Committee on Nutrition emphasized that height deficit in relation to age

Table 3.5.5 Gomez classification of malnutrition

Malnutrition	Body weight (% of standard*)
First degree	75–90
Second degree	60–75
Third degree	<60

* 50th centile of Harvard Standard. (Reproduced from Gomez F et al. *Journal of Tropical Pediatrics*; 1956; 2: 77.)

may be regarded as a measure of the duration of malnutrition.[1] The expression of weight in relation to height gives a measure of nutritional status which is independent of age and of age-related external standards.

Weight for height is an index of current nutritional status while height for age gives a picture of past nutritional history. Seoane and Latham's[4] classification is based on this concept (Table 3.5.6). In this system, malnourished children are classified into three major categories: 1, current short-term or acute malnutrition; 2, current long-term or chronic malnutrition; and 3, past malnutrition or nutritional dwarf.

The term 'stunted' is suggested to describe deficit in height for age and 'wasted' for the deficit in weight for height.[3] Both are the results of malnutrition and most children present a combination of the two. Most community surveys now use 80 per cent weight for age as the level below which 'wasting' malnutrition is defined and 90 per cent height for age as the level below which 'stunting' malnutrition is defined.

Prevalence

PEM is highly prevalent in almost all developing countries. About 1–7 per cent of children below five years suffer from the severe forms of malnutrition like kwashiorkor and marasmus. The occurrence of severe cases even in small numbers is an indication of a much larger number of mild and moderate, frequently unrecognized, forms of malnutrition.

Many community surveys have been conducted over the years to estimate the prevalence of PEM. Unfortunately, most of these cover a limited area or too few children to give accurate information about the size of the problem. Taking only those surveys that cover at least 1000 children, a rough estimate of the prevalence has been made.[5] The results for each continent are given in Table 3.5.7. The prevalence of severe forms

Table 3.5.6 Seoane and Latham's classification of malnutrition

	Weight for age	Height for age	Weight for height
1. Acute or current short-term malnutrition (wasted)	Low	Normal	Low
2. Chronic or long-term malnutrition (wasted and stunted)	Low	Low	Low
3. Past malnutrition or nutrition dwarf (stunted)	Low	Low	Normal

(Reproduced from *Journal of Tropical Paediatrics*, 1971; **17**: 98–104, Oxford University Press.)

Table 3.5.7   Estimated prevalence of PEM (community surveys)

Area	No. children examined	Severe forms Range (%)	Severe forms Median (%)	Moderate forms Range (%)	Moderate forms Median (%)
Latin America	109 000	0.5–6.3	1.6	3.5–32.0	18.9
Africa	25 000	1.7–9.8	4.4	5.4–44.9	26.5
Asia	39 000	1.1–20.0	3.2	16.0–46.4	31.2
Total	173 000	0.5–20.0	2.6	3.5–46.4	18.9

(Reproduced from Beaton GH and Bengoa JM, *Nutrition in Preventive Medicine. The major deficiency syndromes, epidemiology and approaches to control*, Geneva, WHO, 1976, WHO monograph series no 62.)

ranges from 0.5 to 20.0 per cent and that of moderate PEM is 3.5 to 46.4 per cent.

The relative frequency of kwashiorkor and marasmus shows considerable geographic variation.[1] Nation-wide prevalences often are of little value in defining the factors causing malnutrition. Breast-feeding and weaning practices play an important role in determining the age distribution and the type of malnutrition observed. Infantile marasmus is more common in Chile and other Latin American countries where early weaning is common, while in African countries kwashiorkor is more common (Table 3.5.8). Recent reports from Africa, however, indicate a changing pattern with a decline in kwashiorkor and increase in marasmus. This has been attributed to the changing trends in infant feeding practices. In India and other Asian countries where prolonged breast-feeding is common, protein–energy malnutrition is seen after one year of age, kwashiorkor and marasmus being equally common.[6]

Aetiology

Protein–energy malnutrition results from the interaction of several factors of which inadequate diets and

Table 3.5.8   Regional differences in the pattern of PEM (hospital cases)

Country	Percentage of cases classified as: Kwashiorkor	Marasmus	Unspecified
Chile	3	97	—
Iran	33	66	—
Jamaica	32	34	34
Jordan	24	15	61
Senegal	45	55	—
South Africa	96	4	—
Sudan	92	8	—
Thailand	44	46	10

infectious diseases are most important. Children of preschool age are most seriously affected because their nutritional requirements are proportionately higher than those of adults and also for cultural reasons they are frequently given a less nutritious diet than that consumed by older individuals. The incidence of infections is also high in this age group.

Diet

It has long been held that kwashiorkor and marasmus are two separate entities arising as a result of differences in the protein–calorie ratio of the habitual diet. The theory is that a diet predominantly deficient in protein and relatively adequate in calories leads to kwashiorkor, while a diet deficient in calories and adequate in protein results in marasmus. This may be true to a certain extent. In Chile where early weaning is common, the infants are fed diluted milk formulae causing infantile marasmus, whereas in Uganda where young children are fed a traditional diet based on plantain (matooke) which is low in protein, typical cases of kwashiorkor are seen. A number of animal experiments provided confirmatory evidence for the importance of the protein–energy ratio of the diet in the development of these two syndromes. However, this theory does not explain the situation in other parts of the world where PEM is widespread.

In India, where cereals form the staple food, the primary bottleneck in the diets of children is calories and not protein. When the protein intake is adequate but calorie intake is not, some of the protein will be used for energy, leading to conditioned protein deficiency. The term 'protein–energy malnutrition' is, therefore, used to describe the condition.

Careful diet surveys in preschool children revealed no differences between the dietary patterns of children who develop kwashiorkor and those who become marasmic.[6] In view of these observations the earlier theory of two separate dietary aetiologies for these clinical syndromes has been questioned. It has been proposed that these are two facets of the same disease and that the body's ability to adapt to the nutritional stress may determine the course of events.[6, 7] Successful adaptation would result in marasmus while failure to adapt leads to kwashiorkor.

More recent evidence[24] has pointed to excess oxidative stress as a possible cause of the kwashiorkor syndrome in malnutrition. Free oxygen radicals, potentially toxic to cell membranes, are produced during infections or as a result of ingesting aflatoxin (a toxin produced by the *Aspergillus flavus* group of fungi which grow in moist, warm conditions on stored grain and groundnuts). Iron has also been implicated in the production of free oxygen radicals as the iron is reduced. These oxides are normally buffered by protein and 'mopped up' by anti-oxidants, such as vitamins A, C and E, glutathione, zinc and selenium. In the malnourished child, lack of these nutrients, in the presence of infection or aflatoxin, may result in the toxic accumulation of free oxygen radicals. These may then damage liver, epithelial and other cells, giving rise to kwashiorkor. In areas where the aflatoxin content of food is high, appreciable levels of aflatoxin and its toxic metabolites have been found in serum, urine and breast-milk; and much more frequently and in much higher levels in children with kwashiorkor.[25] As yet, all this remains unproven, but would explain some still unresolved questions concerning the causation of kwashiorkor. If proven, it will have considerable implications in the treatment and prevention of kwashiorkor.

Role of hormones

In adaptation to any physiological stress, hormones play an important role. Determination of circulating levels of cortisol and growth hormone could help in understanding the mechanisms involved in a possible adaptation process. Plasma levels of cortisol are raised in severe PEM and are much higher in marasmus than in kwashiorkor. Raised cortisol levels lead to breakdown of muscle protein and the amino acids released are diverted to the liver for the synthesis of plasma proteins. The plasma concentration of β-lipoproteins is well maintained facilitating mobilization of triglycerides from the liver. Thus, the metabolic integrity of the liver remains unimpaired in marasmus (Fig. 3.5.7).

On the other hand, when plasma cortisol fails to reach high levels, muscle protein is not mobilized and plasma concentrations of amino acids remain low. This may operate as a feed-back stimulating the pituitary gland to secrete high quantities of growth hormone. The lipolytic action of growth hormone gives rise to high levels of plasma free fatty acid. Because of reduced synthesis of lipoproteins, fat accumulates in the liver and the impaired hepatic function gives rise to the biochemical changes and oedema characteristic of kwashiorkor (Fig. 3.5.8).

The response of the adrenal cortex may thus be crucial in the evolution of kwashiorkor and marasmus. The failure of plasma cortisol to be maintained at a sufficiently high level to mobilize muscle protein, may represent the major biochemical event concerned with 'dysadaptation' resulting in a transition from marasmus to marasmic kwashiorkor. However, the factors which contribute to the breakdown of adaptation need to be further explored. An abrupt and drastic reduction in the quantity of food consumed, which is already low, may be an important factor. Repeated episodes of infection superimposed on chronic malnutrition may be another.

Role of infection

Kwashiorkor is often preceded by an episode of infection, with diarrhoea and respiratory infection being the most common precipitating factors. Community studies carried out in South India showed that a peak incidence of kwashiorkor was preceded by a peak incidence of diarrhoea. Repeated attacks of diarrhoea were shown to be responsible for poor growth of Guatemalan children and was found to be the most significant infection contributing to malnutrition in Gambian children. Weight faltering was most dramatic during the weaning period, when the diarrhoea incidence was maximum.

Measles is the other common infectious disease affecting children in developing countries. The impact of measles is more than that of other infections because of secondary complications and prolonged illness. In longitudinal studies reported from India, the children not only showed weight loss and hypoalbuminaemia during illness but their growth rate was low for several months after recovery. Frequent episodes of infection were observed in these children for nearly six months after the attack of measles and this could partly account for the slow growth. In Bangladesh, greatest weight loss was seen in children with measles complicated by prolonged diarrhoea. In Zaire, childhood infections, especially measles, were traced in more than half the children in the weeks immediately preceding kwashiorkor.[5] Similar observations concerning the effects of other infections like chickenpox, whooping cough, tuberculosis and malaria have been made in other parts of the world.

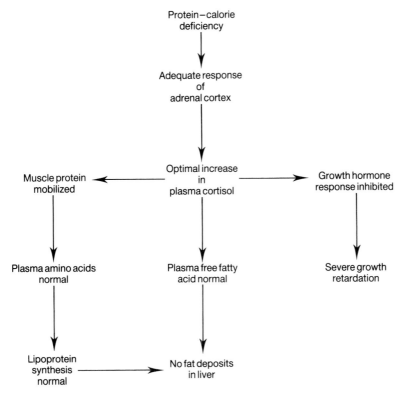

Protein–calorie
deficiency

Adequate response
of
adrenal cortex

Muscle protein
mobilized

Optimal increase
in
plasma cortisol

Growth hormone
response inhibited

Plasma amino acids
normal

Plasma free fatty
acid normal

Severe growth
retardation

Lipoprotein
synthesis
normal

No fat deposits
in liver

Fig. 3.5.7 The evolution of marasmus.

There are several mechanisms by which infection can adversely affect the nutritional status. During acute infection, appetite is usually impaired and the food intake is reduced. Apart from this, dietary restriction is often imposed by the mother as it is generally believed that food intake may aggravate the disease. In Guatemalan children, a significant reduction in calorie intake was observed during diarrhoeal episodes and this was associated with weight loss. Similar observations have been made in Bangladesh. The calorie deficit was found to be more than 30 per cent in children with acute diarrhoea and this could be overcome partially by encouraging them to eat more.

Apart from reduced food intake, malabsorption of nutrients and metabolic losses during infection can aggravate malnutrition. Metabolic studies in patients with acute diarrhoea substantiated malabsorption of fat and nitrogen.[8] There is also evidence of negative nitrogen balance during acute infection. Frank protein-losing enteropathy has been reported in measles enteritis. In a well-nourished child whose dietary intake is adequate, these nutrient losses are of little con-

sequence. In an undernourished child subsisting on a marginal diet, the infective episode can tip the balance towards overt malnutrition.

Socio-economic factors

PEM is primarily a problem of poor countries and of the poorest sections of the community within those countries. Inadequate diets, poor housing and high incidences of infections are the inevitable consequences of poverty. Most women in these communities work in the fields from dawn to dusk and young children are looked after by older siblings or grandmothers. Thus, the children are deprived of maternal care and attention at a critical time. Not surprisingly, higher incidence of kwashiorkor has been reported in children belonging to large families and high birth orders.

While it is undeniable that the major factor responsible for poor diets is the economic status of the families, faulty feeding habits (including infrequent meals after weaning) arising from ignorance and prejudices also

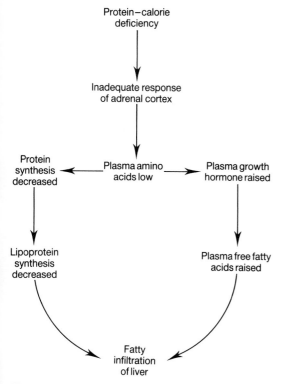

Protein–calorie
deficiency

↓

Inadequate response
of adrenal cortex

↓

Protein synthesis decreased ← Plasma amino acids low → Plasma growth hormone raised

↓ Lipoprotein synthesis decreased

Plasma free fatty acids raised

Fatty infiltration of liver

Fig. 3.5.8 The evolution of kwashiorkor.

contribute significantly. The concept of 'hot' and 'cold' foods is common in India and other Asian countries, for example, eggs are considered hot and avoided during summer. Citrus fruits are believed to cause common colds and coughs. Papaya fruit is avoided during pregnancy as it is believed to produce abortion. These superstitions and taboos concerning food are powerful social factors which influence nutrition.

Pathological changes

Autopsy studies in children dying of severe PEM have shown structural changes in many organs, particularly the liver and pancreas and the thymolymphatic system.[2]

Liver

Fatty infiltration of the liver is characteristic of kwashiorkor, while in marasmus changes are minimal. The fat appears first as small droplets, which coalesce to form large globules filling the cell and pushing the

nucleus towards the cell membrane. Large cysts resulting from fusion of several fatty cells have been observed in severe cases. This change is first noted at the periphery of the liver lobules around the portal tract and then spreads towards the central vein until it affects the whole parenchyma of the liver. Fatty liver is more common in some areas than in others. In Jamaica, severe fatty infiltration was found to be associated with a fatal outcome in kwashiorkor.

The liver cells, though distended, rarely undergo necrosis. Varying degrees of cellular infiltration are seen within the portal tracts and sinusoids, with increased reticulin-staining of fibrous tissue between the lobules. All these changes are completely reversed with treatment.

It has been suggested that malnutrition during childhood may lead to cirrhosis of the liver in later life. However, liver biopsies taken during recovery from kwashiorkor have shown fairly rapid resolution. Long-term follow-up studies have confirmed that fatty liver does not lead to fibrosis. Cirrhosis of the liver has been reported in association with kwashiorkor but this could well be the result of coincidental viral hepatitis.

Pancreas

Children with severe PEM show marked atrophy of the pancreas. Acinar cells shrink, zymogen granules disappear and the nuclei become pyknotic. The extensive acinar atrophy contrasts with the clearly visible inter-calated ducts. A varying degree of duct proliferation is seen, especially in those children who die of severe gastro-intestinal infection.[9]

The pancreas might be expected to suffer permanent damage in the presence of such severe atrophy. Pancreatic calcification often associated with mild diabetes in adults, has been ascribed to childhood malnutrition. However, there is no evidence for the long-term effects on the pancreas. Rapid improvement in the histology with appearance of zymogen granules has been observed following treatment. The enzyme activity in pancreatic secretion also shows rapid increase indicating that the effects of malnutrition can be reversed with adequate treatment.

Kidney

The size of the kidney is reduced considerably in children dying of severe PEM. A variety of pathological lesions have been described in the kidney but these may be related to the associated infection. Pyelonephritic lesions with scarring of the medulla and focal areas of calcification have been observed at autopsy.

Another common finding is cloudy swelling of the epithelial cells of the tubules. This is more marked in the proximal tubules where the epithelium shows hydropic degeneration.[2] Glomerular changes like thickening of the basement membrane and increased cellularity of the capillary tuft have also been described. Follow-up renal biopsy studies after recovery showed marked improvement, suggesting that all these changes are reversible.

Gastro-intestinal tract

The mucosa of the small intestine undergoes atrophic changes in kwashiorkor, reducing the total absorption surface.[2] The villi are shortened and the crypt/villus ratio is increased. This change in mucosal pattern is, however, non-specific and common in most tropical areas of the world. Histologically, the epithelial cells lose their columnar shape to become cuboidal and the brush border loses its fine organization and becomes atrophic. Varying degrees of inflammatory cell infiltration are seen in the lamina propria. In marasmic infants, the mucosal appearance has been found to be normal but the mitotic index is significantly lower than in kwashiorkor and normal controls.

The marked atrophy of intestinal mucosa and the exocrine pancreas, the depletion of enzyme activities and decreased concentration of conjugated bile salts in the upper jejunum may be expected to reduce absorption in kwashiorkor. However, the total mucosal function is still adequate for the absorption of necessary nutrients, allowing rapid and complete recovery on treatment.

Thymolymphatic system

The thymus is greatly reduced in size in children dying of severe PEM. There is a considerable reduction in cortical lymphoid cells and replacement with loose fibrous tissue. The degree of thymic atrophy correlates closely with the depletion of lymphocytes and loss of germinal centres in the lymph nodes of the mesentery, spleen, appendix and Peyer's patches. Tonsil size is significantly smaller in children with PEM. The size of the spleen is also reduced. Decrease in thymus-dependent lymphocytes is associated with impaired cell-mediated immunity in PEM. On the other hand, B lymphocytes responsible for humoral immunity do not seem to be affected.

Muscle

A marked reduction in muscle mass has been observed in children with severe PEM.[2] Comparison of transverse sections of sartorius muscle revealed structural differences between malnourished and well-nourished infants. Both muscle bundles and individual fibres were reduced proportionately. Intermysial connective tissue was increased and crowding of the arterioles and capillaries produced an apparent increase in vascularity. No inflammatory changes were present. Individual muscle fibres showed degenerative changes like swelling, hyalinization and loss of striations.

Biopsy studies of gastrocnemii in children with kwashiorkor, showed a good correlation between the degree of clinical wasting and histological evidence of atrophy. Repeat biopsies one month after treatment did not show much change, despite the general clinical improvement. Loss of muscle fibres in severe PEM has raised the question as to whether the deficit might be permanent. This possibility was contradicted, however, by studies in which muscle DNA used as an estimate of nuclear mass showed no change during malnutrition.[2]

Heart

It has been shown by radiography that heart size is reduced in kwashiorkor. Electrocardiographic changes in the ST segment and T wave suggest non-specific myocardial damage. Autopsy studies reveal atrophic changes in heart as in other muscles. The myocardial fibres show variation in size with vacuolation within the cells and fading of striations. Patchy necrosis of individual fibrils surrounded by scanty cellular infiltration have been observed but these changes are not specific. Following treatment, the heart recovers completely and no late effects of malnutrition on the myocardium have been reported (see p. 781).

Haematological changes

Some degree of anaemia is always found in children with severe malnutrition. In most cases this is moderate with haemoglobin values around $10 \, g \, dl^{-1}$ and the blood picture shows normocytic, slightly hypochromic red blood cells. Allen and Dean found good correlation between haemoglobin levels and plasma proteins.[27] Reticulocyte response and increased erythroid activity on diet therapy alone suggests that the anaemia may be due to protein deficiency. Associated deficiency of other haemopoietic factors like iron and folic acid also contribute to the anaemia in kwashiorkor. Iron deficiency leads to microcytic anaemia with no stainable iron in the bone marrow. Megaloblastic marrow may be seen as a result of associated folate deficiency. Vitamin B_{12} deficiency is, however, rare. Serum B_{12} levels are actually increased in PEM. Anaemias responding to treatment with riboflavin and vitamin E have also been reported. Multiplicity of aetiological factors may explain the variability in the type of anaemia reported from different parts of the world.

Biochemical and functional changes

A number of biochemical changes in the blood and tissues have been described in PEM.[10, 11] These changes vary with the severity of malnutrition as well as type of malnutrition.

Body fluids

Oedema in kwashiorkor implies accumulation of body fluids. Increase in total body water has been estimated by many workers. Most of the excess water lies in the extracellular compartment.[10, 11] With loss of oedema during recovery, there is a marked reduction of extracellular fluid, some of which may shift to the intracellular space. In Jamaica, however, no change was noted in intracellular fluid following recovery. The plasma volume is increased, but it is not clear whether this is a feature primarily of malnutrition or related more to anaemia, since there is a close correlation between plasma volume and venous haematocrit.[11]

The role of plasma proteins in the pathogenesis of oedema is not clear. According to the original theory, an inadequate intake of protein leads to hypo-albuminaemia, which in turn causes oedema. This has been questioned in recent years. Although hypo-albuminaemia is a constant feature of oedematous patients, there is no correlation between serum albumin levels and severity of oedema. During recovery, oedema disappears rapidly long before the albumin concentration is restored to normal. It is, therefore, suggested that apart from hypoalbuminaemia, other factors may be involved in the pathogenesis of oedema. These include hormonal changes, electrolyte imbalance and altered renal function.

Indian workers have suggested that increased secretion, or failure of inactivation, of the antidiuretic hormone (ADH) is an important factor. ADH levels in plasma and urine were significantly higher in children with kwashiorkor than in marasmic children. Following therapy and disappearance of oedema, the hormone levels returned to normal. However, two objections have been raised to this explanation for oedema.[10] First,

increased ADH would lead to concentrated urine while the urine of malnourished children is more dilute than that of well-nourished controls. In addition, there is no evidence that increased ADH activity leads to oedema in any clinical or experimental situations. Aldosterone has also been implicated in the production of oedema but there is no convincing evidence for this.

An alternate theory is that the body fluid changes are basically renal in origin.[11] Inability of the kidneys to excrete the sodium load is believed to be the primary cause of oedema. This possibility is more likely in view of the altered renal function described in PEM. Decreased glomerular filtration rate, lower renal plasma flow and reduced osmolar filtration rate are some of the abnormalities recorded.

Recent evidence that the accumulation of free oxygen radicals can damage cell membranes and may cause oedema has already been mentioned (see p. 339).

Sodium

Several studies of sodium concentration have reported it as low or normal. It is agreed, however, that a low serum sodium level is a bad prognostic sign.[10] The sodium content of erythrocytes has been reported to be higher than normal. Muscle analysis also indicated an increase in intracellular sodium concentration. The cause of this intracellular accumulation of sodium is not known. Estimations of the intracellular concentration of any substance must be viewed with caution, since there is no good evidence that the usual markers such as chloride or bromide maintain their normal distribution when cell function is disturbed.[10]

Potassium

Much more information is available on the potassium status of malnourished children. Potassium concentration of erythrocytes and plasma has been found to be reduced in kwashiorkor. Metabolic balance studies and analysis of muscle biopsy specimens have indicated potassium deficiency in PEM. Studies with the whole body counter have confirmed this. In general, malnourished children have low total body potassium concentration which rises to normal levels after four to six weeks of therapy. After the initial period of treatment, in which any deficits have been corrected, the level of body potassium rises slowly and this rise is now correlated with the protein intake. Approximately 3 mEq potassium are retained per gram of nitrogen.

Although there is a close relationship between muscle potassium and total body potassium this is not a simple linear relationship. It is now clear that in assessing potassium status, the capacity of the body for potassium in relation to the actual body content must be considered. The potassium capacity is a reflection or indirect measure of the intracellular protein which effectively binds potassium. If that capacity is saturated, an individual is in normal potassium balance. Obviously if that capacity is reduced, but still saturated, the individual cannot really be said to be potassium deficient even though the total body potassium is low compared with the normal. These concepts have been proved in protein–calorie malnutrition. When the body potassium is below 30 mEq/kg, there is certainly a genuine potassium deficiency and muscle potassium levels are uniformly very low. However, when the body potassium is between 30 and 40 mEq/kg, i.e. still below 'normal', there is usually a marginal or no true potassium deficiency and muscle potassium is nearly normal. In this situation, body potassium will rise to the normal level of 45 mEq/kg when the child grows and synthesizes enough normal tissue to approximate more nearly to a normal body composition.

Total body potassium is lowest in oedematous children and it has been shown that body potassium is inversely related to extracellular fluid volume. It is generally accepted that potassium deficiency can cause retention of water and sodium but the mechanism is not very clear.

Sodium pump

Low levels of potassium and elevated levels of sodium observed in erythrocytes of malnourished children suggest an alteration in the sodium 'pump'.[12] It is proposed that the intracellular sodium concentration may rise in the initial stages. In response to this and to prevent continued sodium accumulation, the sodium 'pump' is stimulated. Studies showed that ouabain-sensitive Na^+/K^+-transporting ATPase activity in the erythrocyte membrane is significantly increased in oedematous children but not in marasmus. This enzyme facilitates influx of potassium ions into the cell. After dietary treatment, the potassium levels and the enzyme activity were restored to normal and this was associated with loss of oedema fluid.

Magnesium

Serum magnesium is usually normal in PEM but may fall in the presence of severe gastroenteritis. The evidence for magnesium depletion comes from balance studies and muscle biopsies. During recovery from malnutrition, retention of magnesium is greater than would be predicted from the nitrogen balance. Muscle magnesium is low though the reduction is not as great as that of potassium, perhaps because of the large store

of magnesium in bone. Electrocardiographic changes observed in malnourished children have been attributed to severe magnesium depletion.

Copper and zinc

Low serum copper levels have been reported in malnourished children and the reduction appears to be greater in kwashiorkor than in marasmus. Low levels of serum copper are associated with low caeruloplasmin activity. Copper content of hair and liver is also reduced in kwashiorkor. Levels of serum zinc have been found to be low in both kwashiorkor and marasmus. The zinc levels showed a good correlation with serum albumin concentration.

Protein and amino acid metabolism

Serum proteins

Serum protein concentration is decreased in PEM and this is mainly due to hypoalbuminaemia. Serum albumin levels are reduced to a greater extent in kwashiorkor than in marasmus. Since the concentration of globulins (G) is less altered than that of albumin (A) the A/G ratio is frequently inverted. Studies with I^{131}-labelled albumin have shown that the low serum concentration is due to decreased albumin synthesis. This is not a result of the liver's inability to synthesize albumin, but is due to a reduction in the availability of amino acids required for protein synthesis. It has been demonstrated that, even from the onset of dietary therapy, malnourished children had higher rates of protein synthesis and turnover than recovered children.

Serum levels of other proteins, prealbumin, transferrin and ceruloplasmin are also reduced in malnourished children. These proteins have been used for diagnostic purposes. However, their levels are influenced by many factors and serum albumin is a better index of PEM.

Serum enzymes

Since enzymes are proteins, their levels in the bloodstream may be altered, reflecting the rate of protein synthesis in the organ from which they are derived. The activities of serum enzymes like amylase, lipase and cholinesterase have been found to be reduced in kwashiorkor but unchanged in marasmus. These differences suggest that hepatic and pancreatic functions are better maintained in marasmus. On the other hand, certain enzymes like glutamic pyruvic transaminase and isocitric dehydrogenases are increased.

Lysosomal enzymes have also been found to be raised in both blood and urine of malnourished children. These changes, which depend upon leakage from damaged cells, are late events in the progress of the disease.

Serum amino acid pattern

In severe PEM the total serum amino acid concentration is reduced to half the normal value. The pattern of serum amino acids has been found to be remarkably constant in kwashiorkor patients from different countries, irrespective of diet. In general, there is a depression of essential amino acids, particularly the branched-chain amino acids and threonine, while lysine and phenylalanine are less affected. The serum concentrations of the non-essential amino acids are fairly well-maintained or even increased. Whitehead and Dean suggested that the amino acid pattern can be used as an index of protein depletion. A simple chromatographic method was developed to estimate the ratio of non-essential to essential amino acids; the non-essential group consisting of glycine, serine, glutamine and taurine and the essential group consisting of leucine, isoleucine, valine and methionine. The ratio has been found to be greatly increased in kwashiorkor but the changes are less marked in marasmus. The explanation put forward for this is that in calorie deficiency the levels of essential amino acids in the serum are kept up because of the breakdown of muscle protein to supply energy. Since the ratio is high, even in undernourished children subsisting on high-carbohydrate low-protein diet, it was claimed that the test was diagnostic of protein deficiency. Other studies, however, could not confirm this. In Indian children, though total plasma amino acid concentration was reduced, changes in the ratio of non-essential to essential amino acids were inconsistent. In marasmic and undernourished children this ratio was not elevated. More than 50 per cent of kwashiorkor cases had ratios within normal range. Response to protein therapy was also found to be variable. These results imply that the serum amino acid pattern must be used with caution in the detection of protein–energy malnutrition.

Changes in skin and hair

In recent years, studies have been conducted in malnourished children to understand the biochemical basis for some of the clinical manifestations like changes in hair and skin. Analysis of skin biopsy specimens showed a reduction in the nitrogen content, particularly of the dermis. Amino acid analysis revealed a significant decrease in hydroxyproline, reflecting a reduction in the collagen content of the skin. Tyrosine content also was reduced indicating a total impairment of cross-linking of collagen fibrils. These changes were more marked in children who had dermatosis.

The hair protein keratin is rich in cystine and methionine. Copper is necessary for the enzyme tyrosinase which is involved in the formation of melanin. Analysis of hair samples obtained from kwashiorkor cases showed a significant reduction in levels of cystine as well as of copper. However, these alterations were found in all cases of kwashiorkor, whether or not hair changes were present.

Urinary excretion of nitrogenous compounds

The urinary output of nitrogen is low in malnourished children and this is mainly due to a reduction in urea excretion. Studies show that nitrogen is more efficiently utilized in these children, since a larger portion of the nitrogen entering the amino acid pool is used for protein synthesis and a smaller portion is metabolized to urea. These mechanisms of adaptation have been explained on the basis of changes in activity of enzymes concerned with amino acid metabolism.

The excretion of 3-methyl histidine partly reflects myofibril protein turnover and muscle mass. In a malnourished child with both a reduced muscle mass and protein turnover, a reduction of excretion of 3-methyl histidine occurs. Even if protein turnover is increased per unit mass of muscle, this is so much reduced that the excretion of 3-methyl histidine is still reduced in absolute terms.

Urinary creatinine is the sole breakdown product of creatinine and more than 90 per cent of body creatinine is located in skeletal muscle. It has been estimated that one gram of creatinine excreted is equivalent to 20 kg of muscle in children. This estimate is based on the assumption that the concentration of muscle creatinine and its turnover are fairly constant. However, some workers have reported that creatinine turnover can vary and hence caution must be exercised in the interpretation of muscle mass measurements based on creatinine excretion.

Creatinine height index has been used (CHI) for estimating the relative muscle mass of children. This index is defined as 24-hour creatinine excretion of the patient divided by the 24-hour creatinine excretion of a normal subject of the same height. A significant negative correlation between the CHI and N retention is found in malnourished children during recovery, indicating the physiological significance of CHI in estimating protein nutrition. The main limitation of this method is the requirement of 24-hour urine collection.

Urinary excretion of hydroxyproline is also reduced in malnourished children. This may represent a reduction in body collagen due to protein depletion. The hydroxyproline index which is the ratio of hydroxyproline to creatinine per unit body weight has been suggested as an index of protein–calorie malnutrition. Although this index is generally low in kwashiorkor and marasmus, it shows wide variation in undernourished children.

Other doubts about the hydroxyproline/creatinine ratio are concerned with its consistency in random urine samples. Field studies have shown that the use of this index as a measure of nutritional status has several drawbacks.

Carbohydrate metabolism

In general, the fasting blood sugar levels are lower in malnourished than in normal children. Life-threatening hypoglycaemia has been reported in severe PEM in Uganda, but the incidence is relatively low in other parts of the world. In Indian children, blood sugar levels were reported to be normal but glucose tolerance was impaired, suggesting impaired utilization. Others have also found no difference in the blood sugar levels of malnourished and normal children. The past dietary intake of energy and the subject's requirements for energy are uncontrolled variables that affect the actual blood glucose levels after a standard 8-hour fast. Other factors that determine the blood sugar concentration are level of glycogen stores and the rate of its breakdown in the liver and the rates of gluconeogenesis and peripheral utilization of glucose.

Energy metabolism

Many of the clinical features of severe PEM, such as physical inactivity, bradycardia and decreased body temperature are consistent with a decreased metabolic rate.

Many workers have reported low basal metabolic rate (BMR) in kwashiorkor while in marasmus it is normal or high.[13] While discussing his findings in marasmus, Montgomery[14] drew attention to the altered ratio of active cell mass to relatively inactive supporting structures. This would have led to falsely high values for the BMR when expressed on a body weight basis. Jaya Rao and Khan found that the BMR was reduced in both marasmus and kwashiorkor but the value was higher in marasmic children.[28] The reduced BMR in malnourished children could be due to alterations in body composition or to a decreased cellular activity or both.

Fat metabolism

Varying degrees of fat malabsorption have been reported in severely malnourished children.[2] There is a reduction in all the pancreatic enzymes, particularly the lipase activity. The presence of free fatty acids in the stools, however, suggests a defect in the absorptive function rather than in digestion. There is a decrease in the concentration of conjugated bile acids, which are essential for solubilization of lipids in the intestinal lumen and their absorption through formation of lipid micelles. It is important to note that in spite of steatorrhoea, the children recover well with dietary treatment.

In kwashiorkor, plasma levels of free fatty acids are raised, while the levels of triglycerides and phospholipids are reduced with a low ratio of esterified to free cholesterol. After treatment, the levels are restored to normal. The concentration of β-lipoprotein is decreased while that of α-lipoprotein is variable. In marasmus, plasma levels of lipoproteins, triglycerides and free fatty acids are normal or raised.

Fatty infiltration of the liver is the most striking feature of kwashiorkor and is rarely seen in marasmus. Autopsy studies in Jamaican children with malnutrition showed that up to 60 per cent of the weight of the liver may be fat and over 30 per cent of the total body fat may be in the liver. It is now clear that the liver fat originates from the peripheral depots and is not synthesized *in situ*. The major lipid fraction that accumulates in the liver is triglyceride and the defect in transport mechanism arises from reduction in the synthesis of lipoprotein. The marked rise in serum concentration of triglycerides and β-lipoproteins, representing defatting of the liver, following treatment is consistent with this theory.

Endocrine changes

Plasma cortisol levels are raised in all cases of severe PEM but more so in marasmus than in kwashiorkor.

Marasmic children have an exaggerated response to corticotropin (ACTH), while in kwashiorkor this is either inadequate or normal. This would suggest that although children with kwashiorkor are able to maintain their adrenocortical function at satisfactory levels under resting conditions, they are unable to respond to an acute stimulus as well as normal or marasmic children.

Studies from Chile showed thyroid hypofunction in

marasmic infants. There was a decrease in I^{131} uptake by the thyroid and low plasma levels of protein-bound and butanol-extractable iodine. All three showed an increase after an injection of thyroid-stimulating hormone (TSH). In children with kwashiorkor, the I^{131} uptake was found to be normal but plasma levels of protein-bound iodine were low. The perchlorate test was positive in these cases, suggesting an impairment of the organification of iodide. These changes were easily reversible by nutritional rehabilitation.

Conflicting results have been reported with regard to plasma insulin levels. Some workers have reported decreased levels, while others have found normal or increased levels of insulin in kwashiorkor. Blunted insulin response to intravenous glucose and impaired glucose tolerance have been observed in children with kwashiorkor, even after recovery. Administration of glucagon had no effect on plasma insulin, although glucose levels showed a rise.

Perhaps the most surprising endocrine change in malnutrition is the elevation of growth hormone concentration. The hormone levels and their response to stimuli are raised in kwashiorkor but not in marasmus. The action of growth hormone on cartilage is mediated through somatomedins which are generated in the liver. Somatomedin activity has been found to be decreased in kwashiorkor but not in marasmus. The low level of somatomedins may be acting as a feed-back stimulus resulting in high levels of growth hormone in kwashiorkor.

The physiological significance of these endocrine changes is not clear as to which are primary and which are adaptive mechanisms. The hormonal changes may reflect a series of metabolic events arising from repeated periods of fasting to which malnourished children are often subjected. Fasting leads to a fall in blood glucose and consequently a fall in insulin. Reduced levels of insulin and increased levels of cortisol would facilitate the enhanced gluconeogenesis necessary to provide the carbohydrate fuel for tissues, particularly the brain. When glucose levels fall, tissues derive energy from fat breakdown. The real function of growth hormone may be to stimulate lipolysis and thus produce another fuel for brain consumption. In this context, growth hormone and insulin may not be primarily related to growth at all.[11]

Immune response

Frequent episodes of infection in malnourished children suggest that resistance to infection may be lowered (see pp. 449–54). In defence against bacteria, viruses and other pathogens, several facets of immunocompetence come into play. Phagocytic activity and bactericidal capacity of leucocytes contribute the first order of defence. In addition, the two types of immune mechanism that operate against infection are humoral and cell-mediated immunity. There are also other non-specific defence factors such as lysozyme and complement which play an important role in resistance to infection. Studies in children have shown that most of the defence mechanisms are altered in severe PEM.[15]

Phagocytic and bactericidal activities

The major circulating phagocytes involved in these functions are the polymorphonuclear leucocytes. Energy needed for phagocytosis comes from increased glycolytic activity of the cell, while bactericidal function depends upon the activity of the hexose–monophosphate pathway of glucose metabolism.

Using these biochemical parameters, it has been shown that both phagocytic and bactericidal activities of leucocytes are significantly reduced in severe PEM. Direct evidence for altered bactericidal activity has also been obtained by estimating viable bacteria after incubation of leucocytes with *E. coli*. Leucocytes obtained from children with severe PEM showed markedly lowered bactericidal capacity which was restored to normal by nutritional rehabilitation.

The bactericidal system in leucocytes consists of hydrogen peroxide, myeloperoxidase and halide ions. Impaired bactericidal activity of leucocytes of malnourished children has been shown to be due to a reduction in the activity of the rate-limiting enzyme nicotinamide adenine dinucleotide phosphate (NADPH) oxidase, which is concerned with the formation of hydrogen peroxide. There is also direct evidence to show that peroxide formation is reduced in PEM.

Cell-mediated immunity

Cell-mediated immunity is known to be regulated by the thymus. Postmortem studies in children dying of kwashiorkor have revealed severe atrophy of the thymolymphatic system. It has been observed that the Mantoux test is often negative in children suffering from kwashiorkor in spite of clear evidence of active tuberculosis, suggesting that the cell-mediated immune response is impaired. In recent studies, cell-mediated immunity has been assessed by measuring the number of T lymphocytes and *in vitro* incorporation of ^{3}H thymidine into lymphocyte cultures. Using these parameters it has been shown that the cell-mediated immune response is significantly depressed in children with severe PEM. This may partly explain the frequent occurrence of infections such as herpes, candidiasis and

Gram-negative bacterial infections in malnourished children (see pp. 844-5).

Humoral immunity

Humoral immune response has been assessed by measuring circulating levels of immunoglobulins as well as antibody response to specific bacterial antigens. The three major classes of immunoglobulin – IgG, IgA and IgM – have been found to be similar in normal and malnourished children. Antibody response to diphtheria and tetanus toxoids was normal but the response to typhoid antigen was significantly depressed in children with severe PEM. Many children with kwashiorkor failed to develop antibodies against O as well as H antigens. Poor antibody response to typhoid observed in malnourished children may be secondary to depressed cell-mediated immunity since this is a T cell-dependent antigen. Other studies have also shown that the response varies with the antigen tested. While the antibody responses to measles and polio vaccines were found to be normal, the responses to influenza and yellow fever were impaired in severe PEM.

Secretory antibodies of the IgA class play an important role in the protection of mucosal surfaces against infective agents. This local immunity is independent of systemic immunity. In children suffering from severe PEM, secretory IgA levels in duodenal fluid, saliva, tears and nasal secretions are significantly low on admission and return to normal within a few weeks of nutritional rehabilitation. Secretory antibody responses to measles and polio virus vaccines also are significantly reduced in PEM. Alterations in the local immunity can account for the increased incidence of mucosal infections seen in malnourished children.

Complement system

Total haemolytic activity of the serum has been shown to be significantly reduced in children with severe PEM. Studies in Thai children with PEM have shown that all the components of complement, except C4, are markedly low on admission, and after treatment their concentrations rise above normal. The levels of protein and calorie intake have a pronounced influence on the repair of the complement system. Low levels of complement in malnutrition may reflect a general reduction in protein synthesis or an increased consumption of complement proteins in antigen–antibody reactions during infection. The mean haemolytic activity and concentration of C3 have been found to be lower in malnourished children with infection than in those without infection.

Lysozyme

This enzyme is present in high concentrations in polymorphonuclear leucocytes. It is also present in various body fluids, including serum and secretions (particularly tears). Studies in malnourished children have shown that lysozyme content of leucocytes is significantly reduced, and following nutritional rehabilitation, the enzyme levels are restored to normal. Reduced bactericidal activity observed in malnourished children may partly be due to decreased levels of lysozyme in leucocytes.

Clinical features

Kwashiorkor and marasmus are the two well-recognized clinical syndromes of severe PEM. Detailed descriptions of these syndromes have been published by several workers.[9] Although the clinical manifestations may vary from one area to another, certain features are common and constitute the minimum diagnostic crite-

Table 3.5.9 Salient features of severe PEM

	Kwashiorkor	Marasmus
Age of maximal incidence	12–36 months	6–12 months
Essential features		
Oedema	Present	Absent
Wasting	Less obvious	Gross wasting
Growth retardation	Less severe	Severe
Mental changes	Present	Sometimes
Variable features		
Appetite	Poor	Good
Diarrhoea	Present	Present
Skin changes	Present	Infrequent
Hair changes	Present	Infrequent
Moon face	Present	Absent
Hepatomegaly	Present	Absent
Liver biopsy	Fatty infiltration	Minimal change
Biochemical changes		
Serum albumin	Decreased	Slightly decreased
Serum amino acid ratio	Elevated	Normal
Serum enzymes	Decreased	Normal
Blood urea	Decreased	Normal
Blood sugar	Low/normal	Normal
Serum triglycerides	Decreased	Normal
Serum cholesterol	Decreased	Normal
Serum free fatty acid	Elevated	Elevated
Serum cortisol	Elevated	Markedly elevated
Serum growth hormone	Elevated	Normal
Serum insulin	Low/normal	Normal

ria. The main features of kwashiorkor and marasmus are set out in Table 3.5.9.

Kwashiorkor

In most tropical countries infants are breast-fed during the first year of life and kwashiorkor occurs during the second or third year, when the diet is suddenly changed to that of the adult. Because of the bulk, a child cannot consume sufficient quantities of the diet and stops gaining weight. Superimposed infections like diarrhoea and respiratory infection, which are common at this age, may aggravate the deficiencies and precipitate kwashiorkor.

Apathy and anorexia are the early manifestations of kwashiorkor. The onset of the disease is usually insidious but sometimes a child may develop full-blown kwashiorkor suddenly after an episode of infection.

The three essential features of kwashiorkor are oedema, growth retardation, and mental changes. Oedema appears first on the lower extremities and then spreads to the rest of the body. The face looks puffy with sagging cheeks and swollen eye lids. Ascites is very rare. Growth retardation is a constant feature, the body weight being low in spite of oedema. Some degree of muscle wasting is present in almost all cases but it may be masked by the oedema. The distinction between marasmic kwashiorkor and 'sugar baby' kwashiorkor is based on the degree of wasting, which is less apparent in the latter (see Fig. 3.5.9).

Psychological changes are constant and characteristic of kwashiorkor. Most children are apathetic, indifferent to their environment and have an expression of misery. (The look in the child's eyes has been described vividly as the 'radar gaze' focussing not on the immediate surroundings but on infinity.) They resent being disturbed and protest with a weak cry to any stimulus, even when feeds are offered.

Apart from these main diagnostic signs, there are other features which are variable. Skin changes like dryness and scaly pigmentation may be seen over the limbs and trunk (see Fig. 3.5.9). Unlike pellagra, these changes are not limited to areas exposed to sunlight. In the typical 'crazy pavement' dermatosis which is less common, the epithelium eventually peels off, leaving behind depigmented patches with oozing fluid which can be easily infected, resulting in indolent ulcers. This is usually seen in severe cases of kwashiorkor and is considered to be a sign of bad prognosis. Purpuric spots and echymotic patches are also encountered.

The hair shows changes in texture as well as colour. It becomes thin and dry and is devoid of the normal sheen. It can be pulled out easily without causing pain.

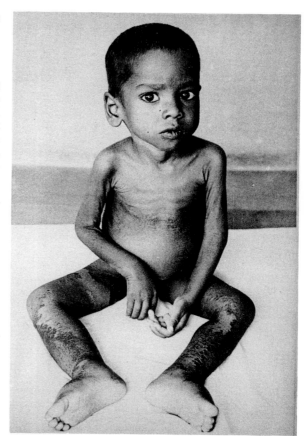

Fig. 3.5.9 Kwashiorkor with oedema and skin changes.

Loss of hair results in diffuse or patchy alopecia. Characteristic change in pigmentation includes brownish or reddish discoloration. These colour changes may be seen throughout the length of the hair, or as alternate bands of depigmentation and pigmentation described as the 'flag sign'. Although uncommon, it is a good record of the nutritional history of the child (see Fig. 3.5.10).

Recent history of diarrhoea is common in children with kwashiorkor. The diarrhoea, which may start some weeks or months before as an acute infectious episode, may become chronic or recurrent. It is usually non-specific and is corrected by diet therapy without specific treatment. The stool volume is large, even when diarrhoea is not present, suggesting intestinal malabsorption. Vomiting may also occur, especially when the child is forced to eat. The abdomen is distended due to flatulence and flaccid abdominal

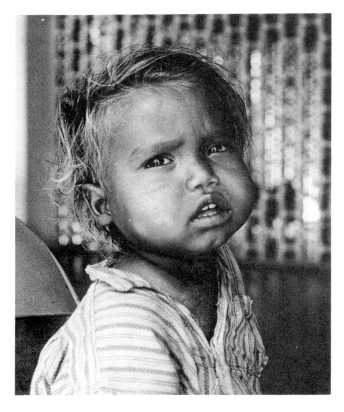

Fig. 3.5.10   Kwashiorkor with hair changes.

muscles. The liver is often enlarged due to extensive fatty infiltration. The consistency of the liver is soft and the margin is rounded. Splenomegaly may be due to malaria in certain parts of the world.

Signs and symptoms of other nutritional deficiencies are common in children with kwashiorkor. They may vary from one region to another, depending upon the dietary pattern. Vitamin A deficiency is more common in South-east Asia. The incidence of xerophthalmia among children with kwashiorkor is as high as 30 per cent in some areas. This is mainly due to the lack of vitamin A in the diet but also to metabolic disturbance resulting from protein deficiency. Clinical signs of B complex deficiencies, such as angular stomatitis, glossitis and cheilosis, are not uncommon. Associated iron deficiency anaemia is also a frequent feature.

There are a few reports describing neurological signs in kwashiorkor. These include coarse tremors, rigidity, exaggerated tendon reflexes, myoclonus and oculogyric crises. They are considered to be the result of extra-pyramidal lesions.

Reports from Mexico have described a 'nutrition recovery syndrome', which is seen about 20 to 40 days after starting the treatment. It usually presents as hepatomegaly, abdominal distension with prominent veins and ascites. This syndrome may be related to the high protein intake, especially with intravenous protein therapy.

Marasmus

Marasmus may be seen in breast-fed infants when the amount of milk is markedly reduced, or more frequently in those who are artificially fed. This is described as infantile marasmus, wherein the diet may be qualitatively adequate but fails to satisfy the minimum requirements of the rapidly growing child. Marasmus is also seen in older children subsisting on inadequate diets for prolonged periods. This is described as 'late marasmus' and is akin to chronic starvation in adults. Growth retardation is one of the early manifestations. When this process is prolonged, the body is forced to utilize its own tissues for metabolic purposes and the child develops full-blown marasmus, characterized by emaciation. The cardinal features of marasmus are severe growth retardation and absence of oedema. In extreme cases, the body is shrivelled with wrinkled skin and bony prominences. The child may be irritable, crying continuously due to hunger or may become apathetic. Skin and hair changes are infrequent. Associated vitamin deficiencies are, however, seen (see Fig. 3.5.11).

In addition to these differences in clinical manifestations, the biochemical profile in marasmus is also different from that in kwashiorkor. Another major difference between the two conditions is that hepatomegaly with extensive fatty infiltration, seen in kwashiorkor, is absent in marasmus.

Marasmic kwashiorkor

Children with kwashiorkor but no preceding calorie deficiency, are extremely rare. Such a situation only

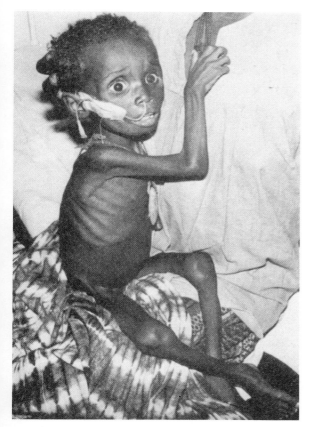

Fig. 3.5.11 Marasmus. (Reproduced from G. Alleyne *et al.* *Protein-Energy Malnutrition*, Edward Arnold, 1977.)

develops when infants are weaned on to a starchy diet very low in protein and are forced to consume large amounts of this diet. This is described as 'sugar baby' kwashiorkor where there is not much loss of subcutaneous fat or wasting.

Much more frequently, however, oedema appears in a child who is chronically undernourished and has not been growing well for weeks or months. Generally the muscles of the upper limbs are wasted while the lower limbs appear swollen. These children are classified as marasmic kwashiorkor as they have clinical features of both marasmus and kwashiorkor. The degree of stunting is significantly greater in these children, suggesting that the duration of illness is longer in marasmic kwashiorkor than in kwashiorkor. Psychological changes and skin and hair changes, as well as other clinical features previously described, are common in these children . Since such presentations are a rule in many areas where PEM is prevalent, they are described simply as kwashiorkor. Some workers feel that distinction between the various forms of severe PEM need not be emphasized as they are different facets of the same disease.

Differential diagnosis

The oedema of kwashiorkor should be differentiated from that in hepatic and renal diseases, hookworm anaemia and cardiac failure. The most common condition with which kwashiorkor may be confused is nephrotic syndrome. Oedema is common to both the conditions but in the nephrotic syndrome, ascites is frequently observed and large amounts of albumin are present in urine.

The dermatosis of kwashiorkor may be confused with pellagra but the distribution is different. In pellagra the skin changes are confined to areas exposed to sunlight.

Children with 'Indian childhood cirrhosis' may also present a picture of kwashiorkor but they often have ascites and hepatosplenomegaly.

Complications

Infections

Most children with PEM are brought to the hospital for associated infections, gastroenteritis and respiratory infections being the major complications. Infections are not only frequent but also occur with greater severity in malnourished children. This has been attributed to their lowered resistance to infection. The prognosis depends on the severity of the condition, the age of the child and the associated complications. High mortality rates ranging from 10 to 30 per cent have been reported from various hospitals. A majority of deaths occur within the first few days after admission.

Diarrhoea is usually mild and responds well to diet therapy but sometimes acute infective enteritis leads to dehydration and electrolyte imbalance. In Jamaica, this is the most common cause of death in the first few days of admission.[2] In malnourished children, dehydration may be difficult to judge because wasting may exaggerate the loss of skin turgor, while oedema may mask the presence of dehydration. In such children, depression of the anterior fontanelle and dryness of mouth and skin are more reliable signs.

Apart from gastroenteritis, other acute infections of the lung, ear and urinary tract are common in severely malnourished children. Infections of the skin and mucous membrane such as severe moniliasis and cancrum oris have been reported from some regions. Bronchopneumonia and Gram-negative septicaemia are the most fatal infections. Difficulties may be encountered in diagnosing infection in malnourished children since the usual responses of fever and leucocytosis are absent. Owing to altered immune response, the Mantoux test may be negative in spite of active tuberculosis. In addition to routine blood and urine examinations, cultures and X-ray of the chest should be taken for proper diagnosis.

Acquired immuno-deficiency syndrome (AIDS) is vertically transmitted in the first two to three years of life, or acquired through contaminated transfusions at any time in infancy or childhood, and presents as malnutrition and repeated opportunistic infections. It should be considered in the differential diagnosis of all malnourished children especially in or from areas of high endemicity or when rehabilitation is repeatedly interrupted by infections, particularly of the opportunistic variety, such as thrush.

Parasitic infections

The incidence of intestinal parasitic infections (notably ascariasis) is high in malnourished children. Hookworm is less common because most of the malnourished children are too young to walk in the fields and contract infection. Malaria, still endemic in many African countries, may be a fatal disease in the malnourished infant, though in general it does appear to be less severe and less common in the malnourished.

Hypoglycaemia

Fasting blood sugar levels may be low but symptomatic hypoglycaemia is uncommon. A child may develop this complication if feeding is infrequent. Hypoglycaemia is more common in marasmus where energy stores are depleted. It is often associated with septicaemia. In severe cases, twitchings and convulsions may occur and the child becomes unconscious. Early and adequate feeding usually avoids this complication.

Hypothermia

Severe cases of PEM sometimes develop hypothermia and shock. It occurs more often in severely wasted children and is associated with high mortality. Hypothermia is a manifestation of impairment of thermoregulatory control and decreased energy stores. In addition, emaciation leads to reduced specific thermal insulation.

Cardiac failure

In Uganda, cardiac failure has been reported in malnourished children during treatment and the incidence decreased when the dietary sodium intake was reduced. This has not been observed elsewhere. Occasionally a child may develop cardiac failure due to severe anaemia.

Treatment

The treatment of severe cases of PEM, especially those with complications, is better carried out in hospital since correction of severe dehydration and control of infections demand special attention. Although treatment of complications can reduce mortality, proper dietary management is important for speedy recovery.

Dietary management

The basic principle of treatment is to improve the nutritional level of the child as quickly as possible by providing a diet with sufficient energy-producing foods and high-quality proteins.[16] Anorexia is a common feature of severe PEM. The child may require tube feeding in the initial stages and the diet must therefore be in a liquid form. When the appetite improves and the child is able to take food, this can be given as small quantities of solid supplements at frequent intervals.

Protein

Both protein and calories are required in larger than normal quantities for rapid recovery. Experience from various countries suggests that a daily protein intake of 3–4 g/kg can meet the requirements of the malnourished child. Milk is an excellent source of protein and reconstituted skimmed milk has been widely used for the treatment of PEM. However, if skimmed milk powder is not available, fresh whole milk can be used. There is considerable evidence that even diets based on vegetable protein foods are effective in the treatment of PEM. The rate of clinical response is similar but the increase in serum albumin concentration is lower with vegetable proteins than with milk protein. However, this can be overcome either by raising the level of protein intake or by prolonging the treatment.[16] The most significant observation made in this connection is that a combination of vegetable and milk proteins in the proportion of 3:1 is as effective as milk protein alone. Thus, a diet providing 3–4 g/kg of protein/day with at least one-fourth of it derived from milk is sufficient to meet the child's needs.

Calories

Although acute manifestations of kwashiorkor can be reversed with protein-rich diets containing about 100 cal/kg, weight gain depends on extra energy intake. The calculated energy needs are about 50 per cent greater than normal during recovery from malnutrition. In Uganda, when diets containing up to 200 cal/kg/day in a skimmed milk, oil and sugar mixture (DISCO) were supplied the children showed rapid weight gain. Dramatic improvement has been demonstrated in Indian children[16] treated with diets supplying 200 cal/kg. As carbohydrate sources are bulky, oil is used as the energy source in these diets. It is generally believed that children suffering from kwashiorkor do not tolerate dietary fat well. However, balance studies in malnourished children indicated that the net absorption of fat was higher on high-fat diets and the beneficial effect of additional fat calories was reflected in better weight gain. About 30–40 per cent of the total calories can therefore, be provided safely through fat in the diet. In addition, feeding at frequent intervals is necessary to achieve high energy intakes.

After the initial period of anorexia, the child usually develops a voracious appetite. It has been observed that when children were fed ad lib, some of them consumed more than 200 kcal/kg per day. The children voluntarily decrease their dietary intakes when expected weight for height is achieved.

Therapeutic diets

A number of workers in different parts of the world have developed special diets to achieve calculated high-energy intakes and to fulfil protein requirements for maximum catch-up growth.[17] They follow the same general pattern. High-quality protein is usually provided by milk, energy is supplied by the oil, and sugar is added for taste and to supply extra energy. These diets can be used for all cases of severe PEM, whether marasmus, kwashiorkor or marasmic kwashiorkor, and should be calculated on the basis of actual weight and not expected weight.

In some areas, malnourished children are fed lower amounts in the initial stages, increasing gradually over the first week until the full quantity is tolerated, while in other places a high-calorie diet is prescribed from the beginning and the children are allowed to take as much as possible. The consensus is that dietary intake should reach full requirements as soon as these can be tolerated.

Vitamin deficiencies

Many children with PEM show clinical signs of vitamin A and B complex deficiencies. Even if there are no clinical signs, it is reasonable to expect that rapid growth during recovery increases vitamin demands. A multivitamin tablet is therefore recommended as a routine along with the daily diet. However, if a child shows evidence of severe deficiency, large doses of vitamins should be given. In areas where vitamin A deficiency is common, kwashiorkor is frequently associated with keratomalacia. Such cases should be treated with an intramuscular injection of 100 000 IU water-miscible vitamin A immediately after diagnosis.

Anaemia

Iron deficiency anaemia is common in malnourished children. Coexisting folate deficiency has also been observed in some areas. Mild to moderate anaemia can be treated with an oral dose of 120 mg elemental iron and 1 mg folic acid/day. A child who does not tolerate oral iron should be treated with intramuscular injection or iron dextran (100 mg). For severe anaemia, blood transfusion (10 ml/kg) may be given as a slow drip. Packed red cells should be used to avoid cardiac failure.

Management of associated complications

Diarrhoea and dehydration

Mild diarrhoea does not require any specific treatment. Sometimes, however, diarrhoea of infectious origin is very severe leading to dehydration and electrolyte imbalance. Replacement of fluid and electrolyte losses is essential in the management of such cases. The use of antibiotics will depend upon the causative organism and its sensitivity.

Management of dehydration depends on the severity of the condition. Mild to moderate dehydration can be treated with oral rehydration solution (NaCl 3.5 g, NaHCO$_3$ 2.5 g, KCl 1.5 g and glucose 20 g dissolved in 1 litre of water). This mixture can be prepared in the hospital and used as a routine in all cases of diarrhoea to prevent dehydration.

For severe dehydration, intravenous fluid therapy is required to improve the circulation and expand plasma volume rapidly. About 100–150 ml/kg of fluid can be given in the first 12 hours. Initial attempts should be directed at correcting the metabolic acidosis. Sodium bicarbonate or Ringer lactate solution can be given at the rate of 20 to 40 ml/kg in the first 2 hours and then 5 per cent glucose–saline in a volume of 100 ml/kg during the subsequent 10 hours. Hypertonic solution should not be used, even if serum sodium levels are low. As soon as urine flow is established, potassium supplements can be given orally (1–2 g/kg per day) as potassium chloride.

In children with severe oedema the quantity of fluid and rate of administration should be lowered to avoid circulatory overload. In a majority of cases, after correcting the deficit of body fluids, maintenance therapy can be instituted with oral rehydration solution. As soon as vomiting subsides, feeding should be started. Early refeeding is essential for rapid recovery.

Lactose intolerance

There have been numerous reports of lactose intolerance and lactase deficiency in children with PEM. However, this has little functional significance. In areas where PEM is endemic the incidence of lactase deficiency is high even in the general population. However, many subjects with lactase deficiency drink milk without any symptoms of intolerance. The incidence of lactose intolerance and low levels of lactase, therefore, are not reliable guides to assess milk tolerance and the use of milk in the diet should not be based on these considerations.

A great majority of malnourished children can drink milk without any problem. The diarrhoea subsides spontaneously with the restoration of the general condition of the child. Only when it persists or becomes worse should the diet be changed. A child who cannot tolerate full-strength milk may be given diluted milk or buttermilk for the first few days, followed by the regular milk diet.

Infections

Apart from gastroenteritis, infections of the respiratory and urinary tracts are common in severely malnourished children. Adequate therapy with antibiotics should be instituted. If the infection does not respond to pencillin or erythromycin, broad-spectrum antibiotics must be used. The choice of antibiotic will depend on the results of blood culture and local experience. Prophylactic antibiotic therapy has been adopted in some hospitals but others do not find any advantages with this procedure.

Intestinal infections such as giardiasis and ascariasis, and in older children ancylostomiasis, are common. Appropriate deworming agents should be given as soon as the child recovers from the acute stage.

In areas where malaria is endemic a suppressive dose of chloroquin is recommended for all children on admission. Acute attacks should be treated as they occur. The drug of choice will depend on local experience.

Hypoglycaemia

Although uncommon, hypoglycaemia can be life-threatening and requires urgent treatment. Intravenous injection of 10 ml of 50 per cent glucose should be given and after the symptoms disappear, two hourly oral feeding should be instituted.

Hypothermia and shock

If hypothermia and shock develop it is important to keep the child warm. The state of shock must be treated promptly with intravenous injections of glucose–saline solution or blood transfusion. This should be done cautiously since there is a risk of cardiac failure. Blood transfusion should not be used as a routine in the treatment of PEM.

Thus, the complications that arise in severe PEM require special therapeutic measures, but it cannot be overemphasized that a suitable diet is the mainstay of treatment. A majority of children show improvement with the type of treatment described above. Other therapeutic measures such as administration of diuretics, anabolic steroids and protein hydrolysates, intravenous infusions of amino acids and plasma are expensive and ineffective.[16] Limited resources available in the hospitals should not be wasted on such unnecessary treatments.

Recovery

Signs of recovery are generally seen within a week of starting diet therapy. The child becomes alert and the appetite improves. A change in emotional responses is also significant. The child becomes playful and shows interest in the surroundings. It has been said that the first smile is the most important milestone in recovery.

Children with kwashiorkor begin to lose oedema soon after dietary treatment is started and in most cases, the oedema disappears completely by 7 to 10 days. During this period, the child may lose weight, but thereafter starts gaining weight. A marasmic child, on the other hand, shows progressive weight gain from the beginning. These children can be given a mixed diet based on local foods after the first two weeks and sooner if appetite permits. They can be discharged from the hospital when they are on their way to recovery. Ideally, they should be referred to a nutrition rehabilitation centre. Where such facilities are not available the children should be followed up at least in the out-patient clinic until they achieve the expected weight for height. It must be ensured that the mother understands how to feed the child with the diet available at home. Nutrition education is an essential component of treatment which is often overlooked.

Out-patient treatment

Since hospital beds are limited, they should be reserved only for the very severe or complicated cases. Experience in different parts of the world has shown that a majority of malnourished children can be treated without hospital admission. Even frank cases of kwashiorkor have been treated successfully in the out-patient clinics and health centres. In a general hospital, the doctor is very much occupied with curative practice and often unable to devote much time to nutrition counselling for mothers. A separate nutrition clinic is therefore recommended, where mothers can be given advice. At the same time recipes based on locally available foods can be used as dietary supplements for the treatment of these cases and thus reduce the need for hospital admission.

In areas where health services are not adequate, treatment of malnutrition in the hospital clinics may not be feasible. Creation of special centres has been suggested for taking care of the children during the day. Nutritional rehabilitation centres were first proposed by Bengoa as cheap convalescent units for children discharged from the hospital after the initial treatment[29], but those with moderate or severe PEM without complications can also be treated in these centres. In addition to providing adequate diet therapy and other medical services in these centres, mothers can be educated by means of direct involvement in the nutritional rehabilitation of their children. Such child-care centres have been established in many places and have proved to be effective in the management of PEM (see pp. 387–90).

Other workers have suggested domiciliary management of PEM which may work out to be cheaper. The mothers have to be instructed precisely regarding the preparation of the diet and other aspects of child-care. Frequent home visits and close supervision by qualified personnel are essential for the success of the programme. Though the nature of the services may vary in different places, the general principles are the same. In all programmes for improving child nutrition, the emphasis is on food supplementation and nutrition education.

Mild and moderate PEM

Milder forms of PEM affect a majority of children in developing countries and constitute a far more serious, problem from a public health point of view. They manifest as varying degrees of growth retardation. Of the various anthropometric measurements, weight for age has been most commonly used to assess growth status of children. On the basis of weight deficit it has been reported that nearly 80 per cent of Indian children are malnourished. Results of the analysis based on the Gomez classification showed that about 40 per cent of children have grade I malnutrition, 35 per cent grade II and 6 per cent grade III. Similar figures have been reported from other developing countries.

In these studies, standards for weight used to judge the extent of growth failure have been those obtained from American children. There is considerable debate as to whether local or international standards are more appropriate. It has been suggested that there may be racial or ethnic differences in the genetic potential of growth. However, results of recent studies have shown that even in developing countries, the growth performance of children belonging to well-to-do communities in whom environmental constraints do not operate, is similar to that of children in affluent parts of the world.[18] The growth retardation seen in children of poor communities thus appears to be due to environmental factors, of which nutrition is an important one (see p. 265ff).

While the reasons for poor growth are fairly well

understood, the real significance of growth failure is not known. It is logical to assume that growth occurs to a level permitted by the nutrient intake and a reduction in body size may therefore be considered as adaptation to nutritional stress. If the reduction in body size does not lead to altered function, it has been argued that the small size *per se* need not cause serious concern. It becomes important, therefore, to determine the level of growth retardation that marks the beginning of functional impairment.

While there is considerable information on the functional deficits in severe PEM, the extent to which biological functions are affected in milder forms of malnutrition is uncertain. The results of a few recent studies have shown that in mild to moderate PEM, intestinal absorption of xylose, fat and vitamin B_{12} is normal. Various functional parameters involved in resistance to infection such as bactericidal activity of leucocytes, humoral and cell-mediated immune mechanisms were found to be unaltered in children with milder grades of PEM.[19] These observations suggest that functional integrity is well maintained in mild and moderate PEM. However, more studies are needed to investigate other functions, in order to understand the physiological significance of growth failure.

Long-term effects

With the increase in the number of children who survive even the severe forms of PEM, there has been a growing concern about the long term sequelae of early childhood malnutrition. A number of studies in experimental animals have shown that malnutrition during the critical stages of growth and development in early life can lead to physical and functional deficits in later life. However, the human situation is much more complex and the long-term effects of early malnutrition are difficult to establish. When children who recovered from kwashiorkor were examined several years later, their heights and weights were found to be significantly lower than those of control children. However, it is difficult to say from these studies whether stunting is the result of childhood malnutrition or due to continued malnutrition during subsequent years. There are other studies to show that malnutrition may not affect the potential for catch-up growth, provided the environment is good. In the 10 year follow-up study reported from South Africa, a majority of children who recovered from kwashiorkor attained normal heights and weights.

An equal or even greater concern has been the suggestion that malnutrition may affect intellectual potential.[20] Disturbances in neurological and psychological functions have been documented both in the acute stage and during recovery. When children who suffered from severe PEM were examined several years later there was impaired cognitive development and neurointegrative competence. Although there are many studies to show such a relationship, the extent to which nutrition influences psychological development is not clear. Malnutrition invariably occurs in children from a poor environment and non-nutritional factors associated with poverty can also contribute significantly to their poor mental function. These include loss of learning time, family environment with particular reference to mother–child interactions and the amount of stimulation which a child receives. Several studies have demonstrated the influence of these factors on the cognitive development of the child.[21]

It is also not known whether the effects of malnutrition are permanent or reversible. In most situations, children treated for severe PEM go back to the poor environment which has had an adverse effect on growth and development. It is possible that if malnourished children receive adequate diet and intellectual stimulation during and after recovery, they could show considerable improvement. A study from Peru illustrates this point very well. Two groups of children who suffered from severe PEM were followed up.[22] One group had been fostered after treatment in a much more stimulating environment, while the other group of children returned to their deprived environment and served as controls. Both groups had shown similar catch-up growth during rehabilitation and fall-off in growth velocities on going to their original or foster homes. However, the study children showed a more rapid growth as measured by height, head circumference and developmental quotients after fostering. The control children maintained a much slower rate of growth and development, chronic undernutrition and poor environmental conditions preventing them from reaching anywhere near the ultimate level attained by the fostered children.

There have been very few studies of the effects of chronic marginal malnutrition which is much more widespread in poor communities. The results of a recent follow-up study showed that adult height and weight were influenced by the nutritional status during childhood. Children who were below the third centile at 5 years of age continued to be so even at 14 years. The physical work capacity of the adolescent boys was related to their current body weight; lighter subjects performed less well than heavier subjects. Impairment in work capacity has been shown to be related to reduced lean body mass. Studies have also been conducted on the relationship between nutrition and work output in real-life situations. Analysis of data on work output of industrial workers showed a direct relationship between body weight and productivity.[23] Similar observations were made of sugar-cane cutters. Productivity was positively correlated with height, weight and lean body mass. These studies indicate that chronic undernutrition leading to low body weight in adulthood may result in reduced work capacity and low work output.

References

1. Joint FAO/WHO Expert Committee on Nutrition. *WHO Technical Report*. 1971; **477**: 34–70.
2. Alleyne GAO, Hay RW, Picou DI, Stanfield JP, Whitehead RG. *Protein Energy Malnutrition*. London, Edward Arnold, 1977.
3. Waterlow JC. Classification and definition of protein calorie malnutrition. *British Medical Journal*. 1972; **3**: 566–9.
4. Seoane N, Latham MC. Nutritional anthropometry in the identification of malnutrition in children. *Journal of Tropical Pediatrics*. 1971; **17**: 98–104.
5. Beaton GH, Bengoa JM (eds). *Nutrition in Preventive Medicine*. Geneva, WHO, 1976. pp. 23–54.
6. Gopalan C. Calorie deficiencies and protein deficiencies. In McCance RA, Widdowson EM eds. *Kwashiorkor and Marasmus: Evolution and Distinguishing Features*. London, Churchill Livingstone, 1967. pp. 49–58.
7. Jaya Rao KS. Evolution of kwashiorkor and marasmus. *Lancet*. 1974; **1**: 709–11.
8. Molla A, Molla AM, Sarker SA. Effects of acute diarrhoea on absorption of macronutrients. In Chen LC, Scrimshaw NS eds. *Diarrhoea and Malnutrition*. New York, Plenum Press, 1982. pp. 143.
9. Trowell HC, Davis JNP, Dean RFA. *Kwashiorkor*. London, Edward Arnold, 1954.
10. Waterlow JC, Alleyne GAO. Protein malnutrition in children: advances in knowledge in the last ten years. *Advances in Protein Chemistry*. 1971; **25**: 117–241.
11. Whitehead RG, Alleyne GAO. Pathophysiological factors of importance in protein calorie malnutrition. *British Medical Bulletin*. 1972; **28**: 72–8.
12. Patrick J. Oedema in protein energy malnutrition: the role of sodium pump. *Proceedings of the Nutrition Society*. 1979; **38**: 61–8.
13. Gardner L, Amachar P. (eds). *Endocrine Aspects of Malnutrition*. California, Kroc Foundation, 1973.
14. Montgomery RD. Changes in the basal metabolic rate of the malnourished infant and their relation to body composition. *Journal of Clinical Investigation*. 1962; **41**: 1653–63.
15. Reddy V, Srikantia SG. Interaction of nutrition and the immune response. *Indian Journal of Medical Research*. 1978; **68**: 48–57.
16. Reddy V, Bhaskaram P. Treatment of severe protein energy malnutrition. *Indian Pediatrics*. 1982; **19**: 243–8.
17. Cameron M, Hofvander Y. *Manual on Feeding Infants and Young Children*. Oxford University Press, 1988.
18. Habicht JP, Martorell R, Yarbrough C *et al*. Height and weight standards for preschool children: how relevant are ethnic differences in growth potential? *Lancet*. 1974; **1**: 611–14.
19. Reddy V, Jagadeesan V, Ragharamulu N *et al*. Functional significance of growth retardation in malnutrition. *American Journal of Clinical Nutrition*. 1976; **29**: 3–7.
20. Hoorweg JC. *Protein–Energy Malnutrition and Intellectual Abilities*. The Hague, Mouton, 1976.
21. Wurtman RJ, Wurtman JJ (eds). *Nutrition and the Brain*. New York, Raven Press, 1977.
22. Graham GG, Adrianzen Blanca. Late 'catch-up' growth after severe infantile malnutrition. *Johns Hopkins Medical Journal*. 1972; **131**: 204–11.
23. Satyanarayana K, Nadamuni Naidu A, Narasinga Rao BS. Nutrition, physical work capacity and work output. *Indian Journal of Medical Research*. 1978; **68** (Suppl.): 88–93.
24. Golden MHN. Consequence of protein deficiency in man and its relationship to the features of kwashiorkor. In Blaxter K, Waterlow JC eds. *Nutritional adaptation in man*. Rank Prize Funds Symposium London. Libbey, 1985. pp. 169–87.
25. Hendrickse RG. Kwashiorkor and aflatoxins. *Journal of Pediatric Gastroenterology and Nutrition*. 1988; **7**: 633–6.
26. Jeliffe DB. *WHO monograph series no. 53*, Geneva, WHO, 196b.
27. Allen JM, Dean RFA. *Trans. Royal Society of Tropical Medicine and Hygiene*. 1965; **59**: 326.
28. Jaya Rao KS, Kahn LN. *American Journal of Clinical Nutrition*. 1974; **27**: 892.
29. Bengoa JM. Nutritional rehabilitation centres. *Journal of Tropical Pediatrics and Environmental Child Health*. 1967; **13**: 169–76.

PREVENTION OF PROTEIN-ENERGY MALNUTRITION
M. G. M. Rowland

Malnutrition is a product of the interaction of man with his physical, biological and social environment. In its most dramatic form, entire nations may be afflicted by famine arising from natural disasters such as drought, or from acts of war. Whilst such disasters are all too common they will not be considered here.

Likewise national and supranational approaches to combat poverty, ignorance and food shortages are beyond the scope of this chapter. It is worth noting, however, that undernutrition has continued to occur in countries which have enjoyed a substantial increase in per capita income, and agricultural programmes aimed at increasing food availability for the poor have not always improved nutritional status in the community. Clearly the prevention of malnutrition on a large scale is complex and difficult.

Nevertheless many health personnel will be concerned with the prevention of protein–energy malnutrition (PEM) which is chronic and endemic in underprivileged communities throughout the less developed countries (LDCs) of the Third World. For this it is necessary to consider the early origins and aetiology of malnutrition.

The clinical manifestations of severe PEM, a spectrum ranging from marasmus to kwashiorkor, are seen most frequently in children under the age of three years; marasmus commonly arises during infancy or early childhood, kwashiorkor tends to arise later and more acutely. Thus malnutrition, as it presents to the health sector, is mainly a problem of young children, of whom some 100 million may be affected, and of their mothers. It normally results from a combination of nutritional deficiency and infection.

Frank malnutrition in childhood has long been recognized as a serious, sometimes life-threatening condition. Only relatively recently has it been realized that lesser degrees of undernutrition or, more precisely, poor nutritional status are associated with a measurably increased risk of death. Thus, when talking of preventing malnutrition it must be clear that we are concerned not just with preventing the occurrence of florid cases but with wider improvements in nutritional status in undernourished populations. If successful on a comprehensive scale, such an achievement may lead to worthwhile improvements in child health and survival. Prevention will therefore be considered largely in the context of family health, with emphasis on maternal and child care, and selected aspects of environmental health.

Malnutrition and low birth weight

Low-birth-weight infants (< 2500 g at birth) comprise about 16 per cent of all births globally but may be as many as half of all births occurring in underprivileged communities in LDCs. Such infants tend to be underweight in later life and may contribute substantially to the prevalence of childhood malnutrition. Indeed one study estimated that up to one-third of malnourished children may have been babies with low birth weights.

Some low-birth-weight infants are born preterm (less than 37 completed weeks of gestation) but probably more than half in LDCs are growth-retarded *in utero* and are born small for gestational age (SGA). Growth performance in the two groups differs during early childhood. Preterm infants of appropriate size appear to continue to grow at a rate compatible with their conceptional age and attain more or less normal size by the end of the first year. By contrast, healthy SGA infants grow more slowly, with measurable differences in mean attained weight in later childhood.

Moreover, immunity is impaired in low-birth-weight infants, particularly those who are small for gestational age. Increased susceptibility to infections, including diarrhoea, could be expected to contribute indirectly to impaired growth and hence malnutrition.

Thus, interventions preventing low birth weight, particularly the SGA category, might contribute to reducing childhood malnutrition. Though the effective-

Table 3.5.10 Selected maternal factors associated with low birth weight

Fertility	Teenage (esp. adolescent) pregnancy
	Extremes of parity
	Short birth intervals
Infections	Urinary tract infections
	Malaria
Nutrition	Severe iron-deficiency anaemia
	Folic acid deficiency
	Acute reduction in food (energy) intake
Occupation	Manual labour
Other	Hypertension, pre-eclampsia
	Alcohol abuse
	Smoking

ness of such an approach is largely unknown we shall consider selected aspects of maternal and reproductive health which appear to be associated with an increased risk of low-birth-weight babies and are at least theoretically avoidable. These are summarized in Table 3.5.10.

Fertility

Adolescent pregnancy

In both developed and developing countries teenage pregnancies result in a higher frequency of low-birth-weight babies for any given parity. Thus, avoiding teenage pregnancy might reduce low-birth-weight outcomes.

It has been suggested that pregnancy coming shortly after the menarche may compete with the nutritional needs of the still-growing mother and even curtail her final attained height. Since birth weight correlates positively with maternal height, avoiding adolescent motherhood could conceivably affect all of a woman's pregnancies.

Large family size and birth order

Large family size is associated with poorer growth of children and with increased risk of malnutrition. The mechanism is not clear: it might be related to reduced food availability in the poorest families or to increased infections, as suggested by the association between crowding, severity of infection and malnutrition found in some studies. In this situation inadequate child-care by the overtaxed mother may be another factor. Related to this, high birth orders have been associated with both low birth weights and with protein–energy malnutrition.

Short birth intervals

Short birth intervals have been found by some to be associated with lower birth weights and with lower weight and height in later childhood, but others have not confirmed this, possibly because of a better overall level of health and nutritional status. An association between short birth interval and malnutrition has also been described in conditions of severe food shortage, but again the relationship appears to be inconsistent. Such inconsistencies are irrelevant, however, in terms of policy-making since short birth intervals are found repeatedly to be associated with higher mortality, even in communities where the association with nutritional status is not clear.

Fertility regulation

Family planning is a major component of many primary health care programmes world-wide and there may be little obviously controversial in advocating small, well-spaced families, born to mothers mainly between the age of 20 and 35 years. Indeed it would appear sound advice in the general context of maternal health. Nevertheless, in many parts of the world, implementing such a policy would require major social change. If achieved, the expected benefits would include lower incidence of low-birth-weight babies and early childhood malnutrition.

Maternal health and nutrition

Infections

Any serious illness during pregnancy may affect the outcome in terms of length of gestation and birth weight; some specific examples are well documented.

Urinary tract infections, particularly common during pregnancy, adversely affect size-for-gestational-age and also length of gestation.

Malaria, which impairs placental function particularly in primiparous women, has a deleterious effect on pregnancy outcome, reflected in low birth weight and stillbirth incidence. In the British Solomon Islands a successful malaria eradication programme was followed by an increase in mean birth weight and a reduction in preterm births.

Nutritional deficiency

Iron and folic acid requirements are increased during pregnancy and anaemia of pregnancy is common in all LDCs. Several studies have shown that severe maternal anaemia is associated with risk of low birth weight, and this relationship may exist even in milder cases with haemoglobin levels of around 8 g/dl.

Several studies have shown a relationship between maternal anthropometry and birth weight. Famine studies suggest that birth weight is markedly reduced during periods of acute food shortage. In less extreme circumstances, pregnant women in LDCs regularly subsist on dietary intakes which are substantially lower than the minimum internationally recommended amounts. Seasonal falls in the already low mean birth weight are commonplace during the pre-harvest lean season typical of many Third World rural communities and it is often stated that the incidence of low birth weight may be reduced by improving maternal nutritional status.

A study in Guatemala suggested that a reduction in low birth weight could be achieved by increasing maternal energy intake during pregnancy but it was unclear whether the situation was one of acute or chronic dietary insufficiency. It seems that under steady conditions chronically undernourished populations may adapt in some way to low dietary energy intake, which some studies have found to be surprisingly low, whilst maintaining relatively normal birth weights. Only when intakes fall further, below such levels, does fetal growth appear to be markedly affected, and perhaps only in situations of acute food shortage are nutrition interventions really effective in increasing birth weight. Thus comprehensive dietary supplementation of pregnant women in a rural community in The Gambia was effective in increasing birth weight only during the hungry season, despite energy intakes below recommended allowances throughout the year.

Re-examination of the relationship between maternal anthropometry and birth weight suggests that fetal growth is related in some way to lean body mass rather than to maternal energy reserves. This may help to explain why energy supplementation, which is effective mainly in boosting fat reserves, might have no impact in mildly malnourished women with adequate lean body mass.

Maternal workload

This subject is understandably usually considered in relation to energy balance. Equal, and perhaps more important, is the effect of hard physical labour, particularly in a hot climate, which results in increased sympathetic nervous activity and may reduce placental blood flow. The importance of this has been discussed in detail in relation to man's upright posture and the biologically distinctive and possibly disadvantageous preterm dip in growth exhibited by the human fetus.

Historically, social laws introduced to limit women's work in the last trimester of pregnancy were the first public health measures taken to reduce low birth weight on a wide scale in the developed countries. The impact of these measures is difficult to assess now, but they are likely to be highly relevant in poor communities where women continue hard physical labour throughout pregnancy, and could be more important than providing extra food. Indeed, one of the benefits described by the pregnant Keneba mothers receiving a dietary supplement was a greater capacity for agricultural labour! This highlights an important problem; in many LDCs rural women form an important part of the labour force involved in food production. Attempting to remove them from this for several months during a critical season could have a substantial economic as well as social impact.

Antenatal care

Considerable concern has been voiced recently about the inadequacy of the maternal component of maternal and child health (MCH) programmes. In many countries little if any regular contact is made between health personnel and women during pregnancy, though all agree that this is necessary for the health of both the mother and the fetus. The problem is compounded on the one hand by real difficulties in gaining access to services and on the other by their limitations when they are available.

Effective treatment of urinary tract infections should be a priority, though in many developing countries it may be difficult to implement systematic screening and treatment, even where antenatal facilities have been established.

In countries where malaria is endemic, chemoprophylaxis should be given to primiparous women throughout pregnancy and to multiparae at least during the last trimester. In combination with folic acid supplements this might also have a beneficial effect in relation to anaemia of pregnancy referred to above. In some countries, particularly in south east Asia where parasite resistance is high and endemicity low, emphasis is now placed on early diagnosis and adequate treatment of malaria during pregnancy, together with vector avoidance, where possible. Chemoprophylaxis has been abandoned.

In many LDCs the routine use of iron or folate supplements during pregnancy may be justified by the high prevalence of moderate degrees of anaemia but it is not clear to what extent this would increase birth weights, unless combined with a programme to detect and effectively treat more severe cases.

Nutrition in pregnancy also is important. Intensive nutrition interventions aimed comprehensively at boosting the energy intake of all pregnant women are likely to be complex and costly. Whilst the problem of chronic undernutrition cannot be dismissed, targeting limited resources at times of acute shortage, particularly during the last trimester of pregnancy, is likely to be the most effective way of reducing the incidence of low birth weight. In parts of East Africa a habit of traditional dieting during the last trimester in particular is common for the very purpose of reducing birth weight; to what extent it is successful is not well documented, but certainly fairly dramatic weight losses are induced in the mothers who practice it. It clearly should be discouraged.

The tradition already exists in many subsistence farming communities of a communal approach to shared labour, which may include working on neighbours' lands when the need arises. This kind of approach offers the only practical hope of rest for many rural mothers in the later stages of pregnancy and the potential benefits make it well worth pursuing.

The reproductive span of women in LDCs is typically around 30 years, though theoretically this might be halved by effective family planning measures. Even so, reproductive health cannot be divorced from general health and the factors affecting it. No maternal health care programme can be entirely effective in communities where practices discriminating against females are commonplace, particularly with respect to diet and food-sharing, educational opportunities and access to preventive and curative health care.

Many of the above measures, and others not previously mentioned, including treatment of hypertension and pre-eclamptic toxaemia and avoidance of smoking, may produce only modest increases in mean birth weight, particularly when incompletely implemented. However, small improvements are compatible with a substantial reduction in the incidence of low birth weight, as described in West Africa and South America.

Postnatal factors

A simple list of factors which influence growth in childhood and the development of malnutrition is shown in Table 3.5.11.

Nutrition–infection interactions

Malnutrition in childhood has two major components, dietary deficiency and infection, which almost always

Table 3.5.11   Selected factors directly or indirectly affecting growth in early childhood

Feeding practices	Bottle-feeding
	Inadequate lactation/breast-feeding
	Inappropriate weaning practices
Infections	Gastro-intestinal infections
	Malaria
	Measles
	Tuberculosis
	Pertussis

coexist and which interact synergistically. The contribution of the latter is so great that, except during periods of acute food shortage, control of certain infections might almost eliminate much of the so-called malnutrition which is so rife in LDCs. Nutritional status in turn can modify the impact of infections which tend to be more prolonged and severe in the presence of severe malnutrition. Thus, any programme aimed at preventing malnutrition must have both nutritional and public health elements if it is to be really effective.

The most important infections in this context are undoubtedly the diarrhoeal diseases. In general, there is a strong negative linear correlation between prevalence of diarrhoea and growth. Though some have found the number of episodes to be the more important factor others, probably more correctly, have found that the prolonged attacks have the greatest impact on growth. In terms of aetiology, the least important episodes appear to be those in which no pathogenic agents can be identified. Of the known pathogens, *Shigella* spp. have the greatest effect. Giardiasis is the most important example of a protozoal gut infection sometimes associated with marked growth faltering, though not always with diarrhoea. One study in rural Gambia suggested that the growth rate in early childhood was halved by the level of diarrhoeal illness experienced there. A more detailed analysis in an urban population showed that the impact was minimal in exclusively breast-fed children and increased four-fold once supplementary feeding was introduced. It seems that the effect of diarrhoeal illness on growth in some children persists long after the illness, possibly due to dietary constraints which prevent catch-up growth, persisting pathology impairing gut function, or a combination of both.

Measles is probably the next most important infection precipitating protein–energy malnutrition, both kwashiorkor and marasmus. High fever and anorexia occur during the acute phase, mucous membranes are extensively affected, producing a protein-losing enteropathy in some children, and lower respiratory tract infection is a common complication. Lower respiratory tract infection and malaria are two other entities which also have a profound effect on growth when estimated on the basis of days ill, but their relatively low prevalence diminishes their contribution to the overall picture of childhood malnutrition.

Two other specific infections of the respiratory tract, tuberculosis and pertussis, particularly the former, are also major causes of malnutrition. The impact on nutritional status of lower respiratory tract infections in general, and of specific infections such as measles, tuberculosis and malaria, has been demonstrated even in communities where they have been actively treated. To an even greater extent than with diarrhoea, prevention must be considered the main strategy in the context of combating malnutrition. The role of HIV infection has already been mentioned and is dealt with more fully on pp. 600–4.

Infant feeding

Breast-feeding

There is abundant evidence that bottle-fed children, particularly those in underprivileged communities in LDCs, suffer significantly more frequent and severe gastro-intestinal infections than breast-fed children. To a lesser extent this may apply to respiratory tract infections. Thus, breast-feeding plays an important role in protecting the infant from gastro-intestinal infection. This may be partly due to the relatively low exposure to gut pathogens of the exclusively breast-fed child and partly to the protection afforded by the various antimicrobial factors demonstrated in breast-milk. There is now evidence to suggest that prolonged breast-feeding up to three years of age may reduce the severity of at least one gastro-intestinal infection, shigellosis, apparently due to this protective effect rather than to any difference in nutritional status.

From the purely nutritional side there is considerable debate as to how long breast-milk alone can adequately meet the needs of the growing infant. Despite a lot of studies we seem unable to do better than to say that this period is usually between three and six months. Prolonged *exclusive* breast-feeding, which in some societies may extend into the second year of life, is itself an important cause of malnutrition.

Lactation

Understandably there has been considerable interest in attempts to improve lactational performance, in other words, to boost breast-milk production. Though somewhat controversial it may be said that dietary supplementation of lactating women has been generally disappointing in this respect. The suckling infant appears to be the main factor controlling the amount of milk produced and the interventions most likely to be effective are those leading to higher-birth-weight babies and improving feeding practices, including avoiding unnecessarily early introduction of complementary feeds which may inhibit milk production.

Weaning

Weaning here is defined as the introduction and regular consumption of additional foods by an otherwise breast-fed infant. The weaning period commences with the first of these regular additions and ends with the cessation of breast-feeding. During this period the child is referred to as the 'weanling'.

Timing of the onset of weaning is obviously a critical factor affecting nutrition both directly and indirectly. If delayed, the child will suffer a shortfall in nutrient intake which may lead eventually to severe malnutrition and in turn be compounded by increasing severity of intercurrent infections. Excessively early weaning, on the other hand, may increase the risk of some infections and their impact on growth and hence nutritional status. This 'weanling's dilemma' is illustrated in Fig. 3.5.12.

One method used to help decide when weaning should be initiated in the individual child is growth monitoring and the use of growth charts. This has also been promoted as a major health care strategy aimed at preventing malnutrition and will be considered here in some detail.

Growth monitoring

The concept behind growth monitoring is that the regular measurement and recording of a child's growth, usually weight, in relation to some normal standard, will enable us to detect minor degrees of growth faltering, so called 'invisible malnutrition', and to intervene to prevent the development of frank malnutrition (see pp. 270–5). For this approach to be successful, we must be able to detect growth faltering, to interpret the cause of growth faltering and to treat the child effectively. In practice none of these is straightforward or easy to achieve in many Third World situations.

To detect weight faltering it is necessary to make regular (usually monthly) contact with the mother and child and to measure and record weight with reasonable accuracy. Because access to clinics is often limited, efforts have been made to introduce simple, low-cost

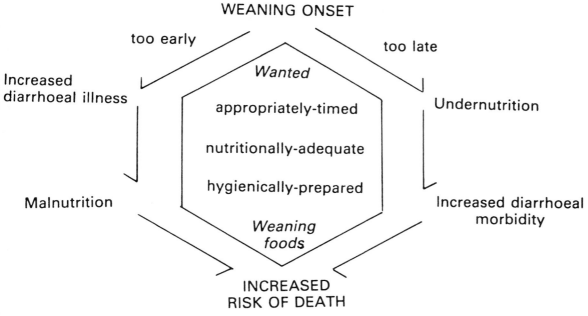

Fig. 3.5.12 The dilemma of weaning.

weighing scales which may be kept and used in the home by the mother. Growth faltering is then identifiable by the weight curve deviating from centile lines of an internationally recognized standard, usually the Harvard or National Center for Health Statistics standard. Unfortunately, at the critical period during the second three months of infancy when most decisions about weaning arise, the shape of these standard curves is inappropriate for breast-feeding populations. The more common practice is to teach people to recognize growth faltering when there has been no weight gain over several measurements or actual weight loss. The problem with this approach is that a period of several months may elapse before the pattern of growth becomes clear and this is incompatible with the concept of detecting the earliest signs of faltering. Often the failure of adequate catch-up after an infection indicates an inadequate diet (see p. 272).

Once faltering is identified, it is necessary to decide whether the problem is one of nutritional shortfall, continuing infection or, more often than not, both. If the former, the interventions required may range from nutritional advice on the best use of existing resources, provision of food supplements in the home or at a day-care centre, or in more serious cases, more intensive nutrition rehabilitation on an in-patient basis. Only the first can seriously be considered in the context of preventing malnutrition.

Nutrition education

Though of considerable general relevance, nutrition education is perhaps most important in relation to weaning. Unfortunately, it is a health intervention which is often implemented inadequately and ineffectively. Nevertheless, working on the premise that faulty weaning practices, rather than food scarcity, are important in the aetiology of malnutrition in young children, it has been concluded that weaning education can improve the nutritional status of infants and young children provided that programmes are appropriately designed with regard to both content of the messages and the method of delivery. Both of these aspects can vary considerably between one community and another, involving social and cultural factors as well as economic and agricultural realities.

The three major aims of general relevance to any weaning education programme have already been set out in Fig. 3.5.12. The first, the question of timing of initiation of weaning, has been dealt with. The question of nutritional adequacy is largely covered on pp. 324–35 but two general points deserve emphasis.

First, many of the traditional weaning foods are dilute cereal gruels with no additional nutrients. Such foods typically have an energy density around half that of breast-milk and are deficient in a range of nutrients. By contrast, foods being consumed by toddlers are often multimixes containing a range of nutrients and an energy density adequate to sustain normal and even catch-up growth. One generally appropriate piece of advice, therefore, may be to keep to a minimum the period during which children are fed the earlier transitional weaning foods. This is a message which needs continual re-inforcement, particularly when children are recovering from illnesses associated with anorexia.

The other generalization that may be made is that gruels, which are the typical early weaning foods in many communities, are very often highly contaminated. The regular consumption of contaminated foods plays an important role in transmission of bacteria and protozoa associated with diarrhoeal disease, and probably also in the pathogenesis of the small bowel contamination syndrome. Measures reducing their incidence can reasonably be expected to improve nutritional status. Detailed studies of the role of food and water hygiene and the way in which weaning foods become bacterially contaminated within the home, including one in The Gambia, have given some indication of the steps needed for improvement.

The management of some infections may be carried out in the home whilst others will require referral to a clinic with diagnostic and curative facilities. Early treatment in the home of gastro-intestinal and even lower respiratory tract infections is possible given good coverage by paramedics trained in the wise use of simple regimens. Because of its strong relationship with malnutrition, diarrhoea merits special mention here.

Diarrhoea management

Oral rehydration therapy with a glucose or sucrose electrolyte mixture is now the cornerstone for the management of watery diarrhoea. Its effectiveness was first demonstrated on a large scale in 1971, during a cholera epidemic among the West Bengal refugee camps during the Bangladesh liberation war. Subsequently, it was noted both in community and ward studies that its use appeared to be associated with a small improvement in nutritional status. This probably stemmed from improved food intake during or shortly after the diarrhoeal episode. Maintaining dietary intake is increasingly recognized as an important part of diarrhoea management, particularly for reducing nutritional sequelae. There is no physiological basis for 'resting' the bowel in acute diarrhoea; fasting

should be avoided, except in the severely dehydrated child who is too ill to eat, a condition which should be actively treated and reversed within four to eight hours.

It now seems that replacing the glucose or sucrose in the ORS formulation by cooked rice powder can also result in a substantial reduction in the diarrhoea stool volume and in the duration of diarrhoea. The use of such a cereal-based ORS furthermore appears to confer a marked nutritional benefit. There are some problems in that the cereal powder must be cooked, packaging is more complex and once prepared the solution may be more prone to overgrowth by bacterial contaminants. Nevertheless, the regular use of such improved formulations for the treatment of diarrhoea in the home, if feasible, may be an effective strategy for combating diarrhoea-induced malnutrition. (Fig. 3.5.13).

Conclusions

Health strategies aimed at preventing malnutrition coincide very closely with those promoted by UNICEF for improving child health and survival referred to under the acronym GOBI-FFF (Table 3.5.12).

This is not surprising given the close link between nutritional strategy, health and mortality in childhood, and serves to emphasize further the role of integrated health services aimed at improving nutrition and health. The need for such a comprehensive package makes it all the more important to examine critically each component in terms of effectiveness whilst also being alert for any important omissions.

Growth monitoring is not *per se* a health or nutrition intervention but the measurement of growth or nutritional status is necessary if intensive interventions are to be targeted on individuals at risk.

Oral rehydration therapy must be widely practised at home if it is to have an impact on malnutrition. Oral rehydration solutions do not constitute a universal panacea. Maximum effectiveness requires improved formulations, properly used and reinforced by appro-

Table 3.5.12 GOBI–FFF

Growth monitoring
Oral rehydration therapy
Breast-feeding
Immunization

Female education
Food supplements
Family spacing

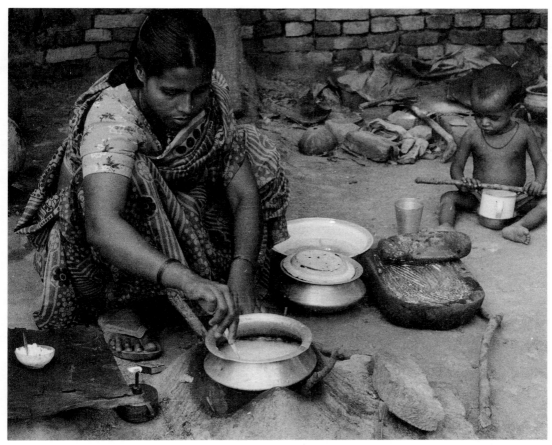

Fig. 3.5.13 Having ground dry rice (approx. 80 g) to a fine powder, a mother brings it to the boil in a litre of water. Next she must cool the mixture and add salt. The procedure can be simplified by providing her with premeasured rice powder and electrolytes but packaging of rice powder ORS is not as simple as with the WHO/UNICEF formulation. (By courtesy of A. Ansari.)

priate nutritional practices. Furthermore, it is of limited relevance for shigellosis which is perhaps the most important diarrhoeal illness in the context of nutritional and other problems. There appears to be a growing epidemic in south-east Asia of highly virulent *Shigella* strains with increasing resistance to a range of antibiotics used in the treatment of the more severe cases.

Effective support must be given to ensure that lactation is successfully established and maintained. Amongst other factors, breast-milk intake correlates positively with birth weight. No breast-feeding programme is complete without advice and support on weaning and this is one of the areas in which growth monitoring is potentially important.

Immunization is an important part of any MCH programme in its own right. BCG and measles immuniza-tion are amongst the most important in terms of growth and nutrition. The currently used Schwartz vaccine for measles prevention suffers two drawbacks in relation to its timing: 15 per cent or more children will have suffered an attack of measles by the age of nine months; and attendance at most MCH clinics has been found to fall off quite markedly in the second half of infancy. If other approaches are adopted, such as the use of the Edmonston–Zagreb strain permitting immunization before the age of six months, we can expect nutritional as well as other health improvements (see however p. 81). Similar benefits should result from progress with vaccines against enteric infections, shigella vaccines again being of particular interest in the context of nutrition.

An important addition was recently made to UNICEF's so-called 'lifelines' which now include combating malaria, acute respiratory infections and a section on iron, iodine and vitamin A. The importance of vitamin A lies partly in its apparent effects on child mortality in chronically vitamin-deficient populations. Its action is thought to be related to host-defence mechanisms at mucosal level, and two of the illnesses which may specifically be influenced are diarrhoeal and respiratory disease, including measles. If it affects morbidity as well as mortality, then it is likely to be of beneficial effect on nutritional status following non-fatal infections.

We are still unable to make more than the most general of recommendations on water and sanitation measures and on hygiene in the home. Nevertheless, this important topic must not be neglected in any comprehensive health care programme which has the improvement of nutritional status as a major objective. Also important is the regular treatment of intestinal parasites, particularly hookworm and giardia.

Food supplementation is a rather controversial subject; used uncritically it is an expensive form of first-aid which many fear breeds dependency and in few situations can it be thought of as a preventive strategy. Nevertheless, it should be available to back-stop more general measures such as nutrition education.

The case for family spacing and limitation of family size is now well established. The problem of preventing adolescent motherhood is far more difficult to tackle, particularly in communities where betrothal and marriage close to the age of puberty is the norm. The need for female education is unlikely to be a simple question of knowledge and is probably related, amongst other things, to status of females in society. Until this is improved much of the potential impact of the integrated package described above will be lost and for this reason many would put this issue at the top of the list. Though not normally within the realms of responsibility of health professionals they should nevertheless seize whatever opportunities may come their way to promote this.

Further reading

Ashworth A, Feachem RG. Interventions for the control of diarrhoeal diseases among young children: prevention of low birth weight. *Bulletin of the World Health Organization.* 1985; **63**(1): 165–84.

Briend A. Normal fetal growth regulation: nutritional aspects. In: Gracey M, Falkner F eds. *Nutritional Needs and Assessment of Normal Growth. Nestlé Nutrition Workshop Series,*

Vol 7. New York, Raven Press, 1985. pp. 1–18.

Church M, Stanfield JP. The weight chart: an invaluable aid in nutrition rehabilitation. *Journal of Tropical Paediatrics.* 1971; **17** (Monograph): 61–5.

Ebrahim GJ. Protein–energy malnutrition. In: *Nutrition in Mother and Child Health.* London, Macmillan Press, 1983. pp. 104–33.

Hytten FE, Leitch I. *The Physiology of Human Pregnancy*, 2nd Edn. Oxford, Blackwell Scientific Publications, 1971.

Lechtig A. Early malnutrition, growth and development. In: Gracey M, Falkner F eds. *Nutritional Needs and Assessment of Normal Growth. Nestlé Nutrition Workshop Series, Vol 7.* New York, Raven Press, 1985. pp. 185–214.

Mahalanabis D. Oral rehydration therapy. In: Gracey M ed. *Diarrhoeal Diseases and Malnutrition: A Clinical Update.* London, Churchill Livingstone, 1985. pp. 145–57.

Mata L. Environmental factors affecting nutrition and growth. In: Gracey M, Falkner F eds. *Nutritional Needs and Assessment of Normal Growth. Nestlé Nutrition Workshop Series, Vol 7.* New York, Raven Press, 1985. pp. 165–84.

Mata L. Role of health services in improving nutrition and health. *Proceedings of the XIII International Congress of Nutrition 1985.* London, John Libbey, 1986. pp. 106–9.

Prentice AM. Variations in maternal dietary intake, birth weight and breast-milk output in The Gambia. In: Aebi H, Whitehead RG eds. *Maternal Nutrition During Pregnancy and Lactation.* Berne, Hans Huber, 1980. pp. 167–83.

Prentice AM, Whitehead RG, Prentice A, Cole TJ. Interventions to improve lactational performance: a practical proposition? *Proceedings of the XIII International Congress of Nutrition 1985.* London, John Libbey, 1986. pp. 618–21.

Rowland MGM. Infant feeding practices. In: Gracey M ed. *Diarrhoeal Diseases and Malnutrition: A Clinical Update.* London, Churchill Livingstone, 1985. pp. 119–27.

Rowland MGM. Bacterial diarrhoeas: contaminated food and water. In: Gracey M ed. *Diarrhoeal Diseases and Malnutrition: A Clinical Update.* London, Churchill Livingstone, 1985. pp. 47–62.

Rowland MGM. The weanling's dilemma: are we making progress? *Acta Paediatrica Scandinavica.* 1986; **323** Supplement: 33–42.

Rowland MGM, Rowland SGJ Goh. Growth faltering in diarrhoea. *Proceedings of the XIII International Congress of Nutrition 1985.* London, John Libbey, 1986. pp. 115–19.

UNICEF. *The State of The World's Children 1987.* Oxford, Oxford University Press, 1987.

Victora CG, Barros FC, Vaughan JP. Mortality, morbidity and malnutrition in relation to birth weight: a longitudinal study of 5914 Brazilian children. *Proceedings of the XIII International Congress of Nutrition 1985.* London, John Libbey, 1986. pp. 96–100.

Whitehead RG, Lawrence M, Prentice AM. Incremental dietary needs to support pregnancy. *Proceedings of the XIII International Congress of Nutrition 1985.* London, John Libbey, 1986. pp. 599–603.

SPECIFIC VITAMIN DEFICIENCIES
V. Reddy and W. H. Lamb

Vitamin A

Vitamin A deficiency and xerophthalmia are among the most widespread and serious nutritional disorders in developing countries. In acute deficiency, many tissues are affected but the most significant lesion is the disruption of the cornea leading to blindness. About half-a-million children become blind every year as a result of this deficiency. Most of them lose their sight before they reach five years of age. The immense social and economic implications of the disease are obvious. The tragedy is that nutritional blindness is easily preventable and need not and should not occur.

Dietary sources

Vitamin A is obtained through the diet as preformed vitamin A or its precursor, β-carotene, Preformed vitamin A is present in animal foods such as milk, butter, eggs, liver and fish. Green leafy vegetables and fruits (like mango and papaya) are rich in β-carotene. Other sources are carrots, yellow corn and red palm oil.

β-carotene is not utilized as efficiently as vitamin A because of its incomplete absorption and conversion into vitamin A. Absorption of β-carotene from different foods varies widely and its availability is generally considered to be about 33 per cent.[1] Since the efficiency of its conversion to retinol is limited, 1 μg of β-carotene is equivalent in terms of biological activity to 0.16 μg retinol. This may, however, lead to an underestimate of vitamin A activity of β-carotene when consumed in small amounts.

The bioavailability of carotenoids depends on the level of intake and its mode of dispersion. Higher rates of absorption has been observed with carotene dissolved in oil. In the studies reported from India, absorption of carotenes from green leafy vegetables was more than 50 per cent, and therefore a factor of 0.25 was suggested instead of 0.16 to convert β-carotene to vitamin A.[2] Thus, if the vitamin is derived entirely from vegetable sources, the intake of β-carotene should be about 4–6 times the recommended level of retinol.

Daily requirements

The dietary allowances of vitamin A recommended for different age groups are given in Table 3.5.13.[1] These estimates are based on two types of data: field observations on human population groups and control depletion experiments carried out in human volunteers. The

Table 3.5.13 Recommended intake (μg retinol/day) for different age groups

0–6 years	300
7–10 years	400
Adolescents	750
Adults	750
Pregnancy	750
Lactation	1200

(Reproduced from *Requirements of Vitamin A, thiamine, riboflavine and niacin: report of a Joint FAO/WHO Expert group. Geneva, WHO*, no. 362, 1967.)

recommended intakes are described here as micrograms of retinol. The international unit is equivalent to $0.3 \, \mu g$ retinol. Adjustments have to be made when the vitamin is obtained from its precursors of plant origin.

Terminology

Xerophthalmia

This term covers all ocular manifestations of vitamin A deficiency including night blindness, conjunctival and corneal lesions.

Vitamin A deficiency

This includes not only xerophthalmia but also other conditions in which vitamin A status is subnormal. It has much wider implications since vitamin A is known to have an important role in many extraocular processes.

Prevalence

Global distribution

Vitamin A deficiency is widely prevalent in large parts of Africa and Asia. There are also scattered foci in the Middle East and Latin America. Results of recent surveys conducted in different countries have been reviewed in a WHO report.[3] Vitamin A deficiency has been identified as a significant public health problem in the following countries:

- Africa: Sahelian and sub-Sahelian regions – Benin, Mali and Mauritania; east and south Ethiopia, Malawi, Tanzania and Zambia
- Americas: El Salvador, Haiti and parts of Brazil and Mexico
- Asia: Bangladesh, India, Indonesia, Nepal and Sri Lanka
- Eastern Mediterranean: Oman and Sudan
- Western Pacific: Philippines and Vietnam

Precise figures are not available for the total incidence of xerophthalmia but a rough estimate has been made using information obtained from Asian countries where the children have been closely followed. A world-wide projection based on these estimates exceeds 500 000 cases of corneal lesions that result in partial or total blindness, and 6–7 million cases of mild xerophthalmia, each year. These figures may be considered conservative since mortality is very high among these children.

Age and sex incidence

Age plays an important role in determining not only the incidence of vitamin A deficiency but also the nature of ocular lesions. Though conjunctival signs are seen in all age groups, serious corneal damage occurs in children below five years of age and is usually associated with protein–energy malnutrition.

The incidence of xerophthalmia has been reported to be slightly higher in males than in females. Seasonal variation has also been observed, which may be related to the availability of vitamin A-rich foods.

Pathogenesis of deficiency

Inadequate dietary intake of vitamin A is the most important cause for the wide prevalence of xerophthalmia in children.[2, 4] Other factors like poor nutritional status of the mother during pregnancy and lactation, the time at which supplementary feeding is started and frequent infections are all important in determining the clinical manifestations of the disease.

Dietary intake of vitamin A

Diets of pregnant and lactating women in poor communities are deficient in many nutrients, including vitamin A. Low serum levels of vitamin A and depleted liver stores have been reported in infants born to undernourished women. During the first few months of life, vitamin A needs of the child are met exclusively from breast-milk and the vitamin content of milk is related to the dietary intake of the mother. However, breast-fed infants rarely show clinical signs of vitamin A deficiency, indicating that the relatively low vitamin content of breast-milk is sufficient to protect them against xerophthalmia.

Once the child is started on solid foods, the amount of vitamin A received depends largely on the types of food given. In many poor communities, supplementary feeding is delayed beyond the age of one year and foods containing vitamin A are seldom given. Diet surveys carried out in Asian and Latin American countries have shown that the daily intake of vitamin A in preschool children is less than $100 \, \mu g$ and most of it is derived from β-carotene.

Role of protein–energy malnutrition

In south-east Asian countries, protein–energy malnutrition and vitamin A deficiency are the major nutritional problems and often coexist among preschool children. The prevalence of xerophthalmia is several fold higher in children with kwashiorkor than in the general population.[2, 5] Serum vitamin A levels are also reduced in malnourished children. These observations suggest that protein malnutrition may aggravate vitamin A deficiency and precipitate clinical manifestations. There is also experimental evidence that protein deficiency can influence vitamin A metabolism by interfering with the absorption and transport of the vitamin. However, the vitamin A content of the diet appears to be more critical than that of protein in the development of ocular manifestations. In some parts of Africa, habitual diets contain red palm oil which is a rich source of β-carotene. In such populations, although protein–energy malnutrition is widespread among children, ocular signs of vitamin A deficiency are extremely rare. Similar observations have been reported in Indonesian children who had low protein intake but good amounts of vitamin A in their diets.[5] In the studies reported from India, undernourished children receiving daily supplements of leafy green vegetables showed a significant increase in serum vitamin A levels.[2] These observations indicate that β-carotene is absorbed and utilized well even in malnourished children.

Dietary intake of fat

Dietary fat is known to influence absorption of β-carotene and vitamin A. In Indonesia, children whose diets contained adequate β-carotene but low fat had low serum vitamin A levels and these could be raised by small supplements of fats. Studies in Indian children have also shown that additional fat in the diet improved absorption of β-carotene.[2]

Diets of preschool children in poor communities are deficient in several nutrients. Though the interplay of these factors is significant, inadequate intake of vitamin A is the primary cause of xerophthalmia.

Role of infections

Xerophthalmia is often associated with infections such as measles, diarrhoea and respiratory infection. During acute infection, not only is the food intake reduced but metabolic alterations are also known to occur. Clinical studies have shown that the intestinal absorption of vitamin A is impaired and serum levels of vitamin A are significantly depressed in children with acute infection. Apart from these metabolic effects, measles seems to have a direct role in the development of corneal lesions. Many reports from Africa document the serious nature of measles and the frequency of keratoconjunctivitis leading to blindness.[6] Intestinal parasitic infections are also common among children in poor communities. Malabsorption of vitamin A has been reported in subjects with ascariasis and giardiasis.

Clinical features

Ocular manifestations

In humans, the most notable effects of vitamin A deficiency are the ocular manifestations. Mild deficiency leads to night blindness and conjunctival changes while severe deficiency results in corneal destruction.[2, 3] The term 'xerophthalmia' includes all these lesions.

Night blindness Deficiency of vitamin A leads to delayed synthesis of rhodopsin and impaired dark adaptation, resulting in night blindness. Testing dark adaptation in young children is difficult, especially in the field. A history of night blindness, although a subjective sign, is more useful for screening xerophthalmia in a community.[5]

Colour vision Although vitamin A deficiency is known to cause disturbance of rod function, there is little information regarding its effect on cone function. In patients with biliary cirrhosis who had impaired dark adaptation and defective colour vision, vitamin A treatment produced significant improvement. Studies in Indian children with vitamin A deficiency, however, revealed no abnormality in colour vision.

Conjunctival lesions Conjunctival xerosis is characterized by dryness, loss of transparency, non-wetability and wrinkling of the conjunctiva. Early stages are, however, not easy to diagnose clinically. Staining with rose bengal or lissamine green has been suggested but recent studies indicate that this is not reliable.

Bitot spots appear as greyish white, foamy patches, raised above the level of the conjunctiva (Fig. 3.5.14). They are usually bilateral and located on the temporal side of the eye. Sometimes they appear black when smeared with kajal (carbon cream) or mascara. Bitot spots generally reflect chronic deficiency and may not be seen in all cases. Some children develop serious eye lesions progressing to keratomalacia and blindness without ever developing Bitot spots.

Some adults and older children have Bitot spots which do not respond to treatment with vitamin A. On this basis, the role of vitamin A in the pathogenesis of Bitot spots has been questioned. The disappearance of Bitot spots in most preschool children following

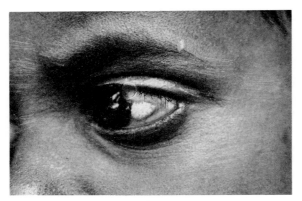

Fig. 3.5.14 Xerophthalmia: Bitot spots.

administration of vitamin A, suggests some correlation in this age group.

Corneal lesions Severe vitamin A deficiency leads to corneal involvement and is invariably associated with protein–energy malnutrition. Even before the clinical lesions become evident, changes occur in the corneal epithelium which can be detected by slit-lamp examination after fluorescene staining. Punctuate keratopathy has been observed in many children with night blindness and conjunctival xerosis whose cornea appear normal on clinical examination.[3]

Loss of lustre, haziness and dryness are characteristic of corneal xerosis. This can be reversed completely with vitamin A therapy but in untreated cases it progresses rapidly to keratomalacia (Fig. 3.5.15). Stromal defects cause ulceration and in advanced stages there is softening, perforation and complete destruction of the cornea resulting in blindness. The healed lesions remain as corneal opacities or staphyloma (Fig. 3.5.16). Loss of vision depends upon the degree of corneal involvement and the extent of scarring.

Extraocular effects

In experimental animals, vitamin A deficiency produces a variety of effects, including growth retardation, sterility and changes in bone tissue and the central nervous system. However, these effects have not been confirmed in humans. Infections and deficiency of other nutrients, particularly protein–energy malnutrition can also impair the appetite and retard growth, and their common occurrence in vitamin A-deficient children has hitherto precluded the demonstration of such an effect of vitamin A deficiency.

Follicular hyperkeratosis has been observed in depletion studies on adults but it is a non-specific sign

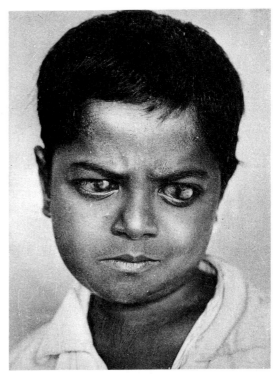

Fig. 3.5.15 Xerophthalmia: keratomalacia.

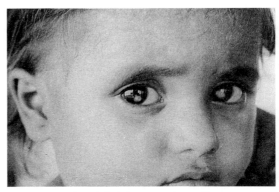

Fig. 3.5.16 Xerophthalmia: corneal opacities.

and rare in young children. In these studies, abnormalities were also observed in taste and smell.

Anaemia Studies in experimental animals as well as in human volunteers have shown that vitamin A deficiency can lead to anaemia. Low haemoglobin levels have been reported in children with xerophthalmia.[2] After treatment with vitamin A, there was a significant increase in haemoglobin as well as serum iron concentration. Since the absorption of iron is not altered in vitamin A deficiency hypoferraemia has been attributed to impaired mobilization of iron from the stores.

These observations suggest that apart from iron deficiency, hypovitaminosis A may also contribute to the prevalence of anaemia in poor communities. This is supported by the data generated from intervention studies. In countries where a vitamin A supplementation programme has been implemented, there was not only an improvement in vitamin A nutrition of the population but also a significant increase in their haemoglobin levels.

Resistence to infection Vitamin A has been called an 'anti-infective' vitamin because its deficiency leads to a variety of infections in experimental animals. Although epithelial changes and reduced mucus production are primary factors, altered immune mechanisms also contribute to lowered resistance to infection. Both the humoral and the cell-mediated immune responses have been shown to be altered in vitamin A deficient rats. There is, however, little information on immunocompetence in human vitamin A deficiency.

In Indian children who had clinical signs of vitamin A deficiency, lysozymal content of leucocytes has been shown to be significantly reduced.[2] Humoral immune response is not altered but there is some evidence that cell-mediated immunity is impaired in human vitamin A deficiency.

Association between vitamin A deficiency and infection has been well documented. In children with severe PEM, mortality was found to be four-fold higher when they had xerophthalmia as well. The effect of vitamin A deficiency is difficult to assess in such cases, since they suffer from severe degrees of PEM that could have contributed independently to high mortality. Studies carried out in Indonesia have shown that even mild xerophthalmia is associated with increased mortality. The mortality rate was eight times higher in children with night blindness and Bitot spots compared to those with normal eyes.[7] Poor survival was attributed to high rates of respiratory disease and diarrhoea.

These observations suggest that inadequate vitamin A nutrition, apart from causing eye lesions, may contribute to other health risks in young children.

Assessment of vitamin A status

Clinical assessment

In most surveys, ocular signs like night blindness and Bitot spots have been used to assess vitamin A status. The WHO expert group has suggested that the presence of one or more of the criteria shown in

Table 3.5.14 Population at risk (%) for criteria indicative of xerophthalmia

Night blindness	>1.0
Bitot spot	>0.5
Corneal xerosis + keratomalacia	>0.01
Corneal scar	>0.05
Plasma vitamin A <10 µg/dl	>5.0

(Reproduced from *Control of vitamin A deficiency and xerophthalmia*: report of a Joint WHO/UNICEF/USAID/Helen Keller International/IVACG meeting. Geneva, WHO, no. 672, 1982.)

Table 3.5.14 in the population at risk should be considered as indicative of a xerophthalmia problem of public health significance.[3]

Biochemical assessment

Serum vitamin A concentration is commonly used as a biochemical index of vitamin A nutritional status. In areas where vitamin A deficiency is widespread the mean serum vitamin A level is around 20 µg/100 ml, while in populations whose dietary intake of vitamin A is adequate, the levels range between 30 and 50 µg /100 ml. Vitamin A deficiency is considered to be a significant health problem if more than 5 per cent of the population at risk show values below 10 µg/100 ml.

Clinical studies have shown that there is a rough correlation between the serum level of vitamin A and clinical manifestations.[2] The mean level was lower in children with clinical signs than in those without. In children with conjunctival lesions vitamin A levels were moderately low, while in those with corneal lesions serum vitamin A concentration was less than 10 µg/100 ml. Although this is true of group averages, in individual cases serum vitamin A levels do not always correspond to the nutritional status of vitamin A as judged clinically.

Storage and transport of vitamin A

The liver is the major site of vitamin A storage. Both in man and experimental animals, no correlation has been found between the hepatic stores and the serum levels of vitamin A. It has been demonstrated in rats maintained on vitamin A deficient diets, that serum levels of the vitamin continued to be normal even when liver stores were almost completely exhausted. It is, therefore, clear that blood levels provide little information about falling hepatic stores.

Vitamin A is present in the liver mainly in ester form and transported in plasma as alcohol. Retinol binding protein (RBP) is essential for the transport of vitamin A. Under physiological conditions, retinol and RBP are present in serum in equimolar ratio and after retinol is taken by the target tissues, free RBP is metabolized in the kidney.

Serum levels of RBP are normally in the range 30–50 μg/ml. The synthesis of RBP is influenced by the protein nutritional status of an individual, while its release from the liver depends on the vitamin A status. Serum levels of vitamin A and RBP have been reported to be decreased in both protein–energy malnutrition and vitamin A deficiency.

Treatment

Night blindness and conjunctival lesions respond well to relatively small doses of vitamin A. Oral administration of 10 000 IU of vitamin A daily for 10 days is sufficient to reverse the changes.[8] Instead of small daily supplements, a single massive dose of 200 000 IU can be used. This dose will not only cure the condition but will also help to build up the liver stores and prevent recurrence.

Corneal xerosis may progress rapidly to keratomalacia with irreversible loss of vision and must, therefore, be treated as a medical emergency. An intramuscular injection of 100 000 IU of water-miscible vitamin A must be given immediately on diagnosis. This will result in a rapid elevation of serum vitamin A levels. The second dose can be given orally on the following day. Parenteral therapy is preferable to oral administration of vitamin A in the treatment of malnourished children who have associated gastroenteritis. Oil-soluble vitamin A should never be injected intramuscularly because the vitamin is liberated extremely slowly from the site of injection. If a water-miscible preparation is not available, oil-soluble vitamin A may be given orally.

To control infection, antibiotic eye ointment should be applied locally until the eye lesions clear. Associated malnutrition and infection should receive appropriate therapy. In areas where keratomalacia is common, a prophylactic dose of vitamin A is recommended for all cases of severe protein–energy malnutrition with or without eye lesions.

Prevention

Since inadequate dietary intake of vitamin A is the most important cause of xerophthalmia, the most rational approach to prevent this condition would be to improve the diet so as to ensure adequate intake of the vitamin.

Nutrition education

Foods containing preformed vitamin A are expensive but alternative cheap sources of provitamin A are easily available. Green leafy vegetables are good sources of β-carotene. In areas where xerophthalmia is a public health problem, various educational measures have been adopted to encourage the production and consumption of vitamin A-rich foods. This approach has the advantage of being a part of the public health programmes directed towards reducing malnutrition in the community and improving health status in general. However, this can be considered only as a long-term approach. Additional short-term measures are necessary to reduce the blinding effects of vitamin A deficiency. Massive dose programmes and vitamin A fortification of foods are the two public health approaches that have been attempted in recent years.

Massive dose programme

Since vitamin A can be stored in the body, periodic administration of massive doses of vitamin A has been recommended for the prevention of xerophthalmia. This approach has been found to be feasible in extensive field trials carried out in India by the National Institute of Nutrition.[9]

Studies in preschool children showed that following a single oral dose of 200 000 IU of vitamin A, about 50 per cent of the dose was retained in the body. Satisfactory serum levels of vitamin A were maintained for nearly six months after a massive dose. Field studies conducted in some of the villages near Hyderabad showed a significant reduction in the incidence of ocular signs of vitamin A deficiency among the children who received the massive dose. On the basis of these studies, it was recommended that all preschool children at risk should be given a single oral dose of 200 000 IU once in six months. Such a programme has been implemented on a national scale in many countries, including India, Bangladesh and Indonesia. Evaluation of the programme has shown it to be associated with a significant reduction in the incidence of vitamin A deficiency signs in the children following the massive dose of the vitamin. There is also evidence to suggest that vitamin A supplementation can reduce child mortality. In a community trial reported from Indonesia, the mortality rate among children receiving vitamin A was 30 per cent lower than in the control population.[10] This gives added impetus to programmes for preventing vitamin A deficiency.

Fortification of foods

Fortification of foods with vitamin A is another approach to prevent vitamin A deficiency.[3] Fortified sugar has been introduced in Central America while fortification of monosodium glutamate, a flavouring agent, has been found to be effective in reducing vitamin A deficiency in the Philippines. Fortification of other foods such as salt and tea has also been attempted. Dried skimmed milk, used in food aid programmes in countries where vitamin A deficiency is widespread, is now fortified with vitamin A.

Hypervitaminosis A

Hypervitaminosis A is usually seen in children fed large doses of vitamin A. The dose required to produce toxic manifestations shows wide individual variation and the age of the child is also important. Infants may develop toxic symptoms with as little as 100 000 IU, whereas older children can tolerate much larger doses.

Acute vitamin A toxicity manifests as malaise, headache, irritability, vomiting and in infants, bulging of the fontanelle. These symptoms are caused by raised intracranial tension. Withdrawal of vitamin A results in rapid recovery.

B-complex deficiencies

The water-soluble B group of vitamins are present in all living cells, typically acting as coenzymes and cofactors for fundamental metabolic processes. There are similarities in the clinical manifestations of deficiency states, often involving tissues with a high turnover, such as epithelia and bone marrow. In most cases of nutritional deficiency, more than one of the B group vitamins are likely to be involved and attention to the general diet is an essential part of the management.

Table 3.5.15 lists the important B vitamins with a brief description of their principal function and the common features of deficiency. Nutritional deficiencies of some B vitamins such as biotin and pantothenic acid are rare and not included (see pp. 867–8).

Beriberi

Beriberi, which is caused by thiamine (B_1) deficiency, was once a major problem among rice-eating populations of south-east Asia. The disease was reported to be common in the Philippines, Malaysia and Thailand. Today, with general improvement of the diet, the prevalence of this disease is greatly reduced, although periodic outbreaks are reported in times of crisis.

Pathogenesis

In rice-eating areas, the thiamine content of the rice is critical. Polishing the grain and washing procedures lower the thiamine level. A considerable amount of the vitamin is also lost during boiling. In Japan and Thailand, the enzyme thiaminase is present in some

Table 3.5.15 Group B vitamins: main function and clinical signs of deficiency*

Vitamin	Main function	Deficiency
Thiamine (B_1)	Cleavage of carbon–carbon bonds	Beriberi: neuropathy and cardiomyopathy
Riboflavin (B_2)	Transfer of hydrogen molecules	Glossitis, angular stomatitis, normocytic anaemia
Niacin (nicotinic acid)	Carrier of hydrogen molecules	Pellagra: glossitis, stomatitis, dermatitis, neuropathy, diarrhoea
Pyridoxine (B_6)	Amino acid metabolism	(Following drug therapy) Neuropathy, siezures, anaemia
Folic acid	Transfer of carbon units	Megaloblastic anaemia, diarrhoea
B_{12}	Conversion of homocysteine to methionine	Megaloblastic anaemia, neuropathy, diarrhoea

* See Herbert V. *American Journal of Clinical Nutrition*, 1987; **45**: 661–70 and Chanarin I, The folates. In: BH Barker and DA Bender (eds) *Vitamins in Medicine* vol 1. 1980, Oxford, Heinemann.

raw fish and vegetables. Antithiamine factor has also been demonstrated in fish and tea leaves.

The effects of thiamine deficiency have been described in various reviews.[11, 12, 13] Deficiency of this vitamin leads to disturbance of carbohydrate metabolism with accumulation of incomplete breakdown products such as pyruvic acid and methylglyoxal. However, their relationship to the clinical picture is not clearly understood.

Clinical manifestations

Infantile beriberi   Beriberi may be seen in breast-fed babies when the diets of mothers are deficient in thiamine. It occurs during the first year of life, usually around three months of age. The earliest symptoms are loss of appetite, pallor and restlessness. Infantile beriberi can be classified into three overlapping syndromes.

Acute cardiac   This type is often seen in plump babies between one and three months of age. The onset is sudden with restlessness and bouts of screaming, similar to those occurring in abdominal colic. There is anorexia and vomiting. Then oedema, dyspnoea and cyanosis may develop. Most of the physical signs are related to acute cardiac failure. These include tachycardia, enlargement of heart, systolic murmur, pulmonary oedema, enlargement of liver and oliguria.

Death may occur within a few hours. A therapeutic test with i.v. injection of thiamine produces dramatic improvement.

Aphonic   This type is less acute and usually occurs in infants between four and six months of age. The striking feature is the tone of the infant's cry which varies from hoarseness to complete aphonia. The usual history is that the child is apparently crying but no sound is heard. This may last for a few days before the patient develops restlessness, dyspnoea and oedema, the common symptoms for which the child is brought to hospital.

Pseudomeningeal   This form has been described in older infants of 6–12 months. There is vomiting and irritability. The infant develops nystagmus, a bulging fontanelle, twitching of muscles and convulsions, followed by unconsciousness. The clinical picture resembles meningitis or encephalitis but the cerebrospinal fluid does not show any abnormality.

It is not unusual to find the features of two or three of these forms in the same patient.

Adult beriberi   In older children and in adults, the disease is usually mild. Two major systems are involved: cardiovascular and nervous systems resulting in two types of disease – wet and dry beriberi. Cardiac symptoms often start with palpitations, breathlessness and peripheral oedema. A rapid pulse, enlarged heart and low diastolic pressure are some of the characteristic features. In some patients, beriberi may develop without evident oedema and neurological signs may be predominant (dry form). Peripheral neuritis is a common feature while the central nervous system is scarcely involved. Paraesthesia is often the earliest sign of the diminished sensitivity and the patient complains of a burning sensation in the feet. In severe cases, the sensory disturbances are followed by lower motor neurone paralysis with loss of tendon reflexes.

Wernicke's encephalopathy may develop with severe restriction of thiamine intake. It is usually seen in association with chronic alcoholism. Mental symptoms and paralysis of cranial nerves dominate the picture. Irritability and forgetfulness are early manifestations. They may progress to confusion and delirium. There may be ptosis and ocular palsies.

Biochemical changes

Urinary excretion of thiamine is low in subjects with thiamine deficiency. Values of less than 65 μg/g creatinine excretion are considered indicative of thiamine deficiency. This test can be done on random urine samples and is therefore useful for population surveys. However, it is not satisfactory for individual assessment.

Transketolase is a TPP (thiamine pyrophosphate)-dependent enzyme. In thiamine deficiency, erythrocyte transketolase activity falls but its stimulation *in vitro* with TPP, referred to as TPP effect, increases.[14] TPP effect is less than 20 per cent in normal subjects and values above this are indicative of thiamine deficiency.

Treatment and prevention

In the acute cardiac beriberi, the patient may die if treatment is not given promptly: 50 mg of thiamine should be given parenterally, at least half the dose by the intravenous route for immediate relief. This should be followed by oral supplements of 10 mg/day for several weeks. Since infantile beriberi always occurs among breast-fed babies, mothers should be treated with 50 mg of thiamine daily for the first few days.

The improvement occurs rapidly with the onset of diuresis. The striking changes are decrease in heart rate, reduction of cardiac size and clearing of pulmonary congestion. Aphonia of the subacute form may persist for several weeks even though other symptoms have disappeared. Other neurological signs also take a long time to recover.

Beriberi is entirely preventable by the consumption of foods containing sufficient amounts of thiamine. The recommended daily allowance is 0.4 mg/1000 cal. Therefore, the intake of infants under one year should be about 0.4 mg/day. For pregnant and lactating women an intake of 1.5 mg/day is recommended.

There are several approaches to the control of this disease in the community. Diversification of the diet or the use of parboiled or undermilled rice are the logical approaches. In some countries a fortification programme has been introduced by adding synthetic thiamine to polished rice.

Riboflavin

The chief dietary sources of riboflavin (B_2) are meats, milk and wholemeal flour, with the vitamin being rapidly destroyed by sunlight. Nutritional deficiency is probably widespread, particularly amongst groups with a low milk and meat intake. The clinical manifestations are angular stomatitis with early cheilosis, glossitis (classically described as 'magenta tongue') and a normocytic anaemia. The symptoms resolve rapidly on treatment with the vitamin (at least 2 mg daily).[15]

There seems to be a general feeling that deficiency is not of great clinical significance but recent work suggests an important role for the vitamin in iron deficiency; more research is needed. Minimum daily requirements are in the order of 1.4 to 1.8 mg per day, with lactating women requiring at least 2.5 mg/day.

Niacin

Meat (but not milk), wholemeal flour, yeast and green vegetables are important dietary sources. Deficiency is more often seen in areas where maize (which contains little niacin) is a staple. However, as the vitamin is also synthesized from tryptophan the development of deficiency is not solely linked to vitamin intake.

Clinical deficiency manifests as pellagra with the three Ds: dermatitis, diarrhoea and dementia.[16] The symmetrical, photosensitive dermatitis has a well-demarcated 'glove', 'boot' and 'necklace' distribution. The skin is dry and scaly becoming erythematous and bullous on exposure to sunlight. Glossitis and stomatitis reminiscent of riboflavin deficiency are common in children but the diarrhoea may be intermittent. Apathy, irritability and dementia develop slowly. If there is any associated neuropathy it is probably due to concurrent thiamine deficiency. Response to treatment with 10–15 mg/day of niacin is rapid. Minimum daily requirements vary according to the dietary intake of tryptophan but are probably about 10 mg.

Pyridoxine

True nutritional deficiencies of this ubiquitous vitamin (B_6) are unlikely[17] but the administration of some drugs, particularly isoniazid[18], cycloserine and penicillamine can lead to deficiency partly through increased urinary losses.

Convulsions, particularly in infancy, peripheral neuropathy, glossitis and stomatitis and a microcytic, hypochromic anaemia are the major manifestations of deficiency. Children on isoniazid therapy should be monitored particularly for neuropathy. Treatment with 1–1.5 mg pyridoxine/day is usually sufficient for both treatment and prevention, although much higher doses may be required in association with penicillamine therapy.

B_{12}

Found in most foods of animal origin, nutritional deficiency of B_{12} is rare[19] and occurs only amongst strict vegetarians (vegans), and occasionally in the breast-fed infants of vegan mothers.[20] The manifestations of pernicious anaemia in the infant and young child include megaloblastic anaemia, anorexia, irritability, glossitis, diarrhoea, hyporeflexia and eventually coma. Response to 1 mg of B_{12} intramuscularly leads to a rapid return of appetite and a reticulocytosis. It is recognized in adults that the neuropathy may not completely revert to normal on treatment and it is recommended that children with neuropathy be given 1 mg daily for one to two weeks.

Scurvy

Scurvy is a manifestation of vitamin C deficiency. The incidence of frank scurvy is surprisingly low even in developing countries, though the dietary intake of vitamin C in these populations is far below the recommended allowances. The possibility of widespread prevalence of subclinical deficiency, however, cannot be ruled out.

Dietary sources and requirements of vitamin C

The best sources of vitamin C are fresh fruits like guava and citrus fruits. Vitamin C is also present in tubers and vegetables like potatoes, tomatoes and green leafy vegetables. Sprouted gram and amla are very rich in this vitamin. Breast-milk contains 4–7 mg/100 ml when the mother's intake of the vitamin is adequate. Cow's milk has a low concentration of vitamin C and this may be destroyed while heating the milk.

The recommended daily allowances are in the range 30–70 mg but these levels are much higher than the amounts needed to prevent the appearance of clinical signs of deficiency. Studies carried out in Indian subjects have shown that an intake of 10–20 mg/day was sufficient to maintain adequate levels of tissue ascorbic acid.[21] However, these levels may be adequate under normal conditions but may not be so under conditions of stress, particularly during infections.

Vitamin C is required for maintaining the activity of mixed-function oxidases – prolyl hydroxylase and lysyl hydroxylase which play an important role in collagen metabolism.[22] Many of the manifestations of scurvy are attributed to a failure of collagen synthesis, especially in skin and bone, which leads to a weakening and failure of repair processes in the extracellular matrix.

Clinical features

Scurvy is usually seen in infants 6–12 months of age who are fed only boiled cow's milk without any supplements. It seldom occurs in breast-fed infants, since breast-milk provides adequate quantities of the vitamin unless the mother is grossly depleted. Sporadic cases are also seen in older age groups, generally after an episode of infection.

Defective formation of collagen is the main pathological feature and can explain most of the signs noted in scurvy. After the initial stages in which there are vague symptoms like anorexia, pallor and irritability, the main features are pain and tenderness in the limbs. The infant may scream when picked up or moved during bathing. There is pseudoparalysis; the pain is so severe that the child can hardly move the limbs and assumes the typical 'frog position' with semiflexion of hips and knees. There may be obvious swelling of the limbs, usually the thighs due to subperiosteal haemorrhage at the lower end of the femur. The swelling may become hard after some weeks due to calcification of the haematoma. Radiological examination reveals a characteristic ground-glass appearance of the bones due to generalized osteoporosis and atrophy of the trabeculae. Subperiosteal haemorrhages are seen as large, dense shadows surrounding the shafts of the bones. Costochondral junctions appear prominent because of the subluxation of the sternal plate. Scorbutic beading is sharp and angular unlike that of the 'rickety rosary'.

Gums are spongy, bluish purple and start bleeding with the slightest pressure. These changes are seen when the teeth are erupted. The swollen gums sometimes completely conceal the teeth, especially the upper incisors. Petechial haemorrhages may occur in the skin and mucous membranes. In severe cases, haematuria, orbital and subdural haemorrhages can also occur. Anaemia and low-grade fever are usually present.

In older children and adults subperiosteal haemorrhages are rare. In human volunteers maintained on vitamin C-deficient diets the most apparent features of scurvy were changes in the skin, such as hyperkeratosis and petechial haemorrhages.[23] Bleeding gums and swelling of the joints may be seen in severely affected patients. Psychological changes like loss of motivation and depression have also been described in scurvy.

Biochemical changes

Plasma levels of vitamin C range from 0.5 to 1.5 mg/100 ml in normal individuals. However, lower levels have been reported in apparently normal subjects whose dietary intake of vitamin C is low. Thus, plasma levels of vitamin C over 0.5 mg/100 ml may exclude scurvy but a lower level does not prove its presence.

Levels of ascorbic acid in leucocytes are accepted as reflecting tissue concentration of the vitamin. Normal levels of ascorbic acid in leucocytes range from 8 to 16 μg/1 × 10^8 cells. Leucocytes obtained from normal subjects belonging to low-income groups have been found to contain approximately 60 per cent of the fully saturated value. This level is obviously high enough to prevent clinical manifestations of deficiency.

The saturation test has also been employed to assess the tissue stores of the vitamin. A test dose of 200 mg vitamin C is administered and the urinary excretion of the vitamin in the next 24 hours is estimated. Normally more than 30 per cent of the dose is excreted in the urine, while in deficient subjects the excretion is much less.

Treatment and prevention

Response to the administration of vitamin C is dramatic in acute scurvy. The pain ceases within a few days but the swelling caused by subperiosteal haemorrhage may take a long time to disappear. Oral administration of 100 mg of vitamin C daily for a week is sufficient to produce complete healing. Since an oral dose of vitamin C is absorbed completely, i.m. or i.v. injections which aggravate the pain should be avoided.

Infants, especially those who are artificially fed, should be given orange juice or tomato juice to provide enough vitamin C. Older children or adults can take fresh fruits and vegetables which are good sources of this vitamin.

Nutritional rickets

Rickets is a disease of a growing skeleton and is characterized by defective calcification of the osseous matrix and epiphysial cartilage. Many factors causing disorder of calcium and phosphorus metabolism result in bone changes but nutritional rickets occurs primarily as a result of lack of vitamin D. Contrary to general belief, rickets is widely prevalent in many tropical and subtropical regions despite abundant sunshine.

Dietary sources and requirements of vitamin D

Vitamin D can be obtained either through diet or by exposure to sunlight. The oil obtained from fish liver contains large amounts of vitamin D. Under normal conditions the most important source of vitamin D is the conversion of 7-dehydrocholesterol in the skin to cholecalciferol by UV radiation. The cholecalciferol thus produced, and that absorbed from food sources is metabolized in the liver and kidney to 1,25-dihydroxy cholecalciferol which is the major mediator of the biological actions of vitamin D.

Dietary requirement of vitamin D will vary with the available sunlight. The recommended intake of vitamin D is 400 IU (10 μg/day) for Western children. In tropical countries, the relative abundance of sunshine may diminish the need for dietary vitamin D. Studies in Indian children have shown that daily intake of 100 IU of vitamin D is sufficient to obtain maximum calcium absorption.[24]

Prevalence

Rickets has been virtually eliminated from the West by improving vitamin D intake through fortification of foods. However, rickets has reappeared as a significant health problem among Asian immigrants in Britain.[25] Nutritional rickets is not uncommon among preschool children in the Middle East and in some Asian countries. Although, rickets is a disease of rapidly growing children, it also occurs in undernourished children. In fact, reports from Iran[26] and India[27] indicate that the incidence is higher in undernourished than in well-nourished children.

Aetiology

Primary deficiency can occur due to lack of vitamin D in the diet or inadequate exposure to sunlight. Secondary deficiency is associated with fat malabsorption and certain diseases of the liver and kidney.

Relationship to diet

Apart from poor intake of vitamin D, low calcium and a high phytate content of the diet have been implicated in the aetiology of rickets. Studies in experimental animals have shown that phytic acid interferes with the absorption of calcium. However, long-term balance studies in humans have shown that adaptation occurs.[28] When children with rickets were given calcium supplements along with a low phytate diet, there was no significant change in biochemical or radiological measures. The response to small doses of vitamin D observed in these cases, suggests that inadequate supply of the vitamin is the major aetiological factor.

Exposure to sunlight

Until recently it was thought that rickets was rare in sunny areas of the world. However, recent reports show that this is not true. Poor living conditions and certain social customs may prevent adequate exposure of children to sunlight. The incidence of rickets is particularly high in slum children who live in crowded houses almost devoid of sunlight.

Clinical features

The peak incidence of rickets is seen in infants 6 and 24 months of age. Preterm infants are more prone to rickets than full-term babies.

Early manifestations are craniotabes, wide fontanelle, enlargement of costochondral junctions and slight thickening of the wrists. In advanced cases, bone changes are more obvious. There is bossing of the frontal and parietal bones giving rise to the so-called 'hot cross bun' skull. There is marked beading of costochondral junctions (rickety rosary). The sides of the thorax become flattened and the sternum projects forward producing a 'pigeon-breast' deformity. There is a horizontal depression across the lower chest (Harrison's groove). The epiphyseal enlargement of the wrists and ankles is more marked (Fig. 3.5.17). In a child who has learnt to sit up resting on the hands, bending deformities of the forearms may be seen. When the child begins walking, bending of the softened long bones results in bow-legs or knock-knees (Fig. 3.5.18). Deformities of long bones, spine and pelvis result in stunting or rachitic dwarfism.

Radiological examination of the bones shows characteristic changes. These include cupping and fraying of the distal ends of radius and ulna, and generalized osteoporosis. Epiphyseal bands of calcification represent the healing stage.

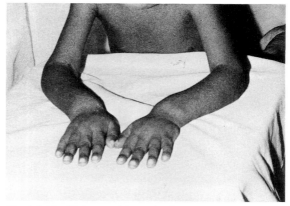

Fig. 3.5.17 Rickets: epiphyseal enlargement.

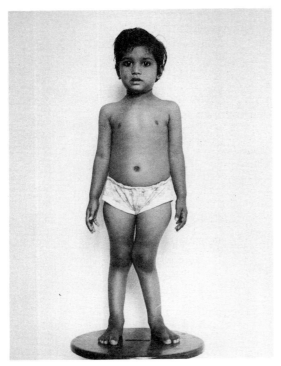

Fig. 3.5.18   Rickets: knock-knee.

Biochemical assessment

Alterations in serum calcium, phosphorus and alkaline phosphatase are the conventional criteria employed for the diagnosis of vitamin D deficiency. Rise in alkaline phosphatase activity is believed to be one of the earliest biochemical changes in rickets. However, studies reported from India show that alkaline phosphatase activity is normal in a proportion of malnourished children who have radiological evidence of rickets.[27] Serum 25-hydroxy-D$_3$ is now recognized as a more sensitive indicator of vitamin D status. In normal subjects, the serum levels are in the range 20–60 ng/ml while in children with rickets, they are less than 10 ng/ml.[29]

Treatment and prevention

In Western countries infant foods are fortified with vitamin D, whereas in developing countries the children depend entirely on sunshine as the natural source of the vitamin. Adequate exposure to sunlight must be ensured to prevent rickets in these populations.

Nutritional rickets can be treated with small daily supplements or a single massive dose of vitamin D. Oral administration of 10 000 IU of vitamin D daily will produce a biochemical response in about 10 days and X-rays show evidence of healing after 3–4 weeks. Administration of a single massive dose of 600 000 IU of vitamin D is followed by more rapid healing.

Toxicity

An overdose of vitamin D causes toxicity that may be very serious. It may occur when parents inadvertently continue to give vitamin concentrates to the infants for long periods. The symptoms include anorexia, irritability, nausea, vomiting, constipation, polydypsia and polyuria. There is hypercalcaemia and hypercalciuria. Chronic toxicity leads to calcification of soft tissues, particularly the kidney. Treatment includes discontinuation of vitamin D and decrease in calcium intake. In severe cases cortisone or calcitonin can be used.

References

1. WHO. *Requirements of Vitamin A, thiamine, riboflavin and niacin*: report of a joint FAO/WHO expert group. *WHO Technical Report Series* No. 362, 1967.
2. Reddy V. Vitamin A deficiency and blindness in Indian children. *Indian Journal of Medical Research*. 1978; **68** (Suppl): 26–37.
3. WHO. *Control of Vitamin A deficiency and xeropthalmia.* Report of a joint WHO/UNICEF/USAID/Helen Keller International/IVACG meeting. *WHO Technical Report Series* No. 672, 1982.
4. Sommer A. *Nutritional Blindness: Xerophthalmia and Keratomalacia.* New York, Oxford University Press, 1982.
5. Oomen HAPC. Clinical epidemiology of xerophthalmia in man. *American Journal of Clinical Nutrition.* 1969; **22**: 1098–105.
6. Sandford-Smith JH, Whittle HC. Corneal ulceration following measles in Nigerian children. *British Journal of Ophthalmology.* 1979; **63**: 720–4.
7. Sommer A, Hussaini G, Tarwotjo I, Susanto D. Increased mortality in children with mild vitamin A deficiency. *Lancet.* 1983; **1**: 585–8.
8. Reddy V. Hypo and hyper-vitaminosis A. In: Rakel RE ed. *Conn's Current Therapy.* London, W B Saunders, 1985. pp. 424–25.
9. Reddy V. Vitamin A deficiency control in India. In: Bauernfeind JC ed. *Vitamin A Deficiency and its Control.* London, Academic Press, 1986. pp. 389–404.
10. Sommer A, Djunaedi E. Tarwotjo I *et al.* Impact of vitamin A supplementation on childhood mortality. *Lancet.* 1986; **1**: 1169–73.
11. Goldsmith. The B vitamins. In: Beaton GH, McHenry EW eds. *Nutrition: A Comprehensive Treatise*, New York, Academic Press, 1964. p. 109.
12. Katsura E, Oiso T. Beri beri. In: Beaton GH, Bengoa JM eds. *Nutrition in Preventive Medicine: The Major Deficiency*

Syndromes, Epidemiology and Approaches to Control. Geneva, WHO, 1970. pp. 136:45.

13. Krishnaswamy K, Gopalan C. Vitamin deficiencies. In: Woodruff AW, Wright SG eds. *Medicine in the Tropics*. London, Churchill Livingstone, 1984. pp. 431–5.

14. Bamji MS. Transketolase activity and urinary excretion of thiamine in the assessment of thiamine nutritional status. *American Journal of Clinical Nutrition*. 1970; **23**: 52–8.

15. Bates CJ. Human riboflavin requirements and metabolic consequences of deficiency in man and animals. *World Review of Nutrition and Dietetics*. 1987; **50**: 215–65.

16. Carpenter KJ, Lewin WJ. A re-examination of the composition of diets associated with pellagra. *Journal of Nutrition*. 1985; **115**: 543–52.

17. Merril AH Jr, Henderson JM. Diseases associated with defects in vitamin B6 metabolism or utilization. *Annual Review of Nutrition*. 1987; **7**: 137–56.

18. Pellock JM, Howell J, Kendig EL Jr, Baker H. Pyridoxine deficiency in children treated with isoniazid. *Chest*. 1985; **87**: 658–61.

19. Herbert V. Nutrition science as a continually unfolding story: the folate and vitamin B-12 paradigm. *American Journal of Clinical Nutrition*. 1987; **46**: 387–402.

20. Sklar R. Nutritional B-12 deficiency in a breast-fed infant of a vegan diet mother. *Clinical Pediatrics*. (Philadelphia). 1985; **25**: 219–21.

21. Srikantia SG, Mohanram M, Krishnaswamy K. Human requirements of ascorbic acid. *American Journal of Clinical Nutrition*. 1970; **23**: 59–62.

22. Bates CJ. The function and metabolism of vitamin C in man. In: Counsell JN, Hornig DH ed. *Vitamin C*. London, Applied Science Publishers, 1981. pp. 1–17.

23. Hodges RE, Baker EM, Hood J *et al*. Experimental scurvy in man. *American Journal of Clinical Nutrition*. 1969; **22**: 535–48.

24. Perera WDA, Reddy V. Effect of vitamin D supplements on calcium absorption in children. *Indian Journal of Medical Research*. 1971; **59**: 961–4.

25. Goel KM, Logan RW, Arneil GC *et al*. Florid and sub-clinical rickets among immigrant children in Glasgow. *Lancet*. 1976; **1**: 1141–5.

26. Salimpour R. Rickets in Tehran. *Archives of Disease in Childhood*. 1975; **50**: 63–6.

27. Reddy V, Srikantia SG. Serum alkaline phosphatase in malnourished children with rickets. *Journal of Pediatrics*. 1967; **71**: 595–7.

28. Bhaskaram C, Reddy V. Role of dietary phytate in the aetiology of nutritional rickets. *Indian Journal of Medical Research*. 1979; **69**: 265–70.

29. Raghuramulu N, Reddy V. Serum 25-hydroxy vitamin D levels in malnourished children with rickets. *Archives of Disease in Childhood*. 1980; **55**: 285–7.

MINERAL AND TRACE ELEMENT NUTRITIONAL DISORDERS

Peter J. Aggett

Nutritional mineral deficiencies rarely occur in isolation; they are commonly accompanied by deficiencies of other essential nutrients. Clinical situations which predispose children to mineral deficiencies can be classified simply (Table 3.5.16), but many mechanisms may simultaneously be influencing nutrient intake, absorption and body losses; superimposed on these are varying systemic requirements for nutrients.

Deficiencies may not appear until the primary cause of malnutrition or associated deprivation of energy, protein and other nutrients are corrected. Recommended dietary intakes and estimated safe and adequate dietary intakes for minerals have been described (see p. 331). In contrast, mineral excesses may present independently, although their clinical features also may be influenced by the supply of other nutrients.

Table 3.5.16 Situations which may predispose to mineral deficiencies

Inadequate dietary intake
  'Protein calorie malnutrition' (especially during recovery)
  Vegetarian diets
  Synthetic diets for management of inborn errors of
    metabolism or malabsorption states
  Subsisting on crops grown on anomalous soils
Malabsorption
  Immaturity of absorptive mechanisms
  Inborn error of absorption (e.g. acrodermatitis enteropathica
    – Zn)
  Inborn error of metabolism (Menkes' syndrome – Cu)
  Enteropathies
  Exocrine pancreatic insufficiency
  Intestinal resection
  Dietary factors forming intraluminal complexes which
    impair absorption
Increased body losses (catabolic status)
  Starvation, burns, diabetes mellitus
  Infections, haemolysis, blood loss
  Diuretic therapy, dialysis
  Exfoliative dermatitis

Calcium deficiency

Although 96–99 per cent of total body calcium is in bone, the most closely regulated pool is the ionized calcium in the extracellular fluid; in plasma, ionized Ca^{2+} (approximately 1.0 mmol/l) comprises 40–60 per cent of the total pool (2.0–2.6 mmol/l). The ionized pool participates in neuromuscular transmission, muscular contraction, membrane-receptor signal transmission, and in extracellular hydrolytic enzyme activities. If plasma ionized calcium concentrations fall, they are maintained by increased intestinal absorption of calcium mediated by 1,25-dihydroxycholecalciferol (calcitriol), and by increased resorption of bone induced by increased secretion of parathormone and reduced secretion of calcitonin. Chronic calcium deficiency therefore causes demineralization of the skeleton; it can also cause osteomalacia and rickets.[1]

The factors influencing the features of chronic calcium deficiency are complex. If the concurrent supply of energy, protein and, possibly, other nutrients (e.g. iodine, vitamin D and copper) is adequate, the protein matrix of bone is made normally and linear growth proceeds but the skeleton is poorly mineralized and appropriate homeostatic increases in plasma parathormone and calcitriol occur. However, if there is accompanying malnutrition (predominantly of energy and/or protein) then, because growth is retarded,

skeletal mineralization is normal, and plasma calcitriol concentrations may be normal or low.

It has been suggested that calcium deficiency by itself can cause growth retardation but this has not been established clearly.[1, 2]

Interactions between calcium supply and vitamin D_3 are discussed elsewhere (see p. 377). Calcium deficiency can arise from an inadequate calcium intake or possibly by impaired absorption of calcium, which in the gut lumen is complexed with phytic acid, oxalic acid, or the uronic acid component of 'non-available polysaccharides' (fibre). However, the metal can be absorbed in the distal small bowel and colon after these complexes have been broken down by the gut flora. Thus, many communities subsisting on vegetable diets rich in fibre and phytate exhibit no untoward effects of calcium deprivation. Additionally, with dietary calcium deprivation, the efficiency of the intestinal uptake and transfer of calcium can increase up to a net efficiency of 80 per cent or more, effectively compensating for any impairment of calcium availability induced by other dietary factors. Thus, although dairy products are the best sources of calcium, vegetables and grains may be adequate sources also, despite concern about the bioavailability of the metal from them. Nonetheless, communities consuming large amounts of unleavened wholemeal flour products may be at risk of developing chronic calcium deficiency, even with adequate vitamin D production.

Assessing the possibility of chronic calcium deficiency is difficult. Plasma calcium levels are maintained, while skeletal demineralization can only be detected radiologically when about 30 per cent of bone radiodensity has been lost. Photon densitometry is more sensitive but this is not universally available. Changes in the plasma concentration of the mediators of calcium metabolism can be monitored to discern clues that the body is trying to maintain ionized calcium levels. Parathormone and calcitriol levels will be increased, and calcitonin concentrations reduced. Other clues include phosphaturia and a hypophosphataemia secondary to hyperparathyroidism. With prolonged secondary hyperparathyroidism, osteoblastic activity is increased and this is reflected by a raised activity in the plasma of bone alkaline phosphatase.

It has been shown in rats that hepatic destruction of calcitriol may occur with calcium deficiency. If this is true for man then this may contribute to the occurrence of rickets and osteomalacia in regions (e.g. Saudi Arabia and Egypt) with abundant sunlight. This is yet another reason for considering vitamin D metabolism and deficiency in patients with evidence of chronic calcium deficiency.[1]

Magnesium deficiency

Magnesium is the second major intracellular cation. It participates in many enzyme activities requiring ATP, and in protein synthesis. About 25–30 per cent of body magnesium is in muscle and 55–60 per cent in the skeleton.[3] Since magnesium is a component of chlorophyll, it is abundant in vegetables and primary nutritional deficiency of the element is rare. However, deficiencies arising from malabsorption, diarrhoea, increased losses from endogenous depots (e.g. renal disease, catabolism, hyperaldosteronism) or increased tissue synthesis[4], can lead to symptomatic hypomagnesaemia with non-specific anorexia, apathy, tremors, carpopedal spasm, facial muscle twitching, fasciculation, altered muscle tone, convulsions, coma and death. Non-specific EEG changes occur and the ECG shows arrhythmias, prolonged QT intervals, flattened and inverted T waves and U waves indicative of secondary alteration in metabolism of calcium and potassium.

Plasma analysis shows hypomagnesaemia (reference range 0.7–1.1 mmol/l) which may be accompanied by hypocalcaemia, hypokalaemia and hypophosphataemia.

Treatment with intramuscular magnesium (0.4–0.75 mmol/kg body weight daily) produces a rapid remission. Oral therapy (up to 2 mmol elemental magnesium/kg daily) can be tailored to match the clinical response. Many magnesium preparations are available – large doses of all of which can cause a secretory diarrhoea.

Potassium

Potassium deficiency

Since 95 per cent of body potassium is intracellular, hypokalaemia (reference range 3.5–5.0 mmol/l) is an unreliable indicator of body potassium, but as a rough measure a fall of 1 mmol/l represents a 5–10 per cent loss of cellular potassium. Potassium deficiency results usually from renal losses, severe diarrhoea and during rapid tissue synthesis, if intake is inadequate. The nutritional importance of potassium is emphasized by the observation that in anabolic states potassium accumulation precedes that of nitrogen. Adequate potassium supply is vital in nutritional rehabilitation.[5]

Potassium deficiency leads to impaired insulin secretion, and impaired glucose tolerance and protein synthesis. Muscular weakness affects progressively the limbs, trunk and respiratory muscles. Deep tendon reflexes are depressed. Intestinal ileus and gastric distension may develop, as may an atonic bladder. Cardiac involvement is manifest by an ECG with low T waves, depressed ST segments and U waves. Proximal renal tubular function becomes defective and a metabolic alkalosis may develop. If renal function is normal, urinary potassium concentrations of less than 15 mmol/l are usually indicative of potassium depletion.

Hypokalaemia should be corrected cautiously. Oral potassium is the preferred approach. If urgent treatment is required, it can be given i.v. in a 5 per cent glucose solution at a rate of 3 mmol/kg daily.

Potassium toxicity

Hyperkalaemia (>5.5 mmol/l) can develop from small increments in total body potassium. It results from renal failure, acute tissue catabolism, adrenal insufficiency and hyporenic hypoaldosteronism. Excessive exogenous potassium from injudicious treatment of hypokalaemia is another important cause.

Hyperkalaemia manifests as hypotonia, paraesthesiae, muscular weakness and a flaccid paralysis. Death may result from cardiac toxicity: at potassium levels above 6.5 mmol/l, the ECG may show either a bradycardia or more usually a tachycardia, with high peaked T waves. The appearance of a prolonged PR interval and wide bizarre QRS complexes presage arrhythmias and are particularly sinister.

Acute treatment with intravenous $NaHCO_3$ (2 mmol/kg body weight) should be given, and if necessary repeated with a two hour infusion of glucose (0.5 mg/kg body weight) and soluble insulin (1 unit/3 g glucose). Sometimes it is necessary to resort to peritoneal or haemodialysis. This acute therapy should be accompanied by efforts to reduce total body potassium with a low or potassium free diet, and oral potassium-binding resins.

Iodine

Iodine deficiency disease

Iodine deficiency disease (IDD) describes better than goitre the extent of iodine deficiency: focusing on the gross extremes, goitre and cretinism, obscures the insidious socio-economic impact of iodine deficiency which affects over 400 million people in Asia alone.[6,7] Although iodine deficiency is classically described as occurring in mountainous areas, it occurs also in alluvial plains and delta areas (especially if seafood is not eaten).

Whereas iodine deficiency is the final precipitant of IDD, other environmental and dietary factors facilitate its pathogenesis. These include ingestion of thiocyanate in cassava, maize, bamboo shoots, sweet potatoes, and lima beans which blocks thyroid uptake of iodine; thioureas in millet, sorghum and ground-nuts which impair the organification of iodine; riboflavinoids, iodide in kelp; bacterial and chemical contamination of the water sources, and exposure to resorcinol.

IDD affects all stages of fetal development causing infertility, abortions, stillbirths, congenital malformations and neonatal morbidity. It is important to realize that while these defects occur in regions where iodine deficiency is known to occur, the affected mother may have no overt evidence of iodine deficiency.

Table 3.5.17, shows a classification of goitre and of endemias of goitre. Endemic cretinism in neonates occurs in populations whose daily iodine intake is less than 20 μg. It comprises two overlapping forms; neurological and myxoedematous cretinism. The former comprises profound mental retardation, deafness, mutism, spastic diplegia, ataxia and strabismus.

Table 3.5.17   Classification of goitre and goitre endemias

Goitre:	A thyroid gland whose lateral lobes have a volume greater than the terminal phalanges of the thumbs of the person examined will be considered goitrous
Size:	0 – no goitre IA – goitre detectable by palpation but not visible with neck extended IB – goitre palpable and visible with neck extended II – goitre visible with neck in normal position III – goitre visible at a distance
Endemic goitre:	Is present in an area if more than 10 per cent of the population or of children aged 6–12 years have goitres
Endemias:	I – Goitre endemias with an average urinary I excretion greater than 50 μg/g creatinine; at this level thyroid hormone is probably adequate for normal mental and physical development II – Iodine excretion 25–50 μg/g creatinine; thyroid production may be suboptimal and there is a risk of hypothyroidism but not of overt cretinism III – Urinary iodine excretion below 25 μg/g creatinine; serious risk of endemic cretinism

(Reproduced from Querido A *et al. Endemic Goitre and Cretinism: Continuing Threat to World Health.* Pan American Health Organization, 1974, no. 292.)

Goitre may not be present; in fact, thyroid function may even be normal. Neurological cretinism is probably caused by a profound iodine deprivation of the fetus occurring in early gestation before thyroid organogenesis.

Myxoedematous cretinism may be caused by a later deficiency of iodine in fetal and neonatal life combined possibly, as occurs in central Africa, with exposure *in utero* to a 'facilitator' such as thiocyanate in cassava. These patients have hypothyroidism with low plasma thyroid hormones and high thyroid stimulating hormone (TSH) levels; many have a goitre, and most have associated features such as delayed skeletal maturation, and growth retardation. The nervous system on gross examination may not seem to be affected; however, more sensitive psycho-motor tests may show some deficit.

In later childhood and adolescence endemic goitre occurs with IDD. The highest prevalance is in 12 to 14-year-old girls.

These are the gross features of IDD. Only recently has its impact on fertility and reproductive efficiency been realized and with this has appeared the demonstration of motor incoordination and possibly other psycho-motor deficits in overtly normal children, which have serious connotations for the socio-economic development of communities. The causative IDD was probably experienced *in utero* or during infancy.

Treatment of IDD

Affected communities need iodine supplementation, but the implementation of such programmes is variably achieved. By the very nature of their IDD, affected populations are geographically and economically underprivileged, and politically apathetic. The expense of iodine supplementation is modest compared with the benefits, which have been shown to be improved fertility, and infant birth weight, survival and development, and an increase in the economic independence of communities.

A common means of supplementation is the provision of sodium chloride which has been sprayed with potassium iodate. This treatment is more stable in hot, humid environments than other forms of iodized cooking salt. Iodinated oil is also used; poppy seed oil containing 400 mg of iodine per ml is commonly used. Of this, 2–4 ml i.m. can maintain daily urinary iodine levels above 50 μg for 4–6 years.

Iodinated oil can be given orally; this is easier and cheaper to dispense, but on an equal dose basis it is only a third as effective as iodized salt.

The benefits of iodine supplementation in pregnancy

are greatest if women are treated before they conceive; their improved iodine intake is reflected in their babies who, up to six months of age, have increased plasma thyroxine levels.

Some governments have iodized water supplies to reduce IDD, but the success of this is yet to be determined.

The selection of communities to treat is still debated. Some authorities only treat endemic goitre areas; others, aware of the subtle effects of clinically covert IDD, treat all members of communities in which only one goitrous person has been found.

Iodine excess

Iodine supplementation programmes are associated with increased incidence of thyrotoxicosis and toxic nodular goitre. These most frequently affect women aged over 40 years and so some policies exclude such women from individual treatment. There may also be more cases of autoimmune thyroiditis and thyroid cancer in populations receiving prophylactic iodine. These disturbances seem only to involve previously iodine-deficient populations, and may spare children.

Endemic goitre occurs in communities with high iodine intake from seafood, seaweeds and iodine-rich water (e.g. in low lying lands in China), but affected people are usually euthyroid and neurologically normal.

Fluoride excess (Fluorosis)

Excess ingestion of fluoride causes a chronic metabolic bone disease and arthropathy. Affected populations occur in Tanzania, Kenya, South Africa, the Indian subcontinent, and the People's Republic of China, where subsoil water high in fluoride is taken up by plants and enters the food chain. This problem has been exacerbated in some areas by elevation of the water table following the construction of dams. Excessive intakes of molybdenum and a resultant impairment of copper metabolism has been proposed as a coprecipitant of this debilitating syndrome. Fluorosis is more frequent in populations subsisting on sorghum rather than maize, because the former retains more fluoride from cooking water.

Children may present with severe fluorosis from six years of age. Males are more often affected than females. The earliest and mildest evidence is dental fluorosis, a dark mottling of the enamel. Asymptomatic skeletal fluorosis radiographically shows focal areas of osteosclerosis, osteoporosis and features of secondary hyperparathyroidism. Patients then develop stiffness, arthralgia, arthropathies (first of the large joints), and limited movement of the cervical and lumbar spine progressing to kyphosis. Tendons and ligaments become calcified with osteophyte formation. Concomitant low calcium intakes predispose to deformed bones manifest as genu valgum, genu varum, bent tibiae and fibulae and, less commonly, bent forearms. Secondary entrapment neuropathies are common with advanced fluorosis.

The pathogenesis of fluorosis is unknown; the condition itself is heterogenous and its features vary with calcium intake. Clinical biochemistry demonstrates a urinary fluoride excretion above plasma fluoride concentrations and evidence of hyperparathyroidism and, because of fluoride interference with iodine metabolism, hypothyroidism.

For a review of recent progress in understanding fluorosis see Ref. 8.

Selenium

Selenium deficiency

The major biochemical role of selenium is in the cytosolic antioxidant enzyme glutathione peroxidase. The risk of selenium deficiency depends on the relative activity of other potential antioxidant factors such as vitamins C, E and A and oxidant stress imposed by exercise, infection and intakes of oxidizable substrates such as polyunsaturated fatty acids.[9]

Populations in an extensive area from the north-east to the south-west of the People's Republic of China are affected by a selenium-responsive cardiomyopathy. The severity of this condition, Keshan disease, varies from acute cardiac failure through to congestive cardiac failure. ECGs have a low voltage, non-specific conduction defects, and arrhythmias. Children, adolescents and pregnant women are most susceptible. Affected regions have a low selenium content in soil and crops; domestic livestock are also selenium deficient and individual selenium intakes are less than 12 μg per day.

Associated precipitants of this syndrome may be intercurrent viral infections, extremes of temperature, and exposure to nitrates. Mild cases respond to selenium supplements, and population prophylaxis with sodium selenite (aged 0–5 years give 0.5 mg; 6–10 years give 1.0 mg weekly) has considerably reduced, if not eradicated, the incidence of this condition. This improves the selenium 'status' of the population so that blood selenium levels are above 10–15 μg/l, the level below which there is a risk of developing the cardiomyopathy. A selenium-responsive increased red cell peroxide fragility has been described in an infant with malnutrition and normal tocopherol levels.[10]

Selenium levels in plasma, blood and tissues are influenced by dietary intakes and vary throughout the world.[11] Gross deficiencies are rarely associated with whole blood levels above 10 μg/l. Although low blood selenium concentrations have been reported in some children this loss does not constitute evidence of selenium deficiency.

Selenium toxicity

This occurs in seleniferous areas of the People's Republic of China and South America, where intakes of selenium may be as much as 15 mg/day or more and blood selenium levels of 3.2–6.8 mg/l have been reported.

The clinical features include dry and brittle body hair, hair loss with new hair that is depigmented, streaked or spotted, brittle nails which may be shed, an erythematous vesiculo-bullous intensely pruritic skin rash, and peripheral neuropathy. Mottled tooth enamel and increased caries are endemic in affected areas.

Selenium uptake into the food chain in these areas is increased by high selenium content in soil and water and controlled by increasing the alkalinity of soil.[12]

Trace metals

The functions of iron, zinc and copper are summarized in Table 3.5.18.

Iron deficiency

This is probably the most common nutrient deficiency. It causes systemic alterations of tissue metabolism which do not relate to the degree of anaemia. Often systemic symptoms respond to iron supplements before any correction of an anaemia.

Iron deficiency is associated with subtle psychological changes, impaired scholastic performance and behavioural changes. Exercise tolerance and sustained efficiency of physical work are similarly impaired. Paraesthesiae, muscular weakness and exertional dyspnoea may develop, and with marked deficiency cardiac function deteriorates and failure may supervene with a low-amplitude ECG.

Chronic deficiencies may cause growth retardation, hepatosplenomegaly, and changes in the finger and toe

Table 3.5.18 Summary of the biochemical roles of zinc, iron and copper

Zinc	Catalytic, structural and regulatory roles in metalloenzymes (involving metabolism of protein, fatty acids, carbohydrate) gene transcription and polymeric macromolecules (e.g. presecretory insulin)
Iron	Haem proteins and iron–sulphur proteins; oxygen transport and storage, redox enzymes (e.g. catalase, peroxidase, phenylalanine hydroxylase), oxidative phosphorylation
Copper	Metalloenzymes; oxidases; oxidative phosphorylation (cytochrome c oxidation); collagen and elastin cross-links; fatty acid metabolism, cytosolic antioxidant (superoxide dismutase)

nails such as flattening, brittleness, and spoon deformities (koilonychia).

The sequence of events with iron depletion is a loss of iron stores in the bone marrow and liver, a fall in serum/plasma ferritin (<10 μg/l), a fall in serum/plasma iron (reference range 10–20 μmol/l) and iron saturation of transferrin accompanied by an increase in its iron-binding capacity, increased whole blood free erythrocyte protoporphyrin (>35 μg/dl) and a hypochromic and/or microcytic anaemia.

Biochemical diagnosis of minor iron deficiency is difficult. Plasma iron concentrations are depressed also by infections and a variety of stresses which may also increase ferritin levels. This reflects a systemic recompartmentation of iron which, with chronic stress, can lead to functional iron deficiency in the presence of a normal or increased body burden of iron.

Administration orally in divided doses of an iron salt providing about 5–6 mg (80–100 μmol) elemental iron/kg body weight daily is, in the presence of normal intestinal function, appropriate treatment.[13]

Chronic iron toxicity

Chronic iron overload from exogenous sources can arise from primary (genetic or hereditary) haemochromatosis, excessive ingestion of iron as a consequence of food prepared in iron utensils (e.g. in Southern Africa), oral iron and transfusional therapy for sideroblastic and haemolytic anaemias, and ineffective erythropoiesis.

Symptomatic chronic iron overload is not a common problem in childhood although overload often starts in childhood. Hepatic iron overload can be detected in children identified as being at risk of hereditary haemochromatosis and prophylactic treatment started. Similarly risks of haemosiderosis resulting from multiple transfusions can be minimized by treating with desferroxamine, children with 80 per cent or more transferrin saturation, or a correspondingly reduced iron-binding capacity.

Zinc deficiency

The individual features of acute severe zinc deficiency are non-specific but the classic combination of neuro-psychiatric changes (jitteriness, anorexia, apathy and irritability), circumoral and acral dermatitis, frequent loose stools and hair loss should alert one to the possible diagnosis. Other important features are failure to thrive, impaired cell-mediated immunity and thymic atrophy. If untreated, progressive weight loss and death from overwhelming infection can occur. The skin lesions range from a vesiculo-bullous dermatitis to hyperkeratotic lesions on extensor surfaces and bony prominences.

Such severe symptoms are rare, but zinc-responsive defects have been demonstrated in malnutrition syndromes[14] and in children with haemolytic anaemias, and protracted diarrhoea. Their responses include improved weight gain, immune function and healing of skin lesions during treatment of protein–energy mal-nutrition, improved dark adaption in patients with haemolytic anaemias, and possibly earlier resolution of infectious diarrhoea. Symptomatic zinc deficiency is being increasingly recognized in three to five month old term and ex-preterm infants.

Zinc-responsive growth retardation[15] has been found in North American children whose only abnormality was short stature (< 10th centile).

A syndrome comprising hypogonadism, growth retardation, hepatosplenomegaly, and rough dry skin, has been described. Although zinc deprivation probably contributes to this, other nutritional deficiencies (e.g. calcium, vitamin D, iron and iodine) may also be contributary.

There is no single reliable indicator of zinc deficiency. Although the plasma zinc (reference range 9–22 μmol/l) may be low, it is depressed by infections and other stresses, and it may even be normal in the presence of symptoms. The zinc content of leucocytes and leucocyte subsets may be useful, as may deter-mination of the activity of a zinc-dependent enzyme such as alkaline phosphatase. None of these, nor hair zinc content, is universally acceptable. If zinc defi-ciency is suspected, the best policy is to monitor the clinical and biochemical response to zinc supplements:

2 mg (30 μmol) of elemental zinc/kg body weight daily is commonly used.

Copper deficiency

This is seen most frequently in preterm infants, in term infants who are fed inappropriate feeds or cow's milk and in children with protracted diarrhoea or those recovering from malnutrition.[16]

The features include low plasma copper (reference range 10–22 μmol/l), and caeruloplasmin (reference range 2–4.5 μmol/l), altered metabolism of iron possibly with a hypochromic microcytic anaemia, neutropaenia, hypotonia, and non-specific skeletal changes including osteoporosis, fracture of long bones, epiphyseal porosis and separation, periosteal reaction, metaphyseal broadening, and cupping with irregu-larities, spur formation and corner fractures. Severe deficiency may cause failure to thrive. A variety of other metabolic and biochemical defects affecting, for example, carbohydrate and lipid metabolisms and cardiac function, have been noted but their precise clinical relevance has not been established. Copper supplementation (80 μg or 1.25 μmol/kg body weight per day) which increases daily copper intake 3–5 fold, reduces the rate of infections in children recovering from malnutrition, and maintains their plasma copper concentrations.[17]

Copper toxicity

This may well be the cause of Indian childhood cirrhosis (ICC). (See pp. 735–6). This presents at one to three years of age; non-breast-fed infants are more sus-ceptible to developing the high hepatic copper content of ICC. This may arise from drinking animal milks which have been contaminated with copper after storage or heating in copper or brass utensils. The pathogenetic role of copper is suggested by the efficacy of penicillamine in reducing the mortality of children with pre-icteric ICC[18]; otherwise progressive hepatic failure leads to death.

Chromium deficiency

Chromium has a role in glucose tolerance and lipid metabolism. It is unclear how important this is. In adults on prolonged parenteral nutrition, chromium-responsive insulin-resistant glucose intolerance, weight loss, hypercholesterolaemia, hypertriglyceridaemia, impaired nitrogen retention, and neuropathies have occurred.[19, 20] Glucose intolerance and retarded growth in some children with malnutrition may respond to chromium.

Minerals and malnutrition syndromes

Different intakes and bioavailability of minerals may contribute to the regional variabilities in malnutrition and stunting syndromes.[21] The intake of anionic elements (e.g. fluorine, iodine and selenium) reflect local geochemical and soil conditions which influence their entry into the food chain.[22] Cations (calcium, magnesium, iron, zinc and copper) may be affected similarly, but this is less easily determined.

In severe malnutrition, losses of endogenous elements may result from tissue catabolism and increased bone turnover. The elements released may be able to maintain their plasma concentrations and the function of the remaining tissues. However, as soon as catabolism is reversed by treating the precipitant causes of the malnutrition, the need for elements such as magnesium, potassium, zinc and copper increases greatly. If these are not met then functional and symptomatic deficiencies develop. Thus, attention must be paid to these and other minerals in the management of malnutrition.

References

1. Fraser DR. Nutritional growth retardation: experimental studies with special references to calcium. In: Waterlow JC ed. *Linear Growth Retardation in Less Developed Countries*. New York, Raven Press, 1988: 127–41.
2. Kanis JA, Passmore R. Calcium supplementation of the diet – I. *British Medical Journal*. 1989; **298**: 137–40.
3. Brenton DP, Gordon TE. Magnesium. *British Journal of Hospital Medicine*. 1984. pp. 60–9.
4. Montgomery RD. Magnesium metabolism in infantile protein malnutrition. *Lancet*. 1980; **ii**: 74–5.
5. Alleyne GAO. Studies on total body potassium in malnourished infants. Factors affecting potassium repletion. *British Journal of Nutrition*. 1970; **24**: 205–12.
6. Hetzel BS. Iodine deficiency disorders and their eradication. *Lancet*. 1983; **ii**: 1126–9.
7. Querido A, Delange F, Dunn J *et al*. In: Dunn JT, Medciros-Nero GA eds. *Endemic Goitre and Cretinism: Continuing Threat to World Health*. Scientific Publication No. 292. Washington DC, Pan American Health Organisation, 1974.
8. Kaur K. Skeletal fluorosis in humans: a review of recent progress in the understanding of the disease. *Progress in Food and Nutrition Science*. 1986; **10**: 279–314.
9. Chen X, Yang G, Chen J *et al*. Studies on the relations of selenium and Keshan Disease. *Biological Trace Element Research*. 1980; **2**: 91–107.
10. Mathias PM, Jackson AA. Selenium deficiency in kwashiorkor. *Lancet*. 1982; **i**: 1312–13.
11. Casey CE. Selenophilia. *Proceedings of the Nutrition Society*. 1988; **47**: 55–62.
12. Yang G, Wang S, Zhou R, Sun S. Endemic selenium intoxication of humans in China. *American Journal of Clinical Nutrition*. 1983; **37**: 872–81.
13. Stekel A ed. *Iron Nutrition in Infancy and Childhood*. New York, Raven Press, 1984.
14. Golden MHN, Golden BE. Effect of zinc supplementation on the dietary intake, rate of weight gain and energy cost of tissue deposition in children recovering from severe malnutrition. *American Journal of Clinical Nutrition*. 1981; **34**: 900–8.
15. Golden MHN. The role of individual nutrient deficiencies in growth retardation of children as exemplified by zinc and protein in linear growth retardation in less developed countries. In: Waterlow JC ed. *Linear Growth Retardation in Less Developed Countries*. New York, Raven Press, 1988. pp. 143–63.
16. Editorial. Copper and the infant. *Lancet*. 1987; **i**: 900–1.
17. Castillo-Duran C, Fisberg M, Valzuela A *et al*. Controlled trial of copper supplementation during the recovery from marasmus. *American Journal of Clinical Nutrition*. 1983; **37**: 898–903.
18. Tanner MS, Bhave SA, Pradham AM, Pandit AN. Clinical trials of penicillamine in Indian Childhood Cirrhosis. *Archives of Disease in Childhood*. 1987; **62**: 1118–24.
19. Gurson CT, Saner G. Effects of chromium on glucose utilisation in marasmic protein calorie malnutrition. *American Journal of Clinical Nutrition*. 1971; **21**: 1313–19.
20. Freund H, Atamian S, Fisher JE. Chromium deficiency during total parenteral nutrition. *Journal of the American Medical Association*. 1979; **244**: 496–8.
21. Aggett PJ. Malnutrition and trace elements metabolism. In: Suskind R and LeWinter-Suskind L ed. *The Malnourished Child*. New York, Raven Press, 1990. pp. 155–76.
22. Sillanpaa M. Micronutrients and the nutrient states of soils. FAO Soil Bulletin 48. Rome, FAO, 1982.

Further reading

Bothwell JH, Charlton RW, Cook JD, Finch CA. *Iron Metabolism in Man*. Oxford, Blackwell, 1979.
Mertz W (ed.). *Trace Elements in Human and Animal Nutrition*. 2 Vols. London, Academic Press, 1986.
Shils ME, Young VR (eds). *Modern Nutrition in Health and Disease*. Philadelphia, Lea and Febiger, 1988.

NUTRITION REHABILITATION
M.A. Church

Philosophy and basic principles

The need to integrate health education with treatment in the management of childhood malnutrition is now widely acknowledged. 'Nutrition rehabilitation' is the term that has been applied to this broad process and to a wide range of centres and programmes based on it that have been developed in many different countries. Although there can obviously be no single method suitable for all places, there are some useful basic principles.

Principle 1: functional analysis

Nutrition rehabilitation requires a thorough functional analysis of the background of childhood malnutrition, with full regard to socio-economic, cultural and clinical factors. From this information both a 'community diagnosis' and 'clinical diagnosis' need to be made. Even at the clinical level this implies an epidemiological as well as individual approach, i.e. information based on individual cases of malnutrition needs to be accumulated to build up a general picture. Data from established young child clinics, as well as hospitals, can provide a useful picture of preclinical and clinical malnutrition.

A simple medical extension process found to be very useful in Uganda, was to make follow-up home visits for individual malnourished children and use these for an assessment of the particular household, as well as a chance to get a wider picture of the community, including making contact with leaders. Specific nutrition surveys may be necessary for a more detailed picture but as these are often expensive, they are probably most valuable when used to refine some existing working hypothesis.

Health workers need to be aware that there are also many other valuable sources of nutritional data and expertise such as agricultural and social science departments and local literature, poetry and art.

Principle 2: intervention strategies

The second principle of nutrition rehabilitation is to plan clear intervention strategies based on this functional analysis. Deciding the appropriate place for health programmes within the nutrition strategy is essential, although this is not often easy because agricultural, economic and health planning are rarely integrated in practice.

Within the health sector, a general working assumption is that it is quite inadequate to rely only on hospitals geared to diagnosing and treating severely malnourished children. That approach alone is not only expensive but can only deal with few children, many of whom die despite intensive therapy. Without effective education of mothers and a good follow-up service, many of the children discharged are likely to become malnourished again.

Thus, a vital purpose of young child clinics and nutrition rehabilitation centres is to complement the hospital service with appropriate nutrition education and follow-up. These services are not only essential for the earlier detection of malnutrition, for appropriate nutritional intervention and for the follow-up of recovering malnourished children, but have also been found to be highly cost-effective.

Principle 3: involving mothers

In a nutrition rehabilitation programme, communicating with mothers is as important as the cure of their children and both must be completely integrated. The most successful programmes have been the ones in which malnourished children are carefully selected clinically and are only included if their condition is likely to be cured with appropriate feeding. Very sick children requiring intensive medical treatment are still admitted to a paediatric ward. In a nutrition rehabilitation centre, mothers need to be involved fully in the preparation of food and the feeding of their children, as the credibility of the nutrition education depends on the experience of cure by feeding.

Principle 4: education

'Each one teach one' is a basic educational principle of nutrition rehabilitation, with mothers both in the residential and follow-up phases. Some programmes have also made natural extensions of the process to involve husbands, other family members and other people from the community. Some centres have deliberately included the training of community leaders within a nutrition rehabilitation programme.

Practice

Organization

Nutrition rehabilitation programmes have been organized in a wide variety of ways. Many have been closely related to an existing health service centre, usually a hospital, but some have been developed independently or related to another service such as agriculture. Some centres provide residential or day-care alone while others provide both, which is probably the best practice.

Staffing

Although nutrition rehabilitation programmes need clear medical and nutrition supervision and support, centres can usually be successfully staffed with nurses and paramedical workers and local people trained in the centre itself.

Rehabilitation diets

Diets suitable for rehabilitation are fortunately the same as those appropriate for weaning. Thus, the successful teaching of mothers in the rehabilitation of a child will also best prepare them for the successful weaning of any further children.

Although the nutrition education needs to be appropriate culturally to a specific situation, a number of useful generalizations drawn from different programmes can be made.

It is a good idea to separate the weaning child's portion of food. Often the weaning child eats from the communal family meal and can easily miss out, especially if weak or ill, which at that age is common. It is particularly beneficial for the child to have his own identified food container.

Available local foods should be mixed and mashed in suitable proportions. Only homely and locally suitable measuring methods should be used, such as handfuls and cupfuls. Foods need to be prepared so that when cooked they can be easily mashed and will be smooth enough for a toddler. For example, beans need to be either ground into flour or soaked and peeled. Foods should wherever possible only be handled and mixed before cooking, so that the mashing process after cooking requires the minimum of handling, reducing the risk of contamination. To be practical and realistic, this whole process needs to be closely integrated with existing cooking practices.

All traditional staple foods are low in fat and high in starch, which means that when cooked they tend to be high in bulk and low in energy. Thus, it is difficult for a weaning child to eat enough of these foods to cover needs for energy and growth. The mixing of foods described can help greatly and in addition, mothers should be encouraged to feed their young children regularly throughout the day.

Probably the most important ways of tackling the problem of bulk is by adding fat or oil to the diet or by providing some of the carbohydrate as sugar. These measures both increase the energy density of the food and reduce viscosity. Fat can either be included in cooking, as for example with palm oil, or can come from naturally high-fat foods such as ground-nuts or sesame. The cooking of legumes with marrow bones, a common practice in many parts of the world, is a cheap and very useful way of gaining the benefits of marrow fat. Sugar, either refined or raw, can be added to the food or it can come from fresh or dried fruits. The malting of cereals is another useful and widely practised process for transforming some of the starch to natural sugars and making gruel or porridge, which is more suitable for young children.

The expensive foods such as meats, fish, milk and dairy produce and manufactured foods should only be used and advocated with great caution in nutrition rehabilitation programmes. For instance, the introduction of milk powder to a mother may not only be of limited use in the longer term rehabilitation of her child at home, but may also inadvertently support the idea of its being used for the next baby, even though the cost of commercial milk powders is likely to be beyond her means.

Teaching methods

Teaching methods need to be culturally appropriate, and different approaches may be required even within the same centre. Maximum use needs to be made of local materials and real things where possible, e.g.

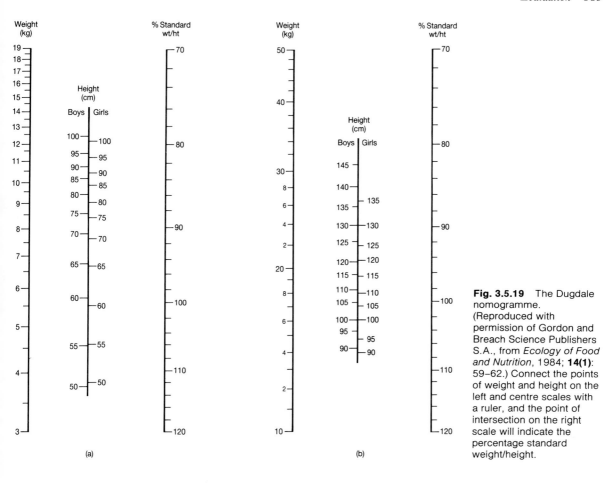

Fig. 3.5.19 The Dugdale nomogramme. (Reproduced with permission of Gordon and Breach Science Publishers S.A., from *Ecology of Food and Nutrition*, 1984; **14(1)**: 59–62.) Connect the points of weight and height on the left and centre scales with a ruler, and the point of intersection on the right scale will indicate the percentage standard weight/height.

foods and plants rather than pictures of them. All food preparation and cooking techniques should be based on local utensils, practices and skills.

Familiar means of communication such as proverbs, stories, songs and plays need to be used and adapted, and visual materials should fit with the local scene. Any text should be related to the appropriate level of literacy. Photographs can be very useful, but are best when any distracting background is cut out to leave the main item clear.

Evaluation

The evaluation of nutrition rehabilitation needs to be faced at the broad general level, as well as at the specific practical level. Important broad issues include:

- How does nutrition rehabilitation fit into existing nutrition policies and services? It has been shown to be cost-effective compared with intensive hospital-based treatment of severely malnourished children. But this should not be assumed to be a cheaper option, because a nutrition rehabilitation programme intervenes earlier in the process of malnutrition and hence involves many more children. The basic assumption is that with a progressive condition such as malnutrition, it is preferable to have systems to intervene early rather than just to wait for severe malnutrition to occur. Young child clinics using growth charts aim, of course, to catch the process of weight faltering at an even earlier stage than do rehabilitation centres.

- How the programme relates to non-medical agencies and policies that affect nutrition, such as in agriculture, development and trade. A nutrition rehabilitation programme can only make sense if it is complementary to these other major forces.

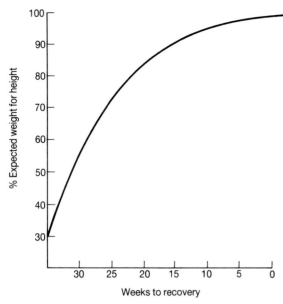

Fig. 3.5.20 Average expected catch-up during nutrition rehabilitation. Weight for height is the assumed target expressed as percentage deficit of the target. (Reproduced from Wallace HM, Ebrahim GJ (eds) *Maternal and Child Health around the World*. London, Macmillan, 1981. pp. 175–82.)

Some important specific practical issues include:

- Setting realistic targets for weight catch-up. The most easily identifiable target for weight catch-up is the expected weight-for-height. The Dugdale Nomogramme (Fig. 3.5.19) is a useful tool for estimating both the existing degree of wasting and the target catch-up weight.
- Estimating a reasonable target rate for weight catch-up and the length of the rehabilitation period relates both to the degree of malnutrition and the intensity of the treatment process. Figure 3.5.20 shows a reasonable expected catch-up curve, based on experience from research centres in Uganda and Jamaica, using energy-rich diets providing in the

order of 200 kcal (836 kJ)/kg per day (see p. 353). However, nutrition rehabilitation programmes based on modified home diets with slower patterns of catch-up, that reached the weight-for-height target in about six months, have been matched by good clinical progress. Height catch-up only occurs slowly and over a much longer rehabilitation period. The regular weight chart is the best means for monitoring long-term progress.

Further reading

Beaudry-Darisme M, Latham MC. Nutrition rehabilitation centres: an evaluation of their performance. *Journal of Tropical Pediatrics and Environmental Child Health*. 1973; **19**: 299–332.

Beghin ID, Viteri FE. Nutrition rehabilitation centres: an evaluation of their performance. *Journal of Tropical Pediatrics and Environmental Child Health*. 1973; **19**: 404–16.

Bengoa JM. Nutrition rehabilitation centres. *Journal of Tropical Pediatrics and Environmental Child Health*. 1967; **13**: 169–76.

Church MA. Educational methods, cultural characteristics and nutrition rehabilitation: experience in Kampala unit. *Journal of Tropical Pediatrics and Environmental Child Health*, 1971; **13**: 43–50.

Church MA. Nutrition rehabilitation: an approach to the management and prevention of childhood malnutrition. In: Wallace HM, Ebrahim GH eds. *Maternal and Child Health Around the World*. London, Macmillan Press, 1981. pp. 175–82.

Church MA. Health education and maternal and child health: newer considerations and the international perspective. In: Jelliffe DB, Jelliffe EPF eds. *Advances in International Maternal and Child Health*, Vol. 3. Oxford, Oxford University Press, 1983. pp. 90–108.

Cook R. Is hospital the place for the treatment of malnourished children? *Journal of Tropical Pediatrics and Environmental Child Health*. 1971; **17**: 15–25.

Hoorweg J, Niemeijer R. *Intervention in Child Nutrition*. London and New York, Kegan Paul International, 1989.

Practical guide to combating malnutrition in the pre-school child: nutrition rehabilitation through maternal education. *Report of a Working Conference on Nutrition Rehabilitation and Mothercare Centers, Bogota, Colombia*. New York, Appleton-Century-Crofts, Educational Division Meredith Corporation, 1969.

CHAPTER 6

Behaviour

EMOTIONAL DEVELOPMENT
A. D. Nikapota and H. G. Egdell

Emotional or behaviour disorders in children are usually due to poor adjustment or faulty interactions between a child and the environment. Behaviour, the observable response to events or circumstances, is greatly influenced by psychosocial development. A knowledge of child development therefore helps in the understanding of child behaviour and the genesis of emotional disorders in children, as well as highlighting children's needs in relation to cultural attitudes, service provision and national policies for child health and welfare. The clinician in a tropical country has an important role in interpreting children's behaviour and emphasizing children's emotional needs to parents and communities, who may be relatively unaware of the importance of healthy emotional development.

Here the major aspects of emotional development in children: infants, toddlers, preschool and school children and adolescents are considered. Although development is commonly subdivided into physical, emotional, cognitive and social, in reality these aspects are interdependent. Hence, a description of emotional development must include the impact of childhood experience on overall development.

Definitions

The following simple definitions are used here:

- *Emotional development* refers to a child's ability to perceive, experience and express feelings such as affection, love, happiness, fear, frustration and anger. It is modified by factors in the child such as intelligence and temperament, in the environment and arising from the interaction of the child and the environment including learning and maturation.
- *Intelligence* is a child's ability to learn, understand concepts and solve problems and is related to cognitive skills.
- *Cognitive development* refers to the development of thought processes in children.

Both intelligence and cognition are developed through learning, the degree of development depending on both the child's innate ability and the opportunities for learning to which the child is exposed. In many communities, parents make considerable efforts to send children to school, but undervalue day-to-day experience in developing children's intelligence and thought.

- *Temperament* refers to the behavioural traits or behavioural style a child exhibits from birth. This will also contribute to the personality of the child.
- *Personality* refers to the specific characteristics of an individual's behaviour and includes the capacity to act independently, cope with conflict and stress and appreciate moral and ethical issues, as well as the individual's knowledge of himself. Family, social and cultural values will greatly affect the development of personality, despite temperamental traits. For example, in some cultures, a girl will be brought

up to be dependent so as to fit into her community. In such circumstances, a liking for independence will be considered unusual and will be discouraged.

Theories of development

There are many theories of child development. Foremost is the work of Sigmund Freud, who pioneered the psychoanalytic approach to development and gave prominence to the effects of early childhood experiences on development and later behaviour.[1] Erik Erikson described development in terms of psychosocial stages[2, 3] while Jean Piaget not only researched cognitive development, but also highlighted the concept that all development is an ordered process resulting from interactions between a child and the environment.[4] Melanie Klein[5] and Anna Freud[6] studied emotions in early childhood and John Bowlby[7] described the importance of the mother–child relationship or 'bond' for healthy development, as well as the harm caused by separation from the mother.

The description of development given here draws on the work of these and other workers.[8, 9] Unfortunately, there is a serious lack of studies on the effects on emotional development of family structures common in the Third World, for example the extended family and multiple-mothering figures for each child.

The developmental process: some important facts

Development is a process of continuous interaction between the growth and maturation of physical (especially neurological) structures, intrinsic qualities and abilities and environmental influences.

The sequence of development therefore is the same cross-culturally, i.e. all children pass through stages of development in the same order. All babies, for example, respond to a friendly face at about four to six weeks with a smile. The meaning of the first smile is interpreted differently according to cultural beliefs. However, although environmental influences cannot alter the developmental sequence, they can alter the quality of development. For example, all children display selective recognition i.e. the recognition of a familiar face at six to eight months. This will be recognition of the mother if the child is looked after almost exclusively by her. On the other hand, a child looked after with love and interest by two or three people in an extended family, will recognize more than one person,

whereas a child looked after by constantly changing staff in an institution may not demonstrate this stage of development. These facts are central to all therapeutic programmes aimed at promoting children's development.

Another important fact is that children interact with their environment and modify environmental factors which affect their development. A baby who is a poor sucker and difficult to feed will produce anxiety in the mother. She will probably spend a long time feeding the baby and will find it difficult to relax, play with and enjoy the baby in a way that she could have done had the baby sucked vigorously.

Individual differences in children are also important in development and behaviour. This may not be understood by families and communities and may lead at times to the rejection of the difficult or different child.

Maturation is the process of coming to full growth and development and applies to emotional, social and cognitive, as well as physical, development. However, these may not be in step with each other. The degree of maturity determines the readiness of the child to experience and learn. For example, the first smile occurs when the baby is able to focus the eyes and has reached the level of maturation required for the smiling response.

The concept of maturational readiness has led to the idea of critical periods and imprinting. Psychological research indicates that certain responses are best learnt at certain or critical periods when the child has reached the appropriate stage of maturation. This has been illustrated in studies of animal development but is less easy to demonstrate in children. Imprinting refers to learning which having occurred at a critical period cannot be easily altered. It is likely that the development of attachment bonds in early childhood is related to critical periods and imprinting, as these are very strong. A child brought up from infancy by an aunt, may always relate most closely to her, even if looked after later by the natural mother.

Stages of emotional development

Infancy

Initially the most easily recognized emotions a baby expresses are anger and frustration in response to hunger and discomfort. The first obvious pleasurable expression by a six-week old baby in response to an external stimulus such as a friendly face, is the smile. In the first few months, babies begin to distinguish objects as being apart from them and to acquire a sense of their own bodies. The efforts of babies to identify objects as being part or apart from them can be observed by watching babies' behaviour towards their hands and feet. Initially these objects are looked at and 'talked to', and then held and brought to the mouth for tasting once the baby realizes that they can be controlled. Emotional feelings towards the mother, or breast, will be of anger or satisfaction, depending on the responsiveness of the mother to the baby's needs and the consistency of mothering behaviour. The temperament of both the mother and the baby will influence mothering and emotional satisfaction even in these early months.

Psychoanalysts call the first year the 'oral' stage since the baby's main preoccupation and pleasure is centred around feeding and, at this age, a baby tends to taste everything encountered. The capacity to trust and feel secure arises from the security and warmth received by the baby. The child who is given warmth and security has an ability to develop close relationships later, whereas a child who does not have this experience is often unable to form such relationships.

Selective recognition of the mother or caring person occurs at about six to eight months, and at this age a baby's feelings of happiness, security, anger, sadness focus on the mother's behaviour in relationship to the baby's needs. Selective recognition gives rise to separation anxiety when the mother is not present, and fear and anxiety in the presence of strangers. Separation anxiety occurs when there is a good relationship between the mother and baby which has led to attachment or bonding. Attachment occurs when there is not only a consistent person looking after the baby but when that person is responsive to the baby. Responsiveness is not just feeding the baby when hungry but interacting with the baby. In an extended family, a baby may develop bonds with a grandmother who carries, cuddles, or talks to him, rather than with a mother if she only feeds him.

Selective recognition, separation anxiety and bonding are very important features of the emotional development of children which can affect later development and behaviour.[10] It has long been recognized that children brought up in an institution may have impaired emotional development since these early experiences do not occur. The effects, if any, on the development of children where attachment is different as a result of growing up in an extended rather than nuclear family have not been very extensively researched, but where there is warmth and consistency it is not likely that having more than one caring person is harmful, so long as the bonds with such carers are not suddenly broken. In many cultures in developing countries this is not realized and a baby may be passed for care from mother to another according to custom or necessity without making allowance for distress in the child.

Rapid motor development during the first year, allows a baby to exert increasing control over the parts of the body, leading to walking towards the end of the first year. This motor development increases the variety of responses a baby can make. Recognition of mother can be followed by holding arms out to her and later, by crawling and finally walking towards her.

Communication also develops. In early infancy, a baby communicates through crying and body language, for example becoming rigid to signify protest when placed in a cot or on a mat. Sounds begin as a form of communication when the baby babbles and makes noises resembling words. This signifies that the baby is acquiring the maturational readiness to learn speech. Language is learnt when the mother teaches the baby words based on the sounds the baby makes. One of the first sounds is 'm', which may be why the word for mother has this sound in virtually all languages.

Toddlers (one to two years)

As the infant becomes a toddler, rapid motor development enables the child to be mobile, independent and explore the surroundings. The toddler also develops increasing control over the body and bodily functions, including bladder and bowel.

The learning that accompanies this control will determine how a child demonstrates control and will vary from culture to culture. A child will learn to feed with the hand or using a spoon, depending upon custom.

Control over feeding and bowel and bladder function will be achieved quickly and happily if the relationship between the child and mother is good. Children, however, may use their power to refuse food, or to empty their bowels, and become difficult over these developmental tasks, if they want more parental attention or want to control the mother.

Emotional security comes from attachment to the mother and separation anxiety is very marked at this age. The child is independent and mobile but needs the security of the mother's nearness. Attachment occurs to the carer or mother or, as in many developing countries, surrogate mother who may be an extended-family member or 'ayah'. This is often not appreciated in young children who are handed over for care when parents need to move away for employment or for study, and then taken back without thought for the distress in the child caused by the breaking of attachment bonds.

Objects such as comforters and soft toys provide

reassurance at this stage. Thumb-sucking has the same effect, as have songs or rituals carried out to make the child feel secure. In many tropical countries, the mother's breast continues to be the comfort producer as part of cultural habit and it is common to see children of one to three years being given the breast to keep them quiet, or to soothe them when they are upset. Children also become very attached to particular objects, a piece of cloth or a toy, which they may clutch constantly.

Speech development provides the principal excitement at this age. It gives a child tremendous pride and satisfaction and enhances the ability to express ideas and feelings. Stimulation from the environment is necessary for speech to develop and children who grow up in very deprived circumstances often develop speech late.

Preschool children (two to five years)

Development at this stage is characterized by rapid advances in speech and social behaviour. The child still needs the mother but attachments occur to other people also and contacts with children and adults become less fearful and more pleasurable. The use of language becomes increasingly complex and children of this age take great delight in exercising their verbal skills. Stammering may occur briefly. This should not be a cause for anxiety, though it does cause alarm in cultures such as in South Asia, where there are traditional rituals associated with speech development or where stammering is mistakenly thought to indicate a 'brain problem'. Learning to speak in more than one language, as occurs when children grow up in bilingual homes, does not lead to language delay where speech development is normal. Parents should not feel anxious about this. However, where children have developmental language impairments or delays, learning to speak bilingually can cause difficulty to the child but does not cause harm in the long-term.[11]

Children of this age are still egocentric and respond only to their own needs and desires. As with younger children, they see themselves as the centre of the world and temper tantrums due to frustration are common. Parents often find tantrums irritating and embarrassing and may threaten, slap or smack the young child in an attempt to control the tantrum, or may give in to the child's demands. Neither method helps control. The child may become upset, angry and frightened when punished physically without appreciating the reasons for parents' anger. Threats especially ones such as 'I will leave you here if you don't stop' or 'I will ask the bogey-man to take you away' will only frighten and make the child feel rejected. Once the child learns that

they are empty threats they will have no impact. Giving in to the tantrum teaches the child that tantrums work. Whenever possible a tantrum should be ignored. If necessary the child may be taken away briefly until quiet if those around are very disturbed by the behaviour. Tantrums normally become less frequent as the child nears school age.

Exploration as a result of curiosity about the environment is marked and results in a considerable amount of behaviour which may be termed meddlesome, and a large number of questions, often repetitive, which can be irritating. The child is simply demonstrating the need for stimulation from the environment. Limits may need to be placed on such behaviour for the safety of the child but punitive measures to limit curiosity may be detrimental.

Play, in particular imaginative play, is important at this age. Fantasy and enactment of events help children to understand the world around them and enable them to practise for the future. Play is often solitary but play with other children becomes possible as social skills mature. Sibling rivalry may also occur at this age. This is normal but is often not recognized as such by parents. In Western cultures, a child of this age will have been encouraged to separate from mother and may be prepared for the birth of a younger child. In many developing countries, however, the youngest child is kept near the mother, sleeps with her and is given the breast for comfort up to this age unless another child is born, at which point the older child is supplanted suddenly by the new baby. This may be associated with abrupt weaning and malnutrition and even the development of kwashiorkor.

Thought processes develop, but children of this age can understand events only as they are seen to have happened. Concepts are not understood. Fantasy and reality, animate and inanimate have limited meaning. Children easily and genuinely become terrified of simple non-threatening events, or as a result of ghost or fairy stories. Distress can occur when events are not understood. For example, a child of three years became very insecure after her shoes were removed before entering a Hindu temple and were subsequently found to be missing. A much-loved and protected child, she could not appreciate the strict religious taboos which dictated this event. To her perception her parents had selected the removal and loss of her shoes as a means of making her unhappy for no good reason.

Awareness of sexual differences also develops at this stage and results in identification with the same sex parent and attachment and possessiveness towards the parent of the opposite sex. Curiosity about genitals and play with genitals is normal and not related to adult sexuality. Parents should be advised not to over-react to this behaviour with distress and anxiety but merely to teach the child to limit such play if it is being done at socially unacceptable times or places.

The beginning of conscience is seen at this age, as the child develops the ability to internalize parental instructions and dictates. The child therefore begins to make decisions about the acceptability of his/her actions based on parental teaching. Where the latter is inconsistent or has not occurred, this aspect of development may also be delayed. Consistency of discipline is much more important in emotional development than whether the carers are strict or lax. Many children do have formal preschool education. The principal value of preschool attendance is not in learning scholastic skills but in learning to live in a new environment, to mix, share and work with other children and relate to adults other than family members. Much social learning also occurs in the group of children in the extended family – perhaps under the guidance of an older sibling or cousin.

Secure family attachments will facilitate performance of the many developmental tasks which occur during this period. Children who are emotionally secure are able to cope with new situations with confidence, whereas children who are insecure and mistrustful tend to withdraw. This difference can be seen when assessing children in clinic or preschool, though the temperamental traits of the child will also affect behaviour. A timid child, even if secure, will tend to withdraw and be anxious in a new situation, but where there is close emotional attachment the child will clearly derive support from the mother or accompanying adult.

It would be useful to consider what role the extended family plays in child development. Extended families often provide care and stimulation. Increasing the social contacts of a child facilitates social development. However, care of the child may be transferred to other family members without considering the child's needs, as is increasingly common in some Third World countries where many parents seek contractual employment abroad. It is important to recognize that this type of separation breaks bonds formed by the child and can be harmful unless a considerable amount of careful preparation and reassurance is given to the child.

School age children

Children of school age enjoy doing things that they are taught and become concerned with achievement and the learning of skills. The main source of instruction for many children is school but the learning of day-to-day life skills from parents, carers and older siblings is also important; ideally teaching should be from both family and teacher. In all cultures and communities, vocational skills are taught at home, many involving considerable responsibilities, e.g. cooking, tending domestic animals and cultivating. The development of cognitive and social skills will be altered by such employment and adult-type responsibilities, particularly where school attendance does not occur.

Selection of children to attend school occurs in some communities. Boys or younger siblings are often favoured as older ones are needed to work. There may be lack of school fees. Selection may aggravate sibling rivalry or produce feelings of rejection, especially when the rest of the family makes heavy sacrifices and those selected may have the burden of high expectations from the rest of the family. It may perpetuate prejudice against women.

School provides opportunities to socialize with peers in work and play, as well as to learn academic skills. Adjustment to school is difficult for children who have been very protected at home, or have no experience of siblings or cousins already attending school, as they have to cope with many new circumstances away from the support of the mother and family. Children begin to develop a sense of their own abilities and skills at this age. Failure in school can cause feelings of inadequacy and it is important that parents and teachers are aware that some children need additional support and encouragement to learn skills such as reading, writing and counting. In most developing countries, high value is placed on education and primary school children are often pushed to achieve higher grades than they are able to achieve. This leads to frustration, feelings of failure and emotional problems. It may be aggravated by school practices of keeping children of limited abilities in the same form year after year. In many developing countries, there is little awareness about the learning problems children may have and how these may be managed, e.g. by understanding the effects of emotional problems and the variety of learning speeds.

Children of this age should have few separation difficulties, although the need for emotional support from the family, particularly mother, continues. They are aware of their sex and should be aware of their position in the family and therefore what is expected of them.

Behaviour may differ according to the temperament and developing personality of the child. Children may be timid or outgoing, like to lead or prefer to be led. These temperamental differences should be taken into account in the management of the child at home and in school.

From about seven to eight years of age, there is a

developing ability to understand concepts, e.g. distinguish animate from inanimate. Children can give reasons for what they do but their thinking depends on immediate perceptions and not on the application of concepts, e.g. of size, shape, colour. They are less egocentric and can play in a cooperative fashion, which increases their capacity to form relationships with peers. Erickson called this the stage of industry versus inferiority. This is a useful description since, at this stage children begin to take pride in learning skills and also become aware of inadequacy.

Adolescence

Adolescents form a small minority in the paediatric clinics of the developing world and health workers may not be very familiar with adolescent development and problems. Children usually accept parents bringing them along to clinics, whilst an adolescent may resent this and the young person's anxiety may present as hostility and suspicion. In addition, older health workers may be out of touch with the adolescent's values, attitudes and interests. It may be difficult for the doctor to be professional and avoid judging the individual. There is a danger of either taking the role of a strict parent or seeing all problems as illness.

Adolescence is usually defined as beginning with the onset of puberty, the most dramatic manifestations of which are in girls the menarche (onset of periods) at about 11 to 13 years, and in boys seminal emissions normally at 13 to 17 years. These are preceded by physical changes and this entire period is one of considerable and critical development both physical and psychological. The physical changes of puberty begin to appear from about 10 years and have an emotional impact on the child. There is often both anxiety and embarrassment associated with physical development. These feelings may be exacerbated by ignorance if parents have been unable to discuss puberty and its implications with the child or traditional group educational practices have been lost. In addition, there are changes in personality. The adolescent develops an awareness of personal and sexual identity. The boy or girl is required to adjust to rapidly altering roles within the family, school and society and to make the transition from dependent child to independent adult. There are many challenges – academic, vocational and social. The boy or girl has gradually to develop an independent life-style and attitude, make mature relationships with peers of both sexes and cope with emerging sexual needs and desires.

The degree of confidence with which an adolescent copes with these changing roles will depend on individual temperament, personality and the security of family relationships. Considerable support is necessary during this period. The very close peer group relationships formed are, in part, due to this need for support, since through relationships the child is able to share experiences with others who face the same problems. Parents too often tend to give the view that they themselves had no difficulties.

Sexual behaviour and the relationships with the opposite sex will develop, varying considerably according to family attitude and social cultural habit. The opportunity to mix with the opposite sex will vary from country to country and society to society. Another important aspect of behaviour is related to the adolescent's ability to develop an independent lifestyle, which will again vary in different cultures. There may often be an inconsistency of attitude in family and school where responsibility is given for some aspects of life but strict limits imposed on others according to tradition. This certainly is so in many South Asian countries where high academic achievement is expected, but the adolescent is allowed very little freedom to form independent relationships and lifestyle. In some societies, Western influences may encourage independence and responsibility to an inappropriate degree, irrespective of the level of maturity and ability of the individual. Rapid urbanization is associated with the breakdown of the extended family, poverty, and parents working long hours out of the home and this may force very young adolescents into an independent life.

Adolescence is recognized as being a difficult period and called by Erikson a crisis of identity. In traditional societies, achieving an identity as an integrated member of a group may be more important than achieving an individual identity. On the other hand, adolescents do not invariably go through a period of difficulty, turmoil and difficult relationships, particularly where the parents are flexible and sensitive whilst still prepared to set clear limits of acceptable behaviour. Where there is an established warm and secure relationship between the adolescent and parent and both sides feel able to accept some compromises, the transition may be smooth and trouble free. In traditional societies the transition from childhood to adolescence and adulthood is marked with clear rituals and very strictly defined changes in role. Whilst this clear definition gives more support and less confusion, it provides little latitude for individual choice and development. This again illustrates the emphasis in traditional societies on group identity as opposed to the individual identity highlighted in the West. Adolescents have problems where the family and home style of life contrasts with that of the surrounding community – for example in migrant families. The young people may have to choose between the two conflicting cultures.

It is important to recognize that difficulties can be easily experienced without there being psychiatric illness, and also that at this age physical symptoms often arise from psychosocial distress.

Adolescents may present to the clinician with attempted suicide. In South Asian countries where the completed suicide rate amongst adolescents is high, studies indicate that these are closely related to stress rather than major psychiatric illness such as depression.[12] Counselling and help with psychosocial stresses for such adolescents will be required.

Conclusion

This description of development highlights children's emotional and developmental needs and the ways their behaviour might change according to their ability to understand and respond to events and feelings. Health workers need to be familiar with the normal range of variation in development. They can help the child, parents and others to allow for such variation and not mistake them for abnormality. This knowledge also enables them to advise the planners of child health and welfare services of children's needs for healthy emotional development. An awareness of developmental needs and the way environmental circumstances can alter development and behaviour should make it easy for the clinician to include in routine assessment of children questions to assess early development and psychosocial circumstances.

References

1. Freud S *Three Essays on the Theory of Sexuality*. New York, Harper and Row, 1982.
2. Erikson EH. *Childhood and Society*. St. Albans, Triad (Paladin), 1978.
3. Erikson EH. *Identity and the Life Cycle*. New York, W.W. Norton, 1980.
4. Piaget J. *The Construction of Reality in the Child*. New York, Ballantine/Random House, 1986.
5. Klein M. In: Greenspan IS, Pollock G eds. *The Psychoanalytic Contribution Towards Understanding Personality Development, Vol. 1: Infancy and Early Childhood*. USA, NIMH, 1980.
6. Freud A. *Normality and Pathology in Childhood*. New York, International University Press, 1966.
7. Bowlby J. *Attachment and Loss in Attachment*, Vol. 1, 2nd Edn. New York, Basic Books, Harper and Row, 1983.
8. Mussen PH, Conger JJ, Kagan J, Huston AC. *Child Development and Personality*, 6th Edn. New York. Harper and Row, 1984.
9. Hetherington EM. Socialisation, personality and social development. In: *Handbook of Child Psychology*, Vol. 4. New York, John Wiley, 1983.
10. Rutter M. *Maternal Deprivation Re-assessed*, 2nd Edn. Harmondsworth, Penguin Books, 1981.
11. Puckering C, Rutter M. Environmental influences on language development. In: Rutter M, Yule W eds. *Language Development and Disorder*. Blackwell Scientific Publication, 1987.
12. Dissanayake SAW, De Silva P. Suicide and attempted suicide in Sri Lanka. In: Headley LA ed. *Suicide in Asia and the Near East*. Berkeley, University of California Press, 1984.

MENTAL HEALTH PROBLEMS

H. G. Egdell and A. D. Nikapota with K. Minde and S. Musisi

Mental health problems in children may be defined as 'abnormality of behaviour, emotions or relationships sufficiently marked and sufficiently prolonged to be causing persistent suffering or handicap to the child himself or distress or disturbance in the family or community'.[1]

Emotional disorder in children can no longer be considered to be an uncommon problem in childhood in developed or developing countries.[2] The study by Giel *et al.*, in four developing countries, demonstrated that 12 to 29 per cent of children from 5 to 15 years attending primary health care clinics suffer from a mental disorder.[3] A cross-cultural similarity with regard to symptoms and associated stress factors was reported in eight national case studies from India, Philippines, Indonesia, Thailand, Sri Lanka, Greece and Nigeria.[4]

Somatic disorders are the most common mode of presentation of emotional problems, perhaps because the parents are most sensitive to physical complaints in such children. Children with emotional problems will therefore often be seen first by the primary health care staff and would need to be diagnosed and managed at this level wherever possible.[5] Such large numbers of children could not all be referred to a child psychiatrist service – even if it were available.

Assessment

What then is the method for assessing a child in a general health setting? The brief outline which follows could serve as a guide for assessment for emotional disorders which are described later. This assessment procedure is basically similar to the rest of the paediatric assessment and should be included as part of the overall examination of the child.

Whilst taking the history of the presenting complaint, it would help to obtain a history of behaviour changes such as irritability, weepiness, disinterest in studies and disobedience. Any history of recent stress, however trivial, that may have caused the child distress would be useful. Questions on school performance should be included to exclude problems such as school failure, parental over-insistence on academic success or difficulties with other children. When taking the family history it would help to know family structure and any history of important events such as separation from the parents. Staff need to know how local culture influences child-care, for example, a boy may be spoilt or expected to be very boyish or a middle girl may feel left out. Some information regarding the child's developmental level, by asking about early milestones, will also help the clinician to understand the child's behaviour and symptoms in relation to age. Questions about the child's ability to make friends, relationships with adults outside the family and the way the child plays, will give some idea of the child's temperament.

The accompanying adult's attitude to the child may be noted as the history is being given and indicates whether the child is accepted, favoured or rejected by the carers. An essential part of an assessment is talking to the child – seeking both history and obtaining the child's ideas about the problem. This aspect of assessment is often overlooked when considering only physical illness. Talking to the child will also give some idea of the child's temperament and, from direct observation, whether confident or fearful, very restless or conforming in the clinic situation. Having some opinion about the child's temperament is important as this has a bearing on the ways in which an emotional problem might manifest. For instance, a timid child may react to stress by becoming increasingly weepy and withdrawing from the situation, whereas an aggressive child when frustrated may become more aggressive. The clinician would also gain some idea of the child's intelligence from the way the child understands or describes recent events.

Emotional problems are very likely to be present in particular clinical situations. Examples are multiple symptoms or repeated attendances in an apparently physically healthy child, chronic physical illness or malnutrition, recent severe and repeated stresses on the child and family and the accompanying adult or the health staff themselves believing that there is an emotional problem.

Additional questions, when included in the usual assessment or examination, particularly when the clinician has become familiar with them, are not as time-consuming as they appear. A nurse, auxiliary or volunteer can be trained to assist by asking some of these questions to save time in a busy clinic. These additional questions are extremely helpful, not only in assessing the presence or absence of an emotional disorder, but also in looking at any psychosocial factors which affect physical illness.

Developmental problems

Enuresis

Enuresis is persistent involuntary micturition without organic cause. In the study of Giel *et al.*, wetting or soiling were the most common complaints in the centre of Sudan; the second most common in Colombia; fourth in the Philippines and sixth in India in an eight-symptom enquiry.[3] Western studies reveal about 10 per cent of children still wetting their beds at the age of about five years, with a steady fall to about 1 per cent in their teens. Obviously, complaints of parents will vary with their expectations of when the child should be dry. This is often influenced by experience of bladder control in other siblings and in the parents themselves.

Daytime wetting in one Western study was about 2 per cent in five-year-olds, but this will vary with the criteria of how often the child wets.

Aetiology

Many factors are involved. A genetic contribution is shown by the higher-than-expected rate in the second of identical twins where the first is wetting and that in Western studies nocturnal enuresis is more common in boys. There is often a familial delay in bladder control.

Only a minority of patients with enuresis have associated emotional disorders. This is more likely to occur with secondary and diurnal enuresis. Whilst most enuretic children do not have an emotional problem, there is evidence that stressful events and circumstances in early childhood have a contribution. Examples of stresses would be parental disharmony, separation from mother, birth of a sibling, hospital admission and neglectful parents. The parents may be indifferent to teaching bladder control. It may be that these stresses interfere with the development of bladder control during the 'critical period' of gaining control from 24 to 36 months.

Clinical features

The most common presentation in the West is nocturnal enuresis (wetting at night-time), though it may occur in the daytime (diurnal enuresis). Primary enuresis is when the child has never been dry, whilst secondary enuresis is when the child has been dry and later begins to wet himself. Urinary infection is more common as a differential diagnosis in daytime wetting, and abnormalities of the urinary tract may cause wetting day and night.

There may be secondary problems arising from the family's reaction with punishment or rejection. The child may be anxious or ashamed.

Management

Urinary infection and diabetes need to be excluded. Further renal investigation is probably not indicated unless there is recurrent infection. This is no evidence that urethral dilatation or bladder neck surgery is helpful.

Any associated behavioural or social problem should be identified and helped if possible. It is important to know the local attitudes to this particular milestone and to toilet training practices. Parents may need to be told that harsh punishment is unproductive and may upset the child. They should be encouraged to continue commonsense measures, for example, 'lifting' the child, that is waking the child in the night to pass urine and restricting fluids at the end of the day. It is important that the child understands what is happening and that the problem is seen as slow development of control rather than bad behaviour.

Behavioural principles underly the three most effective methods of treatment. The first involves breaking the whole process of emptying the bladder into a series of steps when toilet training is necessary. The first step is the child indicating in some manner the need to pass urine. The next step is going to the toilet, and the third, pulling down the pants, passing urine and pulling up the pants. Each successfully completed step is immediately rewarded. Giving large amounts of a favourite drink produces frequent opportunities to practise and be rewarded for success.

Use of a 'star chart' for nocturnal enuresis and toilet training involves a sheet of paper with lines drawn to mark a space for each night of the week. The successful dry nights are marked by a tick or brightly coloured stick-on paper star. The sheet is placed in some conspicuous position so that the child and all the family can be aware of the successes. This is a social reward for the child. The cooperation of the family with the use of a sheet can be a guide to motivation for treatment. It is feasible and effective in a rural African community.

The 'bell and pad method' is effective in nocturnal enuresis, provided the equipment is available and parents and child can fully cooperate. The bell and pad equipment available in the UK has to conform to the Department of Health and Social Services specifications and British Safety Standards and may be provided with a battery. They are available on loan from health and paediatric departments. It would be reasonable for departments of paediatrics in the developing world to possess this equipment and assess its efficacy in their local community. It consists of a mat or pad placed under the child so that on micturating the urine wets the pad and completes an electric circuit. This rings the bell and wakes the child. The child and the carer need a careful demonstration and an opportunity to set up the equipment under supervision. Problems may arise when the equipment is not used properly or the child turns it off or sleeps through the alarm which then disturbs the rest of the family. When properly used it is highly effective with most children over seven years of age. A few have later relapses which usually respond to a further course of treatment. Children of limited intelligence learn more slowly and need longer courses of treatment.

Tricyclic antidepressant drugs have been shown to be effective in the control of enuresis. The benefit is not due to the antidepressant action. Drugs are indicated when there is need for short-term dryness, for example, when the child has to be away from home, when there has been failure of the bell and pad methods or when there are serious problems within the family due to the wetting. Successful patients become dry in a week or two. Unfortunately on stopping the medication there is a high risk of relapse. In addition, there are dangers of fatal overdosage and side-effects such as constipation, dry mouth and headache. Even when successful, the drug should not be given for more than three months. These drugs should not be used in children under seven years of age. Dosage is 25–50 mg at night – no more.

Encopresis

Encopresis or faecal soiling is the persistent, voluntary or involuntary passing of normal or near-normal faeces in inappropriate places.

The accepted age for expected control of the bowels varies. In Western studies, it is between two and four years of age. Up to 1 per cent of older children occasionally soil after this age. It is a more common problem with boys than girls and may be associated with enuresis.

Clinical features

Punishment has probably already been tried and failed by the time the child is brought to the health services. There may be disturbed family relationships secondary to the encopresis and problems of soiled clothing and bed linen. The soiler may be rejected at school and suffer educational retardation.

Hersov[6] suggests the following classification:

- Control achieved but inappropriate defaecation with normal stool. This may follow acute stress (e.g. attending school, separation from parents) or chronic psychosocial stress (e.g. family instability, punitive care). In the West, the child with this form of soiling may deny its existence. The encopresis may be an expression of aggression towards the carers.

- Failure to learn and the bowels are opened at random. This may be associated with low intelligence, physical disability, lack of opportunity to learn and family problems. There may be accompanying enuresis. There may be other evidence of parental neglect in the child's clothing and personal cleanliness. The child may never have gained control due to poor training or stress occurring at 'the critical period' of learning. The stool is normal.

- Abnormal stool associated with gastro-intestinal illness, stress diarrhoea or severe constipation when liquid faeces pass the impacted faeces and leak from the anus. Constipation may be associated with a fissure *in ano*, which helps to perpetuate the problem.

* Fear of the toilet, for example because of fear of the dark, insects, snakes or wild animals associated with an outside toilet.

Management

Physical causes need to be excluded, though these, e.g. Hirschprung's disease are uncommon. Severe constipation may need the temporary use of suppositories and appropriate dietary and training measures. There may be other developmental or family problems requiring explanation and help.

The carer needs guidance in preparing a simple record of toileting. Preparation of this is a test of the motivation of the child and carers to cooperate. 'Star charts' like those used in enuresis are useful. Successful toilet attendance is marked by a star or a tick and publicly exhibited. Other rewards may be added.

Prognosis is usually good with the above measures but this may be largely due to the passage of time. However, it is poor where there are multiple problems and the child is older.

Hyperkinesis

Purposeless and impulsive overactivity often associated with short attention span and distractability is known as hyperkinesis.

Aetiology

Aetiology is still not clear and there is some controversy as to whether hyperkinesis is a distinct entity or an extreme of a normal variation. It may be associated with brain damage but, generally, there are important psychosocial factors.

Clinical features

This problem is commonly present before the age of three years. At this age, there is a poor attention span and a child does not seem to listen or concentrate. There is an inability to finish tasks and the child is easily distracted from these. Impulsiveness and hyperactivity result in behaviour such as excessive running about, restlessness and difficulty in staying seated. There may also be behavioural problems such as bullying, a poor response to discipline, and outbursts of bad temper over trivial matters. Impulsive behaviour is a major problem, especially if associated with aggression and destructiveness as in conduct disorders. In the clinic the child may be fidgety and restless, there may be overactivity without impaired attention, or there may be inattention with little overactivity. In adolescence, there may be depression and poor self-esteem (see p. 407).

The tolerance and ability of carers to cope with difficult behaviour will obviously influence whether the child is brought for health care. The child's behaviour may disturb the family and result in problems in relationships in the family and elsewhere. Some children are hyperactive only in certain situations and it is important to enquire whether the problems are worse in any particular situation, for example, at school. Teachers and parents may disagree about the severity.

At school, restlessness and poor attention interfere with a child's ability to learn as well as the teaching of others. A child can be more of a problem in class when expected to sit for long periods in formal work. Learning difficulties are common and usually persist as the child grows older, even when the extreme restlessness is less. Learning problems may result from impulsiveness, neurological impairment or overactivity interfering with attention.[7]

Management

Psychosocial treatments are very important for these children although drugs can also be used where the hyperkinesis is severe and causing serious problems. Phenobarbitone should be avoided as it may accentuate the symptom.

Family management is important in the short term but even more so in the long term, as the benefits of drug effects wear off or the drugs are withdrawn. It is important to understand how the family have been affected and how they see the problem. It may be necessary to help them to see the child as having a genuine problem rather than being badly behaved. Where the family is unable to cooperate, problems may persist. Hyperkinesis may aggravate other family problems.

Health care staff need to be trained in methods of teaching parents how to cope with hyperkinesis. This training is most effective when parents are well motivated to cooperate, particularly in rewarding desirable behaviour and in avoiding those actions which are known to provoke overactive behaviour.[8]

At school such children perform best in small groups, preferably avoiding long periods sitting at a desk. Individual teaching may be necessary for the persisting learning disabilities. The teacher will be able to report on the effects of drugs if these are used.

Stimulant drugs reduce overactivity and impulsiveness and can help inattention. There may be some improvement of antisocial behaviour. Learning difficulties, however, are likely to continue.

Methylphenidate (0.25–1 mg/kg per day in divided doses) or dexamphetamine in half this dose is useful; pemoline (0.5–2 mg/kg per day) is an alternative. This should be given at the beginning of the day to avoid interference with sleep. If there are problems of the drug wearing off towards the end of the day, a major tranquillizer such as haloperidol may be added at that time.

Problems arising from the stimulant drugs include loss of sleep and appetite, headache and abdominal pain. There is a risk of interference with growth and so weight should be regularly recorded. Growth problems may be overcome by ensuring that there are breaks in drug treatment. Although short-term benefit follows the use of stimulants there is no clear evidence of long-term benefit.

In some countries, prescription of stimulant drugs may be restricted. In these instances, major tranquillizers will have to be used if drugs are needed. Major tranquillizers such as chlorpromazine and haloperidol may be used when stimulants fail. Although these reduce overactivity, the inattention and learning problems do not appear to be affected.

Chlorpromazine may be given as 15–30 mg per day in divided doses for children less than five years old; and for older children 25–100 mg per day in divided doses. Haloperidol dosage is 0.025–0.05 mg/kg per day.

Unfortunately major tranquillizers are associated with the short-term side-effects of tremor, restlessness, involuntary protrusion of the tongue and sometimes acute dystonia and oculogyric crises. There may be a fall in blood pressure and sensitivity to light. A grave risk is long-term and irreversible tardive dyskinesia – widespread involuntary movement of face and body. It is therefore important to plan steady withdrawal of the drugs once symptoms are in satisfactory control.

Prognosis

It should be possible to provide some immediate lessening of acute problems with drugs but long-term benefits will depend more on psychosocial treatments. Problem behaviour persists when the child has low intelligence and learning problems.

Follow-up studies in the West have shown that by adolescence, only half of the children have persisting problems such as restlessness, difficulties in relationships and impulsiveness. In adult life they show some features of restlessness and impulsiveness. A few have lasting antisocial problems.

Isolated speech delay

Sometimes a child may have a significant degree of speech delay which affects both understanding of and ability to speak language, although other abilities such as hearing and motor development are normal and severe mental handicap, autism and child abuse are absent. Causes of this type of speech delay include hereditary factors (there is often a family history) or environmental factors such as neglect or gross understimulation of language development.[9] This condition is quite distinct from elective mutism where the child has a normal ability to speak but remains silent in specific situations due to psychological factors. Elective mutism is a relatively rare condition and may be associated with a history of marked shyness.

Emotional disorders

Anxiety states

Anxiety states are emotional disturbances where anxiety and fearfulness are the main features and are severe, persisting and disabling.

'Nervousness' was one of the five most common complaints in primary health clinics in Colombia, North India, Sudan and the Philippines in Giel's study.[3] Normal anxiety occurs in response to uncertainty or danger. This fear is a normal reaction to stress and is often a useful preparation to taking appropriate action – 'fight or flight'. The physical aspects of fear may be mistaken for a physical illness. A brief, appropriate explanation of physical aspects of emotion can be followed by firm reassurance of the absence of illness.

Clinical features

The most common symptoms of an anxiety state in the developing world are an increase in the physical features of emotion, for example palpitations, breathlessness, tremor, fatigue, frequent micturition, loose stools, pruritus. The child may be timid, cling to the carer and be constantly nervous, especially in unfamiliar situations. This may be aggravated by the child's imagination and limited understanding. The child is unlikely to complain of anxiety. The risk is that the child, family and staff will think that this is a physical illness which may then be expensively investigated.

The common forms of presentations of anxiety are stress reactions, phobic anxiety, panic attacks, school anxiety and the anxiety-prone child. School refusal and its management are described later. All forms of anxiety are eased or aggravated by the attitude and behaviour of carers.

A stress reaction occurs when the child reacts excessively to a single or a number of adverse experiences. This will occur in the normal child if the stress is severe and in the anxiety-prone child with only moderate stress. In Western studies, problems within the home, such as parental discord and poor living conditions, appear to affect a child's mental health more than stresses outside the home.[5]

Common sources of stress in the developing world include the following:

- Physical – for example organic illness, real or imaginary, in themselves or those caring for them, threats or actual violence at home or school or in the community.
- Psychosocial – for example parental disharmony, separation from one or both parents, sibling rivalry, family friction or breakdown, excessive punishment, school anxieties, fears of examinations or failing at school, unwanted pregnancy.
- Spiritual threats – for example fears of bewitchment, the breaking of taboos or offending ancestors.

Children with stress reactions tend to be excessively fearful and timid, they may show immature and 'clinging' behaviour, be frightened by noises and people and may be constantly thinking of the original stress. Sleep may be disturbed with nightmares about the stressful event. They may develop a tendency to over-react to later minor stresses. They may temporarily avoid mixing with other children. Children in disturbed families tend to show more severe reactions. Usually a child responds to stress in the same way as his parents. Management includes understanding the child's view of what has happened and sensitively responding to upset feelings. Bereavement and physical injury are associated with the greatest degree of persistent anxiety. On the whole, children are remarkably resilient and stress reactions are usually brief.

Phobic anxiety is when the child is unreasonably fearful of an object or place. The anxiety is worse when approaching the feared object or situation. There may be fear of animals, insects, being outside alone (agoraphobia), being in enclosed spaces (claustrophobia). A common cause is when the child fears return to a place associated with a frightening experience. Refusal to go to such places, for example the village well or school, is 'avoidance behaviour' and this can seriously restrict a child's life.

Panic attacks are episodes of severe anxiety, perhaps with fears of organic illness or sudden death. There may be sweating, faintness, hyperventilation with associated paraesthesia. Differential diagnosis includes epilepsy and hypoglycaemia.

The anxiety-prone child must be recognized, as the child and carers probably hope for a magical medical solution to the child's life-long tendency to become anxious. The management of these attitudes is crucial. There is a history of repeated anxiety states – often provoked by everyday stresses. The child always finds new situations and tasks frightening and may lead a very restricted life. The child clings to carers and worries excessively about the past, present and future. The origin is the interaction of vulnerability due to genetic factors and temperament and often the experience of chronic environmental stress perhaps aggravated by anxious and overprotective carers.

Management

Community and traditional beliefs are most important. Individuals and communities in the developing world are often intensely aware and concerned about the influence of the religious and spiritual aspects of life in producing symptoms. Child and carer may be more concerned about the underlying origin and meaning of the problems, than learning the Western name for a disease. The scientific view of the cause and pathology may not be accepted by the patient or family. Blaming another person or a spirit is common and traditional healers are frequently consulted, particularly for long-standing symptoms. Their contribution may or may not be therapeutic but their attitudes and treatment are always important to children and carers.

The ability of health carers to provide an explanation in a way which is understandable and acceptable is fundamental to all treatment. It is very difficult to modify longstanding beliefs in an individual or community who expect drug treatment.[10] The carer, and child if able, must be given an opportunity to ask questions.

The first step is to explain that there is no physical illness yet it is still a very real problem. Next there needs to be an explanation of how stress may affect the child in four ways: autonomic nervous system (producing the physical symptoms, for example palpitations), behaviour, feelings, and thinking. Finally, reassurance must be given that the problem will usually settle in time but that this will be sooner if the stress can be identified and removed or lessened. Throughout management there will be a need to remind carers that the child is not imagining the symptoms or making them up for some reason.

In planning reduction of stress the carer and child take a much more active part. They are asked what can be done to reduce the identified stresses. They are encouraged to consider a series of possible actions together with the likely outcomes. Then *they* must decide what to do, possibly after consultation with other family members. A review should be planned to assess success of the action taken and the effects on the anxiety. Explanation and family discussion may be all that is required. At the other extreme, if the child is seriously disturbed by insoluble or grave family problems it may be necessary to establish the child with a member of the extended family.

Chronic anxiety and tension may be helped by teaching a simple method of muscle relaxation in which all muscle groups are tensed and then relaxed.[11] This can be combined with: deliberately breathing out when relaxing; closing the eyes and visualizing a happy or peaceful memory; quietly saying 'calm' or 'peace' or a brief prayer.

Anxiety management is a plan prepared in advance to deal with future episodes of anxiety. It may be practised by child and carer with the health care staff. Each may take turns in pretending to be the child dealing with a situation (role play). At the same time the child may recall past successes and quietly acknowledge future success.

A past stressful experience can be discussed, emphasizing actions which were successful and planning future ways of coping with similar problems. Group story-telling has been used in this way where a community has suffered a natural or man-made disaster.

For phobic anxiety, anxiety management is combined with exposure to the feared object. Avoidance of the feared situation tends to perpetuate the anxiety. Treatment can be by a sudden or gradual approach:

- Implosion (flooding). In the company of the carer, the child is quickly and totally exposed to the feared object or situation and forced to remain there until the anxiety subsides. This is an alarming experience but is effective. It requires full understanding and cooperation by child and carer.
- Desensitization. Whilst accompanied, the child slowly approaches the feared object or situation by small steps. Anxiety management and reassurance

aim to keep the anxiety as low as possible – delaying progress if anxiety begins to rise. Treatment may take many sessions.

Health care workers should discuss community support with carers in planning the management of all mental health problems. This will include the extended family, local chiefs and elders, statutory and voluntary community workers.

Drugs are of limited use but can help the short-term control of severe anxiety and agitation. The drugs should be used to enable the child to plan how to cope with initial stress and control the secondary anxiety.

Failure to respond may occur when the original stress or stresses have not been correctly identified or the child and carers or the rest of the family do not understand or believe the offered explanations. The child may benefit from being considered ill and so avoid difficult tasks. For example, the child may avoid long, lonely days herding cattle and instead has easy tasks at home in the enjoyable company of mother.

The anxiety-prone child cannot be expected to become free of anxiety but both child and family need to understand and adjust to the child's limitations. The child will always tend to be more anxious than others but must face, with support, the inevitable stages towards a normal life and develop a philosophy of living a normal life despite the tendency to anxiety. This lessens the risk of the child leading a severely limited life.

School phobia

Reluctance to attend school associated with anxiety and often depression.

Clinical features

This problem may be less common in the developing world. Although the anxiety is related to attendance at school, the child may be fearful of leaving home, with physical symptoms such as loss of appetite, vomiting, nausea, diarrhoea, frequency of micturition, abdominal or limb pains. Discussion may reveal unhappy experiences at school or with peers, or problems during journeys to and from school. The child may be obviously anxious or miserable. There may be clinical depression requiring treatment. The child may feel a failure by letting down a family who have made heavy financial sacrifices and expect the child to support them in the future. The child may have fears of loss of a close family member. There may be other problems in the family or at school.

Children in developing countries often have the

stress of long journeys to school, perhaps walking alone through potentially hostile areas, in town or country. They may be established away from home at an early age with members of the extended family in order to attend school.

Differential diagnosis Exclude truancy, in which the child is not anxious but goes off to enjoyable or anti-social activities, in contrast to the school refuser who tends to cling to the carer with otherwise good conduct. In older schoolchildren there is also the well-recognized anxious student with 'brain fag syndrome' who complains of difficulties in concentrating, study, seeing the blackboard and keeping awake in lessons. This may be helped by counselling of study problems and relaxation[8] and anxiety management. The syndrome is distressing and may end in student failure.

Older children with school refusal may also have behaviour changes such as avoiding people, loss of interest in usual activities, misery and feelings of worthlessness. The possibility of depression must then be considered.

Management

Active involvement of the carer is essential. This will include discussion with teachers and at first taking the child to and from school. The most effective treatment is firmly taking the child to school and making the child stay there. If this repeatedly fails, then a plan to overcome each of the problems at school and home is made. Family and teachers are involved and a carefully planned return to school is arranged. Residential school may be considered.

Minor tranquillizers have a small place in treatment, for example on the night before return to school. Antidepressants are indicated if there is persistent misery, impaired sleep and appetite, and loss of interest in former activities.

Prognosis

In the West, two-thirds are successfully established back in school. Children who are older, and have personal and family problems do less well. Those failing may become depressed.

Hysteria

Hysteria can be a disorder of physical function (conversion symptom) with no underlying organic cause but related to some environmental stress. It may also present as dissociation – a disorder of mental function, again with no underlying 'organic' cause and related to stress – this is less common.

Whilst the mechanism of hysteria remains unclear, a simplified but practical approach to its understanding is that the child is communicating distress to others by a symptom or change in behaviour. This leads to a response from others which may then relieve the child from the stress. It is important for health staff and family to appreciate that the child is *not* pretending to have a symptom or being deliberately deceiving. The concept of the 'sick role' can also help health staff to understand what is happening. The community decides that the child is ill or disabled and allocates that child to the 'sick role'. This implies that it is not the child's fault, and that the child is entitled to treatment and excused from various duties provided he/she cooperates with treatment. In hysteria, the relief from responsibilities may mean that the child is taken away from the stress which provoked the hysteria. In this way, a particular symptom or behaviour is rewarded and therefore tends to persist.[12]

Clinical features

Although hysteria is uncommon in the West, it regularly presents to health clinics in the developing world. Hysteria formed 11 per cent of the 11–16-year-old group at a child psychiatry clinic in Sri Lanka. In the West, boys are more affected than girls and there is more commonly an underlying physical illness.[13]

Conversion symptoms are usually of sudden onset and include aphonia, paralysis, disturbance of gait and posture, deafness, blindness and 'pseudoseizures'. In dissociation, there is a temporary interference with the child's awareness of surroundings and self-knowledge. There are secondary effects on behaviour. The child may have loss of memory or wander around in a strange fashion. Physical examination and investigations reveal no obvious physical cause, though there is often concern that this is an unusual presentation of a serious or treatable condition. There may be anxiety that the child has epilepsy or encephalitis or has been poisoned.

Diagnosis

A number of clinical features can be helpful in diagnosis. Behaviour may be extremely strange with odd gait or unusual physical limitations such as the inability to raise one foot from the floor.[14] Patient or carers may emphasize the symptoms in an inappropriate way. There may have been previous similar episodes which recovered with no evidence of physical illness. Although a diagnosis of hysteria should never be made lightly, it is reasonable to consider hysteria as a part of the differential diagnosis when there is no obvious physical illness. Patient and carers should be asked about recent or long-term stress. The stress is usually immediately associated with the onset and may be an occurrence at home, in the community or at school, which seriously troubles the child. Conversion symptoms in the adult may be associated with lack of concern about the symptoms. This is not so in children who are usually distressed by both the symptom and the underlying stress.

A particular diagnostic problem is 'pseudo-epileptic seizures' which need to be differentiated from epilepsy. The history may reveal the absence of incontinence of urine, major injury or scarring (pointing to previous injury), for example of the tongue. Lishman suggests the following distinguishing features. The child's behaviour in the attack may draw the attention of observers to some problem, for example anxieties about a particular part of the body. During the attacks there may be a response to a painful stimulus or restraint. Pallor or cyanosis do not occur in the absence of breath-holding. There is no loss of pupillary or corneal reflexes and there are no extensor plantar responses.[15] The child may also be aware of surrounding events which took place during the attack. Finally, epilepsy is usually brief and stereotyped whereas pseudoseizures may be prolonged and are quite different from status epilepticus.

Another diagnostic problem area is where an undoubted organic illness is complicated by a hysterical prolongation of the disability. An example is persisting symptoms or limitations of activity because of fears that the underlying illness is still present or because there are more benefits for the child in continuing to be disabled than in being well again. The child may not be aware of this despite obvious benefit from the situation. It is therefore important that the child is not considered to be deliberately behaving badly and is not punished.

Differential diagnosis

This includes epilepsy, postepileptic states, encephalitis, hypoglycaemia, various poisonings (alcohol, traditional and Western medicines). Rivinus *et al.* reported a series of uncommon neurological conditions presenting as psychiatric disorders.[13] Clinical features pointing to the diagnosis were abrupt change in school performance, loss of vision or definite abnormality of posture. Difficulties occur when a definite physical condition accompanies hysteria, for example epilepsy or hysteria complicating the recovery from encephalitis.

Management

The first stage is for health staff to convince themselves that there is no underlying physical illness. Common and potentially life-threatening illnesses need to be excluded. It may be difficult to know when to stop further investigations. Brief admission to hospital is often very helpful, allowing observation of activities such as eating, dressing and orientation, which may be inconsistent with the findings during examination by the doctor.[15]

The health staff need to help the carers to understand and accept that, although there is no underlying physical illness, it is still a genuine problem and arises from stress. The child is not telling lies and should not be blamed for the symptom or change in behaviour. The family will need an opportunity to understand and discuss the situation. They are likely to have had a different view of the illness and treatment required and need further discussion and explanation. Most families, however, will appreciate that stress can affect a child. Identifying the recent stress which the child finds overwhelming is important.

In management the aim is to give the child an opportunity to recover with dignity rather than to 'catch him out'. The basic principle is to ignore undesirable symptoms of abnormal behaviour and reward (reinforce) any evidence of improvement. The reward can be material (for example fruit, food) or social (praise, encouragement) and should immediately follow the improvement. This can be part of a programme of increased physical activities – bicycling, playing games, depending upon facilities available to health staff and the family.[12]

A family therapy approach to hysteria has been recommended but techniques described by Barker in *Basic Family Therapy*[16] will need to be modified and developed for local use.

Follow-up by out-patient review will help to reassure health staff and others of the continuing absence of organic illness. It will also enable health staff to encourage the patient and carers to persist with effective rewards.

Prognosis

Conversion symptoms and dissociation usually settle rapidly with out-patient explanation and effective management of the stress. Occasionally a brief admission to hospital is helpful. Persisting symptoms will require more careful rewarding of any appropriate improvement and planning the support of carers by village health workers or others who understand this principle of management.

Epidemic hysteria

Clinical features

Epidemic hysteria occurs in close-knit groups of children, usually girls, such as a school or village. There is an outbreak of giggling, laughing or dancing, over-breathing, restlessness, headache, faints, muscle twitching, vomiting or pruritus. The person first affected may have some particular physical or emotional problems and is usually older or a leader or a specially feared girl. The whole community becomes anxious with fears of poisoning by contamination of food or water, witchcraft or spiritual intervention. Reports in the media may provoke more anxiety. Traditional healers are commonly consulted and their interpretations may aggravate the situation. Usually the outbreak quickly settles with no persisting problems. Typical epidemics have been described in Malaysia,[17] Zambia[18], England[19] and the United States[20] illustrating clinical and social features.

Management

Epidemic infections and poisonings must be excluded. Most affected children show no physical or emotional problems but there may be community problems such as discipline or examination or cultural stresses. There should be a clear explanation to all involved that there is no epidemic or poisoning and they should return as soon as possible to normal activities. The individuals at the centre of the epidemic may need particular help with their problems.

Should the epidemic continue despite the above measures, then the school may need to be briefly closed. This is usually effective though there may be an occasional recurrence on re-opening the school. This may indicate a need for more intensive help for those at the centre of the outbreak.

Depression

Depressive illness can be diagnosed when depression is severe, persistent and disabling.[21, 22] To distinguish depressive illness from 'normal' sadness and misery: 'There must be not only at least two weeks of misery and loss of enjoyment but also four out of the following features – loss of appetite, impaired sleep, agitation or withdrawal, loss of interest, loss of energy, self reproach or guilt, loss of concentration, recurring thoughts of death or suicide'.[23]

Clinical features

Depressive moods or feelings are common in children, usually secondary to other problems, in the environment, in the family or the community. Psychological factors, such as losses, or physical factors, such as viral infections, may produce depression when the child is vulnerable. Depression may accompany conduct and emotional disorders or hyperkinesis. It can, however, be the main presenting symptom in older children.

Most depressed children will not complain of depression, but Western studies have found that most parents recognize when their children are depressed. Health staff can seek a history of poor sleep and loss of appetite, weight and concentration, together with the child looking miserable. Young children may present by weeping or angry protest followed by withdrawal, inactivity and clinging to the carer. Even the older child may have difficulty in describing a change in feelings and complain only of boredom and present with difficult behaviour. The older child develops an idea of value as a person (self-esteem). Loss of this is associated with a feeling of worthlessness and uselessness and possibly self-harm. All of these can aggravate the depression.

Bereavement is naturally followed by sadness and misery. Long-lasting problems, however, only occur if there is no adequate person to replace the one lost or if there are additional adverse experiences. Prompt acceptance by a member of the extended family can help to protect a child against harmful emotional effects even when the mother dies. Without this protection the child may be vulnerable to depression in adult life.

Adolescent depression is more common and can present as mood swings and angry rebellion. With increasing age, depression resembles that in adults. Adolescents occasionally present severe depression and retardation with a family history of manic depressive illness. They often respond to the same antidepressants as their parents.

Management

Child and carer need to understand how stresses have affected the child physically and in behaviour, feelings and thinking. A particular difficulty is when the child feels hopeless and is withdrawn and inactive. The child may believe that there is no solution to the problem. The child's past achievements and abilities are emphasized and carers are encouraged to praise any success or activity, however small. The aim is to enhance self-esteem.

Planned reduction of stress will involve discussion with carer and child. A slow return to normal activities is planned. Punishment will not help.

Antidepressants have yet to be proved to be effective in depressed children. They may be indicated for severe illness, when there are most of the features listed in the definition above, together with a family history of depressive illness. Imipramine tablets may be given in slowly increasing amounts of 25 to 125 mg per day in divided doses, depending upon the weight of the child. Serious cardiac side-effects may occur and preferably ECG monitoring should be used. A further difficulty is ensuring adequate therapeutic serum levels.

Suicide and attempted suicide

Fortunately suicide is uncommon before the age of 12. The risk of suicide, however, should be considered in all who are depressed as well as those who threaten or have mentioned suicide. Direct questioning about suicidal thoughts and plans does not increase the danger of suicide. The risk is higher in the older child, the severely depressed, those who feel hopeless and can find no solution to severe problems. There is increased risk in those with detailed plans of self-harm, who have attempted suicide in the past or have a family history of suicide.

Those young persons who have already deliberately harmed themselves may be able to give a clear reason or reasons for this. These include a response to severe depression, deliberately aiming to die, trying to change a difficult situation in the family or community, risk-taking ('I didn't care what happened to me') or an impulsive angry outburst against themselves or others. A 'cry for help' is implied when the attempted suicide is a communication to the family and others that the young person cannot cope with a situation and needs their help. It is essential that these young people are closely supervised by relatives 24 hours a day until the underlying problem has improved.

In the developing world, death is often by hanging and drowning. Half of the young persons in the West who commit suicide have threatened to do so in the previous 24 hours and some faced the possibility of punishment for problem behaviour at school or in the community.

Prognosis

Most depressions will recover spontaneously or with the above management techniques. Very few are asso-ciated with problems persisting into adult life. However, severe prolonged depression with persistent low self-esteem has a poor prognosis. Persistent severe depression with suicidal plans will need referral for specialist care because of the risk of suicide.

Obsessional disorders

An obsession is an unwanted thought which the child realizes is inappropriate and may try to resist. Examples are counting, repeated words, impulses to particular actions. Obsessions are uncommon in childhood.

These persistent thoughts may be accompanied by rituals – that is behaviour which helps to relieve the child's anxiety, for example repeated touching, counting, hand-washing or checking. If these activities are prevented the child may become very anxious. The child may irritate carers by trying to involve them in the rituals. Management is by preventing the child performing such activities, care of anxiety and firm reassurance of child and carer.

Conduct or behaviour disorders

Persistent and serious behaviour (often aggressive or destructive) which is not acceptable in a community or seriously interferes with the lives of others is considered here.

Behaviour arises from the interaction of a child's temperament, abilities and personal problems with the environment in the family, school or community. Communities vary in the strictness of their expectation of standards of behaviour for children. The use of discipline to control behaviour varies from physical punishments to verbal correction or withdrawal of privileges. Some behaviour acceptable to parents and other children may be unacceptable to the rest of the community. Studies in the West have shown that praise, encouragement and rewards are more effective than punishment in the elimination of undesirable behaviour in the home and school.

Conduct disorders are brought to the health services only when the usual controls and punishments have failed. The range of conduct disorders seen by health staff reflect the views and attitudes of the carers involved and the willingness of medical services to help. They do not necessarily reflect the form and frequency of conduct disorders in the community.

Clinical features

Conduct disorders include aggressive behaviour such as disobedience, tantrums, fighting and destructiveness, running away from home, lying, stealing and truancy. There may be particular local problems such as alcohol abuse, inhaling petrol, vagrancy with children living on the streets and emotionally disturbed survivors of disasters, e.g. civil war. Common complaints by carers about less serious problems are that the child is aggressive, disrespectful and disobeys elders or refuses to fulfil allocated duties. Conduct disorders are more common in boys than in girls.

Age has an important influence on presentation. Complaints about younger children are of overactivity, restlessness, perhaps associated with developmental delays. Older children may lie, steal or wander away from home and these are aggravated by school failure, especially delays in reading. Adolescents may be aggressive or antisocial when emotionally disturbed, for example following bereavement.

Stealing may arise in a number of circumstances. If it is within the home it may arise from an emotional or relationship problem. 'Comfort stealing' occurs when a child feels unwanted. Stealing outside the home may be impulsive or a group activity in a casual manner. There may be the influence of friends or a 'delinquent' neighbourhood in addition to a deprived family and inconsistent discipline. Lying should be assessed by enquiring if the child lies to everyone or only in particular circumstances or with certain individuals. Truancy is when the child is deliberately absent from school to undertake some other activity. This is in contrast with school refusal, when it is anxiety which keeps the child away.

Aggression may arise with hyperkinesis or brain damage, or from a child's experience of chronic frustration. Less commonly, a child may learn that this is the way to succeed or is copying an admired member of the family.

Management

Management is based on the behavioural principles of ignoring undesirable behaviour and promptly rewarding the desirable. There should be emphasis on the positive qualities and abilities of the child which are often overlooked when carers are preoccupied with the conduct disorder. It is sometimes necessary to help carers to notice positive qualities in their children.

Particular underlying problems should be sought, such as physical, social and educational factors and any events which provoke attacks of difficult behaviour. This may involve taking the child away from examples of unsatisfactory behaviour and introducing the child to more appropriate examples.

The attitude, cooperation and activities of carers is crucial. The whole family and community elders may need to be involved, particularly where there are other problems in the family or the behaviour has grave effects. If family problems are overwhelming or unlikely to be helped, then it may be necessary to establish the child on a short- or long-term basis with a part of the extended family which can provide greater consistency and warm concern.

The carers need to learn new skills in child management. This may be achieved by verbal advice together with written handouts and teaching sessions, providing practice and rehearsal of difficult situations. A parent may be used to demonstrate skills to a group of others. The aim is to encourage parents to use fewer punishments and more rewards.[8, 24] Carers may raise the objection that management of behavioural principles by rewards and the ignoring of difficult behaviour does not deal with the underlying problems. This is true but in practice such problems may be multiple, difficult to identify and hard to change.

Parents should be warned that, initially, behaviour may deteriorate. Particular episodes of undesirable behaviour such as temper tantrums, which do not respond to ignoring, may be managed by 'time-out training'. This involves taking the child away from the setting in which the tantrum is persisting. The principle is to place the child in some quiet setting where behaviour will not be rewarded in any way. The child should be returned in a few minutes – when there is some satisfactory behaviour. If the child is doing something dangerous for himself or others then he should be firmly physically controlled and told that this behaviour is unacceptable. It is important that as far as possible the child understands the reason for any reward or 'time-out management'. It may be helpful to ask the child to repeat what is expected of him so that there is no doubt of his understanding or lack of it.

Rewards may take the form of food or drink or be social rewards such as praise or a hug or some special activity. 'Star charts', as in enuresis, may be used for identifying periods of the day when there is desirable or undesirable behaviour. Lines are drawn on a sheet of paper to split the day into portions and the child is allocated a tick or star for satisfactory behaviour during that particular portion of the day. This requires persistence by carers and family agreement.

The trainers of carers need not be sophisticated or highly educated individuals. They should be sensitive to the child's needs, well-motivated and have task-orientated training. They can be selected on the same principles as trainers for the mentally handicapped.[25] Teachers can actively influence conduct disorders by group counselling and behavioural treatments.[26]

Prognosis

Management of conduct disorders, particularly aggression, takes time but is worthwhile, as otherwise aggression may persist into later childhood and possibly even into adulthood. There is a risk that the next generation may repeat the same pattern of disturbed behaviour. Carers have been proved to be effective where they are well-motivated and cooperative and are providing care for intact families. If there are multiple family or personal problems or the carers are unable or unwilling to change their management of the child, then the outlook is poor. Nevertheless most children achieve acceptable behaviour.

Persistent difficult behaviour, especially in the family with multiple problems, may need help from the extended family, primary care staff, community elders and teachers.

Prevention

Prevention of conduct disorders is presented in detail as an example of a feasible approach in clinic and community. Acceptable behaviour in the family, school and community is associated with a stable and accepting family background with consistency in the carers. The consistency of discipline is much more important than whether it is strict or relaxed. Varying discipline is particularly likely to occur where a number of family figures share the responsibilities of supervising the child's behaviour. The child needs to understand clearly what is desirable behaviour, what will not be tolerated by others and what will happen if the child does not conform. Any punishment which is promised should be carried out and take place as soon as possible after the undesirable behaviour. There should not be threats which are not carried out. Family rules should be as few as possible and be made clear to the child.

Punishment is seen by many communities as an important part of a child's upbringing and 'correction'. However, withdrawal of privileges, for example from a joint activity with the family, combined with an immediate reward of desirable behaviour is more effective. Severe physical punishments may provoke an angry reaction and may teach a child to behave in this way also. A child needs to understand the reason for punishment. It should also be made clear during punishment that this is not because the carer dislikes or rejects the child or that the child is not wanted in the family. Teaching present and future parents and community leaders these principles can prevent many conduct disorders.

Involvement of schools is important. Teachers should provide particular attention to those with reading retardation, as these children are prone to conduct disorders. This is an example of secondary prevention.

Teachers can reduce conduct disorders by providing good models of behaviour themselves, the use of rewards and praise rather than punishment, allowing children to develop responsibility by taking part in the running of the school and by giving a reasonable balance of attention to both the able and less able children.

Infantile autism

Infantile autism is a severe and uncommon disorder of development starting in early childhood and affecting speech, relationships and behaviour. The child may avoid eye contact, be unresponsive to others, flap his hands up and down, or insist that belongings or food are not changed in any way. There may be associated epilepsy.

Differentiation from severe mental handicap can be difficult as unusual and repetitive behaviour can occur in both conditions. Social relationships are much more normal in severe mental handicap than in autism – the child will look at others and be cooperative in simple activities and play. Severe mental handicap is very much more common. Deafness, delays in language development, encephalitis, lead poisoning and rare progressive neurological conditions need to be considered. In elective mutism and parental rejection or abuse, the child's speech and behaviour is normal at times.

Unfortunately treatment is disappointing. The most effective approach is using special educational techniques. Behavioural methods used with severe mental handicap, and persistent attempts at social interaction, can be tried. A course of chlorpromazine may reduce overactivity.

Other problems

Reactions to chronic illness and disability and death

The attitude of parents is crucial. They may take up extremes of attitudes such as overprotection or rejection and neglect. This will affect cooperation with treatment. Disappointment with progress in medical care may lead to poor compliance with treatments which could otherwise be effective. Disappointed carers turn to other forms of treatments, other hospitals, general practitioners and traditional healers. Overprotection may limit the activities of the child much more than the original illness. Long periods of admission to hospital may further isolate and limit the child's life.

The child must understand as much as possible of the nature and likely outcome of the illness. This must be stated in a way which is understandable and hopeful but realistic. There will need to be particular emphasis on the child's understanding of the necessity of painful procedures or admission to hospital or separations from the family.

Time spent in initial explanation to both the carers and the child is amply repaid by improved compliance and less emotional disturbance in the child. This is of particular importance where the illness interferes considerably with the child's activities, social contacts and also where cooperation of the child is important, for example, in taking regular medication or self-injecting with insulin.

In regular out-patient reviews of chronic illness, not only should the physical symptoms and progress be considered but also the effect this has upon the life of the child and the rest of the family. If there are serious effects on both, then it may be necessary to establish the child with a member of the extended family who can devote more time to the child's care, particularly when the mother has several other young children.

The impact on the child of repeated episodes of hospitalization should always be remembered. The child is separated from home, family and normal life-style. In addition the child has to cope with the experience of hospitalization and treatment. It has been found that factors, such as age of the child, ability to understand the need of hospitalization and treatment, clear and age-appropriate explanations of the purpose of admission, flexible arrangements for visiting by family or provision for close family members to be with the child, reduce harmful psychological sequelae and help the child to extend active cooperation to medical and nursing staff. This is an important aspect of paediatric care which requires a good deal of attention in developing countries.

Long-stay in-patient care will require particular attention to such issues as arranging teaching and grouping children together, making their surroundings more home-like and planning regular visits by parents if they are not resident with the child, as well as volunteers, carers and teachers. Parent self-help groups and voluntary organizations such as 'Friends of the Hospital' can be an important source of both ideas and practical support for the needs of these children.

The child will need help with planning for future problems such as separation from home, the physical limitations of the illness, absence from school, coping with future painful procedures and the threat of death. There can then be an opportunity to plan possible responses to these stresses.

Dying children often have a very practical and realistic awareness of what is happening which may be underestimated by those around them (see p. 125). Their distress may present as difficult behaviour or poor compliance. This in turn may be complicated by the parents' anticipatory grief and distress. Opportunities to discuss this should be arranged to include the likely outcome and complications during the terminal illness. Staff should encourage support for the child and relatives in traditional rituals of approaching death and bereavement. It may be necessary to accept the presence of many members of the extended family and volunteers from the community in the ward. Most children who die in hospital have had an acute illness. Parents often wish to take their dying child home. When hospital staff feel this to be undesirable, they must nevertheless remember the parents' natural grief and confusion and give sensitive support. Where little or nothing can be done, staff should always consider if the child might be more appropriately cared for in the community in this stage of illness. There will need to be a hospital policy allowing staff on duty to make urgent decisions about this.

This is also a stressful time for staff who may have feelings of failure and recurrence of their own unresolved grief experiences. A group discussion by staff on the effects of deaths of children can allow these feelings to be aired and assist staff in this difficult area of child-care. Staff feelings include sadness, guilt, loss and even anger. If there is no opportunity to express such feelings and gain support from others, there is the risk of staff having continued underlying emotional distress. The health worker may show this as 'hardness' and apparent indifference and insensitivity to the sufferings of relatives. Some health personnel may simply leave, as they find such work intolerable. Care of the dying is one of the most stressful areas in health care and insufficient emphasis is given in training and staff support. The whole area of the perception of health care and death in the Third World needs more study. In most traditional societies there is a community response to death which is psychologically very healthy. A hospital community can use this in support of the health staff involved in the terminal care of children.

Tics (habit spasm)

These are repeated brief involuntary movements of muscles or groups of muscles, serving no purpose and affecting the face, especially blinking of the eyes. Western studies show that up to 5 per cent of children have these. They should be distinguished from mannerisms in which there is much more complicated activity, for example, nail-biting. Tics are common in younger children and are made worse by stress at home or school. Usually there is no physical underlying illness though rarely these are associated with types of encephalitis e.g. subacute sclerosing panencephalitis (pp. 755–6).

Treatment is only indicated if the tics are severe and persistent. Many will settle with reassurance. Tics may be reduced if the child deliberately and frequently practises the tic.

Stuttering

Stuttering (stammering) is disorder of rhythm of speech in which the child knows what to say but is unable to say it because of involuntary repetition of sound, cessation of sound or blocking of sound. It may often occur when children begin to speak more quickly. In the West it has been reported in 1 per cent of schoolchildren, usually before the age of 10 years and more commonly in boys. There may be associated stress and anxiety and a history of developmental delays, including speech delay. The child may stutter in special circumstances, for example, when elders are present. There is not usually an associated psychiatric or emotional disorder but there may be secondary anxiety. In some Asian countries parents often bring three to four-year-old children for treatment for stuttering as they regard it as a serious problem.

The major aims are reduction of anxiety in the child and family and encouraging carers not constantly to correct or help the child with his speech, as this aggravates the problem. For very severe problems in school-age children, where speech therapy is not available, a course of haloperidol (0.5 mg three times a day) may be tried. Speech therapy, if available, is indicated for severe and persistent problems.

Prevention of mental health problems

There are three levels of prevention:

- Primary prevention, e.g. immunization preventing measles encephalitis; family planning to prevent child neglect; education of parents, teachers and community leaders in child development and children's needs.
- Secondary prevention, e.g. control of epilepsy to prevent burns.
- Tertiary prevention, e.g. appropriate training of the mentally handicapped.[9, 27, 28]

Training

Changing attitudes

Health staff often believe child mental health problems are uncommon, unimportant and difficult to treat. In fact many of them fulfil the Morley criteria for high priority in being common, disabling, disturbing and treatable.[29] Child mental health problems can be prevented and treated by trained health staff working in and with the community in primary care settings.

Principles of training

Training should be orientated to the needs and demands of the community. An idea of needs can be obtained by studying children with mental health problems presenting to health personnel or identified as disturbing the community by their behaviour or from key informants such as teachers. Demands and expectations can be obtained from the views of health staff, teachers, parents and community leaders, during interviews, informal discussions or local workshops. From this information it is possible to identify priorities for both clinical problems and service development.

Prevention and short-term mental health treatments aimed at a particular symptom or problem have been shown to be the most effective. Training should therefore be problem- or task-orientated. The content will need to be suitable for the level of health worker and the cultural background of the community. It may be necessary to train some staff in a very structured way in particular treatment options. The WHO manuals on child mental health[30] give an idea of basic treatments.

Health staff need supervised experience at an appropriate level of joint problem-solving with the child and carer. This will include identifying areas for treatment, considering possible solutions, choosing one, implementing it and reviewing the outcome. The trainee must be able to assess the understanding and acceptance of the goals of treatment as well as the motivation for cooperation in therapy by patient and carer. Role play is a useful technique. Trainees need practise in the use of special techniques according to their abilities; for example, 'star charts' would be appropriate for most workers whereas training in the use of the 'bell and pad' equipment would be more restricted.

Skills in listening, communication and counselling

are fundamental to all health care. Training should include supervised practise with feedback to the students by trainers, patients, families, and voluntary and community health workers to enable health staff to assess emotions, child behaviour and relationships.

Coordination of community resources is a special skill and requires a sensitive and informed approach, taking into account community attitudes and expectations. Carers are co-therapists who will need guidance in working with elders, community leaders, teachers, village aides, community workers and voluntary organizations. Training should include an understanding of the role and limitations of local traditional healers.

Field training as well as theoretical courses are essential to enable trainees and health staff to develop skills in mental health care in close contact with children and carers.

Visiting specialists and national experts in child and adult psychiatry, psychology, development and education should be used to provide teaching, planning, guidance and support. This approach is more productive than referring problem children to a distant specialist service.

Attitudes towards mental illness

There is little literature available on the subject of attitudes to mental illness in developing countries. For information one must rely on informal discussions, personal experiences and deductions from reading related subjects such as anthropology and sociology. Only recently has it been recognized in the West that mental disorders exist in tropical countries.[31] In 1970, G.A. German wrote: 'On the mile high East African plateau, mental illness flourishes unembarrassed by the relative absence of the trappings of Western civilisation'.[32]

Here the focus is on attitudes to childhood mental illness in East Africa. If psychiatry is neglected in developing countries, its subspecialities are often absent. Consequently, child psychiatric services are minimal or non-existent.[33, 34] The very notion of mental illness occurring in children is usually unappreciated.

Definitions

Western definitions of mental illness are rooted in the cause-and-effect concept of disease as perceived in Western scientific medicine. Traditionally, African societies define health and disease somewhat differently. Since mental illness often causes changes in personality and behaviour, its conceptualization evokes cultural and religious explanations in addition to the usually accepted notions of disease. Thus, mental illness is perceived as abnormal behaviour over which the patient has no control. It is therefore attributed to something going wrong or taking control of one's body or actions. Sometimes it is also seen as 'a disease' in which a particular organ of the body, e.g. the brain or the heart, will be blamed.[32] At other times the whole body, including the personality, is seen as having gone awry. In this case, a supernatural explanation related to religion, sorcery or witchcraft is evoked.[31, 32, 35] Such forces are also said to cause physical disease, e.g. 'ngulu' in Zambia or 'ddogo' in southern Uganda.[35]

Traditional classifications of mental disorders are descriptive and based on the understanding of the illness. In most African societies, there is no clear division between body and mind, spiritual and physical, heavenly and earthly, or health and disease. All are thought to coexist in a complex interplay and on a continuum. The following generalizations are therefore very broad. Diseases are divided into those which occur from birth, those whose causes are known, those with unknown causes, and those which are not usually recognized as mental illnesses.

Mental handicaps present from birth

This category includes genetic and acquired congenital illnesses. Among these are various forms of congenital mental retardation, e.g. chromosomal abnormalities as in Down's syndrome; inborn errors of metabolism or the various brain malformations, e.g. microcephaly. Also included are autism, unrecognized perinatal brain damage[34] and severe speech impairments.

Illnesses of this sort are usually labelled early in childhood as disorders associated with 'deficient brains'. In southern Uganda the term used for them is 'kasiru' meaning foolishness or low IQ.[32] No attempts are usually made to treat these children or teach them any social skills.[34] It is accepted that affected children will always be dependent on their family. As a consequence, such children are usually neglected and their hygiene is poor. Often they are treated as family outcasts,[34] they eat dirt, are infested with worms and die young. The few who reach adulthood exist as the village retardates. In urban areas, they will usually be sent to a regional psychiatric hospital where they live as permanent residents of a child psychiatric ward and later as institutionalized adults. There are few, if any, treatment services available to them.[34]

Mental illnesses with known causes

This category includes mental illnesses associated with fever, alcohol and drug abuse, and brain trauma. They account for many cases of acute brain syndromes, convulsions or epilepsy.[31]

Febrile illnesses Febrile illnesses such as malaria, typhoid fever, bacterial infections (e.g. pneumonia, cellulitis, tetanus, peritonitis) and viral infections (e.g. measles, chickenpox) are common in the tropics and subtropics. These illnesses may cause brain dysfunction either directly (e.g. meningitis and cerebral malaria) or indirectly (e.g. hypoxia in croup). Mental confusion seen in the acute phase of these conditions is usually attributed to the brain being 'mixed up'. It is generally recognized that the delirious state will clear when the associated illness improves. However, the onset of mental confusion is considered an ominous sign which may precede death. Quite frequently, traditional treatment methods will be attempted even when the child is in hospital. This may cause parents to 'steal' their child from hospital or to try traditional treatments which are considered 'stronger' than Western medicines.[32] If permanent brain damage occurs, with associated moderate to severe mental retardation, the affected child will be treated like one who has the congenital form of mental retardation.[34]

Alcohol and drug abuse Alcohol abuse is common in developing countries and on the increase.[31] It is especially prevalent in urban areas and often starts in adolescence. The abuse of chemicals has only recently been described.[37] For example, the use of hallucinogens such as cannabis (also known as marijuana, hemp or bhang), stimulants such as amphetamines (also part of the miraa chewing ritual) or cocaine, is rare in African children compared with those in Western countries. Traditional use of these substances by adults is quite common and often associated with certain forms of religious or job-related practices such as miraa chewing.[37] Dependency on these substances which interfere with a person's social functioning, causes such an individual to lose respect in society. During adolescence, substance abuse is usually associated with other delinquent behaviour and is more common in urban than in rural areas.[37] The abuse may not be considered a form of mental illness but the associated behavioural abnormalities will be attributed to a 'mixed up or spoilt brain'.[32] There are no traditional forms of treatment for chemical dependencies. In modern urban areas, there are hardly any institutions for the treatment of these disorders. Psychotherapeutic counselling is usually left to relatives in the extended family systems or is occasionally done in remand homes. In most cases, however, substance abusers are left alone and degenerate into village or city vagrants. Organic complications of these chemicals, especially alcohol, are on the increase.[31]

Head injury Trauma to the head caused by accidents may occasionally be followed by organic brain syndromes which in turn cause definite changes in the personality and behaviour of the affected individual.[31] Most often the cause of the trauma will be blamed for the personality change. In childhood, however, the affected child will usually be treated like the child with a severe form of mental retardation or epilepsy. Birth trauma is common in the tropics but may not be recognized as a source of mental handicap.[31, 34]

Mental illnesses with no known causes

This group of disorders comprises the classical psychiatric syndromes, including the psychoses (e.g. schizophrenia, affective disorders), epilepsy (usually grand mal) and conversion disorders including mass hysteria. Childhood psychosis is rare. However, the rate of psychosis in adolescence in Africa is similar to the rate in the Western world.[31]

The attitude to psychosis in childhood and adolescence is similar. If the psychosis is associated with violence it is generally referred to as 'true madness'.[32] Such illnesses are said to be associated with possessing exceptional physical strength, violent rages and with other forms of unpredictable behaviour.[32] Their cause is attributed to sorcery, unhappy spirits, ghost possession or witchcraft.[31, 32, 35] Sometimes certain insects or lizards are thought to reside in the brain of the affected individual.[32, 35] Grand mal epilepsy is seen as a violent and horrifying illness and is believed to be caused by similar supernatural forces. In many societies, epilepsy is considered infectious by the froth or urine produced during the convulsion.[32] Febrile convulsions resulting in death or severe cerebral damage were called 'ennyonyi' in Buganda, meaning 'bird'. They were regarded as the result of a bird, representing an evil spirit, casting its shadow on the child whilst flying over it and causing convulsions and death or prolonged brain damage.

Psychosis and epilepsy are greatly feared and cause much distress to families. Gross conversion disorders such as aphonia, paralyses or other 'wild' behaviour disorders are also feared and thought to be caused by supernatural forces. Epidemic mental illnesses are not uncommon in the tropics. In 1979, girls in a Ugandan secondary school were all affected by a 'duck-like gait' following a rampage by soldiers. Such epidemics have also been reported elsewhere, especially in schools.[31, 38] They are associated with severe mass anxiety. Traditional treatment usually involves ritual communal worship, sacrifices or wearing protective amulets, including crosses.

Often, mental illnesses without known causes are regarded as specific to the culture of a particular people and are not believed to be treatable by Western medicine.[31, 32] In Africa, these are referred to as 'African diseases', and are usually regarded as 'very strong' and treatment is generally sought from traditional healers.[32, 35] There is no specific treatment for each particular disease. Treatments used include exorcism, cupping of the head,[32] ritual religious worship, animal sacrifices, spirit appeasements, or the taking of medicinal herbs, smoke inhalations or reciting incantations.[32, 35] Especially violent patients will be seized and tied hand and foot. In the past, such patients used to be held in stocks until they improved or died.[32, 34] Today, most will eventually be arrested and taken to a regional psychiatric hospital. Whatever the treatment, conversion disorders including mass hysteria will usually improve. However, the major psychoses and epilepsy follow a more chronic course and frequently lead to permanent incarceration in a psychiatric hospital. Patients may also be left alone to wander about as unwashed vagrant psychotics. It is generally believed that once truly mad, the brain remains 'spoilt forever' and that one cannot expect anything from such an individual.[32]

Some mental illness, such as epilepsy or violent forms of mania or schizophrenia, carry a special stigma and are handled as individual and family secrets.[34] In the Baganda of Uganda, epileptic children are often isolated, live alone, eat alone and may not be allowed to play with other children.[32] Even when treated, people do not believe that epileptics can ever become totally normal.

Unrecognized mental illnesses

A number of psychiatric disorders such as depression or petit mal epilepsy are not recognized as illness in most tropical societies. Other conditions are misdiagnosed when they present in unusual forms. For example, depression associated with physical complaints is often thought to be a physical illness such as anaemia, hypovitaminosis or malnutrition.[31, 39, 40]

Conduct or personality disorders are considered as unruly behaviour. If they present with violence, they are treated by corporal punishment or by other concrete correctional measures. In children, histrionic, dependent, narcissistic, avoidant, passive–aggressive or other forms of non-violent personality and anxiety disorders are often considered to be forms of laziness or unacceptable behaviour and disciplinary measures are employed. This also applies to learning disabilities which are the cause of much corporal punishment in schools.[32, 34] Psychosomatic illnesses, including enuresis, peptic ulcers, psychogenic pain disorders as well as hypochondriasis and most neurotic complaints, are perceived as true medical conditions and are therefore not considered to be mental disorders. Depression and anxiety may, as stated above, take on various clinical forms.[31, 39, 40] Some are so common that they have become distinct syndromes, e.g. the 'brain fag syndrome' describing student examination anxiety[41] or the 'East African tumbo syndrome', denoting diffuse abdominal complaints.[42] Such symptoms are usually attributed to witchcraft.[31, 32, 35]

In societies where witchcraft, magic and sorcery are believed to be common, paranoid illnesses may go unrecognized. Fortunately, these are rare in childhood. However, one can identify overprotected children by their scarifications and protective amulets. Prolonged bereavement and mild forms of depression are usually attributed to the obvious environmental stressors. Impotence, which may accompany a mild depression, is not considered a mental illness. However, the failure to have erections is worrisome to adolescent boys, as many African societies value machismo, polygamy and many children. Sexual dysfunctions, in general, are therefore highly distressful to individuals, although they are usually considered a family secret and often only traditional methods of treatment are sought.[32] To prevent such problems, mothers sometimes bring their two-year-old sons to doctors complaining that they have not seen them have erections.

Many developing countries have undergone significant social transformations through urbanization and the introduction of Western technology. Associated with this have been violent disruptions of traditional life systems, affecting the family unit. War, famines and urban poverty are often followed by chronic malnutrition and are responsible for the neglected and homeless city street children whose attachment systems have been disrupted.[33, 43] Such disruptions are not usually recognized as causing psychological illnesses and are not addressed in treatment.

After a war or famine, one often finds an increased number of orphans and street children with severe developmental disorders. One particular child, the 'Monkey Boy' in Uganda, was found to have profound physical and psychological handicaps.[44] All his family had been killed in a war and he was left alone in the bush. When found at the age of six years he could only crawl on all fours, had no language, made no social contact, showed no fear and never smiled. He preferred to pick and eat earth, weeds or grass to cooked food. He urinated and defaecated wherever he sat. After some months at a war orphanage in Kampala, his development improved significantly.

A few orphanages and baby homes attempt to care for these displaced children. However, these institutions are often underfinanced, understaffed and overcrowded. Child adoption programmes are inadequate.

Changing attitudes

The mixture of traditional and modern Western attitudes to mental illness found particularly in present-day Africa has been described. The care of mentally handicapped children throughout the developing world is generally poor. In cities there are usually few out-patient and virtually no in-patient facilities for disturbed children. In rural areas psychiatric care is generally unavailable and families resort to traditional healers for the treatment of psychological disorders in their children.

To overcome these shortcomings, it is important to include the teaching of basic psychiatric disorders in the syllabus of all health care workers and to provide seminars in child psychology to all primary school teachers. It is also important to decentralize the provision of medical care and include a psychiatric evaluation in primary health care programmes at village health centres. This would not only make psychiatric care available in rural areas, but also avoid separating psychiatrically disturbed children from their relatives.

Psychiatric illnesses in children are common in developing countries but often go unrecognized. Psychiatric services are generally poor and mentally handicapped children are often neglected.[34, 45] To change the attitudes which contribute to the persistence of such poor care must, therefore, be an important educational goal of health professionals.

Legislation, national policies and aspects of community life affecting mental health and mental retardation in children

National policies for health should identify the needs of children in the promotion of physical and mental health, as well as the prevention of specific conditions and the provision of physical and mental health care. Health staff concerned with contributing to or initiating national policies on mental health and mental retardation will find useful guidelines in *Mental Retardation: Meeting the Challenge*, WHO.[25]

Each country will need to develop a National Coordinating Group for child health, which will include mental health, mental retardation and other disabilities. The group will need contributions from various ministries (e.g. Education, Community Development and Social Welfare), non-government organizations and professionals. They will need to review all other general national policies which affect the welfare of children. Tasks for such a group would include a review of the current services for physically handicapped and mentally retarded children, both in hospital and the community, and the assessment of numbers of children affected perhaps using key informants (e.g. village chiefs, community leaders). A plan with short- and long-term goals to provide for the needs of the children can then be devised which may be used to draw these needs to public attention and to enable them to be placed in the list of national priorities.

The provision of a special service for children with physical handicap and mental retardation is not usually feasible, as it would be very expensive and is often inappropriate. The greatest hope for this neglected population is prevention, with promotion and care being an integrated part of the general children's services, and particular emphasis on rehabilitation in the community.[46]

Doctors and health workers should be alert to the important effects of legislation on child health and development. Examples are the laws relating to marriage, custody of children, child working practices and conditions, and the rights and access to education facilities.

Community life, attitudes and customary practices naturally have a profound effect on the developing child. An awareness of these can allow health workers to consider in what ways helpful practices can be encouraged and how potentially harmful practices can be discouraged. An example of two areas where there is clear evidence of harmful effects upon children are inconsistency of parenting and family breakdown. The response of the community to the break up of families is important. The extended family, self-help groups and other community resources can benefit and develop with prompting and support from health care workers.

Children in prison and young offenders

National policies on offenders

The national committees devising such policies should have paediatric advice. The formal statement of a national policy should include the special mention of very young offenders and also mothers with babies and young children in prison. Medical and nursing paediatric advice is also important for any prison admitting children, probation hostels and approved schools admitting young people.

Mothers and babies in prison

On general humane grounds, as far as possible, non-custodial sentences should be allocated to mothers in late pregnancy or with small children. If this is unavoidable, then the admission of babies and very small children with mothers, at least avoids separation during a period when a consistent relationship with a mother or mother figure is fundamental to normal development.

An important principle throughout is that the community as a whole, and the prison authorities in particular, have responsibility to ensure that the child is not punished along with the mother and that its development is not in any way impaired. There is a need for special facilities for such mothers and babies in prison. The national policy on the care of offenders should include a section on the provision, staffing and monitoring of these facilities. In addition, each prison facility should have its own special committee to assess requirements and ensure that they are provided and maintained. It would be essential for such a committee to include persons with experience in the care of children, such as experienced and mature mothers and professionals in child-care and development. The opportunity for regular visiting by father, siblings and the extended family is also essential for the child's development.

Very young offenders in prison

Young children in prison are at serious risk of being trained in criminal activities and becoming hardened in attitudes and less law-abiding. It is virtually impossible o protect them from physical and sexual abuse. Finally, there are no suitable education facilities for young people.

In summary, prison is an adult situation which is a totally inappropriate environment for normal child development. Much more appropriate provisions for young offenders include community work, supervision by probation officers and the offender making some reparation for those harmed.

Community education

All those dealing with young people, whether parents, elders or professionals, need to understand the principles of behaviour management. The whole community needs to know the limitations of punishment, the effectiveness of reward in promoting good behaviour and the important influence of older persons providing good models of behaviour. Young people need opportunities for positive and productive activities which allow them to improve their valuation of themselves.

Some behavioural disorders arise directly from the experience of failure at school. These can be reduced by the identification of pupils having difficulties and the provision of appropriate remedial education.

Penal authorities and the community need to be aware that most offending children do not grow up to be adult criminals. Punishment, therefore, must avoid producing long-term harmful effects, for example, in prison sentences.

Corporal punishment for young people

Psychological studies show that punishment is most effective when it occurs immediately after the undesirable behaviour, when the young person understands the reason for the punishment and when the punishment is not unduly harsh. Corporal punishment ordered by a court can only be given long after the offence and its administration is a degrading experience for the child, the prison staff and any medical or nursing personnel providing supervision.

Promotion of mental health by teachers

Teachers are important contributors to the mental health of children. Teacher training should stress that this is an integral part of teaching of all age groups. Health staff, both medical and non-medical, can also help to prepare local teaching staff for this part of their work. One important aspect is the effect of family, and physical and psychosocial problems on the learning and behaviour of children.

Health staff may feel hesitant about entering this area of education, but authorities responsible for the education of teachers and the teachers themselves usually warmly welcome such a contribution. Teachers need to be alert to:

- the importance of sensory deficits such as short-sightedness and deafness, which may be helped by treatment;
- their role in the reduction of road traffic accidents;
- the way anxiety and parental expectations affect children's learning ability and what might be done to help this;
- the potential benefit of information, education and counselling in the prevention of teenage pregnancy, abuse of alcohol, drugs, solvents and petrol, and smoking.

References

1. Barker P. *Basic Child Psychiatry*, 4th Edn. London, Granada, 1983.
2. Graham PJ. Epidemiological approaches to child mental health in developing countries. In: Purcell EF ed. *Psychopathology and Youth: A Cross-cultural Perspective*. New York, Josiah Macey Jr. Foundation, 1979.
3. Giel R *et al.* Childhood mental disorders in primary health care; results of observations in four developing countries. *Pediatrics*. 1981; **68**(5): 677–83.
4. WHO. *Report of the WHO Inter-Regional Workshop in Child Mental Health and Psycho-social Development*. Athens, 1982.
5. Nikapota AD. Paediatric symptoms without signs: recognition of functional complaints in childhood. *Tropical Doctor*. 1987; **17**: 108–10.
6. Rutter M, Hersov L. *Child and Adolescent Psychiatry: Modern Approaches*, 2nd Edn. Blackwell Scientific Publications, 1985.
7. Kolvin I, Goodyear I. In: Granville-Grossman K ed. *Recent Advances in Clinical Psychiatry*, Vol. 4 London, Churchill Livingstone, 1982.
8. McAuley R. Training parents to modify conduct problems in their children. *Journal of Child Psychology and Psychiatry*. 1982; **23**(3): 335–42.
9. Graham PJ. *Child Psychiatry: A Developmental Approach*. Oxford Medical Publications, 1986.
10. Minde KK. Psychological problems in Ugandan school children: a controlled evaluation. *Journal of Child Psychology and Psychiatry*. 1975; **16**: 49–59.
11. Yorkston MJ, Sergeant HGS. A simple method of relaxation. *Lancet*. 1969; **ii**: 1319–21.
12. Goodyear IM. Hysteria in childhood. *Hospital Update*. February 1985: 103–10.
13. Rivinus TM, Jameson DL, Graham PJ. Childhood neurological disease presenting as psychiatric disorder. *Archives of Disease in Childhood*. 1975; **50**: 115–19.
14. Dubovitz V, Hersov L. Management of children with non-organic (hysterical) disorders of motor function development. *Developmental Medicine and Child Neurology*. 1976; **18**: 358–68.
15. Lishman WA. *Organic Psychiatry: The Psychological Consequences of Cerebral Disorder*. Oxford, Blackwell Scientific, 1978. pp. 367–9.
16. Barker P. *Basic Family Therapy*, 2nd Edn, Granada Paperback, 1986.
17. Teoh J, Kim-Leng Y. Cultural conflict and transition: epidemic hysteria and social sanction. *Australian and New Zealand Journal of Psychiatry*. 1973; **7**: 283–95.
18. Dhadphale M, Sajihk SP. Epidemic hysteria in a Zambian school: the mysterious madness of Mwinilunga. *British Journal of Psychiatry*. 1983; **142**: 85–8.
19. Mohr PD, Bond MJ. A chronic epidemic of hysterical blackouts in a comprehensive school. *British Medical Journal*. 1982; **284**: 961–2.
20. Levine RJ, Sexton DJ, Romm FJ *et al.* Outbreak of psychosomatic illness at a rural elementary school. *Lancet*. 1974; **ii**: 1500–3.
21. McConville BJ, Bruce RT. Depressive illness in children and adolescents: a review of current concepts. *Canadian Journal of Psychiatry*. 1985; **30**: 119–29.
22. Barrett L, Kolvin I. In: Granville-Grossman K ed. *Recent Advances in Psychiatry*, Vol. 3. London, Churchill Livingstone, 1979.
23. *Diagnostic and Statistical Manual (DSM III)*. American Psychiatric Association, Washington DC, 1980.
24. O'Dell S. Training parents in behaviour modification: a review. *Psychological Bulletin*. 1974; **81**(7): 418–33.
25. WHO. *Mental Retardation: Meeting the Challenge*. Geneva, WHO (Publication No. 86) 1985.
26. Kolvin I, Garside RS, Nicol AR *et al. Help Starts Here: The Maladjusted Child in the Ordinary School*. London, Tavistock, 1981.
27. WHO. *Prevention of Mental, Neurological and Psycho-social Disorders*. A 39/9 25 February 1986. Geneva, WHO.
28. Graham PJ. Possibilities of prevention. In: Graham PJ ed. *Epidemiological Approaches to Child Psychiatry*. London, Academic Press, 1977.
29. Morley D. *Paediatric Priorities in Developing Countries*. London, Butterworths, 1973.
30. WHO. *Manual on Child Mental Health and Psychosexual Development for: I Primary Health Care Physicians; II Primary Health Workers; III Teachers; IV Workers in Children's Homes.* WHO, Regional Office for South East Asia, New Delhi, 110002, India. 1982.
31. German GA. Aspects of clinical psychiatry in sub-Saharan Africa. *British Journal of Psychiatry*. 1972; **121**: 461–79.
32. Orley JH. *Culture and Mental Illness: A Study from Uganda*. Nairobi, East African Publishing House, 1970.
33. Jegede OR, Olatawura MO. Child and adolescent psychiatry in Africa: a review. *East African Medical Journal*. 1982; **59**: 436–41.
34. Brown J. Care of the mentally handicapped (Editorial). *East African Medical Journal*. 1981; **58**: 469–71.
35. Dhadphale M. Attitude of a group of Zambian females to spirit possession (ngulu). *East African Medical Journal*. 1979; **56**: 450–3.
36. Arap-Mengech HNK, Lukwago MG. Psychiatric illness

in Kenyan children with mental handicap. *East African Medical Journal.* 1983; **60**: 827–32.

37. Dhadphale M, Arap-Mengech HNK, Syme D *et al.* Drug abuse among secondary school students in Kenya: a preliminary survey. *East African Medical Journal.* 1982; **59**: 152–6.

38. Kagwa BH. The problems of mass hysteria in East Africa. *East African Medical Journal.* 1964; **41**: 560–6.

39. Njenga FJ, Acuda SW. The clinical presentation of depressive illness in children at Kenyatta National Hospital. *East African Medical Journal.* 1981; **59**: 623–6.

40. Swift CR, Asuni T. *Mental Health and Disease in Africa.* Edinburgh, Churchill Livingstone, 1975.

41. Prince R. Brain fag syndrome. *Journal of Mental Science.* 1960; **106**: 559–70.

42. Otsyula W, Rees PH. The occurrence and recognition of minor psychiatric illness among outpatients at the Kenyatta National Hospital, Nairobi. *East African Medical Journal.* 1972; **49**: 825–9.

43. Minde KK, Minde R, Musisi S. Some aspects of disruption of the attachment system in young children: a transcultural perspective. In: *The Child in His Family.* New York, Wiley-Interscience Publications, 1982. pp. 215–33.

44. 'Monkey Child': a sad victim of war. *African Concord.* 10 July 1986: 23.

45. Acuda SW. Mental health problems in Kenya today: a review of research. *East African Medical Journal.* 1983; **60**: 11–13.

46. Helander E, Mendis P, Nelson G. *Training Disabled People in the Community. A Manual on Community-based Rehabilitation for Developing Countries.* Geneva, WHO, 1983 (RHB/83.1).

Further reading

Bailey RD. *Therapeutic Nursing for the Mentally Handicapped.* Oxford Medical Publications, 1982.

Granville-Grossman K (ed). *Recent Advances in Clinical Psychiatry*, Vols 2, 3, 4, 5. London, Churchill Livingstone, 1976, 1979, 1982 and 1985.

Nikapota AD. Contribution of integrated mental health services to child mental health. *International Journal of Mental Health*, 1984; **12**(3): 77–95.

Rutter M. *Helping Troubled Children.* Penguin, 1984.

WHO. *Child Mental Health and Psychosocial development.* Technical Report Series no. 613. Geneva, WHO, 1977.

Also particularly recommended are Refs 1, 6, 9, 30 and 46.

DELINQUENCY
K. Minde and S Musisi

Definition, incidence and clinical picture	Prognosis and treatment
Aetiology	References

Definition, incidence and clinical picture

Delinquency is a legal and not a psychiatric diagnostic term. A juvenile delinquent is defined as a young person who has been charged and found guilty of an offence which would be labelled a 'crime' in an adult, such as an activity related to theft, vandalism, hold-up or breaking into a building with the intent to steal.

It is obvious from this definition that the incidence of juvenile delinquency will depend to a large extent on the standards of the local law enforcing agency, the age at which youngsters become eligible for prosecution in a particular country, and whether parents or teachers are willing to report incidents to the police. It also depends on what a particular society or cultural group regards as illegal. For example, the legal drinking age of a minor in Canada varies from province to province. Since illegal drinking is one reason for prosecution by a Court of Law, youngsters of the same age engaging in the same activity may be labelled delinquent in one province in Canada, but not in another.

In the developed world, a substantial minority of the male adolescent population can expect to acquire a criminal record. For example, it has been estimated that 22 per cent of all juvenile males and 5 per cent of all juveniles females in England will have a criminal record before the age of 21[1], and figures in the United States are similar.

In developing countries, the label of delinquency is often even more arbitrary. In studies of children in remand homes in Uganda, about 50 per cent of those labelled delinquent had never committed any criminal act but were simply neglected.[2] Many of them had been forced to leave their homes and families because their mothers had either left their husbands or had married other men who were not interested in the children. As a consequence, these children wandered around the country, living off the land until they were finally picked up by police and placed in prison cells, usually together with adult criminals.

Nevertheless, clinical impressions supported by official statistics suggest that fewer children are engaged in delinquent activities in developing countries than in Europe or North America[2, 3]. However, this may be changing with increasing urbanization and other developments which disrupt traditional family life.[4, 5]

Delinquents are usually divided into two categories: socialized and unsocialized. Unsocialized delinquents are poorly adjusted in any situation. They are unhappy, moody, quarrelsome, aggressive and unpopular. Socialized delinquents, in contrast, may be well-integrated into delinquent gangs and may adapt their behaviour to the subculture they have chosen. They may also be loyal to other gang members and have enough self-control to plan long-range activities, such as robbing a bank. Unsocialized delinquents, on the other hand, are often unable to 'bond' even to socially deviant groups because of their pervasive impulsivity and aggression.

In developing countries, delinquent children may steal clothes or other possessions from direct family members and sell them at the market. They may also engage in prostitution and be found among those who abuse drugs such as cannabis, amphetamines or chew miraa.[3, 5] They also frequently abuse alcohol or inhale petrol fumes. Gangs of delinquent youngsters have been known regularly to steal specific merchandise, such as watches, and distribute and sell it through individual market boys. They may also engage in other organized black market activities or work as 'assistants' to corrupt officials or army personnel. This problem occurs more commonly in societies where traditional social customs have been broken down by wars, famines or political instability.

Aetiology

There is good evidence that youngsters who commit one type of crime, e.g. stealing from shops, have also been involved in other offences, e.g. taking illegal drugs. They also frequently have a history of specific behavioural abnormalities such as fighting, poor school attendance or sexual promiscuity.[6] Because of this combination of problems, delinquency has been assumed by some to be due to a particular fundamental psychological or even neurophysiological defect.

Some reported features of delinquents are indeed suggestive of minor neurological impairment. For example, many delinquents show a general restlessness and have other symptoms characteristic of hyperactivity. Significant differences between violent and non-violent delinquents have been documented, the former group showing more specific neurological abnormalities such as choreiform movements or an inability to skip.[7]

However, there is good evidence that inadequate perinatal care and other causes of damage to the brain occur more frequently in poor, neglectful or abusive families, who in turn provide the social milieu in which delinquency is most commonly found.[8] There exists no readily predictable connection between the location and type of cerebral pathology and the type of subsequent psychological abnormality. Furthermore, the great majority of delinquents are physically healthy and neurologically normal.

The most commonly held aetiological theory suggests that sociocultural breakdown as encountered in poor urban neighbourhoods, and uneven distribution of wealth, lead children to delinquency. In one of the few studies which have examined delinquent children in the developing world, Minde[2] found 75 per cent of delinquent children to come from broken homes. However, on other potentially important background variables (e.g. parental death or previous serious medical illnesses) there was no difference between the delinquent and other disturbed, but non-delinquent, youngsters. African workers[3, 4] have made similar observations. They have also confirmed that in traditional societies with intact extended family systems, delinquency is very rare.

While the social theory of causation appears eminently logical and is supported by the apparent increase in juvenile crime among the urban poor in developing countries, there is little empirical evidence to confirm this. The most comprehensive studies in that area suggest that any one theory of delinquency may at best offer a partial explanation. The clinician should therefore be aware of a variety of possible influences such as poor carer–child relationships, delinquent companions, as well as the lack of legitimate educational and occupational opportunities, which may cause delinquent behaviour.

Prognosis and treatment

Studies in developed countries indicate that about 75 per cent of all juvenile delinquents will 'outgrow' their antisocial behaviour once they reach adulthood and get married. Those who do not change have often begun their delinquent careers earlier and have committed more offences both at school and in the community and come from more deprived backgrounds. Data from developing countries are not yet available.

The management of these children is obviously difficult and frustrating, as their behaviour is often associated with social factors over which the health care professional has little control. Since delinquent children are usually in conflict with their families, interventions may be most effective if the family can be persuaded to participate in the treatment. Thus, an important goal would be to give more efficient control over the day-to-day activities of these youngsters to family members. Finding a more meaningful social structure and support system, possibly within the extended family, is often helpful. This is frequently difficult to achieve since these youngsters have usually lost their traditional family roots and may have been exposed to severe and long-standing psychological or physical abuse. For this reason, the physician or health care professional should get involved in educating parents and community representatives about the need for sound discipline and fair occupational opportunities for both the rich and the poor.

To assist government agencies in their daily work and future planning, it is also important to differentiate clearly between the therapeutic requirements of true delinquents and those primarily in need of care and protection. For example, many market boys in African cities are initially not delinquent and respond well to social support measures. Likewise, neglected children who inadvertently have been caught up in the criminal system, may do well in foster homes arranged by local branches of social organizations, such as Save the Children Fund, and should not remain in remand homes or reform school.

Finally, the role of the traditional remand homes and reform schools in many developing countries needs to be re-examined. While there is no empirical evidence that these institutions improve the prognosis of the individual delinquent,[8] they may nevertheless at times be helpful to isolate the truly delinquent youngster by preventing him from inducing other children into illegal activities.

In summary, it is obvious that delinquency is becoming a serious problem in developing countries and that delinquent children are difficult to treat. With the likelihood of even more major changes taking place in these societies in the future, the prevention of associated social disorganization must remain a high priority for each health professional.

References

1. Farrington DP. The prevalence of convictions. *British Journal of Criminology*. 1981; **21**: 173-5.
2. Minde K. Children in Uganda: rates of behavioural deviations and psychiatric disorders in various school and clinic populations. *Journal of Child Psychology and Psychiatry*. 1977; **18**: 23-37.
3. Kagwa BH, Kagwa GW. Juvenile delinquency in Uganda, East Africa. *East African Medical Journal*. 1969; **46**: 376-81.
4. Swift CR, Asuni T. *Mental Health and Disease in Africa*. London, Churchill Livingstone 1975.
5. Dhadphale M, Arap Mengech HNK, Syme D, Acuda SW. Drug abuse among secondary school students in Kenya: a preliminary survey. *East African Medical Journal*. 1982; **59**: 152-6.
6. West DJ, Farrington DP. *The Delinquent Way of Life*. London, Heinemann Educational, 1977.
7. Otnow-Lewis D, Shanok SS, Pincus JH. The neuropsychiatric status of violent male juvenile delinquents. In: Otnow-Lewis D ed. *Vulnerabilities to Delinquency*. New York, SP Medical and Scientific Books, 1981. pp. 67-8.
8. West DJ. Delinquency in child and adolescent psychiatry. In: Rutter M, Hersove L eds. *Child Psychiatry: Modern Approaches*. Oxford, Blackwell Scientific Publishers, 1986. pp. 414-23.

CHAPTER 7

Deprivation

SOCIAL DEPRIVATION
S. N. Chaudhuri

The majority of the present population of the world have been conceived and nurtured under conditions of deprivation, the hallmark of poverty and a hostile environment. As a result of adaptation, many are able to compensate for mild or moderate deficits of food, clothing, shelter and parental care, but severe deprivation wreaks havoc, resulting in morbidity, permanent disabilities or death in the growing child.

Using anthropometric measurements related to the age of the child, such as height, weight and mid-upper-arm circumference, it is estimated that about 60 per cent of children in the developing countries of Asia, Africa and Latin America are failing to reach their potential, and this is largely the result of growing up in situations of deprivation. Such children put pressure on curative and preventive medical services, often fail at school and by swelling the numbers of child labourers, add to the unemployment figures in countries over-burdened with debt, lacking renewable energy sources and in which there may be political and social strife. It is vital for health workers as well as policy-makers and planners, to be aware of the large numbers of deprived children, the underlying causes for their problems and the programmes aimed at improving their lot.

Deprivation is complex, and the result of many adverse influences. The deprived child does not have enough food, clothing, shelter, parental love, education or medical care for many interrelated reasons. Physical well-being at any stage of life is important for emotional and social development, and as it can be measured easily, it is the usual tool for identifying deprived children.

Among deprived children, boys may do better than girls in some developing countries. In parts of India, for example, male children are desired because of the social and cultural advantages which boys enjoy. Earlier referral of boys in case of illness and better opportunities for education, give them an advantage over girls. This bias may be serious enough to reverse the usual sex ratio and lead to more male than female children living in later life.

The hostile environment

With rapid advances in the knowledge of the control of communicable diseases, death rates have dropped in many developing countries over the past few decades. Birth rates continue to be high leading to an increase in the number of children compared with the number of elderly. Aggravating this situation is the early age of marriage, some girls being given away in marriage before they complete adolescence. The large number of children compete for food resources, there is a fall in the per capita availability of food and undernutrition results. The country's health services become increasingly strained and its hospitals overcrowded. If the allocation of scarce resources to the hospitals at the expense of the preventive outreach community health services is increased, the deteriorating health situation is aggravated.

Children of poor communities are born into families who live in overcrowded city slums or in big and small villages in remote areas. In villages the houses may be overcrowded and small, but they usually have some open space in which children may run around and play. Unfortunately, with an increasing trend towards migration of landless rural people to overcrowded city slums, many children are being denied the use of open space for play, so essential to their growth and well-being. Urban mothers often have to leave their infants and toddlers at home as they travel to work. They use hazardous public transport, whilst their counterparts in the villages carry the young children to the fields strapped on their back or front and so are able to continue breast-feeding and to have more body contact.

Ignorance regarding safe child-rearing practices among mothers is common in poor communities. Aggravating this in many parts of the world, are superstitious and harmful beliefs which lead to the restriction of certain types of food from mothers during pregnancy and lactation, and water and food during bouts of diarrhoea in children. Elders in the community such as grandparents, quacks and indigenous medical practitioners, are often a repository of harmful as well as good practices influencing child survival.

In poor communities, children are exposed to the elements from a very young age. They may be born in extreme climates of heat, cold or the rains. Inadequate clothing and shelter due to poverty soon force the child's metabolic processes to adapt to the hostile environment. Close body contact provided by the mother during feeding and sleep spares the child for certain hours of the day. However, extreme temperatures may prove fatal when the adaptation mechanism is overwhelmed.

When children in poor communities are ill, mothers give home treatment based on the advice of elders or neighbours. If there is no response, a mother will take the child to the local medical attendant whose fees she may be able to afford and in whom she may have faith. Sometimes the mother may delay seeking advice during illness, as time and money may not be available. The time required to take a child for medical care may compete with prime earning time for subsistence income which is necessary to procure food for the daily meal. Preventive services such as immunization against 'killer diseases', vitamin A supplements to prevent blindness, periodic growth monitoring and iron supplementation to prevent anaemia, are very often not seen as priorities by poor mothers. Families are so much preoccupied with crises of death and disease in children that very often preventive services, which require periodic visits and long waiting times at overcrowded clinics, do not make sense to overworked and tired mothers living in deprived societies.

During early preschool years, toddlers who are not receiving adequate protection or attention from their mothers are prone to accidents. In overcrowded city slums, children play on the streets, risking injury or death from road accidents. In rural areas, children risk drowning and bites from poisonous snakes and insects. Other common forms of accident in children are burns from household fires during cooking and the swallowing of poisons, such as kerosene oil, pesticides and insecticides left within reach. Overcrowding, poor housing and exhaustion of parents due to overwork, coupled with inadequacy of food, increase the chances of such accidents in poor communities.

Malnutrition and infection

The struggle for survival in the deprived child begins at birth. The newborn child, already often underweight and deficient in protective antibodies, is exposed to a continous heavy dose of infectious agents. Common ailments such as chest, skin and gastro-intestinal infections pose a perpetual risk. Diarrhoea, the biggest killer among preschool children in poor communities, is related to inadequate disposal of faeces coupled with a poor supply of water. The children suffer most, as diarrhoea along with anorexia, malabsorption and a high helminthic load compounds malnutrition. Inadequate observance of personal hygiene such as hand washing after defaecation and before taking food or feeding young children, increase the spread of diarrhoea. Tuberculosis is also very common in both adults and children of deprived communities. Children spend considerable time in close proximity to grandparents who may have tuberculosis. Helminthic infections are another almost universal problem in children of poor communities. Roundworm infestation is the most frequent in many parts of the world, followed by threadworms and hookworms. Very often infested children adapt remarkably to a substantial parasite load without any symptoms, with the exception of anaemia from hookworms. Skin infections due to insufficient washing, scratching of insect bites or scabies are common. Heat, humidity and dust aggravate these and they are spread with ease by flies. The AIDS epidemic is leaving children bereft of one or both parents as orphans in a hostile world.

Intervention programmes for child survival

The sharp differences in the quality of life between the rich and poor within a developing country, increase even more when one analyses the services available to the child fortunate enough to be born in a developed country. It should be the birth right of every child to have access to parental love, food, shelter and education. Even the poor countries are now making increasing efforts to allocate more resources to mother and child, supported by international agencies (such as UNICEF) and bilateral agencies. Intervention programmes improving services to the 'child in need' are of value not only for humane reasons. The future repository of human resources of the country, of scientific knowledge, generation of material resources and the capacity to upgrade the quality of life of the country, is dependent on the quality of its future citizens. Investment in measures to improve infant and child mortality also has a quick outcome in bringing down birth rates and population pressure on scarce resources.

When planning and implementing intervention programmes in child-care, it is important to keep in mind that the prime objective is to improve the capacity of the mother and her skills in child-rearing. Dependency on the government or an external source of funding should be kept to a minimum. Sometimes intervention programmes are addressed to one burning problem of which the country wishes to eliminate, for example malnutrition. A few countries in the past launched elaborate feeding programmes in schools or community centres targeted to vulnerable groups. However, these single-point interventions are usually ineffective and results are better if nutrition is part of a package of preventive and curative services for children, for example the Integrated Child Development Services (ICDS) in India. The best results are seen in integrated programmes of child welfare, in which there is a strong component of community participation, so that the people themselves become convinced of the social input necessary at an early age, for the optimum development of children. Some of the national and world-wide intervention programmes for child survival are described below.

Integrated Child Development Services (ICDS) in India

This national programme is one of the world's largest and now covers approximately 30 per cent of India's population living in villages, tribal and slum areas. Children below six years of age, and pregnant and lactating mothers of the community receive a package of services, consisting of nutrition supplementation, antenatal care, referral of sick children and mothers to the nearest health facility, non-formal preschool education, immunization, and nutrition and health education. One local woman in every 1000 is trained over a three month period about basic concepts of mother- and child-care and helps to provide these services through a community centre. Children are weighed at regular intervals, referred for immunization to the multipurpose government health worker and fed a nutritious diet while they learn through play activities. Through an initial house-to-house survey, children who are malnourished and belong to poor families are given nutrition supplementation. Hopefully, as part of India's new drive to uplift the poor, the ICDS programme will eventually cover the whole nation of 750 million people, and become one of the largest intervention programmes for child survival in the world.

GOBI and the 'Child Survival Revolution'

An analysis of child morbidity and mortality in developing countries indicates the need for mounting some short-term measures (see pp. 26–37, 358–66). These measures could be directed simply to malnutrition and infection in children, or be more broadly based and directed to the malnutrition–infection cycle. If mothers and medical attendants were to follow simple instructions on regular weighing of children to detect growth faltering (G), provide immediate and sustained oral rehydration with onset of diarrhoea (O), continue breast-feeding (B) and immunize children periodically against diphtheria, whooping cough, tetanus, poliomyelitis, measles and tuberculosis (I), according to UNICEF a 'Child Survival Revolution' would be imminent. Even with very little investment or increase in the health budgets, a considerable fall in morbidity and mortality in children may be achieved. The effectiveness of this 'revolution' will be enhanced further by the spread of female literacy, spacing of children, and when necessary, nutrition supplementation. Spread of this GOBI concept among mothers is easily achieved through person-to-person contact during home visits and demonstration, and enhances a community's knowledge of child-care. In the end, the regular use of these simple methods in 'child survival' will improve a mother's capacity to take care of her children effectively, though the phrase itself is unsuitable to describe the need for far more than survival, but for enhancement of quality of life for children.

Measures to improve family income by women

Lack of education and skills and non-availability of agricultural land are familiar stumbling blocks to efforts in improving family income. Organization of women into effective groups is a first step in intervention programmes. Backyard poultry, fishery and kitchen garden activities are now part of development projects for women. As much as possible, women should be able to generate extra income and find more time to take care of their children at home, instead of leaving households and children to elder siblings or elderly grandparents. In urban situations work at home, for example assembly of electronic components, may bring supplementary income to mothers.

Improvement of female literacy

In many parts of the world, young girls either drop out from the formal education system early or never go to school, in order to help their mothers with household duties, including the care of young children. All efforts should be made to keep children of deprived families attending schools, with special emphasis on girls. Since poverty is the main reason for girls dropping out of school, measures such as work education for them which generates income instead of their working as housemaids, should be propagated. Introduction of lessons in mothercraft and healthy child-rearing practices in the school curricula can also play a positive role in child survival.

Training of mother- and child-care workers

Mother and child health (MCH) services form an important component of primary health care but many countries are finding it difficult to implement these services due to lack of trained personnel. 'Grass-roots' level workers with some training are able to motivate mothers to space their children, give proper advice as regards diet, immunization, oral rehydration, etc. In many countries, such workers are provided with a small allowance by the state, and supplement the government's health infrastructure. Training given to women in this way has an influence on the health of their children, their neighbour's children through propagation of the health message and, hopefully, in future decades, their grandchildren. Child health is therefore assured over many generations through training.

Allocation of resources to mother- and child-care

In many developing countries, the allocation of resources for specialist units outstrips investment in preventive aspects of mother- and child-care. As well as investment in paediatric wards and obstetric units of general hospitals, it is essential to establish outreach programmes in antenatal care, training of traditional birth attendants and domiciliary visits by MCH workers to ensure proper growth and development of the child over the vulnerable years of life. When the level of malnutrition is high and the purchasing power small, supplementary nutrition programmes for pregnant and lactating mothers and children even through school years makes sense. It is necessary to integrate such welfare programmes into a development plan for the country with as little external support as possible. Caution should be exercised so that the benefits reach the deprived segments of the population and are not siphoned off by the middle class.

The future

Poverty in many parts of the world, population increases, a rapid depletion of non-renewable energy sources and pressure on land, seemingly hold out a bleak future for the human race and the deprived child in particular. In developed countries, families without income obtain state subsidies and are assured of minimum daily needs for all family members. The help for the deprived child differs sharply from country to country, depending on economic status. In parts of Africa with worsening famine situations, the numbers of children with malnutrition are increasing. In some Asian countries the children suffer the worst consequences of increasing unemployment and a deteriorating economic situation, and swell the morbidity and mortality statistics. Increasing urbanization and sociopolitical unrest in most parts of the developing world take a heavy toll on children. Much of the future improvement for deprived children depends on giving women equal status to men, in terms of employment opportunities, education and legal aid, because their children will benefit indirectly.

The policy-makers and planners of many developing countries have a hard choice to make between a quick return from investments in a steel mill, a cement factory, or a fertilizer factory, which save precious foreign exchange, and an outreach programme of MCH services. The return on investments in children is slow and may not be perceptible for a generation.

Massive investment in a basic health and education infrastructure is a prerequisite before appreciable improvements are noticeable in the quality of future citizens of a country. A strong political will is necessary to make the required investments, sacrificing popular options such as importing cars or luxury items for the rich. Clear thinking, leading to careful planning is the by-product of political stability and peace sadly is rare in the world today. In most of the countries which have improved the lot of children, political stability and lessening of tensions both internal and external have been important contributory factors.

Further reading

Cassen RH. *India: Population, Economy, Society*. London, Macmillan, 1980.

Grant JP (ed.). *The State of the World's Children 1986*. Oxford, UNICEF/Oxford University Press, 1985.

Integrated Child Development Services. A co-ordinated approach to children's health in India: progress report after five years (1975–80). *Lancet*. 1983; **1**: 109–11.

Jelliffe DB. *The Assessment of the Nutritional Status of the Community*. Geneva, WHO, 1966. p. 121.

Morley DC, Woodland M. *See How They Grow – Monitoring Child Growth for Appropriate Health Care in Developing Countries*. London, Macmillan, 1979. pp. 216–42.

UNICEF. A child survival and development revolution. *Assignment Children* 61/62, Geneva, UNICEF, 1983.

UNICEF. *An Analysis of the Situation of Children in India*. Regional Office for South Central Asia, New Delhi, 1984.

WHO. *WHO Programme for Control of Diarrhoeal Diseases, Fifth Programme Report 1984–1985*. WHO/CDD/ 86.16. 1986.

CHILD ABUSE AND NEGLECT WITHIN THE FAMILY

Nigel Speight

Physical abuse
  Diagnosis
  Management
Emotional deprivation and neglect
  Growth failure
  Developmental retardation

Emotional effects
Long-term effects
Institutional deprivation
  Deprivation in hospital
References

In the first part of this chapter, the problem of deprivation is addressed in sociopolitical terms, i.e. deprivation of the child is regarded as the end result of social and economic deprivation acting on the adults. This view is probably the most important globally as it applies to the majority of potentially normal and loving families.

However, experience in the West has shown that even when social and economic deprivation is largely eradicated, there remains a substantial residue of children who suffer physical and emotional abuse and neglect at the hands of their own parents. Societies and professions have been slow to recognize this. In 1962, Henry Kempe had to coin the provocative title 'The battered baby syndrome' to bring home the reality of physical abuse to Western doctors.[1] Subsequently, Western society has also had to come to terms with the importance of emotional abuse and neglect as an entity in its own right. At present, the problem of sexual abuse is being recognized in all its magnitude and complexity. It seems inevitable that developing societies will tread

the same path. At present, it is likely that the majority of children abused or neglected by their parents in the developing world are forming part of the mortality statistics, either through malnutrition or through neglect of medical needs.

The implications of this are disturbing in the extreme. Western societies have developed extremely complicated and costly ways of intervening in cases of child abuse and neglect. These methods are of dubious efficacy in terms of the size of the problem and are quite inappropriate to developing societies. However, it is surely desirable that the professions in developing countries should acknowledge the existence of intrafamilial child abuse and neglect, and to develop as simple and effective a strategy as possible for intervention. The bottom line of this strategy should recognize that in the worst cases children deserve to be removed from their natural parents and provided with an alternative loving family for the rest of their childhood.

Physical abuse

Physical abuse (battered baby syndrome, non-accidental injury, NAI) has been recognized as a major problem in Western society since 1961. It was reported in East Africa as long ago as 1971 by Bwibo. The same author described eight cases with two deaths from Nairobi,[2] and suggested that many cases were being missed. Around the same time, a casualty surgeon from Nigeria reported over a hundred cases presenting to his hospital over a two-year period. It is likely that most doctors working with children in the Third World are seeing cases of physical abuse and that these are just the tip of the iceberg. While the extended family system can be an important factor in reducing the risk of abuse, no system is perfect, and the Kenyan paper stressed the role of uncles, aunts and stepmothers as potential abusers.

Diagnosis

The most important step in the diagnosis of NAI is to think of it in the first place. In the past, doctors tended naively to accept highly implausible explanations from parents and allowed children to go home after treatment. The diagnosis of NAI should be regarded as part of the differential diagnosis of all childhood accidents, especially in the under three years age group. In particular the diagnosis should be considered when a case differs from an innocent accident in the following ways:

- The account given of the 'accident' is not adequate to explain the observed injury. This is the most important element of the diagnosis. Accounts should be viewed with suspicion if they differ between parents and also if the account varies each time it is given. An invented story tends to be vague and lacking in detail.
- There is often an unnatural delay between the injury taking place and the parents seeking medical help. However, this is by no means a diagnostic feature. Some cases of NAI present early, and some innocent accidents present late for innocent reasons.
- The child may look frightened, sad or apathetic compared with a normal toddler, and may not be interacting normally with his parents. A young child who has been subject to repeated abuse may show the full-blown syndrome of 'frozen watchfulness', and almost catatonic behaviour. This feature is virtually diagnostic but it is a very late sign of serious abuse and *its absence in no way excludes the diagnosis of NAI.*
- The parents may behave oddly. They may appear hostile and defensive to the doctor, and lacking in normal concern for their child's injuries. They are often anxious to avoid being questioned and may leave the hospital suddenly without telling anyone.
- The child may disclose the truth. Any child old enough to speak will be an important source of evidence if questioned gently away from the parents. Of course, some parents will have already threatened the child to keep quiet and the child may only be able to tell the truth after being made to feel safe in hospital.

Management

While many countries have yet to develop machinery to tackle this problem, the following principles have been learned by bitter experience in the West:

- Child abuse does not cure itself. If a child is sent home with no action taken, there is a high likelihood that the child will be abused again and possibly killed. The child may suffer lasting emotional damage.
- It is no favour to parents to cover up their abusive behaviour. At worse they may eventually be charged with murder. It is unlikely they will experience much happiness caring for the child they are abusing. The very fact that they have brought the child to hospital is a 'cry for help'.
- Admission of the child to hospital is a reasonable first step. The hospital is a 'place of safety'. The diagnosis of NAI may be further considered at leisure and possibly refuted. For instance, a child with multiple bruises may be found to have a haematological disorder. Skeletal surveys, blood tests and photographs of the injury can be taken. The child's progress in hospital can be monitored, and observing the parents' behaviour and visiting pattern will be instructive.
- The child's growth and development should be assessed. Catch-up weight gain in hospital will suggest previous neglect.
- Some form of family assessment must be made and the welfare of other children in the family safeguarded.
- If the final decision is that the child has been abused, the child should be discharged to a short-term alternative family placement while social workers decide on the best long-term plan. Use of civil legislation based on the child's best interests is better than reliance on criminal prosecution of parents.

As the detection and management of NAI improves, it is usual to find a reduction in the number of severe injuries and deaths, with an increase in the number of 'early' cases.

Emotional deprivation and neglect

The term emotional deprivation covers a wide spectrum of severity, and clinical evidence varies greatly, depending on the age of the child. The younger the child the more likely it is that there will be detectable evidence of deprivation and neglect. Severe long-standing neglect of a preschool child will almost inevitably produce hard evidence of growth failure, developmental retardation and emotional effects.

Growth failure

Poor weight gain will be the earliest sign (see pp. 254–70). Eventually stunting of linear growth will occur. The child will have infantile body proportions (short arms and legs). 'Catch-up growth' on removal to a better environment is virtually diagnostic.

Developmental retardation

Marked deficits in all aspects of development will be present. Marked 'catch-up' of development on placement in a loving, stimulating environment will again confirm the diagnosis. This catch-up will be most marked for gross motor development and will be the slowest for speech and language, where the long-standing deficit of stimulus is less easy to correct. In the long-term there may be significant educational handicap.

Emotional effects

The child will appear dejected, apathetic and pitiable. There will be little ability for spontaneous play, activity or laughter. The interaction between parent and child will be lacking in warmth. The child will tolerate separation from the mother in marked contrast to other children at this age of maximal attachment behaviour. Similarly, the mother is happy to leave the child in hospital for long periods and may show little interest in reclaiming the child.

On removal to a loving environment, the child will rapidly 'blossom', showing a dramatic increase in happiness, liveliness and capacity to play. The child will then develop marked affection-seeking behaviour towards the caretakers.

If all the above features are seen in, for example, a four-year-old child, a confident diagnosis of psycho-social dwarfism can be made (deprivational dwarfism, non-organic failure to thrive, maternal rejection syndrome). This is a very serious diagnosis and unless one can achieve a dramatic change in the family's functioning, the best hope for the child is replacement therapy by a loving, adoptive family.

Of course, malnutrition can produce similar effects to those of emotional deprivation and, indeed, both conditions may coexist and overlap. It is probable that in the past many children were regarded simply as mal-nourished, and the underlying element of emotional deprivation and neglect was missed.

Another variety of emotional deprivation which may be widespread in the developing world is the situation where young children are informally fostered out with harsh, unloving relatives and are, in effect, used as cheap labour.

Long-term effects

A child who is not loved will grow into an adult who is unable to give and receive love. The lack of self-esteem in such a child carries through childhood and leads to educational underachievement and antisocial behaviour. The street children of Brazil are an example of this, with children as young as 12 years of age leading the life of hardened criminals. Any society which allows too many of its children to grow up without love is storing up problems for the future. Deprived children grow up into depriving parents, thus setting up a 'cycle of deprivation' which will run on and on into future generations.

Institutional deprivation

Every child has the right to be brought up in a loving family, either the child's own natural family or an alternative adoptive family if orphaned, abused or rejected. Unfortunately, many developing countries are repeating the mistakes of Western societies by setting up orphanages. These may be pioneered by religious societies or charities, or by revolutionary governments as prestige establishments, e.g. for 'the children of fallen heroes'. However good the motives, it must be stated that no institution can rival a loving family when it comes to meeting the emotional needs of young children. Almost forty years after John Bowlby's famous work[3] this message should not need to be repeated. All attempts should be made to close existing orphanages and to find good adoptive homes for the children.

Deprivation in hospital

Another form of institutional deprivation which the West pioneered was the admission of young children to hospitals without their mothers. This form of emotional abuse is still regrettably common in Europe despite many years of attempts to combat it.[4] Again it is to be hoped that the developing world will not repeat these mistakes. Planners should resist the temptation to build glossy teaching hospitals that are 'too clean' to tolerate resident parents. All children's wards should have mothers' accommodation as an integral feature.

References

1. Kempe CH *et al*. The battered child syndrome. *Journal of the American Medical Association*. 1962; **181**: 17.
2. Bwibo NO. Battered child syndrome. *East African Medical Journal*. 1971; **49**(11): 934–8.
3. Bowlby J. *Maternal Care and Mental Health*. Geneva, WHO Monograph Series No 2, 1951.
4. Robertson J. *Young Children in Hospital*. London, Tavistock, 1958.

CHAPTER 8

Genetics of tropical diseases

J. Burn and A. J. Clarke

Genes and inheritance can be implicated in all aspects of life. The genetic structure of immunoglobulins permits man to mount a specific response to any of the almost infinite range of bacterial antigens, while genetic mutations in the bacteria and other infectious agents serve to produce an ever-changing threat. The study of such genes and their products is now central to the attempts by the pharmaceutical industry to improve on available therapeutic agents. The pace of progress is illustrated by the recent report of a recombinant DNA vaccine to the *Plasmodium falciparum* sporozoite, based on the genetic sequencing of the circumsporozoite protein.[1] Animal and plant breeders attempt continually to 'improve' food sources, now aided by the techniques of genetic engineering. Politically, the minor genetic differences responsible for racial variation are exploited as a justification for tribal conflict.

This chapter is concerned with the practice of genetics as a clinical speciality and is therefore focused on the several thousand diseases, defects and malformations which result from alterations in gene structure and function. A small number of genetic disorders, particularly those relevant to medical practice in the tropics, will be used to illustrate the basic principles of inheritance.

What is a genetic disease?

Most gene defects are so obviously harmful that this might seem a strange question, but the answer is not always simple. The inability of humans to produce ascorbic acid makes this an essential dietary compound – vitamin C. If a majority of humans shared the ability of several other species to produce this vitamin, scurvy would be regarded as a treatable 'inborn error of metabolism'. Lactose intolerance provides another example. The only known naturally occurring source of the disaccharide lactose is mammalian milk. Inability to digest this sugar in infancy due to congenital lactase deficiency, described by Holzel *et al.*,[2] results in severe diarrhoea (see pp. 463, 465). This may cause failure to thrive and possible death. Subsequent to this first report, it became apparent that adult lactase deficiency was common.[3] In a majority of the world's population weaning is followed by a major decline in intestinal lactase. Milk ingestion after infancy in such individuals causes dose-related abdominal distension, borborygmi and pain. However, there is a strong geographical correlation between communities with a long-established dairy industry and a high population incidence of lactase persistence into adulthood. Archaeological evidence of a dairy industry dates back to about 4000 BC in the Sahara. The mutation responsible for persistence of lactase production may have allowed this development. Carriers of the gene would be better able to take advantage of raw milk as a food source; a selective advantage. Family studies have shown the lactose tolerance gene to be dominant to the 'wild type' intolerance[4] so selection in favour of the gene could have caused a rapid rise in gene frequency. Some populations, particularly subgroups with lactose intolerance living in areas of lactose tolerance such as those of Jewish and Arabic origin, became able to circumvent the genetic disadvantage of 'normality' by turning milk into yoghurt or old cheese; the lactose is digested by lactobacilli. It has been suggested that the selective advantage which had previously made milk intolerance the norm was the tendency to discourage weaned young from demanding breast-milk, as this would jeopardize the health of the mother and the prospects for subsequent children. Knowledge of this genetic variant has both improved management of malnutrition in the Third World and given an insight into the genetic factors which underlie disease.

Sickle cell disease is another genetic disorder made common by environmental pressure in certain populations (see pp. 827–31). It will be examined in detail because it provides an insight into genetics at three levels: as a basic science, as an applied science and as a clinical art.

Sickle cell disease was the first genetic disease to be fully understood at the molecular level. The sickle cell gene codes for an abnormal β-globin protein which, along with α-globin, forms the protein element of haemoglobin. Carriers of the sickle cell gene are clinically normal because the other copy of the gene produces normal β-globin in sufficient quantities to ensure health. Carriers are said to have the sickle cell trait and are particularly numerous among certain populations such as those of black African descent. Sickle cell trait is very common in areas where malaria is endemic; it does not offer direct protection against malaria, but seems greatly to reduce the risk of death from cerebral malaria associated with *Plasmodium falciparum*. This selective advantage has made the gene common, despite the fact that inheritance of two copies of this gene causes sickle cell disease. The advantage of malarial resistance outweighed the disadvantage of impaired health among the homozygotes with two copies of the gene. This gene has now become a major disadvantage in populations where malaria is no longer prevalent, such as the black Americans of African descent, where about one in 12 carry this gene.

It is worth noting that another genetic variant in black Africans, absence of the Duffy blood group, confers even more effective resistance to *Plasmodium vivax* malaria because the parasite uses this blood group antigen as its means of fixation to the red blood cell and without it cannot gain entry.[5] Loss of this blood group antigen is not known to be a disadvantage, in contrast to the situation with the sickle cell gene.

To understand the basic biology of the sickle cell gene it is necessary to review the basic structure of genes and chromosomes. Human cells contain in their nucleus 46 chromosomes which come in matching pairs, one of each pair having been inherited from each parent in the ovum and the spermatozoon. The chromosomes are numbered in descending order of size and are identified by their banding patterns at microscopy after preparation with Giemsa stain. These 46 chromosomes together carry an estimated 50 000 genes, each gene being a coded message with the genes arranged along the chromosomes rather like beads on a string. Since the chromosomes come in matching pairs, so do the genes. The two copies of the β-globin gene are carried on the pair of number 11 chromosomes. In the precursors of red cells the two copies of the β-globin gene, together with the copies of the α-globin gene on chromosome 16, direct the synthesis of haemoglobin.

The process whereby proteins are created involves several steps collectively described as transcription and translation. The chemical compound from which chromosomes and genes are made is the molecule deoxyribonucleic acid (DNA) which has a ladder-like structure. The longer sides of the ladder are made up of alternating molecules of phosphate and a sugar (deoxyribose), while the rungs of the ladder are made up from the four bases adenine, cytosine, guanine and thymine (A, C, G, T). Each rung of the ladder has two bases loosely joined by hydrogen bonds in the centre. Adenine is always paired with thymine and guanine with cytosine, and thus the bases ACTT on one side will be matched to TGAA on the other. When cells replicate, the DNA molecule splits along its length, each part acting as a template for the creation of a matching strand. This ability of the DNA molecule to duplicate itself is the basis of all life; it allows the genetic information to be transmitted to daughter cells and subsequently through gametes to the next generation.

About 5 per cent of the DNA in each set of chromosomes comprises the coding sequences that we call genes (Fig. 3.8.1). Each gene directs the production of a chain of amino acids, a polypeptide, which in turn is modified to form an enzyme or a structural protein. To code all the 20 amino acids required for the polypeptide chains, the bases must be read in sets of three. Using four bases there are 64 possible triplet combinations (codons), so the code is said to be degenerate in that most amino acids have more than one codon. Only methionine has a single codon, which acts as the start

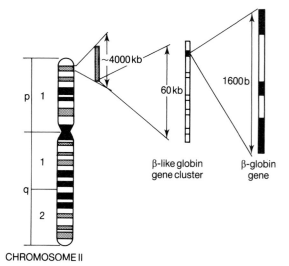

CHROMOSOME II

Fig. 3.8.1 A diagram of chromosome 11 showing the band which contains the β-globin gene. This is about 4000 kb long. The β-globin gene itself is 1600 bases long with three coding sequences (exons) separated by two intervening sequences (introns). (Reproduced from Fraser Roberts and Pembrey, *An Introduction to Medical Genetics*, 1985, by permission of the Oxford University Press.)

signal in all genes. Three triplets do not code for an amino acid and are read as stop signals.

When the β-globin gene is activated in red cell precursors the DNA strands separate. The strand which carries the coded message, the sense strand, is then transcribed by the formation of a matching single-stranded molecule of nuclear RNA (Fig. 3.8.2). RNA (ribonucleic acid) is very similar to DNA, but contains the sugar ribose in the place of deoxyribose along the long sides of the ladder. Apart from being single-stranded, RNA differs from DNA in using the base uracil instead of thymine. Some stretches of DNA within genes do not code for amino acids and are called intervening sequences or introns. These are transcribed along with the rest of the gene into RNA but are then removed within the nucleus, to leave the messenger RNA (mRNA). This is then transferred to the ribosomes in the cytoplasm, where it acts as a template for the polypeptide chain. Here, molecules of RNA called transfer RNA (tRNA) attach themselves to the mRNA in the ribosome, each different tRNA recognizing a specific triplet and bringing with it the appropriate amino acid. In this way, the amino acids are joined end-to-end to form the primary protein.

In β-globin there are 146 amino acids. Analysis of the protein in sickle cell disease reveals a single amino acid change with valine replacing glutamic acid at position

6. This is the result of a single base change in the DNA sequence, from a T to an A. This single point mutation results in a major biological change in the protein. When the haemoglobin molecule is deoxygenated, the valine lies in an exposed position and allows haemoglobin molecules to attach themselves to one another in chains which distort the red cell into the characteristic sickle shape. This causes the red cells to lyse more easily and also to clump together blocking circulation in various parts of the vascular tree. Obstruction of the vascular network of the spleen causes progressive damage to this organ with subsequent increase in sensitivity to infection.

This brief review of the molecular basis of sickle cell disease serves to illustrate the way in which genetics as a basic science can shed light on clinical diseases. Most of this story was deduced by protein chemists in the 1960s, but the complete story only became apparent with the development of recombinant DNA techniques which allow analysis at the gene level. These techniques are discussed in more detail later. First, sickle cell disease will be used to illustrate some aspects of genetics as a clinical science.

Autosomal recessive inheritance

While the details of gene function are complex, the basic principles of inheritance employed in genetic counselling are very simple. Genes come in matching pairs and both copies are normally used to code for the relevant protein or enzyme. When a faulty copy of the gene is inherited, the quantity of gene product is reduced by half. If that is enough for normal health and function, the gene defect is called recessive because its presence is concealed by the normal gene. Disease only then occurs if an individual inherits two bad copies of the gene, one from each parent. In the case of the sickle cell gene, the number of children with two copies of the gene, or homozygotes, is considerable because the gene is so common in certain populations. Where one person in 12 carries the gene, one in 144 couples will both be heterozygotes, with each carrying one normal gene and one sickle gene. When this occurs, each member of the couple has a one in two chance of passing on the haemoglobin S gene, so there is a one in four chance that both will pass on a faulty copy to the same child and thereby cause the disease. Thus, where the frequency of carriers is one in 12 the frequency of homozygotes is one in 576. For any recessive disease the number of carriers in the population can be calculated by reversing this process. For example, in white European populations as many as one in 1600 children has cystic fibrosis, which is the

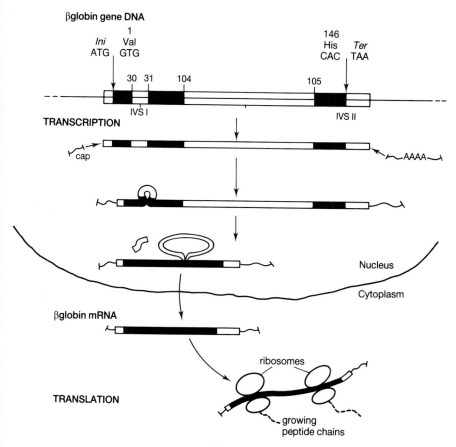

βglobin gene DNA

Fig. 3.8.2 Transcription of the β-globin gene to nuclear RNA and thence to messenger RNA. The bases which initiate (Ini) and terminate (Ter) are shown, together with the base codon of the first amino acid (valine) and the last (histidine). (Reproduced from Fraser Roberts and Pembrey, *An Introduction to Medical Genetics*, 1985, by permission of the Oxford University Press.)

chance of having two copies of the gene. The gene frequency in the whole population must then be the square root of one in 1600 which is one in 40. The chance of being a carrier is one in 20 since each normal member of the population has two copies of the gene and therefore has two chances of having a faulty copy.

It can be seen from this calculation that even rare recessive diseases can be associated with a high carrier rate in the population. It is estimated that, on average, all humans are carriers of one major autosomal recessive gene defect. This is important in those populations where cousin marriage is common. If we start with the assumption that each member of the population has one bad gene, there is a half chance that that particular gene was inherited from the father and a half chance that it came from the mother. There is a one in four chance that the individual shares that particular faulty gene in common with, say, the mother's brother and a one in eight chance of it being shared in common with the mother's brother's child. In other words, there is a one in eight chance that first cousins will share the same faulty gene and hence a one in 32 chance or approximately 3 per cent risk of a child with a recessive gene defect as a result. This is 10 times higher than the risk of recessive gene defects seen in populations where cousin marriage is rare, though in absolute terms it remains a small risk. For this reason, few societies make cousin marriage illegal.

On the other hand, an argument against the practice of cousin marriage can be made in those populations where it has become traditional. One reason for not intervening has been the claim that prolonged inbreeding will lead to the loss of deleterious genes, and hence a decline in the number of recessive diseases. In practice, this effect has not been demonstrated in the populations observed to date.

Before attempting to discourage cousin marriage, it must be remembered that attempts to reduce consanguinity in a society where it has been practised for generations can have serious consequences. Cousin marriage is closely related to the religious and social structure of a society. Only a change in this structure could reduce consanguinity and this would inevitably carry a risk of social disruption. For example, there could be serious economic consequences such as increased fragmentation of property and punitive dowry payments. It is common in some groups for a brother and sister in one sibship to marry a brother and sister in another so that no dowry payment is necessary.

Molecular genetics in clinical practice

The last decade has seen an explosion of knowledge in molecular biology as applied to genetics. It is now possible to identify the carriers of some important diseases and to offer accurate prenatal diagnosis by the use of DNA probes specific for disease genes or closely linked regions of the chromosome in question. The level of expertise of the laboratory staff and the cost of the materials, particularly the restriction enzymes and radioactive label ^{32}P, make these techniques very high technology medicine. On the other hand, newer methods will make the techniques cheaper and easier, and preventive measures are even more deserving of resources when effective care for the chronically sick is limited by financial restraint.

A few basic facts are essential to an understanding of the process. A restriction enzyme cuts a length of DNA into small fragments: a large number of these enzymes are now commercially available. They occur naturally in different bacteria and derive their names from their sources, for example, *Eco*R1 comes from *E. coli* plasmid R. A restriction enzyme is, perhaps, best seen as a pair of scissors capable of reading the DNA code. It will only cut at its own specific sequence of bases, its cutting site. If an individual's DNA is cleaved with a restriction enzyme, it will be broken into many thousands of fragments. Wherever the DNA comes from in the body it will be identical, and so the collection of DNA pieces from that individual will always be the same. The great variability in the base sequence between individuals, however, means that different people will produce different numbers and sizes of fragments with a particular restriction enzyme. Since chromosomes come in matching pairs, one from each parent, there are often many base sequence differences between the two

chromosomes in each pair. Consequently differences in cutting sites and hence fragment sizes are found. Such common differences are called 'polymorphisms'. A polymorphism identified using a restriction enzyme is called a restriction fragment length polymorphism (RFLP). The length of such a DNA fragment is measured by comparison with known lengths of DNA and is recorded as the number of nucleic acid bases in the chain. It is usually expressed as kilobases because most fragments are several thousand bases long.

The two strands of a DNA molecule can be made to separate quite easily under laboratory conditions. If they are allowed to reassociate, each half will find its matching partner thanks to the unique sequence of bases on each strand. An isolated fragment of single-stranded DNA can be used to find its matching base sequence among the multitude of fragments generated by a restriction enzyme. A piece of DNA used in this way is called a gene probe. To identify it in the laboratory, the gene probe is made radioactive by incorporation of ^{32}P into its phosphate-sugar backbone. The gene probe then reveals its position on overlying X-ray film as an autoradiograph.

Reverse transcriptase is a viral enzyme capable of making DNA from mRNA. The product is called complementary DNA (cDNA). It differs from the original in the absence of intervening sequences (see earlier). A cDNA molecule resembles the original closely enough to hybridize strongly with the parent gene. For haemoglobin, the red cell precursors can be used to extract the β-globin mRNA, from which cDNA can then be produced.

To use this piece of DNA for diagnostic purposes it is necessary to produce identical copies in bulk. This is achieved by incorporating the desired DNA molecule into a plasmid, a primitive parasite of bacteria, comprising a piece of DNA formed into a circle. If a piece of human DNA is excised with a particular restriction enzyme and the same enzyme is used to cut the plasmid, mixing these together can generate plasmids which have incorporated the human sequence. This happens because the restriction fragments have the same pattern of 'sticky ends' as the plasmids. Introduction of the modified plasmid into a laboratory culture of *E. coli* allows the plasmid to multiply. Excision of the human DNA using the same restriction enzyme results in millions of copies of the original cDNA.

These various steps can now be put together to outline their first use as a diagnostic process (Fig. 3.8.3).[6] β-globin RNA was extracted and copied with reverse transcriptase to produce cDNA. This was multiplied in a plasmid grown in *E. coli*, and radio-

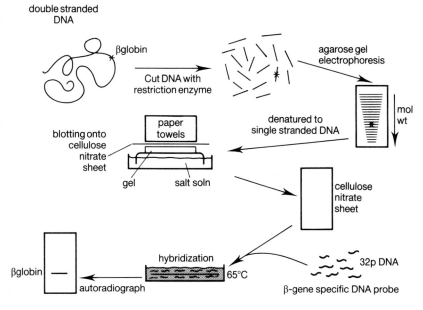

Fig. 3.8.3 An outline of the laboratory steps used to localize the DNA fragment or fragments carrying the β-globin gene. (Reproduced from Fraser Roberts and Pembrey, *An Introduction to Medical Genetics*, 1985, by permission of Oxford University Press.)

activity was incorporated into this to produce a radioactive DNA probe.

The DNA from a patient was then digested with the restriction enzyme *EcoR1*, and the fragments spread out by electrophoresis in an agarose gel (see Fig. 3.8.4). The small fragments travelled further than the larger fragments. These DNA fragments were then absorbed on to a nitrocellulose sheet for permanent fixation (Southern blotting).[7] Addition of the radioactive gene probe to the Southern blot allowed some of the probe molecules to attach to the matching gene sequence on DNA from the patient. Exposure of the blot to X-ray film produced an autoradiograph of the probe. Because the two number 11 chromosomes carrying the β-globin gene in a particular individual had differences in their pattern of restriction enzyme cleavage sites, the two copies of the gene were often attached to fragments of different sizes. These then produced two bands on the final autoradiograph, each band corresponding to one of the chromosome 11s. It so happened that individuals with two bands were carriers of the sickle trait, with one normal and one sickle gene.

The four possible results found in the children of a couple who both carried the sickle trait are illustrated in Fig. 3.8.5. Since this DNA testing may be performed on samples taken from chorionic villi in early pregnancy, antenatal diagnosis of sickle cell disease may be offered, with the selective termination of

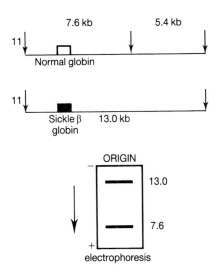

Fig. 3.8.4 The position of a band on the autoradiograph is determined by the size of the DNA fragment that has been recognized by the probe. In the population studied by Kan and Dozy, the sickle gene was associated with the loss of one restriction enzyme site cut by *EcoR1*, so that the sickle gene was generally found on the larger 13 kb fragment. This migrates more slowly from the origin of the gel and is therefore seen at the top of the autoradiograph. The normal gene is found on a 7.6 kb fragment, migrates further along the gel, and is therefore seen further from the origin on the X-ray plate.

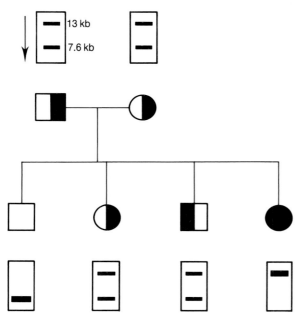

Fig. 3.8.5   An ideal pedigree is shown where the four offspring have the four possible patterns of inheritance of the *Eco*R1 polymorphism detected by the β-globin probe. Each parent has two number 11 chromosomes which differ; one chromosome has the cutting site close to the gene while the other does not. Two bands therefore appear on the DNA blots from both parents. The affected child has inherited the chromosome 11 which has the missing enzyme cutting site, from both parents, resulting in a single band at the 13 kb position. This indicates that the chromosome with the absent *Eco*R1 cutting site is the one with the sickle gene in both parents. The patterns in the three healthy children, two of whom are carriers, are compatible with this explanation. Thus, the linked restriction fragment length polymorphism (RFLP) has allowed the disease gene to be tracked.

affected fetuses. It should be understood that such straightforward testing is not always possible, because the association of one allele with one fragment size of DNA is only rarely as close as was found for sickle cell in the population first studied by Kan and Dozy. This fortunately allowed them to track the faulty gene in their families.

Subsequent research into the genetic basis of sickle cell disease has led to the development of a specific diagnostic test.[8, 9] The restriction enzyme *Msp*II has a cutting site which embraces base 17 in the coding sequence of the β-globin gene. In the sickle cell mutation the cutting site is lost and the effect on the band patterns allows a direct diagnosis of the carrier state and affected homozygote. Similar use of gene-specific probes, particularly those called oligonucleotide

probes derived from short sequences of the gene itself, has been made in β-thalassaemia where production of the whole β-globin is impaired. Such an approach requires a precise knowledge of the abnormality in the gene. It is likely that in many genetic diseases, as is the case in thalassaemia, a great many different mutations within the gene can produce the same clinical defect. Such simple methods as that applied to sickle cell disease, where each case has the same change in DNA base sequence, will not be applicable. The use of RFLPs as linked markers capable of tracking the faulty gene within a pedigree is likely to remain the method of choice in these diseases, where there is no molecular uniformity of the underlying defect.

The laboratory approach outlined for sickle cell can be applied to any disease where RNA from the gene involved can be isolated. Most single gene defects involve unknown genes and this approach is not possible. It is then necessary to use gene probes linked to the same small chromosome region as the disease gene. The advantages and limitations of this approach are discussed in the next section.

A major impact of DNA diagnosis in sickle cell disease, thalassaemia and other serious gene defects is that it makes possible prenatal diagnosis in the first trimester. A piece of trophoblast can be removed from the placenta either transabdominally or transcervically; its DNA can then be extracted and analysed to reveal the genetic constitution of the fetus. If it is shown to be homozygous for the gene defect a termination can be offered. This technique currently involves a risk of miscarriage thought to be in the region of 2 per cent, but is preferred to amniocentesis by most families since it allows selective termination before 12 weeks of pregnancy. This is safer for the mother, is more confidential, and is less distressing than a late termination performed after amniocentesis.

Autosomal dominant inheritance

If one good copy of a gene is not sufficient for normal health, the inheritance of a faulty copy will cause a disease. In this situation the abnormal gene is expressed despite the presence of a normal copy, and is then called a dominant gene defect. If an individual has such a gene defect there is a 50 per cent risk of its being transmitted to each offspring; when gametes are formed a single copy of each pair of genes is transmitted with a random choice being made between the two. Whereas many metabolic defects are transmitted as recessive traits, defects in structural proteins are often dominant traits. By analogy, a house will fall down if half of the bricks used crumble away. In contrast, cellular metabolism may still function even if the quantity of an enzyme is reduced by one half. As with the recessive disorders, a whole range of dominant disorders could be discussed but attention will be focussed on only two: variegate porphyria and Huntington's chorea.

Variegate porphyria

Variegate porphyria is a genetic defect in porphyrin metabolism. The porphyrins are precursors of the compound haem, a structural component of haemoglobin along with the globin chains. The disorder is extremely common in South African Boers due to the founder effect. A Dutch Boer carrying this gene emigrated to South Africa and married a young orphan girl in 1688. He transmitted the gene to several members of his large family. Over the subsequent two centuries, the Boers of South Africa had the benefit of a good climate and excellent farming land, with the result that the population grew almost exponentially and with it, the variegate porphyria gene. This was not a major problem, since the only obvious effect of this condition at that time was to make carriers of the gene light-sensitive. The gene defect became a more obvious disease with the advent of modern medicine because carriers of this gene are sensitive to barbiturates. These drugs can precipitate porphyric crises with bizarre symptoms of psychiatric disturbance, abdominal pains and in extreme cases coma and death. In many cases these would be triggered by short-acting barbiturate anaesthetics and the response would be to repeat the anaesthetic on the assumption that the abdominal pain was due to a surgical emergency. As a result, several carriers of the gene died and the clinical burden of this condition increased dramatically.

Huntington's chorea

This chronic progressive neurological disorder is characterized by choreiform movements and dementia. The gene involved has been localized to chromosome 4. It would seem that mutation at this gene locus is very rare since only one convincing new mutation has been identified and described in the literature.[10] Despite this, the gene has become relatively common in several populations thanks to its variable expression; unlike many genetic diseases which are apparent from birth, Hungtington's chorea rarely manifests before adulthood and in most cases is first diagnosed in the fourth or fifth decade of life. As a result, gene carriers will usually have completed their family before it is realized that they carry the gene. There is even a suggestion that

gene carriers have more children, either because of a direct effect on their reproductive capacity or because the early effects of the dementing process cause disinhibition and more unplanned pregnancies.

This situation contrasts with many dominant disorders in which onset at birth and severe effects in childhood reduce the probability of childbearing. This is described as a reduced genetic fitness since the gene is unlikely to be transmitted to the next generation. In this situation, the population incidence is maintained by new mutations of the gene. Achondroplasia, for example, is relatively severe, so that few affected individuals in the past have gone on to produce children. It is estimated that 80 per cent of children with achondroplasia carry new mutations.

The gene for Huntington's chorea was located using molecular genetic techniques. Since the nature of the chemical defect in the brain was unknown, complementary DNA probes could not be created. Instead, linked intergenic probes were used. Gusella *et al.* in the 1980s set to work to track the Huntington's chorea gene using linked markers.[11] The markers were obtained from a genomic library. It will be recalled that the majority of human DNA does not code for specific genes and appears to have no specific function. Nevertheless, its base sequence contains areas which are unique. If the total human DNA is digested with a restriction enzyme and the fragments used one at a time to produce gene probes, some of these will be shown to produce only a single band or a small number of bands on a Southern blot, suggesting that they are specific to one particular point on one of the chromosomes. Various techniques are then available to map such probes, to discover from which chromosome they derive.

Gusella's group analysed the polymorphisms with several probes in families with Huntington's chorea. One probe, known as G8, was found to be highly polymorphic because it picked up an area with two variable cutting sites, which meant that there were four different fragment patterns on Southern blotting, termed A,B,C and D. In each of the families studied, it was found that a particular letter would always travel with the Huntington's disease; in one large family, for example, the carriers of the disease gene always showed, with the G8 probe, at least one of the chromosomes carrying the C marker. When a marker invariably travels with the disease it is said to be linked to the disease gene locus. It provides clear evidence that the piece of DNA for which the marker is specific lies in close proximity to the disease gene on the same chromosome. This means that they tend to be inherited together, and not independently, as Mendel suggested for single gene inheritance.

It was originally estimated that some 400 markers would be necessary completely to cover the 22 pairs of autosomes (it was already known that Huntington's chorea could not be X-linked because both males and females were affected and because males transmitted it to their sons). Gusella's group were fortunate to find a very closely linked marker almost at their first attempt. Following publication of this report in 1983, the debate on presymptomatic testing became more intense. This debate will be repeated for many diseases but is particularly difficult with Huntington's chorea because of the inevitably progressive nature of the disease and its severity.

It has been argued that it is inappropriate to inform healthy adults that they will develop such a disease later in life. On the other hand, many potential gene carriers who face a one in two risk of having inherited the gene argue that they have already suffered its disadvantages, since they fear having children and are unable to get insurance or to adopt. They argue that if they can show that they do not carry the gene then their life will be greatly enhanced, whereas if they are proven to be gene carriers it will have little impact on them other than meaning that they can use the same techniques for prenatal diagnosis to avoid transmitting the gene to the next generation.

The reason for discussing this particular example is that one of the very large families used to localize Huntington's chorea to chromosome 4 came from Venezuela. Without that large family it may have taken a great deal longer to localize the gene. The important lesson is that there is considerable scope for medical workers in any corner of the globe to contribute to the mapping of the human genome which is now well under way. In almost all cases, localization of a faulty gene will first depend on the use of linked markers in families with a disease resulting from a defect in that gene. In many cases, families with several affected members will be particularly common in less developed societies where selective termination of pregnancy and genetic counselling services are less readily available, or where religious or social practices restrict the use of contraception.

Once a gene has been localized by this approach, it becomes possible to map the area in more detail and ultimately to identify the diseased gene itself. The gene for cystic fibrosis has recently been identified in this way and many more are set to follow.[12] It is likely that effective treatment for genetic diseases will only occur once the gene defect has been identified and its product synthesized.

Sex-linked disease

The transmission of certain harmful traits through females to affect their sons has been recognized since Biblical times. Only in this century, however, has there been an explanation for the phenomenon. The chromosomal constitution (karyotype) of males and females differs; in addition to the 22 pairs of chromosomes that men and women share (the autosomes), a woman has a pair of X chromosomes and a man has one X and one, much smaller, Y chromosome. Whereas a woman's ova all contain a similar set of 22 autosomes plus one X chromosome, a man's spermatozoa contain 22 autosomes plus either an X or a Y chromosome.

There are two consequences of this genetic difference between the sexes. First, the sex of a child is determined by whether the sperm that fertilizes the ovum carries an X or a Y chromosome to produce a girl or a boy respectively. Second, each cell in the female carries more genetic information than in the male, because the X chromosome is much larger than the Y and contains much more DNA. In other situations, when individuals differ in such a large fraction of the genetic material, development is usually disrupted and the pregnancy may miscarry; but for the X chromosome, this does not occur. Instead, only one X chromosome functions in each cell, however many X chromosomes are present. This is true for all mammals, and ensures that the balance of active X chromosome genes to autosomal genes is the same in each cell. The process of X chromosome inactivation seems to occur at a specific time for each tissue in embryogenesis, at the stage of terminal cell differentiation, and is termed Lyonization. Which X chromosome is inactivated in any cell in the embryo is random but once it has occurred, the same X chromosome will be inactivated in all the daughter cells derived from each embryonic cell. Hence the maternal X chromosome will be active in some cell lines of a woman and the paternal X chromosome will function in the other cell lines.

Whether a woman who is heterozygous for an X-linked trait will manifest both her copies of the gene will depend upon two factors. First, the random events of Lyonization may result in one X chromosome functioning in a majority of her cells. Second, it will depend upon the biological nature of the gene; is it expressed locally (independently) by each cell or tissue, or is it a function of the whole organism? A skin disorder may produce a patchy effect on a female's skin, whereas a clotting disorder such as haemophilia may result in below-average plasma levels of coagulation factors that affect the whole body. The terms 'recessive' and 'dominant' are rather less useful in describing sex-linked than autosomal traits.

The inactivated X chromosome in female cells is much more readily stained than the other chromosomes during most of the cell cycle because it remains condensed when the functioning chromosomes have lost much of their structure; this is the reason for the appearance of Barr bodies in epithelial cell nuclei of a woman's buccal mucosa.

The fact that a woman is composed of two distinct sets of cells, which differ in whether the functioning X is derived from her mother or her father, provides some protection in the event of her inheritance of a deleterious gene from either parent; the unfavourable characteristics will be expressed in only some of her cells. A man, in contrast, has no such protection from the ill effects of a gene present on his one X chromosome, which always comes from his mother; if this X carries an unfavourable gene, then it will be expressed.

Sex-linked traits are transmitted through a family in a characteristic fashion. A female carrier will transmit the gene to half her sons (who will manifest the condition) and to half her daughters (who will manifest the condition to a variable extent); a man will transmit an X-linked trait to half his children, to none of his sons and to all of his daughters (who all receive his sole X chromosome). A gene that is transmitted from father to son cannot be X-linked.

Haemophilia

Haemophilia is a sex-linked disorder of coagulation, in which the affected men have a deficiency of one component of the coagulation cascade, either factor 8 (in haemophilia A) or factor 9 (in haemophilia B, Christmas disease). (See p. 836.) Both these clotting factors are encoded by genes located near the tip of the long arm of the X chromosome. Women who carry either disorder will usually produce half the usual quantity of normal clotting factor plus the same quantity of a defective clotting factor; half of the cells producing these factors will be using the 'wrong' gene. This forms the basis for tests that can identify carriers of the haemophilia genes; such carriers produce a normal quantity of clotting factor as identified by radioimmunoassay, but typically only half as much when tested by a bioassay (a test of clotting ability). The ratio of the clotting activity to the clotting factor antigen is half of the normal. Occasionally, sufficient of the women's cells will inactivate the normal allele (the normal copy of the gene) that she manifests a minor bleeding tendency herself.

The genes for both factor 8 and factor 9 have been isolated and gene-specific probes are available for carrier detection and prenatal diagnosis.

Muscular dystrophy

Several muscular dystrophies are inherited on the X chromosome, including the most common variety, Duchenne muscular dystrophy, which affects one in 3000 boys. This is a progressive disorder in which boys may be normal in infancy but then suffer delay in achievement of motor milestones and are unable to run. They develop a waddling gait because of their proximal muscle weakness and have great difficulty in climbing up stairs or standing up from the floor. Calf hypertrophy is typical and so is a grossly elevated serum creatine kinase (CK) activity. Many boys are mildly or moderately impaired intellectually. The usual course is that a boy is confined to a wheelchair by the age of 10 years and that he dies in his late teens or early twenties, often of chest infection; weakness of his respiratory muscles is compounded by scoliosis that may develop once he is confined to a chair. A similar condition, Becker muscular dystrophy, presents later in childhood, and progresses more slowly; confinement to a chair may occur in the 20s or 30s, and death in the 40s from chest infection or cardiac disease.

The gene for Duchenne muscular dystrophy (DMD) is located on the short arm of the X chromosome. Becker dystrophy results from a less disruptive defect in the same gene.

The last decade has seen a dramatic advance in knowledge of the cause of DMD.[13] The mammoth gene is over 2 million bases long. The mRNA of 14 kb is produced from over 65 coding sequences and the protein has been named dystrophin. Using gene specific probes, 70 per cent of affected boys have been shown to have a missing segment.

Women who carry the DMD gene are only rarely clinically affected by it, but they may have elevated levels of muscle proteins such as CK and myoglobin in their serum. By CK testing of the serum of female relatives of males with DMD or Becker, in conjunction with gene probe analysis, it is possible to identify most carriers of DMD with a fair degree of accuracy. When pregnant, carriers may then choose to terminate a male fetus. In most families, it is possible to distinguish male fetuses at high risk of Duchenne from those at low risk, with 95 per cent accuracy; it is then possible for female carriers to give birth to normal boys in relative safety.

If the affected boy displays a deletion, precise prenatal diagnosis is made possible.

G6PD deficiency

This is a common condition in the tropics and sub-tropics (see pp. 221–3, 827–8). The enzyme glucose-6-phosphate dehydrogenase (G6PD) is encoded by a gene located near the haemophilia loci on the X-chromosome long arm. There are many variant forms of the enzyme, most of which have a reduced level of activity compared with the normal protein. G6PD is the rate-determining step of the pentose phosphate pathway, which maintains intracellular NADPH. This is required to maintain adequate glutathione in erythrocytes, protecting the – SH groups of haemoglobin against oxidative damage. Without this protection, haemoglobin can denature to form Heinz bodies and the erythrocytes can lyse. This is thought to happen because the oxidized haem groups directly damage the cell membrane.

Men who carry one of the variant forms of G6PD are susceptible to haemolysis under conditions of oxidative stress, particularly when exposed to certain drugs or infections, and (in the Mediterranean form of G6PD deficiency) when exposed to fava beans (favism). The haemolytic crises produced, may result in hyper-bilirubinaemia, and (in neonates) kernicterus; in adults or older children acute renal failure may be caused by the haemoglobinuria. Some uncommon G6PD variants produce chronic haemolysis and may necessitate splenectomy.

As with many of the thalassaemias and haemo-globinopathies, G6PD deficiency is distributed throughout the world's malarial zones; the large number of variant forms demonstrates that many independent mutations causing G6PD deficiencies have occurred and persisted. Women who are heterozygous for G6PD, with one normal allele and one variant allele, are more resistant to malarial parasites than are normals. They have the best of both worlds, because they are not susceptible to the drug, sepsis, or bean-triggered haemolysis. Men with G6PD deficiencies, and homozygous women, are also at some advantage when infected with malaria, but less so than the hetero-zygotes. One reason for this is that *Plasmodium falciparum* seems able to produce its own G6PD enzyme, but only in individuals who almost totally lack the enzyme activity. However, these individuals suffer the ill-effects of haemolytic crises.

In contrast to haemophilia and DMD, the X inactivation pattern of a heterozygote for G6PD defi-ciency can be determined in small patches of skin. Patches of 1 mm or so diameter are derived from a single embryonic cell at the time of lyonization. G6PD was one of the first markers used to confirm the occurrence of lyonization in humans, and was used simultaneously to demonstrate the clonal origin of neoplasms from a single cell.[14] Even tiny fragments of myometrium ($1\,mm^3$) from G6PD heterozygotes almost always contain both forms of the enzyme; only one form is found in any one leiomyoma, however. Different leiomyomata from the same woman may have different variants of the enzyme, confirming the independent origin of each tumour.

Chromosome Defects

Aneuploidy means 'not good set' and describes any visible defect of the 46 chromosomes. Following the recognition in 1959 of an extra chromosome 21 as the cause of Down's syndrome, a host of chromosome syndromes involving deletion or duplication of all or parts of chromosomes have been described. The technique of chromosome banding introduced in the early 1970s allowed more precise delineation of structural errors (Fig. 3.8.6). The investigation of a retarded dysmorphic child is not complete without chromosome analysis. With the important exception of sex chromosome anomalies such as Turner's syndrome (45X instead of 46XX or 46XY), aneuploidy causes significant mental handicap in virtually all cases. This statement refers to defects visible to the microscopist. With the more subtle techniques of molecular gene-tics, submicroscopic deletions have been shown to be a common cause of 'single gene defects' without retardation.

Chromosome defects are very common; about 10 per cent of recognized pregnancies are affected. The great majority of such defects lead to spontaneous abortion. Among survivors to full-term, trisomy 21 is the most common at one in 700 births. This disorder is more common in older mothers but shows little evidence of geographical variation.

When multiple cases of retardation or spontaneous miscarriage occur in a family pedigree, the possibility of a translocation must be considered. These are of two types. A Robertsonian translocation involves fusion of two chromosomes, usually 14 and 21. If, at meiosis, the 14 attached to the 21 travels with the free 21, the gamete will lead to a child with trisomy 21. The theoretical one in two risk of this error is reduced to about one in 10 for a carrier mother and less than one in 100 for a carrier father, by spontaneous loss between gamete production and birth of the child.

This sex difference in risk is not apparent in reciprocal translocations. These involve exchange of chromosome material between two chromosomes.

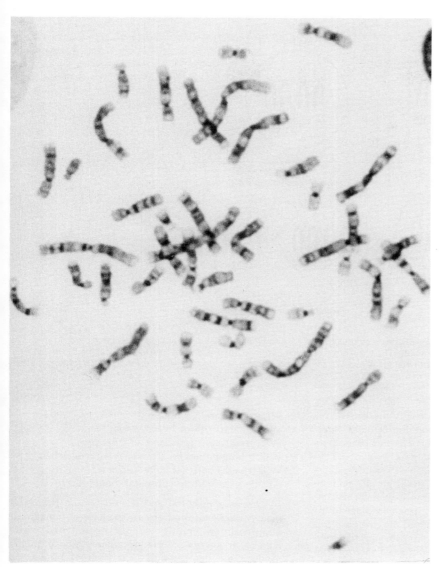

Fig. 3.8.6 A metaphase spread of chromosomes from a single white blood cell (from one of the authors) stained with Giemsa to produce the band patterns which allow the 23 pairs of chromosomes to be identified.

Figure 3.8.7 illustrates a family in which chromosome analysis revealed an extra piece of chromosome on the end of a chromosome 13. The father was found to carry an 8 to 13 translocation. He had passed on in the sperm the normal 8 and the abnormal 13 making the child trisomic for the short arm of 8. Their normal son had received the two abnormal chromosomes making him a balanced carrier like the father. Such carriers have a theoretical one in two risk of abnormal offspring. This is reduced by selective loss of unbalanced embryos to a risk of one in five. This is a high risk which is liable to influence plans for procreation. If available, amniocentesis at 16 weeks can be offered with chromosome analysis of the cultured fibroblasts and termination of unbalanced fetuses.

Malformations and syndromes

Many birth defects do not fit into the categories of autosomal dominant, recessive, X-linked and chromosomal. Heart defects and spina bifida, for example, are

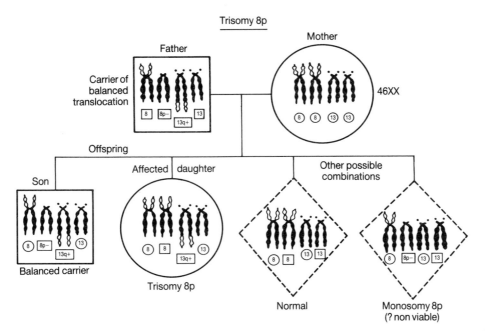

Fig. 3.8.7 The inheritance of two pairs of chromosomes (8 and 13) shown at the metaphase stage when each chromosome has replicated to form identical sister chromatids. The short arms of chromosome 8 are drawn in outline to show clearly the 8p material translocated on to chromosome 13. Note that of the four possible combinations, two were seen in this family. Each form may affect either sex. (Reproduced with permission from *Pediatric Cardiology*, 1984; **5**: 55–60.)

common malformations whose cause is obscure. A discussion of the polygenic threshold model and interactions is beyond the scope of this chapter other than to say that multiple genes are likely to be involved. In the case of heart defects the relatively uniform birth prevalence of six to eight per 1000 in all populations studied[15] favours predominantly genetic causes, whereas the major fluctuations in time and place in the prevalence of neural tube defects and the evidence of a beneficial effect of preconception vitamin supplementation,[16] make it likely that environmental factors contribute in areas of high incidence such as Ireland and the west of Britain.

Practical genetic counselling

Despite the wide variety of problems, it is possible to offer the following simple guide to the structure of a genetic consultation.

- Determine whether the family has requested advice or whether they have been 'sent', perhaps against their will.
- Ask what questions they have. Typically these are:

What is wrong? (diagnosis)
What is the outlook? (prognosis)
What treatment is available? (therapy)
Will it happen again? (family recurrence risk)
Will it be as bad? (clinical burden)
Are there any tests? (prenatal diagnosis)

- Diagnosis is essential and should rest on the usual history and examination. In the case of congenital abnormalities, enquiry should be directed particularly at events in the pregnancy which might account for deformation (e.g. loss of liquor) or disruption. The latter may be caused by mechanical means (e.g. illegal attempts at abortion) or chemical (e.g. drug treatment or alcohol ingestion).
- Taking a family history is at the heart of the consultation. This should include a family tree with males marked as squares and females as circles. It should be extended to children, grandchildren, parents, grandparents, uncles, aunts and cousins of the person presenting at the clinic (known as the consultand). It is important to ask about cousin marriages, miscarriages and all diseases in the family. Sometimes unsuspected problems will be discovered, more important than the presenting enquiry.

- When the diagnosis and pattern of inheritance are deduced, the risk of recurrence should be calculated for the consultand. This may involve reference to family studies, such as have been performed for relatives of cases with neural tube defect, where an empirical risk is given. An empirical risk is used particularly when the mode of inheritance of a condition is not by a straightforward Mendelian pattern. A simple calculation will usually suffice for an autosomal recessive trait, while X-linked inheritance or the use of linked DNA probes may require expert advice.

- When the facts are clear, the consultands should be advised carefully and as quickly as they are able to absorb the information. It must be remembered that most people have little biological training and terms such as chromosome and gene should be explained. (Colourful simplification is permitted: 'We all inherit genes from our parents; in most cases one copy of each gene from each parent. A gene is a coded message that helps to control our growth and development. There are 50 000 to 100 000 genes strung together on chromosomes. Each chromosome is like a long string of beads, with each bead representing a gene. Like the genes, chromosomes come in matching pairs, 23 pairs in all').

- Genetic decisions are difficult and personal. Families should be given information and help to arrive at their own decisions. The question, 'What would you do, doctor?', should be deflected, so that the individual or family is not pushed into a course of action inappropriate or unacceptable to them. Counselling, then, has four major components:

Comprehension of the problem.
Calculation of the risk.
Communication of the facts.
Compassion and caring for the patient.

Conclusion

This chapter has examined a few aspects of modern clinical genetics in the context of health care in the Third World and tropics. Examples of genetics as a basic science, an applied science and a clinical discipline have been touched upon. An observant clinician has much to offer the study of inherited disease even in remote and primitive areas far from sophisticated technology. When disease caused by malnutrition and poor hygiene is less widespread, malformations and chromosome disorders become a major health challenge, especially in paediatrics. Despite poor facilities in an area where the life expectancy is short,

the physician must be receptive to relatives' anxieties about whether a defect will recur and whether it may be more or less severe if it does recur. The availability of prenatal diagnosis gives greater scope for intervention, but sensible and sensitive counselling can do much to dispel superstition and fear and to put recurrence risks in their proper perspective, even when such facilities are lacking.

References

1. Ballou WR, Hoffman SL, Sherwood JA *et al.* Safety and efficacy of a recombinant DNA *Plasmodium falciparum* sporozoite vaccine. *Lancet.* 1987; **i**: 1277–81.
2. Holzel A, Schwartz V, Sutcliffe KW. Defective lactose absorption causing malnutrition in infancy. *Lancet.* 1959; **i**: 1126.
3. Dahlqvist A, Hammond JB, Crane RK *et al.* Intestinal lactase deficiency and lactose intolerance in adults. *Gastroenterology.* 1963; **45**: 488.
4. Ransome-Kuti O, Kretchmer N, Johnson J *et al.* Family studies of lactose intolerance in Nigerian ethnic groups. *Pediatric Research.* 1972; **6**: 359.
5. Miller CH, Mason SJ, Clyde DF, McGinniss MH. The resistance factor to *Plasmodium vivax* in Blacks: the Duffy blood-group phenotype FyFy. *New England Journal of Medicine.* 1976; **295**: 302–4.
6. Kan YW, Dozy AM. Antenatal diagnosis of sickle-cell anaemia by DNA analysis of amniotic-fluid cells. *Lancet.* 1978; **ii**: 910–11.
7. Southern BM. Detection of specific sequences among DNA fragments separated by gel electrophoresis. *Journal of Molecular Biology.* 1975; **98**: 503–17.
8. Chang JC, Kan YW. A sensitive new prenatal test for sickle-cell anaemia. *New England Journal of Medicine.* 1982; **307**: 30–2.
9. Orkin SH, Little PFR, Kazazian HH J, Boehm CD. Improved detection of the sickle mutation by DNA analysis. *New England Journal of Medicine.* 1982; **307**: 32–6.
10. Baraitser M, Burn J, Fazzone TA. Huntington's chorea arising as a fresh mutation. *Journal of Medical Genetics.* 1983; **20**: 459–75.
11. Gusella JF, Wexler NS, Conneally PM *et al.* A polymorphic DNA marker genetically linked to Huntington's disease. *Nature.* 1982; **306**: 234–8.
12. Wainwright BJ, Scambler PJ, Schmidtke J *et al.* Localization of cystic fibrosis to human chromosome 7cen-q22. *Nature.* 1985; **318**: 384–5.
13. Koenig M, Monaco AP, Kunkel LM. The complete sequence of dystrophin predicts a rod-shaped cytoskeletal protein. *Cell.* 1988; **53**: 219–228.
14. Linder D, Gartler SM. G6PD mosaicism: utilization as a cell marker in the study of leiomyomas. *Science.* 1965; **150**: 67–9.
15. Taussig HB. World survey of the common cardiac malformations: developmental error or genetic variant? *American Journal of Cardiology.* 1982; **50**: 544–9.

16. Smithells RW, Nevin NC, Seller MJ *et al.* Further experience of vitamin supplementation for prevention of neural tube defect recurrences. *Lancet*. 1983; **i**: 1027–31.
17. Burn J, Baraitrer M, Hughes DT *et al.* Absent right atrioventricular connection due to an unbalanced familial 8: 13 translocation: a cautionary tale. *Pediatric Cardiology*. 1984; **5**: 55–60.

Further reading

Baraitser M. *The Genetics of Neurological Disorders*. Oxford, 1982.

Emery AE, Rimoin DL. *Principles and Practice of Medical Genetics* (2 vols). Edinburgh, Churchill Livingstone, 1990.
Fraser Roberts JA, Pembrey ME. *An Introduction to Medical Genetics*, 8th Edn. Oxford, Oxford University Press, 1985.
Harper PS. *Practical Genetic Counselling*. 2nd Edn. Bristol, John Wright, 1984.
Smith DW. *Recognizable Patterns of Human Malformation*, 4th Edn. London, WB Saunders, 1988.
Weatherall DJ. *The New Genetics and Clinical Practice*, 2nd Edn. Oxford, Oxford University Press, 1985.
Wynne-Davies R, Hall CM, Graham Apley A. *Atlas of Skeletal Dysplasias*. Edinburgh, Churchill Livingstone, 1985.

SECTION 4

Infectious Diseases

Paget Stanfield

CHAPTER 1

Introduction

Paget Stanfield

Infection pressure
Impaired resistance

Inadequate or inappropriate health services
Changing patterns of infectious disease in children

Infectious disease is the predominant influence contributing to the disparities in child health between the developing and developed worlds. The rapid narrowing of the first five years of population pyramids in Third World countries demonstrates only too clearly the high toll of infant and child life which infection exacts. Mortality represents only the tip of the iceberg, and infectious disease also appears as the chief cause of morbidity and chronic ill health amongst children in the subtropics and tropics.

There are many reasons for this and these are outlined below.

Infection pressure

High environmental contamination and overcrowding ensure optimum conditions for the transmission of microorganisms by contact, droplets, dust, food, water and insect and animal vectors. It is becoming evident that dosage of infection influences severity as well as frequency of infection. In a study in the Ivory Coast, it was found that measles mortality bore a direct relationship to the number of measles cases in each household at any one time. Infection pressure also explains the variation in ages at which infection occurs. High streptococcal infection rates in infancy probably account for the very young age at which rheumatic fever is still seen in some countries. The higher the incidence of measles, the younger the age at which measles begins to appear; the effect of a successful immunization campaign not only reduces the incidence but raises the mean age at which measles occurs.

Impaired resistance

The child in the tropics is often found to have a reduced ability to combat the establishment and severe effects of infection. The impairment may often commence *in utero*, with intrauterine growth failure and low birth weight rendering the infant more vulnerable to infection. Energy–protein malnutrition in the weaning and toddler period reduces immunity and resistance to infection in a number of ways. The major impact is on cell-mediated immunity with less impairment of humoral antibody response.

The effect of infections on nutritional status is equally negative, establishing the downward spiral of ill health and malnutrition which is so difficult to break in many of the situations in which children live in the tropics and subtropics.

Nutritional deficiency, other than energy–protein lack, will increase the morbidity and mortality from infection. Two examples are the adverse effect of anaemia on acute respiratory infection and the loss of epithelial integrity in vitamin A deficiency, especially as it affects the eye. Vicious circles are seen again as infection may well result in anaemia and malabsorption with consequent specific nutritional deficiencies.

Apart from nutritional status, a number of infections themselves impair resistance and suppress immunity. The most notable, the HIV or human immunosuppressive viruses, are by no means the most frequent or lethal for infants and children of the Third World. Measles, malaria and recurrent gastro-intestinal infections in different ways reduce a child's ability to resist infection. Though they may not be mortal in themselves, there may be a very high postinfective morbidity and mortality. The flare up of occult primary tuberculosis infection in a child with measles is a good example. Multiple infections may act synergistically and may be more difficult to diagnose, such as for instance *Trichuris* infestation of the large gut and amoebic dysentery, gastroenteritis and thrush in infancy.

Frequent recurrent infections fail to allow sufficient time between each episode for complete recovery and the child finally succumbs to what might have been a mild infection in health but proves to be the 'straw that breaks the camel's back'.

Inadequate or inappropriate health services

A major reason for the reduction of the threat of infection to the health of children in the developed world is the adequacy of the preventive and curative health services. They are not only supported by adequate resources but are readily accessible. The reverse is often the case in the Third World, where poor resources and long distances limit the impact of health delivery. Infection is often not seen or diagnosed until too late. It has often been treated partially, inadequately or inappropriately, presenting with attenuated and confusing symptomatology or with organisms that are insensitive to available antibiotics.

Single or repeated short courses of treatment in infections which need prolonged therapy lead to chronic ill health and often the emergence and spread of resistant organisms. There is no doubt that this is the danger of distributing antibiotics and antimalarials to voluntary community health workers unless they can be well trained and supervised in their use.

Poor health delivery services not only limit early recognition, proper diagnosis and adequate treatment and follow-up of children with infectious diseases, they also reduce the protection of preventive activities such as full immunization; the insurance of proper weaning practices and if necessary needful supplementation; and the provision of training and resources in rehydration, family planning, etc. It is in the promotion of health of course that community-based health care (CBHC) comes into its own, though CBHC will by no means reduce the need for adequate health services; rather the reverse as an increasingly informed community demand develops.

Changing patterns of infectious disease in children

The understanding of the molecular biology and genetic structure of infectious agents has increased enormously in the last few years. New infectious agents are being identified, mainly amongst the viruses, such as those causing gastrointestinal infection, the retroviruses (HIV) and leukaemia viruses. Furthermore, new vaccine prototypes are now being developed and tested.

Modes of transmission, mainly vertical transplacental passage, of diseases such as in hepatitis and human immunosuppressive viruses, malaria and leprosy, are being recognized. Patterns of perinatal and neonatal infection are beginning to emerge from behind the veil which hides much of this period of life. One simple example is the discovery of the large contribution that neonatal tetanus makes to neonatal mortality.

The capacity of microorganisms to develop resistance to chemotherapy is providing considerable problems as chloroquine-resistant falciparum malaria has continued to increase; penicillinase-producing gonococci have been responsible for ophthalmia neonatorum resistant to penicillin; and as strains of *Shigella dysenteriae* have become resistant to ampicillin – to give but a few examples.

This section of the book provides a comprehensive summary of infectious disease as it afflicts children today in the tropics and subtropics. Where there is overlap with chapters in other sections this will be indicated.

CHAPTER 2

Infections and the immune system

Badrul Alam Chowdhury and Ranjit Kumar Chandra

Our environment contains an array of infectious agents – viruses, bacteria, fungi, and parasites, of diverse size, shape, and subversive characters. Many of these can cause pathological damage and eventually kill the host if allowed to propagate uninhibited. In normal individuals the great majority of infections are of limited duration and leave very little permanent damage. This is due to the immune system which combats the infectious agents and controls or eradicates them before they get a foothold. In this chapter, the mechanisms of host defence, immune response in infections and the effects of some selected infections on immunity are discussed.

Mechanisms of host defence

The human body is provided with a series of defence mechanisms which act as a protective umbrella to prevent the entry and propagation of infection (Fig. 4.2.1). The defence mechanisms are divided into two functional groups, non-specific and antigen-specific. Non-specific defences include the skin and mucous membrane, phagocytic cells, complement, lysozyme, interferon and other humoral factors. All these defence mechanisms are innate in that they are naturally present and are not intrinsically affected by prior contact with infectious agents. They act as the first line of defence and check most potential pathogens before they establish an overt infection. Antigen-specific defences include the B cell system of antibody

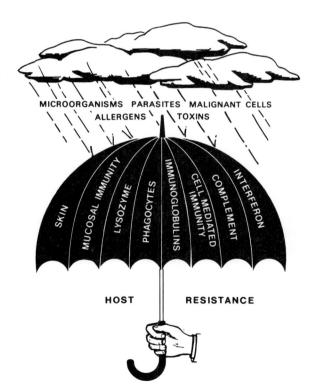

Fig. 4.2.1 Host defence mechanisms. A series of non-specific barriers and antigen-specific immune responses protect man from infectious agents.

production and T cell system of cell-mediated immunity. They are adaptive and acquired in the sense that they produce specific reactions to each infectious agent which are learnt by prior exposure to microbes or their antigenic determinants. They are very effective in eradicating infection, and also remember the particular infectious agent and can prevent it causing disease later. This forms the basis of immunization. In the body, non-specific and antigen-specific defences act in concert to fight off infection.

Non-specific host defences

Skin and mucous membrane

Infectious disease vectors usually enter the body via the skin or epithelial surfaces of the nasopharynx, lung, gut and genito-urinary tract. The mechanical barrier of intact skin and mucosa at these sites prevents organisms from gaining entry into the body. Most bacteria even fail to survive for long on skin because of the direct inhibitory effects of lactic acid and fatty acid in sweat and sebaceous secretions and the low pH that they generate. A variety of physical and biochemical defences protect the mucosal surfaces. For example, lysozyme, an enzyme present in different secretions, is capable of splitting a peptidoglycan bond present in the cell wall of many bacteria. Mucus secreted by the lining membranes blocks the adherence of bacteria and virus to epithelial cells. Microbes and other particulate matter are trapped within the adhesive mucus and removed by mechanical means like ciliary movement, coughing and sneezing. The flushing action of tears, saliva and urine is also protective.

Phagocytes

If an organism penetrates an epithelial surface it is encountered by the phagocytic cells which are distributed richly along the portals of entry. There are two major types of phagocyte – polymorphonuclear neutrophils providing the main defense against pyogenic bacterial infection, and macrophages active against intracellular bacteria, viruses, and parasites. The phagocytes adhere to the microbes by some primitive recognition mechanisms, engulf, and kill them by the generation of lytic enzymes and lethal radicals like superoxide anion, hydrogen peroxide, singlet oxygen and hydroxyl radicals. Phagocytes also have receptors for the carboxyterminal end of antibody molecules (Fc receptor) and the complement fragment C3b (C3b receptor), which aid in homing in on antibody- or complement-coated microorganisms.

Complement

The complement system is made up of over 20 plasma proteins. They have non-specific antimicrobial function and also an effective amplification system which potentiates other non-specific and antigen-specific defence mechanisms. Two parallel but independent mechanisms – the classical and alternate pathways – lead to activation of C3 and a terminal bioactive portion of the complement cascade. The surface carbohydrates of many microbes activate the alternate pathway of complement and split C3 to give C3b, which acts as an opsonin, and C3a, which aids in chemotaxis by releasing chemotactic factors from mast cells. Other complement fragments with antimicrobial properties are also generated in subsequent steps. The same sequence of events can also be initiated through the classical pathway by complexes of antibody and microbial antigens.

Interferon and other humoral factors

Interferons are secreted by virally infected cells and sometimes by lymphocytes. They induce a state of viral resistance in uninfected tissue cells, and also heighten the cytotoxic activity of non-specific natural killer (NK) cells. NK cells are large granular lymphocytes derived from haematopoietic stem cells. They are capable of recognizing cell surface changes on virally infected cells and destroying such cells. They do not need prior sensitization to be active. Other humoral factors which provide non-specific host defence include the acute-phase proteins, C-reactive protein (CRP), α_1 antitrypsin, α_2-macroglobulin, fibrinogen, caeruloplasmin, and Factor B. CRP can bind to bacteria which contain membrane phosphoryl choline and activate complement by the alternate pathway.

Antigen-specific host defences

Antibodies

Antibodies are a class of molecules produced by plasma cells (derived from B lymphocytes) aided by T lymphocytes and macrophages on stimulation by foreign antigens. There are five classes of antibody: IgG, IgM, IgA, IgD and IgE. IgG and IgM are present mainly in the circulation and active against extracellular bacteria and viruses, while IgA is present in mucosal secretions and active in those sites (see pp. 729–30). Antibodies act directly on pathogens and their products to neutralize them, or stimulate non-specific effectors like the phagocyte and complement system. Antibodies help in phagocytosis by acting as an adaptor molecule between the infectious agent, which often evades recognition, and the phagocyte. Antibody molecules of all five classes have the basic structure of two heavy and two light chains linked by disulphide bonds. Amino-terminal portions of both heavy and light chains show considerable variations in amino acid composition, whereas the remaining parts of the chains are relatively constant in structure. Inside the variable region there are three areas where the structural variations are greatest; these are called the hypervariable regions (Fig. 4.2.2). Antigen binding capability of the immunoglobulin molecule resides in these hyper-variable regions. The carboxyterminal end of the heavy chain, called the Fc region, is involved in other bio-logical activities like binding to the phagocytic cells. Antibody molecules bind to microbes by the hyper-variable region, and to the Fc receptor on phagocytic cells by the Fc end. Antibodies also activate the classical pathway of complement activation, the products of which aid in chemotaxis, phagocytosis, and lysis of microbial cells.

Cell-mediated immunity

Cell-mediated immunity is a function of T lympho-cytes. They are particularly important in dealing with infections caused by intracellular organisms like viruses, and some bacteria and parasites. The mechanism of T cell recognition of pathogens is not clear, but interaction through a membrane receptor is probably involved. Sensitized T cells like cytotoxic T cells and antibody-dependent cytotoxic cells recognize virus-infected cells by the presence of viral antigens on their membranes and destroy them. T cells also block cell-to-cell transfer of viral particles, a step which cannot be checked by antibodies. T cells also help in antibody production by B cells and elaborate various soluble factors that stimulate other systems of immune response.

Hypersensitivity reactions

In the normal situation, a second or further contact with antigen leads to secondary boosting of the immune response. In hypersensitivity, the secondary responses occur in an inappropriate or exaggerated form causing inflammatory reactions and tissue damage. Coombs and Gell have identified four types of hypersensitivity reaction (Types I, II, III and IV) which are briefly described below. Often tissue damage in infectious diseases is caused by one or more of these hypersensiti-vity reactions.

Type I or immediate hypersensitivity

In this type of hypersensitivity the antigen reacts with antibody bound to tissue mast cells or circulating

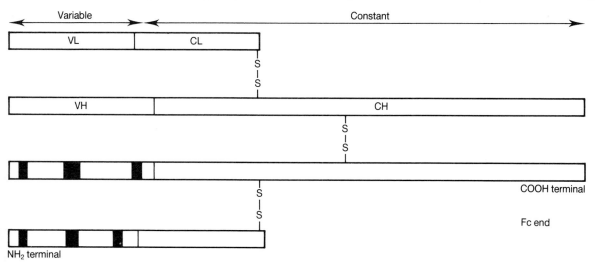

Fig. 4.2.2 Basic structure of an immunoglobulin molecule. The terms V and C are used to designate variable and constant regions and L and H to designate light and heavy chains, respectively. Thus, VL and CL specify variable and constant regions on the light chain and VH and CH specify variable and constant regions on the heavy chain. Shaded areas represent the hypervariable regions.

basophils. The antibody, usually IgE, is attached to cells via its Fc fragment. Combination of antigen to this bound antibody results in activation of the mast cell or basophil and release of various vasoactive amines, such as histamine. The principal effects of the released factors are vasodilation, smooth muscle contraction, and increased capillary permeability.

Type II or antibody-mediated cytotoxic hypersensitivity

In this form of hypersensitivity, antibodies directed against cell surface antigens bind to the cell and bring about its destruction by activating the cytotoxic killer cell, increasing phagocytosis, or causing complement-mediated lysis. The damaging mechanisms are a reflection of the normal physiological processes involved in dealing with pathogenic microorganisms.

Type III or immune-complex mediated hypersensitivity

Immune-complex reactions are induced by deposition of circulating antigen–antibody complexes in tissues, resulting in activation of complement, polymorphonuclear inflammatory response and tissue damage. This type of hypersensitivity is seen in certain persistent microbial infections in which complexes are formed in large quantities and cannot be cleared adequately by the reticuloendothelial system. They become deposited in tissues like the glomerulus, synovium and blood vessel wall, and lead to their destruction.

Type IV or cell-mediated hypersensitivity

This type of hypersensitivity is mediated by sensitized T lymphocytes which on contact with macrophage-bound antigens proliferate and release a variety of soluble mediators collectively called lymphokines. This results in localized accumulation of inflammatory cells and tissue damage.

Immune responses in infections

Viral infections

Immune response in viral infection may range from apparently non-existent (e.g. Kuru) to lifelong immunity (e.g. measles), or chronic immunopathology (e.g. hepatitis B).

Non-specific immunity

Interferons provide the most important non-specific defence mechanism in viral infection. They are produced early in infection, and afford protection before antibody response is mounted. Intact skin and mucosa also offer resistance to viral invasion.

Protection by antibody

Antibodies can neutralize viruses by a variety of means. In influenza, antibody against viral haemagglutinin prevents the combination of virus with receptor sites of host cells, thereby preventing penetration. In measles, similar antibodies that prevent cellular entry are produced as are other antibodies that prevent cell-to-cell transfer of the virus. Antibodies can also directly destroy viral particles through activation of the classical complement pathway, and lyse human cell lines infected with virus responsible for measles, mumps and influenza. Passive administration of antibody can protect against certain infections like measles, hepatitis A and B, and varicella if given before or immediately after exposure.

Cell-mediated immunity

Most viruses modify antigens of the host cell membrane and bud off from the surface as infectious particles. Antibodies alone are therefore inadequate to control these infections. T lymphocyte receptors can recognize the new surface antigens and mount immune response against them. Natural killer cell-mediated and antibody-dependent cell-mediated cytolysis are specially effective in this respect.

Bacterial infections

Bacteria cause a wide spectrum of diseases, many of which are prevalent among children in the tropics. A child's immune system is capable of mounting an effective defence against many bacteria and their toxins.

Non-specific immunity

Intact skin and mucosa prevent entry of bacteria into the body. Phagocytes and complement, aided by antibody, are important in dealing with bacteria which gain entry into the host. The importance of phagocytes is emphasized in a rare congenital disease, called Chediak–Higashi syndrome, in which phagocytes are weakly active and intracellular killing of bacteria is reduced. Patients suffer from recurrent bacterial infections involving organisms with normally low pathogenicity.

Protection by antibody

Antibody can counteract bacterial pathogenicity in a number of ways. Group A streptococci and some gut pathogens have receptors for epithelial surfaces, which are blocked by antibody. Bacterial components which inhibit phagocytosis, like the M-protein of *Streptococcus*, and the capsules of *Pneumococcus*, *Haemophilus influenzae* and *Bacillus anthrax* are inactivated by antibody. Antitoxin antibodies can neutralize toxins of *Corynebacterium diphtheria*, *Clostridium tetani*, *Clostridium welchii*, etc., thus preventing the major damaging effects of these bacteria. Secretory IgA antibodies against *Vibrio cholera* lipopolysaccharide and toxin inhibit adherence of the bacilli to the intestinal mucosa and block the attachment of the toxin to its receptor respectively.

Cell-mediated immunity

Cell-mediated immunity is effective against bacteria which are able to live and grow inside host macrophages, like *Mycobacterium tuberculosis*, *Mycobacterium leprae* and *Legionella*. These microbes evade the killing mechanism of phagocytes by preventing the fusion of phagosome and lysosome (e.g. *Mycobacterium*) or by inhibiting the postphagocytic increase in metabolic activity (e.g. *Legionella*). The macrophages can be activated to kill the bacteria by a T cell lymphokine (lymphokines are soluble factors released by T lymphocytes) called macrophage-activating factor.

Parasitic infections

Parasitic protozoal and helminthic infestations are common among children in tropical countries, and present a major medical problem. The diseases caused are diverse, and the immune responses that are effective against the different parasites vary considerably. Nonspecific host defences are relatively ineffective against parasites. Antibodies, T cells and T cell-stimulated macrophages are mainly active in parasitic infection. In general, humoral responses are important with regard to organisms that invade the bloodstream (e.g. malaria, trypanosomiasis), whereas cell-mediated immunity is elicited in parasites that invade the tissues (e.g. leishmaniasis).

Protection by antibody

Antibodies are produced in various types of parasitic infection, but the parasites develop ways to evade destruction by antibody. Characteristically, levels of IgM are raised in trypanosomiasis and malaria, IgG in malaria and visceral leishmaniasis, and IgE in worm infestation. In trypanosomiasis and malaria, the parasites escape the cytocidal action of antibody by altering the antigenic constitution of their cyclical blood forms. Thus, children in hyperendemic areas suffer repeated attacks for the first few years and then become immune, presumably after developing antibodies against all the antigenic variants. In toxoplasmosis, antibody is effective against the adult form but cannot eliminate cysts. As a result, overt clinical disease is rare but subclinical infection is relatively frequent. In schistosomiasis, antibodies are produced which can effectively block a second infection, but the primary organism lives for years within the blood vessels of the host. It is thought that the worms evade recognition by acquiring the host blood group and histocompatibility antigens on its outer coat. In helminthic infections, particularly *Trichinella spiralis*, very high levels of IgE are produced. IgE may aid in expulsion of the worm by releasing histamine from IgE-coated mast cells which increase peristalsis in the gut and cause exudation of serum containing high levels of protective antibodies from all immunoglobulin classes.

Cell-mediated immunity

T lymphocytes play an important role in the host response against parasites. Lymphokine-stimulated macrophages are effective against infections caused by intracellular protozoa like *Trypanosoma cruzi*, *Leishmania donovani*, *Toxoplasma gondii*, *Plasmodium* spp., and worms like the filarial worms and schistosomes. Cytotoxic T cells directly destroy *T. cruzi*-infested heart cells and fibroblasts. In some infections, like schistosomiasis, where the immune system cannot completely eliminate the parasite, T cells react to antigen released locally by the worms or its eggs, and cuts them off by forming granulomas.

Effects of infection on immune responses

Apart from the direct destructive effect of infectious agents on host tissues, some also alter the host immune responses which in turn exert pathological effects.

Here, immune system alterations and their effects in some infectious diseases common among children in the tropics are discussed. The effects of HIV on the immune system are dealt with on p. 603.

Measles

Clinical and epidemiological data show that measles increases the incidence and severity of secondary infections. This is due to the profound effect of the virus on cell-mediated immunity. In children with measles, delayed skin hypersensitivity to common recall antigens is transiently suppressed during infection, and other *in vitro* functions of T cells are depressed (see pp. 496–501).

Hepatitis

The natural course of viral hepatitis A or B is characterized by sequential appearance of different types of viral antigen in the circulation and their corresponding antibodies. However, in persistent infection, as in hepatitis B, there is long continued low-grade antibody response leading to chronic immune complex formation, with eventual deposition of the complexes in tissues causing a type III hypersensitivity reaction. Immune complexes are the cause of extrahepatic manifestations of hepatitis B virus infection, like the serum sickness-like syndrome occasionally seen early in infection, and glomerulonephritis, nephrotic syndrome, polyarteritis nodosa and other types of vasculitis (see p. 610–14).

Leprosy

Leprosy presents as a spectrum ranging from the tuberculoid form with few viable organisms, to the lepromatous form characterized by abundance of bacteria within the macrophages (see pp. 553–76). In the tuberculoid form, the T lymphocyte system is active, although not good enough to eradicate the bacteria. In the lepromatous form, the T lymphocyte system is suppressed although the plasma cell number and antibody level are very high.

Malaria

In malaria, continuous antigenic stimulation leads to the formation of immune complexes which are deposited in various tissues giving rise to a type III hypersensitivity reaction. The nephrotic syndrome of quartan malaria and brain involvement in malignant tertian malaria are probably caused by deposition of immune complexes (see pp. 660, 662).

Chagas' disease

Some manifestations of Chagas' disease are probably due to destruction of tissue by autoimmune mechanisms. The cardiomyopathy, enlarged oesophagus, and megacolon of Chagas' disease are thought to result from the destruction of nerve ganglia by antibody or cytotoxic T cells that cross-react with *Trypanosoma cruzi* antigen (see pp. 679–82).

Further reading

Capron ARG ed. Immunoparasitology. In: *Clinics in Immunology and Allergy*, Vol. 2(3). London, WB Saunders, 1982.

Chandra RK ed. *Primary and Secondary Immunodeficiency Disorders*. Edinburgh, Churchill Livingstone, 1983.

Cohen S, Warren KS eds. *Immunology of Parasitic Infections*, 2nd Edn. Oxford, Blackwell Scientific Publications, 1982.

Deans JA, Cohen S. Immunology of malaria. *Annual Review of Microbiology*. 1983; **37**: 25.

Hahn H, Kaufmann SHE. The role of cell-mediated immunity in bacterial infections, *Review of Infectious Diseases*. 1981; **3**: 1221.

Jarrett EE, Miller HRP. Production and activities of IgE in helminth infections. *Progress in Allergy*. 1982; **31**: 178.

Mahmoud AAF. Parasitic protozoa and helminths: biological and immunological challenge. *Science*. 1989; **246**: 1015.

Mims CA, White DW. *Viral Pathogenesis and Immunology*. Oxford, Blackwell Scientific Publications, 1984.

Rook GAW. The immunology of leprosy. *Tubercle*. 1983; **64**: 297.

Sissons JG, Oldstone MBA. Antibody-mediated destruction of virus-infected cells. *Advances in Immunology*. 1980; **31**: 1.

Thorne KJ, Blackwell JM. Cell-mediated killing of protozoa. *Advances in Parasitology*. 1983; **22**: 44.

CHAPTER 3

Diarrhoeal diseases

William A. M. Cutting

All children in the world suffer from diarrhoeal disease at some time. For a majority there will be one or a few acute attacks of watery diarrhoea followed by spontaneous and complete recovery. Unfortunately for many children there may be repeated attacks, some of which are serious and result in death. It has been estimated that up to five million children die each year of the immediate or longer term consequences of diarrhoeal disease.[1] The immediate effects are a loss of essential body water and electrolytes in loose stools. This is often associated with an upset in the body's acid–base regulation. There is an important association between diarrhoeal disease and undernutrition. During acute disease the negative metabolic effect may be temporary, but repeated attacks of chronic disease result in varying degrees of protein–energy malnutrition.

Every death is a family tragedy and could be prevented by either simple hygienic measures or early and appropriate management of the illness.

In the last 20 years there have been important

advances in our understanding about diarrhoeal disease. A number of aetiological agents have been identified which are responsible for many of the cases. The pathophysiological mechanisms of some of the agents have been worked out. Management has been simplified and made more appropriate. In particular, it has been recognized that a suitable mixture of salt and carbohydrate in water is readily absorbed from the bowel and can counteract the most serious consequences of the disease. The preventive interventions have also been examined in detail and it is now clear that some methods of prevention are much more effective than others.[2]

Although many individual workers and a number of research teams are responsible for these advances, much credit must go to the WHO programme on the Control of Diarrhoeal Diseases. This has defined the problem, specified the appropriate treatment and preventive interventions, encouraged the production of appropriate instruction and publicity materials, set up numerous training programmes and encouraged the health services of many nations to give this condition a high priority.[3] Despite much progress, for many people now accept the effectiveness of prompt and simple rehydration by mouth, this therapy is under-utilized. The prevention of diarrhoea attacks is a challenge which demands improvements in both primary health care and components of community development.

Definition and classification

Diarrhoea is an increase in the number and volume of stools with an alteration in the consistency, mainly due to an increased water content. Sometimes the fluid stools also contain mucus, pus or blood. The wide range of normal stool pattern makes precise definition difficult. Some breast-fed infants may have a soft stool after each breast-feed, while other children may have a stool only about twice per week. Both of these are compatible with health and normal child growth and development. Therefore it is only the mother, who knows her child's normal bowel pattern, who really makes the diagnosis by noting that her child now has a larger number, volume and altered consistency of stools.

Diarrhoeal disease can be classified in various ways. The first major subdivision is between acute and chronic diarrhoea. *Acute diarrhoea* implies a sudden onset, generally over hours rather than days, and a duration of less than one week. *Chronic diarrhoea* is generally more gradual in onset and lasts for more than one or two weeks (the minimum duration of chronicity is rarely defined). At the beginning of an episode it is impossible to tell if it is going to be acute or chronic, and a proportion of cases with a sudden onset persist and are labelled protracted diarrhoea.

Diarrhoea can also be classified according to the stool consistency. Normal stools in older children and adults, especially on a low-fibre diet, are usually formed, i.e. the excreta has a shape which relates to the dimensions of the lower bowel. In diarrhoea the stools become soft, unformed and eventually completely fluid so they take up the shape of the container into which they are passed. A fluid stool may have a normal colour, but if the diarrhoea is very profuse may be colourless or watery.

Another subdivision of diarrhoeal stools is between *dysentery* and *watery diarrhoea*. Dysentery means diarrhoea with visible blood, and often pus or mucus, in the loose stools. Dysentery is always the result of invasion and damage mainly to the large bowel wall resulting in the loss of blood, and sometimes associated with a cellular reaction in which the leucocytes combat invading pathogens and are excreted as pus. By contrast, secretory diarrhoea is an increase in the water content because the enterocytes lining the small bowel, are not physically damaged, but secrete large volumes of serum-like fluid.

It is sometimes possible to relate the type of diarrhoea to the affected part of the bowel. Small-bowel diarrhoea is usually secretory and therefore watery. Because the whole bowel is available as a reservoir, the stools are generally large in volume.

In large-bowel diarrhoea, the reserve capacity of the bowel is less important and the stools are generally small, frequent and often associated with urgency and cramping pain of the lower bowel known as tenesmus. This type of diarrhoea is more frequently invasive and therefore stools may contain visible blood, pus and mucus. These classifications are not often clear-cut, and shade into each other.

Vomiting is associated with diarrhoea in many patients. Consequently the term *gastroenteritis* is often used to indicate the loss of fluid from both ends of the bowel. In fact, there is rarely inflammation of the stomach and therefore the term is less accurate than using the words diarrhoea and vomiting. *Dehydration* is the physical state in which the consequences of the loss of body water are apparent on clinical examination and will be described later.

Epidemiology

Epidemiology is the study of the dimensions, distribution, duration and determinants of a disease. It is to do with the measurement of the size and importance of a problem like diarrhoeal disease. Epidemiology asks, and attempts to answer, questions about who is affected by the disorder, where and when it occurs most frequently and what factors are associated with it. Epidemiology is not only the study of epidemics, but it is also a problem-solving science which helps to answer questions about the causes and the most effective measures for treating and preventing a disorder like diarrhoea.

Definitions

Morbidity means illness or disease. *Mortality* or death is one outcome of morbidity, but treatment strives for recovery as an alterative outcome.

Epidemiology is concerned with disease in a group of people, each individual illness contributing to the pattern. The word *population* in this context refers to the group of people who are at risk of getting the disorder.

Incidence is the number of new episodes of the disease, for example, new cases of diarrhoeal disease. It is always related to a time period, for example, one year. *Incidence rate* or *attack rate* is the number of new episodes of disease in a population, or a group of individuals at risk over a particular period of time, usually one year. For example, in a group of Bangladeshi children aged between 12 and 24 months, there were 680 episodes of diarrhoea for every 100 children in the group. This gives an incidence rate of 6.8 episodes per child in the second year of life.

Prevalence or *point prevalence* is the number of people suffering from a disease, i.e. the prevailing state of disease, at a particular point in time. For example, the number of children who had diarrhoea on one day when all the homes in a community were visited. *Prevalence rate* is the number of people with the disease compared with the total number in that community at risk from that disease at a particular point in time. For example, in a community of children in the second year of life in an area where diarrhoeal disease is common, on any one day, 15 per cent may have the disease. The prevalence rate for children in such a group is 15 per cent.

Duration of disease is an important measure of illness. In a situation where the occurrence of disease is regular, i.e. where it is endemic rather than epidemic, duration is the link between the incidence and prevalence of a disease. This can be written as a simple formula:

$$\text{Incidence} \times \text{duration} = \text{prevalence}$$

Obviously the longer the duration of an illness, the more likely you are to find a case in a point prevalence survey. The speed of recovery, or the rapidity of death

also influence duration, as both will remove patients from the prevalence state of diarrhoea.

Mortality is a measure of the seriousness of disease in a community. The *case fatality rate* is the number of deaths from a disease compared with the number of cases of the disease. The case fatality rate from diarrhoea varies with the age and the physical state of the subject, and the virulence of the aetiological agent. Estimates of the rate in untreated subjects suggest a figure of about 0.5 per cent or 1 death in 200 diarrhoea episodes in children in tropical countries. Effective treatment will reduce the case fatality rate, so it should be much lower in most communities.

Analytical studies

Analytical studies, particularly use of *controlled clinical trials* are most important in determining what preventive measures are most effective, and what forms of treatment have greatest benefit. All health workers should have an active interest in assessing the size and severity of problems which they are dealing with and the effectiveness of the interventions which they are trying to apply. Large studies are expensive and time consuming in execution, analysis and interpretation. Sometimes small studies can identify key risk factors and appropriate interventions at low cost and with almost immediate application. For example, faecal soiling of a mother's sari when used as a convenient 'bottom wiper', is an important factor in diarrhoea transmission.

Community perception of diarrhoea

The word or words for diarrhoea are varied in different languages and have clinical significance. In Bangladesh, for example, four different words indicate slightly different types of diarrhoea. People associate these with various causes: 'ajirno' – maldigestion, 'dudhaga' – associated with breast-milk, 'amasha' – dysentery-like, and one associated with severe watery diarrhoea, like cholera. Perceptions about cause suggest different remedies, starvation, a change of diet, bulking agents or blocking the outflow. Unfortunately, a number of 'traditional remedies' apply the opposite of modern therapies.

The seriousness of a disease like diarrhoea may depend upon the perspective of an individual. A grandmother looking after a number of grandchildren may notice that from time to time some of the children have diarrhoea, but usually they recover quite quickly and so her attitude may be that this is not a very serious disease. A doctor in a referral hospital will have a different perspective. He may see only the most serious cases, those which have not recovered spontaneously, or have received treatment in their homes or at a local clinic, and only when these measures have failed and the parents are alarmed is the child brought to the hospital. Therefore, the doctor sees mainly serious cases and may believe that diarrhoea is nearly always a life-threatening condition.

Sources of information

From the examples of the grandmother and the referral hospital doctor it is obvious that to get a fair picture of the incidence rate or fatality rate from diarrhoeal disease it is essential to collect information in a systematic and unbiased way. Information is most readily available from hospital records, either admissions or out-patient clinic attendance. Unfortunately, this will only tell you about those who came to the service and not those who were unwilling or unable to reach the facilities.

To answer questions about morbidity and mortality rates accurately it is necessary to set up surveys or longitudinal studies of groups of children in the community and follow them over a period of time. This is expensive and can also introduce a bias, since those who are observing children with disease are morally bound to recommend treatment when children are seriously ill. Therefore, in areas where surveys are conducted, the death rates from diarrhoea can be expected to be lower than in areas without such surveys and advice about treatment. Some simpler survey methods are also available and have been set out by the WHO.

To identify epidemics, it is important to have a reporting system. Then, when there is an outbreak of illness, for example from a single contaminated food source causing an outbreak of food poisoning, the problem can be identified and action initiated. Notification of a cluster of cases, for example cholera, may have important public health implications.[4] A few 'sentinel clinics' which are reliable in their reporting can act as an early-warning system for epidemics.

Health workers who are studying a condition in an area and culture which is unfamiliar to them need to be quite sure that the questions they are asking in any survey are understood correctly by individuals in the local community. For example, as previously described, in Bangladesh, there are at least four types of diarrhoea which are recognized by the people, each with its particular name and association. Appropriate understanding and wording of questions are essential, otherwise wrong information will be collected.

Factors associated with diarrhoea

Diarrhoea affects some groups of people more than others. Age, sex, feeding pattern, environmental hygiene and seasonality are all important.

Age

Infants and toddlers get diarrhoea more frequently than adults. This is mainly because they have never before encountered the common causative organisms and had the chance to build up an immunity.

Feeding pattern

Babies who are breast-fed receive their milk directly from the mother with little chance of contamination and also a variety of agents in mother's milk protect the infants from some potential pathogens. As children get older, particularly once they start crawling in the second six months of life, and toddling and exploring in the second year of life, they frequently find contaminated objects and put them in their mouths. Obviously those who grow up in clean surroundings have fewer episodes than those whose environment is contaminated by faecal pathogens.[5]

Sex

In the first few months of life boys are more vulnerable than girls to diarrhoeal disease, but young women who spend more time with small babies are more likely to contract diarrhoeal disease than young men.

Seasonal patterns

Seasonal patterns of diarrhoeal disease are associated with the rate at which organisms multiply on contaminated food in warm conditions, and the increased risk of person-to-person contact in crowded, indoor situations in cold weather. Some forms of bacterial diarrhoea are more common in the summer months, but as environmental and personal hygiene improve, it is the predominance in cold weather of rotavirus diarrhoea which is the most apparent seasonal variation.

Methods of transmission

Transmission of the disease depends on the interaction of the agent (pathogen), host (man) and the environment. The transmission in most cases of diarrhoeal disease is from the excreta of an infected individual to the food or drink of a susceptible host, the faecal–oral route.

The vehicles or methods of transmission are important. Most diarrhoeal pathogens are transmitted by contamination of food and drink. Shigellosis because of the low number of bacilli needed for infection, can also be transmitted by person-to-person spread. Infection can be spread by contaminated clothing like soiled saris. Salmonella species live naturally in poultry and domestic animals and if their eggs or meat are inadequately cooked these may be a source of infection. Occasionally Salmonella species or *Staphylococcus aureus* multiply on a food producing an enterotoxin. In this instance those who eat the food may be affected by the toxin and get diarrhoea without becoming infected.

Aetiology

Most cases of diarrhoeal disease are due to the action of pathogenic organisms in the small or large bowel. These cause diarrhoea in a variety of ways. The pathogens and the pathophysiological mechanisms are considered here.

Normal defence mechanisms of the bowel

The bowel like other parts of the body is protected by two main systems: the non-specific defence system which acts against all potential pathogens, and the specific or immunological defences. In the alimentary tract, the non-specific defences depend on the integrity of the gut lining; the secretions, saliva, mucus and particularly the acid from the stomach; motility which limits colonization and evacuates agents which irritate, and also the normal bowel microbes which inhibit the multiplication of pathogens.

The immunological system acts against components of particular microbes to which the body is exposed. The mechanisms are both cellular and humoral. The latter include the different classes of immunoglobulins, IgG, IgA and IgM. Secretory IgA is a special form which is important in the bowel since it is excreted from the mucosa to neutralize specific pathogens in the lumen, but it is protected from degradation by the digestive enzymes. The cellular and humoral immune mechanisms complement each other, and are augmented by and interact with the non-specific mechanisms.[6] Breast-feeding exemplifies a number of these immunological and non-specific mechanisms working together.

The infant's gut is colonized shortly after birth. *Lactobacillus bifidus* is the predominant organism in breast-fed infants. Together with the associated acid medium, it discourages the growth of pathogenic organisms. The normal gut flora also inhibit colonization of pathogens by producing growth-suppressing catabolites, such as short-chain fatty acids and by spatial and substrate competition.

Microbial agents

The pathogens which cause diarrhoeal disease include viruses, bacteria and parasites. The most important features of the different agents, their pathogenic mechanisms, clinical and epidemiological effects, are summarized in Table 4.3.1.

Viruses

There was epidemiological evidence for the viral aetiology of some diarrhoea cases many years before organisms were identified and incriminated.

Rotaviruses (family Reoviridae) are double-stranded RNA viruses which affect all mammalian species. The core of the double-shell capsid contains a common antigen, while an antigen of the outer capsid separates rotaviruses into two subgroups. Four human serotypes are recognized on the basis of neutralization assays. Recent advances include culturing the human rotavirus, typing it by electrophoresis of its RNA, and the development of promising vaccine strains. This is world-wide, the most important cause of diarrhoea in small children and the clinical features will be discussed later.

The *Norwalk agent*, and similar small round virus particles, account for outbreaks of diarrhoea in all ages in temperate countries, and episodes (particularly in the second year of life) in some tropical countries like Bangladesh. Other viruses are sometimes associated with diarrhoeal disease. Diarrhoea occurs during measles in a number of cases, and follows the disease in other cases. It is likely that this organism accounts for up to 5 per cent of cases of diarrhoea and 15 per cent of diarrhoea-associated deaths in tropical countries.

Adenoviruses 40 and 41, which have recently been discovered as a cause of infantile diarrhoea, seem to be widespread.

Bacteria

Many bacteria can cause diarrhoea. Identification of the pathogen causing disease in an individual or an out-

Table 4.3.1   Characteristics of the aetiological agents causing diarrhoea

Organisms	Microbiology	Pathogenic mechanisms
Campylobacter jejuni	Special growth requirements, reduced O_2, increased CO_2 and temperature 42°C Various biotypes and serotypes	Mainly invasive in terminal ileum and jejunum Also enterotoxin production
Clostridium difficile	Gram +ve, spore-forming anaerobe	Cytotoxin induces mild to severe features
Escherichia coli Enterotoxigenic (ETEC)	Many serotypes identified with difficulty. Animal and immunological tests for toxins	Toxins cause active secretion. ST (heat stable) the commonest LT (heat labile) least common ST + LT intermediate
Enteropathogenic (EPEC)	Some serotypes implicated. Recognised with difficulty by serotyping e.g. 0:119	Mechanism unclear, possibly secretory but no LT or ST
Enteroinvasive (EIEC)	Different serogroups. Slow lactose fermenters. Detected by animal invasiveness tests	Invades mucosa like shigella, probable cytotoxin
Enterohaemorrhagic (EHEC)	Strains of serotype 0:157:H7	Cytotoxin is the likely mechanism, like Shiga toxin
Salmonellae	Over 1000 potentially pathogenic serotypes • S. typhae and paratyphae • Non-typhae salmonella, many serotypes	Invasive; mild mucosal reaction and blood-borne spread • Typhae • Non-typhae
Shigellae	Four species and 40 serotypes Sh. sonnei Sh. flexneri Sh. dysenteriae Sh. boydii	Invade terminal small bowel and large bowel Multiply in submucosa causing damage and exudate
Staphylococcus aureus	Organisms from skin and nose grow on food	Enterotoxin produced in food. An intoxication, not an infection
Vibrio cholerae 01	Biotypes: Classical and El Tor 01 group are main pathogens in man non 01 groups occur in animals	Enterotoxin, like LT, causes secretion by activating adenylate cyclase in enterocytes
Yersinia enterocolitica	Special culture requirements Slow growth at 25°C	Invasive Probably by an enterotoxin
Rotavirus	Reoviridae family. Double stranded RNA in double shelled capsid, a 70 nm sphere. At least 4 human serotypes	Enterocyte invasion and destruction. Probably both excess secretion and reduced absorption. Viraemia
Norwalk agent and small round viruses	Unclassified small round virus of single polypeptide, 27 nm size	Uncertain
Entamoeba histolytica	Vegetative (amoeboid) and cystic forms. RBCs in vegetative form imply invasion. Pathogenic and non-pathogenic zymodemes. Quite distinct	Invasive infections cause flask-shaped ulcers of colon mucosa, dysenteric stools Cysts in stool do not imply disease

Clinical features	Epidemiology		Other features and modes	Antibiotic treatment
	Incubation period	Age susceptibility		
From mild watery diarrhoea to dysentery. Abdominal pain, fever and malaise. Lasts 2–7 days	2–7 days	All ages	Zoonotic disease. Significant numbers of asymptomatic carriers in Bangladesh	Erythromycin. Only for severe cases
Range from asymptomatic carriage to mild diarrhoea and severe pseudo-membranous colitis (PMC)	?	Adults and elderly	PMC may follow use of clindamycin or ampicillin	Vancomycin
Acute watery diarrhoea	12–48 hours	Children	Affects travellers to the tropics Warm weather	No
Watery diarrhoea with fever and vomiting in some	12–72 hours	Infants	Nursery outbreaks. Role in diarrhoea is controversial	Probably no. Some are antibiotic resistant with R.-factor plasmids
Dysenteric stools with fever	12–72 hours	Adults and older children	Uncommon	Co-trimoxazole
Haemorrhagic enterocolitis	?	Adults and children	Rare	Co-trimoxazole
• Typhoid, fever, systemic upset, slight dirrhoea or constipation. Complications; bowel perforation, haemorrhage • 'Food poisoning' diarrhoea	• Typhoid 7–21 days • Non-typhoid 8–72 hours	Adolescents	• Typhae; food, water and person to person. Hygiene important • Non-typhae, animal foods and caterers	• Typhoid; chloramphenicol, ampicillin • Non-typhae; No antibiotics
Dysentery, much blood in diarrhoea with fever. Occasionally haemolytic-uraemic syndrome or pseudo-membranous proctitis	1–3 days	All except infants	Person to person Hygiene important *Sh. sonnei* more in industrialized countries *Sh. flexneri* more in impoverished places	Co-trimoxazole in children who are toxic with dysentery (Nalidixic acid)
Diarrhoea with sudden onset of abdominal pain, vomiting and prostration	1–4 hours	All ages	Groups eating stored uncooked foods affected	No
Profuse watery diarrhoea with vomiting, acidosis and collapse in severe cases. Only a minority of infections are severe	2–3 days (6 hours to 5 days)	2–5 years in endemic areas. All ages in epidemics	Current 7th pandemic. Seasonal, mostly in warm and wet seasons	Tetracycline decreases duration
Watery diarrhoea or dysentery	3–7 days	Children	Essentially zoonotic Not seasonal	Tetracycline or co-trimoxazole in severe cases
Watery diarrhoea with fever and vomiting in half cases. Severe dehydration and malabsorption in some cases.	1–3 days	Children especially 6 months to 3 years	Maximal incidence in cold months in temperate climates	None
Watery diarrhoea. Short duration. Little vomiting	1–2 days	1–2 years in Bangladesh	All ages in small outbreaks in temperate climates	None
Dysentery of varying severity. Abdominal discomfort, fever, and occasionally hepatic spread, amoeboma or perforation	2–4 weeks	All ages	Person to person spread	5-nitroimidazole derivatives, with diloxanide furoate

Table 4.3.1 *Continued*

Organisms	Microbiology	Pathogenic mechanisms
Giardia lamblia	Motile flagellate vegetative form with sucking disc, and cystic form	Inhabits small bowel. Often asymptomatic. Overgrowth may impair digestion
Cryptosporidium parvum	A coccidian protozoa Both sexual and asexual cycles occur in gut of a host Resistant to chemical disinfectants	Oocysts attach to and invade mucosa of immunosuppressed patients Induce small bowel secretion

break depends not only on a microbiological laboratory, but also on a history of the episode, clinical examination of the patients, inspection of the stools and epidemiological knowledge. A classification of bacteria depends on their morphology, staining, serological reactions, fermentation and culture characteristics. Many can be identified by antigens from their outer layers or flagellae. Many of the pathological factors which enable bacteria to invade, colonize and produce disease are transmitted by extrachromosomal genetic material called plasmids. These can be passed on between bacterial genera, and from virulent to commensal strains, seriously increasing the danger of infection by enteric bacteria. The characteristics which can be transmitted by plasmids include the ability to adhere to enterocytes, to produce secretory toxins, or to resist attack by antibiotics. These last types are known as R-factors.

Parasities

The most important parasites associated with diarrhoeal disease are protozoa. *Entamoeba histolytica* infects hundreds of millions of people, especially in tropical countries, but over 90 per cent are symptomless excretors of the cysts.[7] Invasive intestinal amoebiasis is manifest by trophozoite amoebae with ingested red blood cells visible in dysenteric diarrhoea stools. Few progress to a fulminating colitis, an amoeboma or liver abscess (see p. 739). Serological tests can diagnose invasive disease and zymodeme classification distinguishes pathogenic and invasive from non-invasive trophozoites. (Zymodemes are patterns of isoenzymes used to identify groups of Entamoeba with particular characteristics.)

Giardia lamblia also infects millions of people, in both tropical and temperate climates. This flagellate trophozoite inhabits the small bowel and usually causes diarrhoea with the first infection. In some cases the parasite may damage the mucosa, especially in small children, resulting in malabsorption and failure to thrive and grow. Most infections are benign.[8]

Cryptosporidium is a zoonotic protozoon which is associated with diarrhoea, particularly in the immuno-compromised, but also in normal small children (see p. 730). It probably acts by colonizing and damaging the small bowel, impairing absorption and resulting in watery or mucoid stools for up to two weeks. Helminths, particularly *Strongyloides stercoralis* and *Trichuris trichiura* can cause diarrhoea. The former penetrates the small intestinal mucosa, only causing serious disease in debilitated or immunocompromised patients. Heavy infections of the latter cause inflammation and limit water absorption in the colon.

Parenteral diarrhoea

This is diarrhoea which is not associated with bowel infection, but is an alimentary response to some condition, often an infection, elsewhere in the body. Otitis media, acute pyelitis and malaria are examples of associated infections.

Pathophysiological mechanisms

Diarrhoea results in an increased loss of water in the stools due to inadequate absorption of fluids by the bowel, or to increased fluid poured into the bowel, either by active secretion, or by damage and exudation

Clinical features	Epidemiology		Other features and modes	Antibiotic treatment
	Incubation period	Age susceptibility		
Frothy, fatty stools with abdominal pain and distension	1–2 weeks	Young children Visitors to Leningrad	Food and water-borne Person to person spread	5-nitroimidazole derivatives, e.g. metronidazole, etc
Infection common but normally asymptomatic Chronic watery or mucoid diarrhoea in the immuno-suppressed, especially AIDS Sometimes vomiting and abdominal pain	5–10 days		Reservoir, domestic and wild animals. Animal to person and person to person spread especially in pre-school children and elderly. Water-borne spread also important	Supportive measures to improve defence mechanisms more important than antimicrobials

into the lumen. The mechanisms are summarized in Table 4.3.2.

A knowledge of the physiology of fluid input and output is crucial in understanding diarrhoea. In adults in temperate climates, about 9 litres of fluid enter the alimentary tract every 24 hours. About two litres of this is consumed by mouth and the rest is secreted into the gut in the form of digestive juices. All this liquid is

Table 4.3.2 The pathophysiological mechanisms of diarrhoea

Excessive secretion in small bowel
   toxin induced – eg. V. cholerae toxin.

Impaired absorption
- Maldigestion
  eg. of sugars, lactase deficiency
- Increased osmotic load in the lumen
  eg. also from lactase deficiency or osmotic purgatives, $MgSO_4$
- Damage to the absorptive surface
  eg. gluten enteropathy
- Inadequate mucosal enterocyte replication
  eg. protein-energy malnutrition

Invasion
- Local, with tissue damage and leakage
  eg. Shigella and Entamoeba histolytica
- Local stimulation and systemic spread
  eg. food poisoning Salmonella

Abnormal colonisation
   eg. Large bowel organisms in the small bowel
      (Still not a proven mechanism)

Combinations of these mechanisms

Note: Increased bowel motility and reduced transit time may be more defence mechanisms, voiding pathogens and toxins, rather than pathological mechanisms.

absorbed by the intestines, except 100–200 ml of water per day which is excreted in the stools (Fig. 4.3.1). In children the volumes are all proportionately smaller. In tropical climates, or in those with fever or doing heavy manual work, the fluid intake has to be increased greatly to provide for the insensible losses.

In health, most water from the bowel is absorbed passively through the intercellular spaces in the small bowel mucosa, and a significant amount is actively absorbed through the epithelial cells of the small and large bowels. There are active absorption mechanisms for different essential ions contained in food and drink. For sodium alone there are several absorptive mechanisms in the villus enterocytes. One important method includes a glucose-coupled mechanism which greatly increases saline uptake.[9] Ionic absorption and secretion are controlled by a complex variety of chemical mediators, including intracellular nucleotides, calcium, and neurohormonal substances.

Before a pathogenic microorganism can cause an infection, it must enter the host and overcome a series of defence mechanisms. The numbers ingested must be sufficiently large for a proportion to survive these defences, or they must be resistant enough to inactivation by the gastric acid and other mechanisms. Although individual variations are wide, an infectious dose of enteric viruses or *Entamoeba histolytica* may be only a few hundred organisms, while the dose for Salmonella species or *Vibrio cholerae* is over a million. The pathogens which survive the stomach acid, a fatal environment for many, must multiply in the alkaline lumen of the small bowel and adhere to the lining cells. From this point the various pathogens act in different ways, some producing exotoxins which affect the

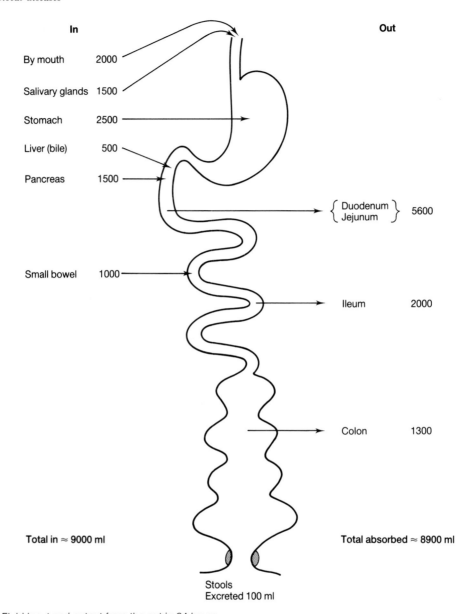

In   **Out**

By mouth   2000

Salivary glands 1500

Stomach   2500

Liver (bile)   500

Pancreas   1500

$\left\{\begin{array}{l}\text{Duodenum}\\\text{Jejunum}\end{array}\right\}$ 5600

Small bowel   1000

Ileum   2000

Colon   1300

Total in ≈ 9000 ml   Total absorbed ≈ 8900 ml

Stools
Excreted 100 ml

Fig. 4.3.1   Fluid input and output from the gut in 24 hours.

biochemical actions of the cells, while others invade and destroy the mucosa.

Toxigenic secretory diarrhoea

Vibrio cholerae and enterotoxigenic *Escherichia coli* (ETEC) cause diarrhoea by toxic stimulation of cell excretion. After multiplication on the microvillous surface of the enterocytes, the bacteria produce enterotoxins which pass through the cell walls and stimulate enzymic reactions in the cells which result in excessive secretion into the bowel lumen. One of the toxins from ETEC is virtually identical with cholera enterotoxin. These stimulate the enzyme adenylate cyclase which converts adenosine triphosphate (ATP) to cyclic adenosine monophosphate (cAMP) on the basolateral walls of the cells. cAMP works through further enzymes, the protein kinases and a calcium-containing substance, calmodulin, which results in the secretion of chloride ions from the enterocytes into the lumen. This is accompanied by water and sodium excretion. Once the toxin has switched on this enzyme mechanism the cell will continue with pathological secretion for the rest of its brief life, which may be some two to three days. However, note that the cells are not structurally damaged, and absorption, particularly glucose-enhanced absorption, is well preserved.

Mucosal invasion with limited spread and local inflammation

The 'food poisoning' group of Salmonella which cause diarrhoea penetrate the epithelial cells but only spread locally as far as the mucosal lining. Local inflammation, a white cell invasion and excessive secretion by some undetermined mechanism results in diarrhoea.

Rotavirus particles invade and destroy patches of enterocytes on the surface of the small bowel. They probably also set up an excessive secretory reaction since they produce a predominantly watery diarrhoea. With rotavirus there is almost certainly systemic spread as well. This may be the cause of the fever and vomiting which occurs with many rotavirus infections.

Mucosal invasion with local damage to cells and villi

Shigella attack the epithelial cells resulting in micro-ulcers which can enlarge to wide areas of inflammation and discharge. The stools contain an exudate including blood and pus cells. In severe cases there will be crypt abscesses.

Microbial contamination and abnormal colonization of the small bowel

The bacterial flora of the duodenum and ileum are controlled by the interaction of a number of chemical, microbial and immunological factors. Contamination and colonization of the small bowel by pathogens, without invasion or toxin production, may be associated with diarrhoea and malabsorption of a range of nutrients. Bile salt and bile acid malabsorption may damage the mucosa and limit colonic water reabsorption. Bacterial colonization may damage the mucosa directly in situations where there is abnormal overgrowth of organisms.

When the body defences are impaired due to malnutrition, after infections like measles, due to infection by human immunodeficiency virus (HIV) as found in AIDS, or during treatment with immunosuppressive drugs, the bowel may be colonized by organisms which do not normally cause disease. These include yeast (*Candida albicans*) and cryptosporidia.

Temporary lactase deficiency and postenteritis diarrhoea

Any form of mucosal damage may impair enzyme production and absorption from the bowel. This may occur for a short period after acute diarrhoea caused by a wide variety of organisms. The most common form is a transient lactase deficiency, as this mucosal enzyme is most readily affected by any infection. Since most infants take milk, lactose (milk sugar) is an important component of their diets. If lactose is not broken down into glucose and galactose and thence absorbed, the colonic bacteria reduce it by fermentation into lactic acid, short-chain fatty acids and gas. The consequences of this are bowel distension, increased osmotic load in the lumen which draws in more water, and acid irritation of the mucosa. The stools are acidic and lactose can be detected by tests for sugar and reducing substances (Fig. 4.3.2).

Severe or recurrent intestinal infection can result in mucosal damage which may proceed to villous atrophy and more general maldigestion with malabsorption. This postinfectious damage is probably the most common cause of chronic diarrhoea. There may be intolerance of other sugars and proteins. Cow's milk protein intolerance occasionally occurs after intestinal infection. This is possibly because intestinal damage permits permeability, with uptake of large milk protein molecules which act as allergens and result in sensitization to milk. These patients often have vomiting and diarrhoea, sometimes with blood and pus.

The pathophysiological mechanisms are briefly summarized in Fig. 4.3.3.

Circulatory and metabolic consequences of fluid and electrolyte loss

The physiological consequences of electrolyte loss depend on the ionic concentration of the diarrhoeal stools, the nature of the dietary and fluid intake and the ionic reserves of the individual.

Hypertonic, particularly *hypernatraemic dehydration* occurs when there is a relative excess of salts (electrolytes) compared with water within the vascular and extracellular compartments. It is important

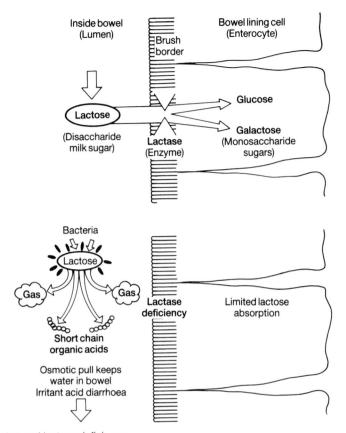

Fig. 4.3.2   Lactose absorption and lactase deficiency.

because shift of fluid into the extracellular compartment causes the brain to shrink. This predisposes to haemorrhages, arterial, venous and sinus thromboses. Because of the fluid drawn into the extracellular and vascular compartments the signs of dehydration are less obvious, but features of CNS dysfunction are important; irritability, lethargy, convulsions and coma. Be alert for conditions which predispose to hypernatraemic dehydration. Children fed on artificial milks which either contain excessive salt or are mixed and given in too concentrated a form overload the body with sodium. This also results from giving rehydration fluid which has been made up with too much salt or too little water. Others predisposed to the condition include infants or the unconscious who are unable to recognize or express thirst, those who have excessive water loss with little solute loss due to dilute watery diarrhoea, hyperventilation or profuse dilute perspiration in fever or a hot climate.

Loss of bicarbonate in stools results in *metabolic acidosis* which causes deep and rapid respiration. Recurrent vomiting with excessive loss of HCl can result in *hypochloraemia* and *alkalosis*. Malnourished children often have a deficit of plasma proteins and potassium. The electrolyte situation is also affected if kidney function is immature or impaired, so they cannot conserve or excrete ions.

In practice, most diarrhoeal stools contain 40–90 Na^+ mmol/l (less than serum) but about 30–40 K^+ mmols/l (more than the concentration in serum, but less than the intracellular concentration).

Hypotonic diarrhoea is the situation when more water than electrolytes is lost in the stools. As already indicated, this is a cause of predominantly intracellular dehydration with relative hypernatraemia.

Isotonic diarrhoea is when fluid with an osmotic pressure similar to that of plasma (270–95 mmol/kg) is lost from the bowel. This is drawn mainly from the

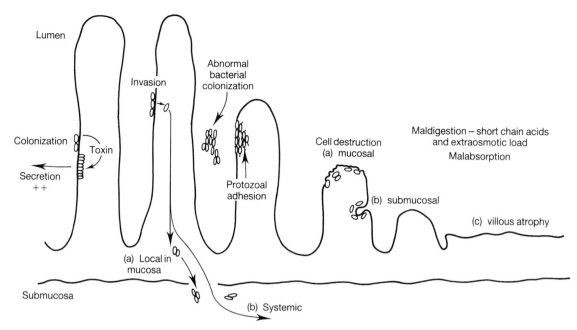

Fig. 4.3.3   Some pathophysiological mechanisms of diarrhoea.

extracellular fluid compartment with the consequences indicated below.

Extracellular dehydration

Extracellular dehydration (ECD) results in a decreased circulating blood volume. The physical consequences of ECD include:

* reduction of skin turgor or elasticity because of dehydration in the interstitial tissues;
* decreased tension of the eyeball and depressed fontanelle in infants;
* weight loss, which accurately reflects the amount of water loss (unfortunately this requires availability of recent weight records).

The haemodynamic consequences of extracellular dehydration include:

* a decrease in the central venous pressure;
* poor right ventricular filling with consequent inadequate cardiac output;
* tachycardia is always present;
* increased peripheral resistance due to vasoconstriction, a mechanism that attempts to maintain blood pressure;
* diminished peripheral and regional perfusion with peripheral cyanosis and cold extremities;

* when these mechanisms fail to maintain the blood pressure cardiovascular collapse is apparent;
* poor renal perfusion leads to oliguria and ultimately anuria.

Intracellular dehydration

During pure intracellular dehydration (ICD) the extracellular volume is little changed. This rarely occurs without some ECD. The direct consequences are weight loss and dry mucosae. The indirect effects are due to brain and hypothalamic dehydration. Thirst is intense and neuropsychic features become apparent. The urine flow is low, even though kidney perfusion is reasonable, due to the release of antidiuretic hormones.

Usually ECD and ICD are associated because water and sodium are lost together. The water loss is generally greater than the sodium loss.

Clinical features

Although the diagnosis of diarrhoea is usually made by the mother, an assessment of clinical features is essential. These will include the degree of dehydration, other indicators of severity and features which may suggest the most likely aetiological agent.

Table 4.3.3 Assessment of dehydration and fluid deficit

Signs and symptoms	Mild dehydration	Moderate dehydration	Severe dehydration
General appearance and condition – infants and young children	Thirsty, alert, restless	Thirsty, restless or lethargic but irritable when touched	Drowsy; limp, cold, sweaty, cyanotic extremities, possibly comatose
– older children and adults	Thirsty, alert, restless	Thirsty, alert, giddiness with postural changes	Usually conscious, apprehensive, cold, sweaty, cyanotic extremities, wrinkled skin of fingers and toes, muscle cramps, giddiness on standing
Radial pulse	Normal rate and volume	Rapid and weak	Rapid, feeble, sometimes impalpable.
Respiration	Normal	Deep, may be rapid	Deep and rapid
Anterior fontanelle	Normal	Sunken	Very sunken
Systolic blood pressure	Normal	Normal-low	Less than 60 mm Hg or may be unrecordable
Skin elasticity	Pinch retracts immediately	Pinch retracts slowly	Pinch retracts very slowly (2 seconds)
Eyes	Normal	Sunken	Deeply sunken
Tears	Present	Absent	Absent
Mucous membranes	Moist	Dry	Very dry
Urine output	Normal	Reduced amount and dark	None passed for several hours, empty bladder
% body weight loss	4–5%	6–9%	10% or more
Estimated fluid deficit	40–50 ml per kg	60–90 ml per kg	100–110 ml per kg

The assessment of patients with diarrhoeal disease should normally follow the classical pattern of history taking, physical examination and laboratory investigations. These are summarized in the WHO guidelines.[3, 10] The main features of dehydration are summarized in Table 4.3.3.

Sometimes a patient arrives in a critical, near terminal condition. In these circumstances, resuscitation should be the first priority and the detailed history, examination and investigations should follow.

History

A careful history should be obtained from the patient or attendant. In addition to the usual information, the following should be specifically ascertained:

- Duration of illness.
- Onset: sudden or gradual.
- Dietary history, especially in relation to diarrhoea.
- Stools: frequency, and volume from onset of illness to indicate the amount of fluid loss.
- Stool character: colour, smell and whether it is mixed with mucus, blood, pus or food constituents.
- Vomiting: frequency, volume and duration.
- Micturition: presence and duration of oliguria or anuria.
- Associated features: the presence of fever, convulsions, altered consciousness, etc.
- Environmental and epidemiological history. Have any other members of the family or contacts suffered from diarrhoea within recent days? Has the child been away from home or fed by someone different?

The socio-economic state of the family may be relevant.

- Previous history of diarrhoea, failure to thrive and other illnesses.

Physical examination

During a systematic physical examination look particularly for signs of dehydration, and give special attention to the alimentary, cardiovascular, urinary and central nervous systems.

Abdominal examination should include examination for distension, palpation for masses, e.g. tuberculous glands or intussusception and auscultation for the presence of excessive or absent bowel sounds. A digital rectal examination is useful if blood has been passed. Insertion of a lubricated tube or drinking straw often provides a sample for stool examination. Examine carefully for other possible sites of infection, like the throat and middle ear, which sometimes cause parenteral diarrhoea.

Assessment of dehydration

Assessment of dehydration requires a great deal of experience. In general the more profuse the stools and vomiting the more severe will be the dehydration. Dehydration may be classified into mild, moderate and severe. Symptoms and signs particularly useful in assessment of dehydration and monitoring of rehydration are: thirst, radial pulse, blood pressure, skin elasticity, anterior fontanelle in infants, appearance of tongue and mucous membranes, eyes, eyeball tension and urinary output. Some of these features are summarized in Fig. 4.3.4.

Weighing the patient

Weighing is not essential but it has definite advantages. It provides a baseline to assess progress and to calculate the dosage of fluids and medicines. If the previous weight of the patient is known, then weight loss associated with diarrhoea is a direct indication of the extent of dehydration.

Interpretation of findings

The findings from history, physical examination and weighing are combined in Table 4.3.3. It would appear that assessment of the degree of dehydration is simple, but in practice this is not so easy, requiring experience and judgement to interpret the true significance of the findings. Referring to dehydration by the percentage of lost body weight gives false exactitude to estimations. One limiting factor is that the proportion of body weight which is water is variable; it is up to 75 per cent in newborn infants, but may be as low as 60 per cent in

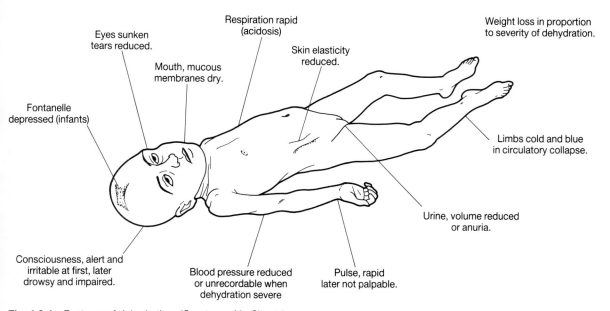

Fig. 4.3.4 Features of dehydration. (Courtesy of L. Skeats).

the elderly. It is more practical to classify dehydration into mild, moderate or severe.

Children are more sensitive to dehydration than adults for the following reasons:

- infants cannot express thirst, the chief symptom of dehydration, so their condition may deteriorate without complaint;
- their relative water requirement is much higher than that of adults;
- dehydration and metabolic disorders more quickly lead to dramatic symptoms such as convulsions or renal failure.

Comparing features of intracellular and extracellular dehydration

Some clinical features are particularly associated with intra- or extracellular dehydration. In fact, because of the physiological mechanisms which attempt to correct and compensate for particular deficiencies, the features of both these conditions normally overlap.

Thirst, dryness of mucosae and central nervous system manifestations are primarily due to reduced intracellular volume. Extracellular fluid deficiency may be predominantly from the interstitial fluid, or from the intravascular compartment, though again both usually occur together. Hypovolaemia is the name given to the decreased volume of fluid within the blood circulation system, and this can have rapid and profound effects. Some of these different features will be considered in more detail.

Thirst is the first important symptom of dehydration. It ranges from a normal desire for water in mild dehydration to an unpleasant craving in the severe state. In young children who cannot express their desire for drinks, crying and restlessness may be the manifestations. In conscious patients the disappearance of thirst indicates the correction of dehydration.

Altered consciousness indicates impaired brain function. *Irritability* may progress to coma, though the coma is rarely due to severe dehydration alone. *Convulsions* may occur at any stage of dehydration in young children, and are particularly associated with high fever, electrolyte imbalance, particularly hypernatraemia and toxaemic states occurring with some infections like Shigella. Sleepy babies are difficult to assess and although attempting to wake them is one manoeuvre, observation over a period of time or asking the parents for their opinion is also important.

Dryness of mouth and other mucous membranes, a reduction in saliva and tears all suggest intracellular dehydration. A dry tongue is not an accurate sign, especially in children who mouth-breathe. Assess this by inserting a clean finger deeply between the lower gum and the cheek.

Three important signs of decreased interstitial fluid are a loss of skin elasticity or turgor, sunken eyeballs, and depressed anterior fontanelle in infants.

Skin elasticity is normally tested in an area where the skin is thin and there is not too much subcutaneous fat. Gently lift a pinch of skin in the subclavicular region: in a normal child this will retract immediately like stretched rubber; in moderate dehydration the skin retraction is delayed; and if the dehydration is severe, a pinched up fold takes more than two seconds to retract. Careful interpretation is needed in marasmic patients and the elderly in whom the natural elasticity is lost, and in obese patients the skin alone cannot be pinched.

With *sunken eyeballs* the eyes appear to retract into their orbits with skin depression at the base of the eyelids. This appears from the stage of moderate dehydration and is more impressive in severe dehydration. In severe degrees, the decreased tension of the eyeballs is detected by gentle finger pressure.

A *depressed anterior fontanelle* may be detected in dehydrated infants. In a healthy child who is sitting upright, there is slight depression and pulsation which is synchronous with the heart beat may be seen. In moderate and severe dehydration the scalp is depressed into the gap between the skull bones.

Extracellular dehydration always decreases the blood volume. Initially all physiological mechanisms act to sustain sufficient perfusion of vital organs. Only when these mechanisms fail are there signs of hypovolaemia. These include the following:

- *Tachycardia*, the first mechanism to maintain cardiac output; the rate is proportional to the severity. However, pyrexia and anxiety also produce tachycardia.
  Collapsed veins reflect hypovolaemia.
- *Vasoconstriction of peripheral vessels*, a mechanism to maintain blood flow through vital organs. The limbs become cold and ultimately sweaty, pale or cyanotic. The radial pulse volume decreases and blood pressure falls. A systolic pressure of 80 mm or less may be found in moderate dehydration.
- *Oliguria*, a renal response to conserve circulating fluid volume; initially due to antidiuretic hormone which increases water reabsorption. Oliguria progresses to anuria when cardiac output decreases and renal perfusion falls.

Laboratory findings in dehydration

Plasma proteins and haematocrit (packed cell volume, PCV) reflect the concentration of the blood, i.e. its water content, and these increase according to the amount of water lost. However, malnourished and anaemic patients have low baseline levels for protein and PCV.

The sodium content of the urine gives an indication of both the mechanism and the degree of dehydration, but it should be interpreted according to other findings. In mild, pure dehydration, urine is concentrated with a normal or high level of sodium. As soon as a sodium deficit occurs, even in mild dehydration, or if the blood volume declines further, the urine sodium concentration drops sharply to less than 10 mmol/l.

Clinical assessment of danger signs

Vulnerable patient groups and virulent pathogens

Groups of patients who develop more severe disease include newborns, infants who are artificially fed, especially bottle-fed, puerperal mothers, elderly patients and those immunocompromised by an underlying disease or chemotherapy. Malnourished children are especially at risk since they have more frequent, more severe and more prolonged episodes. Certain extra-intestinal complications of invasive bacterial diarrhoeas are almost specific to particular host susceptibility or agent virulence. For example, children with a haemoglobinopathy are liable to septicaemia with metastastic osteomyelitis from salmonella enteritis. *Shigella dysenterae* I infection may cause haemolytic–uraemic syndrome.

Indicators of severity

In secretory diarrhoea the severity is directly related to the amount of fluid deficit, the type and degree of electrolyte imbalance and the metabolic and haemodynamic consequences. Some indication of the seriousness of deficit may be gained from a semiquantitative history, for example large 'rice-water' stools and much vomiting, and profound signs of dehydration at initial assessment. Such patients require urgent rehydration.

Invasive diarrhoeas

Abdominal signs and symptoms give warning of progression towards extensive mucosal damage and the consequent complications. These are paralytic ileus with a distended silent abdomen, acute intestinal bleeding with frank blood or melaena in the stools, massive exudation or a protein-losing enteropathy, necrosis associated with perforation and peritonitis, endotoxaemia or septicaemia.

Evidence of complications

Acute complications include convulsions, hypoglycaemia, hypernatraemia, hypokalaemia, especially in malnourished children with chronic diarrhoea, and hypomagnesaemia.

The presence of diarrhoea does not exclude other causes of convulsions and these should be carefully looked for. The most serious chronic complications of acute diarrhoea are postenteritis malabsorption, chronic diarrhoea and protein–energy malnutrition.

Features associated with aetiological agents

Rotavirus

This most often infects young children between six months and three years of age, but asymptomatic infections occur in some children, particularly in newborn nurseries. The incubation period is one to three days and the duration of illness is usually short. In temperate climates there are more cases in the colder months, though it does occur throughout the year. Although in a number of tropical countries rotavirus is found throughout the year, seasonal peaks are observed in some places. Watery diarrhoea may be preceded by vomiting and fever in half the cases. A small proportion become severely dehydrated, mildly acidotic and a few progress to secondary malabsorption.

Cholera

In endemic areas like Bangladesh, this occurs most often in children between two and nine years of age, but it is seen in all ages in newly affected regions. Onset is acute and the duration only a few days, even in those who are untreated. The incubation period is six hours to five days. The disease occurs in outbreaks but these may not be apparent because many cases are mild or asymptomatic. There is definite, but differing seasonality in endemic areas. The clinical features of severe cases are dominated by profuse watery diarrhoea associated with vomiting and abdominal cramps. With acute purging there is severe sodium loss and hypovolaemia can rapidly result in shock.

Escherichia coli

Of the different groups of pathogenic *E. coli*, enterotoxigenic *E. coli* (ETEC) are the most important, commonly causing diarrhoea in children from six months to two years of age in tropical countries. The onset is usually sudden, the duration short, two to four days, and the incubation period six hours to three days. The clinical features are watery diarrhoea, often associated with vomiting, abdominal pain and fever. Some become severely dehydrated. Enteropathogenic *E. coli* have been known to cause serious outbreaks in newborn nurseries but this appears to be less common in recent years.

Salmonella of the non-typhae food poisoning group

These zoonotic infections are associated with outbreaks of diarrhoea. The incubation is short, six hours to three days, depending on the infective dose, and the duration of illness is variable. The condition is most common in warm months and is associated with inadequately cooked meats and unhygienic food handling. The clinical features vary from watery diarrhoea to dysentery, with some vomiting, abdominal pain and malaise. Some cases become dehydrated while others mimic enteric fever. Occasionally there are focal infections in bones, meninges, etc.

Shigella

There are four species of Shigella which produce bacillary dysentery; *S. flexneri*, *S. dysenteriae* and *S boydii* which occur most commonly in developing countries, and *S. sonnei* which is most common in industrialized countries. The disease is most frequently transmitted in crowded and unhygienic circumstances. The incubation period is one to three days, the onset usually sudden and the duration quite short. Secondary cases or outbreaks are quite common, especially in institutions or crowded families. This is because the infective dose is small as few as 100 organisms, there is no animal reservoir and the excretion rate of organisms from patients is high, $10^6 - 10^9$ per gram faeces. The seasonal peak occurs in the warm weather in most countries.

Severity varies with the species; some infections are mild and subclinical, especially those due to *S. sonnei*. *S. dysenteriae* type 1 causes the most severe disease and the usual features include abdominal pain, fever, malaise and tenesmus. Dysenteric stools contain many red blood corpuscles and pus cells. Macroscopic blood is visible in the stools of over half the cases. Loss of plasma protein into the intestine may lead to hypoproteinaemia. In infants there is frequently watery diarrhoea and vomiting, especially in the early stages. Some small children are very toxic and have convulsions. The haemolytic–uraemic syndrome is a rare complication.

Campylobacter jejuni

The incubation period for this organism is two to seven days and the clinical features include abdominal pain (which may be severe), fever and malaise. Some cases have only mild diarrhoea but others have significant dysentery which may last up to a week and cause dehydration. The stools usually contain significant pus and blood cells but the prognosis is good. Animals and birds are the normal reservoir for these organisms but patient-to-patient spread has been described. The condition affects both children and young adults. In India and Bangladesh, asymptomatic carriers have been described, but in temperate climates the organism causes a definitive illness which recovers without a carrier state.

Yersinia enterocolitica

This organism is mainly zoonotic, is transmitted by the faecal–oral route and causes an enterocolitis after an incubation period of three to five days. Most cases are in children, with watery diarrhoea in infants and mesenteric adenitis in older children, mimicking appendicitis.

Entamoeba histolytica

The incubation period after cyst ingestion of this organism is two to four weeks. Infection may be non-invasive or invasive, and in many communities over 90 per cent are symptomless carriers whose only sign of infection is the passage of cysts.[7] Invasive amoebic colitis is diagnosed by the passage of dysenteric stools which contain haemophagous amoeboid trophozoites and macroscopic blood in nearly half the cases. The onset is often insidious and the course chronic with abdominal discomfort, pain and tenesmus, weight loss and recurrent fever. Occasionally the condition is a fulminating colitis with severe systemic upset.

In a few cases an amoeboma, a tumour-like granuloma, may form near the colon or elsewhere after systemic spread. Occasionally, invasive trophozoites from colonic ulcers pass to the liver via the portal system where they form abscesses in necrotic tissue. These can involve the diaphragm, forming subphrenic and pulmonary abscesses (see p. 739).

Giardia lamblia

This is also a common infection, endemic in most tropical and a number of temperate areas. The incubation period is one to three weeks, the onset often insidious and the infection prolonged. Most infections, particularly in adults, are asymptomatic. It can cause chronic diarrhoea associated with malaise, anorexia, nausea, flatulence and abdominal discomfort. In children this is a common and significant pathogen causing malabsorption with greasy, frothy, offensive stools, and resulting in a failure to thrive. It is a treatable disorder that is often missed. It also causes epidemics in some communities.

Examination of stools

Direct visual and microscopical examinations of diarrhoeal stools provide important clues to the nature and cause of the disorder. A few simple biochemical tests provide additional information.

Visual inspection

Watery stool specimens are found in secretory diarrhoea. Unformed, pale, frothy and unpleasant smelling specimens that float in water suggest malabsorption. Frank blood is apparent in dysentery, but streaks of blood may result from perianal bleeding. Altered blood from upper gastro-intestinal bleeding looks shiny black, like tar. Look specifically for parasites, blood, pus and mucus.

Acute dysentery with visible blood in the stools is most often due to shigella infection. It is sometimes seen in cases of *Campylobacter enteritis* and small amounts occur in specimens from patients with amoebic dysentery.

Mucus is also present in the stools of patients with shigellosis, *Campylobacter* and *E. histolytica* infections. It can be distinguished microscopically by the absence of pus cells. 'Current jelly' is the description of the mixture of mucus with blood seen in the evacuations and on the examining finger in cases of obstruction due to intussusception.

Microscopic techniques

Physiological saline preparations are appropriate for visualizing most parasitic pathogens, but eosin and iodine are useful in distinguishing certain parasitic cysts. There are also simple microscopic tests for cholera and *Campylobacter* which are outside the scope of this chapter.

Simple biochemical tests

Testing pH with litmus paper (which turns from blue to red in the presence of a pH less than 7) is used to identify acid stools associated with carbohydrate malabsorption. Acid stools are physiologically normal for most breast-fed babies. Further tests will be considered in the section on chronic diarrhoea.

Malnutrition

There is a serious interaction between diarrhoeal disease and malnutrition. This causes a vicious spiral which results in a high death rate from these conditions, especially in poor communities. Diarrhoea can precipitate clinical malnutrition and, especially if repeated, contribute significantly to the severity of the condition. Malnourished children suffer longer and more severe attacks of diarrhoea and probably these attacks are more frequent than in adequately nourished children.

Weanling diarrhoea, or diarrhoea in the recently weaned child[5] is a term used for the increased attack rates of diarrhoea noticed about the time and stage when children are weaned, i.e. when they are introduced to other items of diet apart from breast-milk. This usually occurs between 6 and 18 months of age in traditional societies, but may be much earlier in urban communities. This is also the age when young children become more active, mobile and often test every item they handle by putting it in their mouth. The risks are naturally much greater if standards of hygiene are poor and there is much environmental contamination.

The weaning patterns are different in different communities.[11] Unfortunately in many poor families, irrespective of the pattern, the outcome is often the same and children enter the dangerous cycle of malnutrition and diarrhoea, as illustrated in Fig. 4.3.5. In traditional Asian homes children are almost exclusively breast-fed until 6 or 12 months of age and sometimes longer. Most mothers, particularly if they themselves are undernourished, will not have sufficient milk to sustain the full rate of growth of their children for more than 3–4 months. Consequently the growth of the infants falters in the second half of the first year of life and they become malnourished with the features of the marasmic form of protein–energy malnutrition (PEM). Even when weaning foods are introduced, they are often gruel, porridge or pap diluted with water to make them liquid and easy for a small child to swallow. Such foods are so low in nutrient and energy concentration that they do not prevent malnutrition.

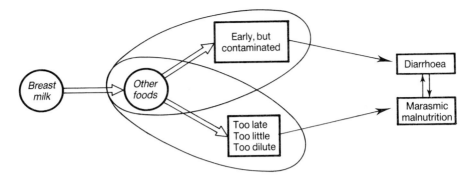

Fig. 4.3.5   Weaning patterns in poor communities and their consequences.

In other societies, particularly in Africa, and also in many urban families in other countries, the practice is to introduce other foods early in the first year. This is often to enable the mother to return to employment. In situations where it is difficult to have high standards of personal and environmental hygiene, the foods given to the infants may be contaminated with pathogenic organisms because it is difficult to store them cleanly. The problem is worse if the baby is looked after and fed by another small child who has no idea about the importance of food hygiene. These infants often have frequent attacks of diarrhoea when they are still quite small and this leads them into the cycle of diarrhoea and malnutrition.

How infections affect nutrition

Diarrhoea contributes to malnutrition by decreasing intake, limiting absorption, damaging tissue and increasing the metabolic rate (see Table 4.3.4).

The amount of food and nourishment taken in is decreased during infections. An illness, especially when associated with fever and bowel upset decreases the natural appetite. This anorexia is probably due to a variety of central and metabolic factors. In many societies it is traditional to withhold food from patients with infections, and this is particularly true in the case of diarrhoeal disease, since eating is considered to aggravate the condition. Even if food is given, some believe that the patient will not be able to digest the ordinary diet, so it is diluted and the amount of real nourishment decreased. A combination of social and pathophysiological factors results in a significant decrease in nutrient ingestion.

The amount of nutrient absorbed from the gut is decreased by bowel infections. Enzymes required for splitting and absorbing disaccharide sugars are formed

Table 4.3.4   How infections affect nutrition

Decreased nutrient intake
 anorexia (multifactorial)
 food withheld
 food substituted by dilute alternatives
 combinations of these

Decreased nutrient uptake by gut
 reduced enzymes required for digestion and absorption
 impaired absorption from damaged bowel
 intestinal hurry and decreased transit time

Tissue degradation
 cell destruction by organisms
 tissue mobilisation for nutrients
 leakage of nutrients through damaged surfaces

Increased metabolic rate
 pyrexia
 increased protein turnover for repair

at the brush-border of mature enterocytes. A high fever and other metabolic disturbances decrease the rate of cell maturation and the availability of disaccharidase. Lactase, the enzyme required to split lactose or milk sugar into glucose and galactose, is particularly sensitive to any adverse factor. When the small bowel is damaged by an infection there will be a decreased area from which absorption can take place. This occurs in any invasive diarrhoea like rotavirus infection or shigellosis.

Infections are catabolic processes that break down and destroy cells and tissues. Because of the negative nutrient balance during infections, the body has to mobilize energy and raw materials for essential metabolism from glycogen, fat and other tissue stores. Not only is there tissue loss due to mobilization of stores and cell destruction, but there is loss of essential body materials like the plasma proteins which exude from a bowel damaged by invasive diarrhoea.

Infections increase the metabolic rate and therefore the requirements of the body. To maintain the essential biological processes in the presence of the increased metabolism, extra energy is required. If intake is reduced at the same time, this obligatory energy must be mobilized from the body tissues.

How severe malnutrition affects infections

Minor degrees of undernutrition probably do not affect the incidence or outcome of diarrhoeal disease. Severe protein-energy malnutrition (PEM), particularly kwashiorkor, is associated with infections which are more severe, prolonged and probably more frequent. Ways in which severe malnutrition affects infections are indicated in Table 4.3.5. The immunological defence mechanisms act against specific organisms. They form a complex system with both cell-mediated and antibody components which are interdependent.[6] In severe PEM, the cell-mediated mechanisms have often been shown to be defective, while there appears to be less depression of the antibody mechanisms. The physical barriers of skin and gut mucosa are cracked and thin in kwashiorkor, so that organisms penetrate more easily. The various secretions into the alimentary tract are reduced in severe PEM. Less gastric acid means that more virulent organisms may reach the small bowel. A number of non-specific factors which kill or inhibit microorganisms have been found in saliva and other secretions. These, and the exocrine secretions from the pancreas and bile from the liver are decreased in severe

Table 4.3.5 How severe malnutrition affects infections

Impaired immune defence mechanisms
  Cell-mediated immunity depressed
  Humoral immunity sometimes depressed
  Interactions in the system impaired

Damaged protective barriers
  Dermatosis with cracks in skin so pathogens can invade
  Intestinal integrity also compromised

Impaired alimentary secretions
  Gastric acid decreased, therefore killing of pathogens in stomach is less effective
  Decreased secretion of various non-specific defence factors in saliva, mucus and other alimentary secretions
  Pancreatic juice deficient
  Bile volume reduced
  These last two factors contribute to the steatorrhoea or malabsorption diarrhoea and an altered bowel flora

Poor tissue repair
  This results in prolonged illness and opportunities for repeated reinfection

PEM. Incomplete fat and protein digestion, an altered bowel flora and overcolonization are associated with diarrhoea.

The deficiency of body-building nutrients in severe malnutrition means inadequate repair to damaged tissues and consequently prolonged diarrhoea.

Chronic diarrhoea

Diarrhoea which persists for more than two weeks may be considered chronic or protracted, though there is no internationally accepted definition. Chronic diarrhoea is a symptom and not a disease. It has a heterogeneous aetiology, is often difficult to manage and still carries a considerable mortality. In young children the condition can be alarming and has sometimes been labelled 'intractable diarrhoea of infancy'. By definition this requires an onset within the first three months of life, a persistence of more than three stools per day for over two weeks and the absence of detectable bacterial pathogens. Chronic diarrhoea is a nutritional disease, with failure to thrive and malnutrition as basic components.

Causes of chronic diarrhoea

The classification of chronic diarrhoea with aetiological subheadings is shown in Table 4.3.6. Even under a single heading there is a variety of potential mechanisms. As with acute diarrhoea, the simplest pathophysiological classification is either absorption failure or excessive enterocyte secretion, or both of these mechanisms together.

Although a single agent or mechanism may initiate chronic diarrhoea, there is a complicated network of factors which can perpetuate the problem. Entrance to the network of possible aetiological factors can be from many points. Mucosal injury can be due to damage by pathogens, dietary protein sensitization and auto-immune damage, or to protein–energy malnutrition. Parasitic infections, like *Giardia lamblia* and *Entamoeba histolytica* can be persistent in themselves, but they also damage the mucosa so that repair and recovery are slow and incomplete. This is exaggerated in protein–energy malnutrition in which nutrients for repair are inadequate and the body's defence mechanisms, particularly cell-mediated immunity, are defective. Maldigestion and malabsorption of nutrients may be due to a deficiency in enteric digestive secretion or mucosal enzymes. Of the mucosal enzymes, lactase deficiency is the most common and most serious because of the dependence of small children on milk. This may be a primary, congenital defect, but more often it is

Table 4.3.6   Chronic diarrhoea, a classification by aetiology and pathophysiological mechanisms

---

Infections • Parasites – Giardia lamblia
                        – Entamoeba histolytica
                        – Cryptosporidia
                        – Strongyloides stercoralis
         • Bacteria – Enteropathogenic Escherichia coli
                        – Clostridium difficile and colitis
                        – Tuberculosis of the bowel
                        – Extra intestinal infections
                          (malaria, otomastoiditis or abscess)

Post-infectious
  • Post-gastroenteritis syndrome (persistent postenteritis diarrhoea), often with abnormal bowel colonisation.
  • Post-measles diarrhoea
These are often associated with secondary lactose and other carbohydrate intolerances.
  • Post-chronic pancreatitis with calcification
  • Post-hepatitis with cirrhosis

Diet related
  • Protein-energy malnutrition and starvation (the diarrhoea-malnutrition syndrome)
  • Excessive carbohydrates, specially sugars
  • Excessive fats
  • Specific intolerances (see below)

Drug associated
  • Antibiotics – altered bowel flora and abnormal colonisation
                  – antibiotic-associated colitis} with Cl.
                  – pseudomembranous colitis} difficile
  • Excessive purgatives

Intrinsic and metabolic errors
  • Protein intolerance
    Hypersensitivity to – gluten from wheat
                          – cows' milk protein
                          – soya protein
  • Carbohydrate intolerance
      Primary lactose intolerance
      Primary lactose/glucose, sucrose/isomaltose (rare)
  • Cystic fibrosis with pancreatic insufficiency
  • Auto-immunity to enterocytes
  • Immunodeficiency syndromes (rare)
  • Inborn errors of absorption – congenital chloridorrhoea, acrodermatitis enteropathica, congenital microvillus atrophy (rare)

Idiopathic
  • Toddlers', chronic non-specific diarrhoea
  • Inflammatory bowel disease; ulcerative colitis, Crohn's disease
  • Psychosocial, irritable bowel syndrome
  • Tumours; ganglioneuroma, lymphoma etc (rare)
  • Familial chronic secretory diarrhoea (rare)

Surgical – Stenosis, malrotation, blind loop etc.

---

secondary to malnutrition, infections or other causes of bowel damage.

'Malabsorption syndrome' is not a well-defined clinical entity, but is manifest as nutritional deficiences, failure to thrive and diarrhoea. Steatorrhoea, or excessive fat in the stools, is due to inadequate digestion or absorption of dietary lipids. There are many possible causes for these conditions and clinical aspects of several of the more important causes of chronic diarrhoea will be considered individually.

Postgastroenteritis syndrome

In 5–10 per cent of children who present with acute diarrhoea due to rotavirus or some other organism, the extent of the bowel damage is so great, or the repair to the bowel structure so slow, that diarrhoea persists for weeks. A similar situation may occur during and after measles which can seriously injure the bowel mucosa. Postinfectious diarrhoea demands careful individual management and in severe cases the prognosis is poor.

Toddlers' or chronic non-specific diarrhoea

This occurs between one to five years of age, more often in boys than in girls, and often in those who are slightly hyperactive. The children generally continue to thrive and the condition usually disappears spontaneously in one to two years. The stools are large, partly formed early in the day but become smaller and looser later in the day, when they contain obvious undigested vegetables. The transit time is decreased but absorption and mucosal biopsy tests are usually normal.

Coeliac disease or gluten-sensitive enteropathy

This is an inherited intolerance to the gluten component of wheat protein, and therefore, only presents after wheat products are introduced into the diet. Children fail to thrive, have abdominal distension, somewhat wasted limbs, are irritable and may have various deficiency disorders. Their stools are pale, loose, bulky and offensive. Bowel biopsy reveals a blunted or flattened villus structure. The diagnosis is confirmed by recovery following gluten withdrawal and a further challenge after one to two years. This condition is rare in tropical countries.

Tropical sprue

This is a form of chronic diarrhoea associated with malabsorption and abnormal colonization of the upper bowel by potential pathogens. Clinical features are those of malnutrition, anaemia and vitamin deficiencies. The diagnosis is more usually made in adults than in children. Epidemic forms have been described in which no aetiological agent has been implicated.

Giardia diarrhoea

This is an important infection in children that is often overlooked. The pathogenic mechanism is unclear and may be due to a combination of mechanical obstruction to absorption, irritation and damage to the microvillus structure and function and poor absorption of nutrients.[8] The clinical picture can start with an acute onset of nausea, anorexia and abdominal discomfort. Watery, foul-smelling diarrhoea with increased flatus may develop. This acute stage may progress to chronicity with more obvious malabsorption, debility and a failure to thrive. Others recover and some may become asymptomatic cyst excretors. Chronic cases have intermittent episodes of loose, offensive stools and abdominal distension with foul flatus. Many adults and children are infected with *Giardia* without any evidence of disease.

Amoebic dysentery

Amoebic dysentery may start acutely or gradually. It may develop suddenly in those who have been long-standing asymptomatic cyst excretors.[7] Features include severe abdominal pain, fever, sometimes with chills, nausea, headache and tenesmus. Stools are liquid and contain blood and mucus but fewer pus cells than in bacterial dysentery. The disorder runs an insidious and chronic course in many patients. In tropical countries, only a minority of those infected with *E. histolytica* develop dysentery.

Strongyloidiasis

This chronic helminthic infection of the small bowel classically causes diarrhoea, upper abdominal pain and urticaria. Diagnosis is made from larvae in the stools and eosinophilia.

Investigation of chronic diarrhoea

The clinical history demands special attention to the feeding pattern, previous illnesses especially diarrhoea, infections, operations and visits to other places. The use of medicines (especially antibiotics), any stress situation at home, school or work and a family history of diarrhoea should all be specifically asked for (see p. 981).

Age is an important factor which partly relates both to diet and possible ingestion of pathogens, etc. In the first four months of life diarrhoea may follow an infection or the introduction of artificial feeding which occasionally induces sensitivity and mucosal injury. In this period some of the congenital forms of chronic diarrhoea make their appearance. Between four months and four years of age, infections and post-infectious diarrhoea are particularly common, and this includes measles. Protein–energy malnutrition is most prevalent in this age group and since feeding with wheat products begins, coeliac disease may be manifest. Toddlers' diarrhoea also occurs at this age.

At over four years of age, the parasitic infections and postinfectious diarrhoea are still problems. Psychosocial diarrhoea begins to appear at this stage.

Physical examination

Physical examination should be general and also particular for the alimentary system. The child's nutritional status, weight and height are compared with standards, and previous measurements. The appearance of skin and hair is important. Look for signs of atopy, allergy and specific deficiencies like xerophthalmia. The mouth, tongue, anus and perianal regions may give clues of vitamin deficiency in sprue-like diarrhoea with malabsorption. The abdomen is often distended. Careful palpation may reveal tenderness from invasive disease of the bowel, glands due to tuberculous lymphadenopathy or the sausage-shape of an intussusception.

Investigations

Stool examination may confirm the diagnosis and give clues to the aetiology. Blood, pus and undigested food may be visible to the naked eye and even more under a microscope. This instrument is essential for the diagnosis of enteric protozoal pathogens. The stool biochemistry should include pH estimation and tests for sugars or reducing substances.

Small bowel biopsy with a capsule which can not only retrieve a mucosal sample for morphology and enzyme activity, but also juice from the jejunum for microbiology and biochemistry, is particularly valuable. However, it does require the right equipment, skill, patience and laboratory back-up. Moreover, the small sample may not be representative of the state of the bowel.

Colonoscopy permits visualization of the lower bowel, biopsy of suspicious lesions and collection of precise samples for microbiological investigations. Modern fibre-optics have added a new dimension to this procedure. Bowel imaging with ultrasound and radiography with contrast media and gas facilitate visualization of the anatomy and abnormal motility.

The hydrogen breath test is a non-invasive method of diagnosing failure to digest sugar. Unabsorbed sugar is broken down by enteric bacteria and the amount of hydrogen exhaled is proportional to the failure of digestion. However, this is a difficult and somewhat unreliable technique. A simple urine test for lactose malabsorption looks promising.

The management of chronic diarrhoea depends on the aetiology and will be considered later in this chapter.

Management of acute diarrhoea

There are four aspects to the management of acute diarrhoea:

- Evaluation
- Rehydration
- Nutrition
- Medication

Evaluation

This is important since it will determine the severity of disease and possibly any specific aetiological agent which may require therapy. The severity of dehydration has already been discussed and was summarized in Table 4.3.3. Other factors which give clues to aetiological agents were also outlined.

It should quickly be apparent if the patient is very dehydrated and shocked. Such a patient requires immediate infusion to expand the circulating blood volume before any further evaluation is undertaken. If the patient's general condition is reasonable a detailed clinical assessment will indicate the most appropriate management for the individual.

Rehydration

The most serious short-term consequences of acute diarrhoea result from the loss of body water and electrolytes. This has been known since O'Shaughnessy's work of 1831.[12] Probably at least 60 per cent of the mortality from acute diarrhoea is because of dehydration. Replacing the water and electrolytes is referred to as rehydration. As these deficits are replaced, the kidneys begin to function normally and the body's pH will also be corrected.

The type of fluid needed for rehydration and the route by which it may be given depends on the clinical state of the patient. Most cases, probably more than 95 per cent, can be adequately treated by providing fluids through the alimentary tract, usually as drinks. This is known as *Oral Rehydration Therapy* (ORT). In the early stages of an attack, or if the disease is very mild, extra household drinks are usually adequate since the body will have reasonable reserves of most electrolytes and kidney function can control losses. In cases of more serious diarrhoea, especially when signs of dehydration are apparent, special oral rehydration fluids are indicated. Even simple formulations are extremely valuable in treating acute diarrhoea. ORT is based on sound scientific principles which should be understood.[13] Only then can the simple solutions be used correctly and patients, relatives and health workers instructed with confidence about how to manage this condition.[14]

Scientific basis for oral rehydration therapy

In many forms of acute diarrhoea the main mechanism is an excessive secretion rather than a primary failure in absorption. Even in the forms of diarrhoea in which organisms invade and damage the enterocytes, for example rotavirus diarrhoea and shigella dysentery, the lesions are only patchy, leaving significant areas of small bowel mucosa available for absorption. Therefore it is reasonable to consider giving water and salts by mouth to replace what has been lost. Unfortunately, the amount of saline the bowel can absorb is rather limited.

Since the late 1960s there have been many studies of the way in which glucose and other carbohydrates enhance the absorption of fluids and electrolytes from the bowel. Figure 4.3.6 illustrates that the addition of

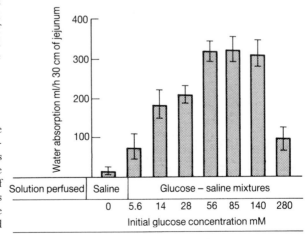

Fig. 4.3.6 Water absorption rates with different concentrations of glucose in saline in gut superfusion studies. (After Sladen and Dawson, *Clinical Sciences*, 1969; **36**: 119–32. © Biochemical Society.)

glucose to saline in a segment of small bowel results in a 25-fold increase in fluid absorption.[9] An important factor which facilitates this dramatic improvement is probably a linked carrier mechanism at the brush-border of enterocytes. An ion of sodium and a molecule of glucose are taken into the cell together and the process is repeated many times. Glucose enters the carbohydrate metabolic pathway while sodium is pushed out of the cell by the 'sodium pump', the colloquial name for the enzyme sodium–potassium ATPase, which is situated on the basolateral membranes of the enterocytes. As sodium accumulates in the lateral intercellular spaces, water is drawn there to prevent an excessive hyperosmolar tension. This results in increased hydrostatic pressure which in turn opens the intercellular pores or 'tight junctions', permitting a paracellular inflow of water and salts from the lumen. In this way the linked mechanism increases both the transcellular and the paracellular pathways of absorption (see Fig. 4.3.7).

It is now recognized that glucose is not the only molecule which can enhance absorption. The amino acid glycine, rice and other cereal powders also increase absorption. There is now good scientific evidence that rice powder rehydration solution is significantly more effective than glucose-based rehydration fluid.[15] The polysaccharides from rice starch are gradually broken down to glucose by the pancreatic amylase. Consequently more glucose is produced over a longer period without increasing the osmolality of the fluid in the lumen. This discovery means that it is possible to prepare a potent rehydration solution from food ingredients found in many homes, though it may not always be convenient to do so.

The composition of appropriate oral rehydration solutions

A patient who has severe diarrhoea with dehydration, probably has a large deficit of sodium, some loss of potassium and an acidosis. An oral rehydration solution should effectively combat all of these factors. In early diarrhoea with little or no evidence of dehydration, almost any fluid will be beneficial as the body stores of electrolytes are not seriously depleted and adjustments can be made by the kidneys. In the most severely ill, especially if the patient is in circulatory collapse, the condition requires immediate intravenous rehydration. If rehydration by mouth is started early in the disease, and continued enthusiastically, there is evidence that relatively few patients will become severely dehydrated.

The most widely tested oral rehydration solution is made up with *Oral Rehydration Salts* (ORS). The amounts of the salts and the concentrations when dissolved in one litre of drinking water are shown in Table 4.3.7. Originally sodium bicarbonate was used as the alkalysing agent, but this has now been replaced by trisodium citrate monohydrate since this gives the powder a much longer shelf-life. The formula contains quite a high concentration of sodium, 90 mmols/litre, for two reasons: it can almost replace the high sodium losses in the most severely purging cases like acute cholera; and it provides a sodium concentration which

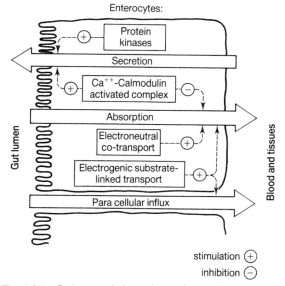

Fig. 4.3.7 Pathways of absorption and secretion across the small intestinal mucosa.

Table 4.3.7 The constituents and composition of oral rehydration salts (ORS)

Sodium chloride-NaCl (ordinary salt)	3.5g
Trisodium citrate	2.9g
(or Sodium bicarbonate-HCO$_3$, baking soda)	2.5g)
Potassium chloride-KCl	1.5g
Glucose (a form of sugar)	20g

Made up in 1000 ml or 1 litre of drinking water.

This should give electrolyte concentrations of:

Na$^+$	90 m mol/litre
K	20 m mol/litre
Cl	80 m mol/litre
Citrate	10 m mol/litre
(or HCO$_3$)	30 m mol/litre
Glucose	110 m mol/litre

N.B. Trisodium citrate has replaced sodium bicarbonate in the current formulation of ORS.

is nearer to the normal blood levels, which facilitates absorption. Potassium is important since this element is deficient in undernourished children and those with chronic diarrhoea. This solution has been widely tested and has been found to be both safe and effective when used properly.[16]

Alternative rehydration solutions have been developed for different reasons. Solutions made with domestic salt and sugar are almost as effective as ORS solution for correcting dehydration, but obviously are not so effective in correcting acidosis and potassium deficits. There have been attempts to develop a 'super solution' which will give even higher rates of absorption from the gut.[17] The most efficient solution tested so far contains the same electrolytes as ORS, but glucose is replaced by 50 g of rice powder, which is boiled and then cooled before administration. This is more effective clinically and is culturally acceptable in some countries.[15] There are several commercial oral rehydration products on the market. Many of these have a lower sodium and a higher sugar concentration than the ORS. Too much sugar can diminish absorption because of the high osmotic tension.

How to prepare and mix ORS solution

Examine the packet of ORS and in particular note in what volume of water it should be dissolved. The WHO packets are generally for one litre of water, but in some countries packets are designed to be mixed in half a litre or in some locally available container. Teach those who prepare the solution to start by washing their hands and rinsing out (with clean water) the vessel in which it will be mixed. Fill the container to the one litre mark (or other volume if appropriate). Pour in all the ORS powder from the packet and mix until the contents are completely dissolved. It is good practice to taste the solution to ensure that it is not too concentrated. It is generally recommended that the solution 'should not taste saltier than tears', but this is a generalization as tears can vary in sodium content. Cover the fluid when it is not being given to the patient.[14]

If packets are not available, the ingredients of ORS can be measured in other ways. They can be weighed if an accurate balance is available, or they can be measured by volume.

How to prepare home-made salt–sugar solution

There are many methods for preparing a suitable salt–sugar solution. Two examples are given here.

For the first use a 5 ml teaspoon and a container for one litre; take salt in the teaspoon and level it with a knife or flat object; pour the level teaspoonful of salt into the container; fill the container to the one litre mark with drinking water; mix to dissolve, and taste the water ensuring that it is not too salty; add eight level teaspoonsful of sugar, and stir to dissolve.[14]

In some countries a system of measuring sugar and salt using fingers and hands has been devised. This is the way in which many women measure cooking ingredients.

With either method there is a risk of inaccuracy unless the method is carefully standardized and taught. Part of the standard instructions should relate to the size of a container available locally. Confusion, wrong mixing and administration of solutions which are too concentrated may cause harm and undermine confidence in what is a very valuable treatment.

How much oral rehydration fluid to give?

The patient should receive enough rehydration fluid to replace the volume lost:

- in previous watery stools;
- in continuing diarrhoeal stools.

In addition the patient must drink as much other fluid as required for daily needs.

Ideally the volume of diarrhoeal stools passed should be measured, and replaced by ORS solution given by mouth. In practice it is impossible to measure stool volume accurately, so estimates are based either on the patient's general condition and weight (method A) or on the patient's age and the number of stools passed (method B).

Method A   A patient with moderate to severe dehydration will have lost about 10 per cent body weight and will require 100 ml of ORS solution per kg of body weight to replace what has been lost. This should be given little by little over 2–4 hours. Thus, a 10 kg child will need 10 × 100 ml ORS solution, i.e. one litre over 2–4 hours. When further watery stools are passed, these volumes will also have to be replaced.

Method B   Stool size and number are the basis for estimating the volume of ORS solution needed. Stool size varies with patient size and the cause and nature of diarrhoea. An approximation is made and a rough guide is to consider that an adult will pass 200–400 ml in a large watery stool, a big child 100–200 ml, a toddler 50–100 ml and a small infant 20–50 ml. Therefore, a toddler who has four large watery stools should drink 4 × 100 ml, i.e. 400 ml of ORS solution in the next two to four hours, and additional lots of 50–100 ml for every additional watery stool. These volumes should be converted into local measures when instructing mothers. Half a 200 ml glass might be an appropriate measure when talking to the mother of a toddler.

Apart from oral rehydration to replace diarrhoea losses, adults and children require fluid for maintenance of ordinary metabolic requirements. This can be given in the form of any ordinary drinks that the individual will usually take; water, fruit juices, tea, breast-milk or diluted cow's milk. These drinks should be offered liberally in tropical countries. Simplified calculations for rehydration and maintenance volumes are set out in Table 4.3.8.

How to give oral rehydration fluids

Patients should be offered ORS solution or other rehydration mixtures in small volumes at frequent intervals; little and often is the rule. This decreases vomiting. Dehydrated children are usually thirsty, but if offered a whole glass of ORS solution they may drink it down and promptly vomit. Patience and persistence are necessary, for an ill and miserable child may at first be reluctant to take ORS solution. A little flavouring from fruit juice or tea is permissible if this helps the child to take the ORS drink. If a child is not fully conscious, or vomiting excessively, and there is no facility for giving intravenous infusions, a naso-gastric tube is a safe and effective way to give ORS solution.

Intravenous rehydration

In severe cases, particularly those in shock, the rehydration fluid should be given intravenously to improve the circulation rapidly (see pp. 1002–7). As the patient improves over the first two to four hours ongoing rehydration ('maintenance therapy') can be given by mouth. Again, for normal metabolic requirements, plain water, breast-milk or simple home drinks like dilute fruit juices and tea should be given. Rehydration therapy by the intravenous route is also required for those few patients with profuse or repeated vomiting, altered consciousness, or occasionally when diarrhoea is truly excessive (greater than 10 ml per kg per hour).

The compositions of four commonly used intravenous solutions are shown in Table 4.3.9. Some regimens recommend plasma, a plasma substitute or blood for expanding the blood volume in cases of shock, but this is not usually necessary.

Table 4.3.8 Fluids and volumes to be given in diarrhoea

Rehydration therapy – replace previous deficits		
Shock or	iv Ringer's lactate	
Severe dehydration	or Darrow's half strength or ORS by mouth if IV not available	100 ml/kg 2–4 hours (iv fast for first hour)
Moderate or Mild dehydration	ORS solution	75 ml/kg over 4–6 hours

Ongoing rehydration for continuing losses (called 'Maintenance therapy' by WHO)		
Measure stool and vomit lost, or estimate	ORS solution	Replace volume lost
For each watery stool replace approximate volumes by age	ORS solution	20–50 ml/stool – small infant 50–100 ml/stool – large infant 100–200 ml/stool – children 200–400 ml/stool – adults

*Daily maintenance requirements**	
Water or	150 ml/kg in 24 hr – small infants
Fruit juice or	120 ml/kg in 24 hr – large infants
Tea or	100 ml/kg in 24 hr – children
Breast or diluted	75 ml/kg in 24 hr – adults
cow's milk, or any other acceptable drink	

* These are approximate volumes.
In a hot climate, or in patients with fever, volumes should be increased substantially.

Table 4.3.9 The ionic composition of four intravenous solutions

Solution	Cations (mMol per litre)				Anions Lactate or acetate*
	Na$^+$	K$^{+\prime}$	Ca^{++}	Cl$^\prime$	
Ringer's lactate	130	4	3	109	28
Half strength Darrow's solution with 2.5% dextrose	61	18	–	52	27
Normal saline	154	–	–	154	–
Dhaka solution (ICDDR,B)	133	13	–	98	48

*Lactate and acetate are converted to bicarbonate which helps to correct acidosis.

- *Ringer's lactate solution* (Hartmann's solution for injection or compound sodium lactate solution) is the best, and is often commercially available. It contains adequate sodium and potassium to correct deficits of those ions and also lactate which yields bicarbonate for the correction of acidosis.

- *Half-strength Darrow's solution* (lactated potassic saline) is often combined *with 2.5 per cent dextrose*. This does not contain enough sodium for adults with severe losses, but has been found very effective in treating children. The dextrose provides some energy and makes the solution almost isotonic.
- *Normal saline* (isotonic or physiological saline). This is relatively high in sodium, but does not contain bicarbonate or lactate to correct acidosis, nor potassium to counter hypokalaemia. These substances are sometimes added into the infusion solution, but this requires careful calculation and monitoring which may not be possible. A sterile technique is required.
- *Fifth-normal saline with 4.3 per cent dextrose*. This is often used as a maintenance solution in patients who cannot drink, but it is too dilute to use for the rehydration stage of therapy, except in hypernatraemia when it should be given slowly.

In any service it is better to have a standard regimen using one or two fluids. Ringer's lactate solution, and with some qualifications, half-strength Darrow's solution, are recommended by WHO.[10] If these are not available, normal saline may be used for the rehydration phase. Ongoing rehydration (maintenance therapy) can normally be given by mouth. If it is necessary to give daily fluid requirements by the intravenous route, fifth-normal saline with 4.3 per cent dextrose is appropriate.

Prompt therapy, even with a solution which does not contain all the correcting agents can be effective. Acidosis can be treated in the absence of an alkali by improving the circulation to the kidneys which then correct the metabolic state. If only normal saline is available, once the patient has passed urine, one gram of a sterile solution of potassium chloride can be added to each 500 ml of normal saline and this will provide 13 mmol of potassium ion.

Guidelines for the rates and volumes of fluid to be given are shown in Table 4.3.10. These volumes are only a general guide, and the condition of the patient will indicate if the speed of the infusion needs to be increased or reduced.

The main advantage of the intravenous route is speed; the rapid expansion of the intravascular volume to restore circulation. There are significant dangers; overloading the circulation, infection and damage to peripheral vessels. Puffiness of the eyes is an early sign of fluid overload in small children. This may progress to other signs of heart failure, cough due to basal congestion and accompanied by fine crepitations in the lungs,

Table 4.3.10   Guidelines for intravenous rehydration therapy

If shocked and severely dehydrated, calculate for 10–15% dehydration, i.e. requiring 100–150 ml fluid per kg body weight.

Example: Use 120 ml/kg weight for calculation.

Infant:
120 ml/kg for replacement
First ⅓ i.e.   40 ml/kg as Ringer lactate I.V.
                         Speed, fast – within 1 hour
Second ⅓ i.e.   40 ml/kg as Ringer lactate I.V.
                         Speed, slower – over 2 hours
Third ⅓ i.e.   40 ml/kg as ORS solution by mouth
                         Little by little – over 2–3 hours

Older children

Adults:
120 ml/kg for replacement as Ringer lactate I.V. at first until pulse steady, then remainder over subsequent 3 + hours. Start ORS solution during later hours of I.V. therapy.

Notes:
1) Continuing diarrhoea losses to be replaced with equivalent volumes of Ringer lactate or ORS.
2) Daily metabolic fluid requirements to be met by drinks of water and domestic fluids.
3) The volumes quoted above are only averages based on theoretical calculations and practical experience. Clinical judgement should be used, so that if rehydration is not achieved the volume should be increased, or if the patient is rapidly hydrated and puffy the infusion should be stopped.

tachypnoea which may be confused with the rapid respiration of acidosis, and enlargement of the liver, especially in small children. When an intravenous infusion has been started the patient should be reviewed after two to four hours, and in the case of infants after one to two hours. This is to check that a patient is receiving neither too much nor too little fluid. Infection at the site of the intravenous needle or cannula and thrombophlebitis are common, but septicaemia from infected infusion apparatus or solution is more serious.

Ongoing rehydration (maintenance therapy) must follow initial rehydration, because diarrhoea does not usually stop suddenly and completely. This requires continuing replacement of the fluids and electrolytes that are lost after the initial rehydration when the deficits were corrected. Ongoing rehydration can normally be achieved by oral fluids as described above. Parents and staff need to be told that ORT does not reduce the diarrhoea suddenly, but it does reduce the danger of the diarrhoea until the body overcomes the infection.

Management of hypernatraemic dehydration

The predisposing factors and the pathophysiology of hypernatraemia in association with dehydration have already been described. Treatment requires caution, as too-rapid correction aggravates CNS dysfunction, probably by causing cerebral oedema.

Rehydration and electrolyte correction should be slower than normal, possibly using a slightly more dilute replacement fluid. Using a very dilute fluid may precipitate rapid fluid shift and cerebral oedema. The simplest regimen is to use the standard WHO oral rehydration regimen (see earlier), but aim to correct the dehydration in 12 hours rather than four to six hours. Others have recommended giving 120 ml/kg over 24 hours of either half-strength ORS solution by mouth, or half-strength Darrow's solution with 2.5 per cent dextrose intravenously.

Cases in hypovolaemic shock are particularly difficult to manage. They need rapid expansion of the circulating volume, and this may be achieved by an initial infusion of a plasma-expander.

Input–output charting

Any patient who is ill enough to require intravenous hydration should have a proper record of fluid input and output for the duration of the procedure. This should clearly show on the input side:

- the fluid ordered;
- the volume ordered;
- the route to be administered;
- the amount actually given/received;
- the times in relation to administration;

and on the output side:

- volume of urine passed;
- any vomits and their approximate volume;
- any stools and their approximate volume and nature.

An example of an input–output chart is shown in Fig. 4.3.8.

The volume on the input and output sides of the chart should be added up to see if the hydration is going to plan or if there is any need for a mid-course correction. Adjustments may be necessary either due to an initial miscalculation, or a change in the patient's condition. This may sound like an impossible counsel of excellence in a busy paediatric service, but careful charting will decrease the risks of overhydration in small children and is also an important aspect of training doctors and nurses.

Nutrition

There is a significant nutritional cost from diarrhoea in all patients (this was discussed on p. 474). The need for nourishment is clear, but the type, method and timing are not so certain.

To feed or not to feed?

There are some theoretical benefits of withholding food. This may decrease problems of maldigestion, particularly lactose intolerance. It might also prevent the gastro-colic reflex.

On the other hand there are practical benefits from feeding during diarrhoea. These have been recognized for many years but have not been actively promoted. Although there is a degree of malabsorption, there is still over 60 per cent of nutrient absorption during diarrhoea. Stimulation of the gastro-colic reflex does not increase the total stool volume, and resting the bowel does not facilitate healing, indeed it promotes villus atrophy. In contrast, food induces enzymic action and secretion which tend to restore the microenvironment and promote healing. The nutritional benefit of feeding during the illness is significant since in communities where diarrhoea is common, children may have the condition for 55 days (15 per cent) of the year and if they are not fed at these times, it will be almost impossible to correct the nutritional deficits. The stopping of breast-feeding is particularly detrimental. Not only will it remove IgA and other factors inhibiting pathogens as well as decreasing the current milk intake but through lack of stimulation it will diminish the production of this important food for the months ahead.[18]

Two critical issues concerning feeding are the nutritional status of the child and the environmental cleanliness. Well-nourished and hygienically protected children who are rarely ill will not be endangered by starvation for one or two days during diarrhoea. However, they do recover and gain weight more quickly with rapid refeeding. For malnourished children in a contaminated environment, repeated starvation as part of the treatment for every episode of diarrhoea may be fatal.

Feeding during and after diarrhoea

As soon as initial rehydration is complete, and this should only take two to four hours, foods should be introduced, with a particular emphasis on high-energy and readily absorbable items which are familiar and acceptable to the child. Breast-feeding should not be

DAILY FLUID BALANCE CHART

DATE_____   WEIGHT_____Kg.

PATIENT'S
NAME   _____   DATE OF BIRTH_____

TIME	OBSERVATIONS –	ORDERS –

TIME	FLUID OUTPUT				FLUID INTAKE				
	VOMIT or ASPIRATE	URINE	STOOL	TOTAL OUTPUT	MOUTH or NG TUBE NATURE	VOL	INTRAVENOUS NATURE	VOL	TOTAL INTAKE
PERIOD TOTAL									

NOTE 1. GIVE EXTRA FLUID IN FEVER OR HOT WEATHER TO COMPENSATE FOR EXCESS SKIN, LUNG
AND SWEAT LOSS.
2. IN ACUTELY ILL PATIENTS, CALCULATE FLUID INPUT AND OUTPUT IN 4 OR 6 HOURLY PERIODS,
NOT ONLY EVERY 24 HOURS.

(a)

Fig. 4.3.8   Example of a fluid chart for a 12 hour period.

DAILY FLUID BALANCE CHART

DATE *15.09.1987*   WEIGHT *8.3* Kg.

PATIENT'S NAME *Mohammed R. Khaled*   DATE OF BIRTH *28.12.'86*

TIME	OBSERVATIONS –	ORDERS –
09.00h.	moderate dehydration.	R ORS solution 600ml. in 6 hours. Extra fluids ad libitum, at least 800 ml in 24 hours.
13.00h.	No signs of dehydration now.	R Continue ORS and fluids

TIME	FLUID OUTPUT				FLUID INTAKE				
	VOMIT or ASPIRATE	URINE	STOOL	TOTAL OUTPUT	MOUTH or NG TUBE NATURE	VOL	INTRAVENOUS NATURE	VOL	TOTAL INTAKE
09.00h admitted 09.30h	V large ≈ 70ml.	—	100 ml.		ORS sol. ORS sol.	100ml 100ml			
11.00	V: ≈ 50ml.	—	50ml.		ORS sol. water	100ml 100ml			
12.00h		30ml.	80 ml.		ORS sol.	100ml			
4 hours	120ml	30ml.	230ml	380ml.		500ml		—	500ml.
15:00h.	—	—	—		fruit juice	150ml			
18.00h.	—	—	50ml.		ORS sol	100ml			
21.00h	—	60ml	—		weak tea	100ml			
		60 ml	50ml	110 ml		350ml			350ml.
	First 12 hours Total – 490ml				First 12 hours Total				850ml.
					Positive balance in 12 h.				360ml.
PERIOD TOTAL									

NOTE 1. GIVE EXTRA FLUID IN FEVER OR HOT WEATHER TO COMPENSATE FOR EXCESS SKIN, LUNG AND SWEAT LOSS.
2. IN ACUTELY ILL PATIENTS, CALCULATE FLUID INPUT AND OUTPUT IN 4 OR 6 HOURLY PERIODS, NOT ONLY EVERY 24 HOURS.

(b)

interrupted, but other milks should be diluted until the diarrhoea stops. This precaution is because some formula-milks contain a large amount of lactose, the sugar which a damaged bowel has the greatest difficulty in digesting and absorbing.

During recovery and convalescence, there is a period of anabolism and catch-up growth. Extra feeding should be given after every episode, but the practicalities of what food, when and how it is provided, will depend on the child's age and the local circumstances. Practical advice about feeding during and after diarrhoea is summarized in Table 4.3.11.

Table 4.3.11 Nutritional management of acute diarrhoea: practical advice about feeding during and after diarrhoea

---

Complete initial rehydration quickly 2–4 hours so that feeding can resume.

Breast fed babies should continue to be fed during diarrhoea.

Babies receiving cows' or formula milks should have these diluted 1:1 with clean water until the diarrhoea stops. (This is to decrease the risk of lactose overload. Note some babies only receive over diluted milk)

Older infants and toddlers should be offered familiar and acceptable food after initial rehydration is complete. Locally available, energy-rich foods high in potassium are particularly valuable.

'Special foods' are not usually required following acute diarrhoea. Soya-based milk or comminuted chicken may be useful in some cases of chronic diarrhoea.

Extra food should be given for 1–3 weeks during the convalescent period of catch-up growth after an episode of diarrhoea. Patience and encouragement may be necessary. (Adopt some easy to remember and culturally acceptable regime, e.g. 'one extra meal per day for as many weeks as the days a child had diarrhoea'.)

Note: Starving patients in order to 'rest the bowel' prolongs negative nutrient balance and encourages mucosal atrophy.

Medication

Man has been described as an animal with a particular desire to take medicines. Expectations have increased since the introduction of antibiotics, like penicillin and streptomycin which have performed miracles in such dreaded diseases as meningitis and tuberculosis. Because of this, people have come to believe that there must be 'a pill for every ill' and surely 'a drug for diarrhoea'. However, diarrhoea is not a single disease and medication is not the most important therapy.

The drugs used in diarrhoeal disease can be divided into those which affect:

- microorganisms;
- motility of the bowel;
- mucosal transport;
- miscellaneous mechanisms.

Antimicrobial drugs

Most microorganisms that cause diarrhoea in children are either not affected by antimicrobial drugs, like the rotavirus, or the natural history of the infection is little influenced by the administration of an antibiotic, for example *Campylobacter jejuni*. Unnecessary antibiotics can damage the bowel (e.g. neomycin), prolong faecal excretion of a pathogen (e.g. non-typhoid salmonellosis), or destroy many of the useful commensal flora (e.g. all wide-spectrum antibiotics).

The efficacy of antimicrobial drugs depends on the fact that they interfere with the metabolism of the cells of the pathogenic organism to a greater extent than that of the cells of the human host. Despite dramatic efficacy and remarkable margins of safety, there is a price to pay in terms of adverse reactions. These reactions are indicated in Table 4.3.12 and should always be kept in mind when a patient is on medication.

Antimicrobial drugs act on bacteria in a variety of ways. They can inhibit the synthesis of different components of the cell structure, the wall (e.g. penicillins), the cytoplasmic protein (e.g. chloramphenicol, tetracyclines and aminoglycosides), DNA (e.g. nalidixic acid and metronidazole) and folate required for metabolism (e.g. sulphonamides and trimethoprim). They may also act on the cell wall either altering function by increasing permeability or by actual disruption.

Bacterial resistance to antibiotics is an important problem. There are a variety of mechanisms by which organisms avoid the effects of the antimicrobial drugs. They may become either drug-tolerant or drug-destroying. Drug-tolerant organisms develop metabolic pathways which are unaffected by the antimicrobial agent. Drug-destroying organisms produce enzymes or other mechanisms which destroy the molecular structure and therefore function of drugs. Penicillinase-producing organisms actively destroy penicillin and most of its analogues.

The bacterial properties of resistance against antimicrobial drugs may become encoded in either chromosomal DNA, or in extrachromosomal plasmid DNA. The plasmid-transmitted R-factor (resistance factor), insensitivity to antibiotics, is more serious. A plasmid in one bacterium that is resistant to an antibiotic can physically transfer the extrachromosomal material to another bacterium which was previously susceptible. Once a resistant strain develops, if much antibiotic is used, that strain is selected, multiplies and can quickly become predominant. Epidemics have occurred in this way due to strains of tetracycline-resistant cholera, chloramphenicol-resistant *Salmonella typhi* and ampicillin-resistant *Shigella dysenteriae* type 1.

Antimicrobials have no value and do harm in most types of diarrhoea. There are diseases for which antibiotics are indicated, for example in dysentery due to *Shigella dysenteriae* type 1, especially in children who become toxic with the infection, and in pseudomembranous enterocolitis due to *Clostridium difficile*. The drugs of choice for severe bacillary dysentery are ampicillin (100 mg/kg/per day, six hourly in divided doses for five days) or cotrimoxazole (TMP 10 mg and SMX 50 mg/kg/per day in two daily doses for five days). Unfortunately, many Shigella species are now resistant to these antibiotics and, where this is the case, nalidixic acid (5 mg/kg/per day in four divided doses for five days) is the drug of choice. In pseudomembranous enterocolitis, vancomycin (44 mg/kg/per day divided into four doses and given with an intravenous infusion) or metronidazole (30 mg/kg/per day in three doses for 10 days) are indicated.

Antimicrobials are a valuable adjunct to ORT in a few types of diarrhoea. In cholera, rehydration is the life-saving factor, but effective antibiotics like tetracycline (50 mg/kg/per day in six hourly doses for three days) and doxycyline (4 mg/kg on the first day and then 2 mg/kg/per day as a single oral dose for a total of three days) can kill off the vibrio and shorten the duration, but not the immediate severity, of disease. In acute invasive amoebiasis, or in severe giardiasis, particularly in children, metronidazole (30 mg/kg/per day in three doses for 10 days) or tinidazole (50–60 mg/kg/per day as a single oral dose for five days) are valuable.

Problems of antibiotic use in developing countries – inflated ideas of efficacy Because antibiotics are highly effective in some conditions, the general public imagines that they are the answer to all infections. People do not appreciate the significant risk of adverse reactions, which are acceptable when drugs are used against life-threatening infections, but not when diseases are self-limiting or non-responsive to treatment.

Insufficient supplies and inadequate dosage Many economic and organizational constraints can contribute to these factors. There is a need for public and medical education with regard to the use of drugs for priority diseases and the use of adequate dosage to avoid either the development of resistant organisms or wastage of valuable medicine.

Incorrect usage of drugs in man This is partly due to wrong prescribing because a precise diagnosis is

difficult even if laboratory services are adequate. The free availability of many antimicrobials without prescription increases this problem.

Indiscriminate use of antibiotics for animals This is more a feature of intensive farming methods in Europe and North America, but is already occurring in a number of tropical and developing countries. It increases the risk of resistant zoonotic strains which can affect man directly or through R-factor transfer.

Undisciplined promotion and frank commercialization Such activities by the pharmaceutical industry, medical shops and individual practitioners must be countered by education, discipline and possibly legislation.

The main danger with regard to antibiotics in diarrhoeal disease, is that they will distract those who are looking after patients from giving the most important treatment, the replacement of lost water and electrolytes by mouth. In most cases, oral or intravenous rehydration, and not antibiotics, will make the critical difference.

Antimotility drugs

Most antimotility drugs are opiates and their analogues. These drugs affect many organs and systems producing, among other actions, analgesia and behavioural changes. They may also cause significant nausea and vomiting due to brainstem stimulation. Within the respiratory system, they inhibit the carbon dioxide sensitivity in the medullary centre which results in respiratory depression. In the cardiovascular system there is some peripheral vasodilatation associated with hypotension. In the bowel, large doses may increase contractions, but smaller doses generally depress motility. This last activity provides the rationale for giving the drug in diarrhoea. Renewed interest in these powerful medicines has followed the discovery of endogenous peptides, endorphins, which mimic the action of opiates. These are particularly located in the pituitary and the bowel.

Tinctures of opium and codeine were previously prescribed to decrease peristalsis and limit the abdominal pain of colic. However, they have significant effects on the central nervous system (CNS) and can cause nausea, vomiting and respiratory depression. Potentially harmful effects of decreased bowel motility are delayed peristalsis with consequent delayed evacuation of pathogens and their toxins.

Two synthetic opiate analogues are diphenoxalate (often combined with atropine as Lomotil) and loperamide (Imodium). These are promoted as antidiarrhoeals and are said to have fewer CNS side-effects.[19] However, there have been accidental deaths

Table 4.3.12   Antimicrobial drugs for the treatment of diarrhoeal disease and alimentary infections

Drug	Indications	Dosage by Mouth Adults	Dosage by Mouth Children	Duration of Treatment	Adverse Reactions	Comments
Ampicillin	*Sh. dysenteriae*	500 mg, 6 hourly	100 mg/kg/day 6 hourly in divided doses	5 days	Maculo-papular rashes (in 5% adults). Occasionally causes pseudo-membranous colitis	Many resistant strains in some countries. Single dose of 4 g is effective and appropriate in some situations.
Co-trimoxazole, Trimethoprim (TMP) with Sulpha-methoxazole (SMX)	*Sh. dystenteriae*	TMP 160 mg and SMX 800 mg twice daily	TMP 10 mg/kg/d SMX 50 mg/kg/d in 2 divided doses (up to a maximum of the adult dose)	5 days	TMP Allergy or toxicity in 5%. Fever, rashes, photosensitivity, GI symptoms. SMX Rashes and GI symptoms.	
Nalidixic Acid	*Sh. dysenteriae when resistant to the antimicrobials above*	*4 g/d in 4 divided doses*	*100 mg/kg/d in 4 divided doses*	5 days	*GI upset, haemolysis in G6PD deficiency, allergic reactions rashes, etc*	*Relatively expensive*
Tetracycline	*V. cholera* 01 (also a support drug in acute amoebiasis and an alternative for *Sh. dysenteriae*)	500 mg 6 hourly	75–140 mg, 6 hourly, or 50 mg/kg/d, 6 hourly (to a maximum of the adult dose)	3–5 days	GI upset, D & V Discolouration of developing teeth and bones. Hepatic toxicity in pregnancy	Some strains are resistant to tetracycline
Furazolidone	*V. cholera* 01 alternative drug	100 mg, 6 hourly	5 mg/kg/d, in 4 divided doses	3–5 days		
Doxycycline	*V. cholera* 01	300 mg once	4 mg/kg/once	Single dose	Inadvisable in renal failure	Single dose convenience
Erythromycin	*Campylobacter jejuni* (Also an alternative drug for cholera)	500 mg, 6 hourly	25–50 mg/kg/d in 4 divided doses	7 days (3 days for cholera)	GI upset, D & V Liver toxicity, but only on long treatment	Reduces duration of bacterial excretion but not symptoms
Chloramphenicol	*S. typhae* (and *H. influenzae*) when these are life-threatening	500 mg, 6 hourly	50 mg/kg/d until apyrexial, then 30 mg/kg/d	14 or more days (5 days in *H. influenzae* infection)	Leukopenia, thrombocytop-enia, and rarely aplastic anaemia	

Drug	Indications	Dosage by Mouth Adults	Dosage by Mouth Children	Duration of Treatment	Adverse Reactions	Comments
Metronidazole	*Entamoeba histolytica*, and *Giardia lamblia*	750 mg 3 times daily	30 mg/kg/d in 3 doses	10 days	GI upsets, D & V CNS disturbances e.g. ataxia, headaches, Disulfiram effect	
Sulphonamides, eg Sulpha-dimadine	In absence of any main drugs for *V. cholera* or *Sh. dysenteriae*	1 g, 6 hourly	100 mg/kg/d in 6 hourly doses	5 days or more	GI upset, rashes, occasional marrow depression	Not recommended because most pathogens are resistant and side effects significant

of children because of respiratory depression due to overdosage of Lomotil. Clinical trials of the efficacy of these drugs have been disappointing. They are not recommended for the treatment of diarrhoea in children, but may be used to produce some symptomatic relief in adults.

Antisecretory and miscellaneous medicines

Many drugs, toxins, humoral factors and food constituents can influence the complex absorption–secretion mechanisms of mucosal transport (see Fig. 4.3.10). The enhancement of absorption by glucose and other food constituents has already been mentioned. Opiate derivatives, particularly loperamide, may also depress secretion, probably by inhibiting the action of calcium–calmodulin which is an important component in the secretion of chloride ions and water from the enterocyte. Phenothiazines, particularly chlorpromazine, the non-specific anti-inflammatory drugs and prostaglandin E inhibitors, aspirin and indomethacin, bismuth and aluminium salts may all decrease secretion. Unfortunately, the pharmacological doses required to reduce enterocyte secretion are so large that there are often significant side-effects on other organs and systems. Laboratory experiments have sometimes looked promising, but in clinical trials it has been difficult to show significant benefits.[19] At present there is no place for the routine use of these medications.

A small injection of phenothiazine may break a cycle

of vomiting in a child, but it will probably decrease consciousness and cooperation in taking adequate fluids by mouth. Rehydration and the correction of acidosis are most effective in reducing vomiting.

The current emphasis is to find a 'super oral rehydration solution' which is so effectively absorbed, that even the bowel secretions will be reabsorbed, reducing the fluid in the stools. So far the most effective compound is a rice powder electrolyte solution.[15]

Management of chronic diarrhoea

Chronic diarrhoea is not a single entity, as discussed on pp. 475–6. An attempt must be made to identify the cause of the diarrhoea, and if possible specific corrective measures should be taken.

Irrespective of the cause, chronic diarrhoea results in malnutrition and a major aspect of therapy is nutritional.[20] Management of cases can therefore be divided into specific, symptomatic and nutritional components.

Specific therapy

Infectious agents, if they are considered to be a significant component in the disorder should be treated. These include amoebiasis, giardiasis and *Clostridium difficile* for which antimicrobials are available and have been discussed. In diet-related chronic diarrhoea, it is important to withdraw the causative item, whether this

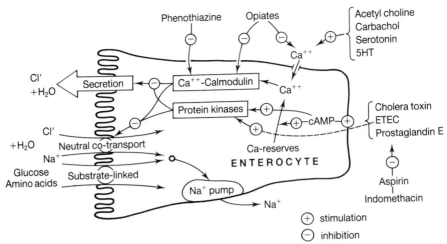

Fig. 4.3.9   Drugs and factors affecting enterocyte absorption and secretion. (Reproduced from A Y Elzouki (ed), *Paediatric Diseases in Arab Countries*, 1987, John Wiley & Sons.)

is wheat containing gluten or cow's milk. Unfortunately for many types of chronic diarrhoea there is no specific intervention because the aetiology is either unknown or a complicated network of factors which have damaged the small bowel.

Symptomatic treatment

The initial step is replacement of fluids and electrolytes as for acute diarrhoea. Drug treatment has been found effective in a number of otherwise intractable cases. Loperamide reduces excessive bowel secretion in some infants with protracted diarrhoea in a dose of 1 mg per kg per day in four doses.

A combination of oral gentamicin (50 mg/kg/per day in six divided doses for three days) and cholestyramine (1 gram every six hours for five days) produced significant improvement in South African children with persistent postinfectious diarrhoea. The addition of metronidazole, which was previously used in combination with the other two drugs, gave no additional benefit. Gentamicin obviously alters the bowel flora and cholestyramine is a non-absorbable basic anion-exchange resin which is believed to act by deconjugating bile salts and binding bacterial toxins. The combination was safe and effective but is not recommended for the treatment of acute diarrhoea or chronic diarrhoea due to specific factors.

Nutrition

Any episode of diarrhoea has nutritional cost, and this has been considered for acute diarrhoea on pp. 474–5.

The need for nutritional therapy is even more necessary in chronic diarrhoea which is a significant nutritional disorder. Without adequate nourishment the condition can only deteriorate.

Following the development of elemental nutrients and the possibility of central venous feeding, total parenteral nutrition (TPN) has been developed and improved. The technique, particularly in children with impaired defence mechanisms, carries a high risk of infection as well as mechanical and metabolic complications. Catheters can slip, fracture, become malpositioned and cause local thrombosis. In services which do not have full facilities the dangers of TPN are greater than the benefits, and the method is contraindicated.

Resting the bowel from the role of absorbing nourishment decreases rather than improves this function. Intraluminal food stimulates the mucosa; it provides nutrients for the enterocytes, enhances proliferation of cells and induces enzymic activity. Feeding also initiates non-luminal factors, both neuronal and hormonal, which stimulate the bowel by mechanisms which are not fully understood. Resting the bowel results not in healing but atrophy.

Controlled comparisons between TPN and different forms of alimentary nourishment suggest that the alimentary tract is both safer and a more effective route. Continuous enteral nutrition (CEN), drip feeding into the alimentary tract, or intermittent oral nutrition (ION) have both been used. The former has advantages in severely ill children and in those who are uncooperative in taking adequate volumes of nourishment.

What are the safest and most effective nutrients to

feed these children? A formula based on comminuted chicken and also elemental diets are being used.[21] Human milk has been found effective in some cases where other enteral nutrients have failed.[22]

The recent research findings about the benefits of enteral nutrition are particularly relevant for the tropical countries with poor environmental hygiene, where chronic diarrhoea is most prevalent and services less sophisticated. Just as giving fluid by mouth has revolutionized the management of acute diarrhoea, giving nourishment into the alimentary tract is an effective way to treat malnutrition of chronic diarrhoea.[20]

Diarrhoeal disease control

The World Health Organization programme on the Control of Diarrhoeal Disease and the national programmes in many countries have the objectives of reducing diarrhoeal disease-related mortality and malnutrition, with the ultimate goal of reducing diarrhoeal morbidity.

The control of diarrhoeal disease can be considered under two main headings; namely the prevention of diarrhoeal disease mortality as a more immediate goal and the prevention of diarrhoeal disease morbidity as a long-term goal.

Prevention of mortality

Effective promotion of oral rehydration therapy

It is generally accepted that ORT is an effective way of reducing the diarrhoeal disease deaths caused by dehydration. The use of this technique depends upon the availability of materials, communication of essential messages, and acceptability of these by the community.

ORT is the method immediately available for the short-term objective of saving lives, but to make this available and effective on a national scale is difficult, and mortality rates from the disease still remain high in most endemic areas. This is for a variety of reasons: either people do not know about oral rehydration; or they do not have the materials for the therapy; or they do not know how to use it; or, last but not least, they are not convinced about its efficacy and so will not use it. There are certain socio-cultural and economic factors responsible for this disparity between the knowledge of how to prevent deaths from dehydration and its implementation by people. There are also socio-cultural factors which can be utilized to facilitate implementation of a diarrhoeal disease control programme.

Essential materials for ORT include clean water, ORS or alternative ingredients like salt, sugar or cereal, and suitable containers in which to measure, mix and store the fluid. In most societies, if not in most homes, the bare essentials are available. The percentage of the world population who now have access to ORS packets has increased from about 5 per cent in 1982 to over 60 per cent in 1988, and is still growing. Clean rather than sterile water is recommended for preparing OR fluid. Boiling drinking water is unrealistic for most poor communities, and if a child shows signs of dehydration, the risks of giving contaminated fluid to drink are much less than the risks of not giving ORT.

Good communication of essential messages is vital to success. The use of ORS packets requires some simple specific instructions. The use of home-made formulae is even more difficult because standardizing the ingredients is necessary. Instruction about ORT should be combined with other messages regarding the danger of diarrhoea, the need for hygiene, especially hand washing, and the importance of good nutrition. This is a large amount of information for any mother to learn on a single occasion. Repetition and reinforcement of the teaching is essential.

The quarterly newsletter, Dialogue on Diarrhoea (available free of charge from AHRTAG, 1 London Bridge Street, London, SE1 9SG), is aimed at all levels of health professionals, administrators and educated lay people. It emphasizes the role of ORT and reviews all other interventions and developments in the control of diarrhoeal diseases. Its circulation exceeds 100 000 in English and it is also translated into French, Spanish, Portugese and Arabic. Other methods to disseminate the messages should be developed and used. Community pharmacies, primary schools, religious organizations and the mass media should be involved.

The training of health professionals in the theory and practice of ORT is essential. The WHO has organized many programmes and prepared materials for various levels of workers, but to retain and convince the army of existing health workers is a major task. The effectiveness and the mystique of intravenous rehydration has been appreciated by health personnel and the public alike. The dramatic results, the professional control and financial rewards of intravenous infusions seem so influential compared with the apparent simplicity of the main message that 'drinking is the right treatment for diarrhoea'. However, the scientific foundation for ORT is sound and the method really works. When promoted vigorously the effects can be impressive, as has been demonstrated in Egypt.

The Egyptian National Control of Diarrhoeal Diseases Project with the support and financial backing of the United States Agency for International Development has run a highly effective promotion programme. In 1982 fewer than 2 per cent of Egyptian mothers had ever heard of ORT and fewer than 1 per cent had used it. In 1983 the project developed appropriate educational materials and messages. ORS was launched nation-wide in 1984 with an intensive mass media campaign using posters, bill boards, newspapers, radio and television. The last two are said to reach 90 per cent of Egyptian people. The television spots starring a popular actress were screened at peak viewing times. In the summer, at the height of the diarrhoea season, the TV film was shown six times a day. Health professionals played a part, as many doctors and nurses were trained in ORT. In rural areas, ORS depot-holders were selected and trained to provide ORS and treatment.

The impact in Egypt has been impressive. The logo of the programme is now the most widely recognized advertisement in the country. Local manufacturers of ORS could hardly keep pace with the demand. Within two years, 96 per cent of mothers with young children had heard of ORT and 82 per cent said they had used it when their child had diarrhoea. Egypt now leads the world in this therapy as a result of what may be 'the worlds most successful health programme'.[23]

Factors limiting acceptability of ORT

False beliefs about what is essential in diarrhoea treatment Intravenous infusions have been seen to be life-saving and appear dramatic. Drugs and injections are so effective in many diseases that they seem almost to have magical powers. Surely there is an effective medicine for diarrhoea.

Response Modern knowledge is clear that infusions and medicines have a useful, but relatively small, place in the management of diarrhoea. Appropriate fluids by mouth should be the first treatment. They are effective, safe and should not be neglected, even if drugs are being given.

Drinking a home-made liquid seems too simple to be effective Can such a commonplace remedy as salt, sugar and water combat a disease that is known to kill many children? Can something as easy and cheap be effective?

Response Yes, surprisingly this treatment is both cheap and effective. The scientific mechanisms have been worked out and its benefits have been proved in many clinical trials.

Drinking will aggravate diarrhoea Drinking large amounts of watery liquid at the very time when there are large losses from the lower end of the bowel as watery stools, appears to be illogical and will aggravate and perpetuate the problem.

Response This misunderstanding is due to ignorance about how the bowel works, and the efficacy of OR fluid. In most types of acute diarrhoea the intestine can still absorb quite effectively, especially if a suitable fluid is drunk. By providing water and electrolytes the body is safe from the serious consequences of dehydration and salt loss. Some diarrhoea may continue for a day or so, but the danger is reduced.

Diarrhoea is so common, it is almost a normal occurrence Diarrhoea is a part of childhood and growing up. Anyway, the outcome is in God's hands, so why rush to give a child special drinks for every watery stool?

Response Diarrhoea may be commonplace, but it still causes many deaths, especially in children from poor circumstances. Probably there is about one death for every 200 cases of diarrhoea if proper treatment is not given. Early in the course of illness it is not possible to know which child will progress to severe disease. Prompt ORT for all is a safe insurance. Of the many children who die from diarrhoea, probably over 60 per cent could be saved by appropriate rehydration fluid given by mouth.

Factors promoting acceptability

Professional knowledge Professional knowledge about the scientific basis and efficacy of the method gives confidence. This is true at all levels from professors and consultants to primary health care village workers.

Personal experience No health worker who has personally helped and supervised the oral rehydration of a moderately or severely dehydrated patient will forget the experience. This should be an essential part of their training. It is a good treatment and, though it may require patience and persistence, it works. Therefore, it is self-authenticating. Personal familiarity with the practical aspects of the technique give workers confidence which is recognized by patients and their families.

Prestige of the method Both the public and professionals should be aware that this method is being promoted by the World Health Organization and is being used in the most influential institutions and by some of the most popular and trusted physicians.

Public awareness Public awareness must be created so that it becomes generally known that new and sound methods of treatment are available for diarrhoea. Also that drinking a special liquid is the modern, acceptable and correct therapy.

Promotion through all channels and media Teaching health workers should be only one of many ways to spread the message. Informal communication networks, gossip and discussion at home, folk songs and drama, the school, the church, the mosque, the radio, the TV, all should repeat the same consistent news about ORT.

Panic Epidemics of diarrhoea and cholera are sometimes the situations in which effectiveness of ORT has been seen most convincingly by the greatest number of people.

Breaking the cycle of transmission

The chain of transmission was considered earlier under the epidemiology, but there are practical implications. In the transmission cycle for any pathogen there may be a link which is vulnerable to attack. If this can be identified and used to break the cycle in a population it is possible to prevent further cases. In the famous cholera epidemic in London in 1850, Dr John Snow observed that most cases were drinking water supplied by one company and especially from a particular pump in Broad Street.[24] By removing the pump handle he broke the cycle and cut short the outbreak.

Prevention of morbidity

Factors facilitating or limiting transmission

These factors can be considered under the headings, agent, environment and host.

Agents which are resistant to adverse environmental conditions, like the cysts of *E. histolytica* are more likely to survive to infect another host. Some agents multiply within a food, thus increasing the potential infecting dose. Organisms which exist in natural reservoirs outside man, like those zoonotic salmonellae which are commensal in many domestic animals, continue their normal life-cycle in their zoonotic host, only infecting man in certain occasional situations. If an agent can live exclusively in man, it must continue to find susceptible human hosts for survival. An agent which can survive and be excreted from a healthy host, the carrier state (for example *Salmonella typhi*) is more dangerous, since such hosts are not apparently ill and may continue to excrete the organism without knowing it. If the agent is very virulent, it will only survive in ill patients and this means that there will be no asymptomatic carriers. (The smallpox virus, variola major, was an example of such an organism.)

Regarding the environment, a warm moist situation with nourishment for bacteria facilitates survival and spread. Communities which are disrupted by natural or man-made disasters permit easy transmission. In these situations there will be crowding, scarce washing water and drinking water may be contaminated by faeces. Insect and animal pests may multiply and spread the infecting agents.

Host factors facilitating transmission of diarrhoeal disease include large numbers of susceptibles, particularly children, living in close proximity. Those with body defences impaired by malnutrition or other infections, such as measles or human immunodeficiency virus (HIV), are more vulnerable. Infants on artificial feeding have a double risk; they are not protected by the anti-infective breast-milk factors, and they may also be fed contaminated milk.

Obviously the pathogen, host and environmental factors overlap and interact. A pathogen may have a potentially long survival time, but if it is in a hot dry environment survival may be brief. A host factor, like the presence of abundant gastric acid, is an adverse environmental situation for a potential pathogen.

Interventions to control diarrhoeal disease

These can be subdivided into clinical and non-clinical interventions. Clinical interventions include appropriate and effective treatment of which ORT is an important component.

Non-clinical interventions can be divided into three groups (Table 4.3.13). The first group comprises interventions for which there is evidence of high effectiveness and practical feasibility. The second group comprises interventions which might be useful, but for which there is still little hard evidence that they are both effective and feasible. The third group comprises interventions which are ineffective, or of limited feasibility, or are too costly to have a major role in poorer countries.

The most effective and practical preventive interventions relate to proper infant feeding, good hygiene and sanitation, and certain immunizations.

Most of these interventions are mentioned elsewhere in this chapter. The following comments indicate the relative importance of different factors and suggest priorities.

Table 4.3.13   Interventions to control diarrhoeal disease

Interventions for which there is evidence of high effectiveness and practical feasibility.

Infant feeding
  Promotion of breast feeding
  Improved weaning practices
Certain immunizations
  Measles immunization
  Rotavirus immunization
  Cholera immunization in certain communities
Hygiene and sanitation
  Improved water supply and sanitation facilities
  Better personal and domestic hygiene

Interventions which might be useful, but for which there is still little hard evidence that they are both effective and feasible.

Preventing low birth weight
Using growth charts to improve services and child nutrition
Increasing child spacing
Vitamin A supplementation
Improving food hygiene
Control of zoonotic reservoirs of pathogens which can
  cause diarrhoea
Epidemic control

Interventions which are ineffective, or of limited feasibility, or are too costly to have a major role in poor countries.

Fly control
Chemoprophylaxis, giving antimicrobial drugs to the
  contacts of those who have diarrhoea
Supplementary feeding programmes for children, and
Attempts to enhance lactation in mothers who are breast
  feeding, in order to improve the nutritional state of babies
  and decrease the need for supplementary food which
  may be contaminated.

Breast-feeding   Children who are exclusively breast-fed have about one-half to one-third of the risk of diarrhoea in the first months of life. Over six months of age and for partially breast-fed babies, the protection is less complete. Breast-feeding should be encouraged by special changes in hospital routine and by giving information and support to mothers (see pp. 95–102).

Weaning   Improved weaning practices can be achieved by appropriate programmes targeted at the mothers of children aged 6–23 months and at secondary school girls. The messages need to be appropriate both in content and method of delivery. Local face-to-face discussions between mothers and locally recruited workers, reinforced by radio and other mass media seem to be most effective. The larger the proportion of malnourished children, the greater the potential impact

and cost-effectiveness of this intervention. (These factors are emphasized elsewhere in this book, see pp. 358–66.)

Immunizations   These have a definite place in the control of diarrhoeal disease. The three priority vaccines are for measles, rotavirus and cholera. Measles vaccine, a live attenuated strain given by injection, effectively prevents the disease and the serious diarrhoea associated with many cases in tropical countries. No vaccine currently available for cholera is entirely satisfactory. The traditional whole-killed vibrio vaccines give a fair protection, but only for a short period. Better vaccines are under development and trial.[25] Heterologous rotavirus vaccines (derived from animal strains) were shown to be effective during trials in industrialized countries. However, subsequent trials in tropical countries failed to confirm this efficacy. Possible reasons for these failures include the high prevalence of enteric viral infections and breast-feeding, which may both limit colonization with the vaccine strain, and the presence of different rotavirus strains. The latest developments of biotechnology can be applied to the preparation of vaccines by probing for specific genes which cause pathological effects and reproducing identical (monoclonal) antigens or antibodies by DNA replication in bacteria, yeasts or mammalian cells. Future prospects for such immunizing agents are good, but only if pharmaceutical companies, research agencies and national governments are willing to invest in this technology (see pp. 78–87).

The relative cost-benefits of the three current candidate vaccines, for measles, rotavirus and cholera, have been reviewed. It has been estimated that these vaccines could be added to an existing immunization programme at the cost of US$2–4 for each vaccine. Assuming a diarrhoea morbidity rate of 220 attacks and a diarrhoea mortality rate of 1.4 per 100 children per year under the age of five, the relative calculated costs of cases and deaths averted are as follows. Measles vaccine would cost US$6 per case averted and US$180 per death averted. Rotavirus vaccine would cost US$5 per case averted and US$220 per death averted. Cholera vaccine in Bangladesh would cost US$220 per case averted and US$2000 per death averted. Many other assumptions are necessary for such estimations, and because attack and death rates vary from country to country average figures have little meaning. In communities where the attack and death rates are higher than those used in the calculation, the benefits indicated above are probably an underestimate. The calculation for measles immunization ignores the important benefit of the reduction of measles and its other complications.

Environmental improvements

- improved water supply;
- improved excreta disposal system;
- hygiene education.

There is evidence that well-designed programmes which combine these factors may reduce diarrhoea mortality by 35–50 per cent. The impact on mortality may be even greater, except where other interventions like oral rehydration therapy have already reduced the risk of death from diarrhoea.[2]

The cost of such improvements vary greatly from place to place and depend on the type of system. It has been estimated that for a rural water supply and latrine, in developing countries the cost is about US$14 per person per year, and in an urban area, in-house water supply and sanitation cost about US$46 per person per year.

Although general education may have some benefit, disease-specific education is more important, especially when related to the hygienic measures. Decontamination of hands by washing with soap and water can reduce diarrhoea attack rates by up to 50 per cent in some countries.

In conclusion, a national diarrhoea disease control programme has to choose the most appropriate set of interventions which suit its circumstances and budget. For example, in Bangladesh, most mothers normally breast-feed, but in urban Latin America breast-feeding promotion could be very important. The opposite may be true for cholera vaccination which has no place in America. The selected interventions must coordinate with other health and development programmes and be promoted with carefully designed and targetted messages.

References

1. Snyder JD, Merson MH. The magnitude of the global problem of acute diarrhoeal disease: a review of active surveillance data. *Bulletin of the World Health Organization.* 1982; **60**(4): 605–13.
2. Feachem RG. Preventing diarrhoea: what are the policy options? *Health Policy and Planning.* 1986; **1**(2): 109–17.
3. WHO/UNICEF. *The Management of Diarrhoea and Use of Oral Rehydration Therapy*, 2nd Edn. Geneva, WHO, 1985.
4. WHO. *Guidelines for Cholera Control.* Geneva, WHO, 1980 (WHO/CDD/SER/80.4).
5. Gordon JE, Chitkara ID, Wyon JB. Weanling diarrhoea. *American Journal of Medical Science.* 1963; **245**: 345–77.
6. Rowley D, Brooy JL. Intestinal immune responses in relation to diarrhoeal diseases. *Journal of Diarrhoeal Disease Research.* 1986; **4**: 1–9.
7. Nanda R, Bavesa U, Anand BS. *Entamoeba histolytica* cyst passers: *Lancet.* 1984; **2**: 301–3.
8. Farthing MJA. Giardiasis: pathogenesis of chronic diarrhoea and impact on child growth and development. In: Lebenthal E ed. *Chronic Diarrhoea in Children.* New York, Raven Press, 1984. pp. 253–367.
9. Sladen GE, Dawson AM. Inter-relationships between the absorption of glucose, sodium and water by the normal jejunum. *Clinical Science.* 1969; **36**: 119–32.
10. WHO. *A Manual for the Treatment of Acute Diarrhoea.* Geneva, WHO, 1990 (WHO/CDD/SER/80.2 REV No. 2).
11. WHO. *Contemporary Patterns of Breast Feeding.* Geneva, WHO, 1981.
12. O'Shaughnessy WB. Experiments on the blood in cholera. *Lancet.* 1831; **ii**: 490–1.
13. Cutting WAM, Langmuir AD. Oral rehydration in diarrhoea: applied pathophysiology. *Transactions of the Royal Society of Tropical Medicine.* 1980; **74**: 30–5.
14. WHO. *Treatment and Prevention of Acute Diarrhoea: Guidelines for the Trainers of Health Workers.* Geneva, WHO, 1985.
15. Molla AM, Molla A, Nath SK *et al.* Food-based oral rehydration salt solution for acute childhood diarrhoea. *Lancet.* 1989; **2**: 429–31.
16. Pizarro D, Posada G, Mata L. Treatment of 242 neonates with dehydrating diarrhoea with an oral glucose-electrolyte solution. *Journal of Pediatrics.* 1983; **102**: 153–16.
17. Mahalanabis D, Patra FC. In search of a super oral rehydration solution: Can optimum use of organic solute-mediated sodium absorption lead to the development of an absorption promoting drug? *Journal of Diarrhoeal Disease Research.* 1983; **1**: 76–81.
18. Hoyle B, Yunus M, Chen LC. Breast feeding and food intake among children with acute diarrhoeal disease. *American Journal of Clinical Nutrition.* 1980; **33**: 235–2371.
19. Candy DCA. Diarrhoea, dehydration and drugs. *British Medical Journal.* 1984; **2**: 1245–6.
20. Editorial. Chronic diarrhoea in children–a nutritional disease. *Lancet.* 1987; **1**: 143–4.
21. Larcher VF, Shepherd R, Francis DE, Harries JT. Protracted diarrhoea in infancy: analysis of 82 cases with particular reference to diagnoses and management. *Archives of Disease in Childhood.* 1977; **52**: 597–605.
22. MacFarlane PI, Miller V. Human milk in the management of protracted diarrhoea of infancy. *Archives of Disease in Childhood.* 1984; **59**: 260–5.
23. Conference Report. Egypt's triumph with oral rehydration treatment. *British Medical Journal.* 1985; **291**: 1249.
24. Snow J. *On the Mode of Communication of Cholera.* London, Churchill Livingstone, 1855.
25. Editorial. Oral cholera vaccines. *Lancet.* 1986; **2**: 722–3.

CHAPTER 4

Common childhood infections

Nimrod Bwibo

Measles

Measles is an infectious viral disease which is an important child health problem in the subtropics and tropics. It is highly contagious and transmitted by droplet infection. Overcrowding of families leads to early contact with the virus in high dosage. This accounts for the earlier age of occurrence and the greater severity of the infection in the tropics. The main features of the disease are a maculopapular skin rash, so characteristic of measles that similar rashes are called morbilliform (measles-like), and generalized mucosal inflammation which in the mouth has an initial appearance of grains of sand each with a red halo, known as Koplik's spots. Complications are frequently encountered, being much more severe in malnourished than in normally nourished children. Mortality is high and on recovery there is lifelong immunity. Treatment is directed to alleviating symptoms and managing the various complications when they arise. The disease is preventable by immunization.

Epidemiology

The incubation period of measles is 10–14 days, usually 11 days. The disease is transmitted as a droplet infection and occurs in seasonal outbreaks.

Children have a gradually waning passive immunity acquired transplacentally from their mothers; this may persist for up to a year, though effectively lost by over 90 per cent of the infants by nine months. Recent work suggests that this passive immunity may vary from place to place in the duration of its effectiveness in preventing measles and thus also of measles vaccine on infection. Owing to heavy and early exposure to the infection, the greatest incidence in children in the tropics occurs in those under two years of age. Children between 6 and 12 months of age account for 20 to 40 per cent of the total morbidity and very few children have escaped infection by the time they reach five years of age, as shown in Table 4.4.1.

There are no sex differences in morbidity and mortality. The disease is severe and carries more complications and mortality in malnourished than in well-nourished children.[1] It is mild in children in North America and Europe as well as in the children of the well-to-do families in the tropics. This difference is due not to the virulence of the virus or race but to nutritional and socio-economic status. Studies in West Africa suggest that the dose of infectious particles (virions) has a bearing on severity. A significant positive correlation was found between severity and the number of cases of measles in each household. Infection pressure probably lowers the age of incidence of the infection to below nine

Table 4.4.1 Incidence of measles and mortality in Kenyan children

Age (months)	No. patients	Percentage of patients	No. deaths	Mortality (percentage)
0–4	47	1.0	5	10.6
5–8	741	14.0	59	8.0
9–12	1636	31.0	171	10.5
13–16	512	10.1	58	11.3
17–20	599	11.0	79	13.2
21–23	107	2.0	6	5.6
24–35	737	14.0	73	9.9
36–47	353	7.0	30	8.5
48–59	187	4.0	15	8.0
60 +	301	6.0	11	3.7
Total	5020	100.0	507	10.1

(Reproduced with permission from O'Donovan C, *East African Medical Journal*, 1971; **48**: 526–32.)

months, a situation in which dose of virions is being titrated against waning maternal antibodies.

Community perception

Various beliefs exist about measles, many of which may hinder treatment and prevention. Measles may be thought to be the will of God, and that nothing should be done to displease God. Like smallpox, measles is only referred to by pseudonyms in some African cultures, lest God makes the disease severe. In India where the disease is thought to be the Goddess Matta, children are kept in dark houses away from the public. Many cultures believe that if the rash of measles is abundant, the disease will not go 'inside the body' to do more harm; sparse rash is associated with severe disease. Efforts are made in many cultures in tropical countries to hasten the eruption of the rash by application of medicinal herbs to the body. Some concoctions are administered orally. In Bangladesh, it is believed that children with measles should be purified.[2] Bathing a child who has measles is believed to reduce the eruption of measles rash in some parts of Africa. Among the Akambas of Kenya, milk and water are withheld during measles.[3] This contributes to dehydration and malnutrition. In any culture it is important to be sensitive to beliefs about the cause of the infection, how they influence lay management and how firmly they are held.

Aetiology and pathogenesis

Measles is caused by an RNA virus of the paramyxovirus family. It is antigenically related to canine distemper and rinderpest viruses. After inhalation, the virus particles invade cells of the upper respiratory mucosa, multiply and spread to adjacent cells. This process continues until the entire mucosa of the respiratory tract is infected. The infected cells tend to coalesce into multinucleated giant cells. By the tenth day of infection, cell dysfunction begins and the first signs of inflammation appear. This corresponds to the prodromal stage of the illness. The cilia of the respiratory epithelial cells are paralysed, rendering the child prone to secondary bacterial pneumonia. By the 12th day of infection many infected cells start breaking apart releasing large numbers of virions into the surrounding environment through coughing and sneezing and the patient becomes febrile. The virus enters the bloodstream and spreads throughout the body. Cell fusion occurs in the reticuloendothelial tissues with the appearance of multinucleated giant cells similar to those in the respiratory tract.

In severe measles, there is marked inflammation of the skin with haemorrhage into the dermis and dark staining of the rash. The mouth is diffusely red with swollen gums. The larynx is often oedematous, causing hoarseness of the voice and varying degrees of respiratory obstruction. Children with severe measles are usually malnourished, as distinct from those with mild measles who tend to be adequately nourished.[4, 26]

Shedding of giant cells containing virus particles, and thus infectivity, usually ceases by 48 hours after the appearance of the rash. In severe measles, giant cells continue to be shed from the respiratory tract for an average of 10 days after the onset of the rash. Patients with prolonged giant cell excretion have prolonged viral infection and remain sick while excretion of giant cells continues. Recovery is accompanied by cessation of the excretion of these giant cells.

Antibodies are produced in significant quantities by the 14th day, reach a peak by the fourth to sixth week of infection and help to neutralize circulating virus. Children with agammaglobulinaemia do not form antibodies against measles and yet recover, thus indicating that antibodies are not essential for recovery. The production of activated lymphocytes is stimulated in thymus-dependent lymphoid tissues. By the 14th day of infection, there are enough of these activated cells to destroy the infected cells. This activity is seen in the skin as the rash of measles. Similar cell destruction occurs in infected cells throughout the body. Cell destruction is accompanied by a peak of fever, malaise and misery. Failure of the cellular immune response, with sparse rash and severe toxaemia presages early death from overwhelming tissue infection. This underlines the validity of the belief of many communities in the tropics that measles without much rash is a deadly disease.

Clinical presentation

The symptoms occurring in the first three to four days, the prodromal phase, are non-specific, consisting of fever, coryza, cough and malaise. There is conjunctivitis associated with lacrymation and photophobia. Coryza increases and there is severe sneezing and watery nasal discharge. The cough, which is mild initially, becomes troublesome, brassy and husky in character, suggesting tracheal and laryngeal involvement and is often associated with hoarseness of the voice and/or a croup. A croup signifies the occurrence of laryngotracheobronchitis, a common problem in children in tropical countries.

Koplik's spots appear on the third or fourth day of the prodromal period. They are characteristically like grains of sand surrounded by narrow red areolae (1 mm diameter) appearing on the buccal mucosa opposite the lower molar teeth. They quickly spread to involve the whole of the buccal mucosa and gingiva. Their presence is a pathognomonic sign of measles. Similar lesions have been found at autopsy along the gastro-intestinal mucosa in the small intestines and may be the basis of the diarrhoea which occurs in measles.

The rash of measles appears on the 14th day at the peak of respiratory symptoms and when the temperature is quite high (39°C or above). The Koplik's spots have reached a peak at this time and over the next three days they disappear leaving a red sand-papery mucosa which continues for at least another two days. Such rawness of the mouth interferes with feeding. The skin rash first appears behind the ears and at the hairline on the forehead, and spreads sequentially to the whole face, neck, trunk, upper extremities, buttocks and lower extremities, completing the whole body by the third day (see Figs. 4.4.1 and 4.4.2). The rash is initially erythematous maculopapular and becomes confluent mainly on the face and trunk, while on the lower extremities it remains discrete. By the third and fourth day the rash begins to clear, following the same sequence of its appearance. Often the clearing is accompanied by fine or sometimes even extensive desquamation (Fig. 4.4.3). The rash usually lasts six to seven days.

The fever, which is high just before the rash, continues to be high during the period of the rash, reaching a peak on the second or third day of the rash. Thereafter it falls by lysis over a 24 hour period. A fever that persists after three or four days of exanthem indicates the onset of a complication. A number of children are quite sick-looking and toxic during the stage of the rash. In early childhood, the patient may present initially with pneumonia or diarrhoea with dehydration and may be treated for those conditions in

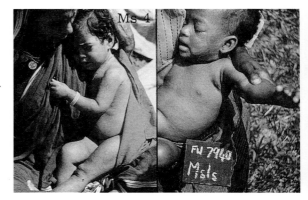

Fig. 4.4.1   Typical measles rash in early stage on dark skin. (© TALC.)

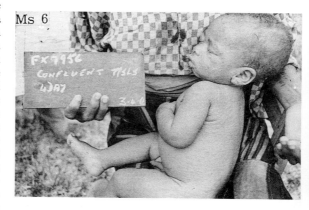

Fig. 4.4.2   Full-blown measles rash with conjunctival infection. (© TALC.)

the out-patient clinic, before the typical features of measles arise. Such children are a danger to the others, as they pass on their disease in crowded clinics. It is not unusual for a child who has been in contact with such cases in hospital to develop measles 10–14 days afterwards.

Conjunctivitis and nasal symptoms usually subside as the fever falls. But nasal discharge may continue as mucopurulent discharge when secondary bacterial infection occurs. This discharge blocks nostrils, interfering with feeding.

Cough normally loosens up with the appearance of the rash, becoming productive in older children but may persist for several days. During the whole of this period the child is anorexic.

Diarrhoea is thought to be a direct effect of viral involvement of gastro-intestinal mucosa, occurring in the early stage of the illness and persisting even after the rash has disappeared. It is often accompanied by vomiting. Secondary bacterial enteritis is possible after the rash has disappeared. Diarrhoea is an important precedent of malnutrition.

Modified measles occur in partially immune children, as in infants under one year who still have transplacentally acquired maternal measles antibody

and children with partial protection from measles vaccination. Immune serum globulin, administered at the time of exposure, also modifies the clinical picture of measles. Measles vaccine sometimes gives rise to an illness resembling modified measles in immunosuppressed or malnourished children. Modified measles is characterized by mild illness that follows the usual sequence of measles infection. The prodromal period is shorter; while cough, coryza and fever are minimal and Koplik's spots are few, often absent, making the diagnosis of measles very difficult. In these cases measles rash is sparse and discrete. Subclinical cases probably occur, as some children are shown to have measles antibodies without having overt signs of measles.

Complications

Respiratory complications are the most common. They include: otitis media, croup, laryngotracheobronchitis, pneumonia, surgical emphysema, empyema, and flaring up of quiescent primary tuberculosis. Bronchopneumonia, which is the most usual single complication, is difficult to distinguish from the interstitial pneumonia of measles virus. Viral pneumonia is complicated by multinucleated giant cell pneumonia, particularly in malnourished children.

Bronchopneumonia due to secondary bacterial invasion usually attacks when the measles rash has subsided, at a time when viral pneumonia should have cleared. It is characterized by increased cough, secondary rise in temperature and bilateral crepitations. Its radiological features are difficult to distinguish from those of measles viral pneumonia. X-ray changes of measles consist of enlarged hilar shadows, increased broncho-vascular markings, patchy opacities, segmental lesions, atelectasis, pleural reaction and emphysematous areas. Bronchopneumonia carries a high mortality. Prolonged bronchopneumonia failing to improve on antibiotics or associated with loss of weight raises the possibility of pulmonary tuberculosis. By depressing cell-mediated immunity, measles flares up quiescent tuberculosis. Radiological evidence for tuberculosis should be sought as the tuberculin test is usually negative up to three months after measles.

Bacterial or viral enteritis is the second most common complication of measles, after bronchopneumonia. This is associated with varying degrees of lactose intolerance and protein losing enteropathy.

Malnutrition is also a common sequel of measles. The factors that contribute to malnutrition are: anorexia; stomatitis; blocked nostrils that interfere with feeding; persistent diarrhoea with loss of nutrients in

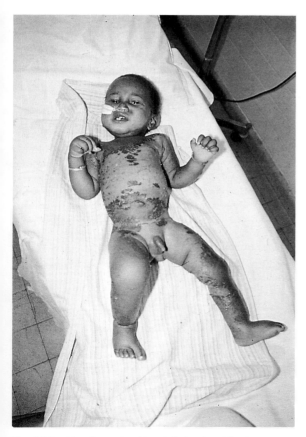

Fig. 4.4.3 Measles rash with exfoliation in a Nigerian child.

stool and a protein-losing enteropathy; increased catabolism due to high fever and depressed enzyme function. A number of children lose as much as 10 per cent of their body weight. Recovery of body weight is often slow following measles, while in some patients measles precipitates acute kwashiorkor.

Severe conjunctivitis may be accompanied by corneal ulcers, especially where vitamin A intake is low. Marked darkening of measles rash with pronounced desquamation occurs in malnourished children with measles and is a serious sign. Bleeding occurs due to thrombocytopaenic purpura but may also be due to vascular damage and disseminated intravenous coagulopathy. Myocarditis is associated with marked tachycardia and may progress to congestive cardiac failure.

The central nervous system is rarely involved but when it is the complications are often serious. Febrile convulsions may occur at the height of the fever and subside as expected. An acute encephalitis may occur (see p. 754), usually during the period of the rash within eight days of the onset of the illness and rarely beyond three weeks after the onset. Encephalitis is due either to measles virus infection of the brain or to an antibody–antigen reaction in the brain. Some of the patients with encephalitis recover but may remain damaged with mental retardation or epilepsy.

Subacute sclerosing panencephalitis (SSPE) is a slowly progressive neurological disorder with insidious onset and characterized by progressive behaviour and intellectual deterioration (see pp. 755–6). The symptoms are complex and bizarre with confusing psychological features. Most characteristic are the myoclonic jerks, visual impairment and difficulty in speech; leading eventually to mutism, central blindness, dementia, stupor, and finally decerebrate rigidity. Death follows in about six to nine months.

The evidence of measles causation of SSPE is the presence of high measles haemagglutinating inhibition antibody (core antibody), titres in CSF and sera and the isolation of measles virus from the brain of these patients. The risk of SSPE in children who have had natural measles and those who have been immunized with measles vaccine is 1 per 100 000 and 1 per 1 000 000, respectively.

Diagnosis

Diagnosis of measles is based on clinical features and the typical disease present no difficulties. If atypical, a smear of the naso-pharyngeal secretion shows the characteristic giant cells containing measles antigen,

identifiable by immunofluorescence technique where available.

The differential diagnosis includes: roseola infantum (exanthem subitum); rubella (German measles) in which fever is not very high and there is a skin rash which in dark skin is not easily visible, and lymph node enlargement particularly the postauricular and those in the posterior triangle of the neck; infectious mononucleosis in which the peripheral lymph nodes are enlarged; adenoviral infections; scarlet fever; and drug rashes. In none of these infections is the child as sick as in measles.

Management

The management of measles is essentially symptomatic and supportive. Specific therapy is directed to the complications. The high fever is controlled by paracetamol or ibuprofen (Brufen) 20 mg/kg daily or tepid sponging. As soon as diarrhoea sets in, oral fluids are administered to avoid dehydration. It is important to ensure that nutritious food is offered during and after the measles attack. This maintains nutriture and helps prevent deterioration of nutritional status. The child's personal hygiene should be maintained by washing the body and cleaning the mouth. There may be thrush in the mouth for which gentian violet or clotrimazole 1 per cent (Canesten) is administered. There is no special treatment for the rash or the cough. The nostrils should be cleared of discharge and saline nasal drops applied to keep them clear and open so as to allow the child to feed.

Complications are treated as they arise. It is important to check the eardrums frequently so as to diagnose and treat early acute otitis media with antibiotics. When discharging ears occur, proper cleaning of the discharge should be done and the child placed on antibiotics. Bronchopneumonia is treated by penicillin and if there is no improvement, broad-spectrum antibiotics such as ampicillin, ampiclox and amoxil are given. One should not wait too long if pneumonia is not resolving. This may indicate an underlying tuberculous infection which should be treated with streptomycin, isoniazid and thiacetazone.

Laryngotracheobronchitis (LTB) presents with croupy cough and respiratory distress, signifying upper airway obstruction. It may be combined with pneumonia in which case both should be managed simultaneously. Management of LTB includes oxygen for very severe cases or just steam inhalation in a croup tent; antibiotics are justified, especially where there is bronchopneumonia as well. Tracheostomy is useful to relieve upper airway obstruction.

Prognosis

Prognosis of measles depends upon age, nutritional status and the severity of the complications, including degree of dehydration and electrolyte imbalance. Children with poor nutritional status have severe and prolonged complications. Hospital fatalities are high since only severely ill children are admitted. Community-based data would give a more accurate case fatality rate.

Prevention

Measles is preventable by active immunization with live measles vaccine. The two vaccines in common usage are attenuated Enders vaccine and further attenuated Schwarz vaccine. Enders vaccine is supplied in 0.5 ml doses with accompanying diluent and syringe. Great care should be taken in reconstituting the vaccine to avoid inactivation of the virus, which is very sensitive to chemicals. Schwarz vaccine is passed many additional times in chick embryo tissue culture. The result is further attenuation with preservation of potency but lessened capacity to causing febrile and exanthematous reactions.

For these vaccines to remain potent, they have to be kept in cold storage from manufacture to use. The vaccine arrives deep-frozen ($-40°C$) and should remain so. At collection from port of entry the vaccine must be put in a refrigerator at $2-5°C$. With the heat of the tropical and subtropical countries and the fluctuating electricity current or non-existence of electricity in some parts, cold chain storage is often broken. It is difficult in field conditions to ascertain how potent the vaccine is. There are no deep-freeze facilities in health centres. One author has estimated that only one in 20 vials used for vaccinating children in one tropical country was viable. In such a case, low conversion and low protection rates are to be expected. There is nothing so disastrous than a measles immunized child getting measles.

Measles vaccine can be combined with mumps and rubella vaccines, to give the MMR vaccine.[5] The right age for measles immunization has been a subject of many studies.[6, 7] The mean age at which children contract measles in the tropics is 17 months versus three to four years in North America and Europe. Immunizing children in the tropics at nine months (as the manufacturers of the vaccine recommend) means that many susceptible infants will miss this protection. Immunizing very early is no advantage either, as many children will still have maternally acquired measles antibodies which will neutralize the vaccine, thus leaving them unprotected. Available figures show that the presence of antibodies at six months ranges from 8 to 56 per cent; rising to over 90 per cent by nine months of age, which still remains the recommended age for immunization. A high coverage and seroconversion rate at nine months results in 'umbrella' protection of infants below nine months by reducing infection pressure. Each region or country may still want to establish its own vaccination age.

Unimmunized children with no history of measles should be immunized if seen between nine months and three years. When used properly, the vaccine gives a 95–100 per cent seroconversion. Malnourished children retain their ability to respond to measles vaccine and hence should be immunized.

Long-term measures for controlling measles include improvement of nutritional and socio-economic status as well as reduction of overcrowding and reduce not only the incidence but also the severity of measles.

Whooping cough

Whooping cough or pertussis is an acute respiratory tract infection caused by *Bordetella pertussis*. The disease occurs world-wide, and is usually seasonal. Unlike measles, there is no intrauterine acquired protection, hence the disease occurs even in the first month of life. Its characteristic clinical picture is that of explosive paroxysmal cough ending in a whoop and vomiting. The whoop gives the infection its name but does not usually c cur in infants, especially those under nine months, hence it is appropriate to call the disease 'pertussis' which means intensive cough. Like measles, whooping cough occurs at an earlier age in the tropics, and in many infants where the characteristic whoop is lacking, it is very difficult to recognize unless there are older children nearby with the classical whoop. Whooping cough is a serious disease in the tropics where it is accompanied by many complications and a high fatality, particularly in very young children. Malnutrition commonly occurs among the survivors.

Epidemiology

The incubation period for whooping cough is 7–14 days. Most patients are under six years old. Overcrowding in communities in the tropics exposes young children early to a high infection pressure. This is even more so in poorly ventilated houses since transmission is by droplet infection.

The highest infectivity is in the early stage of the disease and the attack rate is 80–100 per cent. Since there is no transplacental passage of antibodies against the causative agent, very young children are unprotected. Infection may occur at any age after birth. Severity of the disease decreases with increasing age. The highest mortality is among infants, with females, for unknown reasons, having a higher mortality than males. The median age for whooping cough has been found to be two to three years in Africa and the Middle East. This is much younger than the four to five years reported in North America and Europe.

The infecting agent also contributes to the severity of the disease; *B. pertussis* gives rise to a much more severe illness than *B. parapertussis* or *B. broncho-septica* which cause milder disease of shorter duration.

Aetiology

Most cases of pertussis are caused by *Bordetella pertussis* and *B. parapertussis* though other bacteria, for example, *Bordetella broncho-septica*, a zoonotic infection, and adenoviruses types 1, 2, 3 and 5, can cause an illness indistinguishable from whooping cough. *Bordetella pertussis* is a small Gram-negative rod which grows well on Bordet–Gengou agar (glycerin–potato–blood) to which penicillin is added to inhibit the growth of other organisms.

Pathogenesis

Following inhalation of infected droplets, the bacteria get attached to the ciliated epithelial cells of the respiratory tract by means of their pili or surface appendages and multiply on the lining. Multiplication occurs along the whole respiratory tract from the nasopharynx to the alveoli with particularly severe effects in bronchioles. Inflammation of the mucosal lining is accompanied by the production of much mucus, congestion and infiltration of the mucosal lining with lymphocytes. Congestion and infiltration narrow the lumen of the bronchioles, resulting in atelectasis and emphysema in areas of incomplete obstruction. Inflammation in the bronchioles weakens their walls, and leads to bronchiectasis at a later date.

The organisms secrete an endotoxin at the site of their multiplication. This becomes fixed in the mucosa and is thought to cause the paroxysmal cough.

Clinical presentation

The clinical manifestations of the disease are divided into three stages: catarrhal, paroxysmal and convalescent, each lasting approximately two weeks.

Catarrhal stage

This stage, which lasts about one to two weeks has an insidious onset with no specific features suggestive of whooping cough. It is difficult to diagnose unless there is an older sibling with an established disease. The cough increases in severity and frequency and becomes paroxysmal.

Paroxysmal stage

This stage may last two to four weeks. It is characterized by a repetitive series of forceful coughs in a single expiration. Unlike the child with bronchitis, the child with whooping cough does not take a breath in anticipation of an outburst of coughing.

The cough is associated with choking and vomiting, and production of sticky, stringy sputum. There is thin nasal discharge. The characteristic whoop, which is a massive inspiratory effort as the air is inhaled forcefully through the narrowed bronchial tree, occurs at this stage. This is diagnostic of whooping cough but does not occur in infants below one year of age and not often in children up to the age of two, being replaced by a period of apnoea which may be prolonged and sometimes results in the sudden death of the infant. The whoop is usually followed immediately by vomiting and profuse sweating. Convulsions may occur due to hypoxia or intracerebral haemorrhage.

Feeding or examination of the throat provokes the paroxysmal cough. Poor feeding and vomiting cause loss of weight, dehydration and eventually malnutrition. The intense cough and resulting increased abdominal pressure may result in umbilical hernia, inguinal hernia and rectal prolapse. With the intense cough and increased venous pressure, oedema of the orbits and subconjunctival haemorrhages are often seen. Ulceration of the frenulum of the tongue and epistaxis also occur. Presence of any of these signs is useful in diagnosis. Paroxysmal coughing is exhausting and often keeps the child and family awake. Older children complain of headaches and chest pain due to the intensity of coughing.

Convalescent stage

There is a decrease in both severity and frequency of paroxysms but cough and whoop may persist for several months. Appetite returns, vomiting ceases and the child gains weight. It is usual for a subsequent upper respiratory tract infection to be associated with recurrence of paroxysmal cough and even whoop for months afterwards.

Complications

Bronchopneumonia is the leading complication of whooping cough. Clinical studies done in Uganda in cases of whooping cough revealed that bronchopneumonia accounted for 75 per cent of the complications.[9] The initial pneumonia is an extension of the upper respiratory tract infection. Secondary bacterial pneumonia, as an early or late complication, may cause death in whooping cough. Pulmonary collapse and bronchial wall destruction, especially of the cartilage, leads to bronchiectasis which may be permanent.

As in measles, whooping cough causes severe and prolonged weight loss due to vomiting and the prolonged paroxysmal cough which interferes with food intake. This may develop into frank marasmus or kwashiorkor. Follow-up of the child's weight in the months after whooping cough is important. The slope of catch-up weight gain will indicate the adequacy of the dietary intake, providing no residual infection is present. Clinical malnutrition becomes apparent earlier in children whose diets are marginal at the onset of the disease, and such children may take much longer to regain weight unless this diet is improved. Complications may arise from the rapid rises of venous pressure during the paroxyms of coughing. Among these are convulsions from intracerebral bleeding due to ruptured capillaries or hypoxia during a paroxysm; fortunately this is rare. Hemiplegia may occur due to the same vascular damage. It is difficult to distinguish such vascular lesions from those due to hypersensitivity reactions in the brain.

The explosive nature of the cough is also responsible for rectal prolapse and development of herniae, subconjuctival haemorrhage, epistaxis, oedema of the eyelids (particularly if the child is initially mildly malnourished) and surgical emphysema from the escape of air into the mediastinum and into the subcutaneous tissues. Like measles, whooping cough reactivates quiescent primary tuberculosis which may spread to cause tuberculous meningitis, though this is less likely than in measles, as whooping cough does not affect cell-mediated immunity.

Diagnosis

The characteristic cough, whoop, vomiting and stringy sputum make clinical diagnosis easy in an established case. The disease is underdiagnosed in infants and young children who do not usually whoop. Whooping cough is probably the most frequent cause of sudden apnoea in infancy. History of contact with an elder sibling with whooping cough should aid in the diagnosis of the atypical presentation. A very high white cell count (up to 50 000–100 000 per mm) with an absolute increase in lymphocytes (leukemoid reaction) greatly supports the diagnosis and is common in young children less than six years old. Very low white cell counts of 2500 cells per mm^3 with 72 per cent lymphocytosis have been seen in bacteriologically proven cases. One Kenyan study suggested that the white cell count may not serve as a diagnostic criterion.[10] Chest X-rays show perihilar infiltration and patchy atelectasis or emphysema. These are difficult to distinguish from those of pulmonary tuberculosis which may coexist. Enlarged perihilar lymph nodes from whooping cough do not deform the outline of the air passage as tuberculous lymph nodes tend to do.

The diagnosis is confirmed by positive cultures of *Bordetella pertussis* on Bordet–Gengou medium cough plate or plated postnasopharyngeal swab. Cultures done late in the course of the disease have a low yield. Where facilities permit, fluorescent antibodies can be demonstrated in stained postnasopharyngeal specimens.

Treatment

Antibiotics started early within two weeks of appearance of a whoop or as early as possible in the course of the disease may shorten the duration of the paroxysmal stage and reduce the period of communicability, while antibiotics started late do not alter the course of the disease. Erythromycin is quite effective at a dosage of 20–40 mg/kg/per day as is ampicillin (100 mg/kg/per day) or chloramphenicol (50–100 mg/kg/per day). They eliminate *B. pertussis* from the nasopharynx within three to four days. Antibiotics are also indicated for secondary bacterial pneumonia.

Supportive therapy in the course of the illness significantly reduces morbidity and mortality. This includes skilled nursing and feeding. Infants must be monitored for apnoea which will need immediate clearance of the airway and manual respiratory stimulation or mouth to mouth breathing. It is essential that a child is refed after vomiting a feed or a drink. This helps to maintain hydration and nutrition status. Feeds should be small but frequent. Mild sedation with linctus codeine, phenergan or phenobarbitone rests the child and reduces the paroxysmal cough, thus allowing feeding.

Sedation is also required at night to allow child (and family) to sleep but should not be deep enough to suppress the cough entirely. Gentle suctioning of mucous secretions should be done and the stringy viscid saliva removed by cotton-wool swab. Oxygen is indicated for infants with respiratory distress. If vomiting is severe and there is dehydration, intravenous fluids should be administered.

Prognosis

Hospital-based statistics show that the overall fatality is about 10 per cent. Community studies show about one per cent mortality.[10] Most deaths are due to bronchopneumonia and other pulmonary complications. Forty per cent of deaths occur within the first five months of life, whereas only 10 per cent of all cases occur in the first year of life. For some unknown reasons females are more affected and suffer higher fatality than males, unlike all other infectious diseases where males are more affected than females. This sex difference is not always observed.

Prevention

Active immunization against whooping cough is quite effective in preventing the disease. The vaccine is a suspension of killed *B. pertussis* and does not require the elaborate storage facilities of measles vaccine. The vaccine should be administered as early as possible in infancy so as to protect young infants who normally have protective antibodies. The vaccine is administered in combination with diphtheria and tetanus toxoids in the triple vaccine, DPT (see p. 81). A 0.5 ml dose of the triple vaccine is injected subcutaneously. Early detection of the disease and vigorous treatment prevent the spread of the infection to other children in the family or community.

Adverse reactions such as fever, encephalitis or convulsions may follow whooping cough vaccination. Once a child has developed convulsions or encephalitis with the first whooping cough injection, no further vaccination should be administered, as subsequent vaccination increases still further the risk of convulsion or encephalitis which might lead to permanent neurological disorder. There is no firm evidence that children with a family history of a convulsive disorder, or the child with brain damage such as cerebral palsy or mental retardation or with seizures that antedate immunization, are in greater danger from whooping cough vaccination than the general population.[11]

Whooping cough should be anticipated in younger siblings of an older sibling with the disease. Such young infants who are exposed to pertussis and unimmunized can be given human immune serum globulin in a dosage of 1.5 ml intramuscularly. They should be put on antibiotic treatment at the earliest symptom to reduce the severity of the infection.

Diphtheria

Diphtheria is an acute infectious disease whose symptoms and signs are due to the action of exotoxin produced by *Corynebacteria diphtheriae*. In the tropics and subtropics the disease occurs in two forms: classical and cutaneous.

Classical diphtheria occurs in epidemics in some subtropical and tropical countries, whereas in more temperate climates it is sporadic or absent. This form of diphtheria tends to have complications involving the heart, central nervous system and respiratory system, resulting in high mortality. The cutaneous form is characterized by various types of ulcer which may not be recognized as diphtheritic, unless there is a high index of suspicion. Cutaneous diphtheria maintains a high level of immunity to diphtheria in the community where it is prevalent and may be a source of classical infection. The high fatality rate of classical diphtheria can be reduced by early diagnosis and treatment.

Epidemiology

The extent of diphtheria in tropical countries is difficult to assess. There are case reports of sporadic and endemic faucial diphtheria from various countries. Diphtheria is a health problem in some tropical countries, such as India, Singapore, Philippines and Sudan. If the prevalence of the infection is assessed by the level of antitoxin immunity in the population a different picture emerges. There are two methods of assessing antitoxin immunity. The first is the Schick test and the second is determining antitoxin titre in serum.

In the Schick test, a small dose of diphtheria toxin is injected intradermally. If the subject has sufficient circulating antitoxin to neutralize the dose, there is no reaction and the test is reported negative, i.e. the individual is regarded as having adequate immunity and hence protection against diphtheria. Where there is a positive reaction at the site of injection, the injected toxin is not neutralized and such a subject has no immunity, is not protected against diphtheria and hence is susceptible to the disease. A more accurate measure of antitoxin immunity is the determination of the levels of antibodies in serum.

Surveys in Third World countries using either or both of these methods have demonstrated a high level of immunity, despite the rarity of clinical diphtheria and the low level of active immunization. For instance, Schick testing showed 98 per cent immunity to diphtheria in 474 individuals over 10 years of age in Western Samoa, while haemagglutination tests in Rarotongan children aged five years showed that 90 per cent had antibody titres of over one in 64. Similar high levels of antibodies were found in West Africa. Evidence is accumulating that this immunity is as a result of cutaneous diphtheria. Cutaneous diphtheria is probably more common in the tropics than is realized and is transmitted by direct contact whereas faucial or classical diphtheria is transmitted by droplet infection through close contact. Overcrowded living conditions in the tropics favour the spread of the illness among family members. Active immunization would break the chain of transmission in an outbreak.

Aetiology

Corynbacteria diphtheriae are Gram-positive club-shaped non-motile and non-spore forming pleomorphic bacilli. There are three subspecies: *C. diphtheriae gravis*, *C. diphtheriae mitis* and *C. diphtheriae intermedius* with varying virulence and easily distinguishable in tellurite media. Their ability to cause disease is due to the production of an exotoxin which causes necrosis of tissue. *C. diphtheriae mitis* is the main cause of diphtheria in Africa and, as its name implies, appears to cause less severe disease than do the subspecies *gravis* and *intermedius*; *C. diphtheriae gravis* gives rise to the most severe disease. Significant sources of infection are individuals incubating the disease and asymptomatic carriers.

Pathogenesis

On entry into the body, the bacilli settle on the mucosal surface of the upper respiratory tract where they multiply and produce exotoxin. The toxin is absorbed by the cell membrane causing tissue necrosis in the vicinity of the bacillary colonies. This is followed by an inflammatory response producing a patch of exudate forming a membrane, which is so typical of the disease. Necrosis extends with the membrane, depending upon the amount of toxin produced. The membrane is adherent to the surface of the tissue, and consists of fibrin, inflammatory cells, red blood cells and superficial epithelial cells. Bleeding readily occurs on removal. The membrane is usually grey but may be black if bleeding occurs in it. This and oedema of the soft tissue beneath the lesion cause respiratory embarrassment as they encroach on to the airway. Secondary streptococcal infection may complicate the appearance of the membrane.

The toxin is absorbed and distributed by the bloodstream or lymphatics to many parts of the body; but has a predilection for the heart muscles, nervous tissues and the kidneys where it becomes fixed to the tissues, thus causing damage. While in circulation, the toxin can be neutralized by diphtheria antitoxin, but once fixed the antitoxins have no effect.

Clinical presentation

Classical diphtheria

Following an incubation period of 17 days, symptoms and signs appear depending on:

- the site of the infection;
- the individual's immunization status;
- the amount and distribution of toxin.

There are systemic and local features of the disease. Classical diphtheria presents faucial, laryngeal and nasal lesions. Faucial diphtheria presents mainly with sore throat and a rapidly spreading membrane over the tonsils, pharynx and uvula. In mild cases the membrane may be minimal or absent. Oedema of the soft tissue in the neck and enlarged cervical lymph nodes give rise to a 'bull' neck in severe cases. The disease presents with toxaemia, malaise, anorexia, low-grade fever and sore throat (worse on swallowing). The laryngeal form of the disease is characterized by hoarseness, increasing stridor, respiratory distress and a cough. In severe cases of laryngeal involvement, the membrane extends into the trachea causing increasing obstructive respiratory distress. A detached piece of membrane may block the airways causing sudden death. Laryngeal and pharyngeal involvement may coexist. Toxaemia is less in laryngeal disease. Nasal diphtheria may be isolated or occur as an extension of a pharyngeal lesion. It is characterized by a unilateral or bilateral purulent blood-stained discharge simulating a foreign body in the nostril. There may be excoriation of the skin of the nares. Diphtheria infection may also occur in the middle and external ear as well as in the conjuctiva.

In all forms of the disease, a rapid pulse and toxaemia should suggest the aetiology. Sudden cardiac failure from toxic myocarditis is a much feared complication of diphtheria. It occurs one to six weeks (usually two weeks) after the onset of the disease, and is heralded by enlarging liver and pulmonary congestion. Toxic myocarditis may follow both severe and mild diphtheria and is characterized by tachycardia, muffled heart sounds, murmurs, arrhythmias, bundle branch block, even complete heart block or congestive cardiac failure. Fatality is high with toxic myocarditis; but recovery does not leave permanent cardiac damage.

Symmetrical paralysis of the soft palate occurs in the third week, associated with nasal voice, nasal regurgitation of food and difficulty in swallowing. It is transient, disappearing in 48 hours, but may herald more serious forms of paralysis of the eyes in the third to the fifth week, and of respiratory muscles, pharynx, diaphragm, or limb muscles in the sixth or seventh week of the disease.

Ocular paralysis presents as blurring of vision, difficulty of accommodation and internal strabismus. Paralysis may also affect the diaphragm. Deep tendon reflexes may be depressed with elevated cerebrospinal fluid protein similar to Guillain–Barré syndrome.

Cutaneous diphtheria

Cutaneous diphtheria is common in the tropics. The lesions are quite varied.[12-14] Typically, they are punched-out ulcers with steep sides, thickened edges and a pseudomembrane on the base. More commonly the lesions are superficial, and resemble impetigo, pyoderma or eczema. Lesions may also develop in pre-existing surgical wounds, insect bites, burns and even in deep tropical ulcers. Diphtheria skin lesions are painful and tender, like faucial diphtheria. They may also be followed by cardiac and central nervous complications as in classical diphtheria.

Diagnosis

A high index of suspicion for the disease is necessary in areas where prevalence is low, otherwise many cases will pass unnoticed or be diagnosed as streptococcal throat infection. A prompt diagnosis is very necessary, as delayed therapy increases the risk of complications and fatality. A direct-stained smear shows the typical drum-stick bacilli indistinguishable from non-toxigenic diphtheroids which confirmation is obtained by isolating *C. diphtheriae* from culture on Loeffler's or preferably potassium tellurite media. On tellurite media *C. diphtheriae* grows as easily identifiable black colonies. For the yield of the growth to be high, a swab is taken from areas adjacent to or underneath the membrane and not on the membrane surface. The isolated bacilli are then tested for virulence. A positive virulence test confirms that the bacilli are toxigenic and should not be omitted, except on strains isolated during

a well-defined epidemic. The test is done either by inoculation into guinea-pigs or by precipitation on a gel diffusion agar on Elek's plate. If the bacilli obtained are toxigenic, necrosis occurs at the site of injection in the guinea-pigs and the animal dies within three to five days. Guinea-pigs injected with antitoxin before inoculation are unaffected. Elek's plates are prepared by incorporating strips of filter paper impregnated with 1000 units/ml of antitoxin into a serum agar base. The organisms to be tested are streaked at right angles to the filter paper and the plate incubated at 37°C. If a toxin is produced, a precipitation line is formed where the toxin–antitoxin concentrations are in optimal proportion. The results can be read within 24 hours.

Electrocardiography is a useful tool in the diagnosis of toxic myocarditis; when it shows prolonged PR interval, elevation of ST segment and inversion of T wave. There is also tachycardia or bradycardia in bundle branch block.

The presence of anaesthesia in the skin adjacent to a suspected diphtheritic ulcer is suggestive, but its absence does not rule out the disease. Culture of a swab from the lesion yields the causative *C. diphtheriae*.

Attempts should be made to detect carriers who are symptomless and yet possess virulent organisms in their throat or nose; they are Schick test negative. The carrier state may develop in contacts of patients with diphtheria or during convalescence. About 5–10 per cent of cases with diphtheria may have persistent diphtheria for as long as three months after treatment.

Differential diagnosis

Diphtheria may resemble a common cold in the partially immune. When there is serosanguinous nasal discharge, a foreign body in the nostril should be considered. Membrane occurs with streptococcal pharyngitis but this is associated with severe pain on swallowing and high temperature and the white membrane is non-adherent and limited to the tonsils. Diphtheria should also be differentiated from infectious mononucleosis, Vincent's angina, thrush, sporadic croup, laryngotracheobronchitis caused by various conditions, retropharyngeal abscess, blood dyscrasia as well as papillomata and haemangiomata. Direct visualization of the lesion helps to distinguish these conditions. Cutaneous diphtheria may resemble impetigo or any chronic staphylococcal infection.

Treatment

The primary aim of the treatment is to neutralize the circulating toxin and eliminate the diphtheria bacilli.

The amount of antitoxin administered is based on the severity of disease. The recommended doses are 5000–10 000 units for mild cases, 20 000–60 000 units for moderate and 60 000–100 000 units for severe. Before administration of the antitoxin, a sensitivity test should be done to eliminate the possibility of reaction to horse serum. Antibiotics are supplements, not substitutes, for specific antitoxin therapy, and are aimed at reducing the microbial load at the site of infection thus reducing the amount of toxin being formed. Antibiotics also control any concomitant infection such as β-haemolytic streptococci. Such therapy reduces the length of the carrier state which otherwise may persist for weeks following recovery from the disease.

Penicillin and erythromycin are the recommended antibiotics. Penicillin is given in doses of 600 000 units intramuscularly once daily for seven days. The dose of erythromycin is 40 mg/kg over 24 hours in four divided doses for 7–10 days. A culture should be done at the end of the treatment to confirm eradication of the diphtheria. Three successful negative nose and throat cultures are necessary before discharge.

Supportive therapy is very important. This should include bed rest and serial ECG to determine myocardial involvement. Absolute bed rest is indicated when myocarditis has occurred. Digoxin is contraindicated in diphtheritic myocarditis. Prednisone (1–1.5 mg/kg/every 24 hours) may lower the incidence of myocarditis. Hydration and nutrition should be maintained. Gag reflex should be checked regularly and the throat secretions suctioned. Elective tracheostomy should be done early to reduce strain on damaged heart muscles. Skilled care of the tracheostomy is extremely important. The secretions should be suctioned to reduce blockage of the tracheostomy tube.

Treatment of diphtheritic ulcers is difficult, especially if they have reached a chronic stage. Penicillin and antitoxin are administered as explained earlier for classical diphtheria. Cleaning the ulcers with antiseptic solution is necessary.

Carriers should be given diphtheria antitoxin in a dosage of 10 000 units together with one mega unit of procaine penicillin daily for seven days. Thereafter, nasal and pharyngeal swabs should be taken before discharge. Three successful negative cultures are mandatory before discharge.

In an outbreak in Khartoum, Sudan, a carrier rate of 2.3 per cent was reported following treatment. But many studies report carrier rates of roughly 4–10 per cent. The low carrier rate for Sudan was probably due to wide usage of penicillin. Effective and early treatment of a diphtheria epidemic with penicillin (300 000–600 000 units) or erythromycin (40 mg/kg/per day) reduces the carrier rate.

Prognosis

Prognosis depends upon the strain of diphtheria causing the disease. The site of infection is also significant. Extensive pharyngeal membrane extending into the larynx carries higher mortality. Diphtheria untreated or treated late may end fatally. Some disease is attenuated in the immunized individuals, immunization is very important. Death occurs most commonly in children below four years old from laryngeal obstruction, myocarditis with congestive cardiac failure and respiratory paralysis due to phrenic nerve paralysis.

Prevention

Diphtheria is preventable by active immunization. The vaccine is usually combined with that for pertussis and tetanus to form the triple vaccine (DPT), and is administered as shown in Table 4.4.2.

Cutaneous diphtheria contributes to the immune status of the communities where it occurs. As personal hygiene and nutrition continue to improve, cutaneous diphtheria will disappear leaving indigenous children unprotected against the more serious faucial diphtheria. This calls for more concerted efforts in providing active immunization against the disease.

Table 4.4.2. Immunization schedule

Vaccination	Age	Remarks
Primary		
BCG	Birth	or at first contact with
OPV I		child
DPT I	6 weeks	or at first contact with
OPV II		child after that age
DPT II	10 weeks	4 weeks after the above
OPV III		or at next contact with
		child after that age
DPT III	14 weeks	4 weeks after the above
OPV IV		or at next contact with
		child after that age
Measles	9 months	or at first contact with
		child after that age
Other		
Tetanus toxoid	During pregnancy	Two doses 4 weeks apart; one booster dose every pregnancy
	People with open wound	Two doses 4 weeks apart or one dose if immunized

Tetanus

Tetanus is caused by the exotoxin of *Clostridium tetanus* and is characterized by muscular rigidity and spasms. The disease is world-wide but is a health problem in tropical countries where it causes many deaths in neonates, children and adults. Practices at birth encourage contamination of the umbilical cord with tetanus bacilli, while wounds occurring in children and adults may be associated with contamination from soil and animal sources. Active immunization is an effective method of preventing tetanus.

Epidemiology

Tetanus is responsible for many deaths in children as well as adults in tropical countries. The causative organism, *Clostridium tetanus*, is widespread in the subtropics and tropics. Its spores are distributed in the soil and in atmospheric dust derived from animal and human faeces.

The spores enter the body through wounds. Many children walk bare foot and may be pierced by various objects, allowing spores to enter. Wounds occurring on farms where people and animals live in overcrowded conditions are particularly risky. Such wounds include: compound fractures, penetrating wounds due to rusty nails, thorns, wood splinters, broken bottles, animal and insect bites, jigger wounds, suppurative otitis media, circumcision, tribal scarification, teeth extraction by traditional healers, ear piercing in girls, uvulectomy where practised and the injured post partum birth canal.

The custom of applying medicinal herbs in the treatment of burns or discharging ear introduces tetanus spores on to the raw burnt area of the body and into the ear canal respectively.

In newborn infants where there is great risk of dying from the disease, tetanus spores reach the umbilical cord in the home environment in the following ways:

- Cutting the umbilicus with dirty, unsterilized instruments, such as old razor blades, knives and pieces of reed collected from grazing land.
- Tying the cord with an old piece of cloth. The cloth has probably been lying on the floor for some time with the risk of contamination by dust containing *Clostridium tetanus*.
- Dressing the cord with unhygienic medicinal herbs, animal butter or ghee, or even old talcum powder that has been sitting uncovered in the house for a long time. These can be heavily contaminated with tetanus spores.
- House dust from the floor (which has been hardened with animal dung) reaching the raw umbilical stump. Cow or ass dung is full of tetanus spores.
- Rarely, by direct application of animal dung as a dressing on the umbilical stump. Even babies born in hospitals under hygienic conditions may become infected with tetanus after they are discharged home early from maternity units.

Aetiology

The organisms are Gram-positive, non-capsulated anaerobic bacilli which form terminal spores and so look like drum-sticks. They are sensitive to antibiotics and physical and chemical agents. However, the spores are quite resistant and can survive in a wide variety of conditions. In severe, deep and dirty wounds contaminated with soil and in anoxic conditions, the spores germinate and produce exotoxin which is responsible for the symptoms of the disease.

The secreted exotoxin travels from the local site along the axon cylinders of motor nerves and eventually become fixed in the ganglion cells of the anterior horns of the spinal cord and cranial nerves. The toxin interferes with neuromuscular transmission, probably by blocking inhibitor synapses and preventing release of inhibitory transmitter substance, or by suppressing the action of this substance on the membranes of the motor neurones. The result is excitatory impulses through reflex pathways producing the characteristic tetanic spasms of the muscles to different stimuli.

Tetanus toxin also acts on the cranial nerves producing focal spasms of the larynx and pharynx, on the midbrain vital centres and the autonomic nervous system, though it is difficult to distinguish symptoms of direct tetanus intoxication from effects of anoxia on the central nervous system.

Clinical presentation

The mean incubation period is 7–14 days, but may be several weeks or may be shorter. The onset of symptoms is often heralded by development of painful trismus due to rigidity of masseteric muscles. This pain is worse on opening the mouth, leading to 'lock-jaw', which interferes with feeding. Newborn infants are unable to suck and cry. Rigidity spreads to muscles of neck, vertebral column, face, limbs and abdominal wall (Fig. 4.4.4). Rigidity of the extensor muscles dominates and is a characteristic clinical picture.

Superimposed on this generalized muscle rigidity are the tetanic spasms. These spasms are painful but

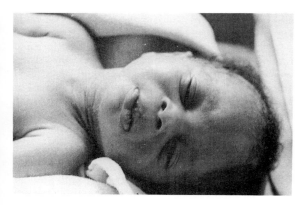

Fig. 4.4.4 Neonatal tetanus in a Nigerian baby.

without loss of consciousness. They vary in frequency and severity and may occur spontaneously but are mostly triggered by movements, touch, sound and even light. Even a light touch provokes attacks of spasms. The face shows typical 'risus sardonicus', a pathognomonic sign of tetanus. In fully developed and severe cases, the neck and back are retracted and there are frequent spasms. Involvement of muscles of respiration, especially the diaphragm, may result in apnoea and asphyxia. In severe cases, laryngospasm occurs leading rapidly to death. Spasm of the pharynx may be associated with increased secretion of mucus, aspiration of vomitus and loss of the swallowing and cough reflex which lead to bronchopneumonia. Constipation and retention of urine are likely to occur and should be anticipated.

Fever is usually mild but may be very high, when it carries a bad prognosis. A persistently raised pulse rate between spasms may occur; normally the pulse falls between spasms. In severe cases, anxiety, restlessness, a rising blood pressure, sweating and cyanosis largely due to impaired pulmonary ventilation may presage a fatal outcome. Reflexes are normal or exaggerated. The site of infection may be visible but in most cases this is healed and cannot be traced.

Clinical examination should be done gently and kept to a minimum to reduce the number of spasms.

Course of illness

The course of the disease is variable. In severe cases, death occurs from respiratory complications, asphyxia or cardiac failure. In favourable cases, the spasms become less frequent, fever subsides, generalized muscle spasms diminish, and the child is able to feed properly and sleep. Finally, the spasms disappear. The patient may, however, remain stiff for some time — the so-called 'stiffman syndrome'. Occasionally the patient may die unexpectedly in convulsions or hyperpyrexia or due to electrolyte imbalance. Many patients are brought to hospital with already established severe tetanic spasms and are dehydrated due to lack of feeding and have a poor prognosis. There are usually no residual ill-effects after recovery, though fractures of the vertebrae can occur and brain damage from prolonged anoxia has also been described. The disease does not confer immunity, hence active immunization should be given after recovery.

Diagnosis

Diagnosis is based on the clinical features of trismus and tetanic spasms. Abdominal muscles are usually rigid early in the disease and this can aid diagnosis. Diagnosis is usually easy, except in a few children with atypical symptoms and signs who may have mild spasm with slight trismus. Differential diagnosis includes causes of masseter spasm due to local conditions such as parotitis, dental abscess, impacted wisdom teeth, infected tonsils and retropharyngeal abscess. Acute fibrositis of the neck or submaxillary lymphadenitis may produce neck stiffness and cause confusion with tetanus.

The spasm of hysteria is easy to distinguish from tetanus in that it is overcome without difficulty. Neck stiffness of meningitis can be distinguished by abnormalities of cerebrospinal fluid, while spasms of tetany are limited to the hands and feet and respond to treatment with calcium. In atypical cases, tetanus may simulate a convulsive disorder, but a thorough clinical examination will fail to elicit muscle stiffness in the case of convulsive disorder. History of previous attacks will support a convulsive disorder.

Treatment

The treatment of tetanus aims at:

- control of spasms;
- maintenance of hydration;
- neutralization of toxin;
- eradication of bacteria by antibacterial therapy;
- maintaining airway;
- providing supportive measures.

Spasms are controlled by various sedatives as soon as the patient is admitted and this is maintained without depressing respiration. Paraldehyde is widely used (0.1 ml/kg) together with phenobarbitone (6 mg/kg), both intramuscularly; these doses are given six hourly alternately.

Chlorpromazine (2–4 mg/kg) and diazepam (0.25–0.5 mg/kg) administered four to six hourly are now used with good results in many centres. The initial dose of diazepam can be given through an intravenous line set up on admission. This not only limits interference but allows the diazepam to be given in 2.5 mg boluses at 5–10 minute intervals until the spasms have been controlled and muscle relaxation and regular breathing established.

Maintenance of hydration and correction of any dehydration can best be achieved by passing a nasogastric tube and giving oral rehydration solution (ORS WHO, see p. 479) or one-fifth strength normal saline in 5 per cent glucose alternating with expressed breast-milk in the case of neonatal tetanus to a total of 160–200 ml/kg in 24 hours. After an initial intramuscular dose, if necessary, the chlorpromazine can be given down the nasogastric tube, alternating with diazepam, so that each is given six hourly. Additional doses may be necessary to control spasms.

After the spasms are adequately controlled, the rest of the management procedures can follow. Where available, human tetanus immunoglobulin (HTIG) (500 units) is given intramuscularly, otherwise anti-tetanus horse serum (ATS) should be used in a single dose of 5000 units intramuscularly, after testing for sensitivity. This dose is given to both neonates and older children. Adrenaline and hydrocortisone should be available for use in the event of allergic reactions. HTIG (250 units) or ATS (50–100 units) can also be administered intrathecally, giving 1 ml after withdrawing 1 ml of CSF. Intrathecal therapy improves survival rates. Some workers recommend infiltration of antitoxin at the entry site such as the umbilicus to neutralize the locally produced toxin.

Penicillin or a broad-spectrum antibiotic is given to eradicate the bacilli from the wound: penicillin G (30 mg/kg daily in four divided doses) or procaine penicillin once or twice daily. Surgical toilet of the wound (umbilical stump in the case of newborn) removes bacteria at the site of entry.

The airway must be maintained. Suction apparatus in working condition must be available, together with a laryngoscope and endotracheal tubes. Mucus should be suctioned from the mouth regularly to avoid aspiration pneumonia. Tracheostomy in older children is considered for severe cases but adequate nursing must be available for its maintenance, otherwise this increases mortality. Indwelling polyvinyl endotracheal tubes are available in place of tracheostomy. Skilful supportive care must be given; survival of patients correlates well with nursing care. Supportive measures include monitoring vital signs and administration of drugs and oxygen. The following should be charted: number and duration of spasms, respiratory rate, pulse rate, temperature, drug administration, fluid input and output, level of consciousness and hydration status. It is important to give support and encouragement to the mother through what must be an agonizing vigil for her. In neonatal tetanus breast-milk should be expressed and given to the baby by intragastric tube until the baby is able to take by mouth or suckle again. In this way mothers milk output is maintained and the baby nourished. If her baby dies, breast-milk production can be suppressed by a short course of stilboestrol.

Prognosis

Prognosis for neonatal tetanus is poor. Case fatality rates range from as low as 20 per cent to as high as 90 per cent. Patients with a short incubation period of less than seven days in the case of the newborn or with rapid evolution of symptoms, i.e. short period from the time of appearance of the earliest symptoms to the onset of spasms, have a poor prognosis. The presence of pyrexia and a high pulse rate between spasms and frequent spasms (more than 20 in 24 hours) indicate poor prognosis. Death may occur due to asphyxia or cardiac failure during spasms. The quality of nursing care and availability of resuscitation facilities greatly affect prognosis.

Prevention

Prevention of tetanus in children is based on active immunization. The vaccine used is alum-precipitated toxoid administered singly or in combination with whooping cough vaccine and diphtheria toxoid (triple vaccine, DPT) according to the schedule in Table 4.4.2. Whenever a dirty wound is sustained, repeat toxoid is given to boost the antibody production if the patient has been vaccinated. In non-vaccinated individuals, antitoxin is given first followed by toxoid; later by two toxoid injections at one month intervals. Patients with such wounds should be given a course of procaine penicillin (300 000–600 000 units daily for three days). Where available, human tetanus immunoglobulin is given in a dose of 250 units intramuscularly and at the same time tetanus toxoid is given in another limb.

Prevention of tetanus neonatorum is based on reducing the chance of the umbilical cord becoming contaminated with bacilli. Traditional birth attendants

(TBAs) should be trained to observe hygienic methods of handling the cord. TBAs should be provided with delivery kits containing a clean pair of scissors (or a razor blade), sterile ligature and gentian violet. These, and nothing else, should be used for cutting, tying and dressing the cord. Immunization of women using tetanus toxoid during pregnancy is increasing in all tropical countries and provides tetanus antibodies in the mother for transfer to the fetus.[15, 16] Ideally two injections of tetanus toxoid are given, one in the first or second trimester and a second a month later. Even when given during the third trimester this is sufficient to elicit adequate maternal antibody response. Trials are underway evaluating single-dose tetanus toxoid to mothers in the control of neonatal tetanus.[16]

The opportunity to immunize pregnant mothers at prenatal clinics is sometimes missed. Where immunization has been carried out, the incidence of tetanus neonatorum has declined. Mothers who are in most need of prenatal immunization protection of their babies from tetanus neonatorum, are least likely to come for prenatal care. Mass immunization of all women of reproductive age with two doses of tetanus toxoid and then continued routine immunization of school girls would also eliminate the incidence of tetanus neonatorum.

Rubella (German measles)

Rubella or German measles is a common viral infectious disease of childhood and young adults (see pp. 163–5). It is usually a mild disease which may not be recognized except for its rash. Enlarged tender lymph nodes, particularly the occipital, retro-auricular and posterior cervical lymph nodes, are a common feature. The infection is particularly serious in the fetus where damage can affect particularly the eye, ear, heart and brain with common presenting features of cataracts, deafness, congenital heart disease and mental retardation. Fetal effects of rubella infection depend upon the stage of pregnancy when a woman is infected. Infection in the first trimester during organogenesis is the most dangerous. Infection later in pregnancy may not affect the fetus. It is desirable for all girls to contract the disease before marriage, to avoid fetal infection. Immunization is available and can be given singly or in combination with other vaccines, as with measles and mumps in the MMR vaccine (see pp. 501, 514).

Epidemiology

Rubella is widespread in the world. It is propagated by droplet infection or by direct or indirect contact with articles freshly soiled with discharge from the nose and throat of the patient. It is less contagious than measles but its period of infectivity lasts from the end of the incubation period to at least one week after the rash has appeared and sometimes longer. The incubation period is 14–21 days, usually 17 days. Epidemiological surveys of immune status at various ages have given direct indication of prevalence of the disease in the community. In most countries where a seroepidemiological survey has been done, rubella immunity is found in 70–95 per cent of females from adolescence to the end of reproductive life. A survey in Trinidad, in contrast, reported a very low level of seropositivity. In such countries, the risk of women contracting rubella and transferring it to the fetus is a big problem.

The infected fetuses have both high levels of specific IgM antibodies and active infection; they secrete the virus and are able to transmit the disease. They are a source of infection to pregnant nursery personnel. Infection of women in the first half of pregnancy carries a risk of fetal infection in as high as 85 per cent of the cases. The highest risk is in the first eight weeks of pregnancy and rapidly diminishes thereafter. Infection in the first eight weeks of pregnancy is severe because:

- the virus interferes with organ formation;
- the fetal cells may provide a fertile tissue culture for the growth of the virus;
- the fetus has not developed antibodies to limit the infection.

In such early infection, multiple organ involvement is the rule. Infection occurring later in pregnancy tends not to affect the fetus because the placenta at that stage acts as a barrier to the virus. The cells of the more mature fetus are less susceptible and less vulnerable to virus replication, and the fetus is able to form antibodies which curtail the invasiveness of the virus and reduce its effects. Minor hearing defects may occur as an isolated feature where maternal infection occurs later. Affected infants are less able to get rid of the virus. A high serum level of haemagglutination inhibiting antibodies persists, with the presence of an active disease process and the shedding of virus particles in urine, stool and nasopharynx for up to 12–18 months. Convulsions and disseminated intravenous coagulopathy (DIC) have also been described in congenital rubella syndrome (CRS). Rubella interferes with fetal growth causing intrauterine growth retardation and low birth weight. Growth retardation continues after birth.

Clinical presentation

There are mild prodromal features with minimal or no fever. The main features are the tender enlargement of the suboccipital, postauricular and posterior cervical lymph nodes, followed in 24 hours by a pink, discrete, macular rash which begins from the face and rapidly spreads to involve the trunk, where it is usually very dense. The rash fades within two days without desquamation. It may be imperceptible in dark-skinned patients. Infection in older children and adults may be severe, with arthralgia, arthritis and purpura. There may be pharyngitis or encephalitis. Neutropaenia and lymphopaenia may occur. Low platelet counts are the basis of purpura.

The clinical features seen immediately after birth differ from those seen later on. For instance, the classical triad of cataracts, congenital heart disease and deafness becomes obvious with age. Clinical features of acute rubella seen in the first week of life include: hepatosplenomegaly, jaundice, hypertonia, lethargy, convulsions, cataracts, cloudiness of the cornea, microphthalmia, congenital heart disease (PDA and VSD), respiratory distress, low birth weight and purpura (Fig. 4.4.5).

Diagnosis

Diagnosis is based on the clinical picture and (where it can be done) on laboratory investigation. Rubella should be distinguished from other exanthematous diseases like measles, drug rash and typhus. The transient nature of rubella arthritis may simulate rheumatoid arthritis with which it shares enlarged lymph nodes. Congenital rubella is one of the 'TORCH' syndrome and should be distinguished from members of this group (see pp. 163–5).

A combination of features as suggested by Ali *et al.*[18] tabulated in Table 4.4.3 can be used to make a diagnosis of rubella in the newborn: any two complications in list A or any one of them with any one from list B should suggest the diagnosis. Where laboratory facilities exist, serial determination of rubella antibody titre (HAI) is useful in the diagnosis of acute infection, if a rising titre of the antibodies is observed. Specific IgM antibodies may be detected in the acute phase of infection and in case of congenital infection, allowing the diagnosis on a single serum sample.

Prognosis

Prognosis of the childhood form of the diseases is good. Poor prognosis is noted where there is severe thrombocytopaenia or encephalitis.

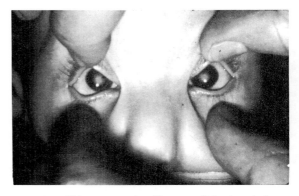

Fig. 4.4.5 Chinese neonate with congenital cataract of rubella. (© Centre for Disease Control, USA/Wellcome Trust.)

Table 4.4.3 Abnormalities compatible with congenital rubella syndrome

List A
  Cataract
  Congenital glaucoma
  Congenital heart disease
  Loss of hearing
  Pigmentary retinopathy
List B
  Purpura, growth retardation
  Hepatomegaly, splenomegaly, jaundice
  Meningoencephalitis, radiolucency of bone
  Microcephaly, mental retardation

(Reproduced with permission from Ali A *et al.*, *Journal of Tropical Paediatrics*, 1986; **32**: 79–82. Oxford University Press.)

Prevention

Female children should be encouraged to contract the natural infection early. This is quite possible in traditional societies with close contacts in large families, where infection can spread rapidly. It is the main cause of high levels of antibodies by 7–11 years of age.[17, 19] The infection is thus acquired early in life due to early exposure. The vaccine should be given selectively to females before or at adolescence. It may be given as a single vaccine or in combination with mumps and measles vaccine, when it is often included in the primary schedule in infancy between nine months and one year (see pp. 501, 514 and ref. 25p.).

Mumps (epidemic parotitis)

Mumps is an infectious disease of world-wide occurrence. The main features are painful swelling of the parotid glands. The other salivary glands may be involved. Insignificant prodromal features precede the swelling of the gland. The disease has a short course lasting about two weeks and carries no fatality. A few complications may arise.

Epidemiology

Mumps is caused by a paramyxovirus similar to the measles virus. The disease occurs in epidemics and is spread by droplet infection. Infectivity is present from two days before the swelling of the gland until 3–9 days after the swelling has subsided. It is estimated that 30–40 per cent of those infected have subclinical illness and this can only be detected serologically by finding elevated complement-fixing antibodies in their sera. Males and females are equally affected. Most infected individuals are under 15 years old. Recovery is followed by life-long immunity.

Pathogenesis

Following entry into susceptible patients the virus multiplies in the respiratory tract, spreading via the bloodstream to reach many tissues of the body. The organs most involved are salivary glands, pancreas, gonads and brain.

Clinical presentation

Incubation ranges from 14 to 24 days, usually 17–18 days. There are minimal prodromal signs of mild malaise and fever. High fever is seen with gonadal involvement and with meningoencephalitis.

The onset of the illness is usually characterized by swelling of the parotid glands. It is common for only one gland to be involved. Where the other gland is affected, its involvement occurs within one to three days of the first. The swelling of the parotid glands may be rapid, reaching a maximum within a few hours. The glands are painful and tender and interfere with opening of the mouth. There is oedema of skin and soft tissue surrounding the gland. The ear lobe is usually pushed upwards and backwards.

Stensen's duct, the parotid duct, is inflamed and any sour liquids like lemon juice reaching it cause pain in the mouth and in the whole gland thus interfering with feeding. The swelling subsides within three to seven days but may last longer. The other salivary glands are involved less often than the parotid glands. In 15 per cent of the patients, submaxillary glands are involved. Least affected are the sublingual glands.

Complications

Meningoencephalitis is the most common complication, occurring in up to 30 per cent of cases and characterized by headache and vomiting, lethargy and high fever (see p. 754). Neck stiffness is present and the CSF shows increased cells of the lymphocyte type with slightly raised proteins. This complication occurs in childhood as well as in adults.

Orchitis is present in about 25 per cent of mumps in adolescent boys and adult males and may be the only evidence of infection. It is characterized by swollen painful testes for four to seven days. Impaired fertility rarely follows. Oophoritis occurs in adolescent girls and adult females but is much rarer than orchitis. It is characterized by lower abdominal pain.

Pancreatitis is a rare complication. It is heralded by epigastric pain, vomiting, fever, chills and prostration. Serum amylase is elevated and this assists in the diagnosis.

Diagnosis

The diagnosis of mumps is easy, based on the characteristic clinical features and the epidemic nature of the disease. There is normally a history of other children from the same school with parotitis. Elevated serum amylase is an important laboratory feature. Blood count shows neutropaenia with lymphocytosis.

Mumps should be distinguished from suppurative parotitis, salivary gland calculus and the painless enlargement of the parotid gland commonly seen in malnutrition.

Treatment

Treatment of mumps is symptomatic. Analgesics are given for pain. For orchitis, the testes are suspended with a special bandage and steroids are often recommended. An adequate fluid intake should be emphasized in children with pancreatitis while bed rest, analgesics and supportive care should be given for meningoencephalitis.

Prevention

Mumps can be prevented by immunization with attenuated mumps vaccine which is a chick embryo-adapted vaccine. It is given at one year of age. It is normally stored freeze-dried. The reconstituted vaccine should be used within eight hours, preferably immediately. Mumps can be combined with measles and rubella in the MMR vaccine, and administered at nine months of age (see pp. 501, 513 and ref. 25p.).

Streptococcal infections

There are two groups of streptococci of clinical importance: group A and group B (see pp. 579–82). Group A is a common pathogen associated with skin, throat and other specific infections. Some of these infections may be mild and of short duration but others are fulminating and life-threatening. The dangers resulting from group A streptococcal infections are delayed, non-suppurative complications of acute nephritis and acute rheumatic fever. Group B streptococci on the other hand are important pathogens causing infections in newborn infants who acquire them from the birth canal of their carrier mothers.

Epidemiology

For group A β-haemolytic streptococcal infections the main diseases are pharyngitis and tonsillitis in the respiratory tract and impetigo and pyodermas in the skin. Transmission of respiratory infection is by droplet while skin infection occurs by direct contact. Contaminated food and milk also transmit infection.

Streptococcal impetigo and pyodermas are very common in preschool children in hot tropical countries throughout the year. In temperate climates these conditions occur in the summer. Pharyngitis and tonsillitis occur commonly in both preschool and school children in winter months in temperate countries while in the tropics and subtropics they occur throughout the year. Both conditions are common in children of families of low socio-economic status. Crowding and close contact in sleeping quarters increase the risk of pharyngeal infection. After the acute disease, some patients remain as nose and throat carriers and can transmit the infection. Nose and throat carriers may be dangerous if employed in nurseries for the newborn, as they can cause epidemic infection.

Mothers who are vaginal carriers of group B streptococcal infections transmit the infection to the newborn infant during childbirth. Mothers also transmit infection to the fetus through amnionitis.

Age distribution of ASO titre shows that high levels of ASO occur quite early in infancy indicating that (as in the case of measles and rubella) infection with streptococci occurs early in children in tropical and subtropical environments.

Pathogenesis

Group A β-haemolytic streptococci invade intact epithelium of the pharyngeal and tonsillar mucosa to multiply and cause disease. In skin disease, the infection needs broken epithelium to gain entry into the skin. The disease may be primary impetigo or pyoderma or secondary infection of skin with scabies, eczema, burns and traumatic or surgical wounds.

Erythrogenic toxin is responsible for the skin rash of scarlet fever. Bacteraemia occurs in infants and young children and patients with leukaemia and other malignancies.

Following pharyngitis and skin infection with group A streptococci, there is a varying latent period before the non-suppurative complications of acute glomerulonephritis or acute rheumatic fever may manifest themselves. The latent period for nephritis is shorter than that for rheumatic fever. The length of the latent period is probably related to the time it takes for antibodies and antigens to react in the site organs and is generally one to three weeks.

Many different types of group A streptococci have been recognized on the basis of serologically distinct surface proteins, the M proteins. The M types causing impetigo and pyodermas differ from those associated with pharyngitis. The M protein renders group A streptococcus resistant to phagocytosis and hence is a major virulence factor. On the basis of M proteins, the group A strains can be subdivided into serological types 1, 2, 3 and so on.

Group A streptococcal pharyngitis stimulates production of antibodies to bacterial antigens some of which are shared with human cell antigens. For instance, antibodies are formed to myocardium — the heart reactive antibodies which cause rheumatic fever (see pp. 776–8). Antibodies for kidney tissue cause acute glomerulonephritis (see pp. 792–3). These antibody–antigen reactions damage the structures involved. Acute glomerulonephritis follows infections with specific serological types of streptococci. It is seen after throat infections with types 1, 4, 12 and 49. Skin infections with types 2, 49, 52, 55, 57, 59, 60 and 61 are also followed by acute glomerulonephritis. In contrast with rheumatic fever, any one of the different types of the group A β-haemolytic streptococci is potentially rheumatogenic but the infection has to be in the nasopharynx. This explains why skin infections are not followed by acute rheumatic fever.

Group A streptococci produce and release extracellular products such as streptolysin O and streptolysin S. These are not group A-specific, as group C and G also produce streptolysin O. These streptolysins stimulate the body to produce antistreptolysin O and antistreptolysin S; the presence of the former is used for diagnosis of group A β-haemolytic streptococci infection.

Clinical presentation

Pharyngitis and tonsillitis have a short incubation period and present with sore throat, pain on swallowing, high fever, malaise, headache and abdominal pain. Inspection reveals an inflamed throat, with or without white follicles or exudate. The exudate may be in patches on the tonsils or appear confluent. The tonsillar lymph nodes at the angle of the jaw become swollen and tender bilaterally. Bacteraemia is uncommon in older children but occurs frequently in infants and children with underlying diseases like leukaemias and other malignancies. Subclinical cases of streptococcal pharyngitis or tonsillitis occur and these can be identified by finding high titres of antistreptolysin O titre in children with no history of sore throat.

Streptococcal pyodermas and impetigo occur anywhere on the skin, but impetigo is most common on the lower limbs, followed by the trunk, upper extremities and face. The lesions are discrete, itchy but not tender. They begin as vesicular eruptions which become pustular, then burst to form crusts with a yellowish exudate with the characteristic appearance of impetigo. The lesion may become secondarily infected with staphylococci. Generally the lesions do not involve the dermis so healing is associated with depigmentation without scarring.

Pemphigus neonatorum is a specific impetigo of the newborn. The whole skin may be involved. The child is very sick, toxic and refuses to feed. There is associated bacteraemia. Pemphigus carries a high mortality.

Pyodermas secondary to scabies, eczema, burns and traumatic or surgical lesions may be a source of bacteraemia and serious metastatic infections.

Scarlet fever is rare and may be difficult to see on dark skins. The rash of scarlet fever is macular and blanches on pressure. It is accompanied by a red tongue resembling the surface of a strawberry. The tonsils and pharynx may only be mildly inflamed.

Group A streptococci also cause otitis media, sinusitis, mastoiditis and pneumonia in older children and also newborn infections such as omphalitis, meningitis and bacteraemia.

Group B infections predominantly affect the newborn. There are two forms of the disease. The common type is characterized by an early or acute infection in infants born prematurely or after prolonged rupture of membranes and maternal infections. The onset is within a few hours of birth and characterized by respiratory distress mimicking respiratory distress syndome in prematurity. Infection is associated with bacteraemia, hence blood cultures are positive. The less common late or delayed onset disease is seen in healthy full-term infants several weeks after birth. Its principal manifestation is bacterial meningitis. Group B streptococci can be isolated at birth in blood and cerebrospinal fluid of affected infants. Group B streptococci are also implicated in septic arthritis, with or without osteomyelitis, but do not cause skin infections.

Diagnosis

The diagnosis is clinical and confirmed by isolation of streptocci from throat, skin lesions or blood as the case may be. Pharyngitis and tonsillitis due to streptococci should be differentiated from viral pharyngitis in which the fever may not be high, and also from diphtheria with the occurrence of a membrane. In diphtheria, the membrane is adherent and tends to extend to the uvula. As the facilities for throat culture to distinguish viral from streptococcal infections are unavailable in most situations in the tropics, some authorities recommend treating all sore throats with penicillin as cost is relatively inexpensive. This removes the subsequent danger of acute rheumatic fever.[20] Impetigo should be distinguished from insect bites and chickenpox. In chickenpox, the lesions tend to be on the trunk. Scarlet fever should be distinguished by its blanching features from drug rashes and the exanthematous disease like measles, German measles and infectious mononucleosis. Scarlet fever is not very prominent on dark skin. Serum antistreptolysin O titre is elevated in group A streptococcal infections.

Treatment

All streptococcal infections respond to penicillin which should be given in full doses. Erythromycin is the drug of choice where there is penicillin sensitivity.

Prognosis

This depends upon the type of disease and the site of infection. Skin infections are mild and of short duration. Skin and respiratory infections are followed by acute nephritis and acute rheumatic fever respectively. Whereas the treatment of throat infection prevents acute rheumatic fever, the treatment of skin disease does not prevent acute nephritis.

Prevention

As streptococcal infections are related to crowding and low socio-economic status, their improvement reduces the disease in the community. Decline of acute rheumatic fever in Europe and North America was due to treatment of streptococcal pharyngitis and tonsillitis with penicillin and to improved living conditions.

It is stressed that vigorous treatment of pharyngitis, tonsillitis and complications like otitis media and mastoiditis forms the basis of preventing acute rheumatic fever.[21, 22] (See also p. 972.)

Chickenpox (varicella)

Chickenpox is a common and a highly contagious disease. The infection is world-wide and generally benign. It occurs in preschool and school-aged children who infect each other at nursery and primary schools. It carries a low mortality and few complications (see p. 616).

Epidemiology

The incubation period for chickenpox is 14–20 days. The disease is transmitted by direct contact, droplets and airborne spread and occurs in epidemics. The patients are most contagious just before and shortly after the skin rash appears. The majority of the patients are aged 2–10 years. The early onset of disease is said to be more likely to be followed by herpes zoster due to persistent and prolonged presence of virus in the body. Adults with herpes zoster can also transmit the disease. Recovery is followed by long immunity. Second infections are unlikely but occasionally occur. By adulthood almost every individual has been infected. Women who get infected as adults during pregnancy are likely to infect their fetuses who are born with the congenital form of the disease.

Aetiology

Chickenpox is caused by varicella-zoster virus. This virus causes chickenpox in children and herpes zoster (shingles) in adults. It is a member of the herpes virus group.

Clinical presentation

In young children, the disease presents with an exanthem of characteristic poxes but with no prodromal signs. Prodromal signs such as fever, malaise, headache, backache and sore throat precede the rash in older children and adults. The rash is centripetal. It is itchy and starts as a macule which progresses into papules, vesicles and pustules which ulcerate becoming crusts. The rash occurs in crops for several days, such that the individual lesions are seen in different stages (macules, papules, vesicles, pustules and crusts) in the affected individual (Fig. 4.4.6).

The rash is mainly on the trunk and spreads outwards to the face and extremities. It is most dense in the axillae; may occur on the mucous membranes, conjunctiva and cornea but spares the hands and soles of the feet. The rash is not umbilicated as is typical of smallpox. The child remains well with no significant systemic features. Atypical cases occur where the rash is not characteristic in its appearance and distribution.

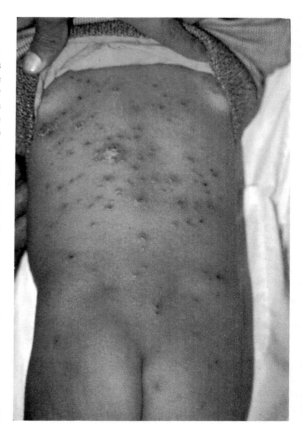

Fig. 4.4.6 Typical sparse chickenpox rash with blisters, pustules and scabs. (Courtesy of Dr P. Rotmil/Wellcome Trust.)

Complications

In normal children varicella is a benign disease. But infection is associated with complications, with fatality in neonates acquiring the disease perinatally and in adults, especially when immunocompromised. In leukaemia the disease may disseminate causing generalized varicella and often death.

Various complications associated with chickenpox are reported from a variety of review and case reports. Cutaneous complications such as bacterial infection, bullous and haemorrhagic lesions, localized gangrene, necrotizing fasciitis and purpura fulminans are reported. Complications involving the central nervous system come next in frequency to the skin disease and include cerebellar ataxia and encephalitis (see p. 754). A cluster of cases of Reye's syndrome has also been reported with chickenpox.[23] Aseptic meningitis and Guillain–Barré syndrome also occur. Pneumonia has been reported, mainly in adults who develop pulmonary nodular infiltration, visible on X-ray of the chest. These may calcify later on in life. Other complications include: keratitis, iritis, conjunctivitis, arthritis, carditis, appendicitis, glomerulonephritis, orchitis, thrombocytopaenia and bleeding tendency. Children with congenital varicella can have congenital malformations such as low birth weight, microcephaly, encephalitis, chorioretinitis and muscle wasting.

Diagnosis

Diagnosis is clinical and based on the distribution and appearance of the rash. During epidemics diagnosis is made even easier. Smallpox is no longer a differential diagnosis of chickenpox following its eradication. Chickenpox may also be confused with impetigo, scabies, dermatitis multiforme and erythema multiforme.

Treatment

Chickenpox is usually a mild disease and does not require treatment. Mild analgesics may be necessary in children with headaches and malaise. It is not advisable to administer salicylates to these children as this predisposes to Reye's syndrome. Application of calamine lotion on the body reduces itchiness of the poxes. Acyclovir has been shown to be useful in the immunodeficient and in neonates if given early, but is expensive and not generally available in tropical countries (see p. 616).

Children on immunosuppressive treatment who are exposed to chickenpox should be given hyperimmune immunoglobulin to suppress the disease. Similar treatment has been tried in the newborn with neonatal varicella.[24]

Prognosis

Prognosis for chickenpox is good as the disease is generally mild with few complications and hardly any mortality, except in children with leukaemia, those with immunodeficiency and those with congenital infection.

Prevention

As the disease is so mild especially during early childhood, one wonders whether it is justified to isolate cases for fear of transmitting infection. Susceptible children have been exposed to chickenpox so that they may contract the infection early, rather than delaying it into adulthood where the disease is known to increase in severity. This argument aside, one can consider keeping children away from school for a period of seven days from the onset of the skin rashes to reduce transmission. By the time the rash is obvious the child has probably already infected his close contacts.

A safe and effective varicella vaccine is now available. Its main use is in the protection of children about to be treated with immunosuppressive drugs and in such conditions as leukaemia. At the moment the cost of such a vaccine is likely to be a factor prohibiting its use in developing countries. The vaccine can be incorporated into measles, mumps and rubella vaccine as MMRV and be administered during infancy.[25] (See pp. 81, 501, 513–4) It is safe not only in normal children but also in leukaemic children. What is not known is the duration of immune protection following the administration of the vaccine. The change of epidemiology of the disease delaying its onset into adulthood when it is more serious is a yet unsolved question.

References

1. O'Donovan C. Measles in Kenyan children. *East African Medical Journal*. 1971; **48**: 526–32.
2. Shahid NS, Rahman AS, Aziz KM *et al*. Beliefs and treatment related to diarrhoea episodes reported in association with measles. *Tropical and Geographical Medicine*. 1983; **35**: 151–6.
3. Maina-Ahlberg B. Machakos project studies. Agents affecting health of mother and child in rural area of Kenya. XII Beliefs and practices concerning treatment of measles and acute diarrhoea among the Akamba. *Tropical and Geographical Medicine*. 1979; **31**: 139–48.

4. Scheifele DW, Forbes CE. Biology of measles. *East African Medical Journal*. 1973; **50**: 168–73.

5. Vesikari T, Ala-Laurila E, Heikkinen A *et al.* Clinical trial of a new trivalent measles-mumps-rubella vaccine in young children. *American Journal of Disease in Children*. 1983; **136**: 843–7.

6. Ministry of Health of Kenya/World Health Organization. Measles immunity in the first year and after birth and optimum age for vaccination in Kenya children. *Bulletin of the World Health Organization*. 1977; **55**: 21–31.

7. Ogunmekan DA, Harry TO. Optimum age for vaccination of Nigerian children against measles. II. Seroconversion to measles vaccine in different age groups. *Tropical and Geographical Medicine*. 1981; **33**: 379–86.

8. Morley DC. Measles vaccine by aerosol: eradication this century? *Tropical Doctor*. 1983; **13**: 90.

9. Bwibo NO. Whooping cough in Uganda. *Scandinavian Journal of Infectious Diseases*. 1971; **3**: 41–3.

10. Voorhoeve AM, Miller AS, Schulpen TW *et al.* The epidemiology of pertussis: Machakos project studies No. iv. *Tropical and Geographical Medicine*. 1978; **30**: 125–39.

11. Prensky AL. Pertussis vaccination. *Developmental Medicine and Child Neurology*. 1974; **16**: 539–42.

12. Rahman KM. Incidence of cutaneous diphtheria in Bangladesh. *Bangladesh Medical Research Council Bulletin*. 1985; **9**: 49–53.

13. Mhalu FS, Lindquist KJ. *Corynebacterium diphtheriae* infection in Tanzania. *East African Medical Journal*. 1974; **51**: 44–50.

14. Bray JP, Burt EG, Potter B. Epidemic diphtheria and skin infection in Trinidad. *Journal of Infectious Diseases*. 1972; **126**: 34–40.

15. Chen ST. Timing of antenatal tetanus immunization for effective protection of the neonate. *Bulletin of the World Health Organization*. 1982; **61**: 159–61.

16. Agarwal K *et al.* Single dose tetanus toxoid: a review of trials in India with special reference to control of tetanus in newborn. *Indian Journal of Pediatrics*. 1980; **51**: 283–5.

17. Najera E, Najera R, Gallardo FP. The seroepidemiology of rubella. *Bulletin of the World Health Organization*. 1973; **49**: 25–30.

18. Ali A, Hull B, Lewis M. Neonatal manifestation of congenital rubella following an outbreak in Trinidad. *Journal of Tropical Paediatrics*. 1986; **32**: 79–82.

19. Hayden RJ. Memorandum on the incidence of rubella in Nairobi children as revealed by antibody study. *East African Medical Journal*. 1971; **48**: 658–61.

20. Jaiyesimi F. Primary prevention of acute rheumatic fever. *Nigerian Journal of Paediatrics*. 1981; **8**: 90–3.

21. Markowitz M. Rheumatic fever in the eighties. *Pediatric Clinics of North America*. 1986; **33**: 1141–9.

22. Strasser T, Dondog N, Kholy EL *et al.* The community control of rheumatic fever and rheumatic heart disease: report of a WHO international cooperative project. *Bulletin of the World Health Organization*. 1981; **59**: 285–94.

23. Hurwitz ES, Goodman RA. A cluster of cases of Reye syndrome with chickenpox. *Pediatrics*. 1982; **70**: 901–6.

24. King SM. Fatal varicella-zoster infection in the newborn treated with varicella zoster immunoglobulin. *Pediatric Infectious Disease*. 1986; **5**: 588–9.

25. Arbeter AM, Starr S, Baker L. Combination of measles, mumps, rubella and varicella vaccine (MMRV). *Pediatrics*. 1986; **78**: 742–7.

26. Dossetter JFB and Whittle HC. Protein losing enteropathy and malabsorption in acute measles enteritis. *British Medical Journal*. 1975; **2**: 592–3.

CHAPTER 5

Tuberculosis

D. H. Shennan and M. A. Kibel

Tuberculosis is today the most serious disease for many developing countries, although it was not originally thought of as a tropical disease. It afflicts largely those in the middle years of life, in the working and caring age-group, including the parents of young children; this is contrary to the natural law followed by other infections, which kill very early and late in life. It leaves many people disabled by lung destruction. It is a great drain on a nation's health finances, since under the conditions generally prevalent in the less wealthy countries, effective treatment requires a long period in hospital. In some countries a third or more of hospital beds are used for tuberculosis.

Children are the tragic victims of tuberculosis. They are infected, but, except on rare occasions, do not infect. The prevention of the disease in children depends entirely on its control in adults.

The root causes of the current tuberculosis pandemic in the Third World have to do with social and economic disadvantage. In the industrialized countries it was seen to wane considerably with an improvement in the standard of living even before the appearance of drug therapy. Poor housing conditions and overcrowding, undernutrition and social stress provide the ideal culture medium for the infection.

Primary tuberculosis occurs in childhood. As the great majority of those presenting have mild forms of disease, the aim in treating such patients is largely to prevent serious disease in later life.

The control of the disease, as opposed to the treatment of individual patients, depends on one key factor: reduction of the number of infectious persons in the community (the 'infector pool'). Infectious people are those suffering from pulmonary disease; they cough up tubercle bacilli in their sputum. Thus when dealing with the problem of tuberculosis, we have to distinguish clearly between measures designed to treat and protect the individual patient, and those aimed at producing an overall reduction of the problem by attacking the infector pool.

Since the introduction of chemotherapy in the 1950s, tuberculosis has become an eminently treatable and controllable disease. Properly administered treatment is particularly effective in childhood. The disastrous failure to control tuberculosis in developing countries has been caused not by the ineffectiveness of drugs but by our inability to organize the taking of tablets daily for the long period required. Factors contributing to this are the problems of arranging treatment in the presence of a poorly financed social organization, the shortage of personnel with the necessary managerial skills and a lack of follow-up staff and staff with the skills and time to make patients and their families and the community aware of the importance of long continued treatment.

Aetiology

Tuberculosis is caused by bacilli of the genus *Mycobacterium* of which the most important species are *M. tuberculosis* and *M. bovis*. *M. tuberculosis* is almost always acquired by inhalation from an infectious person. Rarely, it may enter the body through the mouth, throat, eye or skin. *M. bovis*, the cause of tuberculosis in cattle, occurs in humans through the ingestion of infected milk. In contrast to the human variety, bovine tuberculosis is a 'dead end' disease in man. The infection cannot spread to others because it does not affect the lungs, but is limited to the gastrointestinal tract and the draining lymph glands. The prevalence of bovine tuberculosis varies greatly in different countries.

Because of their waxy outer capsules, mycobacteria do not take up the usual stains for bacteria, but absorb carbol fuchsin stain when it is heated, and thereafter resist decolourization by acid and alcohol. Hence they are often termed 'acid-fast bacilli'. They also absorb a fluorescent stain – auramine–rhodamine – and this staining method, which makes for easier identification of the organism, is now increasingly widely used. The organism shows good growth on solid and liquid media; it may form colonies as early as three weeks, but usually only in the fifth to sixth week.

The tubercle bacillus is tough and slow; slow to stain, to grow, to infect, to spread in the body, and to succumb to treatment. Its hardiness means that it is difficult for drugs to kill off a whole population of bacilli; multiple, prolonged regimens are needed and mutants resistant to particular drugs often survive in viable numbers and multiply.

A variety of other mycobacteria also cause human disease, but with a generally milder clinical spectrum. Their incidence varies widely in different countries. With the waning of tuberculosis in highly-developed countries these are now the commonest mycobacterial infections seen in such settings.

Pathogenesis

On first entering the alveolar spaces of the lung, bacilli are engulfed by macrophages. These unactivated cells cannot destroy all the mycobacteria, so that some multiply within the macrophages causing their death. The release of these organisms attracts more macrophages as well as lymphocytes from the bloodstream, and a small focus of granulomatous infiltration forms – a 'tubercle'. In 10 to 14 days this shows a central area of necrosis or caseation. In this early phase mycobacteria can spread readily along the lung lymphatics to the regional lymph node, and into the bloodstream, to lodge in distant sites, such as the brain, liver, bone or kidney. Small tubercles develop along the lymphatic path and in the gland. The lung focus, lymphatics and involved gland are together termed the 'Ghon complex'. After about six weeks immuno-responsive T lymphocytes induce cell-mediated hypersensitivity with activation of macrophages. This results in greater containment of the infection and most of the organisms lodged in distant sites are killed by these activated cells. However, hypersensitivity also has detrimental effects. In the presence of large amounts of mycobacterial antigen this response causes cell death and tissue destruction, and accounts for much of the symptomatology of childhood tuberculosis.

Healing occurs in most cases. The lesion is walled off by fibrosis and calcification may ensue; the lymph node component takes longer to regress than the pulmonary focus.

In more severe cases there is enlargement and caseation of the nodes. Caseating nodules in the hilum may burst into neighbouring structures. If they burst into the pulmonary vein, miliary disease, tuberculous meningitis or (later) localized organ tuberculosis results; if into a bronchus, progressive tuberculosis of the lung may follow and often the patient, who by this time has become sensitized to the tubercle bacillus, becomes sputum-positive just as in a case of secondary (adult-type) tuberculosis. Pressure on the bronchus by an enlarged lymph node produces emphysema or collapse of a local lung segment or lobe. Consequently not all lung lesions seen in the X-ray of a child with enlarged hilar glands represent progressive disease.

Host factors determine the response of the body to infection. A child who is malnourished or suffering from some other infection or infestation is more likely to acquire overt disease, and more likely also to develop the severe forms such as meningitis, miliary spread or progressive primary tuberculosis. Of the common childhood infections, measles is most clearly associated with this suppression of the immune response. Recently it has become clear that infection with the human immunodeficiency virus (HIV) may also be complicated by rapidly spreading tuberculous disease, as with other opportunistic infectious agents.[15, 16]

Age is also of great importance. The younger the child the greater the danger of progression and the greater the extent of glandular involvement. Frequent intense exposure results in more severe infection. Overcrowding leads to more frequent exposure, and poor ventilation to greater concentrations of bacilli. Children usually acquire tuberculosis from an infectious parent or other close relative.

There is considerable evidence that BCG vaccination gives some protection against the invasive and progressive stages of tuberculosis.

Secondary, 're-infection' or adult-type tuberculosis occurs either when dormant bacilli in the lung again become active or when a patient previously infected is again attacked by tubercle bacilli. By that time the patient has acquired allergy to the bacillus, as a result of which many cells collect at the site of the new infection in the lung, fluid is poured out, and necrosis follows; the patient has also acquired a measure of immunity, which enables the infection to be localized. The result is the formation of cavities, which erode into a local bronchus leading to the expectoration of large numbers of tubercle bacilli. Secondary disease thus does not disseminate through the lymph vessels or blood stream, but by local extension. This can result in bronchopleural fistula and empyema, or if dissemination occurs through the infected sputum, can result in tuberculous laryngitis and intestinal tuberculosis, where again localized walled-off cavities (ulcers) form because of the allergic state.

Tuberculin skin test

The cellular immune response is assessed by the tuberculin skin test. This is a delayed hypersensitivity reaction and skin reactivity indicates that infection with mycobacteria has occurred. Only the tubercle bacillus induces a strong skin reaction, but BCG and other mycobacteria induce lesser skin responses which cause confusion in interpretation.

Mantoux test

This is carried out by injecting 0.1 ml of diluted tuberculin intradermally, using a very small (27 gauge) needle. A suitable dose is 5 tuberculin units (TU) of purified protein derivative (Siebert) (PPD-S). In children it is particularly difficult to insert the needle accurately between the dermis and the epidermis, and care must be taken to see that a wheal appears in the skin as the fluid is injected. If the injection is too deep a false-negative result may be obtained. The test is positive if after 48–72 hours there is an area of induration (not only colour alteration) greater than 10 mm in diameter. Reactions of 6–9 mm diameter are generally regarded as equivocal. The best cut-off point has been determined for some geographical regions by testing groups of children to exclude, as far as possible, the small reactions which occur after infection with atypical mycobacteria.

Heaf test

This is easier to administer than the Mantoux test, but is less accurate. There are various designs of spring-loaded machine which release six points at a constant pressure through a layer of concentrated PPD (100 000 TU per ml) to a skin depth (for children) of 1 mm. The needles should be tested repeatedly for sharpness, and the spring should be in proper working order. The test is done by holding the base-plate firmly against the skin and pressing the trigger. If several tests are being done, the device is sterilized by passing the base-plate and needle points through a flame briefly. The result is read on the third to seventh day as:

- Negative: less induration than Grade I.
- Grade I: three or more indurated bosses at least 1 mm in diameter.
- Grade II: an indurated ring with three or more of the bosses joined together.
- Grade III: the centre of the ring is filled producing a single large boss.
- Grade IV: vesiculation.

Grades II, III and IV are equivalent to a Mantoux test result of about 8 mm diameter or more.

Other multiple puncture tests

Several commercial disposable multiple puncture kits are available. Though expensive, these are convenient when occasional tuberculin tests are required. In some, the antigen is dried on the prongs and in others it is liquid. One example is the Tine test, which consists of a disposable thimble with four sharp points, the tips of which are coated with dried PPD. The test is read after 3–7 days like the Heaf test, using the following criteria:

- Negative: less than 3 mm of induration at each of the four points
- Doubtful: each point shows 3–4 mm induration
- Positive: the induration has coalesced into a papule or blister.

The significance of the tuberculin skin test result is discussed later in the section on diagnosis.

Effect of previous BCG vaccination on the tuberculin test

BCG vaccination induces a delayed hypersensitivity response to tuberculin and consequently may lead to the incorrect diagnosis of natural tuberculous infection. This BCG effect is most dramatic three to six months after vaccination. There is then waning of the skin response and the delayed hypersensitivity response probably returns to its original state about two to three years later in older children and before 18 months in infants.[1].

A well-indurated grade 3 Heaf reaction, a Mantoux test of 15 mm or more or the presence of any vesiculation after any test should be regarded as due to tuberculous infection.

BCG vaccination used as a tuberculin test

A child who is already reactive to tuberculin owing to a natural tuberculous infection will respond to BCG vaccination with an accelerated reaction akin to the tuberculin test itself. This early reaction is characterized by induration, vesication and even ulceration coming on from a few hours to two to three days after vaccination. It is a reliable indicator of past exposure and should always be followed up.[10, 11]

Epidemiology

The epidemiology of tuberculosis is, in essence, extremely simple (Fig. 4.5.1). The disease is spread only by people suffering from tuberculosis of the lung itself – disease of the pleura and hilar glands is non-infectious. They are members of the infector pool from the time when the disease developing in them becomes 'open', i.e. infectious, to the time when they either die or come under treatment, plus any subsequent periods during which they are again infectious due to relapse. The average length of this infectious period in a patient can only be guessed at.

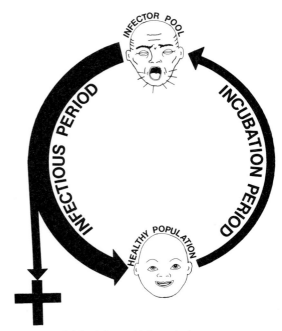

Fig. 4.5.1 Epidemiology of tuberculosis.

Infected individuals are more likely to become infectious themselves if their resistance is lowered by adverse environmental factors. These include malnutrition; poor, unfamiliar or stressful living conditions; and the presence of other diseases or immune deficiency states. Previous BCG vaccination may reduce the likelihood of becoming infectious.

Prevalence

The prevalence of infectious tuberculosis in the population depends on the annual number of new infectious patients (the incidence) multiplied by the number of years for which each is infectious. For instance, if there are 3000 new sputum-positive patients in a year, and the average period for which they are infectious is 18 months, then the total number of infectious patients at any one time is 4500.

There are considerable difficulties in ascertaining the incidence of tuberculosis in children. As most primary tuberculosis is mild, physicians vary widely in their judgement of what is or is not a case. The most useful pointer to the trend of incidence in the population as a whole is the annual number of sputum smear-positive patients recorded, which is more or less *pro rata* with the total number of all forms of the disease. Sputum smear-positive patients are easy to define, and the information can be recorded by non-medical staff. If, however, meaningful figures can be kept of childhood incidence, this index reflects much more closely the prevalence of tuberculosis in the whole population, since primary tuberculosis develops soon after infection and not after many years of incubation, and it is the prevalence trend that gives the most useful information. The incidence of tuberculous meningitis can also be used as a guide to prevalence trends.

Prevalence can be measured directly in three ways: sputum surveys, tuberculin surveys and mass radiography surveys.

Sputum surveys are made of carefully randomized selected samples of the population to discover the number of infectious cases. This is difficult and tedious to carry out, and generally can only be undertaken by a research organization with special skills in laboratory work and statistical methods. To show an upward or downward trend, the survey has to be repeated later in the same area.

Tuberculin surveys of school children provide a relatively simple method of estimating the risk of infection in a given area, which is directly related to the prevalence of infectious tuberculosis.[12] The annual infection rate is the percentage of children found positive in a particular group, such as school entrants, divided by the average age of that group. If such a group is tested at intervals of two or three years, an upward or downward trend may be demonstrated. Moreover, if a large number of children of different ages are tested in a single survey, an indication of the trend in prevalence can be obtained immediately by calculating the percentage tuberculin positive in each age group. If the prevalence in the community is decreasing, the positive reactor rate increases disproportionately with age. If it is increasing, the reverse is found. Figure 4.5.2 shows the rising curve found in 1982 in Transkei, Southern Africa, during the third of three sputum and tuberculin surveys which showed a 60 per cent fall in prevalence over the ten years 1972–82.[1] Of course, to collect information about an entire country, schools in all areas would have to be sampled in a tuberculin survey. In areas where BCG vaccination has been widely used, the interpretation of tuberculin testing is less precise owing to skin reactivity induced by BCG.

Such surveys are useful also to indicate the significance which can be attached to a tuberculin test when used clinically in an individual child. For instance, if the infection rate is 4 per cent per annum, then about 40 per cent of all children will have a natural infection by the age of 10; on the other hand, if the annual rate is only 0.5 per cent, 5 per cent of normal children can be

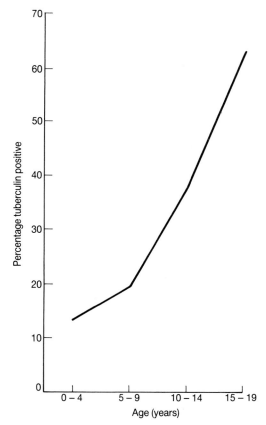

Fig. 4.5.2 Upwardly convex curve of tuberculin reactor rates at various ages, occurring in a South African population which showed a 60 per cent fall in prevalence of tuberculosis during 1972–82. (Reproduced from Fourie PB, *Tubercle*, 1983; **64**: 181–92. Churchill Livingstone, Edinburgh.)

expected to show a positive skin test at age 10, and a positive result to a skin test has a far greater significance.

Mass radiography surveys have not been shown to give an accurate assessment of prevalence unless supported by a referral clinic at which all suspects are properly investigated, including sputum smear examination.

Delay between prevalence and incidence trends

Whether secondary pulmonary tuberculosis (i.e. infectious disease) develops through reactivation of the original infection or from a second infection after healing of the first has long been a subject of controversy. Probably both mechanisms occur.

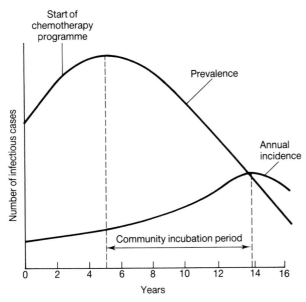

Fig. 4.5.3   Significance of the average interval between infection and infectiousness (incubation period) in assessing progress against tuberculosis.

The interval between initial infection and the time when the person becomes infectious is crucial in control programmes. If the average time between being infected and becoming infectious is long, say 15 years, then even if a tuberculosis programme has successfully reduced the prevalence of infectious cases, the number of new sputum-positive patients occurring can still increase for 15 years afterwards (Fig. 4.5.3). During this period the average age of patients diagnosed rises progressively. The annual number of notifications of new sputum-positive patients may be the only available guide to progress in a control programme. If so, all we can say is that, in the presence of a programme, the quality of which remains undiminished, when the annual number of notifications of infectious patients starts to drop, the prevalence is already falling and may have been doing so for some years. However, the incidence in children will fall at the same time as the prevalence, because primary disease develops very soon after infection.

There is unfortunately no guarantee that the fall in the prevalence rate caused by the introduction of an effective chemotherapy programme will necessarily be followed in due course by a reduction of the total number of infectious patients occurring annually. If the population is increasing rapidly and the average incubation period is long, it is quite conceivable that the number may actually rise progressively into the future.

Clinical features

Tuberculosis is unique among the infectious diseases in the wide spectrum of different clinical manifestations it produces and in the great variation in the time scale of symptomatology.[2] Severity may range from no departure from normal to acute and rampant disease. The diagnosis may be obvious and straightforward or extremely obscure. In some cases it can never be established with certainty as to whether tuberculosis was the sole cause of a respiratory illness or merely an additional component. The reason for this difficulty in diagnosis is that the 'gold standard' – identification of mycobacteria – is seldom possible in children as it is in adults. This is because discharge of bacteria to the exterior occurs relatively late in childhood tuberculosis and because sputum is less easily obtained from children. Diagnosis must therefore generally be established by considering a combination of the following:

- symptoms and signs;
- history of contact with an infectious case;
- presence of skin hypersensitivity to tuberculoprotein;
- radiological appearances.

The tuberculin test, if carried out correctly, will be positive in an infected child unless rendered anergic by severe malnutrition or a serious illness. Measles is the most important infection which induces this anergy – particularly in a child who is already malnourished. A severe tuberculous infection may also induce anergy to the tuberculin test. This is discussed further in the section on diagnosis.

Asymptomatic primary complex

The majority of newly infected children of all ages never display overt symptoms of disease. The tiny nidus of infection in the periphery of the lung and hilar lymph gland is walled off, and the mycobacteria are either killed off totally or lie dormant within the macrophages. Such a minuscule infection is not associated with any disturbance to the child nor is it obvious radiologically. The only indication of its presence is the development of skin reactivity to tuberculin six to eight weeks after entry of the organisms. However, even in these minor and undetected infections dissemination of a few organisms through the bloodstream may occur. They take root in the apices of the lungs or in more distant foci such as brain, bone or elsewhere.

Reference has already been made to the factors which determine progression and dissemination of disease. Age is of paramount importance. Children under five years of age are able to mount far less resistance to the organism and dissemination is especially common in this age group. Those under one year are most vulnerable. There is less risk of progressive primary disease in later childhood, but the adolescent years again represent a high-risk period, with greater chances of progression and breakdown into adult-type disease associated with the period of very rapid growth and with changes in life-style associated with starting work and leaving home.

Poor nutrition induced by dietary deficiencies certainly plays a key role in lowering resistance against spread of the bacilli. Parasitic infections, especially those of the intestinal tract, frequently add to the nutritional drain. Conversely, the added stress of a tuberculous infection may tip a child with borderline malnutrition into the dangerous decompensated state of marasmus or kwashiorkor.

Any infection which lowers general resistance during early primary tuberculosis may result in progression of the disease; measles and whooping cough are particularly dangerous.

Clinical manifestations of hypersensitivity to tuberculoprotein

Tissues far removed from the primary complex may sometimes show the only clinical expression of tuberculous infection.

Phlyctenular conjunctivitis

These distinctive ocular lesions consist of one or more tiny raised nodules on the junction between cornea and sclera, usually in the inner or outer quadrant (Fig. 4.5.4). The nodule is associated with a leash of injected blood vessels in the adjacent bulbar conjunctiva. The lesions cause considerable irritation and photophobia, persist for a week or two and then heal completely. Recurrent attacks are, however, not

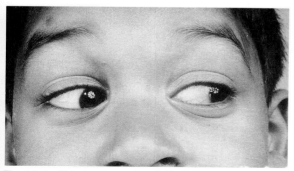

Fig. 4.5.4 Phlyctenular conjunctivitis, left eye.

infrequent. Occasionally the phlyctenule affects the cornea and scarring can result. While phlyctenular conjunctivitis is virtually pathognomonic of tuberculous infection, it may develop long after the primary complex has appeared. It is possible that a second antigenic stimulus in addition to that of the tubercular antigen is required to induce the appearance of lesions. As there is extreme hypersensitivity to tuberculin in these cases, a tuberculin test may aggravate the conjunctivitis, as well as producing a very severe skin reaction. It should only be carried out in high dilution (0.5 TU).

The use of hydrocortisone drops results in rapid improvement. Other ocular manifestations of tuberculosis are rare.

Erythema nodosum

This eruption consists of hot, red, slightly raised, tender areas of induration symmetrically situated over the lower legs, particularly along the shins. The lesions are ill-defined, and measure 1–4 cm in diameter. At the outset there may be some fever. Pain and swelling of the ankles is frequent and occasionally other joints are involved. In severe cases the nodules extend on to the thighs and even the upper limbs. After some days they become less angry, and dusky in colour, and later bruise-like due to the presence in the skin and subcutaneous tissue of extravasated blood (Fig. 4.5.5). In the most severe cases many small subcutaneous or even intramuscular nodules may be palpable in the lower limbs.

Erythema nodosum can be produced by a wide range of antigenic stimuli including fungal and bacterial infections, drugs (sulphonamides), sarcoidosis and autoimmune diseases. Tuberculosis and Group B haemolytic streptococcal infections are the most common inducers of this skin reaction in children. A tuberculin test should be done, using 0.5 TU.

The disorder usually settles after a week or two and can be eased by anti-inflammatory agents such as paracetamol or salicylates and by bed rest, with elevation of the lower limbs.

For the other cutaneous forms of tuberculosis the reader is referred to p. 856.

Poncet's arthritis

Acute arthritis of one or more large joints is occasionally seen associated with exquisite skin reactivity to tuberculin. Erythema nodosum is not present. In such cases pain and swelling may persist for several weeks, seldom for more than two months. The tuberculin test is strongly positive and may also show an early positive

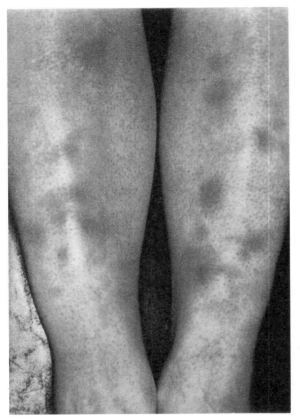

Fig. 4.5.5 Erythema nodosum over anterior aspect of lower legs.

response – at six to eight hours – suggesting the presence of circulating antibody (Arthus phenomenon). Other causes of arthritis require exclusion before the diagnosis can be made. This rare form of joint involvement due to tuberculosis must be clearly distinguished from a true infective tuberculous arthritis (see later). The arthritis responds well to salicylates and bed rest.

Investigation and treatment of hypersensitivity reactions

A chest X-ray should be done in all cases. If positive, appropriate treatment should be given. However, the X-ray is often clear. Although these reactions present a strong immune response to the organism, they indicate the presence of viable bacilli, and treatment should be given as described in the later section on management.

Tuberculosis of the pleura

The most common clinical manifestation is the sudden development of a pleural effusion (Fig. 4.5.6a, b). This usually occurs in the older child (over four or five years), when a subpleural focus, often a relatively small one, touches the pleura and induces a large accumulation of fluid as a hypersensitivity phenomenon. A few tubercles are scattered over the pleura, but they may be relatively scanty. The tuberculin test is strongly positive. The child presents with a sudden onset of dull chest pain or breathlessness associated with cough, but is otherwise relatively well. A small sample of fluid should be aspirated (see p. 1013). The fluid may be clear and 'straw coloured' or moderately blood-stained, and the protein content is usually over 30 g/l. A useful test is the adenosine deaminase assay (ADA), which shows levels well above 35 units per litre. If possible, fluid should also be examined microscopically for organisms and cultured to exclude pyogenic causes. Where facilities and expertise are available, a needle biopsy of the pleura can sometimes provide a rapid diagnosis. Aspiration of a large amount of fluid is unnecessary and indeed inadvisable unless the child's breathing is seriously embarrassed. A purulent fluid should, however, be drained. This will generally indicate the presence of a bronchopleural fistula.

More widespread tuberculous involvement of the pleura also occurs in children. The pleural space is obliterated by a thick layer of fibrocaseous tissue, with relatively little fluid, and generally widespread associated lung disease. This form of pleural involvement is indolent and may take months or years to resolve. Adhesion of the lung to the chest wall and marked restriction of thoracic cage movement on the affected side may be the end result. The addition of corticosteroids to the therapeutic regimen in the early phase appears to improve the outlook in these cases and to obviate the need for later surgical intervention.

Progression of the primary complex

The enlargement of the primary complex to visible proportions causes illness in the child; however, the symptoms and signs may be subtle and often go unrecognized. Mild intermittent fever and slight cough, both persisting for some weeks, are frequent, or the child may simply seem unwell and below par. Most important is flagging weight gain or actual loss of weight. When used correctly with regular clinic visits the Road-to-Health Card is often a valuable tool to demonstrate unsatisfactory progress in growth (Fig. 4.5.7). Tuberculosis should always be suspected

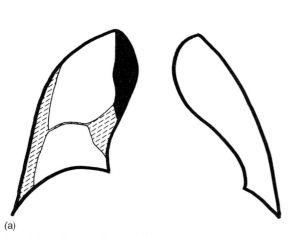

(a)

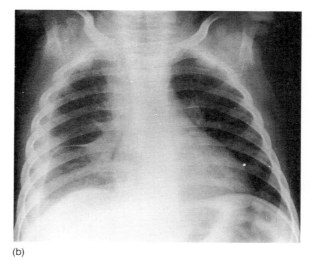

(b)

Fig. 4.5.6 Pleural effusion. (a) Diagrammatic representation. (b) Chest X-ray showing right-sided tuberculosis effusion.

in the infant and child presenting with malnutrition and particularly marasmus who fails to show catch-up on full calorie protein replacement. Chest X-ray will usually reveal either singly or in combination, an area of opacity in the lung together with a prominent hilum or broadened mediastinal shadow, but clinical examination of the chest commonly shows no positive findings at this stage. The right-middle and right-upper lobes are the most common sites to be affected, followed by the left-upper lobe and lingula and the lower lobes. The primary complex is multiple in 10–15 per cent of cases.

Tuberculous glands of considerable size may sometimes not be revealed on a routine X-ray if they are situated deep in the middle mediastinum around the bifurcation of the trachea.[3]

Disease of this order may still resolve spontaneously without the diagnosis being made or effective treatment instituted. Fibrous scarring and calcification will then appear in the lung and/or lymph nodes after about a year as a long-lasting record of the disease. There is, however, a grave risk of progression of disease and dissemination without treatment.

Syndromes associated with enlarged mediastinal nodes

The numerous lymph nodes which surround the structures at the root of the lungs are in direct continuity with a rich lymphatic system from the abdomen, limbs, head and neck. Once tuberculous infection has gained entry into the hilar nodes,

extension can occur not only to other lymph nodes in the chest, but also to those far distant from the primary infection, in the neck, axilla or abdomen.

As nodes enlarge and become adherent to each other, a large caseating mass develops in one or both hila or in the upper or lower mediastinum. The nodes are easily visible in the radiograph as rounded masses, with a well-defined convex outer edge. The pulmonary component is quite often insignificant or invisible (see Fig. 4.5.8a, b).

Such children show significant symptoms. They are ill and debilitated with high fever and clear loss of weight, but a cough and other respiratory symptoms may sometimes be surprisingly inconspicuous.

Tuberculous mediastinal glands may be confused with a normal thymic shadow. However, a lateral radiograph will clearly demonstrate the central situation of the glands around the hila, whereas thymic enlargement is visible in front of the heart in the anterior mediastinum (Fig. 4.5.8c). More rarely mediastinal tumours and lympadenopathy due to other causes require differentation. Sarcoidosis is extremely rare in the first decade of life. In this condition, the hilar glands are usually bilateral and are often accompanied by a symmetrical, fine-scattered infiltration radiating out from the glands in a 'butterfly distribution'. Other manifestations of the disease, such as uveitis, may be present. Lymphoma, Hodgkin's disease and leukaemia can also present difficulties with diagnosis. Gland biopsy and bone marrow examination may be required if there is reason to suspect a malignancy.

Stridor and wheeze Glands often become adherent to

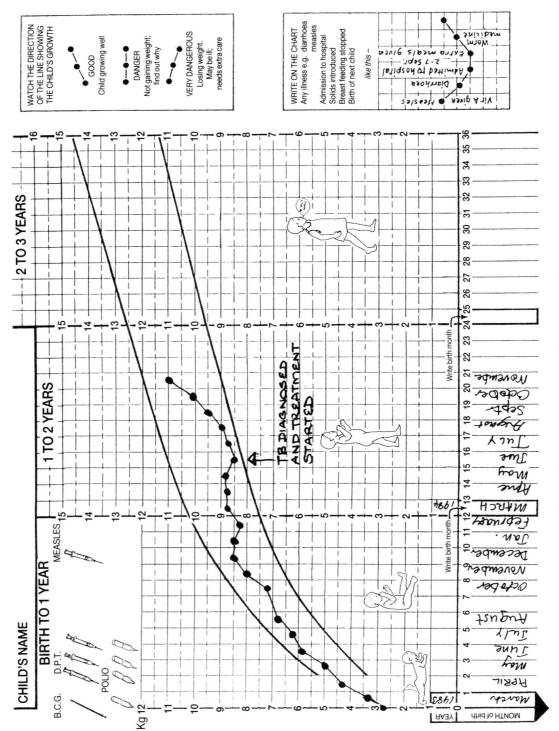

Fig. 4.5.7 Faltering in growth due to primary tuberculosis, as demonstrated on the Road-to-Health Card.

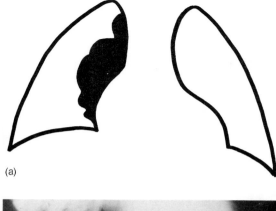

(a)

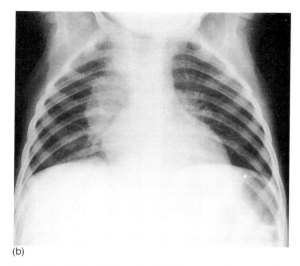

(b)

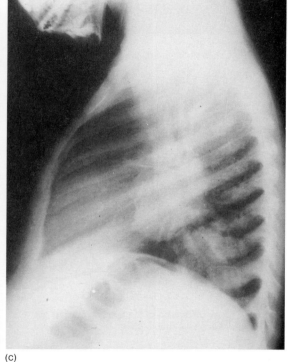

(c)

Fig. 4.5.8 Mediastinal nodes. (a) Diagrammatic representation. (b) Chest X-ray showing massive mediastinal glands without compression. (c) Chest X-ray showing large glands around the hilum in lateral projection.

children the lungs are hyperresonant to percussion due to persistent and generalized air-trapping.

The symptom complex of cough accompanied by stridor and/or wheezing is perhaps the most common manifestation of pulmonary tuberculosis in young children and its presence always justifies investigation for this disease. However, many other conditions can produce these symptoms and require exclusion. Other causes of prolonged stridor include laryngomalacia (benign laryngeal stridor) and foreign body in the larynx. Persistent wheezing is associated with a foreign body in the lower airways, and with asthma, bronchitis, recurrent aspiration, and larval pneumonitis caused by roundworms or other parasites.

Endobronchial disease

Inflammation from adherent tuberculous glands may spread further throughout the full thickness of the bronchial wall, resulting in granulations within the bronchial lumen itself. The clinical syndromes which can result from this process are outlined below.

Over-distended lung Partial obstruction of the bronchus results in air gaining entry to the lung on inspiration but total blockage on expiration – a 'ball valve' effect (Fig. 4.5.10). The segment, lobe or lung involved then shows progressive over-distension, and acute and severe respiratory distress results. Such children require admission to hospital for urgent diagnostic

the bronchi above and below the carina, or to the trachea, so that the bronchial tree itself is involved in the inflammatory process (Figs. 4.5.9a, b). Cough then becomes troublesome and persistent. Inspiratory stridor and brassy cough are a feature of enlarged paratracheal glands. Wheezing results from pressure of glands on bronchi. If only one bronchus is involved wheezing may be confined to one lung only, but generalized wheezing is more common. In such

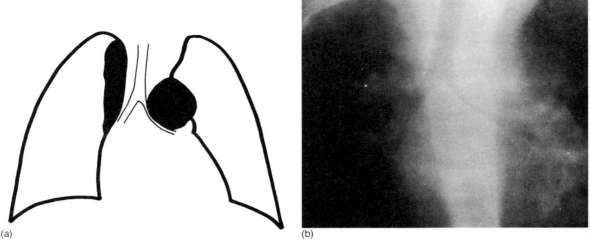

(a)   (b)

Fig. 4.5.9   Compression of the bronchus. (a) Diagrammatic representation. (b) 'High kV' film defining a compression of the left main bronchus.

evaluation and management. The acute distress can be relieved with oxygen and nebulized salbutamol, and oral corticosteroids are beneficial.

Segmental lesion   Complete obstruction of a bronchus results in total atelectasis of that portion of lung distal to the obstruction – usually the right middle or right lower lobe, or a segment thereof. Caseating material may enter the lung, resulting in spread of tuberculous disease. The collapsed areas may also become secondarily infected. In milder cases, re-expansion occurs after about four to six months following successful treatment, but in others segmental collapse is prolonged. Total resolution may eventually occur, but the end result is often a permanently damaged bronchiectatic lobe following years of recurrent secondary infections (see Figs. 4.5.11a, b, c, d).

Rarer manifestations   Tuberculous erosion through the full thickness of the bronchial wall or oesophagus can result in the passage of air, fluid or food into the pleural cavity. Pneumothorax and empyema and broncho-pleural or broncho-oesophageal fistulae are the end results of such advanced disease, and present complex management problems.

Entrapment of the phrenic nerve in caseating tissue can result in paralysis of the diaphragm. There is asymmetrical movement of the lower rib-cage on inspiration and varying degrees of respiratory stress may be produced, depending on the completeness of the paralysis. On chest X-ray there is marked elevation of one dome of the diaphragm on the affected side.

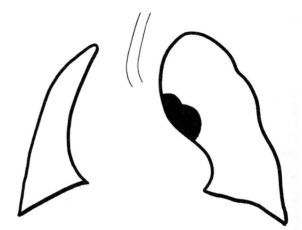

Fig. 4.5.10   Over-distension of the left lung caused by glandular compression of the left main bronchus – lobar emphysema.

Progression of the lung lesion

The tuberculous process spreads rapidly throughout a segment or entire lobe. The appearances may be difficult or impossible to distinguish from those of a simple pneumonia, particularly if hilar nodes are not visible radiologically. With the development of hypersensitivity there is acute swelling within the segment and this leads to bulging outwards of the fissure on which the segment abuts. An area of liquefaction

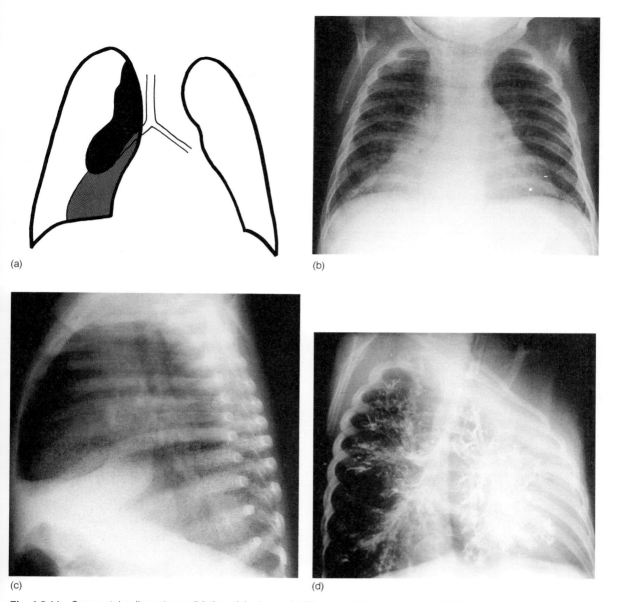

(a)

(b)

(c)

(d)

Fig. 4.5.11 Segmental collapse/consolidation of the lungs. (a) Diagrammatic representation; (b) Chest X-ray showing massive enlargement of mediastinal nodes with segmental collapse/consolidation of the right lower lobe; (c) Lateral chest X'ray showing segmental collapse of the right middle lobe in lateral projection; (d) Bronchogram showing bronchiectasis following primary tuberculosis (predominantly right lower lobe).

commonly develops in the consolidated lung and if this erodes into a bronchus, an air-containing cavity with a fluid level develops (Fig. 4.5.12a, b). Widespread dissemination throughout the lungs may occur if proper treatment is not commenced. The cavity may remain freely connected to a bronchus for some time, allowing infectious dissemination of organisms, as in secondary tuberculosis. Large thin-walled air-containing cysts may develop in the affected lung, probably because of entrapment of air with a 'pumping up' effect. Such cysts may be a long-standing feature at the site of a lung totally destroyed by tuberculous infection.

'Tuberculous pneumonia' in childhood often presents great diagnostic difficulties. Clinical signs may be indistinguishable from simple pneumonia, but on the other hand auscultation over the affected lung may reveal little. The illness should be treated with antibiotics on the basis of a straightforward pneumonia while at the same time instituting investigations for tuberculosis. A high white cell count with a predominance of polymorphonuclear leucocytes is suggestive of 'simple' pneumonia but may also be seen in tuberculosis, perhaps because of secondary infection. A repeat chest X-ray after two weeks is essential. If there has been failure to respond to antibiotics, this will be strong evidence for the diagnosis of tuberculosis.

In an unresolving pneumonia with or without visible adenopathy on X-ray *always consider tuberculosis*. High KV X-rays may help to show up the nodal compression of airways.

Tuberculous bronchopneumonia Massive extrusion of caseating material into the bronchial tree results in widespread dissemination throughout both lungs (Fig. 4.5.13a, b). The picture may ensue quite suddenly with a sudden worsening of fever, respiratory difficulty (widespread crackles on auscultation) and rapid deterioration.

Tuberculous pericarditis

Disease spreads to the pericardial sac either directly from adherent glands or lung or via the bloodstream. It is uncommon in the early years of life, but may be seen occasionally in older children. The disease may be manifest either by a pericardial effusion or with constriction of the pericardium. A combination of both processes is also seen. Cough and dyspnoea are the symptoms produced by both pericardial effusion and constriction. Sometimes evidence of heart involvement may be apparent only from the chest X-ray, showing a globular heart shadow. Signs suggestive of a pericardial effusion are a pulsus paradoxus of 12 mm of mercury or greater, the presence of increased cardiac dullness and a pericardial friction rub. Signs of venous obstruction may be seen, especially where constriction is present. In the latter case, jugular venous pressure will be markedly raised, the liver considerably enlarged with ascites, and probably peripheral oedema will be noted. Pulsus paradoxus is again evident and a distinctive pericardial knock early in diastole is a typical feature on auscultation.

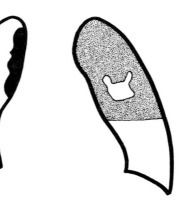

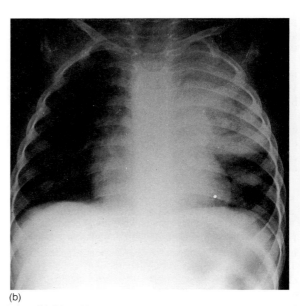

(a) (b)

Fig. 4.5.12 Tuberculous pneumonia. (a) Diagrammatic representation. (b) Chest X-ray showing tuberculous consolidation of the left upper lobe with cavity formation.

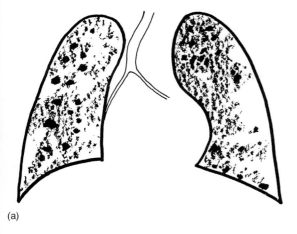

(a)

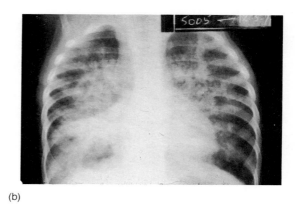

(b)

Fig. 4.5.13 Bronchopneumonic tuberculosis. (a) Diagrammatic representation. (b) Chest X-ray showing right middle lobe consolidation with bronchopneumonic spread.

Pericardial effusion is relatively easy to diagnose on chest X-ray, the heart showing a globular shape and sharp border. Fluoroscopy will show diminished movement. The radiological diagnosis of constriction is less easy. The distended superior vena cava may be evident adjacent to the upper mediastinum. The left cardiac border is usually straight and the size of the heart generally normal. A pleural effusion is often present. An ECG shows generalized low-voltage complexes in both forms, with T-wave inversion throughout.

Pericardiocentesis should be carried out to confirm the diagnosis of pericardial effusion (see p. 1014). Where available, ultrasound provides a simple and highly sensitive diagnostic method.

In tuberculous pericardial effusion, treatment with corticosteroids in association with antituberculous drugs may lessen the subsequent development of constriction.[13] Constriction requires surgical intervention when fully developed.

Glands elsewhere

In areas where tuberculosis is rife, tuberculous glands in the neck are a relatively common childhood problem. These usually originate from an infection within the chest – primary tuberculous infection in the oral cavity or tonsil is far rarer. There is gradual painless enlargement of one or more nodes in the anterior or posterior triangles. These merge and coalesce into masses which become adherent to skin. With time, the glands liquefy and one or more sinuses form, discharging caseous material through the skin. Sometimes glandular enlargement is rapid and massive, leading to the suspicion of malignancy (Fig. 4.5.14). If the diagnosis is in doubt, biopsy of a gland is advisable, to exclude leukaemia, lymphoma or non-tuberculous mycobacterial infection. Wherever possible material should be sent for both microscopy and culture. Glands in the axilla and groin may also be affected by tuberculosis (Fig. 4.5.15). This is usually seen only in children with widely disseminated disease.

Abdominal tuberculosis

In previous times, bovine tuberculosis was the most common cause for such disease, a primary infection developing in the bowel from ingestion of infected cow's milk. However, in most countries bovine tuberculosis has now become rare.

Spread of infection down the lymphatic system from the chest is the most common mode of infection of the abdominal cavity. From caseating glands infection spreads to the omentum and mesentery, and loops of bowel are enmeshed in the inflammatory process.

Children with abdominal tuberculosis usually present with chronic failure to thrive and weight loss. There is generally intermittent vague abdominal pain together with alternating diarrhoea and constipation and progressive distension of the abdomen. Obstruc-

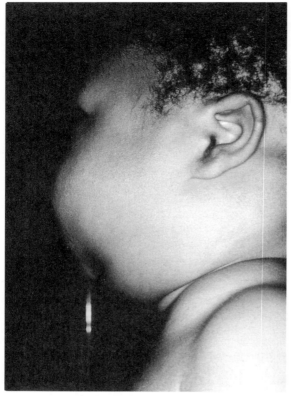

Fig. 4.5.14   Rapid enlargement of neck glands due to tuberculosis.

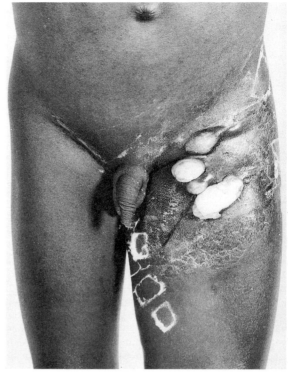

Fig. 4.5.15   Tuberculous glands in the axilla and groin.

tion of the lacteal (lymphatic) vessels of the bowel causes an exudative enteropathy, and this results in extremely low levels of serum albumin and peripheral or generalized oedema. On clinical examination, the abdomen has a characteristic 'doughy' feel, and enlarged nodes or large irregular firm masses may be palpable. The liver is frequently enlarged also, and the spleen may be palpable. Generalized ascites or encysted collections of fluid occur. The disease is generally indolent and of long standing, and calcified glands may be evident on chest or abdominal X-ray.

High levels of protein in aspirated fluid (above 45 g/l) are strongly suggestive of tuberculous peritonitis. A further helpful finding is an ascitic fluid/blood glucose ratio below 0.96. Mycobacteria may also be identified on direct smear or culture. When available, ultrasound examination of the abdomen is of great assistance in demonstrating deep-seated enlarged glands.

Tuberculosis of the small and large bowels are uncommon in childhood and take the same forms as in adults.

Blood dissemination

At a very early stage in the development of the primary complex, before cellular immunity has become established, mycobacteria readily gain access to the bloodstream. Isolated organisms may take root anywhere in the body, the most common sites being the apices of the lungs, liver, spleen, brain, bones and kidneys. A small tuberculous focus established in one of these areas may only manifest many years later.

Miliary tuberculosis   Massive spread of infection into the bloodstream is most common in young infants, when resistance to infection is very much impaired, but can occur at any age. The onset may be abrupt with high fever and severe illness, or insidious with surprisingly little general disturbance. In most cases, chest X-ray appearances show evidence of a primary complex as well, but the highly characteristic miliary picture in the

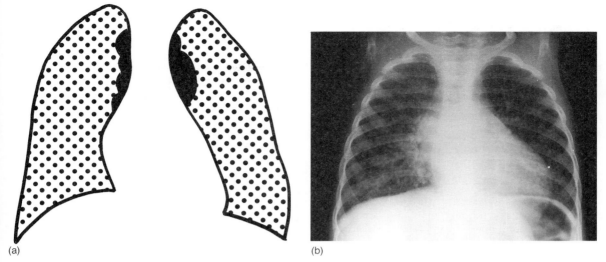

Fig. 4.5.16   Miliary tuberculosis. (a) Diagrammatic representation. (b) Chest X-ray showing miliary changes.

lungs is virtually pathognomonic. Fine nodules of uniform size are seen throughout the lung field, measuring a millimetre or two in diameter. (Fig. 4.5.16a, b) Despite the dramatic radiological appearances there is generally no evidence on auscultation of this widespread infection. Fever and obvious illness may precede the appearance of miliary foci by several days. Such infants almost always show evidence of weight loss, enlargement of liver and spleen or generalized lymphadenopathy. Careful ophthalmoscopic examination of the retina may reveal choroid tubercles – round white to yellow cotton wool-like lesions situated near the retinal vessels.

If allowed to reach an advanced stage, nodules in the lung become far larger and even confluent, cavities form and tubercle bacilli may be isolated from the sputum or gastric washings (Fig. 4.5.17).

In miliary spread, the nodules are usually widely distributed throughout the body. If there has been erosion of a pulmonary artery instead of a vein, however, they may be confined to the lungs, so that liver and splenic enlargement are not noted.

Diagnosis   Virtually no other condition looks like miliary tuberculosis on chest X-ray and the diagnosis can usually be made with confidence. Disseminated malignancies, such as neuroblastoma, multiple septic emboli, tropical eosinophilia (see p. 721), and fungal infection can occasionally cause confusion. Chlamydial pneumonitis in young infants sometimes produces a fine miliary nodulation, but such infants are relatively well and there will be no other evidence of tuberculosis.

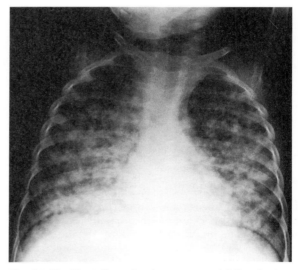

Fig. 4.5.17   Chest X-ray showing coarse nodulation due to miliary tuberculosis, untreated for two months.

Evidence of dissemination into other organs will be found, if sought, but this is seldom necessary. The simplest is examination of the retina. Lumbar puncture may show an increase in white cells – early evidence of meningeal involvement. Bone marrow and needle biopsy of the liver may be resorted to in cases of doubt.

A history of close contact with an infectious case is

more usual in children with miliary tuberculosis than in those with less severe forms of the disease.

The tuberculin test is often negative because of anergy due to the overwhelming infection. However, a repeat test after a month of drug treatment will generally be positive.

'Cryptogenic' haematogenous infection In blood-borne tuberculosis, high continuing fever and marked malaise may very occasionally be seen without any definite radiological or other features to assist in diagnosis. Full investigations for other infections such as malaria, typhoid and hidden sepsis will generally have been undertaken and various antibiotics given without success; the lack of response will raise suspicion of tuberculosis. The syndrome may also account for persistent fever and non-recovery after measles as well as for failure of the marasmic child to respond to adequate diet (the so-called 'stuck marasmus'). Such children pose great diagnostic problems. Slight enlargement of the liver and spleen may be the only positive findings other than fever. The tuberculin test is usually negative. If available, needle biopsy of liver and bone marrow aspiration may provide a rapid diagnosis with the demonstration of typical granulomas on microscopy. Material should also be sent for culture, but treatment cannot await the result and is usually started empirically. A dramatic improvement within 48–96 hours of starting treatment is a sensitive diagnostic test, and in the absence of such improvement the diagnosis is unlikely.

Extrathoracic tuberculosis

Tuberculous meningitis

Tuberculosis of the nervous system is the most common cause of death and long-term disability in childhood infection. The most common form is tuberculous meningitis (TBM), and young children are mostly affected. Single or multiple tuberculomata of the brain may occur in older age groups, but are rare in young children. Very rarely, tuberculosis may involve the brain by direct extension from the spine, skull bones, middle ear or mastoid.

TBM is of particular importance not only because of its catastrophic consequences but also by virtue of its value as a measure of the overall prevalence of TB in the community, and of the effectiveness of control measures. Unlike primary TB in general, children with TBM are readily identified and can be counted.

Tubercle bacilli may be seeded anywhere in the nervous system. The most common sites are the superficial brain substance of the cerebral and cerebellar hemispheres and ventricular system. When the small focus of caseation involves the overlying meninges, infection enters the subarachnoid space. The ensuing inflammatory response is most extensive at the base of the brain, where a steadily thickening grey-white exudate entraps cranial nerves, obstructs blood vessels, and blocks the foramina of the fourth ventricle. The intracranial pressure may also be raised by cerebral oedema of varying degree. The clinical manifestations of TBM therefore result from one or more of the following:

- meningeal irritation;
- obstructive hydrocephalus;
- cerebral oedema;
- cranial nerve damage;
- ischaemic infarction of any part of the brain.

The focus may never reach the meninges; instead, it becomes encapsulated and gradually expands, forming a tuberculoma. This may remain clinically silent indefinitely, or show the symptoms and signs of a slowly growing space-occupying lesion.

Clinical features While TBM can occur at any age, it is essentially a disease of young children. Of a large group of cases under 15 years of age, 50 per cent were under two years and 80 per cent under five years of age.[4] Most of these children probably develop the disease within 6–12 months of first infection. The onset is usually insidious. Over the space of a week to 10 days the child becomes apathetic or excessively irritable, with some pyrexia. The symptoms may be intermittent at first, but there is gradual worsening, with poor appetite, decreasing interest in play, sporadic vomiting, and, if old enough to complain, diffuse headache. Frequently there is some abdominal pain and change of bowel habit. These non-specific early symptoms are often referred to as Stage 1 of the disease. After a week or so, meningeal irritation is usually obvious. The child is incapable of play and prefers to lie curled up away from bright light. There is neck stiffness, and positive Kernig and Brudzinski signs (Stage 2). As the disease progresses there is increasing stupor. Focal signs such as squint, facial weakness or blindness appear and limb tremors or choreoathetoid movements may be evident (Stage 3). Deep reflexes tend to be exaggerated and pupillary responses sluggish. Careful scrutiny of the optic fundi may show small, yellowish or white, rounded woolly lesions along the retinal vessels – choroidal tubercles – which, when present are diagnostic of TBM. Papilloedema is seldom present. In Stage 4 of the disease the child is completely comatose and unresponsive, with signs of long-tract damage in the form of hemi- or quadriplegia. Terminally, the child is opisthotonic or decerebrate, and without treatment, death is inevitable.

Sometimes the whole course may be much more acute. Meningeal symptoms come on rapidly, closely mimicking viral or bacterial meningitis, or the illness may even take the course of an acute encephalopathic illness, with prolonged convulsions and/or coma.

Investigations-Lumbar puncture (see pp. 981, 1011) The opening pressure is raised, unless a complete block is present. The fluid is clear or faintly opalescent and may show a fine, spiderweb-like clot on standing. It shows pleocytosis, with, characteristically, 50 to 500 white cells per mm³, a mixture of lymphocytes and poly-morphs, the former usually predominating. Protein is raised above 0.8 g/l and Pandy's test for globulin is positive. If inflammatory exudate has blocked off completely the cerebrospinal fluid or CSF outflow at the foramen magnum, protein will be raised to very high levels, and the fluid will be yellow or orange in colour and scanty in quality. CSF glucose is fairly consistently low in TBM, usually less than a third of the blood glucose level (below 2.2 mmol/l). The chloride level in the CSF tends to be low also, but this is less constant. Careful scrutiny of the centrifuged stained deposit may reveal mycobacteria, especially if a large sample (5–10 ml) is obtained specifically for this purpose. Eventual culture of the organism confirms the diagnosis.

Adenosine deaminase assay (ADA). CSF levels of this enzyme are generally elevated, levels above 5 units/l being usual.

Bromide partition test. This test utilizes labelled bromide to demonstrate an increased permeability of the blood–brain barrier to bromide in TBM. When positive, the ratio of blood to CSF bromide is reduced below 1.6.

Tests for tubercular antigens. Various attempts have been made to develop tests for the detection of tuber-cular antigen in the CSF, using latex particle, ELISA and other techniques.[5] So far these methods lack the specificity required for practical use in diagnosis.[18]

Diagnosis Diagnosis at the earliest possible stage of the disease is of crucial importance, to ensure the best chances of recovery with the minimum of disability. A few hours without treatment may sometimes represent the difference between full recovery and permanent impairment. Yet diagnosis often poses great difficulties.

This is particularly so in the early phase of the illness when, in the absence of clear signs of meningeal irritation, the need for lumbar puncture is not appreciated. As in all forms of tuberculosis, suspicion of the disease is half-way to diagnosis. It is hardly necessary to emphasize that the CSF should be examined in any child displaying such symptoms with a history of primary tuberculosis or exposure to an infectious case.

Once pleocytosis in the CSF has been demonstrated TBM needs to be differentiated from the following:

- viral meningitis;
- bacterial meningitis (particularly if partially treated);
- other rarer forms of meningitis (fungal, protozoal);
- 'neighbourhood syndromes' – such as tumours, parasitic cysts, abscesses.

Demonstration of mycobacteria in the CSF on direct examination, and/or finding choroid tubercles in the retina are rapid confirmatory tests, but the high rate of positives on these tests in cases of TBM described in the large British studies have not been confirmed in our own, or in other Third World experience. In one study, AFBs were visible in only five of 62 (8 per cent) cases of TBM. Nevertheless, whenever possible a large specimen of CSF (5–10 ml) should be designated specially for this purpose.

Several recent studies have evaluated additional diagnostic aids in TBM.[5] CSF lactate, lactic dehydro-genase and C-reactive protein were of no value in differentiating TBM from the other forms mentioned. Adenosine deaminase levels in CSF clearly different-iated TBM from viral meningitis but not from bacterial causes, and the raised levels in the CSF appeared to correlate simply with those of protein. The various immunological tests for detecting antigen – immuno-radiometric, enzyme-linked immunosorbent assay – lack the necessary specificity. The investigation with the highest degree of both sensitivity and specificity is the bromide partition test, but this would only be available in well-equipped centres.

Radiological evidence of primary infection in the chest, or a positive tuberculin test, provide only indirect confirmation of the diagnosis in a suspected case of TBM but are often the only supporting evidence available. Both are, unfortunately, often negative. In our own experience only 65 per cent of cases showed a positive skin reaction and only 45 per cent positive radiological changes. We have found the following scheme useful in establishing diagnosis in a suspected case; at least three of the findings are required.

- A clinical course consistent with TBM.
- CSF pleocytosis and protein greater than 0.8 g/l.
- CSF microscopy positive *or* adenosine deaminase greater than 5 units/l *or* bromide partition test less than 1.6.
- Radiological changes suggestive of TB *or* sputum or gastric washings positive on direct examination *or* tuberculin test positive.

If in doubt it is far safer to begin treatment at once and at the same time cover with antibiotics for acute bacterial meningitis, rather than refer the child for further investigation elsewhere. The diagnosis can then be reviewed two weeks later after repeating the lumbar puncture. The tuberculin test, if negative at first, will become positive when the child's general condition improves.

In those children presenting acutely with coma or convulsions, other causes of encephalopathy will require exclusion.

Other diagnostic procedures. When available, computerized axial tomography (a CAT scan) provides invaluable information regarding the degree of ventricular dilatation present, and enhancement at the base of the brain strongly suggests the diagnosis of TBM. Sometimes tuberculomata can be visualized in

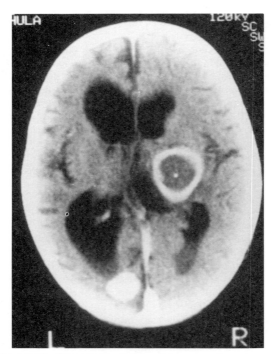

Fig. 4.5.18   CT scan showing two tuberculomata and gross hydrocephalus in a case of tuberculous meningitis.

association with tuberculous meningitis (Fig. 4.5.18). In young children in whom the anterior fontanelle is still patent, ultrasound can also be used to demonstrate ventricular obstruction.

Management   Drug treatment follows the general lines described below. Accepted practice has been to continue treatment for at least 12 months; this period may be excessive, but no controlled study of this aspect has been done. Drugs which cross the blood–brain barrier best are isoniazid, rifampicin, ethionamide and pyrazinamide. The use of intrathecal streptomycin has largely been abandoned in children, perhaps prematurely. There have been no satisfactory trials to establish efficacy of the various regimens used in TBM.[19]

Corticosteroids are considered to reduce the inflammatory response and lower intracranial pressure due to cerebral oedema. Prednisolone (2 mg/kg) is given orally for four to six weeks and then tailed off over a two-week period.

Where pressure is raised as a result of hydrocephalus, it can be reduced by the administration of acetazolamide and furosemide, or by repeated lumbar punctures. When available, early resort to shunting procedures (ventriculoperitoneal or thecoperitoneal) undoubtedly improves the outlook.

Prognosis   The outcome in earlier studies from Europe and the USA was more favourable than more recent reports from the Third World. Not surprisingly, the best results are obtained in children presenting early before neurological deficits are evident. In our own experience a quarter of the cases die within a year of diagnosis and about a half show major or minor degrees of disability.[4, 20]

Tuberculosis of the upper respiratory tract

Tuberculous ulceration of the larynx is a feature of advanced adult-type disease and is rare in childhood. In contrast, tuberculosis of the middle ear and mastoid is not uncommon. It is not known whether infection reaches the middle ear via the bloodstream or from the eustachian tube; probably both occur. The usual scenario is that of a child with extensive pulmonary disease who also shows a chronic aural discharge on one side. The tympanic membrane will be perforated with exuberant pale granulations and often exposed bone. Paralysis of the facial nerve is often an added complication. Extensive bone destruction may be evident on X-ray. The finding of acid-fast bacilli in an ear swab does not in itself constitute a diagnosis, as concomitant organisms may stain in this way and cause confusion. Atypical mycobacteria such as *M. kansasi* and *M. chelonei* can also cause disease. Diagnosis rests on histology and culture.

Tuberculous disease of the middle ear usually responds quickly to chemotherapy alone.

Tuberculosis of the spine

Tuberculosis of the spine is still a relatively common problem to orthopaedic surgeons working in developing countries. The disorder was first described by Potts in 1779. He noted that symptoms referable to the spine usually preceded the development of deformity. All health professionals need to be on the alert for early signs of this disfiguring and potentially devastating form of the disease. It may occur at any age, but tends to be most common in the elderly and in children, in whom it may be seen even in the first year of life.

Pathogenesis Spread to the spine is usually via the bloodstream. The disease starts in the vertebral body, usually in the area supplied by the posterior spinal artery. By far the most common site is the mid-dorsal region, but any vertebrae may be involved. Commonly, multiple sites are involved. There is progressive destruction of bone, and vertebral end-plate collapse allows the intervertebral disc to herniate into the body of the vertebra with apparent loss of the disc space on X-ray. Later, spread to the disc itself occurs and there is collapse of adjacent vertebrae. The normal curvature of the thoracic spine aggravates the tendency to forward angulation, with the formation of a gibbus. At the same time caseation and abscess formation results in pus tracking in various directions along soft tissue planes. In the thoracic region there is tracking along the ribs with pointing of the abscess anywhere on the chest wall. In the lumbar region pus tends to track down the psoas sheath and point in the lumbar region or groin. The vertebral arches are usually spared, but the spinal cord may be compressed by granulations and caseating tissue, resulting in paraplegia.

Clinical features Pain and stiffness in the back together with withdrawal from activity are early symptoms. In addition there may be loss of weight and appetite, crying at night, low-grade fever and easy fatigue. Most children already have a gibbus (kyphosis) at the time of diagnosis.

Early radiological signs are loss of bone substance and narrowing of the intervertebral disc space. Later, angulation and destruction of bone are clearly evident (Fig. 4.5.19). When a soft tissue mass adjacent to the

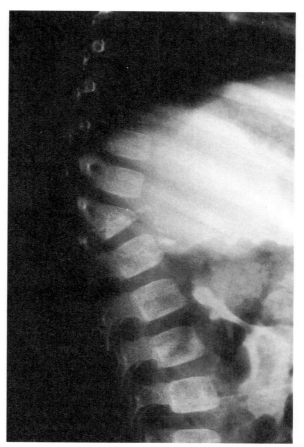

Fig. 4.5.19 Tuberculosis of the spine: lateral approach showing collapse of the 12th thoracic vertebra.

involved area can be seen, a diagnosis of tuberculosis is almost certain.

Diagnosis is straightforward in the common case where a gibbus accompanies active lung disease. In early cases, direct surgical biopsy may be required for confirmation.

Paraplegia This most commonly occurs with mid-thoracic lesions where the spinal cord is most easily compressed by the soft tissue mass. Paralysis can occur with relatively small lesions. Sustained clonus is often the earliest sign of spinal cord involvement. It may be accompanied by muscle weakness, spasticity, a positive Babinski sign and sensory changes. In lower lesions paralysis may be confined to the bladder and/or the lower bowel.

Treatment Wherever possible the child should be admitted to hospital for full evaluation and to ensure proper treatment until progress in the direction of healing has been obtained. Chemotherapy comprises the standard regimens described below. A high-protein, well-balanced diet with adequate vitamins is essential to prevent osteoporosis, which could aggravate vertebral collapse. The results from simple ambulant therapy alone are very good. The value of prolonged bed rest, immobilization of the spine by applying plaster of Paris jackets, radical resection of the lesion with bone graft, and simple debridement have been studied in a series of multicentre trials by the British Medical Research Council, but no clear-cut advantage from these procedures has emerged.

Complications Abscesses may require draining if there is a danger of chronic sinus formation.

For paraplegia, conservative treatment alone results in improvement in many cases, but if progress is unsatisfactory after six to eight weeks the child should be referred to a surgeon for decompression.

Tuberculosis of other bones and joints

Tuberculosis of other bones is encountered occasionally in childhood. The bones of the phalanges are the most common sites – tuberculous dactylitis. The clinical picture is one of tense, relatively painless fusiform swelling of one or more fingers. Circumscribed tuberculous foci may also develop in the ribs, skull and long bones (Fig. 4.5.20). The child presents with a mass localized to one (or more) of these areas. There is expansion of the bone involved and an overlying soft tissue mass, which may be fluctuant. Such lesions often

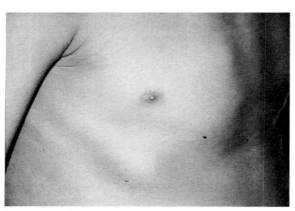

Fig. 4.5.20   Chest wall swelling due to tuberculous osteitis of a rib.

pose diagnostic dilemmas which can only be resolved by needle or open biopsy.

Tuberculosis of peripheral joints is even rarer in childhood. Most commonly involved are the weight-bearing joints of the lower extremities, particularly the knee or hip. A vague history of trauma to a joint with soft tissue swelling that does not resolve rapidly should raise suspicion of tuberculosis. The disease may closely mimic the pauciarticular form of juvenile chronic arthritis; however tuberculosis is usually mono-articular, while in juvenile chronic arthritis more than one joint is involved.

In both bone and joint tuberculosis loss of bone substance together with soft tissue swelling are seen on X-ray. Where a joint is involved, narrowing of the joint space will be seen. Synovial biopsy is generally required to establish the diagnosis of tuberculous arthritis.

The hypersensitive type of arthritis (Poncet's disease) was described earlier in this chapter (see p. 525).

Tuberculosis infection of the skin in children is dealt with on p. 856.

Genito-urinary tuberculosis

Renal disease Bacilli are probably seeded to the cortico-medullary region of the kidney fairly frequently, but this seldom leads to clinically apparent disease. At a large children's hospital dealing with hundreds of cases of tuberculosis every year, only 12 renal cases were recognized in 19 years. With established disease a cavity develops, usually in the central part of the kidney, involving the papilla. Disease spreads downwards to affect the ureter and bladder. In the late stages, the entire kidney and ureter are reduced to a functionless sac.

Painless haematuria may first draw attention to the renal lesion. Other children have shown varying degrees of loin pain or dysuria. The presence of 'sterile' pyuria should suggest tuberculous pyelonephritis or bladder involvement.

An intravenous pyelogram will show deformity of the collecting system suggestive of ulcerocavernous disease or complete non-function on one side. Calcification may be visible within the kidney. Where available, ultrasound is extremely helpful in demonstrating renal and bladder pathology. Culture of mycobacteria from the urine will establish the diagnosis.

Treatment Chemotherapy and general measures follow the usual lines. Surgical removal of the kidney is required in advanced disease.

Involvement of the testes and associated epididymis

in males and ovary and tubes in females are extremely rare in childhood.

Tuberculosis and HIV infection

HIV infection in children is most commonly caused by vertical transmission from an infected mother. Childhood cases have recently increased dramatically in number in many countries. Respiratory involvement occurs in a high proportion of children in the symptomatic phase of HIV infection, and various opportunistic infectious agents may be responsible.[15] An association between HIV infection and TB has been documented in several studies and is especially striking in communities with a high prevalence of both infections.[16] It is clear that HIV infection is playing an important role in the re-emergence of tuberculosis in communities where it was previously uncommon.

In HIV victims, both adults and children, TB infection is often clinically atypical. Infiltrates may be seen in any lung zone, often with mediastinal and/or hilar lymphadenopathy. In addition to pulmonary lesions there may be extrapulmonary disease in 40–75 per cent of cases.[17]

The diagnosis of TB may thus be difficult to establish in known HIV cases because of the atypical features. Other opportunistic infections may be present concomitantly. Only culture can distinguish TB from non-tuberculous mycobacterial infections. Thus, a high level of suspicion of mycobacterial infection must always be maintained.

Equally, HIV should be suspected, and if necessary tested for, in any child with TB who fails to show the expected improvement after a month or two of anti-tuberculous therapy. Children with symptomatic HIV infection usually show severe failure to thrive, and recurrent or chronic diarrhoea is a common finding.

Diagnosis

History and clinical evidence

A great responsibility rests with the provider of primary health care – usually a clinic or out-patient nurse. It is at this point of first contact that the disease may be recognized and investigated further. Suspicion of tuberculosis is half way to diagnosis. Health professionals must be sensitized to the suggestive symptoms – loss of weight (Fig. 4.5.7) and lassitude or cough, wheeze or stridor which have lasted for more than two to three weeks, or failure to rehabilitate or catch up in severe malnutrition.[14]

A history of contact with an infectious case should be sought in all patients. Of particular significance are close contacts, affected parents or affected individuals who sleep in the same room as the child.

Tuberculin test

The tuberculin test is an essential part of the diagnosis of childhood tuberculosis. The test is highly reliable if properly performed with active tuberculin and properly maintained equipment. Anergy, resulting in a negative test, occurs from certain well-defined causes, namely very severe infection with *M. tuberculosis*, serious malnutrition, severe viral infections or any condition that suppresses the immune system. As stated earlier, measles is the most important infection inducing this anergy, which may persist for up to two months after the infection. Similar, though less prolonged, suppression occurs following measles vaccination. Other infections which cause temporary suppression of the tuberculin reaction include rubella, scarlet fever, pertussis, infectious mononucleosis, influenza and malaria. Infection with human immunodeficiency virus (AIDS) will also need consideration in view of its rapid international dissemination. If treatment for tuberculosis is started on the assumption that anergy is present, the test must repeated after a month or two months following measles, when all these factors will have been corrected, to confirm the diagnosis. Previous BCG vaccination may render the tuberculin test positive. A positive reaction indicates that infection with the tubercle bacillus has occurred. It does not necessarily mean that active disease is present.

Radiology

The presence of nodal enlargement or miliary changes will make diagnosis likely or near certain. However, equivocal changes will justify the administration of an antibiotic for 7–10 days, with a repeat X-ray after this period. Resolution of the changes and improvement of symptoms will then exclude tuberculosis, while their persistence makes the diagnosis more likely.

One is often hampered by the difficulty of obtaining good radiographs of children in rural conditions. In these circumstances it may be difficult to decide whether the hila are abnormally large or not; where possible, a lateral film is helpful. It is important to be guided by the tuberculin test result. Where the quality of radiography is good, a high-kV exposure may be taken to show an 'air bronchogram', in which the bronchi are seen to be compressed by enlarged hilar glands[6] (Fig. 4.5.9b).

Microbiological tests

Wherever possible, three early morning sputum specimens (or in small children gastric washings) should be obtained (see p. 1016). In addition to immediate microscopic examination, the material may be cultured. The presence of atypical mycobacteria or other organisms in the gastric secretions results in an unacceptably high false-positive rate in direct examinations of gastric washings, and positive tests must always be confirmed by culture. As stated earlier, a positive yield from culture is low in children – less than 10 per cent.

The production of bronchial mucus can be enhanced by the prior administration of nebulized hypertonic saline (3 per cent).

Histology

Biopsy of the liver, bone marrow, pleura or superficial lymph node (see p. 1014) may assist in diagnosis in exceptional cases. Material must be sent for both histology and culture.

Haematology

The white cell and differential counts are seldom helpful in diagnosis. The erythrocyte sedimentation rate (ESR) is generally elevated, but this investigation is of little value in diagnosis or assessment of progress. Many children have a raised ESR for a variety of reasons, including infections and anaemia; in particular patients with any chest infection may show a raised ESR. As guides to progress, the child's symptoms, weight and chest X-ray give more reliable information.

Chemical tests

If possible liver function tests should be obtained as a baseline before starting therapy. In this way the occasional hepatotoxic effects of drugs may be distinguished from prior liver disease.

Management

Antituberculosis drugs

The discovery in 1948 of the first effective antituberculosis drug, streptomycin, was the beginning of a whole new era in chemotherapy, and it was only slowly and painfully that the medical profession came to understand the new rules that applied to drugs used against tuberculosis.

Apart from streptomycin, the first big discoveries were of *para*-amino salicylic acid (PAS) in 1950 and isoniazid in 1952. It must be emphasized that these three together still make a highly effective combination of drugs for patients whose organisms are sensitive to them. Isoniazid is as good a killer as rifampicin, and streptomycin is better than ethambutol. The main role of PAS was to prevent the emergence of resistance to isoniazid. Later, thiacetazone took the place of PAS in African countries, where trials showed that it was as effective and no more toxic; it was also cheaper and much more convenient to take. In some other areas, however, an unacceptably high toxicity rate has been reported and it is not used.

The regimen of streptomycin with isoniazid and thiacetazone or PAS lost some of its effectiveness as isoniazid-resistance became more widespread. Recent surveys of isoniazid resistance in untreated patients have shown figures of 22 per cent in Madras, 30 per cent in Pakistan, 6 to 8 per cent in East and Central Africa, 13 to 20 per cent in southern Africa, 2 to 5 per cent in southern and eastern South America, 11 per cent in Venezuela and 30 per cent in Bolivia. During the 1960s, pyrazinamide, rifampicin and ethambutol were introduced and it became possible to cure patients with isoniazid-resistant bacilli; rifampicin, however, remained very expensive until 1984, when the price was approximately halved. Recently short-course regimens which include rifampicin have been devised for the first-time treatment of pulmonary and other established tuberculosis. These are discussed further below.

Mode of action

There are bactericidal or killing drugs, and bacteriostatic or paralysing drugs. The function of the latter is largely in support of the former, particularly in preventing the emergence of resistance to them.

The bactericidal drugs are isoniazid, rifampicin, pyrazinamide and streptomycin. Isoniazid and rifampicin are the two most powerful killers and to be effective, any regimen must include one or both of them. Pyrazinamide is most effective inside the macrophage cells where the environment is more acid, while the other drugs act mainly outside the cells. Pyrazinamide has its greatest effect in the early stages of treatment. Short-course chemotherapy (discussed below) kills off almost all the bacilli in the first two months by a combined attack with the four bactericidal drugs working simultaneously within and outside the cells. Rifampicin and pyrazinamide have, in addition, a sterilizing effect on the few semi-dormant bacilli remaining after the initial bactericidal onslaught. The usefulness of pyrazinamide is mainly limited to the early months of treatment, but if rifampicin can be continued throughout the 6 months its sterilizing effect reduces the relapse rate.

The bacteriostatic drugs ethambutol, ethionamide and thiacetazone form effective combinations with the bactericidal drugs but are much less useful when combined only with each other. Isoniazid, pyrazinamide and ethionamide penetrate the meninges well, rifampicin and ethambutol to a lesser extent, and streptomycin only during early, severe inflammation.

The conventions used for indicating drug regimens are:

S = Streptomycin   H = Isoniazid
R = Rifampicin   T = Thiacetazone
Z = Pyrazinamide   El = Ethambutol
Ee = Ethionamide

The figure before the letters represents the number of months for which the regimen is given. An oblique divides the regimen into two stages; if the second stage excludes rifampicin it is given as out-patient. Brackets indicate regimens for use in areas where thiacetazone is not tolerated.

Principles of drug treatment

In cases of pulmonary, progressive primary and established organ tuberculosis, rigid rules must be followed to prevent the emergence of drug resistance:

- Drugs must never be given singly.
- Treatment must be continuous, and long enough to kill off the bacilli; this period varies from 6 to 18 months, depending on the drugs used.
- At the outset at least three drugs should be given in case there is already resistance to one of them. By the end of two months the bacterial population is greatly reduced, so the hazard posed by drug-resistance is less.
- Once a drug regimen has been decided upon and started, it should not be altered in any way unless there is toxicity.

Where the bacterial populations are small these principles can be relaxed in some respects. Where a child aged five or less is found to be tuberculin-positive but X-ray negative and symptomless, the bacterial population is so small that treatment may be given with isoniazid alone (usually for six months). Adult studies have also shown that following a two-month short-course regimen with four drugs (to be described later)

the bacillary population is reduced to a very low level; when this is followed by six months of isoniazid alone the results are as good as those following isoniazid/thiacetazone. This finding is of particular value in areas where thiacetazone is poorly tolerated.

Short-course regimens

Extensive studies in adult patients with drug-sensitive organisms have shown that if isoniazid and rifampicin are given together, the period of treatment for pulmonary or other organ tuberculosis need be no longer than six months. The regimen should be supported in the early stages by two months of pyrazinamide and two months of either streptomycin or ethambutol. These short-course four-drug regimens have certain other advantages. The relapse rate after the end of treatment is very low, and even when relapse takes place the organisms are still sensitive to the same drugs as before treatment started, so they can be used again with confidence of success.

Many regimens using shorter courses of rifampicin either continuously or spread out over two or three doses a week or even weekly in the later stages have also been shown to be effective in adults.

The use of streptomycin, isoniazid, rifampicin and pyrazinamide (SHRZ) daily for two months followed by isoniazid/thiacetazone (HT) or isoniazid alone (H) daily for six months (2SHRZ/6HT) was found in two small trials to be about 98 per cent effective.[7] The regimens are therefore especially useful where a two-month in-patient stay is already customary, and where out-patient attendance tends to be poor, since they reduce the period of compliance required from 10–16 months to six months. In practice, the results though better than with the old drug combinations, are not as good as those obtained in these trials because patients may miss some or all of the follow-up treatment. For patients harbouring bacilli resistant to isoniazid or streptomycin or both, a good cure rate was achieved with six-month regimens which included rifampicin throughout.

Whereas with the old regimens the purpose of using multiple drugs was to prevent resistance, with the SHRZ regimen the aim is to achieve a rapid kill, leaving only a few bacilli to be 'mopped up' during the six-month period of treatment with HT or H.

The most recent studies have indicated that if the 60 doses of rifampicin are spread out, for instance giving three doses weekly (together with streptomycin and increased doses of isoniazid and pyrazinamide) for two months, followed by one dose weekly for the next four months, results approaching those given by a daily six-month rifampicin-containing regimen can be achieved. Such a regimen can be given on a fully supervised domiciliary basis from the start. It is, however, only practicable for patients who live near the treatment centre and who can be expected to attend regularly; it is also necessary to have a good record-keeping and patient control system. Alternatively, supervised weekly rifampicin with other drugs can be used after a two-month in-patient period of a daily short-course regimen.

It must be emphasized that no similar controlled studies on short-course regimens have been carried out in children, because the lack of a clear end-point in terms of a negative sputum test makes such studies extremely difficult. However, extensive clinical experience in childhood tuberculosis indicates that such regimens are adequate or more than adequate for all childhood disease, other than tuberculous meningitis.

Policy of chemotherapy and hospitalization

Policy regarding both the duration of in-patient stay and the drugs used depends very much on the finance available.

In countries where the population is predominantly rural, hospital accommodation is considerably more expensive than drug costs. On the other hand, experience in rural areas has shown that a policy of treating all patients with pulmonary tuberculosis on an out-patient basis leads to such a high proportion of failures that the problem is not reduced, but instead the prevalence of isoniazid-resistance is increased. A period of guaranteed intensive therapy lasting two months will serve to kill off a high proportion of the bacilli and gives the patient a reasonable chance of cure if then released to a further period of out-patient treatment. The additional cost of using rifampicin and pyrazinamide during this initial two-month period is relatively small, and this regimen yields a much better cure-rate. In addition the required out-patient period is reduced from 16 to 6 months.

Faced therefore with the twin problems of financial constraint on the one hand and the long duration of treatment required for an effective programme on the other for patients with established tuberculosis of the lungs or other organs it is reasonable to aim at two months of treatment initially with rifampicin, isoniazid, streptomycin (or ethambutol) and pyrazinamide – which for rural patients means two months in hospital.

Although sputum-positive relapses are relatively rare in childhood, the occurrence of such a case suggests the presence of resistance to isoniazid. It is a great advantage, if the budget can stretch to it, to have a six-month second-line fully-supervised regimen which will cure a high proportion of these patients, who are unlikely to respond to a two-month rifampicin regimen unassisted by isoniazid. This means six months in hospital. Not only will this regimen cure patients who otherwise have little or no hope, but it will in the course of time reduce the prevalence of isoniazid-resistant bacilli.

Isoniazid-resistance has become so severe a problem, that in some countries as many as 20 per cent of patients who have never been treated for tuberculosis before, are excreting isoniazid-resistant organisms. In treated patients the rate is often well above 50 per cent. The cause of this is the widespread misuse of isoniazid in the past, with patients taking it for inadequate periods, intermittently, or on its own without other drugs. For this reason there is a strong case for limiting the use of rifampicin to in-patients or to patients who can report to a clinic or hospital for each dose.

Recommended regimens

Progressive primary tuberculosis, miliary tuberculosis, pericarditis, organ tuberculosis outside the chest, glandular tuberculosis and pleural effusions.
I. Full supervision possible (generally in urban communities): out-patient regimens.

2HRZE1/4HRE1

Ethambutol is sometimes withheld because of the difficulty in detecting defects of vision in young children. However, a fourth drug is advisable because of the high prevalence of INH-resistance in many developing countries. We have used E1 extensively without encountering any permanent visual damage.

An alternative regimen now used in several countries is 6HRZ. The drugs are given separately in young children, or as a fixed combination tablet (Rifater) in older children and adults. The constituents of Rifater vary in amount in different countries. It should be obtained from a reputable manufacturer to ensure proper absorption of rifampicin.

A very cost-effective regimen which has undergone satisfactory trials in both adults and children in 2HRZ followed by 4HR given twice weekly (H 10–15 mg/kg and R 20 mg/kg). These regimens are only advisable where good attendance for treatment is expected.
II. Supervision not possible: regimens which include an initial period of in-patient treatment.

2HRZE1/6HT (or 2HRZE1/6HE1 or 2HRZE1/6H)

If a moderate degree of reliable supervision is possible,

such as weekly or fortnightly visits, the use of rifampicin as out-patient treatment may be considered, e.g. 2HRZE1/4HRE1.

Children who relapse with progressive lung tuberculosis

3SHRZE1/3HRZE1, all six months in hospital.

Tuberculous meningitis

6HRZEe/6HEe is an ideal regimen. The optimal length of treatment with rifampicin-containing regimens has not been established; many would continue rifampicin for 12 months or even longer, but this is usually impracticable in developing countries.

Ethionamide is not now manufactured in some countries. If it is not available ethambutol may be substituted.

The dosages during the first three months are generally larger in order to achieve an effective concentration in the CSF (in mg/kg/day): H 15–20, R 20, Z 40, Ee 15, E1 25.

Protection of tuberculin reactors and contacts

Children aged five years or less who have a positive tuberculin test but no enlarged glands or other clinical findings, and a normal chest X-ray, may be treated with isoniazid for six months. Some doctors give 6HEl. Children with symptoms of hypersensitivity, such as phlyctenular conjunctivitis or erythema nodosum, may be treated similarly.

The management of tuberculin-negative contacts is discussed later.

Management of TB in HIV infected individuals

The recommended drugs and dosages are no different from those used in straigthforward TB cases, but treatment should be continued for a minimum of nine months. BCG vaccination is not contraindicated in HIV positive children except those with established disease (AIDS).

Doses

All drugs are given in a single morning dose except for ethionamide, which is given twice or three times daily because of its tendency to induce nausea.

Streptomycin: 15–25 mg/kg
Isoniazid: 10–15 mg/kg
For TB meningitis 15–20 mg/kg; maximum 500 mg/day
Rifampicin: 10–15 mg/kg
For TB meningitis 20 mg/kg; maximum 600 mg/day
Pyrazinamide: 30 mg/kg
For TB meningitis 40 mg/kg

Ethambutol: maximum 2 g/day
15–25 mg/kg
Thiacetazone: 2.5–3.5 mg/kg
In practice this is always used in combination with isoniazid. The tablets commonly contain H 100 mg and T 50 mg. A child of average size should have: under 1 year half a tablet; 2–6 years 1 tablet; 7–12 years two tablets; 13 years or more three tablets
Ethionamide: 15 mg/kg daily in divided doses, twice or three times a day.

Toxic effects

Whenever possible liver function tests should be done before starting treatment, as a baseline in case of later toxic effects. All the drugs are potentially toxic to the liver, except streptomycin and ethambutol. It is remarkable, therefore, how well they are tolerated in those parts of Africa where liver function may be impaired by protein–energy malnutrition.

A wide variety of toxic effects may be caused by the antituberculosis drugs. The doctor should be aware of the more common of these, and at the same time should be on the look-out for any unusual symptoms occurring in a child on antituberculosis treatment. A drug formulary can then be consulted as required. The common toxic effects are listed in Table 4.5.1.

Corticosteroids

In considerable degree the ill effects of primary tuberculosis are due to hypersensitivity and the inflammatory response which results from the cellular immune reaction to tuberculoprotein, rather than from a direct toxic effect of the organisms. This reaction can be modified by corticosteroids, which have an important place in therapy in certain circumstances.[8] Compression of airways by enlarged glands represents the most common indication for steroids. If wheeze or stridor are of recent onset their introduction with standard chemotherapy is often dramatically effective. The use of steroids is also standard practice in tuberculous meningitis to lessen cerebral oedema, meningeal thickening and cisternal block. They are used similarly in tuberculous pericarditis to diminish serosal inflammation which leads to constriction.[13] The use of steroids is not standard in tuberculous pleural effusions, as recovery in this condition is generally rapid. However, they may be of benefit in the thickened

Table 4.5.1   Toxic effects of anti-tuberculosis drugs

Toxic effect	Likely drug(s)	Management recommended
Fever and/or rash (4–8 weeks after starting the drug)	Any	Re-start isoniazid first, then other drugs at six-hourly intervals. Exclude any drug which causes a reaction
Liver toxicity, including jaundice	Rifampicin Pyrazinamide Thiacetazone Isoniazid Ethionamide	Continue treatment with streptomycin and ethambutol. After 3–4 days when the condition has improved, re-start isoniazid, then re-start rifampicin, if needed, 4 days later
Dizziness	Streptomycin	Substitute ethambutol (25–30 mg/kg) for streptomycin
Purpura	Rifampicin	Discontinue rifampicin
Visual disturbance	Ethambutol	Discontinue ethambutol
Orange-coloured urine	Rifampicin	Rifampicin stains urine (and other body secretions) an orange colour; this should be disregarded
Peripheral neuritis	Isoniazid	Stop isoniazid for a few days and give pyridoxine (10–15 mg kg/day). When improved re-start isoniazid and continue pyridoxine in a dose of 2–3 mg/kg/day
Mental confusion (not present before starting treatment)	Isoniazid	Stop isoniazid. Exclude other causes of confusion. If isoniazid is essential re-start it after 3–4 days and observe the child
Diarrhoea and nausea	Thiacetazone	Persist with treatment using a short course of anti-emetic drug; the symptoms usually go away
Nausea	Ethionamide	Try giving full dose at night instead of divided doses twice daily or an anti-emetic before each dose
'Flu'-like syndrome, with general malaise	Rifampicin, if given intermittently, especially once weekly	Increase frequency of dosage to daily, or change to another out-patient regimen

plastic type of pleurisy, which often leads to contracture of the affected rib-cage and spinal deformity. Finally, corticosteroids may be of some benefit in miliary and other extensive forms of disease to lessen general toxicity and restore well-being. Prednisone at 2 mg/kg per day should be given for a period of two to four weeks and then tailed off gradually over 7–10 days. Remember that rifampicin lowers tissue levels of corticosteroids by speeding up their metabolism. The tuberculous aetiology of the lesion should be clearly established before steroids are used.

Assessment of progress

Sometimes the condition of a child due for discharge after two months in hospital is thought not to be satisfactory. The key is the general state of the patient: does he/she feel well and has he/she gained weight? In support of this a chest X-ray can be very helpful. This usually shows definite clearing over the two-month period. However, massive multiple enlargement of the glands, including cervical glands, may take many months to resolve, and segmental lesions may remain unchanged for long periods. It is very seldom that a child does not improve after two months in hospital on antituberculosis drugs, and this is even more true when the regimen includes rifampicin. In older children, the decision that drug-resistance is present should be based on a persistently positive sputum smear result (strongly positive, if graded) combined with loss of weight, no improvement of symptoms and clear evidence of radiological deterioration after two or more months of treatment. A positive sputum smear alone is not a contra-indication to discharge. It is very rare for drug-resistance to be present in children with non-pulmonary forms of tuberculosis, and even rarer for it to be diagnosed reliably. Its rarity is probably related to the relatively small number of bacilli present, the high rate of spontaneous healing of primary tuberculosis, and the fact that isoniazid-resistant bacilli become relatively avirulent.

Out-patient treatment

Children depend for their attendance on the compliance of their mothers. There is a temptation to keep them longer in hospital in case the mother does not attend, but one should rather aim to educate the mothers. The possible ill-effects of maternal deprivation should never be forgotten when deciding how long to keep a child in hospital for the treatment of tuberculosis.

Unsupervised   A new form of paramedical skill brought

into being by the antituberculosis drugs is the art of getting patients to take tablets for a long time. This art we have signally failed to master as yet. Our efforts to do so must not slacken with the introduction of short-course regimens, because out-patient treatment will continue to be a vital part of the course. It is a question of education of the patient or parents on admission and discharge, of organization, and of seeing that the tablets and the clinics do not default from the patient. Community-based out-patient treatment, using either community volunteers selected by the community or cured patients who have been trained in the vital importance of long-term treatment, has not yet provided an adequate solution. It has not yet been possible to provide enough supervision, without which such community-based long-continued treatment becomes progressively less effective. Lines of authority become too long and the necessary control of the patients becomes looser and less than adequate.

As mentioned already, the doctor should hold a second discussion with the mother, if possible, about the child's out-patient treatment before the child leaves hospital. Detailed arrangements should be made, with her agreement, as to where she is going to fetch the tablets and how often. She should be consulted and not coerced. The centre agreed should not be a mobile unit unless its attendance is absolutely reliable. If there is difficulty in reaching a treatment centre the mother should be given up to three months of supplies.

It is an advantage to have a simple regimen for out-patients receiving monthly supplies of drugs, using only one kind of tablet (HT or H), which is easy for clinics to order, issue and ensure that it is kept in stock.

When issuing treatment, nurses should be on the look-out for signs of relapse such as loss of well-being and cough. It is a good policy for children to be weighed every time the tablets are issued.

Supervised As mentioned, patients may have treatment from the start with daily or thrice- or twice-weekly rifampicin-containing regimens, if they live near the treatment centre and can be depended upon to attend regularly. Record-keeping should be good, and there should be arrangements for tracing patients who fail to attend. Generally this method is only applicable to urban patients.

Reviews

The parent should be asked to bring the child for review if possible every three months until treatment is completed, and once three months after stopping the drugs. Thereafter the parent should be told to report back if the child's condition deteriorates. At the reviews the child should be weighed, a chest X-ray done if possible, and symptoms and general condition considered, the object being to decide whether there is any evidence of relapse. An X-ray is an advantage but it is not essential, and reviews can be done at peripheral clinics.

Stocks of drugs

Nothing is more disastrous to the control of tuberculosis than the sapping of patients' confidence that results when a medical unit runs out of drugs. All hospitals and clinics should carry a three-month reserve of all the antituberculosis drugs they need, in case of a failure of supply.

Other aspects of management

General measures

Although the most important aspect of therapy is the administration of a full and continuous course of drugs, other forms of treatment should not be neglected. The child should receive a well-balanced and nutritious diet and vitamin supplements should be given routinely. Prolonged bed rest leads to a loss of calcium and a tendency to rickets. Any evidence of specific nutritional deficiency should be treated. Pyridoxine is not necessary with the standard isoniazid dose of 10–15 mg/kg per day. It is expensive and there is always the possibility that the tubercle bacillus as well as the patient is protected from the toxic effects of isoniazid. Severe anaemia should be investigated or, if this is not possible, iron therapy may be given to those having a haemoglobin level of 8 g/100 ml or less. If intestinal parasites are present, appropriate treatment should be given. The immunization programme should be brought up to date.

Education

On starting treatment the doctor should tell the mother that the child has tuberculosis and explain the nature of the disease. The exact duration of treatment should also be clearly and simply explained and arrangements should be made with the mother as to where she is going to obtain the medication after discharge to out-patient treatment. This should be noted in the case sheet. When discharging the child, time should be taken to repeat in detail the plan of treatment. This procedure does much to prevent default. Every opportunity should be taken by all concerned, particularly the nursing staff, to explain the nature of the disease and the object of treatment to the family and to the patient if old enough to understand. Bizarre notions about the causation of tuberculosis are very common in unsophisticated communities, and can discourage attendance or compliance, especially if accompanied by fear of the disease or doubts about the treatment.

Stimulation, diversion and schooling

In the majority of cases the purpose of admission to hospital is not to ensure bed rest or special treatment, but simply to ensure that drugs are taken correctly. The mother, together with any breast-feeding infant she may be carrying, should preferably be admitted to hospital with the patient if under five years of age. If this is not possible, a relative should accompany the child and the mother should be allowed to visit.

Toys, games, picture-books, reading matter, drawing and colouring materials and special occasions such as Christmas parties do much to ease the tedium and strain of a long period in hospital.

Older children can engage in a wide variety of activities, including leather-work, bead-work and helping in the ward. At many hospitals, formal education is arranged and sometimes a full-time school teacher is employed. The importance of adequate stimulation of children in hospital cannot be over-stressed.

Organization of tuberculosis services

A tuberculosis programme should extend as deeply as possible into the community which it serves. That is, it should be mediated by the district hospitals, rural and urban clinics, by health workers and by members of the community. Diagnosis and the prescribing of drugs, however, require many complex clinical decisions, and should be done at a level where there are medical skills, a reliable laboratory service, radiology and authoritative supervision.

The role of the peripheral centres is twofold:

- To recognize the symptoms and outward signs of tuberculosis (which it shares with other forms of long-term lung disease) and refer the patient to the district hospital for investigation. In some countries the number of attendances at medical units annually is several times the whole population of the country; vigilance for tuberculosis suspects at these units is clearly by far the most useful form of case-finding.
- To carry out, supervise and record the domiciliary

treatment of patients when they are referred back, usually after a period as in-patient, and to take measures to trace and recover non-attenders.

Of all the functions of a health department, none requires more organization and capable management than the tuberculosis service. Indeed, there are few things more harmful to patients and the public, or more expensive, than a tuberculosis service which has gone out of control.

Record-keeping and patient handling

An early casualty when the finance available for a health service decreases is the efficiency and uniformity of record-keeping. This affects tuberculosis work especially badly, since it is of a routine nature and requires much repetition. It is important therefore to establish a uniform system of record-keeping and of patient handling. Case records, for instance, should always be pinned together and should be in a prescribed order. The essential facts about a tuberculosis patient can be recorded on a single sheet. A well-trained nurse or assistant who handles the patients and their records systematically can be invaluable.

It is possible for a properly instructed nurse to take much of the history. Apart from details of the present illness, one needs to know whether the child has ever been treated for tuberculosis before, whether anyone else in or close to the family has the disease, and about any previous BCG vaccination.

The diagnosis of tuberculosis in children hinges on the tuberculin test. Every suspect should be tested routinely, and this again can be done by a properly trained nurse, whether the Heaf or the Mantoux test is used.

It is common and proper practice in well-financed health services for patients' records, or a summary of them, to be sent on discharge to the intended out-patient review centre, and used there. In less fortunate areas, however, this process exists only in theory. In such countries, a patient-based record system should be used. The patient should carry, on an out-patient card, all the relevant details of the disease. In addition, it is unfortunately often the case that hospital out-patient departments cannot organize sufficiently to produce the records of patients who return for review; in this case it is very important for the patient to return with the card. Where this has become the normal practice patients learn to keep their records. If miniature (e.g. 100 mm) X-ray films are used, they can be clipped to the out-patient card and produced at the next review.

At the time of discharge the out-patient card must be completed with dates of admission and discharge, diagnosis, tuberculin test result and any sputum test results, treatment given and further treatment required with its duration. It is then not necessary for the next reviewer, if any, to make a new clinical assessment provided the child is well, and it is also possible for the clinic nurse to stop treatment at the right time if the child cannot be medically reviewed. In addition, the card must bear the name and address of the hospital and the patient's hospital number, so that if necessary the receiving hospital, if different, can write for X-rays or more details.

Monitoring

An effective central register of sputum-positive patients fed by information on new cases and on discharges, transfers and other changes in patients' status, is a powerful tool for detecting and correcting faults in the running of the tuberculosis service, as well as providing epidemiological information. A practical and economical register can now be maintained on a microcomputer with a high-capacity hard disc drive, provided that the paper input from the districts can be organized. To develop such a register requires a marriage of tuberculosis management skills and programming ability, either in the same person or through close liaison.

Similarly, district tuberculosis registers can be set up which will receive information about patients immediately. The main value of a district register is the monitoring of attendance for treatment and the means to contact the patient as soon as he/she fails to attend.

Prevention

The prevention of tuberculosis has three aspects:

- Maintenance of general health and nutrition.
- Protection against tuberculosis by means of BCG vaccination and the examination of child contacts.
- Control of tuberculosis and its elimination from the community, which depends on finding and treating infectious people.

Maintenance of general health

Nutrition

This is important in preventing the onset of tuberculous disease in children after they are infected. It is covered by a nutrition rather than a tuberculosis programme.

Avoiding exposure to infection

This is achieved by adequate housing and ventilation, which limits the amount of exposure to infection that children will have. It is partly a social problem and partly a matter of health education.

Protection of individual children

BCG vaccination

In 1886 Marfan pointed to the existence of immunity to tuberculosis by noting that pulmonary tuberculosis was rare among those with healed lupus or healed tuberculous adenitis. Calmette later suggested preventing tuberculosis by using live attenuated tubercle bacilli to create an infection 'light enough to remain indefinitely isolated to some remote corner of the lymphatic system' in order to confer immunity to tuberculosis. The product of his researches with Guerin was eventually introduced in the 1920s as BCG vaccine. Over the past 50 years BCG vaccination has been practised widely throughout the world. It is compulsory in 64 countries and officially recommended in a further 118 countries and territories. Despite this, the evidence for a protective effect from BCG in children remains conflicting, claims for its efficacy varying from 0 to 80 per cent. The only recent large-scale trial showed no protective effect in terms of the distribution of new cases of tuberculosis in a population after seven-and-a-half years of follow-up, but did not address the question of protection of infants and young children. A recent critical review of a number of controlled trials and retrospective studies carried out in the 1930s and 1940s concluded that BCG does indeed offer protection against the invasive forms of the disease – tuberculous meningitis and miliary tuberculosis – in infancy and childhood.[9] A WHO study group has recommended that the use of BCG should be continued and has stressed the importance of international cooperation and efficient coordination in future research.

BCG is given intradermally or percutaneously, the latter employing a more concentrated suspension of bacilli. A Japanese-made 'needle-planted cylinder' is a convenient multi-puncture method of BCG administration. It consists of a plastic cylinder fitted with nine pointed needles, and is rotated and re-applied to give a total of 27 punctures. It has the advantage that there are no moving parts to become worn or damaged. It can be sterilized and re-used about 100 times, compares in cost with spring-loaded devices, and is probably the best instrument to use.

For occasional use the best form of BCG is freeze-dried vaccine supplied in small amounts such as 10-dose vials together with diluent. With the intradermal method a small papule gradually develops at the site of the injection, reaching maximum size at six to eight weeks. Where the multiple puncture method is used the reaction is usually less marked; tiny papules appear at the site of each puncture. Sometimes, particularly with the intradermal method, a small abscess appears at the vaccination site and there may be associated lymphadenitis, which may suppurate. Such severe reactions should be treated with a course of isoniazid (one month) or erythromycin (two weeks). A rarer complication is an area of osteitis of the humerus beneath the vaccination site.

BCG is best given at birth as all infants born in hospitals and clinics may be reached at this time. As newborn infants have a rather poorly developed immune system, vaccination should be repeated at the first clinic visit (3–4 months) unless there is an ulcer or scar at the site of the vaccination. BCG should be given again on entering school, and in countries where infection is less widespread, on leaving school.

BCG is of no value if given to a child who has already been exposed to tuberculous infection. A disadvantage is that it interferes with the diagnosis of tuberculosis in children by rendering the tuberculin test positive. BCG will produce an accelerated response if given to a child reactive to tuberculoprotein. Such early reactors should be questioned about symptoms (see p. 522). Although a large ulcer may result from vaccinating a child who has had a previous natural infection, it is not necessary to do tuberculin tests before giving BCG in mass programmes. All health workers and their children should be vaccinated with BCG.

Conclusion   The objective of using BCG in control programmes is to prevent the serious forms of childhood tuberculosis. It may protect the individual, but does not confer significant benefit on the community as a whole. The powerful instruments for tuberculosis control are case-finding and effective chemotherapy.

Management of child contacts of infectious patients

Where a member of a household has infectious tuberculosis it is very likely indeed that others will be harbouring tubercle bacilli. It is thus important that all child contacts under the age of 15 years should be examined and protected. All child contacts should be tuberculin tested, and where the result is positive a chest X-ray should be obtained. After investigation, children under five years who show no other abnormality should be given isoniazid for six months. Those who react negatively should, if possible, receive isoniazid at 10 mg/kg daily for two to three months. The tuberculin test is then repeated: if negative, BCG vaccination is given; if positive, INH is continued for a further three months.

A small tuberculin-negative child who remains in hospital with a mother who is being treated for infectious tuberculosis should have isoniazid until the mother leaves hospital, and then be given BCG on the day of discharge, not less than 24 hours after the last dose of isoniazid (see also p. 201).

Contact tracing is difficult to achieve in rural settings. Nevertheless it is a vital ingredient to the control of the disease in children, and if properly carried out would prevent many cases of tuberculous meningitis and other tragic consequences from the disease in childhood.

Notification   Where a preventive staff infrastructure exists, all child and other tuberculosis patients should be notified promptly on diagnosis to enable such contact tracing to be carried out. Notification, if done comprehensively, is also of course of value for obtaining national information about tuberculosis.

Control of tuberculosis in the community

The control of tuberculosis in children depends entirely upon its control in adults. The strategy required is simple. It is the identification of all infectious patients who present themselves at medical units (with the careful exclusion of patients who do *not* have tuberculosis) and their complete treatment, thereby removing them from the infector pool. Figure 4.5.21 shows how the cycle of tuberculosis illustrated in Fig. 4.5.1 is broken by this policy of diagnosis and treatment. There is no other technique whose efficacy can approach this. Case-finding by tuberculin testing, mass radiography or sputum surveys in the population, and chemoprophylaxis, all require more work for much less return. The rewards from BCG vaccination, in terms of preventing infectious cases, are so few and so remote in time that it cannot count as a control measure – though it is of value to individual children. Common problem areas in carrying out the primary strategy are:

- to ensure full identification and referral of suspects;
- to have sputum smear examination immediately available at all hospitals;
- to make sure that out-patients take their treatment regularly until the course has been completed.

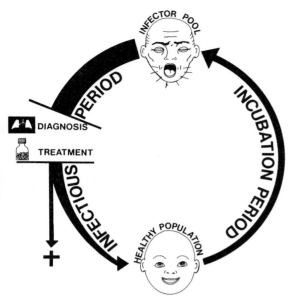

Fig. 4.5.21   Breaking the cycle of tuberculosis.

The numbers of infectious patients found can be increased by questioning for symptoms the family contacts of all children and others who are found to have tuberculosis, and investigating them where indicated.

Education of the public about the symptoms, danger and availability of treatment of tuberculosis, and of patients in the nature of the disease and the regimen of treatment required, are valuable adjuncts in achieving the two primary objectives. It is important to remove the stigma that attaches to the disease, and to educate employers to realize that treated patients are cured, non-infectious and able to continue their work, so that employees do not conceal their illness.

Voluntary organizations should be interested so that the public participates in the control of this very universal disease. Such organizations can do much by producing pamphlets and posters and providing welfare, diversional and occupational therapy, and schooling, to make a long stay in hospital more tolerable.

Confidence of the public in the tuberculosis service is essential, and is most quickly built up by the readily ascertainable facts that sick patients are restored to long-term health, and that people attending hospital with trivial complaints are not apprehended and hospitalized for a long time for non-existent tuberculosis. An efficiently run service is its own advertisement.

As has been convincingly demonstrated in many countries, the root causes of tuberculosis lie in poor social, economic and environmental conditions, and the ultimate total conquest of the disease will be achieved by attacking these deep-seated human problems.

References

1. Fourie PB. Prevalence and annual rate of tuberculosis infection in South Africa. *Tubercle*. 1983; **64**: 181–92.
2. Miller FJW. *Tuberculosis in Children: Evolution, Epidemiology, Treatment and Prevention*, 2nd Edn. Edinburgh, Churchill Livingstone, 1982; 4–17.
3. Lamont AC, Cremin BJ, Pelteret RM. Radiological patterns of pulmonary tuberculosis in the paediatric age group. *Paediatric Radiology*. 1986; **16**: 2–7.
4. Deeny JE, Walker MJ, Kibel MA *et al.* Tuberculous meningitis of children in the Western Cape: epidemiology and outcome. *South Africa Medical Journal*. 1985; **68**: 75–8.
5. Coovadia YM, Dawood A, Ellis ME *et al.* Evaluation of adenosine deaminase activity and antibody to *Mycobacterium tuberculosis* antigen 5 in cerebrospinal fluid and the radioactive bromide partition test for the early diagnosis of tuberculous meningitis. *Archives of Disease in Childhood*. 1986; **61**: 428–35.
6. Slovis TL, Haller JO, Berdon We *et al.* Non-invasive visualization of the paediatric airway. *Current Problems in Diagnostic Radiology*. 1979; **8**(1): 1–67.
7. Fox W. Short course chemotherapy for pulmonary tuberculosis and some problems of its programme application with particular reference to India. *Lung India*. 1984; **11**(2): 161–74.
8. Horne NW. A critical evaluation of corticosteroids in tuberculosis. *Advances in Tuberculosis Research*. 1966; **15**: 1–54.
9. Clemens JD, Chuong JJH, Feinstein AR. The BCG controversy: a methodological and statistical reappraisal. *Journal of the American Medical Association*. 1983; **249**(17): 2362–9.
10. Chandra K, Choudhury P, Choudhury U. Evaluation of Mantoux and BCG test in the diagnosis of childhood tuberculosis. *Indian Pediatrics*. 1977; **14** (2): 99–102.
11. Samai GC. Efficacy of BCG test in diagnosis of childhood tuberculosis. *Indian Journal of Pediatrics*. 1979; **46**: 279–82.
12. Ly HM, Trach DD, Long HT *et al.* Skin test responsiveness to a series of new tuberculins of children living in three Vietnamese cities. *Tubercle*. 1989; **70**: 27–36.
13. Strang JIG, Kakaza HHS, Gibson DG *et al.* Controlled trial of prednisolone as adjuvant in treatment of tuberculous constrictive pericarditis in Transkei. *Lancet*. 1987; **2**: 1418–1422.
14. Edwards K. The diagnosis of childhood tuberculosis. *Papua New Guinea Med. J.* 1987; **30**: 169–178.
15. HIV infection in childhood. Report of a British Paediatric Association Working Party. 1989. pp. 2–11.

16. Center for Disease Control. Tuberculosis and human immunodeficiency virus infection: recommendations of the Advisory Committee for the Elimination of Tuberculosis (ACET). *MMWR*. 1989; **38**(14): 236–250.

17. Sunderam G, McDonald RJ, Maniatis T *et al.* Tuberculosis as a manifestation of the acquired immunodeficiency syndrome (AIDS). *JAMA*. 1986; **256**: 362–366.

18. Wu CH, Fann MC, Lau YJ. Detection of mycobacterial antigens in cerebrospinal fluid by enzyme-linked immunosorbent assay. *Tubercle*. 1989; **70**: 37–43.

19. Parsons M. The treatment of tuberculous meningitis. *Tubercle*. 1989; **70**: 79–82.

20. Arens LJ, Deeny JE, Molteno CD *et al.* Tuberculous meningitis in children in the Western Cape: neurological sequelae. *Paediatric Reviews and Communication*. 1987; **1**(3): 257–275.

CHAPTER 6

Leprosy

M. Elizabeth Duncan

Foreword

"In most communities social attitudes play an important part in the persistence of the endemic compounded of ignorance and prejudice and reinforced by cultural, linguistic and religious factors – the stigma of leprosy is real and persistent. This stigma leads to concealment of people with suspicious lesions until advanced disease and peripheral ulcerations can no longer be hidden. It denies treatment to leprosy sufferers that would rapidly render them non-contagious and hence is responsible for infection of household contacts. Social attitudes exert pressure on teachers and school authorities demanding the exclusion of children suspected to have leprosy sometimes on grossly insufficient grounds. The irony is that the child with a few symptomless hypopigmented macules may be shedding millions of leprosy bacilli every day from the nasal mucosa, whereas an elderly man who has a malodorous ulcer on his foot has not been infectious for years, yet the child still goes to school while the adult is driven from house and home by angry fellow villagers."

"The psychological trauma inflicted on a child growing up in an atmosphere of open hostility and 'untouchableness' has serious and persistent consequences. Many such children become either aggressively antisocial or resignedly acquiescent, some drift into beggary following a family pattern or into a life of prostitution."

"Leprosy in children is thus not simply an infection with a known mycobacterial agent but is in many countries the consequence of the interplay between host and invading parasite in a social environment of poverty, domestic overcrowding, undernourishment and lack of hygiene. Leprosy has largely disappeared from the West concurrently with improvement in socio-economic levels and not as the result of specific therapy or specific preventive measures."

S.G. Browne

Extracts from a preliminary draft which Dr Browne had written for this chapter at the close of a life devoted to the care of leprosy sufferers.

Introduction

To those who have not met leprosy, it may still be thought of as a disease known only in earlier centuries from Biblical times, a disease of the unclean, outcast and beggar. However, today it is one of the six diseases selected by the World Health Organization (WHO) for special study on the grounds that the overall mortality and morbidity caused by them pose vast problems to economic development and growth.

Estimates for total numbers of leprosy sufferers are 11, 15 and 20 millions, but accurate statistics are not available, and the numbers may well include patients 'treated and presumed cured'. The majority of sufferers live in tropical or subtropical zones (Fig. 4.6.1) where an estimated 5.5 million are registered patients and receiving treatment. It is suggested that for every diagnosed sufferer, there are two undiagnosed.

Although there have been tremendous advances in our knowledge of leprosy, and it has been said that the advances in the immunology, bacteriology, epidemiology and treatment are far greater than for any other disease, we are still a long way from eradicating leprosy. The reasons for this include ignorance and the effect of culture, religion and superstition resulting in stigma and fear; lack of medical services and trained workers; difficulties in transportation and obtaining treatment; shortage of money to provide integrated services (much of the money for leprosy treatment is provided by voluntary agencies); problems associated with inadequate housing, overcrowding, deficient food supplies, unsafe water, and the infections which go with these and can themselves reduce resistance to mycobacterial infections.

Epidemiology

The earliest reliable references to leprosy come from India and go back to the sixth century BC. These descriptions, along with those from China, are surprisingly accurate, and clearly describe the disease known today as leprosy and caused by *Mycobacterium leprae*. Leprosy was brought from India into the Mediterranean basin and Europe in the fourth century BC. It spread along the routes of invading and retreating armies, and along trade routes by land and sea. The epidemic of leprosy in Europe in the Middle Ages, following the return of the Crusaders, and the establishment of leper hospitals outside towns is evidence that leprosy was then regarded as an infectious disease.

Leprosy went from Africa to the Americas with the slave trade 400 years ago. When slaves were emancipated and released from their slavery, those who had leprosy took it with them and released the infection among the American Indians. Chinese traders and labourers took the disease with them throughout Australasia. Leprosy was spread in Iceland by the itinerant farm labourers who sheltered for the winter in different farms around the island. In Norway it was endemic until the early twentieth century amongst those who shared crowded single-roomed houses throughout the long northern winter: but interestingly, the children of leprous parents who had the opportunity to emigrate to America and live in spacious houses, with plenty of good fresh food and fresh air, did not develop leprosy.

Clearly leprosy was an infection that was spread by close contact, overcrowding, poor housing and probably amongst those who were undernourished. Tuberculosis thrived in the same conditions. (For an historical review see Ref. 1.)

Influence of culture and religion

The knowledge that leprosy is infectious has made many people afraid of leprosy, and afraid of having anything to do with those who suffer from it. The word 'leper' meant 'outcast'. Today there are many who believe that the term 'leprosy' should be replaced with 'Hansen's disease' or 'HD' after the man who first described the leprosy bacillus, so that 'HD' sufferers are not rejected by society.

In parts of the world where leprosy is endemic the leprosy sufferers are accepted as members of the community. In places where there is very little leprosy, the sufferer has to keep the affliction hidden, or face the consequences of being cast out of society to live the life of a street beggar. There are some places in Africa where the Orthodox Church teaches that it is praiseworthy to give alms (money) to beggars, especially those who are less fortunate, so those with leprosy go to the churches to beg and some become quite rich compared with the ordinary population; for these people there is no financial incentive to get better and to stop begging.

In other countries there are those who although highly educated have developed leprosy – leprosy can affect anyone, poor or rich, educated or illiterate. Some have been so distressed at becoming leprous beggars after holding a university or administrative post, that they have committed suicide. It is ironic that those who, through the misfortune of lack of specialist services or through their own neglect, have deve-

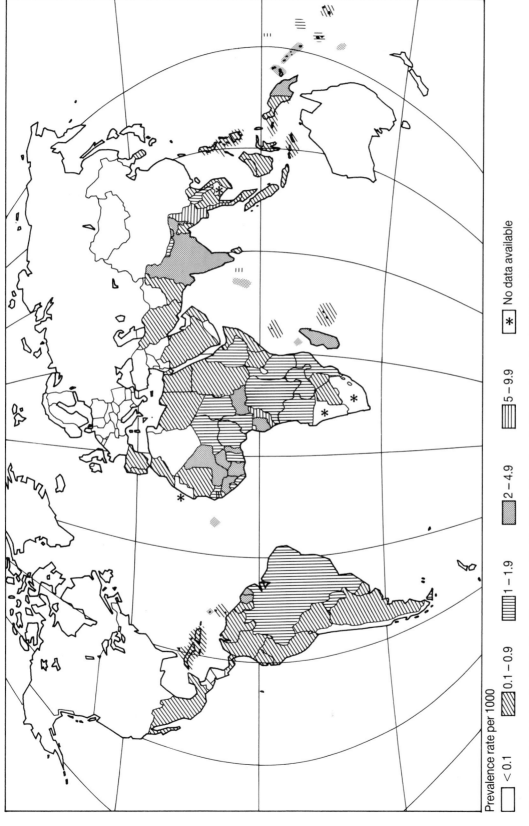

Prevalence rate per 1000

☐ < 0.1	▨ 0.1 – 0.9	▥ 1 – 1.9	▦ 2 – 4.9	▥ 5 – 9.9

✳ No data available

Fig. 4.6.1 Map showing the distribution of leprosy world-wide (1988). (Reproduced with permission from *WHO Expert Committee on Leprosy: sixth report*. Geneva, WHO, 1988. (WHO Technical Report Series no. 768.)

loped leprosy neuropathy and the ulceration of feet and hands associated with it, are regarded as highly infectious and are evicted from their homes, while a healthy child with early infectious lepromatous leprosy can be infecting his siblings and school friends without prejudice.

From earliest times two themes ran side by side: leprosy was highly infectious, and leprosy could result from incurring the anger of supernatural powers or gods. In Judaio-Christian circles it used to be generally understood that leprosy was God's punishment for sin. However, while Biblical references to leprosy (possibly because of a mistranslation of the Hebrew text) have done much to instil the ideas of uncleanliness, incurability and communicability of the disease, Biblical teaching, in particular the words of Jesus Christ 'Heal the sick . . . cleanse the leper', has prompted and inspired a tremendous outpouring of aid and research in the field of leprosy.

In Chinese tradition, leprosy was regarded as a punishment for sexual misconduct and transmissible within the family to the third and fourth generations. In India, children who contract leprosy are believed by some people to have committed a terrible crime or sin in a previous existence.[2] While according to Islamic teaching, it is part of a Muslim's duties to console the ill and help them whenever possible – this is not practised widely towards those with leprosy. In many Islamic communities a medieval type of persecution is still practised. The leprosy patient is not accepted as a member of the community and even his family tend to isolate him.[3] In some Muslim countries, there is legally enforced segregation or deportation of leprosy sufferers. In other communities, it is thought that by treating leprosy sufferers, the faithful may be going against the just will of Allah: moreover, the faithful should not be deprived of the opportunity of giving alms to leprosy beggars, so gaining merit in Paradise (S. G. Browne, personal communication).

The effect of these traditions, cultural attitudes, ignorance, fatalism and fear of ostracism has been that many leprosy sufferers tend to hide the disease instead of coming for treatment in the early stages when the late consequences and deformities can be prevented or treated.

Bacteriology and immunology

Mycobacterium leprae, the causative organism of leprosy is an obligate intracellular acid-fast and Gram-negative bacillus, 3–8 μm in length and 0.3 μm in diameter. It has an affinity for skin, particularly in the cool areas of the body, and a unique ability to invade peripheral nerves. It is found in the skin predominantly in macrophages, and in peripheral and dermal nerves in Schwann cells.

M. leprae has a division time of about 12 days and an incubation time of 2–10 years, on average four to five years, although periods of up to 27 years have been recorded. The host may harbour up to 10^{13} bacilli in body tissues and have a bacteraemia of 10^5/ml without showing signs or symptoms of septicaemia. A patient with active leprosy may thus remain active and apparently healthy. It has been said that leprosy *per se*, even in advanced cases, is rarely a cause of death.

M. leprae has not yet been successfully cultured *in vitro*, but will multiply in the footpads of mice (more widespread infection occurs in animals thymectomized after birth, or nude mice), in the nine-banded armadillo and in the European hedgehog which have low body temperatures. *M. leprae* from armadillos is used for the production of vaccines and for experimental work.

The complex internal structure of the bacillus has been revealed by electron microscopy. Advanced immunological techniques, including crossed immuno-electrophoresis, have been used to identify the various antigenic components (89 to date). While many of these antigens are shared with other mycobacteria, one specific factor, phenolic glycolipid I (PGL-I), appears to be a highly valuable chemical marker for *M. leprae*. The different antigens stimulate the production of specific antibodies, in the IgG, IgA and IgM classes, against various antigenic components of *M. leprae*; non-specific antibodies such as anticardiolipin antibody (giving a false positive WR or VDRL); and auto-antibodies such as antinuclear factor, rheumatoid factor and thyroglobulin antibodies.

The non-specific antibodies and autoantibodies tend to be present during leprosy reactions (see pp. 453, 557). The specific anti-*M. leprae* antibodies present in the serum of leprosy patients, especially those with lepromatous or multibacillary leprosy, do not appear to play any part in defence against the infection. In other words, presence of antibodies does not equate with 'immunity' but, on the contrary, may damage such targets as peripheral nerves and the uveal tract of the eye by immune complex formation as occurs in erythema nodosum leprosum (ENL) (see p. 558). However, demonstration of anti-*M. leprae* antibodies has been shown to be of value in the prediction of relapse due to dapsone resistance, and the evolution of subclinical and indeterminate leprosy.

At present, tests for antigens and antibodies can only be made in relatively sophisticated laboratories.

Antigens originating from *M. leprae* are demonstrable in the urine of patients with untreated multibacillary leprosy and the amount can be correlated with the total bacterial load in the patient. This test, based on radio-immunoassay (RIA) may have prognostic value. Research is currently being directed towards the development of tests using selected monoclonal antibodies. Such tests could be valuable in diagnosing subclinical leprosy and for epidemiological purposes.[4]

Resistance to infection is by cell-mediated immunity (CMI), in particular by activated macrophages and sensitized T lymphocytes. Exposure to *M. tuberculosis*, BCG-immunization and other environmental myco-bacteria may augment natural resistance that has been partly inherited from parents. This inherited resistance or, conversely, susceptibility to and type of response after infection with *M. leprae*, appears to be genetically determined, at least in part. Determination of HLA types in patients and children with and without leprosy has shown that the segregation of HLA haplotypes among healthy children occurs randomly. While children with tuberculoid leprosy shared HLA haplotypes more frequently than expected, children with lepromatous leprosy showed the same pheno-menon to a lesser extent.[5] Study of the genetic markers indicates that the genetic effects operate mainly through immunological mechanisms.

Resistance may be diminished by any factors which decrease CMI. Of these, by far the most important are the nutritional factors. Chronic protein–calorie malnutrition/deprivation causes thymic and lymphoid atrophy which results in suppression of CMI, with subsequent increased susceptibility to infections such as tuberculosis and leprosy. However, the situation is frequently more complicated as viruses, in particular, HIV and measles, and protozoa (especially *Giardia intestinalis* (*G. lamblia*) and to a lesser extent *Strongyloides stercoralis*, *Entamoeba histolytica* and *Leishmania tropica*) also may cause both generalized and specific immuno-suppression. Furthermore, the acute gastroenteritis and diarrhoeal diseases, so prevalent in the tropics and subtropics as secondary causes of protein–calorie deprivation, themselves cause suppression of CMI. Other manifestations of generalized suppression of CMI are increased susceptibility to and occurrence of skin infestations and infections, especially those due to *Candida albicans* and *Staphylococcus aureus*, increased carriage of *Salmonella* species, and re-infection with *G. intestinalis*.

The degree of protective immunity provided by sensitized T cells (CMI) may be affected by exposure to the infection *in utero* or in early infancy, the route of infection, duration of exposure and 'dosage' of the infecting organism. Minimal degrees of resistance may

be overcome by massive and repeated exposure to infection in the overcrowded sleeping quarters of many families in the cities and villages of the developing world.

CMI is also affected by the hormonal status of the individual. In particular, increased levels of oestrogen (as occur at puberty and during pregnancy) cause suppression of CMI. Leprosy may thus first appear at these times. It has been noted that there is a sudden increase in the number of girls compared with boys with leprosy at puberty (Fig. 4.6.2). In adult life it is generally the case that the sex ratio for leprosy is 2 male: 1 female. This may be because males by movement outside the immediate home/village environment run increased risk of exposure to the infection.

Leprosy is a chronic disease where the clinical mani-festations of the disease are not due to the bacillus (which is virtually non-toxic) but to the immune reponse of the host. When there is a powerful cell-mediated immune response, lesions are localized and there are very few bacilli found chiefly in nerves: this is tuberculoid leprosy (TT). Where the cell-mediated immunity is low, probably because of a specific defect of T lymphocyte reactivity to *M. leprae*, the disease is diffuse and generalized: this is lepromatous leprosy (LL). Between these two polar forms of the disease lie the immunologically unstable borderline forms of the disease – borderline tuberculoid (BT), borderline lepromatous (BL) and borderline leprosy (BB) which exhibits features of both BT and BL leprosy. A spectrum of the disease has been defined in terms of bacteriological load, immunological response/status, histology and clinical features (Fig. 4.6.3).[22]

Leprosy reactions

Reactions in leprosy are clinical phenomena caused by alterations in the immune status of the patient. They are most likely to occur in the immunologically unstable borderline forms of the disease (BT, BB and BL) and are responsible for many of the damaging and deforming complications of leprosy. There are two types of reaction.

Type 1 leprosy reaction (reversal reaction). An example of the Coombs and Gell type 4 reaction, this type gets its name because in immunological and clinical terms the course of the disease is apparently 'reversed' from the natural evolution of the disease. Untreated, it would progress from BT to BB to BL and eventually to LL (Fig. 4.6.4). Diminished CMI can cause increased bacillary multiplication, progress of leprosy and down-grading of classification, which is a shift towards the lepromatous end of the leprosy scale. Increase in CMI will tend to cause upgrading or shift towards the

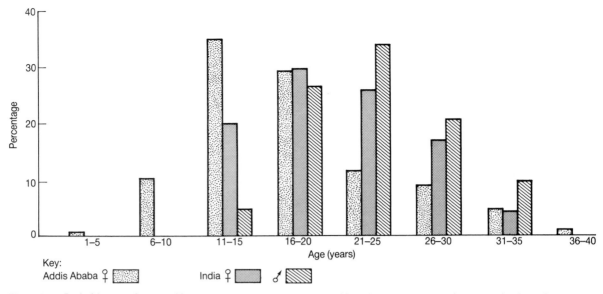

Fig. 4.6.2 Probable age of onset of leprosy as percentage of a group. Note the very small number occurring in early childhood, increasing sharply with onset of puberty. Figures and percentages for males and females in Addis Ababa are comparable. In India, the peak onset in females occurs between 15 and 25 years, while for males it is 5 years later.

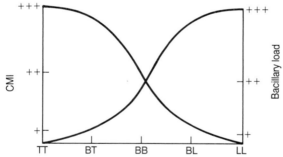

Fig. 4.6.3 The spectrum of leprosy in terms of cell-mediated immunity (CMI) and bacterial load.

tuberculoid end of the leprosy scale (reversal reaction: RR),[6] which may involve either skin (Figs 4.6.5 and 4.6.6) or nerves with resulting neuritis, nerve damage (Fig. 4.6.7) and permanent deformity.

Type 2 leprosy reaction (erythema nodosum leprosum (ENL)). An example of the Coombs and Gell type 3 reaction,[7] this is a form of immune complex disease which may be localized or generalized, depending on whether the immune complexes (antigen/antibody/complement) are fixed in the tissues or circulating. ENL is characterized by the appearance in the skin of crops of painful red nodules lasting three to five days. Frequently there is systemic illness and a variety of clinical manifestations, the most important being neuritis and iridocyclitis. ENL occurs in BL and LL patients as antigen is released from dying *M. leprae* after the start of treatment, or during relapse, when it is associated with bacterial multiplication, increase in antigen load and possibly downgrading. ENL may also occur during a coincidental infection such as typhus or tuberculosis.

HIV infection and leprosy

Because of the important role of CMI in determining the evolution of leprosy, and the well-documented appearance of new cases and exacerbation of established leprosy in immunosuppressed patients, one could anticipate that HIV infection would have very serious consequences for the leprosy patient as it has done for the tuberculous. The few reports of HIV seroprevalence in leprosy patients[8] may reflect coincidental exposure to HIV rather than overt leprosy resulting from HIV immunosuppression. Downgrading and increase in multibacillary leprosy have not yet been documented nor has there been a change in pattern of clinical leprosy, possibly because of the long division time of *M. leprae*, although HIV may contribute to

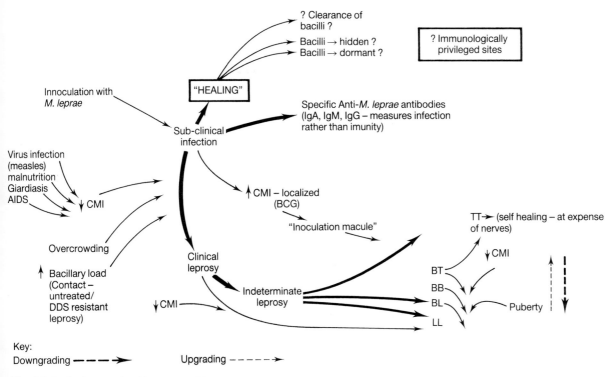

Fig. 4.6.4 Pathogenesis of leprosy and factors influencing the evolution of the infection.

relapse in treated patients as has been observed with tuberculosis.

In practical terms, as most leprosy patients live in parts of the world where HIV infection is endemic, there is a potential risk of transmission of the virus during biopsy, or skin smear preparation. Standard precautions should be taken, including the use of disposable scalpel blades if possible, careful sterilization of blades which have to be re-used, and the use of gloves by health workers, especially if they have sores on their hands.[9]

Pathogenesis and classification

After *M. leprae* has entered the body, it may lie dormant (probably in nerve or muscle) for a variable period of time before division starts. At a certain point after multiplication starts, the bacilli become detected. Macrophages move in to engulf the bacilli which then multiply freely within them. Further development depends on the CMI of the patient and is shown in Fig. 4.6.4. Initially there is a subclinical infection; this may progress to spontaneous healing, or indeterminate

or lepromatous leprosy. Indeterminate leprosy itself may undergo spontaneous healing or progress to clinical leprosy, depending on the host's immune response, and factors influencing it.

Tuberculoid leprosy may undergo spontaneous healing, but at the expense of the patient's nerves, i.e. the patient may during a strong upgrading reaction (RR) destroy the bacilli in the skin and nerve lesions, but develop leprosy neuritis due to granuloma formation within, say, the lateral popliteal nerve. The resulting foot drop will be permanent unless high doses of steroids are given for several months in addition to antileprosy drugs.

BT leprosy may upgrade to TT and undergo spontaneous healing, or, if there is suppression of CMI, there will be a progressive downgrading to BB, BL and ultimately LL. BB and BL may upgrade to BT, but this is less common. While LL may appear to be a homogeneous group, it does comprise two separate groups, LLs (subpolar) and LLp (polar). The chief difference between these two is that LLp cannot upgrade through LLs to the rest of the spectrum.

It has been taught that the type of leprosy most frequently seen in children is indeterminate or tuber-

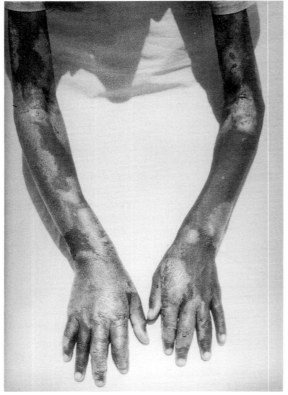

Fig. 4.6.5 BT leprosy showing the appearances of type 1 (reversal reaction) in the skin lesions. (Courtesy of Dr AC McDougall.)

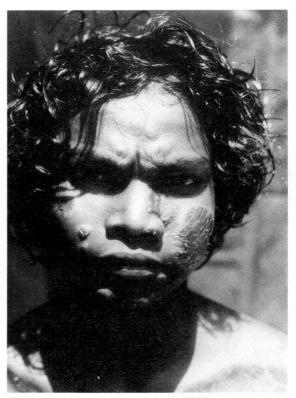

Fig. 4.6.6 Indian child with active BL leprosy with subsiding reversal (upgrading) reaction.

culoid. However, there is a series of papers from the Philippines describing the clinical features, histology and evolution of leprosy in children[10-20] in which it is clear that indeterminate, tuberculoid and BB (with only a few lesions) leprosy underwent spontaneous healing. The observations prompted the following question 'Had the children sterilized their systems of leprosy bacilli, or had the bacilli gone into hiding, e.g. in lymph nodes, nerve tissue or testis or other body tissue to reappear later?'[17]

A new presentation of leprosy in children has recently been observed: a single tuberculoid macule in the vicinity of a BCG scar. It is thought that a localized aggregation of sensitized lymphocytes, and macrophages, as would result from BCG immunization ('localized increased CMI') effectively 'mops up' the circulating *M. leprae* in a child with subclinical or early indeterminate leprosy, causing the appearance of a single lesion. The subclinical/indeterminate leprosy

would become overt tuberculoid and self-healing. This is probably the reason for an apparent increase in tuberculoid leprosy following mass BCG campaigns, with a decrease in the incidence of ensuing lepromatous leprosy (Figs 4.6.4 and 4.6.8).

Ethnic origin influences the prevalence of different classifications of leprosy. In those with darker skins (e.g. Africans) tuberculoid, especially BT leprosy is more commonly seen, while in those with lighter skins (e.g. Indians) BL and LL are more common. Also, in India, there is a form known as polyneuritic, in which there is nerve involvement without visible skin lesions.

Diagnosis and classification of leprosy on the Ridley scale is usually made on clinical grounds backed up by laboratory findings, of which slit-skin smears for bacteriological index (BI) and morphological index (MI) are the most important of all the diagnostic tests, and can be done with very little equipment under field conditions (see pp. 569–70).

In 1982, WHO introduced a new classification for

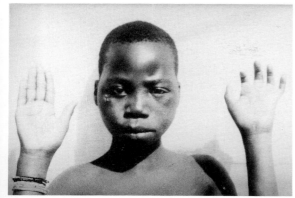

Fig. 4.6.7   BT leprosy. Nerve damage – left facial and ulnar palsy. (Courtesy of Dr AC McDougall.)

therapeutic purposes under field conditions in which patients are divided into two groups.

- Paucibacillary: those with a low bacillary load – BI less than 2 + on the Ridley scale.
- Multibacillary: those with a high bacillary load – BI more than 2 + .[21]

It should be pointed out that after treatment with dapsone (DDS) is begun, some upgrading is usually noted histologically. Furthermore, treated 'cured/inactive' leprosy from TT to LL may show the same histological picture as indeterminate leprosy, from lesions of leprosy that have undergone spontaneous healing (TT and BT), or have burnt out (BB and BL) after many years. In such cases, classification of leprosy can only be made on clinical grounds and by reviewing the case history.[22-24] Moreover, a patient who has had some treatment, e.g. two years DDS monotherapy for BL may well have a low BI, but may deliberately conceal the early treatment when attending a new centre, in order to get better treatment.

Spread of infection

Using the technique of lymphocyte transformation, it has been shown that staff in contact with leprosy patients have been sensitized to *M. leprae*. Most developed a subclinical infection, a situation analogous to that in tuberculosis. Thus, the infectivity of leprosy was confirmed, but the prevalence of clinical leprosy in Ethiopia was only 0.5 per cent or 1 in 200.

M. leprae has been identified not only in skin and nerves but also in virtually every form of human

secretion and excretion. It is generally accepted that the most important means of spread is by droplet transmission from the nose of infectious lepromatous patients (Fig. 4.6.8). The 'nose blow' can be used to assess the infectivity of patients. Skin-to-skin transmission may be of relevance, chiefly in the transmission from mother to child. Sexual transmission has been suggested to explain unusual presence of mycobacteria in amniotic fluid. Of greatest significance for the child, however, is the possibility of transplacental transmission and transmission through the mother's breast-milk.

More frequent transmission and recognition of infection in families are common features in leprosy. Analysis of 271 registered child leprosy patients (age ≤ 15 years) in Ethiopia (P. Bahiru and M. E. Duncan, unpubl.) showed that of all the children 53 per cent had a relative with leprosy. For the children aged ≤ 7 years at onset of leprosy, 48 per cent had a leprous mother and 64 per cent had one or more relatives with leprosy. For the children aged 8–15 years, 44 per cent had a leprous mother and 21 per cent had one or more relatives with leprosy. The average age of onset of leprosy was 7.7 years if the mother had leprosy, 8.7 years if only the father had leprosy, and earlier if both parents had the disease. Sixty per cent of the children presented for treatment within one year if there was leprosy within the family, but those living with healthy relatives came later.

Leprosy in infancy and early childhood, a congenital or acquired infection?

Historical aspects

Hitherto leprosy in children under the age of five years has been regarded as very rare, and congenital infection never established, although a number of cases of leprosy in very young children have been described and reviewed.[25] The earliest cases were described in 1890, but since few had biopsies or bacteriological examination, many modern leprologists have tended to discount these as not being due to leprosy, although clearly there was a risk that children born to leprous parents could develop leprosy.

In the nineteenth century large numbers of abortions occurred in women with leprosy. These were attributed to septicaemia with *M. leprae*, resulting in placental infection and leading to fetal infection and abortion. In 1897, Zambaco[26] considered that the reason for these abortions not being diagnosed as due to fetal leprosy, was that in many cases of abortion both fetus and placenta were discarded without being properly

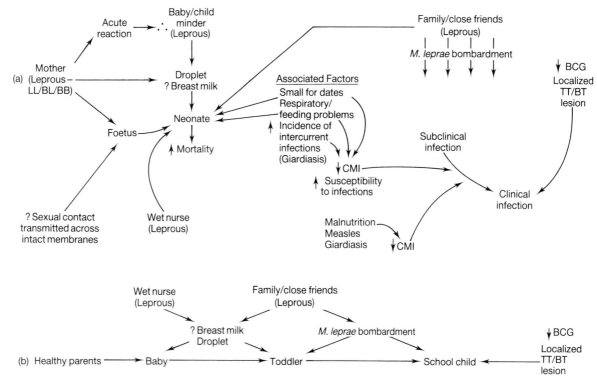

Fig. 4.6.8 Mode of infection and factors influencing the development of leprosy in children born to mothers with multibacillary (BB, BL and LL) leprosy (a) or healthy parents (b).

examined, an observation repeated 30 years later by Montero. Evidence for the maternal bacteraemia and transplacental infection of the fetus was acid-fast bacilli observed in the fetal heart blood at autopsy of an untreated lepromatous woman who was six month's pregnant. A similar situation occurred with tuberculosis. While congenital tuberculosis is not common, it is well documented. In the cases recorded there was little correlation of placental pathology with the degree and type of infection in the infant, because most of the placentae were discarded soon after being recorded as macroscopically normal – an unfortunate habit too frequently practised by midwives and doctors.

The placenta in leprosy

Studies of placentae from leprous women have shown the presence of acid-fast bacilli, by concentration methods only, in approximately one-half of placentae from women with very active, untreated or drug-resistant, lepromatous leprosy. It is impossible to say whether the acid-fast bacilli identified in placental tissue had originated from the maternal or fetal circulations.

Only one placenta from an accumulated series of more than 250 placentae from leprous women showed granulomatous lepromatous lesions in the villous tissue. The long division time of *M. leprae* is thought to account for the lack of histological lesions. A recent study of 81 placentae from leprous women with detailed macroscopic, light microscopic, ultrastructural, immunopathological, microbiological and biochemical examination showed no evidence of abnormality or infection of the placenta due to *M. leprae*. Although placental weights were found to be reduced in mothers with leprosy, particularly in lepromatous leprosy (Table 4.6.1), there is no recent evidence of abortion, stillbirth, or prematurity in leprosy patients who have had proper antenatal care, nor is there evidence of low birth weight or small placenta size being due to active leprosy.

The infants of mothers with leprosy

Relatively little has been recorded of the general state of health of children born to mothers with leprosy, although it was observed by Schilling in 1778[27] that

Table 4.6.1. Infant birth weight, placental weight and placental coefficient according to the clinical classification of the mother

	Birth weight (g) Mean and SEM	Placental weight (g) Mean and SEM	Placental coefficient Mean and SEM
Healthy controls	3280.6 ± 87.6 (18)	595.0 ± 35.4 (13)	0.184 ± 0.01 (13)
Tuberculoid or borderline tuberculoid leprosy	3075.0 ± 61.1 (30)	569.4 ± 19.4 (25)	0.181 ± 0.05 (25)
Borderline lepromatous leprosy	2985.6 ± 69.9 (33)	521.0 ± 26.4 (26)	0.173 ± 0.01 (26)
Lepromatous leprosy	2558.1 ± 60.5 (21)	362.0 ± 19.1 (15)	0.144 ± 0.01 (15)

Numbers of observations are shown in parenthesis. SEM = standard error of the mean.

babies born to leprous parents were healthy at birth, but would not remain free of leprosy unless they were separated from their parents at birth and brought up in a healthy environment with wholesome feeding. This observation was confirmed 100 years later and led to the practice of separation of children from leprous parents, and, to prevent pregnancy, segregation of the sexes unless the leprosy had become quiescent or, in certain cases, voluntary sterilization had been carried out.

In 1897 Zambaco[26] described infants of leprous mothers as small 'like an abortion at term' and 'born like little old men, they do not develop but succumb to athrepsie without showing any sign on their body of leprosy. This foetal cachexia which leads to death *in utero*, or shortly after birth without diagnostic lesions is certainly due to leprosy.' In 1922, it was noted that the children of leprous parents, in addition to the common ailments, had many skin diseases and a very high infant mortality, with 42 per cent of the children dying of infections, debility, and marasmus.[11]

Recent reports from Vietnam and the USA record 30 and 23 per cent premature births in women with leprosy, especially lepromatous leprosy. Retrospectively, it is impossible to assess whether what is reported is true 'prematurity' or 'dysmaturity', namely infants born 'small for gestational age'.

In a comprehensive prospective study, it was noted that the babies of mothers with leprosy grew more slowly *in utero* than did the babies of healthy mothers living in the same environment. This intrauterine growth retardation (IUGR) was most marked in the babies of mothers with lepromatous (LL and BL) leprosy and was detected as early as the sixteenth week of pregnancy. The clinical observation was confirmed by the oestriol excretion.

Babies of mothers with leprosy weighed less than those of healthy mothers: the placental weights and coefficients (placental coefficient = weight of trimmed placenta divided by the birth weight of baby) followed

the same trend. There was no statistical difference between the different groups of mothers with regard to their age, height, weight, skin fold thickness, haemoglobin level or gravidity. The reduced feto-placental weight and reduced oestriol excretion was not related to the severity of the mother's leprosy in terms of bacterial infection nor to her antileprosy drug treatment, but to her immune status. The smallest babies were born to mothers with inactive, quiescent lepromatous leprosy. Fetal distress or Apgar scores of less than 4 at one minute after birth were recorded in 20 per cent of the babies of BL and LL mothers.[28]

Babies of mothers with leprosy grew more slowly, were more susceptible to infections and had a higher infant mortality rate than babies of healthy mothers. This was most marked in babies of mothers with lepromatous leprosy. Two children developed overt leprosy, with histological confirmation and spontaneous healing.

The clinical and pathological evidence so far reviewed falls short of clear proof of the intrauterine transmission of infection. The occasional diagnosis of leprosy in children aged three years or less might indicate either very heavy exposure or infection *in utero*. Possible routes by which these children were infected are skin-to-skin contact, breast-milk, inhalation of droplets from the mother's nasal secretions, or transplacentally. Droplet infection is now considered to be the usual route of spread of *M. leprae*. However, one could expect this 'normal' transmission of infection to cause leprosy with a normal incubation period. For babies aged 12–17 months to develop a disease whose incubation period is usually about four years predicates very heavy exposure, an unusual route of infection, or both. The placenta is highly vascular, and even minor breaches of its integrity might allow the passage of large numbers of *M. leprae* to the fetus.[29]

Hitherto, it has been almost impossible to evaluate placental transmission of *M. leprae*. Now, however, antibody tests are available and used as diagnostic tests for leprosy before there are any clinical manifestations of active disease.

In a recent prospective study[29] it was shown that cord blood immunoglobulin A (IgA) was significantly increased in babies of mothers with lepromatous leprosy. IgA anti-*M. leprae* antibodies were present in 30 per cent of cord sera of babies of mothers with active lepromatous leprosy. There was evidence of active production of specific IgA and IgM anti-*M. leprae* antibody during the first six months of life of babies of mothers with active lepromatous leprosy.[30] The prevalence of leprosy in children under two years of age whose mothers had active lepromatous leprosy was 5 per cent (2/38), a figure comparable with that reported by other workers.[19]

Clinical diagnosis of leprosy in the two children who developed leprosy in this study[29] was confirmed by biopsy. Both children had positive skin tests to *M. leprae*, and a marked increase in IgA and IgM anti-*M. leprae* antibody activity during the first three years of life. A third baby with a transient skin lesion of leprosy of four months duration but no biopsy, and a negative skin test also showed a rise in antibody activity. These children were thought to have been infected *in utero*.

In view of the association between intrauterine growth retardation, low birth weight, failure to thrive, increased infant mortality and maternal leprosy, particularly LL and BL, one might postulate that, in the past, those children who should have developed leprosy at an early age following infection *in utero* had died before the disease could be made manifest. This would then explain the lack of case reports in the early literature.

Other reasons for the failure to report early cases in children are:

- Leprosy may be present without the parents being aware that anything is wrong.
- The lesions may be so small and transient that they are missed unless special efforts are made to find them.
- Leprosy in young children is often self-healing and therefore overlooked.
- Nerve involvement causing sensory or motor loss, so often an early symptom in adult leprosy, frequently does not occur in children.
- Leprosy may masquerade as other skin diseases and *vice versa*.

Breast-feeding in leprosy

Maternal milk may be a possible source of infection for babies. There have been isolated reports of a child born to healthy parents who was 'wet-nursed', i.e. breast-fed by a nurse or another woman who later was found to have leprosy, after the child she cared for developed the disease. In the pre-antibiotic era children separated from their leprous parents at birth, or breast-fed by their mothers who were carefully gowned and masked, were less likely to develop leprosy, indicating that droplet infection from lactating mothers may be equally important.

While high counts of *M. leprae* in breast-milk were reported for a few patients with active, untreated lepromatous leprosy, a larger study failed to corroborate this.[10] Two recent studies show what at first glance may be conflicting results. But one thing is clear, when a woman is receiving effective treatment for her leprosy, breast-feeding causes minimal risk to the child. It appears that heavy breast-milk infection requires advanced leprosy with the disease involving the nipple and milk ducts. What is probably of more significance is the level of defence factors in human milk. Recently, in studies on breast-milk it was shown that there was no significant variation in levels of secretory IgA, lactoferrin, albumin or total protein between women with leprosy and healthy controls. Specific anti-*M. leprae* antibodies were not measured. (For review see Ref. 31.)

It is important to note that when a child in the tropics or subtropics is *not* breast-fed by its mother it stands a very good chance of dying of gastroenteritis.

Women with leprosy should be encouraged to breast feed their children whenever possible, even using expressed breast-milk, especially during the early puerperium when the levels of secretory IgA and other defence factors are at their highest. They should be told that:

- They must continue to take their antileprosy antibiotic treatment regularly.
- The leprosy drugs do not harm the baby.
- The antibiotics will be transferred through the breast-milk to the baby.
- Clofazimine (Lampren) will have the effect of turning the mother's milk pink (the colour of strawberry icecream). This will be especially noticeable when expressed milk is stored in a refrigerator, or when the baby vomits the milk up after a feed. There is nothing whatever wrong with this; the baby is not being harmed.

If a woman with leprosy cannot, or will not breast-feed her baby, the paediatrician should enquire 'Why not?' It may be that the woman has some problem with her leprosy which needs urgent attention.

The effect of pregnancy on the mother's leprosy

Pregnancy causes a non-specific immunosuppression, therefore:

- The first signs of leprosy may appear in association with pregnancy or during lactation.
- Pre-existing leprosy is made worse, new lesions may develop, BI and MI may increase.
- Patients with 'cured' leprosy relapse with active disease.
- There is a tendency to 'downgrade' during pregnancy.
- Even patients taking apparently effective treatment for leprosy are affected.
- Approximately half of pregnant leprosy patients show this phenomenon, which is most marked during the last three months of pregnancy.

Pregnancy is associated with alteration of immune status, suppression of CMI during pregnancy and recovery of CMI afterwards. Therefore, one must look for leprosy reactions in pregnant and lactating women:

- Type 1 (reversal) reaction occurs typically in the puerperium, often about 40 days after delivery. There may be a dramatic onset. Literally overnight, the mother may have facial, ulnar or median palsy or foot drop. These conditions will be permanent unless treated promptly, and affect her ability to care for her child.
- ENL occurs in early pregnancy, and then from the third trimester onwards for up to one-and-a-half years. During the acute episodes the mother may feel very ill indeed, and be unable to care for her child.
- Leprosy neuritis is a very serious complication of both of these forms of reaction. It may present as acute nerve pain or tenderness, in which case it is easy to diagnose.
- Leprosy neuritis may occur as a 'silent' condition with only one warning symptom 'rheumatic pain' or 'limb pains'. This pain may be so severe that the mother cannot hold or carry her baby.
- Immediate treatment is necessary to prevent permanent nerve damage and deformity, prednisolone being required for many cases of reversal reaction and most cases of leprosy neuritis.

As the mother may be too busy caring for her baby/children to attend the leprosy hospital/clinic for her own treatment, the paediatrician is a key person in the supervision of mothers with leprosy. The paediatrician should be aware of the problems and check that:

- The pregnant mother is receiving multidrug therapy.
- She is attending for regular follow-up, and has told the leprosy health workers that she is pregnant.
- She is receiving treatment for reaction/neuritis.
- She is not receiving thalidomide, however indicated for the treatment of leprosy (especially ENL), because of its serious teratotoxic effect.
- If the condition is worsening despite treatment, she is referred back for:
  - urgent review
  - possible steroid treatment/admission
  - exclusion of other diseases, e.g. TB which may be the cause of very persistent ENL.

Clinical presentation

The purpose of this section is to provide the basic essentials for the general practising paediatrician.

Symptoms

In early leprosy there may be no symptoms whatosever, other than a small patch of recent origin which may be paler or redder than normal skin. Even this may not have been observed by parent or child and may be picked up at a routine examination such as at a school health clinic. Other early symptoms include:

- anaesthesia (numbness) in the patch, hands or feet;
- paraesthesiae (pins-and-needles or tingling) in hands or feet;
- burning sensation in the skin;
- slight weakness in hands, feet, face (including eyes).

Later symptoms include:

- more and larger skin patches;
- skin nodules, singly or in crops;
- more weakness or obvious paralysis of muscles of hands, feet and face;
- painless injuries, cuts, cracks, burns or ulcers of hands or feet.

Constitutional symptoms, headaches, general malaise, etc. are not symptoms of leprosy. A few patients may present with leprosy in reaction. This is not common among children, but for the sake of completeness the symptoms include:

Reversal reaction

- painful red, shiny skin patches (Fig. 4.6.6);
- limb pains or 'rheumatism' which may be very severe;
- muscle weakness or paralysis of recent onset.

ENL

- general malaise;
- fever, up to 41°C;
- crops of painful red nodules in the skin;
- symptoms last for 3–5 days and recur at intervals of 2–3 weeks.

Signs

Skin lesions

The skin lesions of leprosy in a light-skinned child appear redder than normal skin. In a deeply pigmented child the lesions may be hypopigmented or sometimes copper coloured. Look for:

- Hypopigmented patches with margins which may be hazy and ill-defined, or well-defined, usually single but occasionally multiple, without sensory loss, transient, self-healing (indeterminate leprosy, Fig. 4.6.9).
- Patches (macules), large or small, paler or redder than normal skin. Usually in children, on the trunk, thigh, or upper arm (tuberculoid, Figs 4.6.5 and 4.6.10).
- Small or large areas of diffuse hyperaemia with no loss of sensation (prelepromatous).
- Smooth shiny skin (early lepromatous).
- Patchy hypopigmentation (early BL).
- Numerous symmetrical copper coloured or reddish macules (early macular LL leprosy, Fig. 4.6.11).
- Nodules singly or in crops, on lower third of earlobes, extensor surfaces of arms and legs (elbows, knees, backs of hands, buttocks), (late lepromatous, Figs 4.6.12 and 4.6.13).

Evidence of nerve involvement/damage

- Loss of light touch sensation (using a wisp of cotton wool), in hypopigmented patches (TT or BT, early or late).
- Dry and/or insensitive hands and feet (late tuberculoid or lepromatous).
- Palpably thickened (enlarged, tender, visible) nerve trunks, especially facial, great auricular, radial, median, ulnar, radial cutaneous, peroneal and posterior tibial (Fig. 4.6.14).
- Obvious paralysis/contractures (late, Fig. 4.6.7).
- Obvious cracks/ulceration of hands and feet (late).
- Eyes: loss of sensation of conjunctiva, conjunctivitis, lagophthalmos, iritis, keratitis, blurring of vision – refer immediately to a specialist.

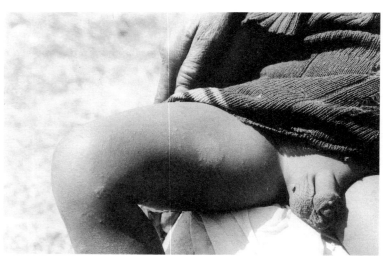

Fig. 4.6.9 Ethiopian child born to mother with active BL leprosy during pregnancy. A hypopigmented slightly raised macule with a clearly defined margin. Lesions of a generalized scabies infection are also visible. Classification strictly indeterminate, but histological features pointed to tuberculoid leprosy.

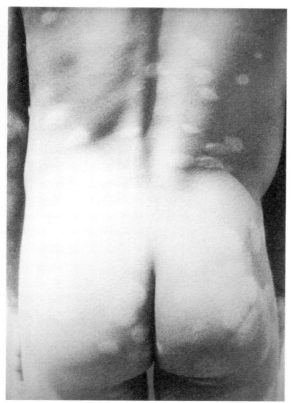

Fig. 4.6.10   Zambian child with numerous dry, well-defined, hypopigmented, anaesthetic lesions. Several nerves were also involved. BT leprosy. (Courtesy of Dr AC McDougall.)

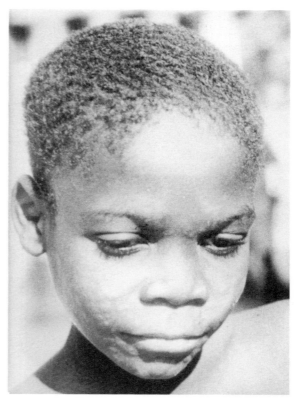

Fig. 4.6.12   Sudanese child with active lepromatous leprosy (nodular LL). (Courtesy of Dr AC McDougall.)

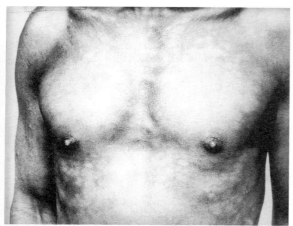

Fig. 4.6.11   Numerous coalescing, symmetrical copper coloured macules. Early lepromatous (macular LL) leprosy. Treatment at this stage will prevent development of nodular LL (Figs 4.6.12 and 4.6.13). (Courtesy of Dr AC McDougall.)

Examination of the child

The child must be examined in reasonable privacy in a well-lit room or in full daylight. The child's clothes should be taken off as far as local customs permit, ideally leaving on only the underpants which can be drawn down to allow examination of the buttocks. The child should be turned slowly so that the skin can be examined with full lighting, also with side-lighting, essential to pick up small differences in pigmentation or shininess of the skin, and slightly elevated skin lesions. The skin should be palpated with the flat of the hand and fingers, to detect changes in skin texture, and dryness of palms of hands or soles of feet.

Loss of light touch sensation is detected using a wisp of cotton wool for the centre of patches and the surrounding skin. Loss of protective sensation is detected using a nylon bristle with sufficient pressure to indent the skin of the palm or fingers, and for the feet, a ball point pen to indent the skin of the soles and the toes.

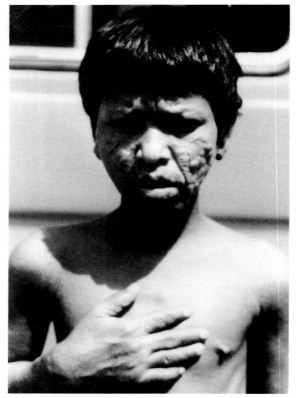

Fig. 4.6.13   Indian boy with active nodular lepromatous leprosy (LL) just beginning treatment. (Courtesy of Dr AC McDougall.)

Peripheral nerve trunks are palpated where they lie close to the skin (Fig. 4.6.14).

All health workers can be trained to carry out this examination and they become expert in following up little hints dropped by parents that indicate some departure from normal.

If the child has a generalized skin infestation such as scabies masking the skin lesions of leprosy, it is advisable to treat the generalized skin infestation/infection first and then to re-assess the child a week or two later for signs of leprosy.

The three pathognomonic features of leprosy

There are three cardinal signs of leprosy. Usually more than one is present, but the diagnosis is certain, even if only one of these signs is definitely there:

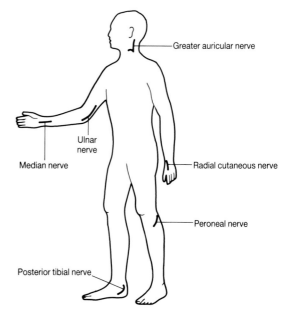

Fig. 4.6.14   Places where enlarged nerves can be felt. (Courtesy of Drs HW Wheate and JMH Pearson from *A Practical Guide to the Diagnosis and Treatment of Leprosy in the Basic Health Unit*, German Leprosy Relief Association for ALERT.)

- Loss of or diminished sensation in a skin patch/macule tested using a wisp of cotton wool.
- Enlargement of peripheral nerves.
- Presence of acid-fast mycobacteria in the skin, as demonstrated with a skin smear (BI, MI).

The flow-chart used at ALERT, Addis Ababa, is helpful (Fig. 4.6.15).

Whenever there is a suspicion that a child may have leprosy, it is helpful to draw the initial lesions on a body chart. The chart should show front and back views of the body. There should be a space to record the state of the nerves (normal/tender/enlarged). Any evidence of nerve function deficit (sensory/motor), i.e. anaesthesia, paralysis, injury or deformity due to these should be recorded. The chart should also show the sites of the skin smears and biopsy (if any).

Diagnostic tests

Slit skin smears for bacteriological index (BI) and morphological index (MI) are the most important of all and can be done with very little equipment under field conditions. Smears are usually made from both ears, and four other sites, edges of patches, or nodules if possible, otherwise elbows, knees, dorsal aspect of middle finger.

Patient's complaints Early – small patch. Numbness or tingling burning sensation in the skin. Slight weakness.
Later – more, larger patches. Injuries etc. Obvious nodules. Severe weakness, paralysis.

Main clinical
findings in
skin:

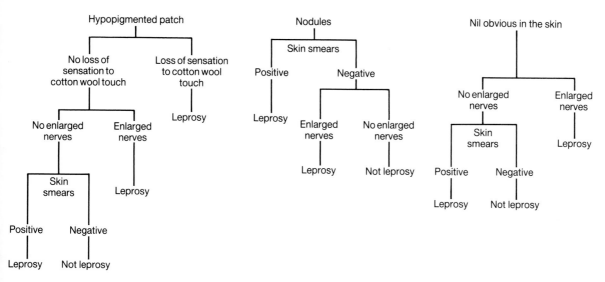

Fig. 4.6.15 Flow chart for diagnosis of previously untreated cases of leprosy. (Courtesy of Drs HW Wheate and JMH Pearson from *A Practical Guide to the Diagnosis and Treatment of Leprosy in the Basic Health Unit*, German Leprosy Relief Association for ALERT.)

Skin biopsy, either an elliptical scalpel biopsy taken from and at right angles to the margin of a macule (TT and BT), or a punch biopsy taken from a nodule or macule of a BL or LL patient, e.g. from the buttock where no scar will be visible.

Nerve biopsy for difficult cases with nerve involvement where skin biopsy is uninformative or unexpected. Note that the biopsy should be a longitudinal biopsy of a nerve bundle not a transverse section.

Lepromin skin test. Read at 48–72 hours this is known as the Fernandez (or early response) reaction. Read after three or four weeks, it is known as the Mitsuda (late) reaction.

Serological, lymphocyte transformation/migration tests are available only in research institutions.

Other tests which should be done at the first visit, or as soon after diagnosis as possible, are tests of sensory and motor function, especially for the eyes, hands and feet to provide a disability grading.[32]

Classification of leprosy

This is made on grounds of clinical findings (Table 4.6.2) and BI. Classification of leprosy at the earliest possible occasion is important because:

- The course and progress of the disease, and type of reaction, if any, can be anticipated.
- Correct treatment can be given from the outset, and for the appropriate duration.
- Infectious cases can be identified and treated quickly, thus preventing disruption to schooling.
- Specific health education can be given.

Special features of leprosy in children

- In young children the lesions are often very small and may only be seen using a hand lens (magnifying glass).
- In young children leprosy tends to be of the indeterminate or tuberculoid form (Fig. 4.6.9). The patches are often single and tend to disappear spontaneously (undergo self-healing) after four to six months. In very young children these lesions may be watched, but in older children a full course of treatment should be given.

Table 4.6.2. Clinical classification of leprosy

Classification	Indeterminate	TT	BT	BB	BL	LL
Skin lesions:						
Number	1–3	1–5	5–25	>25	Innumerable	Innumerable
Type	Patch pale	Patch pale/red	Patch pale/red, satellite	Patch/dome	Patch red/ Nodules	Nodules/ flat patch raised patch thick skin
Edge	Ill-defined, irregular hazy	Defined regular/ irregular	Defined regular/ irregular	Defined	Defined/ill-defined	
Centre		Healing	Some healing	'Punched out'		
Profile	Flat	Raised/flat	Raised/flat	Raised	Raised/flat	Raised/flat
Surface		Dry	Dry			
Distribution		Asymmetrical	Symmetrical	Less symmetrical than BT	Less symmetrical than LL generalized (late)	Symmetrical generalized (late)
Sensory loss (lesion)	±	+ + +	+			
Nerve trunk involvement	No	1–2 (early)	Often (early)	Yes/No (variable)	Yes (asymmetrical)	Yes many (late)
Deformity			Severe: face/hands/ feet			
Other organs						Eyes/hands feet/ testicles
Skin smears	−	−	− usually	+	+ + + (lesions) − (elsewhere)	+ + +
Lepromin reaction	±	+ + +	+ + +	−	−	−
Leprosy reaction		Type 1* (reversal) reaction	Type 1 (reversal) reaction	Type 1 (reversal) reaction	Type 1 (reversal) reaction Type 2 reaction (ENL)	Type 1† (reversal) reaction Type 2 reaction (ENL)

* Occurs in TTs (subpolar tuberculoid leprosy).
† Occurs in LLs (subpolar lepromatous leprosy).

- Following the BCG immunization campaigns, it has been observed recently that the first sign of leprosy may be the appearance of a tuberculoid macule in the vicinity of the BCG scar.
- A child with a large number of patches (>25) with negative skin smears (BI = 0) should have a biopsy done as the child is likely to be BL or LL.
- A safe rule in children is to err on the side of classifying the child one step further along the scale towards the lepromatous end of the spectrum, compared with the classification of an adult with the same lesions, to ensure that the child receives adequate treatment (R. G. Cochrane, unpublished observation).
- Children with leprosy, especially early leprosy, usually do very well and tolerate treatment without problems.
- Children who do not have any disability grading when they start treatment, are very unlikely (<2 per cent) to develop any disability if they are put immediately on to full multidrug therapy, with prednisolone should they develop neuritis.
- Any child who has a disability grading (evidence of loss of sensory or motor nerve function) should be referred to a leprosy treatment centre for treatment under supervision. If the disability has been present for less than six months it is likely that there will be very considerable improvement with steroid therapy in addition to multidrug therapy. Thereafter surgical treatment for deformities can be

carried out, as a planned procedure once the disease is quiescent.

- If the disease is neglected, except in the early self-healing indeterminate form, peripheral nerves are liable to extensive damage, even in young children. Insensitive hands and feet easily become traumatized, ulcers develop, deep infection involves small bones of the hands and feet. Fingers and toes become progressively shortened as sequestra from the phalanges are extruded, and bony absorption occurs. Muscle paralysis leads to contractures. Paralysis of the eye muscles results in lagophthalmos, exposure keratitis and eventually blindness. When a child who has lost sensation in his hands becomes blind, his future is bleak – he becomes a beggar (Fig. 4.6.16).

Management

As long as the child's general health is good, he/she should be treated in the community and allowed to mix with family and friends. The child will be non-infectious within a few days of first taking rifampicin and so is not a danger to other people. There is no need to report to school authorities that the child is receiving treatment for leprosy.

If the child has neuritis or sensory loss associated with leprosy reaction when the disease is diagnosed, a short period of time in hospital is advisable:

- to watch the initial response to drug treatment;
- to assess the response to steroids;
- to teach the child how to care for insensitive hands and feet, exercises to mobilize stiff joints, and other health education.

When leprosy is diagnosed, specific antibiotic treatment should be started. Until recently, treatment has been dapsone monotherapy. However, with low dosage and irregular therapy together with poor patient compliance and initial misclassification of leprosy, e.g. BL as BT, dapsone resistance both primary and secondary has become a world-wide problem. The basis of modern treatment is multidrug therapy (MDT). The objectives of MDT are:

- to make the patient non-infectious as quickly as possible;
- to cure the disease and prevent nerve damage;
- to prevent the emergence of drug resistance;
- to deal as far as possible with dormant but drug-sensitive bacilli.

Since it is impossible to predict which cases of early leprosy will proceed to self-healing, all children with a

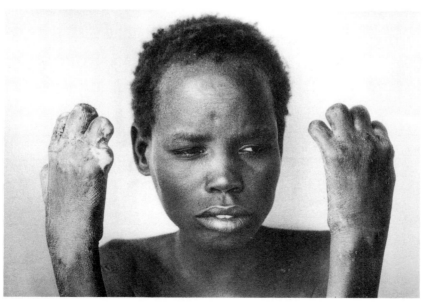

Fig. 4.6.16 Sudanese child, partially blind and with neuropathic hands – late results of neglected nerve damage in BT leprosy. (Courtesy of Dr AC McDougall.)

definite diagnosis of leprosy should be treated. While this may not always be strictly necessary, the boost to the leprosy service and the advertising value of cured disease is considerable.

Treatment regimens

Paucibacillary leprosy – two drugs

- rifampicin, monthly, supervised;
- dapsone, daily, unsupervised;
- duration of treatment – six months.

Multibacillary leprosy (including biopsy proven cases of BB, BL and LL even though their BI is zero) – three drugs

- rifampicin, monthly, supervised;
- dapsone, daily, unsupervised;
- clofazimine, monthly, supervised and daily/weekly according to age, unsupervised;
- duration of treatment – at least two years and for six months after the BI = 0 (i.e. leprosy bacilli are no longer found in the routine skin smear).

For details see Table 4.6.3.[33]

These regimens should not be interrupted (as happened frequently in the past) for leprosy reaction. Episodes of acute reaction should be treated with anti-inflammatory drugs (see below).

The child and/or accompanying relative should be told:

- Leprosy is not the dreaded disease it used to be.
- Tablets are better than injections for curing leprosy.
- The duration of the treatment.
- If there is no disability present at the start of treatment, it is unlikely to develop.
- In lepromatous (BL and LL) patients, anaesthesia of hands and feet without deformity is very likely to recover if full treatment is taken.
- Anaesthesia with deformity present before the start of treatment may not be cured by drug treatment alone, but there are other forms of treatment available.
- The patient must report immediately if anything seems to be wrong, in particular if pain develops in patches, arms or legs.
- Any other member of the family who has a condition that might be early leprosy should come immediately for examination/treatment.

Any questions the child or mother may have should be answered.

Routine clinic observations

At each monthly visit check:

- that the treatment prescribed is being taken, if not,

Table 4.6.3. Recommended dosage of antileprosy drugs in milligrams based on age of children. (Reproduced with permission from Rees RJW, *Leprosy Review*, 1984; **32**: 79–82, LEPRA.)

Paucibacillary leprosy (2 drugs – dapsone and rifampicin)

Age groups	Dapsone: daily dose, unsupervised	Rifampicin: monthly dose, supervised
Up to 5 years	25	150–300
6–14 years	50–100	300–450
15 years and above*	100	600

Multibacillary leprosy (3 drugs – dapsone, rifampicin and clofazimine)

Age groups	Dapsone: daily dose, unsupervised	Rifampicin: monthly dose, supervised	Clofazimine	
			Unsupervised dose	Monthly dose supervised
Up to 5 years	25	150–300	100 once weekly	100
6–14 years	50–100	300–450	150 once weekly	150–200
15 years and above*	100	600	50 daily	300

The MDT is as recommended by WHO; it is assumed that clofazimine is acceptable for young children and therefore no children will require ethionamide/prothionamide.

Where a range of doses is given this relates to age range of the children; those near the lower age range receive the lower dose and those near the upper age range receive the higher dose.

* i.e. use adult doses.

why not. A random urine test to measure dapsone is of use to confirm that treatment is being taken – do not tell the child in advance why the test is being done.[34, 35]

- for evidence of reaction:
  – redness or swelling of the skin lesions
  – painful swelling of the hands and feet
  – painful red eyes, tearing (lacrimation) or photophobia
  – loss of sensation, or new dryness of hands or feet
  – weakness of muscles of face, hands or feet, or foot drop
  – tender nerves

If yes, the child needs careful assessment – refer to a specialist leprosy clinic (see below).

- Is there evidence of trauma to insensitive skin: ulcers or cracks on hands or feet? Refer for surgery.
- Does the child need special shoes?
- If the child has special shoes, are they being worn?
- If insoles were prescribed, are they being used?
- Do the shoes show signs of wear and tear, indicating that they are being worn? Do they need replacing?
- Is the child taking good care of eyes, hands and feet?

Skin smears for BI and MI should be repeated at six month intervals, more frequently if new lesions appear.

If a mother brings a child for leprosy treatment, the paediatrician should automatically enquire of the mother:

- Has she got leprosy? If yes:
  – is she on treatment? Which antileprotics is she taking?
  – does she have drug-resistant leprosy? Her child could have the same.
- Is she pregnant again?
- Is she lactating?
  – is she carrying a baby on her back?
  – is another child carrying the baby for the mother because the lactating mother is too sick to carry the baby herself?
- Has she got any other children? They need to be examined for signs of leprosy.

Treatment of reactions

Ideally refer to specialist leprosy clinic. If this is not possible treat as follows:

Type 1 (reversal) reaction If there is severe neuritis, or marked loss of motor/sensory function:

- admit to hospital;

- keep on full MDT regimen;
- start corticosteroids, dosage 1 mg/kg per day (prednisolone); give this high dose for four weeks, or until symptoms and nerve function show improvement, then gradually reduce the dosage over 4–6 weeks;
- splints may be required to maintain the position of paralysed hands or feet, until motor function recovers;
- eyes may require special protection and treatment.

Type 2 reaction (ENL) With the routine use of clofazimine, there should be less ENL than was formerly seen. Most cases of ENL can be treated as outpatients, but more severe cases require admission:

- continue MDT treatment regimen;
- use simple analgesics, e.g. aspirin;
- if ENL is very severe or persistent try thalidomide, or if the child is not on clofazimine, start clofazimine in high dosage 25, 50 or 100 mg three times a day according to age <5, 6–14, 15 years, gradually reducing to standard MDT dosage when the child is free of ENL for 4–6 weeks;
- if there is loss of nerve function, prednisolone should be used (normally it should not be used for skin ENL although it is very effective).

Health education

At an early age and stage, the child should be taught the following:

- Eye exercises, closing the eyes 15 times three times a day.
- Dry hands and feet must be soaked in water every day, patted dry, then petroleum jelly, baby oil (or cooking oil) is applied to retain moisture.
- If the feet are insensitive, footwear must be worn – sandals with a microcellular insole, and a 1.5 cm microcellular rubber sole, to protect against damage from thorns, broken glass, etc.; alternatively, canvas shoes two sizes larger than required can be fitted with microcellular insoles.
- Plastic shoes should not be worn.
- Care should be taken regarding hot cooking stoves, pots and utensils, and with garden, agricultural and building implements and thorny branches.
- Minor injuries should receive prompt first-aid.
- Girls should be watched particularly carefully as they reach the menarche, as the hormonal effects may adversely affect their leprosy if it is not well controlled.

Prognosis

If the diagnosis of leprosy is made early, and the child adequately treated, cure can be confidently expected and deformity prevented. As in the treatment of tuberculosis, patient compliance is very important. This may be improved by increased doctor–patient contact. It is particularly important that the medical staff, doctors, nurses and health workers speak to, touch and handle the child.

Nerve damage in lepromatous leprosy, due to direct damage to dermal nerves by *M. leprae* dividing within Schwann cells will tend to get better with drug treatment, and full recovery of sensation may well occur. Even when irreversible nerve damage is present at the first attendance, much can be done to prevent extension of the results of nerve damage and to minimize its consequences. Protective footwear, physiotherapy, reconstructive surgery and vocational training may all help to preserve the personality of the child and to ensure that the child takes, or resumes a place in society (S. G. Browne, personal communication).

Prevention and control

The best means of control is to identify the people, adults and children, with infectious disease, and treat them as quickly as possible with MDT to ensure that they are non-infectious.

Contact tracing and regular examination of babies of mothers with leprosy may well enable the detection of early leprosy. This, however, needs to be done very sensitively so that fear is not aroused. Examination of siblings is worth doing at 3–6 month intervals.

A great deal of research work is going on to produce a vaccine that is both specific and safe. While BCG alone may induce some degree of protection, it is more likely to result in children who have early indeterminate leprosy presenting with tuberculoid leprosy. At present a combination of (live) BCG and various antigenic components of armadillo-derived *M. leprae* seems to offer the best hope of inducing CMI, as shown by lepromin skin test conversion. Other possible vaccines made from some of the naturally occurring mycobacteria are under investigation.

Chemoprophylaxis, with an antimycobacterial drug like dapsone has no place in the modern approach to leprosy control.

The unborn child receives antileprosy drugs transplacentally, as well as *M. leprae*. Hence, it is of the utmost importance to ensure that every pregnant woman with leprosy is receiving MDT during her pregnancy. No teratotoxic effects have been recorded with any of the three standard drugs, although the manufacturers do not advocate their use during the first trimester. Dapsone has been safely used in thousands of pregnancies and therefore should be given throughout pregnancy. Clofazimine and rifampicin should be given from the start of the second trimester. This would effectively reduce the relapse rate, and the number of viable bacilli which could pass the placental barrier to the fetus in the second half of pregnancy. At the same time it would probably reduce the amount of ENL seen in the third trimester and after delivery. The problem of drugs in the first trimester is probably more hypothetical than real, as it is very likely that many women would have received MDT (where this is routinely given) in the first trimester of pregnancy, before they realized that they were pregnant.

Many women, especially in rural Africa, continue to lactate well into the next pregnancy and thus are amenorrhoeic during much of their reproductive lives. Antileprosy drugs are also passed into the breast-milk and thence to the baby. It should be noted that the breast-fed baby of a mother receiving clofazimine frequently has a reddish skin, as the crystals of clofazimine are stored in fat cells of the baby's skin.

Clearly, in an ideal situation, one would like to see reduced numbers of children in each family, better spacing (wise use of contraception) and better diet with increased total protein for both mother and child. In turn this would ensure better quality of maternal milk for the baby. Furthermore, as already discussed, there is clear evidence that pregnancy is a major hazard for the woman with leprosy – the women themselves recognize this. Thus, an overall reduction in the family size would benefit not only 'healthy' women living in the tropics and subtropics, but especially those women with leprosy. Because of the additional risk of a leprous woman infecting her child during and immediately after pregnancy, these measures would have a beneficial effect on leprosy control.

Primary health care includes leprosy. Health workers should not only have a basic knowledge of leprosy, and be able to diagnose it, but should have ready access to expert diagnostic assistance and advice. The more the community is involved, the better the patient compliance. Thus, the primary health worker is a key person in the treatment of leprosy. Such a person can travel by mule or bicycle from market to market, covering a wide area of the community in places where the weekly market is the chief meeting place, or the health worker can work within a more restricted area. On the whole, however, the primary health worker, especially the conscientious one, has far too much to do to carry the major burden of leprosy treatment in addition to his other regular duties.

Acknowledgements

I wish to thank Mrs Wilma Nicholson for secretarial assistance; Dr G. A. Ellard for details of testing for dapsone in urine; the Medical Photography Department of Edinburgh University; and Drs W. H. Jopling, A. C. McDougall, R. B. Mackay and C. R. Maddock for helpful criticism.

Further reading

Bryceson A and Pfaltzgeff RE. *Leprosy* 3rd edn. Edinburgh, Churchill Livingstone, 1990.

Jopling WH. *Handbook of Leprosy*, 4th edn. London, Heinemann Medical Books, 1988.

Hastings RC (ed.) *Leprosy*. Edinburgh, Churchill Livingstone, 1985.

The above are standard texts which deal with general aspects of leprosy, but do not deal with leprosy in children. Hastings's book is a much more detailed text, more suited as a reference book than a handbook for daily use.

Ridley DS. *Skin Biopsy in Leprosy*, 2nd edn. Basle, Documenta Geigy, Ciba-Geigy, 1985.

This is a short, well-illustrated handbook of the histopathology of leprosy, unique in that it also correlates the histopathology with the clinical features; essential for anyone having to do their own leprosy histopathology.

Further details of referenced material can be obtained from references 1, 25 and 31 listed below. References to historical aspects of leprosy and child-bearing and leprosy in young children are to be found in Ref. 1 (93 refs) and Ref. 25 (50 refs). Ref. 31 is a short review of the effects of the mother's leprosy on her child, including some basic perspectives in leprosy (162 refs).

References

1. Duncan ME. Leprosy and procreation: a historical review of social and clinical aspects. *Leprosy Review*. 1985; **56**: 153–62.
2. Rastogi N and Rastogi RC. Leprosy in Ancient India. *International Journal of Leprosy*. 1984; **52**: 541–3.
3. Haidar Abu Ahmed Mohamed. Leprosy – the Moslem attitude. *Leprosy Review*. 1985; **56**: 17–21.
4. Melsom R. Serodiagnosis of leprosy: the past, the present and some prospects for the future. *International Journal of Leprosy*. 1983; **51**: 235–52.
5. Serjeanson SW. HLA and susceptibility to leprosy. *Immunological Reviews*. 1983; **15**: 33–48.
6. Ridley DS. Reactions in leprosy. *Leprosy Review*. 1969; **40**: 77–81.
7. Wemambu SNC, Turk JL, Waters, MFR *et al.* Erythema nodosum leprosum: a clinical manifestation of the arthus phenomenon. *Lancet*. 1969; **ii**: 933–5.
8. Léonard G, Sangare A, Verdier M *et al.* Prevalence of HIV infection among patients with leprosy in African countries and Yemen. *Journal of Acquired Immune Deficiency Syndromes*. 1990; **3**: 1109–13.
9. World Health Organization. Guidelines for personnel involved in collection of skin smears in leprosy control programmes for the prevention and control of possible infection with HIV. WHO/CDS/Lep/87.1.
10. Rodrigues JN. Studies on early leprosy in children of lepers. *Philippine Journal of Science*. 1926; **31**: 115–45.
11. Gomez L, Basa JA, Nicolas C. Early lesions and the development and incidence of leprosy in the children of lepers. *Philippine Journal of Science*. 1922; **21** (3): 233–56.
12. Solis F, Wade HW. Bacteriological findings in children of lepers, with special reference to nasal lesions. *Journal of the Philippine Medical Association*. 1925; **5**: 365–9.
13. Chiyuto S. Early leprotic changes in children and their bearing on the transmission and evolution of the disease. *Monthly Bulletin of the Bureau of Health (Manila)*. 1933; **XIII**: 5–48.
14. Lara CB, De Vera B. Clinical observations with reference to leprosy in children of lepers. *Journal of the Philippine Medical Association*. 1935; **15**: 115–29.
15. Lara CB, De Vera B. Early leprosy in infants born of leprous parents with report of cases. *Journal of the Philippine Medical Association*. 1935; **15**: 252–7.
16. Nolasco JO, Lara CB. Histopathology of early lesions in fourteen children of lepers. I. Analysis of previous skin blemishes in relation to sites of biopsies and other positive and probable lesions. *Philippine Journal of Science*. 1940; **71**: 321–58.
17. Nolasco JO, Lara CB. Histology of clinically healed 'primary' lesions of leprosy in children of lepers. II. Their clinical progression and final resolution into healed scars: report of thirteen cases. *Monthly Bulletin of the Bureau of Health (Manila)*. 1948; **24**: 97–128.
18. Lara CB. Leprosy in infancy and childhood. *Monthly Bulletin of the Bureau of Health (Manila)*. 1948; **24**: 61–89.
19. Lara CB, Ignacio JL. Observations on leprosy among children born in the Culion leper colony during the pre-sulphone and sulphone periods. *Journal of the Philippine Medical Association*. 1956; **32**: 189–97.
20. Lara CB, Nolasco JO. Self-healing, or abortive and residual forms of childhood leprosy and their probable significance. *International Journal of Leprosy*. 1956; **24**: 245–63.

21. World Health Organization. *Chemotherapy of Leprosy for Control Programmes*. World Health Organization, Technical Report Series, 1982; 675.

22. Ridley DS, Jopling WH. Classification of leprosy according to immunity: a five-group system. *International Journal of Leprosy*. 1966; **34**: 255–73.

23. Ridley DS, Waters MFR. Significance of variations within lepromatous group. *Leprosy Review*. 1969; **40**: 143–52.

24. Ridley DS. Histological classification and the immunological spectrum of leprosy. *Bulletin WHO* 1974; **51**: 451–65.

25. Duncan ME. Leprosy in young children: past, present and future. *International Journal of Leprosy*. 1985; **53**: 468–73.

26. Zambaco DA. *Les Lepreux Ambulants de Constantinople*, Paris; Masson et Cie, 1897: 317.

27. Schillingii GG. *De Lepra Commentationes*. Batavorum, Lugduni. 1778; 34.

28. Duncan ME. Babies of mothers with leprosy have small placentae, low birth weights and grow slowly. *British Journal of Obstetrics and Gynaecology*. 1980; **87**: 471–79.

29. Duncan ME, Melsom R, Pearson JMH *et al*. A clinical and immunological study of four babies of mothers with lepromatous leprosy, two of whom developed leprosy in infancy. *International Journal of Leprosy*. 1983; **51**: 7–17.

30. Melsom R, Harboe M, Duncan ME. IgA, IgM and IgG anti-*M. leprae* antibodies in babies of leprosy mothers during the first 2 years of life. *Clinical and Experimental Immunology*. 1982; **49**: 532–42.

31. Duncan ME. Perspectives in leprosy. In Jelliffe DB, Jelliffe EFP eds. *Advances in International Maternal and Child Health*. Oxford University Press, 1985; **5**: 122–43.

32. World Health Organization WHO Expert Committee on Leprosy: Fourth Report. Classification of disabilities resulting from leprosy, for use in control projects. 1970. Technical Report Series 459. 26–31.

33. Rees RJW. The dosage of anti-leprosy drugs for children. *Leprosy Review*. 1984; **55**: 309.

34. Ellard GA. Profile of urinary dapsone/creatinine ratios after oral dosage with dapsone. *Leprosy Review*. 1980; **51**: 229–36.

35. Cheesbrough M. Microbiology Vol. II in *Medical Laboratory Manual for Tropical Countries. Tropical Health Technology*. Guildford, UK, Butterworths. 1984: 307–10.

CHAPTER 7

Bacterial, spirochaetal, chlamydial and rickettsial infections

David Mabey

Meningococcal disease

Epidemiology

Meningococcal disease occurs sporadically in all parts of the world. The infection is spread by droplets and the majority of those infected become asymptomatic naso-pharyngeal carriers. Outbreaks of disease frequently occur in communities where people live in close contact, for example Koranic schools, where the carriage rate may be extremely high.

In 1963, Lapeyssonnie described the 'meningitis belt' which extends across the savannah region of sub-saharan Africa from the Sudan to The Gambia.[1] Major epidemics of meningococcal meningitis occur in this region every few years, invariably in the dry season, and terminate abruptly with the onset of the rains. Those aged between 5 and 15 years are particularly at risk during epidemics, whereas at other times the majority of cases are aged less than 5 years.

Aetiology and pathogenesis

Neisseria meningitidis is a non-motile, oxidase-positive Gram-negative diplococcus. The majority of isolates from cases of invasive disease have a polysaccharide capsule. Since the capsule is often deficient in isolates from nasopharyngeal carriers, it is assumed to play a role in pathogenesis, probably by inhibiting phagocy-tosis. Nine capsular serogroups have been identified. Whereas most cases of meningitis in European countries are caused by serogroup B organisms, sero-group A is usually responsible for the major epidemics in Africa and South America.

The factors which determine whether invasive disease occurs in a nasopharyngeal carrier are poorly understood, but a hot dry environment appears to favour invasion. It is probable that complement plays a role in protection, since individuals deficient in the lytic components of complement are prone to recurrent meningococcal disease.

Clinical features

Invasive disease may lead to a fulminant septicaemia, in which death occurs within a few hours of the onset of fever; adrenal haemorrhage may be seen in such cases at postmortem. Alternatively, a chronic meningococcaemia may ensue with fever, a petechial rash best seen in the mucous membranes of dark-skinned patients, and sometimes arthritis. (Fig. 4.7.1) The majority of cases, however, result in meningococcal meningitis.

Meningococcal meningitis is characterized by headache, fever, photophobia, vomiting and neck stiffness. Petechiae are frequently present and herpetic oral lesions are often seen. Untreated, the mortality may be in excess of 70 per cent but with early appropriate treatment this may be reduced to 5 per cent or less. Thus a high index of suspicion is needed in an infant or child with any of these symptoms. Following treatment, recovery is usually rapid. Five to ten days after the onset of symptoms, as the antibody titre rises, an immune complex arthritis may occur, often accompanied by a petechial rash. This usually resolves spontaneously.

Complications

With late or inadequate treatment, neurological sequelae may be frequently seen, usually blindness or deafness due to cranial nerve damage.

Diagnosis

The diagnosis can usually be made by Gram stain of a CSF specimen; large numbers of polymorphs and Gram-negative diplococci are seen. Where facilities are available, CSF should also be cultured on chocolate agar at 37°C in a candle jar, and sensitivity determined.

A latex agglutination test has been developed for the detection of meningococcal polysaccharide antigen in CSF. This test is cheap, rapid and simple to perform, and has been used successfully in rural Nigerian hospitals lacking trained staff during an epidemic.[2]

Treatment

The majority of meningococcal isolates in most countries are now resistant to sulphonamides, which have no place in the treatment of meningococcal disease. Parenteral penicillin or chloramphenicol are the treatments of choice. If possible, penicillin should be given at a dose of 0.2 mg/kg per day in six divided doses i.v. or i.m. for five days; alternatively chloramphenicol may be given, 75 mg/kg per day in four divided doses, parenterally for 48 hours and then by mouth if there is no vomiting.

If this is impractical, comparable results have been obtained with a single-dose regimen in which an oily suspension of chloramphenicol (Tifomycin, Roussel) is given in the following dosage: 0–2 years, 1 g; 3–6 years, 1.5 g; 7–10 years, 2 g; 11–14 years, 2.5 g; 15 + years, 3 g.

Prevention

This falls into two categories: treatment of carriers and contacts, and vaccination.

Treatment of carriers and contacts In the past, sulphonamides have been successfully used to control outbreaks of meningococcal disease. They eliminate

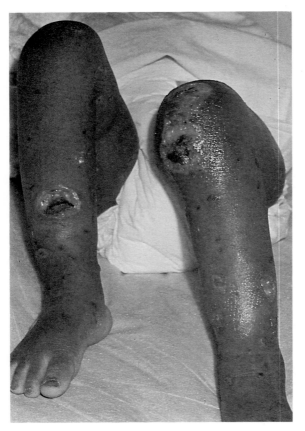

Fig. 4.7.1 Petechial rash and haemorrhage ulceration of the skin as a result of a vasculitis from chronic meningococcal septicaemia.

nasopharyngeal carriage of sensitive strains. Unfortunately the majority of isolates in tropical areas are now resistant to them, which has greatly limited their effectiveness. Rifampicin 10 mg/kg twice daily for two days will eradicate nasopharyngeal carriage. Resistance may develop, however; it is expensive and it is doubtful whether short courses of rifampicin should be widely dispensed in areas where tuberculosis is prevalent.

An alternative is to administer penicillin to close contacts. This does not eradicate nasopharyngeal carriage but has been shown in Norway to reduce the number of secondary cases. Preliminary results from The Gambia suggest that a single dose of long-acting penicillin (Triplopen) is effective.[3]

Vaccination Meningococcal types A and C polysaccharide vaccines have been used widely and effectively to limit the spread of epidemics in Africa, Nepal and South America. Mass campaigns are, however, expensive. Selective vaccination, e.g. of residents of a village in which a case has been reported, has been advocated, but clearly this will only be effective where a well-organized surveillance system is in operation.[4] In the face of an epidemic, probably the most effective means of control is to vaccinate all those aged between one and 25 years with serogroup A and C vaccine, available through the WHO.

Unfortunately polysaccharide vaccines are not available for all serogroups, are poorly immunogenic in those children aged less than two years, and may only protect for a short period.

Streptococcal infections

The streptococci are Gram-positive cocci which are classified according to their ability to haemolyse blood agar as non-haemolytic, α-haemolytic (green discoloration) or β-haemolytic (clear zone of haemolysis). (See also pp. 514–16).

Beta-haemolytic streptococci

These have been classified serologically into Lancefield groups. Group A streptococci (*S. pyogenes*) are major pathogens of man which may cause pharyngitis or skin infections, e.g. cellulitis, impetigo. Scarlet fever was formerly a common complication of streptococcal infections but for unknown reasons is now rare.

The virulence of *S. pyogenes* depends on the presence of a protein (the M protein) in the fimbriae of the cell wall. Some 70 antigenically distinct M proteins have been described; certain M types infect the throat and others the skin. M types vary in their propensity to cause glomerulonephritis, and probably also rheumatic fever. These sequelae are major causes of morbidity in tropical countries.

Poststreptococcal glomerulonephritis is due to the deposition of immune complexes, whereas an antigen common to the streptococcus and cardiac muscle is believed to stimulate the immunopathological process responsible for rheumatic carditis.

Streptococcal pharyngitis

The classical picture is of a follicular tonsillitis with spots of white exudate, fever, leucocytosis and enlargement of the anterior cervical lymph nodes. This picture is not often seen among young infants, who are frequently infected in tropical countries and may be asymptomatic or have a mild pharyngitis only. Antistreptolysin O (ASO) titres have been shown to rise rapidly in the first six months of life in Uganda.

Impetigo

This is highly prevalent among preschool and schoolchildren in most tropical countries. Characteristic golden brown crusts are seen usually on the face or scalp.

Cellulitis

Skin infections due to β-haemolytic streptococci may spread rapidly causing local erythema, oedema and pain, with fever and toxaemia (see p. 855). This condition is potentially fatal and should be treated vigorously.

Rheumatic fever

The classical features of acute rheumatic fever (flitting arthritis, nodules, rash and chorea) are rarely seen in tropical countries, possibly because of the early age at which infants are exposed to streptococcal throat infections. Nevertheless rheumatic carditis is extremely common among children in many areas, and advanced disease may be seen at a relatively young age. (For clinical features of rheumatic carditis, see pp. 776–8.)

Poststreptococcal glomerulonephritis

In tropical areas poststreptococcal glomerulonephritis usually follows a streptococcal skin infection, often associated with scabies.[5] Some two weeks after the onset of skin lesions the patient presents with oedema, haematuria, proteinuria and in some cases hypertension and congestive cardiac failure. The diagnosis in tropical areas is usually clinical, since the ASO titre may not rise following skin infections; high titres of antiDNAase B antibody may be found if this can be measured. Since the course of poststreptococcal glomerulonephritis is usually benign (95 per cent make a full recovery), renal biopsy is seldom indicated (see pp. 792–3).

Management of group A streptococcal infections

All group A streptococci remain highly susceptible to penicillin. Pharyngitis and impetigo can be treated with a single dose of long-acting penicillin (e.g. Triplopen) i.m. or with oral penicillin V 250 mg six hourly for five days. Cellulitis should be treated with full doses of parenteral penicillin.

Acute rheumatic fever should be treated with bed rest and aspirin (in sufficient doses to relieve symptoms). All patients with acute or chronic rheumatic carditis should be started on penicillin prophylaxis because of the high probability of a second attack. Benzathine penicillin may be given i.m. monthly (0.6 mega units up to age 12 years, 1.0 mega units thereafter), or oral penicillin V 250 mg twice daily if possible at least until the patient is 20 years old (see pp. 776–8).

Poststreptococcal glomerulonephritis should be treated with penicillin if skin lesions are still present. Hypertension should be controlled and fluid overload avoided (see pp. 792–3).

Group B streptococci

It has become clear in recent years that these organisms are an important cause of neonatal morbidity and mortality in industrialized countries. Contracted from the mother's vagina at delivery, they are particularly likely to cause septicaemia in premature or low-birth-weight infants, or following premature rupture of the membranes. The prevalence of group B streptococcal infections in developing countries is not known (see p. 234).

Streptococcus pneumoniae

Some 30 per cent of all deaths in children aged less than five years are due to pneumonia. Lung aspirate studies in tropical countries have shown that *S. pneumoniae* and *Haemophilus influenzae* together account for more than 50 per cent of hospitalized cases, with *H. influenzae* the more important before the age of 18 months, and *S. pneumoniae* thereafter.[6-8] *S. pneumoniae* is also a major cause of otitis media and an important cause of meningitis.

Epidemiology

The pneumococcus is spread by inhalation of droplets, and asymptomatic carriage is common. It is endemic in all areas. Pneumococcal disease is more common in overcrowded conditions, e.g. in South African gold mines, where an incidence of 20 per cent per annum has been reported.

Aetiology and pathogenesis

Streptococcus pneumoniae can be distinguished from other α-haemolytic streptococci by its sensitivity to optochin, a derivative of quinine. A zone of inhibition is seen surrounding an optochin-impregnated disc on a blood agar plate. Virulent strains have a polysaccharide capsule, antigenic differences in which have led to the description of 84 serotypes. Strains can be serotyped by the Quellung reaction in which capsular swelling is seen following exposure to specific antiserum, or by countercurrent immunoelectrophoresis.

Following nasopharyngeal colonization, pneumococci may spread locally, to cause otitis media, or via the bloodstream. Invasion is favoured by damage to the respiratory epithelium, for example due to viral infection. Those with defective antibody, complement or splenic function, e.g. sickle cell disease or postsplenectomy patients, are particularly prone to systemic infection. Patients with nephrotic syndrome are predisposed to pneumococcal peritonitis.

Clinical features

Pneumonia   See pp. 713–19.

Otitis media   Presents with irritability and fever. The ear drum is red and bulging, or perforated with a purulent discharge.

Meningitis   Features are similar to meningococcal meningitis (p. 578), except that a rash is not seen. Signs of pneumonia are present in some 25 per cent of cases. The prognosis is poor, with a mortality of up to 50 per cent even with optimum treatment. Poor prognostic features include impaired consciousness, associated pneumonia, low CSF white cell count and high CSF bacterial count.[9]

Complications

Pneumonia   See pp. 713–19.

Otitis media   Chronic otitis media may lead to

conductive deafness, or occasionally to mastoiditis, cerebral abscess or meningitis.

Meningitis   Relapse may occur following apparently successful treatment, or subdural empyema may develop. Some 50 per cent of survivors are left with neurological sequelae, e.g. deafness, hemiparesis.

Diagnosis

Pneumonia   Because asymptomatic carriage of the pneumococcus is common, its isolation from sputum is of no significance. Isolation from blood culture is diagnostic, but is not achieved in more than 30 per cent of cases of pneumonia. There is, therefore, a need for a more precise diagnostic technique. Culture of lung aspirate material is the most sensitive method, but in view of the possible complications is not suitable for routine use. Pneumococcal antigen can be detected in the serum of 30 per cent of cases of pneumococcal pneumonia by countercurrent immunoelectrophoresis (CIE). Serum to be tested and antipneumococcal antiserum are placed in adjacent wells in an agarose gel. An electrical field is applied, causing them to migrate towards each other. If antigen is present in the serum, a line of precipitation is seen. Antigen is also present in the sputum, where its detection is of more diagnostic significance than isolation of the organism.[10]

Otitis media   The only certain method of diagnosis is isolation following aspiration of an intact drum. This procedure should only be carried out by an ENT specialist and the diagnosis is usually clinical.

Meningitis   Gram-stain and culture of CSF, followed by sensitivity testing, should be carried out where possible. Detection of pneumococcal antigen, by CIE or latex agglutination, is a simple and rapid technique, which remains positive for up to 72 hours after the administration of antibiotics.

Management

Pneumonia   F. Shann and colleagues have drawn up guidelines for the management of acute respiratory infections at the primary health care level in Papua New Guinea, where most severe cases have been shown to be caused by *S. pneumoniae* or *H. influenzae*. These depend on the respiratory rate, degree of chest indrawing, cyanosis and the ability to feed.[11] (See pp. 718–19.) Since a bacteriological diagnosis cannot usually be made outside hospital, treatment regimens are empirically decided on the basis of severity of illness

Table 4.7.1.   Management of children with cough and fever

Respiration	Treatment
<50 per minute	Symptomatic
>50 per minute, no indrawing	Aqueous procaine penicillin 50 000 units i.m. daily for 5 days OR Sulphamethoxazole 20 mg/kg + trimethoprim 4 mg/kg twice daily for 5 days by mouth
>50 per minute, indrawing	Admit. Benzyl penicillin 0.5×10^6 units/kg per day in four or six doses (i.m. or i.v.)
Cyanosed, unable to feed	Chloramphenicol 100 mg/kg per day in four divided doses, i.v. or i.m. initially, then orally.

All febrile children receive antimalarials.
Empyema or pericardial effusions to be drained.

(Adapted from *Bulletin of the World Health Organization*, 1984; **62**: 749–53.)

and, if possible, the pattern of antibiotic sensitivity in the area. Their recommendations are shown in Table 4.7.1.

Pneumococcal isolates partially resistant to penicillin have been reported from many countries, but most such strains (MIC 0.1–1.0 μg/ml) respond to a full therapeutic dose of penicillin. Multiply-resistant pneumococcal isolates have been reported from South Africa. Nevertheless penicillin remains the treatment of choice for pneumococcal infections in most areas. In severe pneumonia chloramphenicol has also been shown to be highly effective.[12]

Meningitis   The maximum possible dose of penicillin (0.5×10^6 units/kg per day in six divided doses) should be given intravenously for two weeks. Lumbar puncture should be repeated two days after treatment is stopped before the patient is sent home. If the CSF has not returned to normal, the possibility of a subdural collection of pus should be considered.

Prevention

Mass administration of polyvalent polysaccharide vaccines has been shown to be effective in preventing mortality due to pneumonia in Papua New Guinea.[13] Before this approach can be widely applied it is necessary to determine the capsular serotypes prevalent in different areas to ensure their inclusion in the vaccine.

Polysaccharide vaccine is poorly immunogenic in children aged less than two years. Oral penicillin (125 mg twice daily) has been shown to reduce the incidence of pneumococcal disease in children under three years with sickle cell disease and in children following splenectomy. Since pneumococcal septicaemia accounts for many fatalities in these patients, penicillin prophylaxis should be followed by administration of pneumococcal vaccine at the age of three years.

Staphylococcal infections

The staphylococci are Gram-positive cocci which are often seen in clusters. The pathogenic *S. aureus* can be distinguished from the generally harmless *S. epidermidis* by its ability to coagulate human plasma (coagulase test). Both organisms are common skin commensals, but *S. aureus* produces a number of toxic extracellular enzymes and may become invasive.

Skin infections

These are particularly prevalent in hot humid environments (see pp. 853–5).

S. aureus. This is a common cause of impetigo, which cannot be distinguished clinically from that due to *Streptococcus pyogenes* (qv). Frequently it infects a hair follicle to cause a boil or furuncle. These are usually benign but may enlarge to form a carbuncle or abscess. If they arise near the eye they may lead to orbital cellulitis or cavernous sinus thrombosis, a rare but serious complication.

S. aureus may cause more deep-seated infections at the site of skin trauma. Breast abscesses are common in the puerperium and may interfere with breast-feeding, and palmar and plantar space infections are frequently seen in the tropics.

Osteomyelitis. This is usually caused by *S. aureus* and is common in tropical countries. Local pain and tenderness develop in the affected bone, sometimes at the site of minor trauma, and may be accompanied by swelling and fever. If not diagnosed and treated promptly, chronic disease develops with discharging sinuses, requiring surgical intervention. Infants with staphylococcal septicaemia may develop osteitis and/or septic arthritis at several sites.

Staphylococcal pneumonia. This is less common than that due to *S. pneumoniae* or *H. influenzae* but is important because it has a poor prognosis. It is a well-recognized complication of measles. The onset is sudden and chest X-ray reveals extensive patchy consolidation, often with abscess formation. Tension cysts and pneumothorax may also be seen.

Pyomyositis. This is a disease apparently confined to the tropics. Multiple intramuscular abscesses are seen, new ones frequently developing after the institution of antibiotic treatment. It has been suggested that viral myositis may predispose to staphylococcal invasion in this condition.

Treatment

Minor skin infections may be treated with antiseptics. Small boils generally resolve spontaneously, but larger collections of pus should be drained.

Flucloxacillin is the mainstay of treatment in more severe staphylococcal infections. Penicillin and ampicillin are useless in most areas since the majority of strains now produce penicillinase. Depending on the local pattern of sensitivity, chloramphenicol or cotrimoxazole may be effective if flucloxacillin is not available.

Osteomyelitis should be treated with full doses of fusidic acid, 10 mg/kg eight-hourly, i.v. or orally, in addition to flucloxacillin, since it penetrates bone more effectively; treatment must be for at least six weeks.

Staphylococcal pneumonia should be treated with gentamicin, 2 mg/kg eight-hourly, in addition to flucloxacillin; this dose should be reduced if there is impaired renal function and serum gentamicin levels determined.

Gonococcal infections

Ophthalmia neonatorum

Gonococcal ophthalmia neonatorum (ON) is probably a major cause of blindness in tropical countries; its true importance is not reflected in blindness surveys, since blind infants are unlikely to survive in poor communities.

Epidemiology

The prevalence of gonococcal infection is high among antenatal clinic attenders in many tropical countries, ranging from 3 to 40 per cent,[14] and some 30 per cent of exposed infants acquire gonococcal ON. Thus, in many parts of Africa more than 2 per cent of infants are likely to be affected.

Community perceptions

The connection between maternal infection and ON is seldom appreciated in tropical countries. In West Africa, for example, ON is commonly believed to be due to excessive maternal consumption of pepper during pregnancy.

Aetiology and pathogenesis

Neisseria gonorrhoeae is a Gram-negative diplococcus which does not survive desiccation and therefore cannot survive more than a few minutes outside the body. ON is contracted during passage through the infected cervix at delivery.

It is a disturbing fact that penicillinase-producing strains (PPNG) have become highly prevalent in the tropics in the past 10 years; in many African countries more than 50 per cent of isolates now produce penicillinase.

Clinical features

The incubation period is three days or less. At presentation there is a copious purulent discharge from the eyes and oedema of the eyelids; this is occasionally so gross that the cornea cannot be visualized (Fig. 4.7.2). Corneal ulceration occurs in a proportion of cases. This may resolve leaving a scar with consequent visual impairment, or progress to corneal perforation in which case the eye may be lost.

Diagnosis

Gram stain of the purulent exudate is usually diagnostic. Large numbers of intra- and extracellular Gram-negative diplococci are seen. Where facilities allow, isolation should be attempted on Thayer Martin selective medium, preferably by direct inoculation at the bedside followed by incubation at 37°C in a candle jar, and sensitivities determined. The chromogenic cephalosporin test is a simple and cheap method for identifying PPNG strains. Paper strips impregnated with this reagent are obtainable from Oxoid Ltd, Basingstoke, Hampshire, UK. When a β-lactamase producing colony is applied to the strip a red colour appears, due to the splitting of the β-lactam ring.

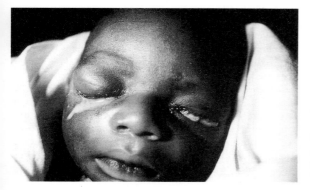

Fig. 4.7.2 Gonococcal ophthalmia neonatorum.

Treatment

Penicillin was formerly the treatment of choice, by single i.m. injection (procaine penicillin 50 000 units/kg) and by frequent topical application (1 per cent drops applied every few minutes for several hours then six-hourly for five days). This can no longer be recommended in areas where more than 5 per cent of isolates are PPNG. Effective alternatives are a single dose of kanamycin 75 mg i.m. with gentamicin 1 per cent drops six hourly for five days, or ceftriaxone as a single i.m. injection (125 mg).[15, 16] Where these alternatives are not available, frequent application of tetracycline 1 per cent drops combined with careful removal of purulent exudate may be effective (see also p. 930).

Prevention

Antenatal screening for gonococcal infection is not practical in many developing countries. Prophylaxis with 1 per cent silver nitrate was introduced by Crede in the nineteenth century and is effective, if applied at birth after careful cleaning of the eyes. Unfortunately if silver nitrate is not properly stored it may cause a chemical conjunctivitis, and this technique has been abandoned in many of the countries in which it is most needed. Use of single-dose ampoules (available from WHO) may circumvent this problem. The application of 1 per cent tetracycline at birth has also been shown to be effective against both gonococcal and chlamydial ON.

Vulvovaginitis

Gonococcal vulvovaginitis is not infrequently seen in prepubertal girls and does not necessarily imply sexual abuse; it may be contracted from the mother or other close relative with whom the patient shares a bed. Treatment depends on local sensitivity patterns. Single-dose procaine penicillin (20 000 units/kg) may be used where PPNG strains are uncommon. Elsewhere, ceftriaxone 125 mg i.m. as a single dose is the treatment of choice.

Gram-negative septicaemia

Septicaemic infections, particularly those due to *Escherichia coli* and non-typhoid strains of *Salmonella* are commonly seen in paediatric practice in the tropics. There are three groups of children particularly at risk:

- Neonates, especially low-birth-weight and premature infants and following prolonged rupture of the membranes.

- Severely malnourished children.
- Sickle cell anaemia children.

Clinical features

Gram-negative septicaemia should be suspected in any ill child in any of these categories. It is important to note that the temperature is often normal or subnormal in Gram-negative septicaemia in such children.

Neonates   Clinical features in neonates are all non-specific. The infant will suck poorly and may be drowsy, hypotonic, anaemic or jaundiced. Diarrhoea, vomiting, abdominal distension, convulsions and cyanotic attacks may occur. The impression of a sick baby, although difficult to define, will be apparent to the experienced paediatrician and should prompt urgent investigation and treatment.

Malnourished children   Severely malnourished children with marasmus or kwashiorkor are particularly prone to serious infections because their immune system is impaired; the impairment is most severe in those with kwashiorkor and marasmic kwashiorkor.

   The clinical features of Gram-negative septicaemia are again non-specific. The child appears ill and will often have diarrhoea and vomiting, which may lead to severe dehydration. The child may be drowsy and hypotonic, or comatose. Acidotic respiration is sometimes seen.

Sickle cell anaemia   The most common organisms isolated in osteitis are Salmonellae. A salmonella infection found in an unusual site (e.g. empyema) or a salmonella septicaemia in an anaemic child should alert the clinician to the possibility of sickle cell disease (see pp. 828–31).

Investigation and management

Any child in whom septicaemia is suspected should have blood and urine specimens taken for culture before antibiotics are administered. Lumbar puncture should also be performed in neonates.

   Treatment should be started as soon as these specimens have been taken. Fluid and electrolyte disturbances should be corrected if possible by intravenous infusion, and anaemia by transfusion. Broad-spectrum antibiotics should be given parenterally, if possible i.v. A suitable regimen is ampicillin 100 mg/kg per day in four divided doses plus gentamicin 6 mg/kg per day in

three divided doses. Alternatively, chloramphenicol 100 mg/kg per day may be given in four divided doses.

Escherichia coli

This group of organisms forms part of the normal flora of the large intestine. Certain strains cause diarrhoea; these are discussed on pp. 455–95. In addition to their important role in neonatal septicaemia and meningitis (see earlier), *E. coli* are the commonest cause of urinary tract infection (UTI).

   The features of UTI are often non-specific in children. It may present with vomiting, failure to thrive or unexplained fever. Older children may complain of dysuria, or may present with enuresis.

   It is often impossible to collect a midstream urine from a child, so that urine cultures may be contaminated with perineal organisms. The presence of white cells in the urine lends greater significance to a positive culture result.

   Male children with UTI, and females with repeated infections, are likely to have renal tract abnormalities and should be investigated by intravenous urography where possible. Treatment of UTI depends on the sensitivity pattern of local isolates. Ampicillin or trimethoprim/sulphamethoxazole are generally the antibiotics of choice, given in standard dosage for five days.

Enteric fever (typhoid)

Epidemiology

Enteric fever is endemic in most tropical countries. *Salmonella typhi* infects only humans and is spread by the faecal–oral route. Other salmonellae are zoonotic and frequently infect domestic animals.

Aetiology and pathogenesis

The salmonellae are non-lactose fermenting, Gram-negative rods. They possess O (somatic) and H (flagellar) antigens, on the basis of differences in which more than 1500 serotypes or species have been described.

   Enteric fever is usually caused by *S. typhi* or *S. paratyphi*. Other species commonly cause 'food poisoning' in temperate countries but in the tropics are also important causes of septicaemia in children. Factors predisposing to invasive disease include malnutrition, sickle cell disease, malaria, relapsing fever and bartonellosis.[17] A chronic form of typhoid is associated with schistosomiasis.

   In enteric fever a transient bacteraemia follows oral

ingestion of the organism, which then multiplies in the reticuloendothelial system of the liver and spleen. After an incubation period of 10–14 days *Salmonellae* disseminate via the bloodstream. They are secreted in the bile and hence reinvade the intestine, where they multiply within Peyer's patches; necrosis may occur at this site leading to intestinal perforation or haemorrhage.

Clinical features

Enteric fever should be suspected in any ill febrile child in the tropics. The presenting clinical features in a series of 316 children with typhoid in Durban, South Africa, are shown in Table 4.7.2.[18]

Fever is almost invariably present but may be absent in severely malnourished children. Once malaria has been excluded or treated the most important differential diagnosis is pneumonia, since cough and chest signs are commonly found. Chest X-ray showed bronchopneumonic changes in 35 per cent of cases in the Durban series.

Older children complain of headache and may be drowsy or withdrawn, occasionally presenting with frank psychosis. Younger children often present in coma following a convulsion. CSF is usually normal but salmonella meningitis is occasionally seen in infants. Typhoid osteitis may also occur, sometimes in unusual sites such as the spine.

Jaundice may be present but hepatosplenomegaly is not a helpful diagnostic feature in malarious areas. Rose spots are sometimes seen in pale, but not darkskinned patients. They are erythematous macular lesions seen mainly on the trunk, usually about 2 mm in diameter.

The most important complications of enteric fever are intestinal perforation or haemorrhage, usually occurring in the second or third week of the illness (Fig. 4.7.3a–c).

Diagnosis

Blood culture is positive in at least 50 per cent of cases and is the only certain way to make the diagnosis. Positive stool culture in an ill febrile child is also strongly suggestive.

The Widal test, an agglutination test for antibodies to the O and H antigens, is simple and quick to perform. It can only be interpreted, however, if the 'normal' range of titres in the local population is known. As with any serological test, a rising or falling titre in paired samples is of more significance than a single value.

S. typhi may be isolated from the urine of patients with coexisting *Schistosoma haematobium* infection. If typhoid is suspected in a patient with schistosomiasis it is important that the laboratory should be asked to look for it in the urine; *S. typhi* will not be detected on routine processing of urine.

Management

Dehydration and anaemia should be corrected and the temperature lowered with paracetamol and sponging.

Chloramphenicol is the antibiotic of choice. It should be given for three weeks, initially 100 mg/kg per day in four divided doses, which may be reduced after one week to 75 mg/kg per day. Chloramphenicol-resistant *S. typhi* have been reported from Mexico but fortunately remain rare in other areas. Alternative antibiotics are ampicillin and trimethoprim/sulphamethoxazole. Treatment for three weeks is said to reduce the likelihood of relapse.

Intestinal perforation should be managed surgically wherever possible (see p. 897).

Prevention

Enteric fever has been controlled in industrialized countries by improvements in hygiene and living standards, and by excluding chronic carriers from high-risk occupations. In many tropical areas this is not feasible, though known carriers should be advised not to prepare food. The eradication of persistent carriage is difficult. Cholecystectomy may be effective if the patient can be persuaded to agree to it. A few recent

Table 4.7.2 Clinical manifestations in 316 children with typhoid

Manifestation	Percentage
Fever	99
Headache	58
Cough	48
Diarrhoea	46
Anaemia	46
Tender/tumid abdomen	43
Hepatomegaly	42
Abdominal pain	37
Splenomegaly	35
Bronchitis	33
Vomiting	32
Delirium	19
Leucopaenia	18
Meningism	17

(Reproduced from Scragg J *et al.*, *Archives of Disease in Childhood*, 1969; **44**: 18–28.)

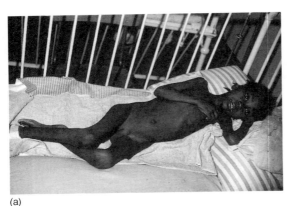

(a)

Fig. 4.7.3 (a) Child with typhoid, toxic and dehydrated. (b) Straight X-ray of abdomen of a child with typhoid after one week, showing distended loops of small bowel. (c) Same child as in (b) shortly afterwards, showing air in the peritoneal cavity following perforation of a typhoid ulcer.

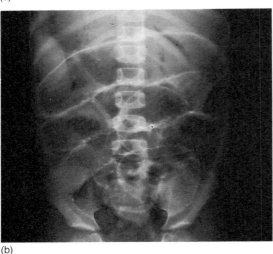

(b)

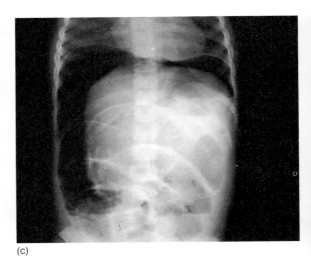

(c)

case reports suggest that the new quinolone antibiotic, ciprofloxacin, may be effective, but its use in children is not recommended.

Parenteral killed vaccines do not induce lasting immunity and frequently cause local side-effects. Recently an attenuated oral vaccine has become available which appears to be well tolerated and effective.[19]

Haemophilus influenzae

Epidemiology

H. influenzae is a ubiquitous upper respiratory tract commensal. Serious disease due to this organism is practically confined to children aged three months to four years; in the tropics the majority of cases occur in infants aged three months to one year. Circulating antibody is presumed to protect older children and adults, since serum bactericidal activity against *H. influenzae* increases after the age of five years.

It is the most important cause of pneumonia and meningitis in children aged three months to two years in many countries.[7, 8] It is also a major cause of otitis media in children.

Aetiology and pathogenesis

H. influenzae is a fastidious Gram-negative bacillus which requires both X and V factors (haemin and nicotinamide adenine dinucleotide) for growth. Some strains possess a polysaccharide capsule on the basis of which serotypes a–f have been defined. The majority of commensal strains are non-capsulated.

H. influenzae may cause disease in two ways. It may spread locally from the nasopharynx to cause otitis media or sinusitis, or it may cause a bacteraemic illness with pneumonia, meningitis, septic arthritis or epiglottitis. It is generally stated that only serotype b causes invasive disease, but recent reports indicate that other serotypes, and even non-capsulated strains may cause pneumonia or meningitis in the tropics.[7, 8]

Clinical features

Meningitis Meningitis due to *H. influenzae* cannot be distinguished clinically from that due to other bacteria. Meningitis should be suspected in any febrile irritable infant even in the absence of neck stiffness. A tense or bulging fontanelle is commonly seen in infants with bacterial meningitis.

Pneumonia Lobar consolidation is usual, with fever and neutrophilia as in pneumococcal pneumonia.

Epiglottitis This is an uncommon manifestation of *H. influenzae* infection which carries a high mortality (see p. 710). The onset is sudden with fever, sore throat and signs of toxaemia. Stridor may develop and difficulty in swallowing leads to characteristic dribbling of saliva from the mouth. Respiratory obstruction may ensue and if this condition is suspected the throat should not be examined unless facilities for tracheostomy are available. Examination of the throat reveals a red oedematous epiglottis said to resemble a strawberry.

Otitis media See under pneumococcal disease.

Complications

If adequate treatment is instituted soon after the onset of symptoms, the mortality of *H. influenzae* meningitis may be as low as 5 per cent. In practice, due to delay in obtaining medical treatment, the mortality is considerably higher in most tropical countries. Up to 50 per cent of survivors are left with neurological sequelae.

Empyema commonly complicates pneumonia due to *H. influenzae*. Local extension may lead to a purulent pericardial effusion. Septic arthritis, affecting one or more large joints, may occur with invasive infections due to *H. influenzae*.

Diagnosis

A presumptive diagnosis of *H. influenzae* meningitis can be made when Gram-negative bacilli are seen in the CSF of an infant aged between three months and two years. CSF should also be cultured on chocolate agar for identification and sensitivity testing. *H. influenzae*

pneumonia can be diagnosed by blood culture or by culture of material aspirated from the affected lung; the latter method is more sensitive but should not be routinely performed unless an empyema is believed to be present. Blood cultures are frequently positive in epiglottitis.

Treatment

Chloramphenicol is the treatment of choice for invasive disease due to *H. influenzae*. 100 mg/kg should be given daily in four divided doses for at least one week, if possible parenterally. Ampicillin was often recommended in the past, but an increasing proportion of isolates world-wide now produce β-lactamase and are therefore resistant to it.

Prevention

A vaccine prepared from the capsular polysaccharide of serotype b has been shown to be well tolerated but is unfortunately not immunogenic in children aged less than two years, the group who are particularly at risk. Coupling of the polysaccharide to a protein, e.g. the major outer membrane protein of *N. meningitis*, has been shown to increase its immunogenicity in young babies.[20] The potential benefits of such a vaccine in the tropics are not clear, since (as mentioned above) invasive disease may not always be due to serotype b.

Anthrax

This is caused by the spore-forming Gram-positive organism, *Bacillus anthracis*. The spores are highly resistant and can survive in soil for many years. It is primarily an infection of domestic cattle and sheep, man being infected by contact with these animals; human to human spread may occasionally occur, e.g. by the communal use of washing materials.

The skin is the site of infection in the majority of cases. A pustule develops at the site of inoculation which enlarges and acquires the characteristic black centre from which the disease derives its name (Greek: anthrax = coal). There is considerable oedema surrounding this lesion, and local lymphadenopathy. Fever and constitutional symptoms may be present.

Pulmonary and gastro-intestinal infections are less common but carry a mortality approaching 100 per cent. Pulmonary anthrax is contracted by inhalation of spores, e.g. from wool, and gastro-intestinal by eating contaminated meat. Both diseases are of sudden onset with either cough or abdominal pain and distension as the principal manifestation. Death usually occurs within 48 hours of onset with or without treatment.

Diagnosis

Direct smear of material from a skin lesion or of sputum (pulmonary) or peritoneal fluid (gastro-intestinal) may reveal typical Gram-positive bacilli with subterminal spores. *B. anthracis* grows readily on blood agar but should be handled with extreme care in the laboratory.

Treatment is with parenteral penicillin in full dosage. Cutaneous anthrax responds well to this treatment but pulmonary and gastro-intestinal disease do not. Equine antisera have been used in pulmonary and gastro-intestinal anthrax but results have been disappointing.

Prevention

Prevention of human anthrax involves the control of the disease in animals. An animal vaccine is available. Contaminated carcases should be incinerated or buried in lime, and unhealthy animals should not be eaten. Unfortunately, once contaminated, pastures are extremely difficult to decontaminate because of the persistence of spores. A human vaccine is available from the Michigan Department of Public Health, Bureau of Disease Control and Laboratory Services, 3500 North Logan Street, POB 30035, Lansing, Michigan 48909, USA. It should be given to those particularly at risk, e.g. vets in endemic areas and laboratory workers.

Plague

Plague is a zoonotic infection caused by the Gram-negative coccobacillus *Yersinia pestis*. The domestic rat (*Rattus rattus*) is the most important reservoir, because of its close relationship with man, but other small mammals may harbour the infection, e.g. the ground squirrel which maintains foci of sylvatic plague in the USA. Man is an incidental host, being infected by the bite of the rat flea *Xenopsylla cheopsis*. Pneumonic cases may infect their contacts directly.

A number of devastating epidemics of plague have been recorded in history. Epidemics arise from enzootic foci, and are thought to follow changes in the behaviour, numbers or susceptibility of rodent populations. Transmission is more efficient in warm humid climates; it is curtailed by very hot weather (30°C or more) and by drought, due to changes in flea behaviour and physiology. Plague remains endemic in many countries in Africa, the Americas and South East Asia.

The characteristic feature of plague is the bubo, an extremely painful haemorrhagic lymphadenitis affecting the glands in the groin, axilla or neck. There is usually no lesion at the site of inoculation and no ascending lymphangitis.

The onset of disease is acute, with high fever often accompanied by convulsions in children, and the simultaneous appearance of a bubo. The disease is fulminant with hypotension, purpura and other signs of disseminated intravascular coagulation, and in the absence of treatment leads to death within 2–4 days in at least 50 per cent of cases. Haematogenous infection of the lungs may lead to so-called pneumonic plague, which carries a high mortality; such patients are highly infectious since bacteria are present in their sputum in large numbers. Occasionally plague causes a septicaemic illness in the absence of a bubo or pneumonia.

Diagnosis

The diagnosis can be confirmed by Gram-stain and culture of a needle aspirate from the bubo. Because pus is not present in the acute stage it may be necessary to inject a few millilitres of sterile saline into the bubo before aspiration. Gram stain reveals polymorphs and Gram-negative coccobacilli 1–2 μm in length. Bacteria are present in large numbers in both the bubo and the peripheral blood, where they may be seen on a blood film. Pneumonic plague can be diagnosed by Gram stain and culture of sputum. *Y. pestis* grows readily on blood agar but should be handled with extreme care in the laboratory.

Treatment

Streptomycin 30 mg/kg per day in two divided doses for 10 days was shown in 1948 to reduce the mortality to below 5 per cent. Chloramphenicol 100 mg/kg per day in four divided doses is probably equally effective; if possible it should be given i.v. for the first 24 hours. Pneumonic cases should be isolated for 48 hours after the initiation of antibiotic treatment and masks should be worn by their attendants.

All cases of plague should be notified to the national health authorities and to the World Health Organization as soon as possible.

Prevention

Urban plague has been successfully controlled in many cities by a combination of quarantine, rat control and insecticides. A formalin-killed vaccine is available from the Cutter Laboratories, Berkely, California 94710,

USA, but the above measures remain the most important in the face of an epidemic.

Brucellosis

This is a zoonotic infection generally contracted from infected milk or milk products, or by direct contact in pastoral peoples. The genus *Brucella* are fastidious slow-growing Gram-negative rods. Two species are prevalent in the tropics: *Br. melitensis*, which infects chiefly goats, and *Br. abortus*, which infects cattle. They are intracellular parasites which multiply in macrophages of the reticuloendothelial system causing a chronic granulomatous reaction without caseation. The disease may be of insidious onset or may present acutely with fever. It often runs a chronic relapsing course. The most important clinical features are fever, malaise and musculo-skeletal involvement. Arthritis affects principally the sacro-iliac or intervertebral joints or the hips. The knees are sometimes involved, with obvious swelling. Splenomegaly may be marked in chronic cases.

There is characteristically a moderate anaemia and neutrophil leucopaenia, and a raised sedimentation rate.

Brucellosis in pregnancy appears to carry no increased risk of abortion over and above that of any acute infection.

Diagnosis

The disease has no pathognomonic features but should be suspected in any febrile child who herds livestock and/or drinks unpasteurized milk. Blood culture is only positive in 20 per cent of *Br. abortus* infections and 70 per cent of *Br. melitensis*. A higher yield may be obtained from bone marrow culture but since the organism is slow growing it may be several weeks before the result is obtained. Diagnosis is therefore usually serological. Agglutination tests which are simple to perform and reliable are available for both species. Enzyme-linked immunosorbent assays for IgM and IgG antibodies have recently been developed.

Management

A combination of tetracycline and streptomycin has been used for many years in the treatment of brucellosis. Mild cases may be treated with tetracycline alone. The recommended doses for adults are tetracycline 2 g daily for three weeks and streptomycin 1 g daily for two weeks. There is little information available on the treatment of brucellosis in children. In those under six years of age, trimethoprim/sulphamethoxazole should be given for four weeks in conventional dosage. If available it may be combined with rifampicin (10 mg/kg per day) since this has good cellular penetration. Rifampicin should not be given alone because resistance readily develops.

Prevention

The incidence of brucellosis could be greatly reduced by the widespread pasteurization of milk.

Treponematoses

According to the unitarian hypothesis of Hudson,[21] which is widely but not universally accepted, the treponematoses are all caused by essentially the same organism, *Treponema pallidum*. Under conditions of poor hygiene the organism is transmitted among children, infecting chiefly the mucous membranes in dry climates and the skin in warm humid climates, causing endemic syphilis or yaws respectively. As hygienic conditions improve, the organism can only be transmitted by sexual contact or from mother to fetus, resulting in venereal or congenital infection.

Epidemiology

Following the mass treatment campaigns of the 1950s and 1960s the prevalence of the endemic treponematoses declined dramatically in many tropical countries. Unfortunately, in some African countries endemic syphilis was never controlled, and in others yaws has re-emerged as a public health problem in recent years.

The incidence and prevalence of venereal and congenital syphilis is unknown in most tropical countries. Seroprevalence studies have been undertaken in several areas but are bedevilled by the frequency of biological false-positive reagin tests in the tropics and the inability of the treponemal tests to distinguish between venereal, congenital and endemic disease. There is evidence that untreated endemic disease protects against venereal infection, and it is likely that the incidence of venereal syphilis has increased following the decline of the endemic treponematoses.

In Lusaka, Zambia, 12.5 per cent of 202 antenatal patients were found to have serological evidence of active syphilis, as were 6.5 per cent of 469 infants delivered in hospital.[22] These figures may well be representative of urban populations in Africa.

Aetiology and pathogenesis

The treponematoses are caused by the spirochaete *Treponema pallidum*. This is a delicate spiral organism less than $0.2\,\mu m$ in diameter and $5-20\,\mu m$ in length, with a characteristic motility. Because of its small diameter it can only be seen with the light microscope under dark field illumination; it can only be cultured in laboratory animals. Some authorities refer to the organism which causes yaws as *T. pertenue* and that causing pinta as *T. carateum* but these are morphologically indistinguishable from *T. pallidum*.

Treponemal infections typically have primary, secondary and tertiary stages. The primary lesion occurs at the site of inoculation after an incubation period of three to six weeks and consists of a painless ulcer. The secondary stage follows dissemination of the organism throughout the body; skin lesions contain large numbers of organisms and the patient is highly infectious.

T. pallidum can survive for many years in the human body in spite of a vigorous humoral and cell-mediated immune response directed against it. The mechanism of this persistence is not clear, although intracellular organisms have been occasionally observed. Untreated subjects are immune from superinfection, as reported by clinicians in the nineteenth century (so called 'chancre immunity'). In a proportion of cases a tertiary stage is seen after a number of years. The gumma, the characteristic lesion of tertiary disease, contains chronic inflammatory cells and few organisms.

In Europe, tertiary vascular or neurological lesions occur in 30 per cent of untreated patients, but disease at these sites is rarely seen in Africa. It is said that cardiovascular and neurological complications do not occur in the endemic treponematoses.

Congenital syphilis

Venereal syphilis acquired in pregnancy frequently leads to stillbirth. In the absence of treatment, subsequent pregnancies may result in repeated stillbirths or in the delivery of congenitally infected infants.

The primary lesion is rarely seen in congenital syphilis. Occasionally infected infants have an extensive bullous rash at delivery; fluid from these bullae contain numerous *Treponemata* and these infants have a poor prognosis (Fig. 4.7.4).

More usually, infected infants appear normal at birth. They present aged one to three months, usually with failure to thrive in association with some of the features listed in Table 4.7.3.

The rash in postneonatal cases can take many forms but almost invariably affects the palms and soles, where

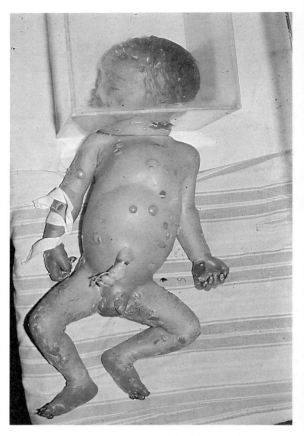

Fig. 4.7.4 Congenital syphilis with bullous eruption.

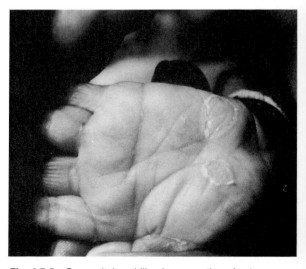

Fig. 4.7.5 Congenital syphilis, desquamation of palms.

Table 4.7.3 Clinical features in 202 infants with early congenital syphilis

Feature	Neonates (percentage)	Postneonates (percentage)
Hepatosplenomegaly	91	87
Radiological changes*	95	91
Anaemia	64	89
Rash	31	55
Jaundice	48	7
Snuffles	12	50
Mortality†	54	8

*Chiefly metaphyseal dystrophy and periostitis.
†Following adequate treatment. (Adapted from Hira SK *et al.*, *British Journal of Venereal Diseases*, 1982; **58**: 355–8.)

it causes desquamation (Fig. 4.7.5). A bloodstained nasal discharge in infancy is strongly suggestive of congenital syphilis.

The late features of congenital syphilis, which affect principally the bones, joints and eyes, are rarely seen in the tropics, probably because untreated the condition carries a high mortality.

When the bones are affected, the infection usually takes the form of a syphilitic epiphysitis and periostitis (Fig. 4.7.6). Clinically there is swelling and pain in the affected epiphysis and the infant becomes reluctant to move the limb so involved, giving rise to the so-called 'pseudoparalysis'.

Diagnosis

In the presence of any of the above clinical features an X-ray of the long bones can rapidly provide supportive evidence of congenital syphilis, since characteristic changes are seen in more than 90 per cent of cases (Fig. 4.7.7).

If a bullous rash is present, the demonstration of *T. pallidum* on dark-ground examination of bulla fluid confirms the diagnosis.

Serological tests for syphilis are either non-specific 'reagin' tests, e.g. the venereal diseases laboratory test (VDRL), or rapid plasma reagin test (RPR); these may give false-positive results with other infections, e.g. malaria; or specific treponemal tests, e.g. the *Treponema pallidum* haemagglutination assay (TPHA) or the fluorescent treponemal antibody test (FTA–Abs). None of these tests can distinguish between venereal, congenital and endemic treponemal diseases. A modification of the FTA–Abs test, the FTA–Abs IgM test, measures only IgM antibody and is therefore useful in distinguishing congenital infection from passively acquired maternal antibody, since IgM does not cross the placenta.

Any positive serological test is sufficient grounds for treatment in infants displaying any of the above clinical features. In the absence of clinical abnormalities it is generally said that infants with positive serology should be followed up for at least six months; in those who are not infected, titres will decline as maternal antibody wanes. Such long-term follow-up may not be possible in tropical countries, in which case all such subjects should be treated. If available, an IgM test such as the FTA-IgM is said to distinguish infected infants from those with passively acquired maternal antibody. Tests for congenital syphilis will also be combined with those for HIV infection (see p. 603).

Management

Lumbar puncture should be performed in all cases. If the CSF is normal, a single intramuscular dose of benzathine penicillin G (50 000 units/kg) is sufficient. If the CSF is abnormal, aqueous procaine penicillin G should be given (50 000 units/kg i.m. daily for 10 days). The mother and, if possible, the father must also be treated.

Pregnant women with syphilis may be treated with a single dose of benzathine penicillin (2.4×10^6 units i.m). Their partners should also be treated to prevent reinfection. If possible they should be followed up to ensure a falling titre by the VDRL or RPR test, and their infant followed up after delivery.

Prevention

General methods for the control of sexually transmitted diseases include education and the provision of easily accessible clinics with adequate supplies of drugs. Wherever possible all antenatal patients should be screened serologically; unfortunately economic constraints often prevent this in the very areas where it is most needed.

Since *T. pallidum* remains fully sensitive to penicillin, it remains possible in theory to control venereal syphilis by mass campaigns similar to those mounted against the endemic treponematoses; this approach has not, however, been evaluated.

Yaws

The primary lesion is a papule, usually on the legs, which enlarges to form an ulcerated papilloma. This is painless unless secondarily infected.

Secondary lesions may appear before the primary has healed. Papillomata are seen particularly in the moist areas of the body (axilla, natal cleft) but may be seen elsewhere (Figs 4.7.8 and 4.7.9). Macular or

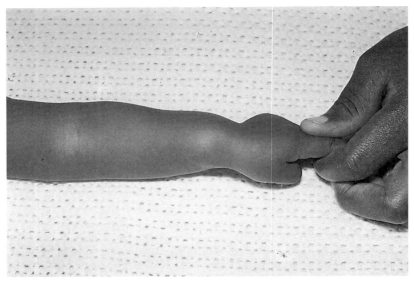

(a)

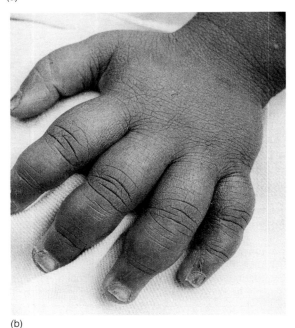

(b)

Fig. 4.7.6   (a) Typical wrist appearance of congenital syphilis. Multiple dactylitis (b).

papulosquamous lesions may also be seen; involvement of the soles of the feet may lead to painful hyperkeratosis. Periostitis may be seen in secondary yaws, affecting usually the long bones; occasionally the fingers or maxilla are involved (Fig. 4.7.10). Tertiary yaws develops in 10–20 per cent of cases, at least five years after infection. Gummata may involve the skin, bone or cartilage. Destructive lesions may affect the palate or nasal cartilage (Fig. 4.7.11).

Endemic syphilis

Primary lesions are rarely seen. Indurated mucous patches appear in the mouth or on the lips; papillomata are seen, as in yaws, in the moist areas of the body, (Figs 4.7.12 and 4.7.13) and painful periostitis of the long bones may occur. The late complications are identical to those of yaws.

Pinta

This condition is seen mainly in South and Central America. A painless erythematous papule slowly enlarges to form a slightly raised scaly lesion known as a 'pintid'. Satellite pintids appear at the margin of the original lesion, which continues to enlarge and may become blue or violaceous in colour. Any part of the body may be involved. Ultimately the affected skin becomes depigmented and atrophic; the deep tissues are not involved.

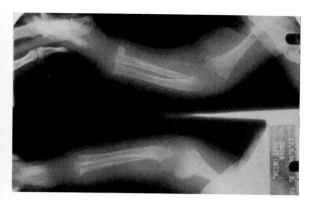

Fig. 4.7.7 X-ray reveals a syphilitic epiphysitis and periostitis.

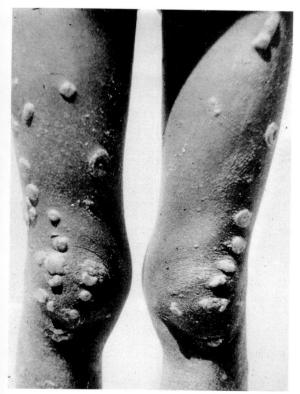

Fig. 4.7.8 Secondary yaws. (Courtesy of Dr CJ Hackett/Wellcome Trust.)

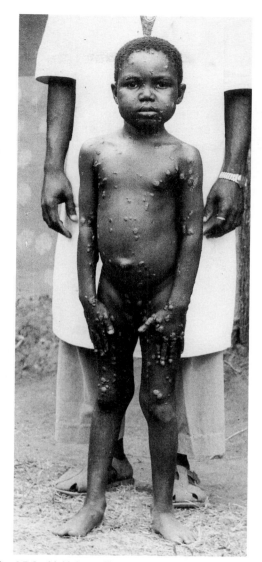

Fig. 4.7.9 Multiple papillomata in a girl with secondary yaws.

Diagnosis

Dark-field examination of exudate from lesions is the method of choice. Treponemes are present in large numbers in the early stages. Serological tests become positive by the secondary stage. Both treponemal (TPHA, FTA) and non-treponemal tests (VDRL, RPR) are positive and the various treponematoses cannot be distinguished serologically. The treponemal

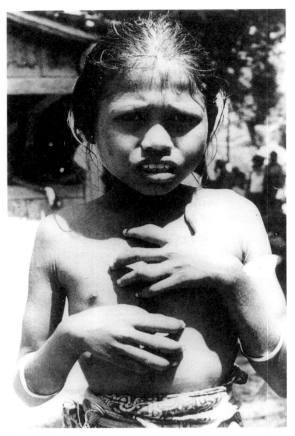

Fig. 4.7.10 Bilateral polydactylitis characteristic, when it does appear, of secondary yaws. (Courtesy of Dr CJ Hackett/Wellcome Trust.)

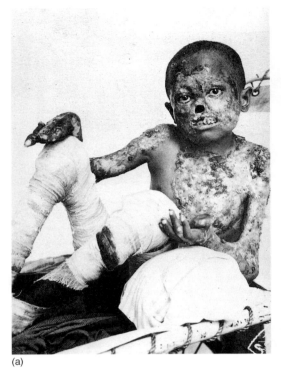

(a)

Fig. 4.7.11(a, b) The hypertrophic and destructive lesions affecting the palate, nasal cartilage and bone in tertiary yaws. (Photo (b) courtesy of Dr CJ Hackett/Wellcome Trust.)

tests may remain positive for many years after treatment.

Treatment

Benzathine penicillin G should be given as a single i.m. injection; 600 000 units to those aged less than 10 years and 1.2×10^6 units to those aged 10 years or over.

Prevention

Treatment of active cases alone will not control the endemic treponematoses since incubating and latent cases maintain a reservoir of infection. When the prevalence of clinically active disease exceeds 10 per cent, as determined by a clinical survey, the entire population should be treated (total mass treatment). In the past this has been achieved by mobile mass campaigns. When it is between 5 and 10 per cent, all children under the age of 15 years and all household contacts of active cases should be treated (juvenile mass treatment). When the prevalence is less than 5 per cent, only active cases and household and other obvious contacts should be treated (selective mass treatment). The recent re-emergence of yaws in West Africa emphasizes the need for continued surveillance and control measures against the endemic treponematoses.

Relapsing fever

This is an acute febrile illness caused by spirochaetes of the genus *Borrelia*, transmitted to man by lice or ticks. The causative organisms of louse and tick-borne disease have been designated *B. recurrentis* and *B. duttoni*, respectively, but are morphologically indistinguishable, measuring 10–30 μm by 0.5 μm with 5–10 irregular coils. They can be cultured in animals or chick embryos.

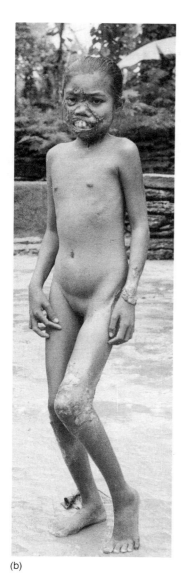

(b)

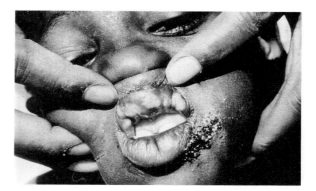

Fig. 4.7.12 Primary endemic syphilis showing the indurated patches on the membrane of the lips and ulcerated papules around the mouth. (Courtesy of Dr CJ Hackett/Wellcome Trust.)

organisms in faeces and saliva. Small rodents provide an animal reservoir in some regions.

Clinical features

After an incubation period of two days to two weeks there is a sudden onset of fever, headache and myalgia, sometimes with vomiting and cough. Hepato-splenomegaly and jaundice, largely due to haemolysis, may be present, as may purpura and other haemorrhagic manifestations. Neurological involvement, e.g. cranial nerve palsy, accompanied by neck stiffness is occasionally seen. Typically there is a peripheral blood leucocytosis, and there may be a raised lymphocyte count in the CSF. Mortality may be up to 40 per cent in untreated louse-borne disease but is considerably lower in the tick-borne disease.

Relapse occurs in about 30 per cent of cases of louse-borne disease; up to three relapses may be seen at weekly intervals. In tick-borne disease, relapse is more common and up to ten relapses may be seen at intervals of a few days. Relapse is due to the emergence of a new antigenic variant; it is usually less severe than the initial attack.

Diagnosis

This depends on detection of the organism which may be seen on examination of a Giemsa-stained thick blood film prepared to look for malaria parasites. Dark-ground examination of fresh blood is a more sensitive technique if available.

Epidemiology

Louse-borne relapsing fever is found, like epidemic typhus, at times of war and famine. Endemic foci also occur in cool areas where living standards are poor, e.g. Ethiopia, Bolivia. Human infection occurs when an infected louse is crushed, organisms entering the body through an abrasion or through intact skin.

Tick-borne relapsing fever occurs sporadically in many tropical and subtropical countries. The vectors are ticks of the genus *Ornithodorus* which are found in cracks in poorly constructed buildings and excrete the

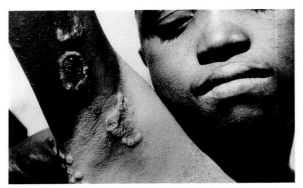

Fig. 4.7.13 Secondary endemic syphilis showing multiple ulcerated papillomata in the axilla. (Courtesy of Dr CJ Hackett/Wellcome Trust).

Management

In louse-borne relapsing fever a Jarisch–Herxheimer reaction invariably follows treatment, but is less severe following treatment with penicillin than with tetracycline. Patients should be admitted and treated with a single dose of procaine penicillin (600 000 units for those aged over 10 years and 300 000 units for younger children). Hypotensive shock should be treated with cautious fluid replacement and heart failure by digitalization. Steroids do not diminish the severity of the reaction and should not be given. A single dose of tetracycline 250 mg should be given the following day, as this reduces the likelihood of relapse.

Tick-borne relapsing fever should be treated with tetracycline (250 mg six-hourly for those aged over 10 years and 125 mg six-hourly for younger children for one week). Single-dose doxycycline (200 or 100 mg) is also probably effective and is more easily administered in the field. Penicillin should not be used, as resistance has been reported.

Prevention

Delousing is essential for the control of epidemics of louse-borne relapsing fever. It is best accomplished by DDT and the issue of new clothes to the community involved. No effective vaccine has as yet been developed.

Leptospirosis

This is an acute febrile illness caused by spirochaetes of the genus *Leptospira*. It is a zoonotic infection, humans being infected by contact (usually indirect) with the urine of infected rodents. Organisms can survive for some time in water and exposure is usually occupational, e.g. in rice fields. Children may be infected in this way or when houses are infested with rodents.

The disease has no pathognomonic clinical features and is probably underdiagnosed. It presents as an acute fever often with severe headache and meningism, myalgia and arthralgia. Conjunctival injection may be present. In severe cases, jaundice develops after a few days, and there is evidence of renal impairment. Protein and blood are commonly found in the urine and death, which occurs in up to 30 per cent of jaundiced cases in the absence of treatment, is usually due to renal failure.

Diagnosis

Dark-ground examination of fresh blood may reveal leptospires in the first week of the illness; they may be present in the urine for several weeks, but are often scanty and may be confused with fibrils in the urinary deposit. Special media are available for isolation of the organism. Serological diagnosis can be reliably achieved with a microscopic agglutination test provided the antigen contains the locally prevalent serovars.

Treatment

Benzyl penicillin should be given parenterally (100 000 units/kg per day in four divided doses for one week). It is important that treatment is started as soon as possible, since it may not be effective if given late in the illness. Peritoneal dialysis may be life saving if renal failure develops.

Chlamydial infections

Chlamydia trachomatis

The Chlamydiae are bacteria which are obligate intracellular parasites. *C. trachomatis* has a predilection for columnar epithelial surfaces and is an important pathogen of the eye and genital tract.

Trachoma is believed to affect at least 400 million people, almost all of them in tropical or subtropical countries. It is particularly prevalent, and more severe, in hot arid regions. There is evidence that its prevalence and severity are inversely related to the frequency of face washing in a given community. The active disease, a chronic follicular conjunctivitis, is seen mainly in children, in whom it usually causes mild discomfort only. In older children and adults it may progress to conjunctival scarring; if this is severe, distortion of the lid margin may cause the eyelashes to abrade the cornea (trichiasis), leading eventually to blindness (see pp. 935–6).

Neonatal infections

Chlamydial ophthalmia neonatorum (ON) affects some 30 per cent of infants born through an infected cervix.[24] It is usually less severe than gonococcal ON but may progress to scarring trachoma. The prevalence of cervical chlamydial infection has been little studied in the tropics, but one study in Nairobi, Kenya, found 29 per cent of parturient women to be infected.[25]

Of exposed infants 10–20 per cent develop chlamydial pneumonia.[24] This usually presents at the age of two to three months with a paroxysmal cough in the absence of fever. Chest signs are scanty on clinical examination but X-ray reveals extensive diffuse changes. Eosinophilia and raised levels of serum IgG and IgM are typically seen. A history of ON may suggest the diagnosis but is not always given (see pp. 183–4).

Diagnosis

In the past, laboratory diagnosis of trachoma has depended on isolation of *C. trachomatis* in tissue culture or on the detection of inclusions in iodine-stained conjunctival scrapings. Newer methods of detecting chlamydial antigen with monoclonal antibodies (immunofluorescence or enzyme-linked immunosorbent assays) appear more promising and are well adapted to field conditions. Chlamydial ON may be readily diagnosed by iodine or Giemsa stain of a conjunctival scraping, since large numbers of inclusions are usually present. Chlamydial pneumonia is best diagnosed serologically since isolation from the nasopharynx is of doubtful significance. High levels of circulating antichlamydial IgM are found.

Management

Active trachoma usually responds to a three-week course of tetracycline 1 per cent ointment twice daily, accompanied by a course of oral tetracycline (or erythromycin for children aged less than six years). Oral therapy is recommended because a nasopharyngeal reservoir of infection may be present. Chlamydial ON should be treated with oral erythromycin in addition to topical tetracycline, since this is believed to prevent progression to pneumonia. Chlamydial pneumonia should be treated with erythromycin (50 mg/kg per day in four divided doses for three weeks).

Prevention

Trachoma has disappeared from more affluent societies. It is probable that its incidence and severity could be greatly reduced in many areas of the world by providing a piped water supply. In arid situations, the provision of leaky tins hanging in appropriate places can afford a trickle of water with which to wash the eyes. The leak can be stopped by an appropriate bung and allows the most economic use of any water available. This method together with tetracycline 1 per cent eye ointment administered by village health workers has resulted in the eradication of trachoma in some nomadic and seminomadic communities in Kenya. Vaccines consisting of live or inactivated whole organisms were unsuccessful and in some cases exacerbated the disease.

Chlamydia psittaci

C. psittaci is a zoonotic infection to which many species of bird and mammal are prone. Man is occasionally infected, suffering an atypical and often severe pneumonia. Recently an atypical strain of *C. psittaci* has been described, the so-called TWAR strain, which also causes pneumonia but appears to be spread from man to man without the involvement of animals.[26] It is said to be prevalent in the United States but its importance in tropical countries has not yet been evaluated. Diagnosis of these infections is serological and treatment is with tetracycline (or erythromycin in children aged less than six years).

Rickettsial infections

The *Rickettsia*, like the *Chlamydia*, are bacteria which are obligate intracellular parasites. With the exception of *Coxiella burneti*, the causative organism of Q fever, they are transmitted to man by arthropods. All, apart from *R. prowazeki* (epidemic typhus) and *R. quintana* (trench fever), have an animal reservoir.

Epidemic typhus is seen in times of war and famine, e.g. in refugee camps. It is transmitted from man to man by the body louse, *Pediculus corporis*. Endemic typhus, by contrast, is seen wherever man comes into contact with the domestic rat; it is transmitted by the rat flea *Xenopsylla cheopsis*, and is probably underdiagnosed in tropical countries, since the characteristic rash may not be apparent in dark-skinned patients.

Although the diseases caused by different species of

Rickettsia vary in severity, they have many features in common and will be described together.

The common pathological lesion is a disseminated focal vasculitis and perivasculitis involving principally the skin, brain, myocardium and kidneys.

The illness is of sudden onset with high fever and headache, following an incubation period of 7–14 days. In scrub typhus and the Eastern hemisphere tick-borne rickettsioses, an *eschar* may be present at the site of inoculation. This begins as a papule which ulcerates and is covered by a black scab with a surrounding area of erythema and local lymphadenopathy.

A rash normally appears on days three to seven. Initially macular, this later becomes purpuric and on occasion confluent; the extent of the rash is related to the severity of the disease. Major thrombotic or haemorrhagic phenomena may be seen in severe cases, in whom hypotension, renal failure and coma may ensue. Pneumonia may be seen in epidemic typhus, scrub typhus or Rocky Mountain spotted fever. Details of the major rickettsioses are given in Table 4.7.4.

Diagnosis

Rickettsial infection should be considered in any ill febrile patient once malaria and typhoid have been excluded. The Weil–Felix test is a serological test which depends on the sharing of antigens between rickettsial species and certain strains of *Proteus*. *Proteus* are agglutinated by the serum of patients with rickettsial infections from the second week of the illness. This test is cheap and simple to perform but is not 100 per cent specific. Isolation of *Rickettsia* is not attempted routinely.

Treatment

Tetracyclines and chloramphenicol are highly effective in conventional doses. A single dose of the long-acting tetracycline, doxycycline, has been shown to be effective in epidemic typhus (200 mg in adults; half this dose should be given to children aged less than 10 years). Delousing is essential in the face of an epidemic. Vaccines are not generally available.

Q fever

Q fever is a disease caused by *Coxiella burneti* which is acquired by inhalation. Sheep and cattle are the usual reservoirs and the disease is seen chiefly in farmers and their families. It presents as an atypical pneumonia, sometimes accompanied by hepatitis. There is no rash. It is diagnosed serologically and treatment is with tetracycline or erythromycin.

References

1. Lapeyssonnie L. La meningite cerebrospinale en Afrique. *Bulletin of the World Health Organization*. 1963; **28** (suppl.): 3–114.
2. Whittle HC, Tugwell P, Egler LJ *et al.* Rapid bacteriological diagnosis of pyogenic meningitis by latex agglutination. *Lancet*. 1974; **ii**: 619–21.
3. Wall RA, Hassan-King M, Thomas H *et al.* Meningococcal bacteraemia in febrile contacts of patients with meningococcal disease. *Lancet*. 1986; **ii**: 624.
4. Greenwood BM, Wali S. Control of a meningococcal meningitis outbreak by vaccination of affected villages. *Lancet*. 1980; **i**: 729–32.
5. Whittle HC, Abdullahi MT, Fakunle F *et al.* Scabies, pyoderma and nephritis in Zaria, Nigeria: a clinical and epidemiological study. *Transactions of the Royal Society of Tropical Medicine and Hygiene*. 1973; **67**: 349–63.
6. Berman S, McIntosh K. Selective primary health care. Strategies for control of disease in the developing world. XXI. Acute respiratory infections. *Reviews of Infectious Diseases*. 1983; **7**: 674–91.
7. Shann F, Gratten M, Germer S *et al.* Aetiology of pneumonia in children in Goroka Hospital, Papua New Guinea. *Lancet*. 1984; **ii**: 537–41.

Table 4.7.4.   Rickettsial infections

Disease	Agent	Vector	Reservoir	Distribution	Course
Epidemic typhus	R prowazeki	Louse	Man	World-wide	Severe
Endemic typhus	R. mooseri	Rat flea	Rat	World-wide	Moderate
Rocky Mountain* spotted fever	R. rickettsi	Ticks	Ticks and small mammals	Americas	Severe
Fievre boutonneuse†	R. conori	Ticks	Dogs and rodents	Africa, India	Moderate
Scrub typhus	R. tsutsugamushi	Mites	Rodents	India, South East Asia	Moderate

*Western hemisphere tick-borne rickettsiosis.
†Eastern hemisphere tick-borne rickettsiosis.

8. Wall RA, Corrah PT, Mabey DCW *et al.* The etiology of lobar pneumonia in The Gambia. *Bulletin of the World Health Organization.* 1986; **64**: 553–8.

9. Baird DR, Whittle HC, Greenwood BM. Mortality from pneumococcal meningitis. *Lancet.* 1976; **ii**: 1344–6.

10. Greenwood BM, Whittle HC. *Immunology of Medicine in the Tropics* London, Edward Arnold, 1981.

11. Shann F, Hart K, Thomas D. Acute lower respiratory tract infections in children: possible criteria for selection of patients for antibiotic therapy and hospital admission. *Bulletin of the World Health Organization.* 1984; **62**: 749–53.

12. Shann F, Barker J, Poore P. Chloramphenicol alone versus chloramphenicol plus penicillin for severe pneumonia in children. *Lancet.* 1985; **ii**: 684–5.

13. Riley ID, Lehmann D, Alpers MP *et al.* Pneumococcal vaccine prevents death from acute lower respiratory tract infections in Papua New Guinean children. *Lancet.* 1986; **ii**: 877–81.

14. Piot P, Meheus A. Epidemiologie des maladies sexuellement transmissibles dans les pays en developpement. *Annales de la Societe Belge de Medecine Tropicale.* 1983; **63**: 87–110.

15. Fransen L, Nsanze H, D'Costa L *et al.* Single dose therapy of gonococcal ophthalmia neonatorum. *Lancet.* 1984; **ii**: 1234–6.

16. Laga M, Naamara W, Brunham RC *et al.* Single dose therapy of gonococcal ophthalmia neonatorum with ceftriaxone. *New England Journal of Medicine.* 1986; **315**: 1382–5.

17. Mabey DCW, Brown A, Greenwood BM. *Plasmodium falciparum* malaria and salmonella infections in Gambian children. *Journal of Infectious Diseases.* 1987; **155**: 1319–21.

18. Scragg J, Rubidge C, Wallace HL. Typhoid fever in African and Indian children in Durban. *Archives of Disease in Childhood.* 1969; **44**: 18–28.

19. Sutton RGA, Merson MH. Oral typhoid vaccine Ty21a. *Lancet.* 1983; **i**: 523.

20. Einhorn MS, Weinberg GA, Anderson EL *et al.* Immunogenicity in infants of *Haemophilus influenzae* type b polysaccharide in a conjugate vaccine with *Neisseria meningitidis* outer membrane protein. *Lancet.* 1986, **ii**: 299–302.

21. Hudson EH. *Non-venereal syphilis.* Baltimore, Williams and Wilkins, 1958.

22. Ratnam AV, Din SN, Hira SK *et al.* Syphilis in pregnant women in Zambia. *British Journal of Venereal Diseases.* 1982; **58**: 355–8.

23. Hira SK, Bhat GJ, Patel JB *et al.* Early congenital syphilis: clinicoradiologic features in 202 patients. *Sexually Transmitted Diseases.* 1985; **12**: 177–83.

24. Alexander ER, Harrison HR. The role of *Chlamydia trachomatis* in perinatal infection. *Review of Infectious Diseases.* 1983; **5**: 713–9.

25. Laga M, Plummer FA, Nsanze H *et al.* Epidemiology of ophthalmia neonatorum in Kenya. *Lancet.* 1986; **ii**: 1145–9.

26. Grayston JT, Kuo C-C, Wang S-P *et al.* A new *Chlamydia psittaci* strain, TWAR, isolated in acute respiratory tract infections. *New England Journal of Medicine.* 1986; **315**: 161–8.

Further reading

Bijlmer HA, van Alphen L, Greenwood BM *et al.* The epidemiology of *Haemophilus influenzae* meningitis in children under five years of age in The Gambia, West Africa. *Journal of Infectious Diseases.* 1990; **161**: 1210–5.

CHAPTER 8

Viral infections

Patrick Goubau, Jan Desmyter and Roger Eeckels

AIDS and other retrovirus diseases

Retroviruses are enveloped RNA viruses characterized by the presence of a RNA-dependent DNA polymerase (reverse transcriptase). After infection of a cell, this reverse transcriptase translates the viral RNA genome into DNA. This DNA needs to be integrated into the host cell genome, and is then called the proviral genome.

The first human pathogenic retrovirus to be discovered was the *human T-cell lymphotropic virus type I* (HTLV-I), a transforming virus, i.e. a virus giving rise to malignant growth of infected cells (T4 lymphocytes). Although HTLV-I has been found world-wide, there are two areas of high prevalence: Japan and the Caribbean. HLTV-I is transmitted by sexual contact, by transfusion and from mother to child. The virus has a long latency and will usually give rise to disease in adults: adult T-cell leukaemia and tropical spastic para-

paresis. A second retrovirus, HTLV-II, which is close to HTLV-I, was first isolated from a patient with hairy cell leukaemia, but no pathology has yet been causally linked to this virus.

The third human retrovirus is the causal agent of AIDS and related syndromes, named *human immunodeficiency virus* (HIV or HIV1) (formerly LAV, HTLV-III or ARV). It was discovered in 1983, only two years after the first description of the disease in American homosexuals. A second AIDS virus, HIV2, which is antigenically different from HIV1, was isolated in 1986 from west African patients. In a number of African patients, antibodies have been found which cross-react with both viruses, suggesting the existence of intermediate virus types. The HIVs primarily infect helper-inducer T4 lymphocytes.

In contrast to the Oncovirinae, represented in man by HTLV-I, HTLV-II and other viruses under study, the Lentivirinae are non-transforming, cytopathic retroviruses which were known to produce slowly progressive disease in sheep, goats and horses. Since the discovery of HIV, related lentiviruses have been found in monkeys (simian immunodeficiency viruses (SIVs)), cats and cattle. HIV2 is more closely related to the SIVs than HIV1, but there is no evidence that the SIVs, found in Old World monkeys, may infect man under natural circumstances.

Human immunodeficiency virus infection

Since its first description in 1981, AIDS has spread in a pandemic fashion and has now been reported from all over the world. AIDS is only the severe fatal end of a wide spectrum of disease manifestations, ranging from asymptomatic virus carrier state through chronic lymphadenopathy to the opportunistic infections, malignancies and encephalopathy of AIDS. The final evolution of the disease is due to the fact that HIV selectively affects the immune system and the central nervous system.

A case definition of AIDS has been developed by the Centers for Disease Control (CDC, USA).[1] The purpose of this definition is to arrive at a reliable and comparable reporting system. Therefore only severe and specific disease manifestations are included. As AIDS manifests itself only months to many years after infection (median incubation period over five years), the reporting of AIDS cases lags behind the real evolution of the epidemic and must be completed with sero-epidemiological studies. The major disadvantage of the CDC case definition is that many diseases which indicate AIDS can only be reliably diagnosed with sophisticated diagnostic tools. Therefore a provisional case definition was worked out by WHO for use in countries with limited diagnostic resources (Table 4.8.1).

Transmission   As HIV gives a lifelong infection with a long asymptomatic latency period there are many healthy virus carriers. Their infection often goes unnoticed and therefore they are a major risk for the dissemination of the disease. HIV is present in blood, seminal and cervical secretions and less constantly and at lower concentrations in saliva, tears and breast-milk. HIV is transmitted through sexual contact, by blood-to-blood contact and vertically from mother to child before birth or during delivery. Sexual transmission was first observed among homosexuals in the USA and in Europe. It is now clear that HIV is also transmitted by heterosexual contact like any other sexually transmitted disease (STD) and that this is the predominant mode of transmission in most developing countries.

Table 4.8.1.   Provisional clinical case definition for AIDS in countries where diagnostic resources are limited. Paediatric AIDS is suspected in an infant or child presenting with at least two of the following major signs associated with at least two of the following minor signs in the absence of known causes of immunosuppression such as cancer or severe malnutrition or other recognized aetiologies

---

Major signs
  Weight loss or abnormally slow growth
  Chronic diarrhoea >1 month
  Prolonged fever >1 month
Minor signs
  Generalized lymphadenopathy
  Oro-pharyngeal candidiasis
  Repeated common infections (otitis, pharyngitis, etc.)
  Persistent cough
  Generalized dermatitis
  Confirmed maternal HIV infection

Adapted from WHO, *Weekly Epidemiological Record*, 1986; **61**: 72.

Transmission by blood-to-blood contact occurs by needle sharing among drug addicts, and by transfusion of infected blood or certain blood derivates. The transmission through blood and factor VIII has been halted in western countries by systematic testing of all blood and plasma units, but transfusion is a major problem in many developing countries. It is certain that unsterilized needles and syringes are a source of nosocomial transmission in scarcely equipped health care facilities, but the importance of this transmission is unknown and different studies have yielded conflicting results. The risk of infection for health care workers after a needle stick accident is extremely low. Only a few cases of HIV infection of health care workers from patients have been reported world-wide, notwithstanding follow-up of thousands of hazardous incidents.

The vast majority of paediatric infections are due to intrauterine or perinatal transmission from the mother, and to transfusion with infected blood.

HIV is *not transmitted* by any other form of social, professional or family contact, even in primitive hygienic circumstances.

Epidemiology   Retrospective studies show that the pandemic spread of HIV started at the end of the 1970s. Among tropical and subtropical areas, HIV is now endemic in the whole of Africa south of the Sahara, with a widely varying prevalence from one place to another, in the Caribbean and in the large cities of South America, particularly Brazil. A growing number of AIDS cases is also being reported from different Asian countries. Only sporadic cases are reported from North Africa. In Africa the large cities, where social circumstances favour the rapid spread of STDs, are most affected. Successively lower prevalences are observed in smaller cities, in peripheral commercial centres and finally in the bush where the prevalence is mostly low, but increasing. The disease is introduced in a new area through travelling men (merchants, drivers, military and civil servants) and first affects prostitutes, who always remain the most affected group. When freshly introduced, HIV infection therefore shows a female predominance which progressively wanes. Infection through transfusion is a major problem in Africa, where the indications for transfusion are numerous, particularly in children and in women of childbearing age. The prevalence of HIV infection among blood donors in some cities approaches 20 per cent. HIV2 is at present predominantly observed in West Africa and is only sporadically observed elsewhere.

AIDS has far-reaching implications on all aspects of life. The burden of the chronic and recurrent diseases due to HIV infection may jeopardize medical services which already face many other problems. HIV also influences the epidemiology of other diseases, e.g. tuberculosis. Tuberculosis in the HIV-infected patient is often symptomatic, difficult to cure and infectious to others. Women have a central role in the family; HIV infection of a pregnant woman, who has a high risk of symptomatic disease, is therefore not only a threat to the woman and the unborn child but also to the structure of the family and the survival of other young children. Finally, the economically most active groups are at special risk for AIDS, having more opportunities for multiple sexual contacts, but all socio-economic classes become involved rapidly.

Clinical features   In adults the infection with HIV, which may be clinically manifested by an acute infectious mononucleosis-like syndrome and sometimes by an acute meningoencephalitis, is followed by a long latency period. After months or years general symptoms develop: chronic lymphadenopathy, a chronic diarrhoea with fever, weight loss and asthenia, a chronic encephalopathy, usually manifested by progressive dementia, and finally the various opportunistic infections and malignancies of AIDS. The most typical malignancy associated with AIDS is generalized Kaposi's sarcoma. It has an aggressive course and should be differentiated from the indolent classic Kaposi's sarcoma, which is endemic in areas of Africa and is not associated with AIDS. The complex of important and prolonged weight loss, diarrhoea and fever, while in principle still reversible, is usually present well before opportunistic infections develop, and has been called ARC (AIDS-related complex). The severe form of weight loss and wasting, or 'slim disease', has now been included in the AIDS case definition.

In children the latency period is often short and the disease often progresses rapidly, particularly in infants. Intrauterine and perinatal HIV infection nearly always become clinically manifest within the first two years. Most children with a later onset of disease have a history of transfusion. The most commonly observed clinical manifestations are failure to thrive, loss of developmental milestones, protein-energy malnutrition, chronic diarrhoea, chronic fever of unknown origin, generalized lymphadenopathy, hepatosplenomegaly, chronic cough, oral thrush, recurrent common infections and in African patients a generalized pruritic rash. Perivasculitis of peripheral retinal vessels is a common finding before the onset of opportunistic infections.

Opportunistic infections occur during the latest and fatal stage of the disease. Some, like chronic ulcerating mucocutaneous herpes simplex virus (HSV) infection and recurrent or extensive herpes zoster (uncommon in children), can be diagnosed clinically. A presumptive diagnosis of candida oesophagitis can be established in a patient with oral candidiasis and retrosternal pain on swallowing. The chronic diarrhoea of AIDS is sometimes due to *Cryptosporidium* or to *Isospora belli*, which can be readily diagnosed by simple laboratory procedures, but most often no cause is found. Chronic cough with interstitial pulmonary infiltrates on X-ray and variable dyspnoea, can be due to cytomegalovirus (CMV) pneumonitis, *Pneumocystis carinii* pneumonia or lymphocytic interstitial pneumonia. Specific diagnosis requires bronchoscopy. Lymphocytic interstitial pneumonia is typical of childhood AIDS and may be a lymphoproliferative response to Epstein–Barr virus. Disseminated infections with *Cryptococcus neoformans*, *Coccidioides immitis* (in the Americas), *Histoplasma capsulatum* and atypical mycobacteria (particularly *M. avium-intracellulare*) can only be diagnosed by culture or histopathology, but the microscopic diagnosis of cryptococcal meningitis is accessible to the laboratory of the rural hospital. Further opportunistic infection, like cerebral toxoplasmosis and generalized CMV and HSV infections, and some malignancies (cerebral lymphoma or non-Hodgkin B-cell lymphomas in other sites) require sophisticated diagnostic techniques.

Children with AIDS are also frequently affected by other non-opportunistic infections: repeated common infections, deep-seated infections (pneumonia, meningitis, osteomyelitis), septicaemia (particularly with non-typhoid salmonellas), refractory tuberculosis (often extrapulmonary).

HIV encephalopathy is manifested in children by one or two of the following: loss of developmental milestones, acquired microcephaly due to impaired brain growth, and progressive symmetrical motor deficits.

Kaposi's sarcoma is only rarely seen in children and then often presents as a pure lymphadenopathic form, which can only be diagnosed by lymph node histopathology. Lymphadenopathic Kaposi's sarcoma of African children also occurs independently of HIV infection.

Dysmorphic craniofacial abnormalities together with growth failure and microcephaly in infants and small children have been attributed to intrauterine HIV infection. However, later prospective studies could not confirm these findings.[2]

The provisional WHO case definition (Table 4.7.1) should allow the diagnosis of AIDS even at the primary care level where no laboratory facilities are at hand. It must, however, be emphasized that the signs which are listed are also seen in many other conditions in tropical areas. Therefore the value of this definition may vary from one place to another, depending on the disease pattern and on the prevalence of HIV in a particular area. Before being introduced into clinical practice and in epidemiological reporting in a particular country or area, the definition should be evaluated locally by laboratory confirmation of a sample of cases. A classification system for HIV infection in children has been proposed for use in industrialized countries.[3] An adapted classification and staging system is clearly needed for clinical and epidemiological studies in developing countries.

Laboratory diagnosis The diagnosis of HIV infection is established by the detection of antibodies to HIV. These become usually detectable two to six weeks after infection and, in almost all cases, before three months. A seropositive person should be considered as infected and infectious. The tests most used at present are enzyme-linked immunosorbent assays (ELISA). Although these tests are highly sensitive and specific, false-positive results may be a problem, particularly where the HIV prevalence is low.

Therefore, supplementary tests are often needed to confirm the positive results. Simple tests, as reliable as ELISA in good hands, are now available, and should be widely used in developing countries if cost permits. It is essential to define clearly what will be done with positive results, before introducing serological tests, as a test is not in itself a solution to the AIDS problem. Clear indications for testing are the screening of blood

donors, epidemiological surveillance and the evaluation of diagnostic criteria. In any testing programme thorough consideration should be given to ethical, psychological and pragmatic problems which might arise.

Virus isolation is not a routine procedure. Direct antigen detection on serum has been found a useful prognostic marker in industrialized countries, a positive test being associated with evolution to overt disease. Unfortunately, antigen detection is seldom positive in African patients, even with full-blown AIDS.

In the infant the serological diagnosis may be difficult owing to the presence of passively transferred maternal antibodies. The infection will be confirmed when compatible clinical symptoms appear or if antibodies persist beyond the age of 15 months.

The immunological test abnormalities reflect a depression of both cellular and humoral immunity with a selective destruction of T-helper/inducer lymphocytes (T4) and a polyclonal B-cell activation. Commonly observed abnormalities include an absolute lymphopenia, a low T4 lymphocyte count ($<400/mm^3$), an inversed helper/suppressor (T4/T8) ratio, hypergammaglobulinaemia and cutaneous anergy. Neutropenia, thrombocytopenia and anaemia are also common findings.

Treatment In developing countries, it is of prime importance to diagnose and treat opportunistic and associated infections with all means at hand.[4]

There is no doubt that the antiretroviral agents zidovudine (azidothymidine, AZT) and dideoxycytidine (ddC) prolong life and the quality of life in AIDS patients. However, they do not cure, are very expensive, and have important side-effects (bone marrow depression and neuropathies, respectively). It is not yet known whether these or newer antivirals may delay evolution of HIV infection towards AIDS. In 1991, a protective vaccine is nowhere in sight.

Public health measures Three lines of action must be taken in the face of the AIDS epidemic: cope with the additional burden on health services; control the spread of the disease; prevent the social consequences of AIDS.

The treatment of chronic and recurrent diseases in HIV-infected people place an increasing burden on health services. Regular evaluation of the HIV-related supplementary needs in manpower, drugs (particularly antibiotics and parenteral fluids) and laboratory equipment should help budgeting and policy decisions.

Appropriate psychological support of HIV-infected people and their families and terminal care of AIDS patients are difficult to achieve in crowded and under-equipped health services. Original solutions should be developed for each society, taking into account the cultural aspects of disease and the ways the society and the family cope with chronic illnesses. The impact of AIDS is more important when social and medical structures are weak. The strengthening of basic medical structures remains a priority and funds for this should not be diverted to 'AIDS' programmes.

In the absence of a vaccine, the only means of direct prevention are the serological screening of all blood donors, the appropriate sterilization of all syringes and needles and education of the public to diminish sexual spread.

The risk of sexual transmission can be lowered by diminished sexual promiscuity with a stable and faithful monogamy or polygamy as ideal situations. The use of condoms as a preventive measure was shown to be feasible in limited high-risk groups (prostitutes in large cities). The theoretical and unproven risk of trans-mission through breast-feeding is far outweighed by the risk of bottle-feeding. 'Breast is best' remains the message. Appropriately organized immunization campaigns are not a risk for the spread of AIDS. No recommended vaccine has up to now been shown to represent a risk for HIV-infected people. The theoretical risks of live vaccines are certainly much lower than the risks of the diseases against which they protect. Only BCG should be withheld from *symptomatic* HIV-infected children.[5]

Discriminatory attitudes against AIDS patients and their family should be countered by objective and simple information which puts the disease in its real perspective. This information must also be directed towards health personnel, whose attitude is important for the credibility of the message. Appropriate legal measures should protect the respective rights of the individual and of the community.

Adenoviruses

Adenoviruses are DNA viruses named after the adenoid tissue from where they were first isolated in 1953. There are more than 40 known serotypes with a world-wide distribution. Some of the higher numbered types (8 and above) have more frequently been isolated in developing countries. Adenoviruses are very stable, with prolonged survival outside the host cells, and may therefore spread from person to person by many different direct or indirect ways. After infection, adeno-

viruses may persist in lymphoid tissues and viral shedding in the stool may recur for prolonged periods of time. Most infections occur in childhood and have a subclinical course in 50 per cent of cases. Small epidemics may occur in closed communities.

The most frequent clinical picture is an *upper respiratory tract disease* of progressive onset with moderate fever in children under five. *Acute follicular conjunctivitis* is the most common and benign adenoviral infection of the eye. *Pharyngoconjunctival fever* is a more typical illness with high fever of abrupt onset, pharyngitis and con-junctivitis (unilateral in 70 per cent of cases). In temperate climates it is seen at school age. *Keratoconjunc-tivitis*, mostly due to type 8, is an acute pronounced con-junctivitis with superficial erosions of the cornea and often subepithelial opacities. There are no general symptoms but marked photophobia. It heals usually without sequelae but symptomatic treatment should be aimed at preventing bacterial infection. Epidemics centred on an eye clinic are regularly observed. *Lower respiratory tract disease* manifested by bronchitis, bron-chiolitis or pneumonia, usually has a favourable course. In young children it may, however, have a serious, occasionally fatal evolution. It is sometimes com-plicated by encephalitis, myocarditis and gangrene of the fingertips. Bronchiectasis may be a sequel. Fatal adenoviral pneumonia has also been seen in mal-nutrition or in the aftermath of severe measles. Adeno-virus infection occasionally mimicks *whooping cough* and is then clinically indistinguishable from *Bordetella pertussis* infection. The fastidious (difficult to grow) adenoviruses 40 and 41 are a cause of *diarrhoea* in infants and young children with little seasonal trend. *Acute haemorrhagic cystitis* is a rare adenoviral self-limited disease of children, and is frequently due to type 11.

Arboviruses

The arthropod-borne animal viruses or arboviruses form a large and heterogenous group of viruses. The common characteristic to which their name refers is their multiplication in, and transmission by, haemato-phagous arthropods (essentially mosquitoes, sandflies and ticks). Over 400 arboviruses have been dis-tinguished up to now, but only about one-fifth of these have been linked to human disease. Most of these human arbovirus diseases are in fact maintained in a zoonotic cycle, man being only an accidental host. Transovarial transmission of arboviruses in arthropods has been demonstrated. The arthropod vector might therefore also be the reservoir, at least in some instances.

On the basis of their antigenic relationship, arboviruses are divided into 48 groups. The most important ones in human pathology are the alphaviruses which are taxonomically part of the Togaviridae, the Flaviviridae and the bunyamwera supergroup, belonging to the Bunyaviridae.

Arboviruses have a world-wide distribution but are most prevalent in tropical and subtropical countries. Many arbovirus diseases only occur sporadically and go mostly unnoticed, while some can be endemic with many human cases (e.g. dengue in South-east Asia) or cause epidemics (e.g. dengue in the Americas or yellow fever in Africa). The surveillance role of peripheral primary health care facilities cannot be overemphasized in this setting. Any upsurge of dengue-like cases (see later) or any case of fever with haemorrhagic diathesis, of fatal acute hepatitis (where yellow fever is endemic) and of aseptic meningoencephalitis should be promptly reported to the health authorities and be considered as a public health priority.

Among the numerous vectors of arboviruses one deserves special mention: *Aedes aegypti* which transmits urban yellow fever, dengue and chikungunya. *A. aegypti* is an anthropophilic mosquito, breeding in mostly man-made containers (old tins, tyres, open water jars, etc.) in the direct vicinity of houses. The eggs can withstand prolonged desiccation. The control or eradication of this mosquito is a public health priority in many countries. Control is achieved mainly by destruction or treatment with larvicides of breeding places. Education of the public, who should be aware of the importance of small-scale environmental sanitation, and a continuous entomological surveillance by well-trained teams are essential parts of any control programme.

The clinical picture of arbovirus infection varies from a clinically inapparent infection to a frequently fatal haemorrhagic fever or meningoencephalitis. Single viruses may be responsible for several distinct clinical diseases, while the same symptomatology may be caused by various arboviruses. An aetiological diagnosis is therefore impossible on clinical grounds and can only be established by laboratory techniques, which are seldom available on the spot. In isolated cases the diagnosis will therefore seldom be possible, but it is of the utmost importance that a precise diagnosis be established as fast as possible in epidemic circumstances. The following clinical pictures are possible, although they should not be seen as separate entities but rather as a continuous spectrum.

Asymptomatic infections are frequent with most arbovirus infections. These are only demonstrated by seroconversion.

An undifferentiated febrile illness accompanied by aspecific flu-like symptoms is more often observed in small children than in adults, who tend to have a more typical and severe illness. It is impossible to distinguish these infections from the numerous other viral illnesses of childhood.

A dengue-like syndrome typically starts abruptly with high fever and aches in joints and muscles. After defervescence a maculopapular rash develops, which sometimes heralds a second rise in temperature.

Haemorrhagic fevers are possibly fatal diseases with haemorrhagic manifestations and frequent signs of circulatory collapse. Hepatic and renal involvement are possible, as is the case with yellow fever.

Meningoencephalitides are caused by a group of neurotropic arboviruses. They vary in severity from fairly mild, such as in California encephalitis, to severe with a high case-fatality rate, as in Japanese or Russian spring–summer encephalitis. Viral encephalitides are reviewed on pp. 749–56.

The convalescence of arbovirus infections is usually prolonged with persistent aches, asthenia and sometimes depression. Still these diseases present as acute fevers and are no part of the differential diagnosis of prolonged fever of unknown origin.

Antibodies appear early during the disease and often persist throughout life. These are protective against infection only with the homologous virus, although many cross-reactions exist with other viruses from the same group. Due to these cross-reactions, it is important to perform serological tests against a panel of different antigens: the highest titre will be observed against the causative virus. Neutralization tests are more specific than complement fixation or haemagglutination-inhibition. In the 1930s an attenuated live vaccine against yellow fever (17 D-strain) was developed which is still successfully used. The only other vaccines which have come into use since are against Japanese encephalitis and European tick-borne encephalitis. Active research is going on for the development of a dengue vaccine.

When caring for patients possibly suffering from arbovirus disease, especially when handling blood or blood-contaminated needles, one should be aware of the possible nosocomial transmission of these viruses.

The main characteristics of some arbovirus diseases are now briefly reviewed. Dengue and yellow fever are discussed later in this chapter under 'Haemorrhagic fevers'.

Chikungunya presents as a dengue-like illness, sometimes with mild haemorrhagic signs, the latter particularly in Asia. Severe haemorrhagic phenomena or shock seldom occur. The virus is transmitted to humans by *Aedes aegypti*. The disease is present in Africa and in parts of Asia, where dengue is also endemic. Epizootics of chikungunya among monkeys have been observed in Africa but have not been carefully investigated in Asia.

Congo-Crimean haemorrhagic fever is a febrile disease with haemorrhagic phenomena which has been observed in southern USSR, Balkan countries, Pakistan and in central Africa, but its exact boundaries are not well defined. The virus is transmitted by ixodid ticks. Haemorrhage is rare in Africa.

O'Nyong Nyong occurs in central and east Africa where it caused a large epidemic from 1959 to 1962. The virus, which is closely related to chikungunya, is transmitted by *Anopheles* mosquitoes. The clinical disease is indistinguishable from chikungunya.

Rift Valley fever (Africa and Middle East) causes epizootics among cattle, with abortion in cows and neonatal mortality of lambs (up to 90 per cent). Human cases are often associated with these epizootics and are contracted by the bite of mosquitoes or by direct contact with carcasses. The disease usually presents as a dengue-like syndrome but severe cases are complicated by a haemorrhagic diathesis. Epidemics of haemorrhagic yellow fever-like disease have been associated with Rift Valley fever.

Sandfly fever (phlebotomus fever/pappataci fever/three-day fever) is a benign flu-like disease transmitted by phlebotomine sandflies. It is endemic from the Mediterranean and Nile basin to Central Asia with sudden outbreaks during summer among newcomers to the area. Local sporadic cases mostly go unnoticed among the many viral diseases of childhood.

West Nile fever is widely distributed in Africa, the Mediterranean basin and Central Asia. The virus is transmitted by different *Culex* mosquitoes. Infants and young children experience a mild febrile illness, while older children and adults more often present with a dengue-like syndrome.

Enterovirus diseases

Together with the rhinoviruses, which are frequent causes of common cold, the enteroviruses belong to the Picornaviridae, a family of small RNA viruses (22–30 nm). There are about 70 serotypes of enterovirus which have been divided into different groups: the three polioviruses (see pp. 750–2), Coxsackie A and Coxsackie B viruses, and echoviruses; further enteroviruses have not been grouped but numbered from 68 onwards. Hepatitis A virus has the characteristics of an enterovirus but is discussed under Hepatitis later in this chapter. We only deal here with the non-polio viruses and the term enterovirus should here be understood as such.

Enteroviruses are transmitted by the faecal–oral route and by droplet infection. In a particular location and period a number of serotypes are endemic, constantly circulating among the few non-immune people, particularly very young children. Owing to the very large number of enteroviruses, specific serotypes may be absent from a particular area during long periods of time. From time to time a newly introduced serotype rapidly spreads in this susceptible population, reaching a large proportion of all age groups. Dissemination of different serotypes thus occurs in waves, with one predominant type succeeding another, sometimes in a short period of time. In tropical and subtropical countries, widespread circulation of enteroviruses occurs throughout the year with a very high incidence among young children. In poor hygienic conditions up to 80 per cent of children under the age of two may harbour one or more enteroviruses at any one time. Large-scale epidemics may occur, e.g. the pandemic spread of acute haemorrhagic conjunctivitis (see later).

Enteroviruses may give rise to many more or less clear-cut clinical pictures. The same virus may cause different syndromes and the same syndrome can be caused by several distinct enteroviruses. Moreover, certain epidemics seem to show that the appearance of a particular symptomatology might be a temporary manifestation of a given virus, not reappearing during later epidemics caused by the same serotype.

Asymptomatic infections and mild disease which passes almost unnoticed occur with all enteroviruses in variable frequency, depending on the virulence of the strain involved.

Non-specific febrile illness is the most common clinical presentation. Respiratory involvement may be present, usually as pharyngitis, sometimes as croup, bronchitis, bronchiolitis or pneumonia, mostly with a benign course. Enteroviruses are not a cause of isolated rhinitis (common cold) except Coxsackie A 21.

Exanthematous febrile illnesses are frequently observed with enteroviruses. The rash is usually maculopapular but may be urticarial, petechial or vesicular. A particular form is *herpangina*, mostly caused by Coxsackie A viruses, which begins abruptly with fever and sore throat (see p. 731). The soft palate and the fauces show a small number of vesicles (no more than 10) progressing after 12–24 hours to shallow ulcers. The disease is self-limiting and lasts for about one week. In the case of *hand, foot and mouth disease*, oral vesicles are more numerous and vesicles also appear on hands and feet, together with maculopapular lesions.

Gastro-intestinal symptoms may accompany other signs of enteroviral illness: abdominal pain, loose stools, nausea and vomiting. But enteroviruses are not considered to be a cause of isolated infantile diarrhoea.

Pleurodynia or Bornholm disease starts usually with a stabbing pain in the epigastrium, shifting to the thorax and making respiration difficult. In children abdominal pain is common. The extremities may also be affected. High intermittent fever appears, mostly after the onset of pain. Usually cough is conspicuously absent. The disease may be biphasic in course. Serofibrinous pleuritis, pericarditis and orchitis are possible complications. Pleurodynia is almost exclusively caused by Coxsackie B viruses.

Acute myocarditis has a significant mortality in neonates and small children. In older children and adults benign pericarditis and myocarditis are seen with a usually favourable outcome.

Infection of newborns may follow transplacental transmission but is more often acquired during delivery or postnatally from the mother or from horizontal spread within a maternity unit. The disease is often severe with a clinical picture resembling bacterial sepsis.

Aseptic meningitis has been found associated with more than 50 enterovirus serotypes. As a group the enteroviruses are the most frequent cause of viral meningitis with a good prognosis. Rarely non-polio enteroviruses will give rise to more severe neurological disease and may cause paralytic poliomyelitis (see p. 752).

Acute haemorrhagic conjunctivitis is characterized by sudden painful swelling and redness of the conjunctivae accompanied by subconjunctival petechial or ecchymotic bleeding. It was first described in West Africa in 1969. The disease was due to a previously unknown enterovirus (serotype 70) and has spread in pandemic waves during the following years. A variant of Coxsackie A 24 has since also been found to cause widespread epidemics of acute haemorrhagic conjunctivitis. The disease has affected mainly tropical countries on all continents and has its highest incidence among adults. Transmission is from eye to eye via hands and fomites.

Coxsackie B viruses (and cytomegalovirus) are under study as possible causes of *juvenile diabetes* in genetically predisposed individuals.

The *diagnosis* of enterovirus infection can be confirmed by virus isolation from faeces, nasopharynx aspirates, throat swabs or spinal fluid. In most cases, faeces have the highest yield of positive cultures and virus may still be detected several weeks after the onset of the acute phase of infection. When a specific serotype or group of viruses is suspected, serology on paired serum samples will be helpful. A fourfold titre rise over a period of two to four weeks is diagnostic.

Haemorrhagic fevers

Haemorrhagic fevers are viral febrile diseases with haemorrhagic phenomena, most obvious as purpura, ecchymoses, epistaxis, and gastro-intestinal bleeding. In some of these, renal failure or hepatitis may be prominent. Although some features of the disease and the geographical location may be helpful in distinguishing these diseases from one another, a firm aetiological diagnosis is only possible by serological or virological means. Furthermore, other febrile haemorrhagic diseases, bacterial (meningococcaemia, relapsing fever, leptospirosis) or rickettsial (typhus) should be excluded. Handling of autopsy material and attempts at virus isolation on samples from haemorrhagic fever patients can be dangerous procedures and should only be performed in laboratories with adequate containment facilities.

Dengue

Dengue virus is a single-stranded RNA virus belonging to the Flaviviridae. There are four types. It is mostly transmitted by *Aedes aegypti*. Human disease presents in two clinical forms: most often the benign dengue fever syndrome and sometimes dengue haemorrhagic fever and dengue shock syndrome (DHF/DSS). Dengue is highly prevalent in South-east Asia and the Pacific and epidemics occur regularly in the Americas and the Caribbean. Dengue has also been observed in several parts of Africa.[7]

Dengue fever is characterized by a biphasic fever with rash. Typically the disease starts suddenly after an incubation of two to seven days with high fever, headache, flushing of the face and sometimes a transient macular rash. Myalgia and pains in joints and bones are prominent and increase in intensity over the days. After two to six days the fever wanes. A second rise in temperature often occurs one to two days later with a generalized maculopapular rash. Asthenia and pains may persist for several weeks after defervescence. In infants and small children, dengue is more often an atypical fever with pharyngitis, rhinitis and mild cough lasting for two to five days.

DHF/DSS starts as benign dengue fever but after two to five days there is a rapid deterioration with often circulatory collapse. The child is restless with cold clammy extremities, scattered petechiae, bruising and easy bleeding at puncture sites. At this stage there is an elevated haematocrit, due to haemoconcentration, thrombocytopaenia, hypoproteinaemia and a positive tourniquet test. Bleeding from the intestinal tract occurs and hypovolaemia due to capillary hyperpermeability, with evolution to irreversible cardiovascular collapse. If untreated, the fatality rate may be as high as 50 per cent. DHF/DSS has a bimodal age distribution, occurring in infants (3–11 months old) with a primary infection and in children older than one year with a secondary infection with a different dengue virus type (most often dengue 2). This could be due to an enhancing effect of cross-reacting passively or actively acquired antibodies. DHF/DSS is not observed in all the endemic areas of dengue. DHF/DSS is endemo-epidemic in South-east Asia and was observed recently during dengue epidemics in the Caribbean.

For public health reasons it is important to confirm the diagnosis. For serological diagnosis an acute-phase serum sample should be taken, preferably before the fifth day, and a second sample two to three weeks later. A fourfold rise in the antibody titre is diagnostic. The results allow the distinction of a primary from a secondary infection. It is not always possible to make a difference between the dengue virus types on the basis of serology alone.

There is no specific antiviral treatment but careful symptomatic treatment lowers the fatality rate of DHF/DSS to 5 per cent. As antipyretic and analgesic acetaminophen (paracetamol) is preferable to salicylates which may worsen acidosis and the haemorrhagic phenomena. Patients should be carefully observed for early signs of shock and fluid replacement therapy instituted when indicated with glucose-electrolyte solutions. Plasma or plasma expanders (10–20 ml/kg/hour) are indicated in case of profound or prolonged shock. The degree of haemoconcentration and the effect of fluid therapy can be simply and reliably followed by regular haematocrit determinations. Where laboratory facilities exist, treatment should be monitored on the basis of electrolyte and acid–base balance.

The prevention of dengue is through control of the vector (see p. 605).

Yellow fever

Yellow fever virus, a flavivirus, is transmitted among monkeys in the canopy of rain forests by zoophilic mosquitoes (*Haemagogus* species in South America and *Aedes africanus* in Africa) in an enzootic cycle. The mosquito is the true reservoir and is infected for life (six to eight weeks) and transmits the virus to its offspring. Monkey and man act as amplifiers by allowing more mosquitoes to become infected. Sporadic infections occur when man enters the forest or is bitten by an anthropozoophilic mosquito in the fields bordering the forest (jungle yellow fever). In some moist savannah areas of Africa yellow fever is endemic with up to 50 per cent of the population having antibodies. Epidemics occur when the virus is introduced into an area with abundant 'wild' *Aedes* mosquitoes (jungle yellow fever) or peridomestic *A. aegypti* (urban yellow fever) and a low immunity in the human population. During epidemics the highest morbidity and mortality are observed among children.[8, 9]

In South America, yellow fever is enzootic in the forests of the Amazon, Orinoco, Catatumbo, Atrato and Magdalena river basins, with sporadic human cases. No urban yellow fever occurred since 1942, but the danger has again increased as *A. aegypti* has reinvaded several areas and invaded some new places. In Africa, yellow fever is considered to be present from 15° North to 10° South, on the basis of serological surveys carried out in the 1930s. Single cases up to severe epidemics occur in West Africa with attack rates of up to 50 per cent or more in the affected areas (Burkina Faso and Ghana, 1983; Nigeria, 1986–7).

The fatality rate is about 5 per cent when all infections are considered but may be as high as 50 per cent among hospitalized patients. Often the infection is inapparent or gives a mild aspecific febrile disease or a dengue-like syndrome. The typical full-blown disease is a haemorrhagic fever with hepatonephritis. After an incubation of three to six days there is an abrupt onset of high fever and violent headache and lumbar pain. The patient appears agitated and anxious with flushing of the face and congested mucosae. After three days the fever drops and the clinical condition improves. This is followed soon by a second bout of fever with vomiting, intense abdominal pains, icterus and quickly increasing proteinuria. Severe central nervous disturbances appear, together with petechial haemorrhage and profuse bleeding from the gastro-intestinal tract. Death occurs between the fourth and eleventh day and is due to shock (haemorrhagic or cardiac), hepatic or renal failure. In non-fatal cases recovery is complete without sequelae.

The aetiological diagnosis of yellow fever, which is important in all suspected cases, can be confirmed classically by serology on paired serum samples or by virus isolation. Newer techniques allow a rapid diagnosis on a single serum sample: the detection of specific antibodies of the IgM class and direct viral antigen detection in serum. Postmortem diagnosis on the histopathological appearance of the liver is also possible, although not entirely specific, but liver biopsy is strictly contra-indicated.

Treatment is symptomatic and not very efficient in severe cases. A more aggressive intensive care approach might lower the lethality, but the means for this are seldom, if ever, available where yellow fever occurs. Patients should be transported under a mosquito net and nursed in a mosquito-free environment when there is a risk of introducing the virus in an uninfected area.

Yellow fever can be efficiently prevented by the vaccine. The extended programme on immunizations offers the opportunity to reintroduce vaccination in high-risk areas where it has been neglected. Control of *A. aegypti* in urban areas remains important.

Arenavirus diseases

Arenaviruses are enveloped RNA viruses. Four have been associated with human disease: lymphocytic choriomeningitis virus (LCM), Junin virus, Machupo virus and Lassa virus. The reservoirs of these viruses are rodents which excrete the virus in the urine. The exact mechanism of transmission to humans has not yet been fully unravelled but it seems likely that infection occurs through inhalation or ingestion of material contaminated with rodent urine. LCM is present worldwide in mice but human cases are infrequent. Infection usually gives rise to a flu-like syndrome, sometimes with aseptic meningoencephalitis with a generally good prognosis.

Argentinian and Bolivian haemorrhagic fevers (AHF and BHF) occur in limited areas of South America. The reservoirs for Junin and Machupo virus, the agents of AHF and BHF respectively are small rodents of species *Calomys*. Since its first description in 1958, AHF has extended its area from the north-west of Buenos Aires province to sections of Cordoba, Santa-Fe and la Pampa. The peak incidence of AHF coincides with the harvest of maize in autumn (May). BHF, which was described in the department of Beni, was more village-associated and has been effectively controlled by rodent trapping and poisoning. Person-to-person transmission is exceptional in both diseases. Both clinical diseases are similar, presenting as a febrile disease of gradual onset. In severe cases, haemorrhagic signs appear as well as encephalitic signs with a high mortality. Rising haematocrit values herald severe hypovolaemic shock. Treatment is mainly supportive. Convalescent immune plasma significantly improves survival if given early.

Lassa fever is known to occur in rural areas of Sierra Leone, Liberia and Nigeria, but seroepidemiological evidence suggests that it is more widespread in an area extending from the Central African Republic to Senegal. The virus is enzootic among peridomestic *Mastomys natalensis* rats. Person-to-person transmission

also occurs. Familial clustering and particularly lethal hospital epidemics have been observed.

In endemic areas, Lassa fever appears to be a frequent cause of benign febrile disease, also among children. The onset is gradual with fever associated with cough, vomiting, abdominal pain, diarrhoea, proteinuria and an exudative pharyngitis, which seems more frequent in children than in adults. Haemorrhagic signs are limited and in one series occurred in only 15 per cent of hospitalized children. An aspartate aminotransferase level of more than 150 IU at hospital admission is an ominous sign associated with a fatality rate of over 50 per cent. Death occurs during the second week due to hypovolaemic or cardiac shock, renal failure and pulmonary oedema.

The aetiological diagnosis is by virus isolation on serum (viraemia can persist for as long as three weeks), urine, throat aspirates or by serology with indirect immunofluorescence. The presence of specific IgM or a high titre of IgG on a single serum sample is diagnostic as well as a fourfold titre rise on paired samples taken three to four weeks apart (seroconversion occurs during the third week). All material for serology or virus isolation must be packed safely and shipped cooled to a reference laboratory after arrangements have been made by telex or telephone.

Specific treatment with intravenous ribavirin for 10 days has lowered the fatality rate of severe cases from 55 to 5 per cent if started before the seventh day of the disease and to 26 per cent if given later.[10] The efficiency of convalescent plasma is controversial. Further treatment is supportive. Strict barrier-nursing is essential and effective in preventing nosocomial spread even in peripheral hospitals without strict isolation units.

Ebola haemorrhagic fever

Ebola virus is a rod-shaped RNA virus. It caused three outbreaks (Sudan, 1976, 1979; Zaire, 1976) of a haemorrhagic fever with sudden onset and a very high case-fatality rate (53–88 per cent). The epidemics were centred on large hospitals where they probably originated from one or a few sporadic cases. Transmission was either by close contact in the course of patient care or by contaminated syringe and needle. The institution of patient isolation and basic hygienic measures stopped the epidemic in all cases.[11]

Marburg virus, the only other member of this group of viruses (proposed name: Filoviridae), caused a similar disease in laboratory workers in Europe, who became infected from Vervet monkey cells. In 1975, a cluster of three cases infected by the same virus occurred in South Africa. The index case became infected during a trip to Victoria falls (Zimbabwe). When a similar disease is suspected the same precautions for patient care and handling of biological specimens should be adopted as for Lassa fever. Reservoirs and vectors of Filoviridae are not known.

Hantavirus disease

Hantaviruses, a group of related viruses belonging to the Bunyaviridae, are enzootic among several species of rats and mice, which may contaminate humans. Human disease, also known as haemorrhagic fever with renal syndrome, has been observed in eastern Asia (Korea, China, eastern USSR) and in Europe. The more severe Asian disease is characterized by fever, proteinuria, renal failure, diffuse haemorrhages and sometimes fatal shock. The European form presents as a flu-like disease with abdominal symptoms, followed by acute renal failure with a spontaneously favourable outcome. Serological surveys of rodent populations have shown that these or related viruses are enzootic on all continents, suggesting that human disease may perhaps exist and go unrecognized outside the known distribution area.[12]

Other haemorrhagic fevers are also caused by arboviruses: Kyasanur forest disease (India) and Omsk haemmorhagic fever (Siberia).

Hepatitis virus diseases

Hepatitis A

Hepatitis A is caused by enterovirus type 72. A single serotype is prevalent world-wide. The incubation period is two to six weeks, usually four weeks. As with other hepatitis viruses, it is not known whether the acute hepatitis is due to effects of multiplication of the virus within hepatocytes, an immunological reaction, or both. Hepatitis A virus (HAV) is spread by faecal shedding, which is highest at the end of the incubation period, and generally ends within two weeks after the onset of illness. Viraemia is brief, and transmission by blood transfusion is extremely rare. Man and the apes are natural hosts. Marmosets and other New World monkeys can be experimentally infected. Strains of HAV have been made to grow in primate cell lines, without cytopathic effects. Cell culture-derived, formalin-inactivated (Salk type) vaccine is in advanced clinical trial.

In the pre-icteric phase, fever, headache and gastro-intestinal complaints are more common in hepatitis A than in hepatitis B, but they are less common in children than in adults. In the icteric phase, fever subsides, but gastro-intestinal complaints may become exacerbated, although usually not in children. Pruritus, bradycardia, and mental depression are common in adults but not in children. The liver is enlarged and tender; the spleen may be palpable. In children, the icteric phase on average lasts 10 days compared with one month in adults. Occasionally, icterus is biphasic and complete healing may take months, but HAV has never been reported to cause chronic liver disease. No long-term excreters are known. Compared with the other hepatitis viruses, HAV is a rare cause of fulminant hepatitis (acute yellow atrophy of the liver). It is believed that hepatitis A tends to be more severe in persons who are poorly nourished; this may particularly apply in pregnant women and in those with sickle-cell anaemia. In children, anicteric forms are common and constitute a majority of cases; anicteric forms are the general rule under the age of three years.

HAV is transmitted by the faecal–oral route and direct contact. Food (not only shellfish) and water can be faecally contaminated and are sources of important epidemics. Hepatitis A usually occurs as definite outbreaks, with always a higher incidence in children. Day-care centres for younger children are at particular risk.

The laboratory diagnosis is made by liver function tests (aminotransferases, bilirubin and others) and by the detection of IgM anti-HAV by ELISA or radioimmunoassay (RIA). IgM anti-HAV is always present when the patient first feels ill and persists for at least six weeks, up to nine months. IgG anti-HAV persists lifelong, indicating protective immunity. In most tropical and subtropical countries, about 90 per cent of adults have anti-HAV; most infections occur in children under 5–10 years of age. In several industrial countries, not more than 25 per cent of young adults have anti-HAV, indicating effective faecal hygiene. Under certain circumstances in the tropics, it will be necessary to exclude other hepatitis viruses, yellow fever, malaria, leptospirosis and other diseases which may affect liver function.

There is no specific treatment. Bed rest and a balanced diet with adequate protein supply are less important than previously believed in normal persons developing hepatitis, but might be particularly valuable in the undernourished.

Normal, pooled human immunoglobulin contains anti-HAV antibody which prevents either jaundice or infection in 80 per cent of those not previously exposed to HAV, for four to six months after i.m. injection of not less than 0.02 ml/kg. If exposure continues, the same dose is repeated usually only once. It is likely that in the meantime inapparent infection will have been acquired, resulting in active immunity.

Epidemic non-A hepatitis (hepatitis E)

Following the availability of specific assays for hepatitis A during the 1970s, it was realized that some large water-borne hepatitis epidemics which had been observed for many years in the Indian subcontinent and in Central Asia were not due to HAV. 'Epidemic' hepatitis is therefore no longer synonymous with hepatitis A, and the term epidemic or enterically transmitted non-A (or non-A, non-B) hepatitis has been coined. Recently the name hepatitis E has been proposed. The area where this infection has been identified now extends from North Africa to China; Mexico has also been implicated.[13] A considerable proportion of acute non-A hepatitis in countries with poor sanitation may ultimately be found to be due to the same agent. The disease is thought to have disappeared in industrialized areas with improved faecal hygiene and, particularly, water hygiene.

The disease has almost exclusively been identified in young and middle-aged adults, with increased morbidity and a case fatality of up to 20 per cent in pregnant women. There is no evidence for chronicity.

The virus has been identified with the use of convalescent sera in human stools, and in hepatocytes of *Cynomolgus* macaques to which it can be experimentally transmitted. There is no proof for more than one serotype so far. Although the nucleic acid has not been definitely identified, the 33 nm round particle (i.e. larger than enteroviruses) has features of caliciviruses, a group of naked RNA viruses with pathogenicity for animals. Human caliciviruses have not been cultured, but other caliciviruses have been observed in stools, and implicated in winter vomiting disease. At present, all reagents for diagnosis are experimental.

Hepatitis B

Hepatitis B virus (HBV) is the human representative of the hepadnaviruses, a newly recognized group of DNA viruses with tropism for hepatocytes and strict host specificity. Hepadnaviruses are exceptional because in spite of the presence of an envelope or shell (hepatitis B surface antigen or HBsAg in HBV), they are highly resistant, and because during their replication cycle their DNA polymerase also acts as a reverse transcriptase, i.e. for transcribing RNA into DNA. This

mechanism relates them to some extent to the RNA retroviruses, and the name 'reversoviruses' has been proposed to cover both groups.

The infectious virion or Dane particle of HBV is a round particle of 42 nm. Under the shell of HBsAg made in the cytoplasm, it contains a core particle of 27 nm made in the nucleus, and consisting of the nucleocapsid of core antigen (HBcAg) enclosing a circular, partially double-stranded DNA and the polymerase. In the blood, there is always an excess of HBsAg under the form of 22 nm round and sometimes tubular particles. There can be up to 1×10^8 infectious virions, and up to 1×10^{13} HBsAg particles per millilitre of blood. In practice, measuring HBsAg in the blood means measuring the non-infectious 22 nm particles. It should be assumed that when HBsAg is found, infectious virions are also present. This, however, is highly variable, and much HBsAg-positive blood has little or no infectivity, except when given in large amounts such as in blood transfusion. Infectivity, i.e. the presence of Dane particles, strongly correlates with the finding of circulating HBeAg in the blood. HBeAg is a byproduct of the manufacture of HBcAg by the liver; HBcAg in the blood is so tightly encapsulated in the virion that it is difficult to detect. Other measures of the infectivity of blood are the HBV DNA polymerase assay, and particularly the measurement of HBV DNA itself.

HBV cannot be cultured *in vitro* in the classical sense, i.e. infectious virions are not produced. HBsAg can be recovered from cultures of primary hepatocellular carcinoma. There are numerous 'subtypes' of HBV and its HBsAg, denoted for example as *adw, ayw, adr. d* and *y* are mutually exclusive alleles, and so are *w* and *r*. Subtypes have geographical predilections – *r* used to be restricted to East Asia and *y* is predominant in Africa. However, there are no proven differences in pathogenicity between subtypes, and there is cross-immunity due to the universal presence of the *a* determinant. Subtypes are epidemiological tools.

Hepatitis B has an incubation period between six weeks and six months. About one-half of the cases, and more in children, are asymptomatic. The prodromal stage is somewhat different from that in hepatitis A, 40 per cent having serum sickness-like urticaria, exanthem, polyarthralgia or arthritis. HBsAg in the blood may precede hepatitis or even the prodrome by several weeks, to be followed by an increase in aminotransferases and by the appearance of anti-HBc. By the time the patient seeks help, HBsAg is almost invariably present. In the rare instances where anti-HBc is still absent, it will be found after a short time. In the acute period, there is HBeAg; the latter invariably disappears before HBsAg disappears, and HBeAg is closely followed by anti-HBe. In acute infection, HBsAg usually wanes after one or two months. With few exceptions, and sometimes with an interval of several weeks, the waning of HBsAg is followed by the appearance of anti-HBs, considered the 'protective' antibody. Anti-HBc and anti-HBs remain present for years, frequently for life.

When HBsAg is present for more than six months, the patient is considered a carrier of HBsAg. Carriers are healthy or have minimally disturbed liver function, and some have or will develop chronic hepatitis. HBeAg correlates with high infectivity and a progressive course; conversion to anti-HBe, which may take place any time even after many years, heralds low infectivity, resolution and, in a minority of cases, future disappearance of HBsAg. Of adults with acute HBV infection, 5–10 per cent become chronic carriers; the figure is higher in children and exceeds 50 per cent in infants. In all countries, a considerable proportion of all cases of non-alcoholic chronic persistent or aggressive hepatitis, with or without cirrhosis, is associated with HBsAg. Extrahepatic manifestations other than the prodrome are ascribed to immune complex formation, and may occur both in the acute and the chronic stage. These include papular acrodermatitis (Gianotti–Crosti syndrome) in children, membranous glomerulone-phritis, Henoch–Schönlein syndrome, cryoglobuli-naemia, periarteritis nodosa, and possibly polymyalgia rheumatica.

HBV is the principal agent of primary hepatocellular carcinoma in man (see p. 886). In males in Africa and parts of Asia, it is the most frequent malignancy. Most cases are associated with HBsAg, and the remaining cases mostly have other HBV markers. HBsAg is demonstrable in the cancerous cells and, regardless of serological status, it has been claimed that HBV DNA is present in almost all primary hepatomas. The HBV DNA is integrated in the cellular DNA. This, however, is not peculiar to hepatoma, since it is a frequent event in all HBV infections, and it can be most efficiently detected in chronic hepatitis. The carcinoma rarely arises in the absence of chronic hepatitis or cirrhosis. There are clearly cofactors, but these are poorly recognized; alcohol abuse, aflatoxin and chronic schistosomiasis may play a role. The risk for a HBsAg carrier of developing primary hepatocellular carcinoma is more than 100-fold higher than for a non-carrier. Persons who have become carriers by perinatal trans-mission or during childhood, are at higher risk than those who have acquired HBsAg as adults.

The diagnosis, apart from the liver function tests, is made by the finding of HBsAg and anti-HBc during acute or chronic infection. Acute infection can be distinguished from exacerbations of chronic infection by the usually rapid disappearance of HBsAg and by the presence of IgM anti-HBc in the former. IgM anti-HBc is, however, not a totally reliable criterion, but is valuable when a patient with hepatitis is only seen after HBsAg has already subsided. Most assays for HBV markers are presented under the form of ELISA or RIA assays. Cheaper versions of the HBsAg assay, such as certain haemagglutination tests, may be acceptable. The older cross-immunoelectrophoresis assays should be abandoned.

Transmission and epidemiology In practice, HBsAg-positive blood is the only source of infection, and trans-mission is parenteral, i.e. via skin or mucous membranes. This includes, however, blood on objects, and micro-amounts transmitted via micro-trauma. This is probably the major way of transmission of HBV between children in developing countries. The small traumas and lack of blood hygiene in children in developing countries are sufficient for transmission of the highly infectious and stable HBV, but not of the much less infectious and more labile HIV. In industrialized countries, improved hygiene has virtually halted HBV transmission between children. Although arthropods can take up infectious amounts of HBV, there is little or no evidence that they have a significant, if any, role in HBV transmission. Sexual partners of HBsAg carriers are at increased risk of being HBsAg-positive or having other HBV markers, especially in the tropics. In industrialized countries, there is no rule, and many partners of HBsAg carriers remain free of HBV markers. This is strongly related to anti-HBe positivity in the HBsAg-positive partner, who is then not very infectious.

About 5 per cent of the world population carries HBsAg, and 50 per cent become infected with HBV during their lifetime. In African and Asian countries, it is common to find 10 per cent or more HBsAg carriers, and up to 80 per cent with other HBV markers (anti-HBs, anti-HBc) in the general population. The rates are lower in Latin America; in Northern Europe and most of North America, less than 0.5 per cent have HBsAg and 90–95 per cent of the total population remains free of HBV infection. HBeAg rates among HBsAg carriers are generally 20 per cent or less world-wide, except that it is higher in China and adjacent areas where a racial factor could be involved. Perinatal transmission, mostly occurring during birth, is much more frequent from HBsAg-positive mothers in East Asia than in other parts of the world, including Africa. Since infection in infancy usually leads to a chronic carrier state, a considerably greater proportion of HBsAg carriage is due to perinatal transmission in East Asia than in other parts of the world.[14] In Africa, most HBV infections result from horizontal transmission during childhood.[15] The net result is about equal numbers of HBV carriers in both areas, and an equal risk of hepatocellular carcinoma. Breast-feeding is of uncertain significance in transmission of HBV from the mother to the infant, and should not be avoided in developing countries because of the high risk of bottle-feeding (see pp. 95–102, 153–7). It has been estimated that over one-third of HBsAg carriers infected during early childhood will develop serious liver disease as adults.

Apart from children, certain groups with impaired immunity are prone to develop inapparent infection with long-term persistence of HBsAg (Down's syndrome, leukaemia, lepromatous leprosy, thalassaemia, and haemodialysis and transplant patients). Others are at increased risk of HBV infection: users of unsafe needles and skin-piercing practices, the medical professions, homosexuals, haemophiliacs, etc.

Treatment There is no specific treatment for acute hepatitis B. Chronic hepatitis B is sometimes treated with corticoids and immunosuppressive drugs; long-term results are uncertain. Present long-term trials with antiviral drugs (interferon, adenine–arabinoside, etc.) may show an advantage.

Control Control of hepatitis B should be inspired by the notion that it is HBsAg-positive and particularly HBeAg-positive blood which is infectious, that it is particularly so on direct inoculation, that minute amounts of serum can be infectious, and that the virus is highly resistant to physical and chemical destruction. Iatrogenic transmission by soiled instruments can be dealt with by standard practice, but has its counterpart in many other incidents which may occur in low-hygiene populations. Hypochlorite is the only common disinfectant with proven efficiency; detergents have cleansing but no sterilizing value.

Screening of blood donors for HBsAg virtually eliminates this previously most common source of severe post-transfusion hepatitis, and is universal since the 1970s in most industrialized countries. In developing countries, cost has frequently been prohibitive, and the gain has been less apparent, given the fact that many recipients are already immune or would soon have become infected through other sources anyway.[16] Whenever HBsAg screening on blood donors can be performed in developing countries, it should be done, but it should never receive priority over anti-HIV screening (see pp. 603–4).

Hepatitis B vaccine has been available since 1982 as particles of HBsAg, derived from blood of asymptomatic carriers (see p. 85). Infectious HBV is eliminated during purification and by treatment with formalin or heat. An alum adjuvant is added. Most injection schemes are 0–1–2–12 months, or 0–1–6 months, with possible booster injections after five years. Anti-HBs is formed. Efficacy is over 90 per cent in normal individuals with the various vaccines and schedules. Children in developing countries have been shown to profit even from two doses, started at the age of three months or later. If the mother is known to be HBsAg-positive, a full schedule should be preferred, starting at birth. In the latter case, there may be some advantage in adding 1 ml of hyperimmune HB human immunoglobulin, administered at the same time but in another body area as the first vaccine dose.

This vaccine, because of its mode of preparation and the need to use chimpanzees for safety tests, has been safe but prohibitively expensive for most developing countries, which are precisely those who should consider it for general use in children. A few remarkable programmes are going on in some countries.[17, 18]

Since 1986, vaccines have been available in which HBsAg is produced by the DNA recombinant technology in yeast cells. Others are now available which are made in mammalian cells, and some of those may include, in addition to the S part of the HBsAg, which is standard in all vaccines, pre-S2 and perhaps pre-S1 polypeptides; the latter are present to various extents in natural HBV and HBsAg. At this time, there is no known advantage for the recipient of any of these and other foreseeable vaccines over existing vaccines. However, the DNA recombinant technology has provided an essential step in the future lowering of the cost of the vaccines.

Apart from its use in neonates mentioned above, there is at present little use for passive immunization with hyperimmune globulin. It is partially active in needle-stick accidents with HBsAg-positive blood, but professionals at risk should now be preventively vaccinated, unless they are known to have HBV markers.

Deltavirus (hepatitis D)

The infectious virion of hepatitis D virus (HDV) is a 35 nm particle in the blood, in which a small piece of RNA is embedded in delta antigen (HDAg) and HBsAg. HDV is a defective virus multiplying only in hepatocytes already infected with HBV. Coinfection is simultaneous introduction of HBV and HDV; most infections are probably superinfection of HBsAg carriers with HDV. HDV production goes on as long as the person is HBsAg-positive. Anti-HD, for which diagnostic tests are available, appears a few weeks after infection and it subsides soon after the person has stopped producing HBsAg.

Coinfection with HBV and HDV is clinically similar to infection with HBV only. Superinfection manifests itself as acute hepatitis in a HBsAg carrier. HDV does not increase the chances of becoming a HBsAg carrier, but it significantly increases evolution to chronic hepatitis in HBsAg carriers. HDV may lower HBsAg and anti-HBc titres, although not below the level of detection by sensitive methods.

Global distribution of HDV is extremely scattered. The highest prevalence is certainly in the Middle East, and in parts of South America. In industrialized countries, HDV was first detected in parenteral drug abusers and in haemophiliacs. Little is known about children and perinatal transmission, but one should assume that their risk parallels that of HBV.

The control of HDV is synonymous with the control of HBV.[19]

Parenterally transmitted non-A, non-B hepatitis (hepatitis C)

Non-A, non-B hepatitis is hepatitis which is not caused by HAV, HBV, other known viruses, drugs, or ischaemia and is not an expression of other known non-viral disease. This definition by exclusion may include a variety of causative factors, infectious or not. Epidemic non-A hepatitis (see earlier) was the first entity which was defined within the complex. In 1988 a long-elusive agent of parenterally transmitted non-A, non-B was identified.

Following HBsAg screening of blood donations and the recognition that HAV had almost no role in post-transfusion hepatitis, transfusion continued to be followed by hepatitis detected by aminotransferases in about 10 per cent in the United States, and 3 per cent in Northern Europe. Some of these cases could be ascribed to rare effects of known viruses (Epstein–Barr virus and cytomegalovirus), but 90 per cent were 'genuine' non-A, non-B, with incubation periods of 15–150 days, usually 50 days. The same donors were a source of non-A, non-B hepatitis in several recipients, and their blood transmitted the disease to chimpanzees. The risk of this hepatitis was also increased in contacts with other patients, in recipients of blood derivatives such as Factor VIII, in frequently hospitalized patients, in parenteral drug abusers and in the sexually pro-

miscuous. It was also increased in haemodialysis and transplantation patients, although not to the same degree as for hepatitis B. In industrialized countries, 15–50 per cent of sporadic cases of hepatitis are non-A, non-B and could be due to the same transmissible agent.

The acute phase of this non-A, non-B hepatitis is frequently less severe than in hepatitis A or B; 75 per cent of the aminotransferase-proven cases are anicteric or asymptomatic. In 30 per cent, however, liver function remains chronically disturbed, which may lead to chronic hepatitis and cirrhosis, although resolution in the long term seems more frequent than with similar stages of HBV disease.

After many false claims that the virus of parenterally transmitted non-A, non-B hepatitis, or its antigen or antibodies had been identified, work on materials from experimentally infected chimpanzees has now succeeded. From their plasma, an RNA genome has been molecularly isolated, and part of the genome has been expressed by DNA recombinant technology. This antigen binds with antibody in the sera from convalescents of non-A, non-B post-transfusion hepatitis, as well as with sera from chronic carriers. For the first time, samples from a coded American panel of non-A, non-B sera of known pedigree have been correctly identified. The genome resembles that of flaviviruses, which is consistent with the known sensitivity of the virus to lipid solvents. This virus is now named hepatitis C virus.[28]

Tests are now available for the detection of antibodies against the agent, or at least a principal agent, of parenterally transmitted non-A, non-B hepatitis. This should replace testing of 'surrogate markers' – alanine aminotransferase and anti-HBc – which, because of their partial association with non-A, non-B hepatitis, has been initiated with great difficulty and loss of donor blood in some industrialized countries.

The new technology is also expected to reveal the extent of parenterally transmitted non-A, non-B hepatitis in developing countries. This is an area where there is virtually no information and where, if parenterally transmitted non-A, non-B hepatitis parallels hepatitis B as it does in the industrialized countries, a major source of liver disease could be unveiled. Recent evidence suggests an association between hepatitis C virus and some cases of hepatocarcinoma.

Herpesvirus diseases

Herpesviridae are a family of morphologically similar DNA viruses with an envelope.[20] Five herpesviruses cause human disease: herpes simplex viruses type 1 and type 2 (HSV1 and HSV2), varicella-zoster virus (VZV), cytomegalovirus (CMV) and Epstein–Barr virus (EBV). After a primary infection, herpesviruses remain present in a latent form and may give rise over the years to recurrences. Herpesvirus infections have a very high prevalence (up to 100 per cent) all over the world, even in the most remote areas. Herpesviruses, which have a potential for causing severe and recurrent infection in the immunocompromised patient, are important opportunistic pathogens in AIDS.

A virus first called human B-cell lymphotropic virus (HBLV) and now human herpesvirus-6 (HHV-6), has been first isolated from AIDS patients. Recent evidence implicates HHV-6 as the cause of roseola infantum (exanthema subitum).[21] Finally, rare cases of monkey herpes (B-virus) infection have been contracted from the bite of monkeys and have led to a lethal encephalitis.

Herpes simplex

HSV1 is usually associated with oral herpes and HSV2 with genital herpes, but this distinction is not strict and both viruses can be recovered from any site. Primary herpes occurs after an incubation of three to nine days and may be asymptomatic or give rise to muco-cutaneous vesicular lesions. After this primary episode the virus becomes latent in the ganglion cells inner-vating this area. Reactivation of the virus, elicited by various stimuli (e.g. fever, trauma, heat) will lead to asymptomatic virus shedding or to recurrent lesions in the same body area as the primary infection. Herpetic lesions are more infectious than asymptomatic virus shedding. Recurrent herpes tends to be more localized and heal more rapidly than primary herpes. In primitive living conditions 90 per cent of children below the age of 10 become infected with HSV1, one-fifth symptomatically, and by adulthood all have acquired the infection. HSV2 is commonly acquired through sexual contact and is the usual cause of neonatal herpes. The association of HSV2 with cervical cancer is no longer believed to be causal.

Herpetic gingivostomatitis, usually seen in children between three months and six years, is the overt form of primary herpes of the mouth. Crops of small vesicles appear on the oral mucosa which rapidly coalesce to aphthous lesions. In some cases there are few with minimal discomfort while in others numerous confluent lesions are observed, with intensely red, swollen, easily bleeding gums, cervical lymphadenopathy, skin lesions around the mouth and high fever. The condition may last for 12–14 days. Children with malnutrition or recovering from measles are particularly prone to the more severe form, which is dangerous by interfering with normal nutrition. *Labial herpes* (fever blisters) is the benign recurrent form of oral herpes.

Pharyngitis is a less typical presentation of HSV infection. *Eczema herpeticum* is a severe primary infection in children with eczema and other dermatoses. It may involve extensive areas of skin and may occasionally disseminate to deep organs. *Herpetic whitlow*, most often seen in medical practitioners but which may complicate primary oral herpes, is indistinguishable from pyogenic infection. *Herpetic keratoconjunctivitis*, primary or frequently recurrent, may lead to permanent corneal scarring. The linear or dendritic acute corneal lesions are best observed with topical fluorescein dye. *Herpetic encephalitis*, either primary or due to reactivation, has no preference for a given age and is the most frequent form of non-epidemic encephalitis (see pp. 754–5).

Generalized or disseminated herpes is an infrequent complication which arises in immunocompromised patients, particularly with AIDS, and in patients with widespread burns. In AIDS, HSV infection often presents as chronic mucocutaneous herpes, with extensive necrotizing lesions.

Neonatal herpes infection has an incidence of 1 in 2500 to 35 000 newborns (see pp. 165–6). Infection by HSV2 is acquired from the mother during birth, while HSV1 is acquired postnatally from the mother or other people caring for the child. Primary genital herpes of the mother during pregnancy, particularly during the last trimester, may also lead to retarded fetal growth, abortion or prematurity. The risk of neonatal infection is rather low from recurrent genital herpes, symptomatic or not (2–4 per cent), and still lower from labial herpes, but the risk is important in case of primary genital herpes. Primary genital herpes is characterized by painful, numerous, bilateral lesions with systemic symptoms often lasting for more than two weeks and sometimes accompanied by lesions at distal sites. Symptoms in the child may appear up to three weeks after birth. Seventy per cent of neonatal herpes cases will lead to disseminated or central nervous system disease if untreated with high mortality and frequent sequels. Symptoms are fever, poor feeding, respiratory difficulties, cyanosis, hepatosplenomegaly, icterus and herpes lesions of the skin. Skin symptoms are absent in more than 20 per cent of the cases.

The diagnosis of HSV infection can be confirmed by culture of the virus from a lesion. Direct antigen detection by immunofluorescence obviates the need for cell culture but is less sensitive than isolation and requires skilled microscopists. Cytological examination of scrapings or biopsies shows typical cells with intra-nuclear inclusions (also seen in chickenpox). Serological tests have limited usefulness in the diagnosis of HSV infections.

Two drugs have substantially lowered the incidence of complications and fatalities in life-threatening HSV infections: acyclovir and vidarabine. As vidarabine has important toxicity, acyclovir has become the drug of choice for severe infections (see Table 4.8.2). The major drawback of all antivirals is their cost. For herpetic keratitis, scarring may be prevented by carefully scraping the superficial epithelial layer and, if available, by applying an antiviral product (see Table 4.8.2). In case of gingivostomatitis the main point is to maintain adequate nutrition. In severe cases it may be necessary to pass a naso-gastric feeding tube.

The prevention of neonatal herpes is a matter of concern and there is no agreement on the best attitude in all circumstances. In industrialized countries Caesarean section is generally recommended when the pregnant woman has extensive primary genital herpes at the end of pregnancy. No Caesarean section is recommended in case of a history of genital herpes without lesions, but samples for HSV detection should be taken from mother (genital) and child (pharynx) at birth to allow rapid diagnosis and treatment if the child

develops symptoms. Caesarean section in cases of limited recurrent or first genital herpes is controversial. In developing countries our attitude should be based on the following: the risk of Caesarean section for the mother or for later pregnancies, the availability of acyclovir and of diagnostic facilities, the risk to the child under the given circumstances. To prevent postnatal infection of the neonate by HSV1, handwashing and the wearing of a mask is recommended for those caring for the child while having fever blisters.

Varicella-zoster virus

Primary infection with VZV presents as chickenpox (varicella), a mostly benign disease, characterized by a vesicular pruritic rash with few systemic symptoms (see pp. 516–8). Moderate fever lasts for two to three days during the onset of eruption. The lesions are seen in different stages of evolution on the same skin area (papules, vesicles, crusts) and are mainly located on the scalp, face and trunk. In industrialized countries it is essentially a childhood disease. In the tropics and subtropics fragmentary evidence suggests that the disease often occurs at an older age with many adult

Table 4.8.2.   Indications for antiviral treatment

Indication	Drug and route	Dosage	Comments
HSV* encephalitis HSV infection in immunocompromised	Acyclovir – i.v. infusion Vidarabine – i.v. infusion	10–15 mg/kg t.d.s. 10 mg/kg daily by slow infusion	Life-saving; acyclovir more efficient and fewer side-effects than vidarabine
Neonatal HSV infection HSV keratitis	Acyclovir ointment – local Trifluorothymidine solution – local	– –	Second choice: idoxuridine (IDU) and vidarabine have corneal toxicity
Severe primary HSV	Acyclovir – i.v. infusion Acyclovir – p.o.	10–15 mg/kg t.d.s. i.v. 100–200 mg 5 times /day p.o.	Treatment of acute episode does not prevent recurrences; no paediatric oral suspension marketed
Chickenpox – immunocompromised – neonate	Acyclovir – i.v. infusion Vidarabine – i.v. infusion	10–15 mg/kg t.d.s. 10 mg/kg daily by slow infusion	Prevent complications if given <6 days after onset; vidarabine toxic; both less effective than in HSV infections
	Varicella-zoster immune globulin	0.1 ml/kg	Alters the course if given <4 days after exposure
Zoster in immunocompromised	Acyclovir – i.v. infusion Vidarabine – i.v. infusion	10–15 mg/kg t.d.s. 10 mg/kg daily by slow infusion of solution	Accelerated healing if treatment <6 days after onset; no effect on post-therpetic pain
Severe RSV† infections	Ribavirin – aerosol	of 20 mg/ml for 12–18 hrs/day for up to 7 days	Moderately useful; not a substitute for O_2 and other supportive treatment
Lassa fever	Ribavirin – i.v. or p.o.		Life-saving in severe cases; highest efficiency if given early

* HSV = Herpes simplex virus.
† RSV = Respiratory syncytial virus.

cases. Severe varicella with organ involvement (hepatitis, pneumonia, encephalitis) is a dreaded complication in immunocompromised children and in neonates (see pp. 517, 754). Intrauterine infection occurs and the risk of congenital abnormalities has been estimated at about 2 per cent when the mother has varicella (not zoster) during the first trimester. Owing to the age distribution in the tropics this might occur quite often, but firm data are lacking.

Shingles (zoster), the clinical form of recurrent VZV infection is uncommon in children, sometimes occurring after malaria and in children who became infected *in utero*. Clinical signs are pain, usually moderate in children, and grouped vesicles on an erythematous base in the area of one to three sensory nerves.

Acyclovir is active against VZV although less than against HSV. When given within three days after exposure, hyperimmune VZV, but not standard immunoglobulin, may alter the course in children at special risk, e.g. a neonate whose mother develops chickenpox within five days before or after delivery. In uncomplicated chickenpox only symptomatic treatment is needed: application of calamine lotion or eosin solution to lesions and trimming of the nails to avoid excessive scratching.

There is an effective live attenuated varicella vaccine but apart from its usefulness in children with malignancies, its indications are not yet well defined, and it needs to be kept frozen.

Epstein—Barr virus

The classical picture of acute EBV infection is mostly seen in young adults as *infectious mononucleosis* with exudative tonsillopharyngitis, lymphadenopathy, splenomegaly, disturbed liver function tests and sometimes hepatomegaly, rash and jaundice. The blood picture shows an elevated number of atypical lymphocytes. Heterophil antibodies develop which can be detected by the Paul–Bunnell–Davidsohn test or the easier rapid slide tests. In children, *asymptomatic EBV infection* without heterophil antibody is the rule and, even in clinical EBV-induced infectious mononucleosis in young children, heterophil antibody is absent in most cases. Only the detection of specific IgM antibodies (not generally available) allows the diagnosis in these cases. An infectious mononucleosis-like syndrome may also be due to CMV and to HIV (AIDS-virus). In tropical countries, EBV infection is acquired very early in life with a peak incidence before three years of age. Infectious mononucleosis is therefore relatively rare.

EBV is linked, probably together with other factors, to the development of childhood *Burkitt's lymphoma* which is endemic in areas of tropical Africa and New Guinea (see pp. 877–80) and of adult *nasopharyngeal carcinoma*.

Lymphocytic interstitial pneumonitis, a common finding in children with AIDS, most probably reflects a lymphoproliferative reaction to EBV.

Cytomegalovirus

Most primary infections with CMV are subclinical and are followed by lifelong latency with frequent recurrences of asymptomatic viral shedding (urine, saliva, breast-milk, genital secretions). In developing countries all have acquired the infection during childhood and most even before five years of age. Acquisition is through intrauterine infection, from genital secretions during birth, from breast-feeding and later through horizontal transmission from other children. Horizontal transmission depends more on intensive contact between children and their habit of 'mouthing' objects than on general hygienic conditions, as has been shown in day-care centres in industrialized countries.

Although congenital infection often follows recurrent infection of the mother during pregnancy, congenital *cytomegalic inclusion disease* (CID), a serious disease of neonates, is only seen after primary infection of the mother (see p. 165). As almost all adults are seropositive (have antibodies), CID will rarely if ever be seen in developing countries. For the same reason neonates will be protected against serious post-transfusion disease, which is seen in premature babies from seronegative mothers.

In normal subjects, CMV is a rare cause of *infectious mononucleosis-like disease* occurring spontaneously or as a post-transfusion syndrome three to seven weeks after administration of blood. The risk is proportional to the volume transfused.

In AIDS and other immunodeficient states, CMV is a frequent cause of severe life-threatening infections, commonly seen as *interstitial pneumonia, hepatitis, chorioretinitis* or *disseminated disease*.

The diagnosis may be confirmed by finding cytomegalic inclusion cells in urine, scrapings of buccal mucosa around Stenson's duct or biopsy specimens. Virus isolation, mainly from urine or throat washings, gives more valid results but does not distinguish between primary infection and recurrent viral shedding. The same is true for the finding of antibodies (simple latex agglutination tests are now available). Specific IgM-class antibodies, which may be detected by ELISA, are more often seen in primary infections and are never present in passively acquired antibody.

A new antiviral, gancyclovir, is useful in the immune compromised patient with severe CMV infection.

Ortho- and Paramyxoviridae

Ortho- and Paramyxoviridae are pleomorphic enveloped RNA viruses. The orthomyxoviruses consist of the *influenza* A, B and C viruses. The paramyxoviruses group the four *parainfluenza* viruses, *respiratory syncytial* virus (RSV), *mumps* virus (see pp. 513–15) and *measles* virus (see pp. 496–501).

Influenza

Influenza A virus has an important antigenic variability. Isolates from successive epidemic waves show minor antigenic changes. This phenomenon is called antigenic *drift*. An antigenic *shift* occurs when there is a complete switch from one subtype to another. The immunity against the new influenza A subtype is then very low in the world population and this provokes a pandemic spread of the virus. Influenza B is only subject to antigenic drifts and causes more localized outbreaks. The epidemiology of influenza C, which is sporadically isolated, is less well known.

Influenza is a disease of acute onset with high fever, general malaise, headache, myalgia and upper respiratory tract symptoms. Pneumonia, viral or by bacterial superinfections, is a well-known complication. In children, abdominal pain and gastro-intestinal symptoms may be prominent features of influenza ('gastric flu'). Influenza is also one cause of acute laryngotracheobronchitis (croup) in young children. Annual epidemics of influenza are less pronounced and less season-bound in tropical than in temperate zones. Under usual circumstances influenza vaccines should be no part of public health policy in tropical countries.

Parainfluenza

There are four distinct types of parainfluenza viruses. Primary infection occurs at a young age and gives rise to respiratory disease which may be severe. Reinfections occur throughout life; they are often sub-clinical or manifested by benign upper respiratory symptoms (common cold, pharyngitis). In young children the most characteristic syndrome associated with parainfluenza viruses is croup, with possible laryngeal obstruction, most often caused by types 1 and 2 (see p. 710). Other manifestations are febrile upper respiratory tract disease, tracheobronchitis, bronchiolitis and pneumonia. The last two are mostly due to type 3. The pathology due to type 4 is less well known but seems more benign.

Respiratory syncytial virus

In all geographical areas RSV is the major cause of bronchiolitis and pneumonia in infants and young children (see pp. 712–13). Most people become infected during infancy or early childhood but reinfection, with a mostly benign course, is common throughout life. Primary infections are usually symptomatic with fever and respiratory symptoms. A number of these patients will develop bronchiolitis or pneumonia, and less often bronchitis or laryngotracheitis. The incidence of RSV infections requiring hospitalization before one year of age has been estimated at 1:200 to 1:70 infants. These infections are often followed by chronic abnormalities of pulmonary function and by recurrent episodes of lower respiratory tract disease through the following years. Ribavirin in aerosol is effective in lowering the severity of the acute disease.

In industrial countries, RSV infection gives yearly epidemics in late autumn and in winter, but few data are available about the seasonality of RSV infections in the tropics. The present availability of sensitive and specific ELISA and immunofluorescence techniques for the detection of RSV-antigen in respiratory secretions, obviates the need for cell culture and should allow a better understanding of the epidemiology in developing countries.

Parvovirus diseases

Parvoviruses belong to the smallest viruses known (18–25 nm). They are widespread among animals. A human parvovirus was discovered fortuitously in healthy blood donors in 1975, but only in the 1980s could it be linked to human disease. The human parvovirus, now designated B19 virus, causes erythema infectiosum, aplastic crisis in chronic haemolytic anaemia and congenital infection. In industrialized countries 80 per cent of adults have serological evidence of past infection. No serological data have been published from tropical countries, but erythema infectiosum is believed to occur world-wide. In Jamaica, clustering of aplastic crises in sickle cell anaemia patients occurs every three to five years.[22]

Erythema infectiosum (fifth disease) is a well-known exanthematous childhood disease. The aetiological role of B19 virus was discovered during a London epidemic in 1983. After an incubation period of about one week a fiery red rash develops on the cheeks ('slapped-cheek' appearance). General symptoms are usually mild. One to four days later a rubelliform exanthem appears on the proximal extremities, trunk and buttocks, and then becomes reticular and lacy in appearance. After a few days the rash has disappeared but may reappear after exercise, bathing or sunlight exposure for a week or two. *Arthralgia* and *arthritis* may occur but are more common in the adult, particularly female patients than in the child. *Subclinical infections* and mild non-specific *upper respiratory tract disease* also occur, particularly in children.

Aplastic crisis in patients suffering from chronic haemolytic disease is characterized by a fall in haemoglobin concentration and a reticulocytopenia, accompanied by general symptoms (headache, shivering, abdominal pain with nausea and vomiting). The association with B19 virus infection was first shown in 1981 in sickle cell anaemia patients in London and Jamaica. The observation was later extended to other chronic haemolytic conditions. B19 virus replicates in dividing erythroid precursor cells with a resultant transient arrest of erythropoiesis. In normal people this has no clinical consequences, but in patients with haemolytic anaemia, whose erythrocytes have a shortened life span, a fall in haemoglobin concentration ensues.

Congenital infection is a frequent occurrence in animal parvovirus infections and has been demonstrated in humans. B19 virus infections during the first and second trimesters have been associated with spontaneous abortion, often with hydrops fetalis, and during the third trimester with stillbirth. Although there is no doubt about the causal relationship, the extent of the problem is as yet unknown. No birth defects in viable infants have been attributed to B19 infection.

The *diagnosis* of B19 virus infection is only possible in a few laboratories, usually by detection of specific IgM antibodies.

Poxvirus diseases

Poxviruses are large (250–300 nm) brick-shaped DNA viruses. There are two strictly human poxvirus diseases: smallpox, which has been eradicated, and molluscum contagiosum (see pp. 863–4). Other animal poxviruses may sporadically cause human disease like cowpox, tanapox, orf and monkeypox. Most of these infections give a self-limited disease with one or a few skin lesions, except for monkeypox which is clinically similar to smallpox (see later).

The global eradication of smallpox

The last case of endemic smallpox was Ali Maow Maalin who fell ill on 26th October 1977 in the town of Merca, Somalia. This was the endpoint of 10 years of continuous efforts by thousands of people coordinated by WHO.[23]

A number of features of smallpox, which are not shared presently by other diseases, allowed total eradication. Smallpox gives no subclinical disease and contagiousness, which is of a relatively low level when compared with diseases like influenza or measles, accompanies the skin lesions. It is thus easy to identify contagious patients, even for lay people, and to contain the disease by isolation. Furthermore, there is no prolonged carrier state nor recurrence of illness and no animal reservoir from where the virus may reinvade the human population. Finally, there is an effective and cheap vaccine with an incredible stability, obviating the need for a cold chain.

Some experience from the eradication campaign may be relevant to other situations. First of all the feasibility of eradication had already been demonstrated before the programme began, as the disease had already been eradicated both from the industrialized countries and from a number of developing countries. Political and managerial aspects were of utmost importance. All countries were interested to support the programme: endemic countries because they were faced with the problem, the other countries because of the continued financial burden of vaccination and surveillance. Experience showed that there is a great deal more trained manpower available in developing countries than is generally assumed. The collaboration of the general public, who were informed about the disease and the goals of the campaign, was essential to identify new outbreaks. From the beginning, epidemiological and clinical research by those involved in the programme and strong links between field workers and research scientists appeared essential as specific and unexpected problems arose. This is striking for a disease which was already so thoroughly known. In the most difficult situations the key strategy to eradication was the identification and containment of smallpox foci rather than 100 per cent vaccine coverage. For every country, surveillance continued until certification of eradication several years after the last case. Research on animal poxviruses is continuing to make sure no unexpected problem can arise from possible oversight. Important stocks of vaccine are kept under supervision of WHO, in case of emergency. A final unsettled question is whether to keep or to destroy the two remaining virulent virus stocks.

Monkeypox

In the era after smallpox eradication, monkeypox has become the most important orthopoxvirus infection of humans, requiring continued epidemiological surveillance and research. It is a rare sporadic zoonosis that occurs only in the remote tropical rainforest areas of Central and Western Africa. Squirrels probably play an important role as reservoir. Person-to-person transmission is limited, with an attack rate of 12 per cent among unvaccinated household contacts, which contrasts with a high 37 to 88 per cent for smallpox. The vast majority of patients are children less than 10 years of age. This points to the protection given by smallpox vaccination in the older age groups. As immunity wanes in the population, the age distribution should change. The longest chain of transmission observed consisted of four serial cases.

The illness usually starts with fever accompanied by severe headache, backache, general malaise and prostration. The rash starts one to three days later. The skin lesions usually first appear on the face as small macules, then extend to the arms, the trunk and the legs. The lesions vary from a few to thousands and are more numerous on the face and extremities than on the trunk. In general, the lesions develop more or less simultaneously and evolve together in the same body region through the stages of macules, papules, vesicles and pustules before umbilicating, drying and desquamating. Painful oral lesions, sore throat, conjunctivitis and oedema of the eyelids may occur. The fever falls at the onset of the rash or during the following days but a second febrile period, lasting two to three days occurs in a third of the patients when the skin lesions become pustular during the second week. The course of the illness lasts two to four weeks. The only clinical sign differentiating human monkeypox from smallpox and some forms of chickenpox is the *pronounced lymph node enlargement*, which appears early on the second or third day of the illness.

Complications are quite common: secondary bacterial infection of the skin, bronchopneumonia, vomiting and diarrhoea leading to dehydration, keratitis and corneal ulceration sometimes leading to blindness, and uncommonly encephalitis and septicaemia. Pock scars are common sequelae seen in most cases. Death only occurs in children under 10 years of age (case-fatality rate is 15 per cent from 0 to 4 years and 6.5 per cent from 5 to 9 years).[24]

In people who have been vaccinated against smallpox but lost part of their immunity, the disease runs often an atypical and more benign course.

Chickenpox can be a diagnostic problem in some cases: in chickenpox the lesions appear on the first day of illness and become rapidly vesicles over a few hours, they are mainly located on the trunk, pustulate within four days, are not umbilicated and are seen in several stages in one area of the skin.

Cases of suspected monkeypox should be promptly reported to WHO or a specialized surveillance team who will confirm the diagnosis and take appropriate samples. The virus can be demonstrated in the vesicular or pustular fluid and in scabs by electron microscopy or by culture on chorioallantoic membrane or tissue culture. Laboratory confirmation is also possible by serology.

Rabies

Rabies is an acute encephalomyelitis occurring as a world-wide zoonosis in a great variety of warm-blooded animals, including man. Many wild animals may be infected, e.g. foxes, wolves, jackals, skunks, weasels, mongooses. Vampires as well as insectivorous bats may be infected asymptomatically for long periods of time. This extensive wildlife reservoir results in constant reinfection of domestic animals, particularly dogs, but also cats, horses and cattle. In tropical countries dogs are the cause of most human exposures. In India rabies causes an estimated 40 000–50 000 deaths yearly, and the magnitude of the problem is similar in many other developing countries.

The aetiological agent is a neurotropic bullet-shaped RNA virus, belonging to the Rhabdoviridae. A number of rabies-related viruses have been described, two of which have been associated with a few human infections: Mokola strain in Nigeria and Duvenhage strain in South Africa. Duvenhage strain virus has also been found in European bats. The antibodies elicited by rabies vaccine are also neutralizing for the Duvenhage strain.

Rabies virus is present in the saliva of infected animals and is transmitted by bites or by licks on mucosa or abraded skin. It progresses from the site of entry through peripheral nerves and the spinal column to the brain. Shortly thereafter the virus may also be detected in many extraneural sites.

The incubation period in man varies between 10 days and more than a year, and is usually one or two months. Multiple bites, bites of hands and face, and young age are associated with shorter incubation periods. More than 80 per cent of patients develop the classic form of 'furious rabies'. Apprehensiveness and restlessness are the first signs which are frequently accompanied by paraesthesiae at the site of the wound. The patient complains of excessive thirst and is feverish. After less than 48 hours, restlessness grows into periods of maniacal behaviour and anxiety. Visual, olfactory and auditory hyperexcitability appear with violent reactions to the slightest exterior stimuli, especially the sight of water (hydrophobia). Dysphagia and painful spasms of the oropharynx are caused by attempts at swallowing. Repeated generalized convulsions with asphyxia and hyperpyrexia herald death. This may be preceded by quickly progressing flaccid paralysis and coma. The excitation phase may be very transient. A number of patients develop 'dumb rabies', the purely paralytic form of the disease, often but not exclusively seen after bat bites. Flaccid paralysis starts in the limb that was originally bitten and spreads to the other limbs and to the cranial nerves. Death from rabies occurs usually within five days of onset, but may be somewhat delayed in the paralytic form.

Typical cases with a clear-cut history present no diagnostic difficulties. In some cases, the differential diagnosis will include other viral encephalitides, tetanus and delirium tremens. In regions where the signs of rabies are well known, hydrophobia may be a sign of hysterical behaviour. Dumb rabies should be differentiated from Guillain–Barré syndrome, poliomyelitis and the neuroparalytic reactions to rabies vaccine. There are no distinctive clinical laboratory signs of rabies and the cerebrospinal fluid is mostly normal.

The diagnosis can be confirmed by immunofluorescent antigen detection on corneal impressions or neck skin biopsies (positive in 50 per cent of patients) virus isolation (takes three weeks) or antibody detection in spinal fluid or serum (but the patient often dies before having detectable antibodies). It is unlikely that any of these tests will be available in the rural hospital. Negri bodies, intracytoplasmic eosinophilic inclusions, are the classic postmortem findings at histological examination of the brain.

Patients should be barrier-nursed because of the theoretical risk of nosocomial rabies transmission. Treatment is only symptomatic and unsatisfactory as the disease is almost universally fatal. Up to now, three survivals have been reported after aggressive intensive care support, but this clearly remains the exception. Prophylactic treatment remains our sole weapon. Owing to the long incubation period it is possible to mount a protective immune response through vaccination after exposure.

Rabies vaccine is classically derived from virus grown in mammalian brains (mostly in sheep) and inactivated with phenol (Semple-type vaccine). These vaccines have a low and variable potency, requiring many large and painful doses with resulting poor patient compliance. Furthermore, they contain high amounts of myelin and give rise (in about 1:2000 vaccinees) to serious neuroparalytic reactions. Vaccines from suckling mouse brains have a higher potency and contain less myelin, resulting in a lower incidence of neurological side-effects (1:8000). The adaptation of rabies virus to avian tissue allowed the development of duck embryo vaccine which has a lower potency, but less side-effects, although rare allergic reactions occur. The best vaccines, with very high potency and negligible side-effects, are now produced in cell cultures, primary mammalian cells and particularly human diploid cells, but are very expensive. A vaccine produced in continuously growing Vero cells could be less expensive and has the same efficiency as human diploid cell vaccine (HDCV) when used by the intramuscular or intradermal route.

As vaccine confers protective antibody levels after 7–10 days, passive immunization is necessary to prevent rabies with a short incubation period. A single intramuscular (i.m.) dose of human rabies immunoglobulin (HRIG) is preferred when available. Alternatively, antirabies serum of equine origin (ARS) may be used but it carries a high risk of serum sickness and important skin reactions.

Management

In case of exposure the suspected dog or cat should be captured and observed for 10 days (unless obviously rabid at the time of exposure), while prophylactic measures are started. Vaccination may be stopped if the animal remains healthy after five days.[25] Rabies in dogs may be furious or of the paralytic type. This procedure is not reliable for wild animals. Reference laboratories can rapidly confirm the diagnosis by immunofluorescent antigen detection on the brain of the sick animal. When the animal is unavailable it should be considered as rabid.

Contact without lesions and indirect contact with a rabid animal are no indications for treatment. Prophylactic treatment should be started whenever an exposure occurs by bite, through scratches and abrasions and by licks of skin or mucosa. If the animal is not suspected as rabid (healthy; no unprovoked bite) and exposure was only light (licks of skin; scratches and abrasions; minor bites on covered body areas) vaccination and passive immunization may be delayed while the dog is being observed.

Immediate thorough washing of the wound with soap and water is essential. After rinsing with water one should apply either alcohol (40–70 per cent), tincture or aqueous solution of iodine or quaternary ammonium compounds (1 per cent) The wound should not be sutured. Tetanus prophylaxis should be updated. For passive rabies immunization (HRIG 20 IU/kg or ARS 40 IU/kg) half of the dose is infiltrated carefully around the wound if anatomically feasible, and the other half is given by deep i.m. injection at a distance of the vaccine. For vaccination, HDCV (or a similar cell-derived vaccine) is recommended at the usual dose of 1 ml given i.m. in the deltoid (not the buttock) on days 0,3,7,14 and 28. Infants can be given the vaccine in the anterolateral upper thigh. In some countries a booster is given on day 90 but the usefulness of this sixth dose is unproven.

In developing countries, Semple-type vaccines and suckling mouse brain vaccines are still widely used for economical reasons and ARS or HRIG are seldom available. As full-dose HDCV is expensive, alternative regimens have been looked for and are widely used. HDCV may be used as 0.1 ml doses given by the intradermal (i.d.) route following the day 0,3,7,14,28 schedule with good resulting immunity. This may still give a problem because the vaccine should be used as soon as possible after reconstitution. Grouping of the patients may be a solution. It can be done in areas where the incidence of exposure is high, by establishing fixed vaccination days, e.g. Tuesday and Friday, and departing from the recommended five dose schedule (four doses on days 0,3,7,10). The patient joins in on the nearest vaccination day. Another schedule which has been used with good results involves eight or even four i.d. doses of 0.1 ml HDCV given at one time on different sites of the four extremities. This is particularly useful when only one patient has to be treated and where patients often do not come back for spaced injections. Intradermal immunizations should only be performed by health personnel who have been trained for this technique. When applied correctly a bleb with an 'orange peel' appearance should be seen. Incorrectly given doses should be repeated. Although these alternative i.d. regimens of HDCV have been shown to provoke a satisfactory immune response, they will not offer the same efficacy as five i.m. doses of HDCV, but under the circumstances they may be the best compromise achievable.[26, 27] Recently, vero cell vaccine was shown to be efficacious by the intradermal route.[29] Exceptional failures have been recorded even after full i.m. regimens of HDCV.

Pre-exposure vaccination can be considered for people at special risk, e.g. veterinary personnel and health care workers often caring for rabies patients.

Vaccination of domestic dogs and elimination of stray dogs are important public health measures. Where canine rabies has been controlled, the number of human cases has dropped dramatically.

References

1. WHO. 1987 Revision of CDC/WHO case definition for AIDS. *Weekly Epidemiological Records*. 1988; **63**: 1.
2. Embree JE, Braddick M, Datta P *et al*. Lack of correlation of maternal human immunodeficiency virus infection with neonatal malformations. *Pediatric Infectious Disease Journal*. 1989; **8**: 700–4.
3. Centre for Disease Control. Classification system for human immunodeficiency virus (HIV) infection in children under 13 years of age. *MMWR*. 1987; **36**: 225.
4. Klein RS. Prophylaxis of opportunistic infections in individuals infected with HIV. **AIDS**. 1989; **3(1)**: 5161–73.
5. WHO. Consultation on human immunodeficiency virus (HIV) and routine childhood immunization. *Weekly Epidemiological Records*. 1987; **63**: 297.
6. WHO. Provisional WHO clinical case definition for AIDS. *Weekly Epidemiological Records*. 1986; **62**: 72.
7. Halstead SB. Selective primary health care: strategies for control of disease in the developing world. XI. Dengue. *Reviews of Infectious Diseases*. 1984; **6**: 251.
8. Bres PLJ. A century of progress in combating yellow fever. *Bulletin of the World Health Organization*. 1986; **64**: 775.
9. WHO. Present status of yellow fever: memorandum from a PAHO meeting. *Bulletin of the World Health Organization*. 1986; **64**: 511.
10. McCormick JB, King IJ. Webb PA *et al*. Lassa fever: effective therapy with ribavirin. *New England Journal of Medicine*. 1986; **314**: 20.
11. Pattyn SR (ed.). *Ebola Virus Haemorrhagic Fever*. Netherlands, Elsevier, 1978.
12. van Ypersele de Strihou C, Van der Groen G, Desmyter J. Néphropathie à Hantavirus en Europe Occidentale. Ubiquité des fièvres hémorragiques avec syndrome rénal. In: *Actualités Néphrologiques de l'Hôpital Necker*, Paris, Flammarion, 1985. pp. 133.
13. Ramalingaswami V, Purcell RH. Waterborne non-A, non-B hepatitis. *Lancet*. 1988; **i**: 571–3.
14. Ghendon Y. Perinatal transmission of hepatitis B virus in high incidence countries. *Journal of Virological Methods*. 1987; **17**: 68–79.
15. Maupas P, Chiron J-P, Barin F *et al*. Efficacy of hepatitis B vaccine in prevention of early HBsAg carrier state in children. Controlled trial in an endemic area (Senegal). *Lancet*. 1981; **ii**: 289–92.
16. Ryder RW, Whittle HC, Wojcie Cowsky T *et al*. Screening of hepatitis B markers is not justified in West African transfusion centres. *Lancet*. 1984; **ii**: 449–52.
17. Chen DS, Hsu NHM, Sung JL *et al*. A mass vaccination program in Taiwan against hepatitis B virus infection in infants of hepatitis B surface antigen carrier mothers. *Journal of the American Medical Association*. 1987; **257**: 2597–603.
18. Coursaget P, Yvonnet B, Chotard J *et al*. Seven-year study of hepatitis B vaccine efficacy in infants from an endemic area (Senegal). *Lancet*. 1986; **ii**: 1143–5.

19. Bomino F, Smedile A, Verme G. Hepatitis Delta virus infection. *Advances in Internal Medicine*. 1987; **32**: 345–58.
20. WHO. *Bulletin of the World Health Organization*. 1985; **63**: 185–90.
21. Yamanishi K, Okuno T, Shiraki K *et al*. Identification of human herpesvirus-6 as a causal agent for exantham subitum. *Lancet*. 1988; **i**: 1065.
22. Anderson MJ. Human parvovirus infection. *Journal of Virological Methods*. 1987; **17**: 175.
23. Fenner F. A successful eradication campaign. Global eradication of smallpox. *Review of Infectious Diseases*. 1982; **4**: 916.
24. Jezek Z, Szezeniowski M, Paluku KM *et al*. Human monkey pox: clinical features of 282 patients. *Journal of Infectious Diseases*. 1987; **156**: 293.
25. WHO. WHO Expert committee on rabies. *Technical Report Series, World Health Organization*. 1984, No. 709.
26. Monson MH. Practical management of rabies and the 1982 outbreak in Zorzor district, Liberia. *Tropical Doctor*. 1985; **15**: 50.
27. Turner GS, Aoki FY, Nicholson KG *et al*. Human diploid cell strain rabies vaccine. Rapid prophylactic immunisation of volunteers with small doses. *Lancet*. 1976; **i**: 1379.
28. Choo QL, Kuo G, Weiner AJ *et al*. Isolation of a cDNA clone derived from a blood-borne non-A, non-B viral hepatitis genome. *Science*. 1989; **244**: 359–62.
29. Chutivongse S, Wilde H, Supiche S *et al*. Postexposure prophylaxis for rabies with antiserum and intradermal vaccination. *Lancet*. 1990; **335**: 896–8.

Further reading

Evans AS (ed.). *Viral Infections of Humans: Epidemiology and Control*. London, Plenum Medical. 1988.
Feigin RD, Cherry JD (ed.). In: *Textbook of Pediatric Infectious Diseases*. London, WB Saunders. 1981: 1061.
Wood MJ, Geddes AM. Antiviral therapy. *Lancet*. 1987; **ii**: 1189.

Mycotic infections

R. J. Hay

Fungi cause a variety of human infections. The most common are those affecting the skin or mucous membranes, the superficial mycoses, which include conditions such as dermatophytosis or ringworm, superficial candidosis and pityriasis versicolor. Superficial fungal infections are distributed world-wide. By contrast, the subcutaneous mycoses, which because of their presumed route of infection are often called mycoses of implantation, are largely confined to the tropics and subtropics. Examples are diseases such as mycetoma, sporotrichosis and chromomycosis. The systemic mycoses include both serious opportunistic infections (those occurring in compromised patients) such as systemic candidosis, aspergillosis and mucormycosis. In addition, there are systemic infections of otherwise healthy individuals affecting deep sites, including histoplasmosis, blastomycosis, coccidioidomycosis and paracoccidioidomycosis, which are confined to endemic zones determined by the distribution of the causative organisms in the natural environment. The systemic opportunistic mycoses have a world-wide distribution.

While the mycoses occur at any age, some are particularly prevalent or show characteristic clinical features in children. Of the superficial mycoses, scalp ringworm and oral candidosis or thrush are examples. Subcutaneous infections are less common in children but two are often seen in this age group – sporotrichosis and basidiobolomycosis, a form of subcutaneous zygomycosis. The systemic mycoses can occur at any age but chronic pulmonary forms, for instance, are most often seen in adults.

Superficial mycoses

Dermatophyte infections

These are dermatophytosis or ringworm (see also pp. 857–61). Dermatophyte fungi invade the keratinized structures of the skin, the stratum corneum, hair and nails.[1] Many of them elaborate specific proteinases – keratinases. The dermatophytes originate from one of three sources – other humans, animals or soil. These infections are known as anthropophilic, zoophilic and geophilic respectively. Frequently, anthropophilic infections are chronic and non-inflammatory whereas the zoophilic infections are often highly inflammatory.

Transmission of ringworm may occur via direct contact with infected humans or animals or from infected material in the environment. For instance, animals shed infected hairs which are a potential source of human infection. The factors which affect the invasion of the skin by fungi are little understood, although the skin surface moisture and carbon dioxide tension have been shown to be important. In addition, medium-chain fatty acids which are produced in sebum by bacterial lipolysis are inhibitory to the growth of dermatophytes. However, these are present in higher concentrations after puberty, a factor which may be reflected by the predominance of scalp infections in children. Immunity to infection is thought to be largely mediated by T lymphocytes. The development of delayed hypersensitivity often correlates with the recovery phase of the infection; and this phenomenon may account for the development of marked inflammatory changes in previously quiescent ringworm lesions. Neutrophil invasion is also an important factor in some infections.

Infections caused by dermatophytes are usually given the name tinea followed by the appropriate part of the body in Latin, e.g. tinea pedis (foot), tinea corporis (body). The most important dermatophyte infections of children are tinea capitis (scalp) and tinea corporis.

Tinea capitis

Tinea capitis or scalp ringworm may be transmitted from animals or other children.[2,3] The most frequent cause of zoophilic scalp infection is *Microsporum canis* from cats or dogs. Other sources include *Trichophyton verrucosum* (cattle) and *T. mentagrophytes* (rodents). In most parts of the tropics zoophilic scalp ringworm is not very common and mainly confined to cities or large towns. Anthropophilic scalp ringworm may be very widespread, occuring in 10–20 per cent of school-children in some surveys in Africa. Endemic scalp ringworm is also prevalent in conditions of over-crowding, e.g. in refugee camps, as well as in residential schools. The main causative organisms vary in different parts of the world. The common varieties are shown in Table 4.9.1. The situation is most complicated in Africa where different organisms predominate in specific areas.[3]

The main clinical features are diffuse or circumscribed hair loss, scaling and itching (Fig. 4.9.1). Hair may be shed in small circular patches, although in some children diffuse hair loss is seen. Itching is variable, but many children appear relatively asymptomatic. The infected hairs often break at scalp level in anthropophilic *Trichophyton* infections, the swollen and fractured hair shaft appearing prominent (black dot ringworm). In *M. canis* and *M. audouinii*

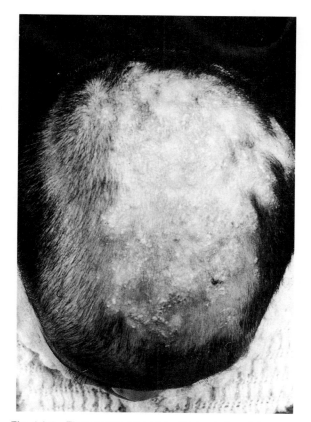

Fig. 4.9.1 Tinea capitis caused by *Trichophyton violaceum*.

infections, hairs break 2–3 mm above the scalp. Scaling may be diffuse or absent. In some children, scales adhere to an erythematous base resembling severe dandruff. Less commonly the infected area becomes swollen and inflamed with, in severe cases, pustule

Table 4.9.1. Sources and distribution of common dermatophytes

	Source	Distribution	Common sites of infection
Trichophyton rubrum	Man	World-wide	Body, feet, groins
T. violaceum	Man	India Middle East	Scalp, body
T. interdigitale	Man	World-wide	Feet
T. mentagrophytes	Rodents	World-wide	Body, scalp
T. tonsurans	Man	USA, Central America	Scalp
T. soudanense	Man	Central Africa	Scalp
T. verrucosum	Cattle	World-wide – usually temperate climates	Scalp, body
T. schoeneinii	Man	World-wide	Scalp
Microsporum canis	Cats, dogs	World-wide	Scalp, body
M. audouinii	Man	Africa (West)	Scalp
Epidermophyton floccosum	Man	World-wide	Groins, feet

(kerion) formation. Kerions are more commonly seen with zoophilic infections but can occur with those of human origin.

Scalp ringworm can be confused with other conditions, mainly seborrhoeic dermatitis, where there is no hair loss, or alopecia areata. In the latter there is no inflammation and characteristic exclamation mark hairs are seen.

Favus is the name given to scalp ringworm caused by *Trichophyton schoenleinii*. It is mainly seen in parts of North and Southern Africa, the Middle East and scattered foci in the USA and Central and South America. In favus, hair loss often occurs later. A characteristic of the disease is the accumulation of epithelial debris and inflammatory cells around hairs. These become matted together to form a crust or scutulum which is said to have a characteristic mousey smell. The crust has a whitish or grey appearance and may cover extensive areas of scalp. Hair loss may be predominant.

Generally, the more inflammatory the scalp ringworm the shorter the course. Chronic endemic anthropophilic forms may persist for years, although remission at puberty is usual. Hair loss is usually reversible although some permanent loss may follow kerion and favus.

The diagnosis can be confirmed in the laboratory by taking samples of infected hair. *Microsporum*, but not *Trichophyton* infections fluoresce greenish under filtered ultraviolet radiation (Wood's light). This procedure is useful for screening children as well as selecting hairs for microscopy and culture. Hairs are examined in 5–10 per cent potassium hydroxide solution. Most of the endemic scalp infections caused by anthropophilic *Trichophyton* species show fungal invasion of hair shafts in which spores form inside hairs (endothrix). Both anthropophilic and zoophilic *Microsporum* infections result in fungal invasion in which spores form outside hairs (ectothrix). In favus, invading fungal elements regress leaving air spaces in the hair. These features can be useful for establishing a diagnosis and the likely source of infection. Definitive identification of organisms can be accomplished by culture.

While in many instances accurate laboratory identification is unrealistic, it is useful to know either by screening with Wood's light or by carrying out a limited survey the likely organisms involved, as these will indicate the source of infection which is important for choosing appropriate control measures (see later).

The treatment of choice for scalp ringworm is the oral antifungal drug griseofulvin given in a daily single or split dose of 10–15 mg/kg with food. This treatment should be continued for six weeks, although in some cases up to four months is necessary. While this type of regimen is ideal and usually produces remission in over 90 per cent of cases, the only main alternative is oral ketoconazole (4 mg/kg daily). The latter has only been assessed in some infections (e.g. *T. tonsurans*). However, as ketoconazole is potentially hepatotoxic care should be taken. While individual cases may respond to topical therapy with antifungal preparations such as Whitfield's ointment, selenium sulphide or imidazole agents (clotrimazole, miconazole), responses are generally unsatisfactory.

The measures just described are ideal for treatment of individuals. However, they may be limited by expense if applied to large outbreaks. It is possible to obtain reasonable (over 80 per cent) cure rates by giving griseofulvin in a single larger dose supervised by a nurse or auxiliary staff, e.g. 1.5 g or 30 mg/kg. This may be repeated three weeks later. Using such modified regimens the cost and administration of effective therapy to a large group of children is optimized.

If the infection is of animal origin it is not necessary to keep infected children away from school, although it is useful to give them a topically active compound in addition to griseofulvin. If the infection is anthropophilic, children should not return to school until treatment has been given for at least three weeks. Relapse, as opposed to reinfection, after successful treatment is unusual. If a group (4–5) of children in a class are clinically infected it is useful to screen all class mates for evidence of infection and treat those with scalp lesions. There is no form of immunization against scalp ringworm.

Reaction by parents to scalp ringworm ranges from concern to indifference. This often depends on the clinical appearance of lesions, and in many cases the presence of mild scaling and hair loss will be ignored. However, most children with severe inflammatory lesions will be brought for treatment.

Tinea corporis

Ringworm affecting the body or proximal parts of the limbs may be associated with scalp infection or occur in isolation.[4] In children the common causes in tropical zones are *T. rubrum*, *T. violaceum*, *T. soudanense*, *T. tonsurans* and *M. canis*. In addition, *M. gypseum*, which is a dermatophyte isolated from soil may cause tinea corporis, particularly in parts of Central America and the West Pacific. Tinea imbricata, a geographically restricted form of dermatophytosis, is discussed later.

The archetypal lesion of tinea corporis is a round or irregular ovoid plaque of scaling with a prominent margin.[1] There is usually some hyperpigmentation and the edge may show follicular prominences or even pustule formation. In *T. rubrum* and other anthropophilic infections, lesions can be extensive and irregular with minimal inflammation. By contrast, lesions caused by *M. canis* and *M. gypseum* are often inflamed. It is important to examine children with tinea corporis for evidence of infection elsewhere. The presence of itching and absence of sensory loss helps to distinguish localized tinea corporis from tuberculoid leprosy.

The diagnosis can be confirmed by direct microscopy of scrapings and culture. In localized infections, treatment with benzoic acid compound (Whitfield's ointment) or an imidazole antifungal (see earlier) or tolnaftate is usually effective. Griseofulvin or intraconazole is required for more extensive lesions.

Tinea imbricata (Tokelau ringworm)

Tinea imbricata is the name given to infections caused by *T. concentricum*. They are typically found in remote humid parts of the tropics in the West Pacific, Southeast Asia, Assam and Central and South America. Infections may occur in infants as young as six months and usually persist for years into adult life.

The most characteristic lesion is a plaque composed of concentric rings of scales.[5] Plaques fuse to cover an extensive body surface area (Fig. 4.9.2) Hypopigmentation is usual. Other morphological variants include large, loose scales, lichenification or solitary uniformly scaly plaques.

The treatment is either a topical azole or antifungal antiseptic (e.g. brilliant green/salicylic acid mixture), but oral griseofulvin is more effective. However, relapse is inevitable unless the patient leaves the endemic area. As individuals shed large numbers of infected scales into the environment, control measures have to involve the treatment of all infected cases plus surveillance to detect and treat early cases of reinfection.

Other forms of dermatophytosis

Tinea pedis (athletes foot) is most often caused by *T. rubrum* and causes interdigital itching as well as more generalized scaling on the sole. This may spread to the palms and elsewhere. However, it is not common in childhood. Likewise, spread of infection to the nails to cause thickening, and onycholysis (separation of the nail from its base) is not common in the tropics. Tinea cruris (groin) is mainly seen in male teenagers and young adults. The most common causes are *T. rubrum* or *Epidermophyton floccosum*. In this infection, lesions are confined to the groin area and spread down the thighs. Itching may be severe. Plaques usually have a prominent distal margin. Treatment consists of topical antifungal therapy (see p. 860) and griseofulvin is reserved for chronic resistant cases.

Pityriasis versicolor

Pityriasis versicolor is an infection caused by *Malassezia furfur*, a normal skin commensal which under appropriate conditions invades the stratum corneum. While

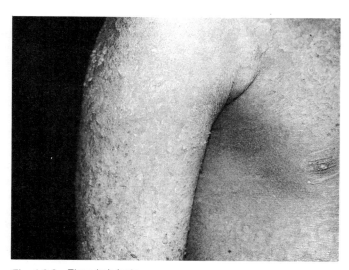

Fig. 4.9.2 Tinea imbricata.

it is the most common superficial mycosis of the tropics, cases are most often seen in teenagers or adults. The trunk, neck and face become covered with discrete, ovoid or confluent scaly macules which are either hypo- or hyperpigmented. The demonstration of scaling by gently scratching distinguishes pityriasis versicolor from early vitiligo. The diagnosis can be confirmed by direct microscopy. Treatment consists of topically applied 1–2 per cent selenium sulphide, 20 per cent sodium thiosulphate, or azole antifungals. The first two treatments are considerably cheaper. Relapse is common in a tropical environment.

Superficial candidosis

Candida albicans is a yeast which is normally a commensal in the oral cavity and gastro-intestinal tract. Infections follow changes in host immune status or local epithelial abnormalities. Immunodeficiency, malnutrition, diabetes mellitus and oral epithelial disease (e.g. herpes gingivostomatitis) may predispose to candida infections. In adults a range of conditions may result from invasion of candida – paronychia or nail fold infections, intertrigo (groins or finger webs) as well as vaginal infection (see p. 860).

In children there are two main sites of invasion. In the first, oral candidosis or thrush, infants are most commonly affected.[6] Prematurity and bottle-feeding predispose. The main symptom is refusal of foods caused by soreness of the oral mucosa which appears red and glazed or covered with soft white plaques (Fig. 4.9.3). Angular cheilitis is usual. In the second form of superficial candidosis seen in infancy[7], candida is a secondary invader in the perianal area in children with napkin dermatitis (Fig. 4.9.4). It is often difficult to prove its involvement but one helpful clue is the appearance of small 'satellite' pustules distal to the edge of the rash.

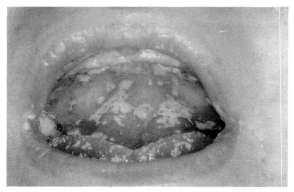

Fig. 4.9.3   Oral candidosis or thrush.

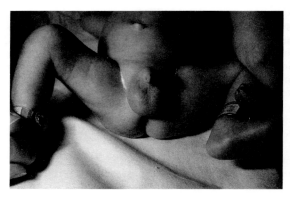

Fig. 4.9.4   Cutaneous candidosis in napkin area.

Treatment of superficial candidosis consists of topical applications of gentian violet or amphotericin or nystatin cream suspension and pastilles (mouth). For skin infections azole antifungals are also helpful.

The rare syndrome of chronic mucocutaneous candidosis usually develops in early childhood (three to seven years).[8] Affected children develop severe and persistent oral candidosis, nail dystrophies and in the worst examples skin and scalp involvement characterized by erythema and crust formation.[9] The characteristic crusts are often referred to as 'granulomas'. While a number of affected children can be shown to have specific immunodeficiencies affecting T-lymphocyte transformation to candida or neutrophil killing, their importance is hard to gauge as they may revert to normal with therapy. However, it is important to screen affected children for hypoadrenalism, hypoparathyroidism and hypothyroidism, inherited as an autosomal recessive trait. Pernicious anaemia may also occur. In some families, autosomal recessive or dominant inheritance of this condition without endocrinopathy is found. Persistent superficial candida infections may also occur in children with other recognizable immunodeficiency states such as chronic granulomatous disease. However, here the development of other systemic infections is a prominent feature.

The treatment of choice for chronic mucocutaneous candidosis is ketoconazole (4–5 mg/kg daily) which is used to induce remission and relapses are common. Fluconazole and itraconazole are alternatives. Severely affected children are prone to develop bronchiectasis and other superficial infections such as ringworm or viral warts.

Oral candidosis is a feature of acquired immunodeficiency syndrome in both children and adults. Lesions tend to respond poorly to topical therapy and it may be necessary to use oral ketoconazole. The clinical situation may be complicated by coexistent herpes simplex infections (HSV) which must be treated. In some patients, oesophageal candidosis may develop and this should be suspected in a patient with AIDS who develops dysphagia. By contrast, systemic candidosis is not common in patients with AIDS.

Subcutaneous mycoses

The subcutaneous fungal infections are largely restricted to the tropics or subtropics. In most cases infection follows traumatic implantation of organisms from the environment. Many of the fungi associated with these infections are found in soil, decaying plant material or thorns. While in adults mycetoma and chromoblastomycosis are prominent amongst the subcutaneous mycoses, in children sporotrichosis and basidiobolomycosis are more common.

Sporotrichosis

Sporotrichosis is a cutaneous or systemic infection caused by *Sporothrix schenckii*.[10] The systemic form is rare and results in disseminated or localized infections of joints, lungs or meninges. Cutaneous sporotrichosis is widely distributed in the tropics and subtropics, such as the southern USA, central and northern South America, southern Africa, Japan and Australasia. Scattered cases occur elsewhere. *S. schenckii* can be isolated from plant debris in endemic areas, however, it has been particularly associated with material used for packing, e.g. straw, moss and thorny plants. Infection is thought to follow traumatic implantation of the organism through an abrasion. All ages may be affected by cutaneous sporotrichosis.

There are two main patterns of infection – fixed or lymphocutaneous.[11] In the fixed type, which in many parts of the world is more common in childhood, the lesion is a soft papule or nodule which enlarges and breaks down to form a deep irregular ulcer. The face and distal limbs are often involved. There may be local lymphadenopathy. Although spontaneous remission can occur, treatment is normally advisable and residual scarring is common. In the lymphangitic type the initial lesion is often localized on an extremity such as the hand. Secondary nodules and lymphangitis occur along the lymphatic channels which may break down to form ulcers. Rarer variants include chronic extensive ulceration, granulomatous plaques and verrucous (warty) dermatitis.

The most important differential diagnosis is cutaneous leishmaniasis (see p. 685). Although the lesions in this infection are less friable, they may be difficult to distinguish and hence it is useful to take smears to exclude *Leishmania* infection. *Mycobacterium marinum* infections, chronic superficial infections caused by marine mycobacteria, may also mimic lymphangitic sporotrichosis.

Where possible it is ideal to confirm the diagnosis by taking smears, curettings or biopsies for culture. Organisms are often sparsely distributed in lesions and, where present, may be surrounded by a refractile eosinophilic fringe to form 'asteroid' bodies.

The treatment of choice is a saturated solution of potassium iodide. In children, the starting dose is 0.5 ml three times a day and this is increased slowly dropwise to three 2–3 ml doses. Treatment is continued for one month after clinical resolution. Potassium iodide commonly produces nausea, hypersalivation and salivary gland enlargement. Alternative forms of treatment are the local application of heat and the new oral triazole, itraconazole, which in initial assessments has produced encouraging responses in this condition. There is no danger of cross-infection with sporotrichosis.

Basidiobolomycosis

Basidiobolomycosis (subcutaneous phycomycosis) is a chronic subcutaneous infection mainly seen in Central and East Africa, more rarely elsewhere.[12] The causative organism, *Basidiobolus haptosporus*, has been isolated from vegetation as well as reptiles in endemic areas.

The disease is mainly seen in children over the age of seven and involves a progressive and painless subcutaneous swelling of a limb or girdle region (shoulder, pelvis) (Fig. 4.9.5.). The swelling is usually hard and may cause considerable disability. The diagnosis is confirmed by skin biopsy which shows large strap-like hyphae in the subcutaneous tissue and a mixed granulomatous and eosinophil infiltrate.

Conidiobolomycosis (rhinoentomophthoromycosis)

A similar infection to basidiobolomycosis is caused by *Conidiobolus coronatus*. It is mainly confined to young adults and occurs in West Africa as well as parts of India and the Caribbean. Conidiobolomycosis involves facial tissues. It arises from the region of the internal turbinates and causes chronic facial swelling, particularly around the nose and upper lip.

The main treatment for basidiobolomycosis and conidiobolomycosis (both forms of subcutaneous zygomycosis) is a saturated solution of potassium iodide

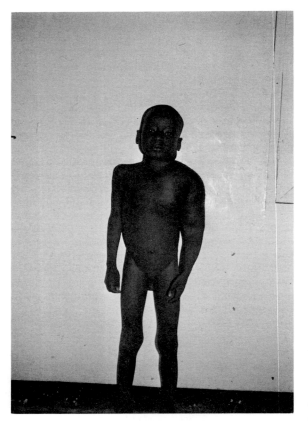

Fig. 4.9.5 Subcutaneous phycomycosis of the shoulder.

given orally in doses similar to those used in sporotrichosis. Cotrimoxazole is usually added for conidiobolomycosis. Ketoconazole can be considered as an alternative for both.

Mycetoma

Mycetoma is a chronic subcutaneous fungal or actinomycete (filamentous bacteria) infection causing osteomyelitis.[13] The organisms form into characteristic aggregates or grains in the inflammatory mass (see p. 861). Cases are mainly seen in the drier tropical areas such as central regions of Africa, Middle East and India as well as parts of central and northern South America. Mycetoma is uncommon in children. The infection present as a painless subcutaneous swelling which with time expands to produce a mass of abscesses and sinuses with bony destruction. Exposed sites such as feet, lower legs or hands are most often involved. The infection is best diagnosed histologically, or by culture

and microscopy of grains. The histological features of grains are often characteristic and differentiate actinomycete (actinomycetoma) infections from those caused by fungi (eumycetoma). The former are treated with cotrimoxazole or dapsone plus a second-line drug such as rifampicin or streptomycin. Eumycetomas may respond to griseofulvin or ketoconazole, but otherwise surgery is indicated.

Chromomycosis and phaeohyphomycosis

Chromomycosis (chromoblastomycosis) is a chronic fungal infection of the skin and subcutaneous tissue caused by pigmented organisms of the genera *Fonsecaea*, *Phialophora* and *Cladosporium*. These can be isolated from the soil or decaying vegetation. Chromomycosis is mainly seen in Central and South America, Southern Africa, South-east Asia and Australasia and the disease is mainly seen in adults (see p. 861). Lesions develop as small nodules with a verrucose or warty surface which enlarge over exposed sites to produce flat plaques or extensive cauliflower-like protuberances.[14] The main treatments are flucytosine (oral), thiabendazole (oral), itraconazole (oral) and local applications of heat.

Less commonly pigmented fungi cause subcutaneous granulomas which develop central necrosis to become fibrous encapsulated cysts (phaeohyphomycosis). These lesions are most often seen in tropical areas and have been described from most parts of the world. The diagnosis is usually made histologically after surgical excision.

Systemic mycoses

Systemic opportunistic mycoses

Generally systemic fungal infections in children caused by opportunists are rare in the tropics. Systemic candida infections, which occur in immunocompromised patients or in those on long-term parenteral feeding, usually produce non-specific features of septicaemia. Rarely endocarditis, endophthalmitis or meningitis can occur. The patients most at risk from systemic candidosis are those with neutropenia associated with leukaemia chemotherapy. Here systemic candidosis should be suspected in patients with unexplained fever which fails to resolve on antibacterial antibiotics. Unfortunately, blood cultures are frequently negative in this group and treatment with intravenous amphotericin B may have to be initiated 'blind'.

Neonatal candida septicaemia is particularly associated with early prematurity (below 30 weeks). This sometimes differs from septicaemia seen in other groups in that there is a high risk of associated meningitis. Also renal infection may be very aggressive in this age group leading to a non-functioning kidney. Outbreaks of neonatal candida infection may occur in nurseries and in these cases it is worth swabbing staff and others concerned with the care of babies to exclude carriage of the organism on hands.

Systemic aspergillus infections, usually caused by *Aspergillus fumigatus* or *A. flavus* cause rapidly fatal disease in neutropaenic patients associated with pneumonia and lung cavitation. Alternatively, aspergilli may cause superinfections in children with cystic fibrosis or cause chronic lung, bone or skin infections in patients which chronic granulomatous disease. Zygomycosis, an acute invasive fungal infection caused by fungi of the general *Absidia*, *Rhizopus* and *Rhizomucor* is rare in childhood. However, severe infections have been reported in malnourished children in Africa presenting with gastro-intestinal invasion.[15] These organisms often produce vascular occlusion.

Systemic pathogenic mycoses

The main infections due to the systemic pathogenic fungi are histoplasmosis, blastomycosis, coccidioidomycosis and paracoccidioidomycosis. In all cases the main route of invasion is via the lungs but disseminated extrapulmonary disease may be a major feature. Most individuals inhaling the organisms are subclinically sensitized without developing overt disease.

Histoplasmosis

Classical histoplasmosis due to *Histoplasma capsulatum* var. *capsulatum* is widely distributed in the tropics in Africa, the South East Asia and Central and South America.[16] The fungi are found as small yeasts $2-4\ \mu m$ in diameter in infected tissue (see p. 861). The organism is found in soil, particularly if there has been contact with bat or bird droppings; in the tropics exposure may also follow entry into a cave. Histoplasmosis is not common in children but may present with widely disseminated infection in infants.[17] This form can also develop in AIDS patients. Here the organisms spread to affect organs of the reticuloendothelial system including liver, spleen and bone marrow. Patients are acutely ill with fever, weight loss, hepatosplenomegaly and purpura. Miliary shadowing of the chest is often seen. The organism can be demonstrated in or isolated from affected sites, particularly bone marrow aspirates. Serology (double diffusion, complement fixation) is helpful. The treatment of choice is amphotericin B given in a dose of 0.8 mg kg^{-1} daily intravenously for at least six weeks depending on response. Ketoconazole or intraconazole are alternative. Other clinical forms such as chronic lung disease or localized dissemination to oral mucosa and adrenals are mainly seen in adults.

A variant of histoplasmosis caused by *H. capsulatum* var. *duboisii*, African histoplasmosis, occurs in central regions of Africa. The organism is identical mycologically to var. *capsulatum* but produces large yeast forms *in vivo* (up to 15 μm in diameter) and it may be called large-form histoplasmosis. Clinically the disease disseminates to skin and bone or it may involve other sites such as gastro-intestinal tract or lymph nodes. Skin lesions resemble cold abscesses or, in widespread infections, molluscum contagiosum.

Other systemic mycoses

Coccidioidomycosis, an infection caused by *Coccidioides immitis*, a soil organism found in arid parts of the New World may present in childhood with meningitis or disseminated infection of the skin, bone or joints.[18] The organism produces a characteristic spore-like structure or spherule *in vivo*. Cryptococcosis due to *Cryptococcus neoformans* is usually associated with meningitis or lung infections.[19] In tropical areas it can affect healthy individuals as well as those with T-lymphocyte defects such as AIDS. Cryptococcosis is found in 4–15 per cent of AIDS patients usually presenting as meningitis. The organism can be demonstrated in India ink preparations of cerebrospinal fluid and can also be cultured. Therapy with intravenous amphotericin B and oral flucytosine is normally used. It may be necessary to treat AIDS patients with intermittent (weekly) amphotericin B when their meningitis goes into remission to prevent relapse. In AIDS, intraconazole and flucanazole have proved useful for initial therapy and long term prevention of relapse. The other two major systemic mycoses, blastomycosis and paracoccidioidomycosis (which is unrelated to coccidioidomycosis), show a variety of pulmonary and mucocutaneous manifestations. The former is found in the USA and Africa, whereas paracoccidioidomycosis is confined to the New World from Mexico to Argentina. In all the latter infections childhood disease is rare. Acute pulmonary forms of blastomycosis[20] and widely disseminated paracoccidioidomycosis may occur in childhood.

References

1. Rebell G, Taplin D. *Dermatophytes: Their Recognition and Identification*. Miami, Florida University of Miami Press, 1970.

2. Kamalam A, Thambiah AS. Tinea capitis in Madras. *Sabouraudia*. 1973; **11**: 106.

3. Verhagen AR. Distribution of dermatophytes causing tinea capitis in Africa. *Tropical and Geographical Medicine*. 1974; **26**: 101.

4. Soyinka F. Epidemiologic study of dermatophyte infections in Nigeria (clinical study and laboratory investigations). *Mycopathologia*. 1978; **63**: 99.

5. Hay RJ, Reid S, Talwat E *et al*. Endemic tinea imbricata – a study on Goodenough Island, Papua New Guinea. *Transactions of the Royal Society of Tropical Medicine and Hygiene*. 1984; **78**: 246.

6. Schnell D. The epidemiology and prophylaxis of mycoses in perinatology. *Contributions to Microbiology and Immunology*. 1977; **4**: 40.

7. Leyden JJ, Kligman AM. The role of microorganisms in diaper dermatitis. *Acta Dermatologica*. 1978; **114**: 56.

8. Cleary TG. Chronic mucocutaneous candidiasis. In: Bodey GP, Fainstein V eds. *Candidiasis* New York, Raven Press, 1985. pp. 241–52.

9. Aronson IK, Soltani K. Chronic mucocutaneous candidosis: a review. *Mycopathologia*. 1977; **60**: 17.

10. Auld JC, Beardmore GL. Sporotrichosis in Queensland: a review of 137 cases at the Royal Brisbane Hospital. *Australian Journal of Dermatology*. 1979; **20**: 14.

11. Valasquez JP, Restrepo A, Calle G. Experiencia de 12 anos con la esporotrichosis polimorfismo clinico de la entidad. *Antioquia Medica*. 1976; **26**: 153.

12. Burkitt DP, Wilson AM, Jelliffe DB. Subcutaneous phycomycosis: a review of 31 cases seen in Uganda. *British Medical Journal*. 1964; **1**: 1669.

13. Mahgoub ES, Murray IG. *Mycetoma*. London, William Heinemann Medical Books, 1973.

14. Londero AT, Ramos CD. Chromomycosis: a clinical and mycological study of thirty five cases observed in the hinterland of Rio Grande do Sul, Brazil. *American Journal of Tropical Medicine and Hygiene*. 1976; **25**: 132.

15. Michalak DM, Cooney DR, Rhodes KH *et al*. Gastrointestinal mucormycosis in infants and children: a cause of gangrenous intestinal cellulitis and perforation. *Journal of Pediatric Surgery*. 1980; **15**: 320.

16. Rhandhara HS. Occurrence of histoplasmosis in Asia. *Mycopathologia*. 1970; **41**: 75.

17. Goodwin RA, Des Prez RM. Histoplasmosis. *American Reviews of Respiratory Diseases*. 1978; **117**: 929.

18. Drutz DJ, Cantanzaro A. Coccidioidomycosis: state of the art. *American Review of Respiratory Diseases*. 1978; **117**: 559, 727.

19. Pillay N, Simjee AE. Cryptococcal meningitis: our experience in 24 black patients. *South African Medical Journal*. 1976; **50**: 1604.

20. Laskey WK, Sarosi GA. Blastomycosis in children. *Pediatrics*. 1980; **65**: 111.

Helminthiasis

John Vince

The term helminthiasis indicates infection of man by species belonging to either the nematode (roundworm) or platyhelminth (flatworm) phylum. Within the platyhelminth phylum there are two classes, the cestodes (tapeworms) and the trematodes (flukes). Infection may be with helminths for which man is the prime host, or with those for which man is an accidental host, the prime host being a non-human vertebrate (zoonosis).

Viewed in detail, the term helminthiasis thus covers a very large, and to the non-parasitologist, bewildering, array of parasitic infections. These infections are responsible for much ill health throughout the world – particularly the non-industrialized world.

Table 4.10.1 lists the important helminthic infections of humans. Schistosomiasis caused by the schistosomes or blood flukes, and filariasis, caused by insect-borne nematodes are considered in detail on pp. 650–6, 686–91. This chapter considers epidemiological and clinical aspects of the other most commonly occurring helminthic infections – the human gut nematodes and cestodes – with less detailed reference to some of the less common, but nevertheless important infections.

Epidemiology

The distribution of parasites of man depends on his behaviour, the environment in which he lives, and his manipulation of that environment. Helminthic infections are spread, in general, by faecal contamination of the environment and by inadequate food preparation. Thus, whilst the five most commonly occurring helminths of man, *Ascaris lumbricoides* (affecting 1300 × 10^6 people), hookworms (400–800 × 10^6), *Trichuris* (500 × 10^6), *Enterobius* (500 × 10^6), and *Strongyloides* (80 × 10^6) are found world-wide, they are endemic with high prevalence in much of the tropical and subtropical world where conditions of poor hygiene and sanitation coexist with environmental factors favouring survival of the extra-human parasitic stages.[1]

Among the factors determining the survival of the non-human parasitic forms – and thus the prevalence and intensity of infection (the number of parasites per person) – are environmental temperature and humidity and the nature of the soil. Thus, hookworms require moist warm sandy or loamy soil for the development of the infective larvae. The eggs of *Ascaris lumbricoides* can survive for more than six years in a temperate climate but for only a few hours in conditions of extreme high temperature or low humidity – this

Table 4.10.1. Helminth infections of man

Parasites which complete life-cycle in man, with spread from man

Nematodes
  'Soil borne' gut nematodes
    Primarily human parasites
      Ascaris lumbricoides – roundworm
      Ancylostoma duodenale ⎫
      Necator americanus ⎭ – hookworm
      Trichuris trichuria – whipworm
      Enterobius vermicularis – threadworm, pinworm
        (*Oxyuris*)
      Strongyloides – *S. stercoralis*
             – *S. fulleborni*
    Zoonoses
      Trichostrongylus (domestic herbivores)
      Ternidens deminutus (monkeys)
      Oesophagostomium (monkeys and apes)
      Strongyloides fulleborni (monkeys and baboons)
      Capillaria philippinensis (? marine mammal)
  Anthropod borne 'tissue' nematodes
    Human parasites
      Filarial worms (pp. 686–91)
      Dracunculus medinensis (guinea-worm)
Cestodes
  Primarily human parasites

Taenia saginata	(beef tapeworm)
Taenia solium	(pig tapeworm)
Diphyllobothrium latum	(fish tapeworm)
Hymenolepis nana	(dwarf tapeworm)

  Zoonoses

Hymenolepis diminuta	(rat)
Dipylidium caninum	(dog)

Trematodes
  Blood flukes – schistosomes (pp. 650–6)
  Flukes of the biliary tract
    Primarily human parasites
      Clonorchis sinensis (Chinese liver fluke)
      Opisthorchis viverrini (Thailand and Laos)
    Zoonoses

Fasciola hepatica	(sheep)
Dicrocoelium dentriticum	(sheep)

  Flukes of the gut
    Primarily human parasites
      Fasciolopsis buski
      Gastrodiscoides hominis
    Zoonoses

Echinostoma	(fish)
Heterophyes heterophyses	(fish)
Metagonimus yokogawa	(fish)

  Flukes of the lung
    Primarily human parasites
      Paragonimus – *P. westermani*
             – *P. africanus*
             – *P. uterobilateralis*

'Tissue' parasites with incomplete life-cycles in man (zoonoses)

Nematodes

Angiostrongylus cantonensis (rat)	Eosinophilic meningitis
Monerastrongylus costaricensis (cotton rat)	Mesenteric arteries
Ancylostoma braziliense (dog hookworm)	Cutaneous larvae migrans
Toxocara canis/cati (dog/cat roundworm)	Visceral larvae migrans
Anasakis spp. (fish)	Gut wall
Gnathostoma spinigerum (fish)	Dermis, viscera, brain
Dirofilaria sp. (dog)	Pulmonary artery, dermis, conjunctivae
Trichinella spiralis (pig)	Trichinosis (muscle)
Capillaria hepatica (rat)	Liver

Larval cestodes

Spirometra (dogs/cats)	Sparganosis
Taenia solium (man as intermediate host)	Cysticercosis
Multiceps (dog)	Subcutaneous/orbital cysts
Echinococcus granulosus (dog)	Hydatid disease
Echinococcus multilocularis (fox)	Liver

explains the seasonal breaks in transmission in some parts of the world. A suitable aquatic environment is necessary for those parasites (e.g. trematodes and guinea-worms) requiring an aquatic intermediate host, whilst biological factors affecting the prime host are important in the diseases of animals transmissible to man (zoonoses).

Various aspects of human behaviour and manipulation of the environment have a major bearing on parasite transmission. These include population density, the availability and use of clean water and adequate faeces disposal.

Population movement may increase or decrease the risk of parasitic disease. Thus, migration to overcrowded, underserviced urban squatter settlements may increase, whilst the nomadic life tends to limit parasitization. The use of 'night soil' for fertilizer, especially if improperly stored, is a potent source of infection, particularly with *Ascaris*. Animal husbandry and other close contact with animals exposes humans to some of the zoonoses. Dietary habits, in particular the eating of uncooked or partially cooked fish, meat and snails may be responsible for infection with *Taenia*, *Diphyllobothrium*, *Trichinella*, *Anasakis*, *Capillaria* and *Angiostrongylus*. Whilst inadequate washing of fruit and vegetables is the major source of infection with *Ascaris*, careful washing of watercress and waterchestnuts may fail to prevent infection with the firmly attached metacercariae of *Fasciola* and *Fasciolopsis* in endemic areas.

In the light of the main factors involved in parasitic transmission the high prevalence of parasitic disease throughout the non-industrialized world is not surprising. Nor is it surprising that polyparasitism is common. Thus, it is not unusual to find children infected with three or more of the most common intestinal helminths, usually *Ascaris*, hookworms, and *Trichuris*, with or without *Enterobius*. In certain parts of the world other 'local' parasites may coexist.

Community perceptions

The ubiquity, size and behaviour of *Ascaris lumbricoides* make it inevitable that infection with this parasite should be perceived as 'worms' by most sections of the tropical community. Adult hookworms and *Strongyloides* are very unlikely to be seen, although the appearance of a few threadworms (*Enterobius*) or whipworms (*Trichuris*) in the stool may excite some attention. Intestinal symptomatology also being very common, it is therefore not surprising that infection with 'worms' is perceived as being responsible for such symptoms as vomiting, abdominal pain of various types, diarrhoea, abdominal distension, and flatulence. The dramatic expulsion of *Ascaris* from the nose or mouth by sneezing or vomiting in a febrile child as a result of temperature-induced increase in motility may result in *Ascaris* being blamed for the fever itself, or for symptoms such as cough and dyspnoea which may accompany it. The association of 'worms' with weight loss is common to both sophisticated and unsophisticated societies throughout the world. Ideas regarding the mode of infection will clearly vary with the level of education of the population concerned. At one end of the scale, worm infection will be attributed either directly or indirectly to eating 'dirty' food or to other unhygienic practices, whilst at the other, sorcery may be believed to be the cause.

Aetiology and pathogenesis

In common with other infectious diseases, the effects of helminthic infection depend on factors relating both to the parasite (the infective load and virulence) and to the host (the state of the body's immunological and other defence mechanisms). Thus, a healthy, well-nourished child may carry low worm burdens with no clinical manifestations whatever – a situation termed helminth infection, rather than helminth disease. Heavy worm burdens are likely to produce effects even in otherwise well individuals, whilst for those children whose body defences are already weakened by malnutrition and other infections, heavy infestations may be catastrophic, and even light to moderate infections are likely to compromise the child's health and nutritional status further. In these instances the term helminth disease is therefore more appropriate. The clinical manifestations of helminth disease are the result of both local and systemic effects.[2]

Local effects

Mechanical damage – biting and burrowing

The adult hookworm bites into the small bowel mucosa and secretes an anticoagulant to help in its appropriation of the host's blood. Local tissue reaction forces the worm to abandon the site of attachment for a new area after about 24 hours. Thus, multiple bleeding points may result from a single worm. In very heavy infections, this feature of hookworm infection may produce frank blood in the stool. Penetration of the gut wall by adult or larval helminths may result in severe effects, particularly if the gut wall is already damaged. Thus, the penetration of the upper gut by *Trichinella* may result in acute and painful gastroenteritis. *Ascaris* may penetrate a gut wall weakened by typhoid or tuberculosis, resulting in peritonitis. The adult *Fasciola hepatica* burrowing though the liver may cause extensive mechanical damage and intrahepatic bleeding. At the other end of the spectrum, the pruritus ani of *Enterobius vermicularis* infection is at least partly caused by the mechanical stimulation of the skin resulting from the wandering adult worms.

Inflammatory response

Although the adult *Trichuris* does not bite into the mucosa of the colon, it does form points of attachment and these are associated with an intense inflammatory response. This is likely to be at least part of the mechanism responsible for the chronic diarrhoea, tenesmus and occasional dysentery seen in heavy infections. *Anasakis* infection results in the development of eosinophilic granulomas in the wall of the small intestine and stomach which may present as acute abdominal pain.

Luminal obstruction

Heavy ascariasis is a well-recognized cause of acute and subacute gut obstruction. Much less common is the obstruction of smaller lumina (the bile duct, pancreatic duct and the larynx) caused by ectopic migrating *Ascaris*. *Fasciola*, *Clonorchis* and *Opisthorchis* may all produce biliary obstruction.

Stimulation of reflex peristalsis

Large parasites, such as *Ascaris*, *Fasciolopsis*, *Taenia* and *Diphyllobothrium*, may all stimulate reflex peristalsis, producing recurrent and sometimes severe abdominal pain.

Malabsorption

True malabsorption syndromes result from strongyloidiasis and capillariasis, and probably from primary hookworm infection. In the first two infections, the adult worms are embedded in the mucosa setting up local inflammatory responses resulting in a malabsorption syndrome similar to tropical sprue. In immunocompromised patients, hyperinfection with *Strongyloides* is frequently fatal.

Immunological response

Localized immunological responses are more directed at larval stages than the adult worm and are responsible for the pulmonary pathology and symptoms seen in those helminth infections in which larvae migrate through the lungs. Thus, in *Ascaris*, hookworm and *Strongyloides* infection, such reactions may be more or less severe. Similar mechanisms combined with mechanical damage and local inflammatory response probably play a part in the reactions seen in cutaneous and visceral larvae migrans, in *Dracunculus* infection and in the myositis of trichinosis. They are also fundamental to the pathogenesis of eosinophilic meningitis caused by *Angiostrongylus cantonensis*. Local immunological responses may be combined with severe systemic responses in situations where there is a sudden release of antigen, such as occurs in a ruptured hydatid cyst.

Space-occupying lesions

Space-occupying lesions resulting from helminthic infection can occur in almost any tissue. Thus, hydatid cysts (*Echinococcus*) and cysticercal cysts (*Taenia solium*) may produce symptoms in liver, lung or brain of patients from endemic areas.

Induction of malignancy

Clonorchis and *Opisthorchis* are associated with biliary tract carcinomas, but this is unlikely to be a problem in children.

These local effects explain many of the common symptoms and signs seen in helminthic disease. Whilst some of these may be of considerable severity, the systemic effects of helminthic infection are more important, but often less obvious.

Systemic effects

Malnutrition and growth impairment

Allusion has already been made to the malabsorption syndromes caused by *Strongyloides*, *Capillaria*, and probably, by acute hookworm infection. However, even in the absence of a specific malabsorption syndrome, helminthic infections of the gut are likely to produce a situation of negative nitrogen balance – and hence of malnutrition or growth failure – where food intake is inadequate for the needs of the host and the parasites. Reasons for this are varied. Loss of proteins and cells occurs not only from the feeding of worms such as hookworms and *Strongyloides* but also from local tissue reactions such as have been discussed for *Trichuris*. The proteins include the normal serum proteins and immunoglobulins, whilst the cells include epithelial cells, red blood cells and lymphocytes. In strongyloidiasis a severe protein-losing enteropathy may occur, particularly in the hyperinfection syndromes seen in immunocompromised individuals and in young infants heavily infected with *Strongyloides* spp., cf. *S. fulleborni* in parts of Papua New Guinea.[3] At the same time, protein and energy requirements are increased in infected patients – particularly in the larval migratory stages – to manufacture immunoglobulins, cells and acute-phase reactants, and to replace losses of blood and protein from the gut. Worm infections themselves, particularly with *Ascaris*, decrease appetite because of the often severe colicky pain following a meal. In heavy ascariasis there must be significant competition for the child's food. It has recently been suggested that even relatively low infective *Ascaris* loads may be associated with impaired growth.

Anaemia

Continuous losses of blood from the gut in the absence of adequate iron replacement will eventually lead to iron-deficiency anaemia. Blood loss from the gut is most common in hookworm infection but may occur also with *Trichuris* and *Strongyloides*. Much less commonly, a megaloblastic anaemia may result from competition for and interference with absorption of vitamin B$_{12}$ by *Diphyllobothrium latum*.

Generalized immune response

Mention has already been made of the generalized immune reactions such as an anaphylaxis that may occur in conditions such as the sudden bursting of a hydatid cyst.

For the majority of the world's children living on a borderline or inadequate diet and affected by a multitude of infectious diseases, helminthiasis – particularly infection with the gut nematodes – is a major burden. Not only does it produce specific signs and symptoms, but it also decreases nutritional status, contributes to anaemia, and plays a large part in maintaining the 'vicious cycle' between malnutrition and infection.

Life-cycles and clinical manifestations

Common gut nematodes

The life-cycles of the five common gut nematodes are shown in Fig. 4.10.1. Three (*Ascaris*, *Trichuris*, *Enterobius*) enter the body in the form of ova – faecal–oral or in the case of *Enterobius* anal–oral routes. The other two (hookworm and *Strongyloides*) enter the body by larval penetration of the skin.[1, 2, 4]

Ascaris lumbricoides – roundworm

The adult *Ascaris* is by far the largest of the gut nematodes, reaching 30 cm or more in length. It lives in the small intestine where it remains by pressing against the gut walls and constantly moving against peristalsis. It secretes a trypsin inhibitor which prevents it from being digested. A single female may produce 200 000 eggs a day, and it has been estimated that as many as 9×10^{14} new *Ascaris* eggs contaminate the world environment each day! The ova embryonate in the soil and by way of contaminated food or fingers are then swallowed by the human host. Within the small intestine the ova hatch and the *Ascaris* larvae thus released begin the process of maturation, penetrate the gut wall, and travel via the portal and then the systemic blood to the capillaries of the lungs. From here they break into the alveolar space and thence migrate up the bronchi and trachea, into the oesophagus and hence into the small intestine. Here they complete their maturation into adult worms.

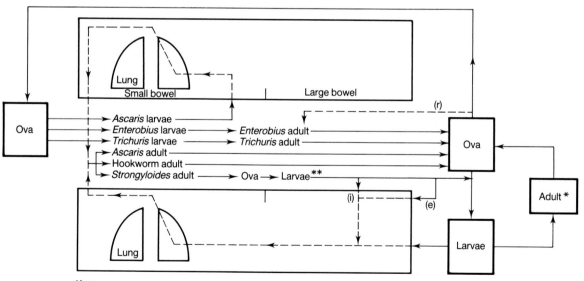

Key:
* Free-living adult — *Strongyloides* species.
** Larvae in gut — *Strongyloides stercoralis* only.
(r) Retro-infection — *Enterobius*.
(i) Internal autoinfection — *Strongyloides stercoralis*.
(e) External autoinfection — *Strongyloides stercoralis*.

Fig. 4.10.1   The life-cycles of the five common gut nematodes.

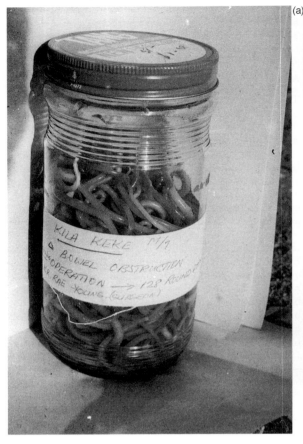

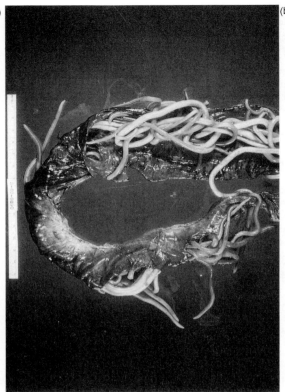

Fig. 4.10.2   (a) *Ascaris* worms which had caused an intestinal obstruction. (Courtesy of Prof J Biddulph.) (b) Obstruction from a heavy infection of Ascaris causing gangrenous rupture of the intestine. (Photo by WH Sternberg, courtesy of Dr PC Beaver.)

The clinical features of ascariasis relate to both larval and adult stages and depend on the intensity of infection. Migration of larvae through the lungs, particularly in heavy infection, may cause a severe immune-mediated inflammatory response resulting in pneumonitis, liver enlargement and generalized toxicity. The effects of large numbers of adult worms in the gut have already been discussed but include competition for nutrients, depression of appetite, colicky abdominal pain and abdominal distension. Intestinal obstruction (Fig. 4.10.2) may be relatively common in areas of intense infection, and occasionally migrating worms may cause obstruction to bile duct, pancreatic duct or larynx with appropriate effects (see pp. 895–6). *Ascaris* worms may also appear from abdominal wounds (following migration through a damaged gut) and may perforate the gut damaged by illnesses such as typhoid.

Ingestion of eggs of the dog roundworm (*Toxocara*

canis) may be followed by visceral larvae migrans, the larvae causing intense tissue reactions, mainly in the liver (Fig. 4.10.3).

Hookworms: *Ancylostoma duodenale* and *Necator americanus*

Both these nematodes are widespread throughout the tropical world, although *Ancylostoma* is better adapted to temperate climates with seasonal transmission, and *Necator* to tropical climates with perennial transmission. Their life cycles are identical. *Ancylostoma duodenale* is longer and fatter than *Necator americanus* (females 10–13 and 9–11 mm long respectively), consumes more host blood (0.15 and 0.05 ml per worm per day) and produces more eggs (30 000 and 10 000 eggs per day). *Ancylostoma* bites on to the small bowel mucosa using teeth, while *Necator* does so using cutting plates, and both feed directly on villous tissue as well as ingesting

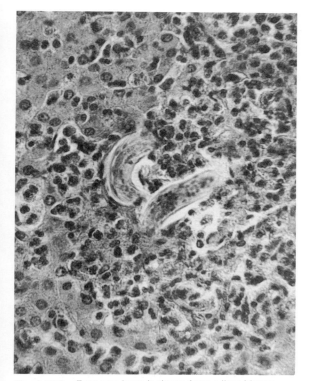

Fig. 4.10.3 *Toxocara* larva in tissue from a liver biopsy ×286. (Courtesy of Dr PC Beaver.)

blood. The worms produce an anticoagulant and, since they change attachments every 24 hours or so, leave multiple bleeding points. The eggs are passed in the faeces, and hatch within 48 hours under favourable conditions. The rhabditiform larvae (morphologically resembling the free-living nematode, *Rhabditis*) released feed on bacteria and moult twice to become the infective filariform larvae, which lie in wait for contact with human skin, frequently ascending surface vegetation in the surface water film. Once on the skin, they penetrate into the subcutaneous tissue and hence travel in the blood or lymphatics to the lung capillaries. Here, like *Ascaris* and *Strongyloides* larvae, the hookworm larvae break into the alveoli, travel up the bronchi and trachea and down the oesophagus continually maturing as they go and undergo their final moult to adult worms in the small intestine. It is likely that some infections may occur perorally, the filariform larvae being ingested in contaminated vegetables.

As with *Ascaris* infection, clinical manifestations may result from both larval and adult stages and are dependent on the intensity of infection and the host's general health and wellbeing. Repeated larval penetra-

tion of the skin in patients in endemic areas may produce itching, whilst a heavy load of migratory larvae may produce respiratory symptoms similar to those occurring in ascariasis.

A heavy primary infection may produce a genuine malabsorption syndrome, but this is not a feature of repeated infections. In patients already iron deficient because of inadequate diet, even moderate infections may result in iron-deficiency anaemia, and hookworm infection is a major factor in the aetiology of anaemia in the non-industrialized world. The anaemia is frequently profound, the affected children presenting with oedema and other signs of heart failure in addition to severe pallor. Great care is required in their treatment, particularly when blood transfusions are used. The absence of skin and hair changes helps to differentiate these children from those with kwashiorkor, but both conditions may coexist in the same patient. Indeed the continuous loss of serum proteins, immunoglobulins and cells consequent on infection is likely to be a contributory factor in tipping the balance from borderline nutritional status to frank malnutrition.

Penetration of the skin by larvae of the dog hookworm *Ancylostoma braziliense* causes intense itching of the feet or buttocks – cutaneous larvae migrans (Fig. 4.10.4). (See p. 850).

Strongyloides

Strongyloides stercoralis *Strongyloides stercoralis* is found primarily in warm, humid climates and where sandy, loamy soil supports its life-cycle. It is unique among the common human nematodes on two counts. Firstly, it has the capacity for internal autoinfection, and thus replication within the host, although under normal circumstances this is not an important aspect of its life-

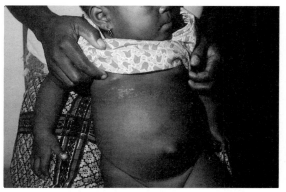

Fig. 4.10.4 Cutaneous larva migrans.

cycle. Secondly, under favourable conditions, it demonstrates a free-living as well as a parasitic life-cycle.

The parasitic adult worms, about 2 mm in length, lie embedded in the jejunal mucosa. The ova hatch near to or on the mucosal surface and release rhabditiform larvae, which in normal circumstances are passed in the faeces on to the soil. There they may develop either into infective filariform larvae or into free-living adults – whose ova in turn may develop either into infective larvae, or continue the free-living cycle. The infective filariform larvae penetrate the skin and continue via the bloodstream, lungs, trachea and oesophagus to the small intestine in almost identical manner to those of hookworms.

Autoinfection may occur either externally or internally. Filariform larvae on faecally contaminated perianal skin may penetrate the skin of the buttocks – one form of cutaneous larvae migrans. Internal autoinfection is much more serious. Under conditions of depressed body defences – naturally or iatrogenically acquired – large numbers of infective larvae within the gut lumen may penetrate the gut wall and hence travel via the portal and then the systemic circulation to the lungs, so to complete the internal cycle back to the gut. Massive infections may build up in this way – producing a 'hyperinfection' syndrome.

As with *Ascaris* and hookworm infections, heavy larval loads may lead to pulmonary signs and symptoms which may be of extreme severity in the hyperinfection syndrome. In the normal host, strongyloidiasis is manifested primarily by watery, mucousy diarrhoea. In heavy infections, a malabsorption syndrome occurs and protein losses from the bowel are significant. The grossly oedematous wall of the small bowel may become atonic with subsequent obstruction and profuse vomiting. Perforation and peritonitis is a well-recognized complication. The hyperinfection syndrome in immunocompromised hosts consists of severe mucousy diarrhoea, malabsorption, protein-losing enteropathy, pulmonary signs and symptoms and systemic bacterial infection resulting from the carriage of bacteria from the gut into the circulation by the invasive larvae. It is frequently fatal.

Strongyloides fulleborni   It is now well-recognized that *Strongyloides fulleborni*, originally thought to be a parasite of non-human primates exhibiting zoonosis, is well adapted to human transmission. *Strongyloides fulleborni* differs from *S. stercoralis* in that embryonated ova rather than larvae are passed in the stool – although once passed the eggs hatch very quickly. Thus, internal auto-infection does not occur. As with *S. stercoralis*, a free-living cycle may occur. Signs and symptoms in the normal host are similar to those produced by *Strongyloides stercoralis*.

A species of *Strongyloides* very closely resembling (if not identical with) *S. fulleborni* occurs in Papua New Guinea, in the absence of any known animal reservoir and is regarded as a primary human parasite. Under certain specific conditions, massive infections may develop in babies between three and six months of age. This is analogous to the hyperinfection syndrome described for *S. stercoralis*, and consists of respiratory signs and symptoms, diarrhoea, abdominal distension with ascites ('swollen belly', Fig. 4.10.5) and hypo-proteinaemic oedema, often with pleural or pericardial effusions. Without treatment the condition is almost invariably fatal. Postmortem examination on three infants showed pneumonia or peritonitis. The precise pathogenesis of heavy *Strongyloides* infection in these young infants remains unsolved. Infection in neonates makes primary postpartum acquisition of the parasite by skin penetration unlikely.

Isolated reports from Zaire of the finding of *S. fulleborni* larvae in breast-milk indicate at least the possibility of transmammary transmission in this species. There are no reports of 'swollen belly' syndrome from Africa though *Strongyloides fulleborni* has been found in many different human populations in widely separated areas of Africa with those residing in heavy rainforest areas being most heavily infected.

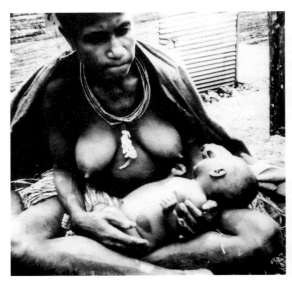

Fig. 4.10.5   An infant showing the abdominal swelling associated with *Strongyloides fulleborni* infection.

Trichuris trichuria – whipworm

Trichuris has the simplest life-cycle of the human gut nematodes. The adult worms, between 30 and 50 mm long, live in the large intestine, primarily in the caecum, but extending to the rectum in heavy infections. The thin anterior ends of the worms lie embedded in the mucosa, where they provoke an inflammatory reaction. The worms are not blood feeders, but bleeding may occur from attachment sites. The very characteristic ova are passed in the stool. Under favourable conditions of warmth and moisture, the eggs embryonate and are ingested via contaminated fingers and food.

The larvae hatch from the eggs in the small intestine and continue their maturation in the mucosa of the terminal ileum and caecum. The immature adults emerge from the mucosa and are carried into the large intestine where they attach themselves and complete their maturation.

The clinical manifestations of *Trichuris* are usually only seen in heavy infections. Chronic diarrhoea is a major feature, but it is important also to exclude other coexistent parasites such as *Entamoeba histolytica* (which may invade the mucosa through the sites of *Trichuris* attachment) and *Giardia lamblia*. Frank dysentery may occur and severe rectal bleeding is a rare complication. Abdominal pain may be a feature and may mimic appendicitis. Tenesmus is an important manifestation, resulting from colitis, and proctitis and recurrent straining, particularly in a debilitated child, may lead to prolapse of the rectum (Fig. 4.10.6a, b). Although a direct causal relationship between trichuriasis and malnutrition and anaemia is difficult to prove, it is hard to escape the conclusion that heavy *Trichuris* infections are contributory.

Enterobius (oxyuris) vermicularis – threadworm or pinworm

The adult worms, the female about 8–13 mm long, live in the caecum where they make loose attachments with their mouth-parts to the mucosa. The gravid female migrates through the anus at night and deposits her embryonated eggs on the perianal skin. Usually the female worm dies following this but sometimes it may migrate back into the large intestine or occasionally into the vagina. The normal route of infection is by carriage of the eggs by fingers either directly or indirectly to the mouth. Eggs may also be carried in dust. Once ingested, the eggs hatch in the small intestine where they moult several times before entering the caecum as immature adult worms. It is known that an alternative route of infection (retro-infection) occurs, in which the eggs hatch on the perianal skin, releasing larvae which then migrate back through the anus into the large intestine. Occasionally the larvae may migrate into the vagina.

Enterobius infections are manifest primarily by intense pruritus which may cause sleep disturbance. Scratching may result in secondary infection. Occasionally migrant adult worms (or larvae) may produce a vulvo-vaginitis with vaginal discharge, and ectopic migration has also been reported to cause appendicitis, endometritis, salpingitis and granuloma formation in the peritoneal cavity. *Enterobius* probably also predisposes to urinary tract infections in girls. It is likely that *Enterobius* plays a role as a vector of *Dientamoeba fragilis*, an amoebic species which can cause a self-limiting diarrhoeal illness in man, and which may be transmitted in *Enterobius* ova.

Common human cestodes

Taenia solium and T. saginata – pig and beef tapeworms

The life-cycles of *Taenia solium* and *T. saginata* are essentially similar, the differences being in the intermediate hosts. The large adults (several metres in length) inhabit the small bowel where they are attached by suckers and/or hooks.

The terminal mature segments, or proglottids, break from the adult and either disintegrate within the bowel lumen, releasing eggs into the faeces, or are themselves passed in the faeces (sometimes appearing as 'clotted cream') with subsequent disintegration. The eggs are ingested by the intermediate host in which the larval stages develop.

Infection in man is acquired by eating infected undercooked meat. Symptoms of infection are few and mild – usually limited to feelings of epigastric fullness. Very rarely, obstruction may occur. In the case of *Taenia solium*, ingestion of the eggs through faecal contamination may lead to man being the intermediate host, the larval cysts developing in the tissues of the body (cysticercosis) with very serious consequences when vital organs such as the brain are involved. Occasionally, internal autoinfection, occurring consequent on the disintegration of gravid proglottids in the bowel, may produce cysticercosis.

Diphyllobothrium latum – fish tapeworm

Diphyllobothrium latum is the largest of the human tapeworms – up to 15 m in length. Its life-cycle involves

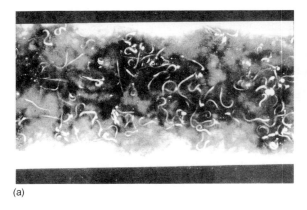

(a)

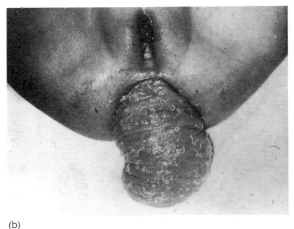

(b)

Fig. 4.10.6 (a) Rectal mucosa infected with *Trichuris*. (b) Rectal prolapse associated with *Trichuris* infection. (Photo courtesy of Dr P.C. Beaver and Dr R. Platou.)

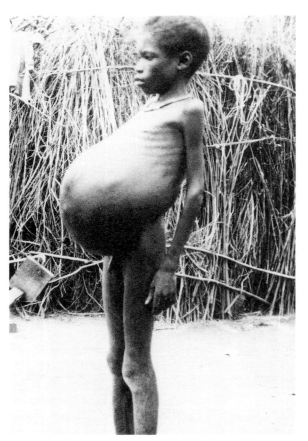

Fig. 4.10.7 Child with large hydatid cysts in the liver.

the production of non-embryonated eggs which embryonate in water before infecting fish – the intermediate host. Clinical symptoms are uncommon and vague, but abdominal pain may occur and vitamin B_{12} deficiency causing megaloblastic anaemia, and occasionally neurological symptoms, develops in a small percentage of infected persons.

Hymenolepis nana – dwarf tapeworm

Hymenolepis nana, a small tapeworm up to 45 mm long and with no intermediate host, is the most common cestode infection in man but is relatively unimportant. Internal autoinfection may result from ova developing into adults in the same host. Clinically, diarrhoea, abdominal pain and urticaria have been described in heavy infections.

A common zoonotic cestode — Echinococcus granulosus (hydatid disease)

Dogs and other carnivores are the definitive hosts of this tapeworm, which has a world-wide distribution (see also p. 738). Sheep are the principal intermediate hosts, but larval forms mature also in other domestic animals such as cattle, goats, water buffalo and camels. Dogs acquire infection by eating dead animals or by 'scavenging' offal from slaughtered livestock. Man is an accidental, but frequent, intermediate host in areas where animal husbandry is common and particularly where man has a close relationship with the dog and where standards of hygiene are poor. Contamination of hands and food by the ova originating in dog faeces may lead to their ingestion, larval penetration of the gut wall and deposition in the body tissues via the bloodstream. Larval cysts develop and gradually enlarge over a 5 to 10 year period. The liver (Figs 4.10.7 and 5.3.2) and lungs are the most frequent sites of these cysts which may measure up to 30 cm in diameter (Fig. 4.10.8). The symptomatology of hydatid disease relates to the site of the cysts and the effect of compression of surrounding structures, and to immune responses consequent on leakage of cyst contents. These vary from an urticarial reaction to a fatal anaphylaxis.

Human trematodes

The lumen-dwelling hermaphroditic flukes have similar life-cycles. Eggs are produced by the adults and excreted in embryonated or non-embryonated forms in the faeces (and sputum in the case of *Paragonimus*). All have snails as intermediate hosts – in most cases aquatic or amphibious species (*Dicrocoelium* being the only exception). The embryonated egg may be ingested by the snail or the non-embryonated egg may embryonate in the aquatic environment and release a miracidium which burrows into the snails. Cercariae are released from the snail and become encysted as

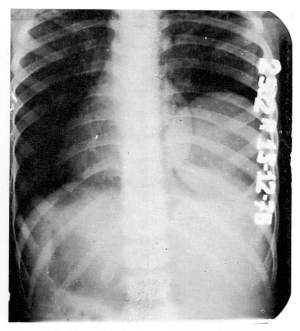

Fig. 4.10.8 X-ray showing large hydatid cyst in the left lung.

metacercariae on plants (*Fasciola, Fasciolopsis, Gastrodiscoides*), in fish (*Clonorchis, Opisthorchis, Heterophyes, Echinostoma*) in crustacea (*Paragonimus*), molluscs (*Echinostoma*), or ants (*Dicrocoelium*). In this form, they are ingested by the human host where they mature in their target tissues.

Clinical symptoms may result both from the effect of larval migration and from the effect of adult worms – particularly from those species that invade the liver (*Fasciola* – see pp. 736–8) and the lungs (*Paragonimus*).

Paragonimus – the lung fluke

Infection with the lung fluke *Paragonimus westermani* is endemic in many parts of South-east Asia and China. Other species, principally *P. uterobilateralis* and *P. africanus*, occur in parts of Africa, while several other zoonotic species with incomplete development in man occur in South and Central America and South-east Asia (see p. 721). The adult flukes live in pairs surrounded by a fibrous capsule forming a cyst, usually close to the bronchi. The characteristic golden brown, operculated eggs pass to the bronchi by a process of infiltration through lung tissue or through direct communication from older cysts and are coughed up in the sputum, to which they give a characteristic rusty appearance. Sputum may be coughed out or swallowed, with consequent dissemination of eggs either directly or via the faeces. Hatching occurs after two to three weeks in water, and the ciliated miracidia released eventually penetrate the host snail in which metamorphosis occurs and from which cercariae are released. These in turn penetrate fresh-water crabs and crayfish and become encysted as metacercariae in which form they are ingested by man. Within the gut the metacercariae excyst and burrow through the gut wall into the peritoneum and thence through the diaphragm and lung tissue.

The main clinical features of paragonimiasis relate to pulmonary damage caused by the fluke and to the host response to infection. Cough with the production of plentiful sputum, often rusty brown in colour, dyspnoea and haemoptysis are major features. Weight loss is common, and the clinical and radiological findings may easily be mistakenly attributed to tuberculosis. Inflammatory reactions round the flukes and their eggs lead to scarring with eventual bronchiectasis, whilst atelectasis, secondary infections, pleural effusions and pneumothorax may all occur. Less commonly, larvae migrate to ectopic foci in abdominal organs, subcutaneous tissues or brain with the production of granulomas which may have very serious consequences, such as epilepsy, hemiplegias, features of a space-occupying lesion, and death.

Diagnosis

Microscopic examination of fresh stool – or if necessary of preserved stool – is, and will remain, the most appropriate and accurate way of detecting the great majority of helminth infections.

A simple, saline preparation of faeces is usually adequate for detecting moderate to heavy infections with the common helminths that produce large numbers of eggs – *Ascaris*, hookworms and *Trichuris*. The ova are quite characteristic (Fig. 4.10.9). For less heavy infections and for the detection of helminths which produce low numbers of ova, concentration methods are required to improve the sensitivity of the smear examination. Quantitative methods may be used to give estimates of worm load.

The finding of nematode larvae in fresh stool is diagnostic of *Strongyloides stercoralis*. However, it must be realized that the ova of *Strongyloides fulleborni* hatch very quickly after the passage of faeces, and that hookworm eggs may also hatch in stale faeces. The larvae of the different nematodes have characteristic features which the parasitologist will recognize.

Where the suspicion of *Strongyloides stercoralis* infection is high but careful stool examination fails to detect larvae, duodenal juice may be sampled for microscopy – when both larvae and ova may be detected.

The ova of *Enterobius vermicularis* are most easily demonstrated by the 'sellotape' method whereby sticky tape is placed on the perianal folds and then stuck on to a microscope slide. The adherent ova are readily seen through the transparent tape by microscopic examination.

The presence of eosinophilia (>600 eosinophils/mm^3) in a blood film is very suggestive of worm infestation. Very high levels may be found in conditions with an invasive larval stage such as *Ascaris*, hookworms, *Strongyloides* and the invasive zoonoses such as visceral larvae migrans (*Toxocara canis*) and *Fasciola hepatica*. High levels are, however, not diagnostic of a specific infection.

In general, immunological techniques of diagnosis are hampered by problems of low specificity and the inability to differentiate current from previous infection. Such techniques may, however, be helpful in the diagnosis of fascioliasis, trichinosis, toxocariasis and in hydatid disease, and may be of value in epidemiological work.[5]

X-ray (Fig. 4.10.8) and, more recently, ultrasonic scanning are important in identifying helminth pathology, especially in ectopic sites and in hydatid disease, cysticercosis and paragonimiasis (see Fig. 5.3.2).

Management

In an ideal situation individuals with signs and symptoms suggestive of helminth infection should be investigated and treated on the basis of the particular parasite or parasites present. In such circumstances, treatment can be tailor-made to the individual and his or her parasites, in order to achieve at least a temporary eradication of infection. Suitable and well-established drugs for the various parasites are listed in Table 4.10.2.

In the conditions prevalent in most of the tropical world, it is impracticable to make an individual diagnosis. It is thus important to choose a treatment regimen which is the most likely to be effective against the parasites which the child is most likely to harbour.[1,6,7]

A single-dose, broad-spectrum anthelminthic highly effective against all the common gut nematodes has yet to be developed. Albendazole, a recently developed benzimidazole, comes reasonably close to this ideal and has some larvicidal and ovicidal effects in addition to its primary vermicidal action. It is being used increasingly in many countries at a single dose of 400 mg (200 mg in small children) and, if available, is the drug of choice. A three-day (six-dose) course of mebendazole (100 mg twice a day) is likely to be highly effective, as is a three-day course of pyrantel (10 mg/kg per day) and oxantel (10–15 mg/kg per day), but problems of compliance make such regimens less than ideal. In situations where only single-dose regimens are practical, and where albendazole is not available, single doses of mebendazole (400, 200 mg in small children), levamisole (3 mg/kg), or pyrantel (10 mg/kg with or without oxantel 10–15 mg/kg) may be used.

Follow-up examination of the individual child and examination of his/her stool after several weeks is ideal but usually impracticable.

Thiabendazole is largely restricted to use in strongyloidiasis, because of its relatively high incidence of side-effects. However, since it is absorbed and achieves relatively high serum levels, it is also the drug of choice in tissue helminthiasis such as visceral and cutaneous larvae migrans and in trichinosis.

In general, anthelminthics should be avoided in children less than one year of age and in pregnancy,

Hookworm: ovoid, thin,
uncoloured shell

Strongyloides: ovoid, thin, uncoloured
shell contains first stage larva

Ascaris: ovoid,
thick brown shell

Trichuris: thick brown
shell — bipolar plugs

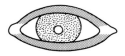

Enterobius: thin shell
flattened on one side

Taenia: spherical thick shell,
radial striation

Trematode: non-embryonated,
operculated e.g. *Paragonimus*, *Fasciola*
Cestode: *Diphyllobothrium latum*

Trematode: embryonated,
operculated
e.g. *Clonorchis*

 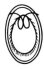

Fig. 4.10.9   Normal microscopic
appearance of helminth ova (not to
scale).

although exceptions should certainly be made on adequate clinical grounds.

It should be stressed that worm infestation cannot be dealt with in isolation. It must be viewed in the context of the child's overall health and social background. Thus, treatment of worm infestation forms a part of the management of anaemia and of malnutrition and proper attention must be focussed on these and other problems in each child. For example, in children in whom there is severe 'hookworm' anaemia and in whom there are signs of heart failure, treatment requires great care. Blood transfusions with packed cells may be life-saving but should be given slowly together with diuretics. The anaemia is not a contra-indication to anthelminthics, which should be given.

Haematinics are usually indicated, as are antimalarials in malarous areas.

Efforts to prevent reinfection for the individual must focus on health education on basic hygiene and sanitation for the family and community in general.

Prevention and control

In no other area of medicine is the inextricable link between prevention and control more clearly demonstrated than in helminthic infections. The problems to be overcome in achieving adequate control of helminthiasis are formidable and it probably must be accepted that eradication of infection is an unrealistic goal in

Table 4.10.2. Drugs used in the treatment of individuals with helminthiasis (number of doses in parentheses; letter indicates dosage given in footnote)

Nematodes				
Ascaris	Albendazole (1) a	Mebendazole (6) b	Pyrantel (1) e	Levamisole (1) h
Hookworm	Albendazole (1) a	Mebendazole (6) b	Pyrantel (3) f	Tetrachlorethylene (1) i
Trichuris	Albendazole (1) a	Mebendazole (6) b	Oxantel (3) g	
Enterobius	Albendazole (1) a	Mebendazole (1) b, r	Pyrantel (1) e, r	
Strongyloides	Thiabendazole (6) c	Albendazole (3) d		
Capillaria		Mebendazole (20–60) r		
Trichostrongylus		Mebendazole (6) b	Pyrantel (1) e	Levamisole (1) h
Cestodes				
Taenia sp.	Praziquantel (1) j	Niclosamide (1) k		
Diphyllobothrium	Praziquantel (1) j	Niclosamide (1) k		
Hymenolepis	Praziquantel (1) j, r	Niclosamide (5) k		
Echinococcus	Albendazole (28 × 5) l			
Trematodes	Praziquantel (3) m (liver, lung and intestinal flukes)	Tetrachlorethylene (3) n (intestinal flukes)		

(a) Albendazole 400 mg (200 mg small children); (b) mebendazole 100 mg twice daily for 3 days (single dose for *Enterobius*); (c) thiabendazole 25 mg/kg twice daily for 3 days; (d) albendazole 400 mg daily for 3 days; (e) pyrantel 10 mg/kg; (f) pyrantel 10 mg/kg daily for 3 days; (g) oxantel 10–15 mg/kg daily for 3 days; (h) levamisole 3 mg/kg; (i) tetrachlorethylene 0.1 mg/kg. Taken on an empty stomach. Unsuitable for use on its own if *Ascaris* is also present; (j) praziquantel 10–25 mg/kg; (k) niclosamide 2 g (1 g in small children). Taken on an empty stomach. (5 days for *Hymenolepis*); (l) albendazole 800 mg daily for 28 days. 5 courses with 2-week intervals; (m) praziquantel 25 mg/kg for 3 doses; (n) tetrachlorethylene 0.1 ml/kg daily for 3 days; (r) repeat after 2–3 weeks.

most parts of the tropical world in the forseeable future. It has, however, been clearly demonstrated that partial control is currently practicable within non-industrialized communities resulting in a reduction both in prevalence and in individual worm burden. Such partial control is likely to have very important beneficial implications in terms of the children's growth, and of the overall physical, mental, and economic health of the community.[9,10]

There are three aspects to prevention and control of the common helminth infections within any community.

Prevention of spread of infection

Since the common gut nematodes (with the exception of *Enterobius*) are faecally disseminated, the provision of adequate faeces disposal systems, i.e. latrines, seems at first to be an easy and obvious control measure. Such measures have been implemented since the beginning of the twentieth century in some tropical areas but have proved disappointing for a number of reasons. The provision of a latrine does not by itself ensure that the population for which it is intended will use it. Unless kept clean, a village, settlement, or town latrine rapidly becomes a repulsive place – smelly, dirty and insect-ridden – and the heavily contaminated soil around it becomes a very potent source of infection, particularly with hookworm and *Strongyloides*. In this situation,

latrines may contribute to increased, rather than decreased prevalence and worm load and it is well recognized that hookworm infection rates are often very high in periurban squatter settlements. Safe and efficient disposal of the effluent or sludge from latrines remains a problem even in sophisticated societies. Children, the most potent source of *Ascaris* infection, are unlikely to use latrines and are likely to continue to defaecate at random in the environment. Worm infections may cause diarrhoea resulting in infected persons having to defaecate where there is no latrine, often near bush tracks and gardens. Infective forms are then spread in the environment through rainfall and drainage. Thus, the provision of latrines is extremely important but, even where they are kept in good condition, is not a complete control measure. Attempts to use chemical agents and biological methods to decrease dissemination have been partially successful but are impracticable on a large scale. Correct composting of night soil for fertilizer is an obvious control measure.

In other helminthic infections, different approaches to control are needed. In the trematode infections, whilst proper disposal of faeces (and sputum in the case of paragonimiasis) is important, attempts may be made to control the snail intermediate hosts, directly with the use of molluscicides, or indirectly by environmental control measures such as drainage, or with both methods. In the case of the zoonotic infections, a number of approaches are applicable. Attempts may be made to reduce the population of the definitive or reservoir hosts. In many instances this is either unacceptable or impracticable. Alternatively, the infectivity of the host may be reduced with chemotherapy. For example 'working' dogs used in sheep husbandry and as 'scavengers', and the definitive hosts for *Echinococcus* and other parasites may be regularly dewormed. In addition, close domestic contact between man and the definitive host may, if practicable, be reduced.

Prevention of infection

The ova of *Ascaris*, *Trichuris*, *Enterobius* and *Hymenolepis nana* (the commonest human tapeworm) enter the body via the oral route. The larvae of hookworms, in particular those of *Ancylostoma*, may also enter by this route. Thus, the provision and use of adequate quantities of clean water for washing hands after defaecation, before preparing and eating food, and for washing soil-contaminated fruit and vegetables is extremely important, and for some infections is equally or more important than adequate faeces disposal. Thorough cooking of meat and fish will prevent the animal tapeworm diseases by killing the larval stages and will also help in preventing trematode diseases.

Since hookworms and *Strongyloides* infections usually occur by larval penetration of the skin of the feet, the wearing of shoes is likely to be an efficient preventive measure. In most situations in which worm infestation is highly prevalent, however, such a control measure is at present of more theoretical than practical value.

Reduction in community worm load – chemotherapy

Reduction in community worm load can be achieved, at least on a temporary basis, by the application of chemotherapy with anthelminthics. Such chemotherapy may be directed either at a specific parasite or parasites, or at achieving a general reduction in parasite load. Mass chemotherapy implies the treatment of all members of the community. Selective chemotherapy implies the use of treatment only in those proven to be infected – and this involves screening of the population. Targeted chemotherapy implies treatment of those with the highest intensity of infection, who thus constitute an important source of infection and are at high risk of morbidity. This in its complete form also implies a preliminary screening of the population. In practical terms, either mass chemotherapy after a preliminary survey to indicate the common helminths present, or chemotherapy of a section of the population

assumed to be heavily infected are most likely to be used. For example, *Ascaris* infections are usually most prevalent and heavy in preschool children – and this is therefore a good and relatively captive target group for chemotherapeutic control of this infection.

A drug used for such control, should ideally be effective against all the commonly occurring parasites in that area in a single dose, should be inexpensive, and should be completely free from side-effects – particularly as it will inevitably be given to a few persons who are not infected. As previously discussed, such a drug does not yet exist, although some come reasonably close to this ideal. At the present time, albendazole is probably the drug of choice, but may not be readily available in all areas. In its absence, mebendazole or a combination of oxantel and pyrantel or of all three are reasonable single-dose regimens (see p. 646). Levamisole is effective against *Ascaris* infection, and praziquantel and niclosamide are effective against the cestode infections, whilst praziquantel is likely to have a major place in the treatment and control of trematode infections (see Table 4.10.2).

While results can be achieved quickly with chemotherapy, they are only temporary, and in the absence of other control measures already discussed, prevalence rates and loads can only be kept low by repeated chemotherapy, usually three or four times during a year. The frequency and spacing of drug doses required to have a long lasting impact on the community when other measures are taken are not known with precision and will vary from one location to another. Mathematical models taking several variables into account have been proposed to help with the construction of adequate control programmes.[11]

As with any control programme, efforts to impose a helminth control programme on a population which is unaware of the reasons for it, or unwilling to accept it are doomed to failure. In the long term, control will only be achieved by the improvement of sanitation, provision of adequate water to each home and education of communities – solutions which are as much political as medical. In the short term, the use of widespread chemotherapy is most likely to succeed when existing health or community structures are used for distribution and administration and where treatment of worm infestation is viewed as an essential part of primary health care and health education (see also p. 972).

The future

There are unlikely to be any very dramatic breakthroughs in the field of helminth infection. Improved diagnostic methods will probably increase the speed and accuracy of diagnosis both for individuals and communities. The search for the ideal control drug will doubtless continue and it is prudent to note that veterinary medicine has led the way in research and application of new drugs, such as the ivermectins. The main advances, however, are likely to lie in the far less glamorous fields of public health education and practice. Health workers and the communities they serve need to be more fully informed of the existence, prevalence and effects of the parasites in the area, and of the means to prevent and control them. Communities can thus themselves come to understand that helminth infection adversely affects health and to be positive in their wish to deal with it – an essential prerequisite for the success of any health improvement plan. How this health education is achieved will depend on variables such as the literacy of the community and the availability of 'teachers' at various levels. The provision of adequate water, and improved sanitation are likely to continue to pose problems for health departments and governments, and efforts need to be made to educate politicians and decision makers as to the necessities of these basic commodities. The crowded periurban squatter settlements are as worthy of attention in this regard as are rural communities.

Decisions need to be taken as to the best way to use chemotherapy using a cheap and effective drug or drug combination, and methods of administering such a programme need to be based on the circumstances of each community. In many instances, existing structures such as under-five clinics or community schools can be utilized.

Helminthic infections are certainly interesting, but are never likely to occupy positions of 'glamour' for the medical profession or the lay public for long. The battle to control them is likely to be long, drawn out and difficult but the rewards are likely to be great.

References

1. WHO. *Intestinal Protozoan and Helminthic Infections.* Technical Reports Series 666. Geneva, World Health Organization, 1981.
2. Knight R. *Parasitic Disease in Man.* Edinburgh, Churchill Livingstone, 1982.
3. Vince JD, Ashford RW, Gratten MJ *et al. Strongyloides* species infestation in young infants of Papua New Guinea: association with generalised oedema. *Papua New Guinea Medical Journal.* 1979; **22**: 120–7.
4. Katz M, Despommier DD, Gwadz R. *Parasitic Diseases.* New York, Springer-Verlag, 1982.
5. Higashi GI. Immunodiagnostic tests for protozoan and helminthic infections: review. *Diagnostic Immunology.* 1984; **2**: 2–18.
6. Sturchler D. Chemotherapy of human intestinal helminthiases: a review with particular reference to community treatment. *Advances in Pharmacology and Chemotherapy.* 1982; **19**: 129–54.
7. Sharma P. Broad action anthelminthics against intestinal helminthiases. *Tropical Gastroenterology.* 1983; **4**(3): 137–54.
8. Rossignol J-F, Maisonneuve H. Albendazole: a new concept in the control of intestinal helminthiasis. *Gastroenterologie Clinique et Biologique.* 1984; **4**: 569–76.
9. Stephenson LS, Crompton DWT, Latham MC *et al.* Evaluation of a four year project to control *Ascaris* infection in children in two Kenyan villages. *Journal of Tropical Pediatrics.* 1983; **29**: 175–84.
10. Stephenson LS. Methods to evaluate nutritional and economic implications of *Ascaris* infection. *Social Science and Medicine.* 1984; **19**, 610: 1061–5.
11. Anderson RM, May RM. Community control of helminth infections of man by mass and selective chemotherapy. *Parasitology.* 1985; **90**: 629–60.

DRACUNCULIASIS
H. Taelman

Dracunculiasis (dracontiasis, guinea-worm infection) is an infection caused by the nematode *Dracunculus medinensis*. Its area of distribution includes western Africa, the Middle East, Pakistan and India. About 50 million people are estimated to be infected.

Epidemiology

Man becomes infected by drinking water contaminated with *Cyclops* crustaceans harbouring larvae of *Dracunculus medinensis*. These are released in the stomach, cross the intestinal wall, and migrate into the abdominal or thoracic cavity where they mature. After about one year the female worm migrates to the subcutaneous tissues, usually of the legs, where it lays its larvae through an ulceration of the overlying skin. When the infected area comes into contact with water, the larvae are discharged in vast numbers, disseminate and are ingested by cyclops. These are found mainly in pools, wells and cisterns. The most important epidemiological feature of dracunculiasis is that its transmission proceeds only by ingesting contaminated water.

Clinical manifestations

The pathology is produced only by the adult female worm when it emerges through the skin after an incubation period of 10–14 months. A painful blister develops at the point of emergence followed by a painful ulcer. Several weeks will be necessary for the worm to be expelled completely. The stage of expulsion is often accompanied by secondary infection of the wound, abscess or arthritis. Another potential complication is tetanus. Because of the prolonged incapacity resulting from these complications, the impact of the disease on socio-economic aspects of life is very important.

Diagnosis

The diagnosis is established when the female worm emerges through the skin.

Treatment

Extraction of the worm from the tissues is performed by rolling it out progressively on to a stick. Niridazole (12.5 mg/kg twice daily for 10 days), thiabendazole (25 mg/kg twice daily for three days) and metronidazole (5 mg/kg twice daily for 10–20 days) may all help to resolve the inflammation produced by the worm and facilitate the extraction procedure. Supportive treatment to relieve the symptoms and appropriate antibiotic therapy for secondary infections should be given when required.

Control and prevention

The most effective control measure is the provision of safe drinking water. International agencies have planned to eradicate dracunculiasis by improvement of water supplies. Treatment of cases and health education are useful additional measures. Individual prevention includes boiling or chlorinating water or sieving it through a cloth before using it for drinking.

Further reading

Hopkins DR. Dracunculiasis: an eradicable scourge. *Epidemiologic Reviews*. 1983; **5**: 208–19.
Muller R. Guinea worm disease, epidemiology and control. *Bulletin of the World Health Organization*. 1979; **57**: 683.

CHAPTER 11

Schistosomiasis

H. A. Wilkins

At least 200 million people are thought to be infected with trematode worms of the genus *Schistosoma*. Although the more serious consequences of infection are frequently found in adults, children are often the most heavily infected subjects and they usually have an important role in transmission of the infection. Schistosomiasis must be seen as a problem that concerns all who care for children in endemic areas, particularly since treatment is now simple and effective.

The parasites and their life-cycle

The three major species of schistosome infecting man have similar life-cycles. A sexual generation of the adult schistosome occurs in man and an asexual stage in a molluscan intermediate host, with transmission between these two depending on larval forms which are free-swimming in freshwater. Infections are sometimes found in other mammalian hosts but these are of little or no epidemiological importance in maintaining transmission, except perhaps in the case of *S. japonicum*. The adults, 1–2 cm long and about 1 mm across, are found in the venules of the large and small intestines, in the case of *S. mansoni* and *S. japonicum*, or the vesical and ureteric plexus, in the case of *S. haematobium*. The males and females remain *in copulo* producing eggs for many years – up to 3000 per day in the case of *S. japonicum* and perhaps a tenth of that number in the other species. The ova, which vary in size and morphology between the species, pass through the wall of the intestine or urinary tract and reach the exterior in faeces or urine. Contact with freshwater causes the ova to develop into miracidia which survive for a few hours during which time they are capable of infecting the snail intermediate host, which must be of a species susceptible to the strain of parasite. Development takes place over some weeks, giving rise to first- and second-stage sporocysts and ultimately to cercariae. A single snail may produce over a thousand cercariae each day which are short-lived, fork-tailed motile larvae up to 200 μm long. On contact with unbroken skin, cercariae attach with a sucker and penetrate with the aid of enzyme secretions, shedding their characteristic tail. The resultant schistosomulum migrates through the lungs and liver developing as it does so. The time between contact with cercariae and the subsequent detection of eggs in the excreta varies and is as long as 12 weeks in *S. haematobium*.

Epidemiology

S. mansoni is a significant infection in the majority of countries in Africa, parts of the Middle East, some islands in the Caribbean, Venezuela and Brazil. *S. haematobium* has a wider distribution in Africa and the Middle East but is not found in the New World. *S. japonicum* occurs in parts of China, Japan, Taiwan, the Philippines and the Celebes.

    Within an endemic area, schistosome infection

characteristically has a very patchy distribution. Large areas of a country may be free from infection and, where it occurs, the prevalence of infection may vary considerably between villages a few kilometers apart. This reflects the distribution and population dynamics of the snails which transmit the local parasite strain and variation in man's contact with, and contamination of, the water bodies where intermediate hosts occur.

In an endemic area there is considerable variation in the egg output of infected subjects with the distribution of egg counts in infected subjects often approximating to log-normal within an age group. In foci of low prevalence light infections predominate. Infections are likely to be heavy in areas of high prevalence. The prevalence and intensity of infection are usually low in toddlers – reflecting their relatively limited contact with water. Intensity and prevalence of infection increase with age often reaching a peak between the ages of 10 and 15 years before falling to much lower levels in middle-aged subjects. As a consequence, children are responsible for a high proportion of the ova that are passed by the community. Studies of the pattern of water contact in endemic areas lead to the conclusion that children's play in water, particularly swimming, is often an important factor in transmission. Children are also often in contact with water at transmission sites when they accompany their mothers to wash clothes and carry out other domestic tasks. Variation in patterns of water contact is partly responsible for the variation in intensity of infection between and within age groups. However, there is increasing evidence that man gradually acquires a significant degree of protective immunity to schistosome infections and this appears to be an additional factor responsible for the lighter infections of older subjects and for variation between children in intensity of infection.

Schistosome worms do not multiply in the individual human host but the worms can survive and produce eggs for more than 30 years. However, cohort studies have shown that the egg output of infected children tends to fall by 50 per cent in two or three years in the absence of further infection or treatment. The intensity of schoolchildren's infection has been found to be a relatively persistent individual characteristic; an adolescent in an endemic area with a high egg count may have been heavily infected for some years and therefore is likely to have significant pathology. The prevalence of hepatomegaly and splenomegaly has been shown to be related to egg output both in *S. mansoni* and *S. japonicum* infection and bladder and renal tract abnormalities show some association with egg output in *S. haematobium* infection.

Clinical manifestations and pathogenesis

The early stages of invasion and maturation of the parasites produce similar manifestations in the three species but once infections become established, with egg production, the pathological consequences depend on the site the adult worms occupy. A characteristic immunological response is the granuloma, or pseudotubercle, around the egg which is a localized collection of epithelioid cells, plasma cells, lymphocytes and eosinophils. Later in the course of infection, when egg output may be reduced, fibrosis at affected sites can have important consequences. The immunopathological mechanisms in *S. mansoni* and *S. haematobium* appear similar but the composition of the cell population in the *S. japonicum* granuloma differs from that of the other two species, possibly reflecting the role of immune complexes. Intensity of infection is an important determinant of severity of disease. In an affected community, infected children usually show a spectrum of disease ranging from asymptomatic light infections to the advanced pathology which is associated with intense infection.

Initial responses to infection

The earliest pathological manifestation of schistosome infection is schistosome dermatitis. Previously exposed and sensitized subjects who come into contact with human schistosome cercariae may develop a pruritic papular rash lasting at most one or two days. Contact with non-human schistosome cercariae can also give rise to a 'swimmers itch'. However, in the resident population of endemic areas such cutaneous symptoms are rare.

Between four and ten weeks after exposure to infection, often before the passage of eggs is detectable, a syndrome known as Katayama fever may develop. The term originates from the name of a village in Japan where *S. japonicum* gave rise to the condition but a similar response can occur to the other species. Antibodies to the parasite are detectable in patients' serum and the condition appears to be a form of immune complex disease. The symptoms are non-specific and may include fever, anorexia, urticaria, arthralgia and gastro-intestinal symptoms. The spleen, liver and lymph nodes may be enlarged and there may be bronchospasm. Eosinophilia is often marked. There are reports of serious complications including jaundice, coma, spinal cord lesions and even death during this phase of infection which may be related to intensity of exposure to cercariae. However, the condition is seldom seen in children living in the endemic rural areas of Africa. The diagnosis is more often made in patients from urban elite groups or visitors from developed countries who may become symptomatic when they have returned to their home.

S. mansoni and S. japonicum infection

In established *S. mansoni* infection, the passage of the ova from the site of egg production into the lumen of the intestine can lead to pathological changes. The mucosa may be granular, haemorrhagic or ulcerated and polyps may be present which can cause protein and iron loss. Patients may present with bloody diarrhoea and tenesmus. However, case control studies have shown that many infected subjects are asymptomatic.

S. mansoni eggs also pass via the portal system to the liver where they elicit a granulomatous response. In heavy infections this may ultimately lead to the characteristic 'clay pipe-stem cirrhosis' in which the liver is traversed by bands of fibrotic tissue in and around the portal venous radicals. The fibrosis is interstitial and the liver parenchyma is relatively unaffected – in contrast to cirrhosis proper. The reaction to the ova leads to a presinusoidal intrahepatic obstruction to the portal blood flow and thus to portal hypertension. Hepatomegaly, often predominantly of the left lobe, is a common clinical finding which has been shown to be related to the intensity of infection. Splenomegaly may also be present, particularly in heavier and more long-standing infections.

The hepatosplenic late stage of heavy *S. mansoni* infection may present to the clinician with discomfort due to splenic enlargement, but haematemesis from oesophageal varices associated with portal hypertension is a more important cause of morbidity. Hepatosplenic disease may also be associated with anaemia, some-times due to hypersplenism. Although the characteristic pathology leaves the liver parenchyma relatively unaffected, children with hepatosplenic disease may present with ascites and oedema – and sometimes with jaundice. The incidence of such signs may vary between areas, possibly reflecting the effects of viral infections. The hepatosplenic stage may also be associated with a glomerulonephritis, which can lead to impaired renal function and renal amyloidosis has also been reported in *S. mansoni* infection. Endocrine abnormalities leading to growth retardation and delay in the development of secondary sexual characteristics, have been attributed to *S. mansoni* infection in children.

The consequences of *S. japonicum* infection are essentially similar to those of *S. mansoni*. However, the liver parenchymal cells are more likely to be affected by the pathology with consequent impairment of liver function. Affected children can develop ascites and hepatic coma may be a terminal event.

S. haematobium infection

The passage of *S. haematobium* through the structures of the urinary tract can cause a wide variety of pathological changes, all of which are related to the granulomatous response. Initially the only change may be hyperaemia of the bladder but subsequently nodular and polypoid lesions may develop by coalescence of the tubercles, mucosal hyperplasia and fibrosis. These may be visualized radiologically as filling defects. Subsequently, fibrosis may become the dominant response giving rise to the characteristic 'sandy patches' on the bladder mucosal surface which are seen at cystoscopy. In longer standing infections, egg output declines but *S. haematobium* ova, often calcified, appear to persist in the tissues longer than those of *S. mansoni*. As a consequence, radiology may show calcification of the bladder wall in children passing few or no ova in the urine – a reflection of their early heavy infection.

The ureters may be directly affected in a comparable way or as a consequence of changes in the bladder. These lesions can lead to abnormalities of ureteric peristalsis and dilatation or stricture of the ureters and thus to hydronephrosis. Ureteric and renal pathology may be present in a significant proportion of heavily infected children in endemic areas. The abnormalities of the bladder and ureters may lead to a urinary stasis and residue and thus predispose to bacterial infection. Whilst bacteriuria does occur it is only present in a small minority of children, but postmortem studies have shown that hydronephrosis may be associated with pyelonephritis. Other complications, including urinary calculi and bladder cancer, occur but these are mainly of importance in adults. Ultimately, obstructive uropathy, particularly when bilateral, can lead to gross impairment of renal function and death due to renal failure. However, while children are the most heavily infected age group, the mortality attributable to the infection is mainly in adults.

Children with *S. haematobium* infection may present with a variety of urinary symptoms. Haematuria is often present in infected children; it may only be apparent as terminal haematuria but in heavily infected subjects the entire specimen may be grossly blood-stained. Such symptoms may be very common and recognized as a specific disease entity. In some communities they may be considered a normal part of development around puberty. Dysuria is also a common symptom and infected children may complain of frequency and nocturia due to contracted bladders. Occasionally the infection leads to incontinence of urine. Lower abdominal pain may be present, or pain in association with a hydronephrosis.

Other manifestations of schistosome infections

Older descriptions of the consequences of schistosome infection give the impression that generalized constitutional disturbance is a common feature of the established infection with symptoms of 'debility' and 'lethargy'. This impression was supported by studies suggesting that infection may have an adverse effect on scholastic performance. These effects have not always been demonstrated in careful field studies and children with heavy *S. haematobium* infection and gross haematuria frequently seem unaffected by their infection. However, recent detailed studies in Kenya have shown that heavy *S. haematobium* infections can lead to anaemia associated with diminished exercise tolerance and that treatment of infection can be associated with a gain in weight (see also p. 845).

Schistosome infections, as well as having effects at the normal sites of egg laying, can lead to pathology elsewhere when worms are present at unusual sites. Worms and/or ova have been found virtually everywhere in the body. The consequences of ectopic egg deposition in the nervous system may be serious. *S. mansoni* and *S. haematobium* can effect the spinal cord, sometimes causing a paraplegia. *S. japonicum* is well recognized as sometimes affecting the brain and is a significant cause of epilepsy in areas where it occurs. The lungs may also be affected. Although *S. haematobium* ova can be found in the lungs, significant pathology is more likely in *S. mansoni* and *S. japonicum* infection when a portosystemic collateral circulation is established. The immune response to the ova which then pass to the blood vessels of the lungs may lead to pulmonary hypertension and the picture of cor pulmonale. Pathology may be found throughout both male and female genito-urinary systems. In the latter it is possible that damage to the Fallopian tubes may lead to infertility but demographic changes in endemic areas suggest that this is uncommon.

A potentially fatal complication of schistosome infection is chronic *Salmonella* infection. Schistosome infections predispose to this since the worm itself is a site where the bacteria persist. It is difficult to eradicate *S. typhi* infections from patients with schistosome infections and relapse is likely unless their schistosome infection is eradicated (see pp. 583–4).

Diagnosis

The diagnosis of schistosome infection is often suggested by knowledge of the pattern of endemicity in the area and a history of the child's movements – urinary schistosomiasis is very likely to be the cause of haematuria in a schoolchild from a known endemic area. Clinical examination is usually unrewarding in urinary schistosomiasis, but it has recently been suggested that the presence of obstructive uropathy in infected subjects may be indicated by the finding of hypertrophy of the seminal vesicles on rectal examination. However, the finding of enlargement of the liver and spleen may suggest the diagnosis of *S. mansoni* or *S. japonicum* infection in areas where these occur. Ancillary investigations may also point to the diagnosis. Characteristic pathology in the urinary tract may be shown by radiological or other imaging techniques – or the urologist may recognize a characteristic cystoscopic appearance. On occasion, biopsy material will lead to the diagnosis. Eosinophilia, which is usually present, may suggest the diagnosis in subjects in elite groups but is of little significance in subjects from rural areas who are exposed to other helminth infections.

The definitive diagnosis of schistosome infections usually depends upon examining excreta for ova which have a characteristic morphology for each species. In recent years the realization that pathology is related to intensity of infection has led to increasing emphasis on quantitative techniques. Urine may be examined for *S. haematobium* ova with filtration techniques that allow the enumeration of the number of ova in a given volume of the specimen. A variety of filter supports, filters and stains give comparable results. Details of these techniques can be obtained from a WHO report on diagnostic techniques in schistosomiasis control.[1] Egg output in urine shows diurnal variation and maximal numbers are present in the middle of the day when specimens should be collected if possible. Faeces may be conveniently examined using the cellophane or glass sandwich thick smear technique. It has been suggested that *S. haematobium* counts of more than 50/10 ml and *S. mansoni* counts of more than 800/g may be regarded as heavy infections. But the distribution of counts given by these techniques varies between areas and in some areas it may be appropriate to consider *S. haematobium* egg counts of more then 1000/10 ml as heavy. Where formal quantitative techniques are not available, every effort should be made to standardize methods of examining faeces and urine, with ova being carefully counted and reported in terms of an agreed semiquantitative scale.

In endemic areas these relatively simple microscopical techniques are appropriate for clinical practice in most circumstances. In areas where *S. haematobium* infection is endemic, a useful indication of infection may also be the finding of haematuria and proteinuria and, even when ova are not demonstrated, urinalysis may provide an indication for a monitored trial of treatment. In some circumstances alternative concentration techniques may be needed for examining excreta but even these may be inadequate, particularly when a light infection is suspected in a traveller from a non-endemic area or in *S. japonicum* infections. Rectal snips may then show ova when examination of excreta fails to do so. Alternatively, immunodiagnostic techniques may be used. An increasing variety of methods and antigens are being described with high specificity and sensitivity. The ELISA technique, using an antigen prepared from *S. mansoni* ova, has been found of value for the diagnosis both of *S. mansoni* and *S. haematobium*. Serological methods have an important role in the diagnosis of the Katayama syndrome and the manifestations of ectopic infections.

Chemotherapy

In recent years the treatment of schistosome infections has become transformed by new drugs which are highly effective and relatively free from side-effects. Although alternative drugs are available there is increasing reliance on three compounds. The most recently introduced is praziquantel (Biltricide, Bayer) which is active against all species of schistosome. It is used in a single oral dose of 40 mg/kg to treat *S. haematobium*. This does may also be used to treat *S. mansoni* – though two doses of 30 mg/kg four hours apart may sometimes be needed to treat heavy infections. Three doses of 20 mg/kg four hours apart are advised for *S. japonicum* infection. The drug can lead to gastro-intestinal symptoms and other subjective side-effects but these are sufficiently mild and short-lived so as not to exclude the drug being used by paramedical personnel in mass campaigns. However, as with any chemotherapy, it is sensible to postpone treatment of children who are ill from other causes. Treatment should also be avoided during pregnancy.

S. mansoni may also be treated with oxamniquine (Vansil, Pfizer). The dose needed varies with the strain of parasite for in South America a single dose of 15 mg/kg may be adequate, while 60 mg/kg in divided doses over three days may be needed in Africa. Oxamniquine has been widely used in large-scale mass treatment programmes.

S. haematobium may also be treated with metrifonate (Bilarcil, Bayer). The drug is usually used in three fortnightly doses of 7.5 or 10 mg/kg, though in some areas the effect of a single dose has been considered adequate when there is continuing exposure to infection. Side-effects from the drug are mild and transient. The drug is an anticholinesterase and overdosage or simultaneous exposure to organophosphorous insecticides can lead to cholinergic side-effects which must be treated with atropine. However, the drug is sufficiently safe to have been used in several large-scale control programmes. Although the three-dose regimen may be difficult to secure compliance with, metrifonate has the advantage of currently costing less than the more recently introduced praziquantel – a fact of importance in many endemic areas.

Clinical management

The clinican's approach to schistosome infections will be influenced by the circumstances in which he/she practices. The clinician working in a non-endemic area should be able to use sensitive diagnostic techniques and to monitor the result of treatment with careful parasitological follow-up. Infection should be eradicated and ancillary investigations carried out to establish the extent of possible pathology and to follow its resolution. These can include appropriate radiological techniques, computer-assisted tomography, renography and ultrasound. Investigation of suspected infection may sometimes lead to serological evidence of exposure to infection in subjects without demonstrable ova. In the past, it has been considered inappropriate to treat such subjects but the increasing safety of the newer drugs suggests there may some justification for a more flexible approach.

The more usual situation in which schistosome infections are seen is in endemic rural areas where there are likely to be very different problems. Careful microscopy may show that the majority of children of school age in the area are infected but any children who are treated may continue to be exposed to infection. The speed of their reinfection after treatment is unpredictable and widely differing observations have been published. In general, reinfection is likely to be quicker and more intense in younger children under 10 years of age and possibly in those who were initially the most heavily infected. While some studies have shown that many participant children lost the benefit of treatment in less than a year, in other studies remarkably little reinfection took place over a two-year period. An additional factor which often must be considered in clinical practice in rural areas is the effect of economic constraints on drug supplies. In these circumstances some system of priorities is called for and attention may be concentrated on treating the most heavily infected and symptomatic children in the hope of preventing the worst long-term consequences of the disease.

It is increasingly apparent that successful treatment may be followed by the gradual resolution of much of the pathology attributable to schistosome infections. Liver enlargement can resolve and radiological abnormalities of the renal tract may improve. Haematuria and proteinuria usually resolve in a few weeks. Failure to improve after successful treatment may be an indication for re-investigation for it may be that additional pathology is present – persisting proteinuria, for example, perhaps indicating the presence of non-schistosomal renal pathology. However, reinfection is likely to be associated with the progression of the original pathology.

The advanced pathology of schistosome infections is sometimes an indication for surgery as in the reconstruction of the renal tract in severe obstructive uropathy with functional impairment. However, in children, considerable improvement is likely to follow successful chemotherapy and a conservative approach is usually appropriate. Detailed urological investigation and the demonstration of persisting obstruction, as distinct from dilatation of the ureter, and impaired function is needed before there is any consideration of surgery.

Control

With the advent of drugs that are suitable for mass administration the control of schistosomiasis has become a more practical proposition than was once the case. The aims of control programmes are also changing and a reduction in the prevalence and severity of pathology is seen as a realistic goal in circumstances where a major effect on the intensity of transmission may be unlikely. A variety of mass chemotherapy strategies have been advocated. These include treating all subjects found to be infected or only those with high egg counts, dispensing with individual examination and treating *everyone* in communities with a high prevalence or limiting treatment to schoolchildren. The choice will depend on the local epidemiological situation and the resources that are available.

Chemotherapy should be supplemented by health education. This should aim to reduce environmental contamination, improve excreta disposal and reduce water contact. Where resources are adequate, improvement in water supply can have a considerable effect on transmission. The local situation needs to be taken into account; for example it may prove to be important to provide facilities for clothes to be washed away from transmission sites. Today less emphasis is placed on snail control than before but molluscicides may have an important role in an integrated control programme reducing the intensity of transmission and reinfection rates after initial chemotherapy. The habitat in which transmission occurs also needs to be considered. Simple modifications may be worthwhile, including the clearing of weed and adjustment of water flow and depth in irrigation systems.

There is an increasing number of examples of successful large-scale control of schistosomiasis from countries as diverse as China, Egypt and Brazil. Many control programmes have been carried out by specialized organizations but today the trend is for control to be increasingly integrated with and dependent upon the existing health infrastructure. The decision to allocate a share of limited resources to schistosome control must be made in the context of the overall needs of the community, the existing pattern of health care, and the relative costs and benefits of schistosome control and alternative programmes. It should be realized that eradication of infection is an unrealistic goal in most areas and that major control schemes should not be introduced without a realistic prospect of adequate long-term financial support. Although the initial effects of mass chemotherapy and molluscicide application can be dramatic, the reproductive potential of the parasite and the snail may bring about a rapid return to the original state once control measures are stopped. It should also be realized that there are examples of considerable sums being spent on control schemes which careful assessment has subsequently shown to have limited effect. Any measures must be carefully evaluated in a pilot project before large-scale implementation.

The rural paediatrician may lack the resources to initiate a large-scale formal control programme, but much may be possible in small-scale local schemes in communities which actively participate in primary health care programmes. Health education should be possible and sanitation may be improved. If an adequate drug supply can be obtained, village health workers and schoolteachers should be able to help in screening and treatment of schoolchildren which may need to be repeated every year or two. Whilst there is no substitute for microscopy in the diagnosis of *S. mansoni*, urinalysis reagent strips, or even simple visual inspection for haematuria, may be suitable to select children for treatment in *S. haematobium* foci. It may be difficult to administer the correct dose of a drug if assistants have limited numeracy. One successful response to this problem has been a simple modification of bathroom scales to give a direct reading of 'pills of praziquantel' instead of weight. If scales are not available local height and weight standards may perhaps be used, so that the dose can be read directly from a height-measuring device as has been practised in Papua New Guinea for antimalarial therapy.[2] The community and the paediatrician must act on the realization that transmission of infection depends on man's actions and that disease due to schistosomiasis is preventable.

References

1. WHO. *Diagnostic Techniques in Schistosomiasis Control.* WHO/SCHISTO/83.69. Geneva, World Health Organization, 1983.
2. Moir JS, Jolley DJ. Determining drug doses by height – a simple method for village based health workers. *Journal of Tropical Paediatrics.* 1986; **32**: 162–7.

Further reading

Jordan P, Webbe G (eds) *Schistosomiasis.* London, Heinemann, 1982.
Mahmoud AF (ed.) Schistosomiasis. *Clinical Tropical Medicine and Communicable Diseases.* 1987; **2**: 2.
Rollinson D, Simpson A (eds) *The Biology of Schistosomes.* London, Academic Press, 1987.

Malaria

Tan Chongsuphajaisiddhi

Malaria is a serious disease of childhood and is one of the top five causes of child mortality in many countries, especially in tropical Africa. According to the statistical information reported to WHO, the overall world malaria situation has not improved in the last 15 years.

About 2772 million (56 per cent) of the world's 4950 million (1986) population live in countries or areas where malaria is still a health risk; 2310 million in areas where a reduced level of infection is maintained by continued application of antimalarial measures and 462 million in areas where no specific measures are taken to control malaria transmission. The number of clinical cases occurring on a global scale is very difficult to assess accurately, owing to under-detection and/or under-reporting of cases. On the other hand, in areas where malaria is diagnosed clinically without blood examination for the malaria parasites, the problem is over-reporting due to presumptive diagnosis of fever as malaria. According to estimates, the total incidence of malaria is of the order of 100 million cases annually.

The mortality due to malaria is virtually unknown in many parts of the world. Studies carried out in hyperendemic areas of Kenya and Northern Nigeria have indicated that between 6 and 8 per cent of infants die from malaria. On this basis, and assuming that approximately 3.5 per cent of the population exposed to moderate and high risk are infants, the malaria deaths in Africa south of the Sahara in the mid 1970s were estimated to be of the order of 750 000 annually. However, recent studies indicate large variability in infant mortality rates and fever/malaria mortality which in several areas are much lower than suspected. This may be attributed to the widespread use of antimalaria drugs.

Malaria is caused by four species of *Plasmodium*: *P. falciparum* (malignant tertian, subtertian or falciparum malaria), *P. vivax* (benign tertian or vivax malaria), *P. ovale* (ovale tertian or ovale malaria) and *P. malariae* (quartan or malariae malaria). The name tertian implies that fever recurs every third day and quartan every fourth day. Malaria is widely distributed throughout the tropics and subtropics and in some temperate areas (Fig. 4.12.1). Falciparum malaria is found most commonly in the tropical regions but also in some temperate areas. Vivax malaria is widespread in the tropics and subtropics, and in some temperate regions. Ovale malaria is uncommon, occurring in Africa predominantly in its western parts, and

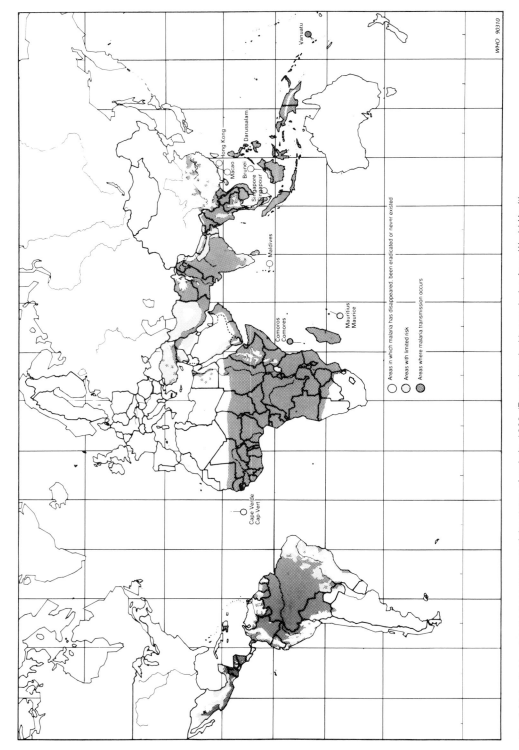

Fig. 4.12.1   Epidemiological assessment of the status of malaria, 1988. (Reproduced with permission from *World Health Statistics Quarterly*, WHO, 1990; **43(2)**: 68–79.)

sporadically in New Guinea, the Philippines and Indonesia. Malariae malaria occurs throughout the tropics, particularly in Africa, South America, India and the Far East.

Life-cycle

An infected female anopheline mosquito injects sporozoites into the hosts's tissue during a blood meal. Sporozoites disappear from the bloodstream within one hour and develop further in the liver parenchymal cell (pre-erythrocytic stage) into tissue schizonts containing thousands of merozoites. Development in liver cells requires about one week for *P. falciparum* and *P. vivax* and two weeks for *P. malariae*. In *P. vivax* and *P. ovale* infections, some sporozoites grow into trophozoites and remain dormant (hypnozoites) in liver cells for months to years before undergoing proliferation responsible for relapses of vivax and ovale malaria. At the end of this phase, merozoites are liberated into the bloodstream and invade erythrocytes, starting the erythrocytic phase. In the erythrocytes, the parasites grow from trophozoites into schizonts containing 6–24 merozoites, the number determined by the species of malaria. The merozoites liberated from the ruptured infected erythrocytes attach to other erythrocytes by specific receptors and start the erythrocytic cycle all over again. Some erythrocytic merozoites develop into sexual forms of the parasites (gametocytes) awaiting ingestion by the mosquito.

When the mature male and female gametocytes in the peripheral blood are ingested by the vector anopheline mosquito, they unite and a fertilized cell (ookinete) penetrates the stomach wall and develops beneath the lining membrane into an oocyst. Within the matured oocyst, thousands of sporozoites develop. After 7–20 days, depending on the external conditions, the cyst ruptures and sporozoites are released into the body cavity of the mosquito. Most of the sporozoites then migrate to the salivary glands and are injected into the new human host during the next blood meal of the mosquito.

Epidemiology

Malaria exists where effective anopheline vectors breed in nature and where human carriers of the sexual forms of the parasites are available to these mosquitoes. Man is the only source and reservoir of human malaria parasites.

There are certain genetic variables in the human response to malaria. It has been shown that sickle-cell trait (AS haemoglobin) reduces the level of *P. falciparum* parasitaemia and thus decreases the morbidity and mortality from malaria. However, this protection is not present in homozygous children (SS haemoglobin) with malaria who have high parasite rates and counts and the infection can be fatal. Because children with AS haemoglobin have a survival advantage in falciparum endemic areas over homozygous children (SS or AA haemoglobin), the frequency of genes for S and A haemoglobin reaches a fixed level called balanced polymorphism. Although the high frequencies of thalassaemia, HbE and HbC in malarious areas of the world suggest a selective advantage to malaria by possession of the genes, there is no direct evidence yet. In Thailand, HbE and thalassaemia have been found to confer no advantage in respect of parasite rate, parasite density or mortality of falciparum malaria in children.

The association between the distribution of G6PD deficiency and falciparum malaria suggests that this enzyme deficiency may offer protection against malaria. Studies of the parasite counts in groups of normal and enzyme-deficient children gave contradictory results. Resistance to malaria may require another factor such as the interaction of favism and G6PD deficiency, since oxidant stress reduces the survival of parasites in culture in G6PD-deficient red cells. Drug-induced intravascular haemolysis with haemoglobinuria may occur in G6PD-deficient children with malaria. The degrees of haemolysis differ among those with different variants of G6PD deficiency.

Most black Africans are refractory to *P. vivax* infection. The vivax-resistant factor is a blood-group determinant, the Duffy-negative genotype, $FyFy$. Other populations who are susceptible to *P. vivax* infection are either Fy^a or Fy^b. A Duffy blood-group determinant is probably involved in attachment between vivax merozoites and red cells.

In highly endemic areas, falciparum malaria infection of indigenous children during the first five years of life causes severe and potentially fatal illness. Infection in the early months of life is usually mild with a low grade of parasitaemia, probably because of passive immunity acquired from immune mothers. The parasite rate increases with age and the mortality rate is hyperendemic areas is highest during the first two years of life. By school age, a considerable degree of immunity has been developed and asymptomatic parasitaemia can be as high as 75 per cent in primary school children. In areas of low endemicity, however, where the immunity in the indigenous population is low, severe infections occur in all age groups including adults.

Malnutrition does not appear to increase susceptibility to malaria. On the other hand, it has been shown that well-nourished children are more likely to develop severe disease than those who are malnourished. In Nigeria, it was found that convulsions and cerebral malaria were more common in well-nourished children than in children with marasmus or kwashiorkor. One of the factors concerned may be that well-nourished children have not been exposed to malaria as frequently and therefore not developed the same degree of immunity as the malnourished children. The other possible factor may be that well-nourished children with higher haematocrit and plasma protein levels are more vulnerable to stagnant anoxaemia in falciparum malaria.

Bionomics of the mosquito vector are the primary determinants of malarial epidemiology. Mosquito density, man-biting habit and longevity are three important characteristics of the anopheline mosquito. Malaria transmission is proportional to mosquito density (in relation to human population). The man-biting frequency and choice of human or animal host are relevant to malaria transmission. The mosquito with longer life (longer than the extrinsic cycle of the parasite) is more effective as a malaria vector.

Malaria endemic areas may be classified into stable and unstable. In stable malaria, the malaria transmission is intense and occurs throughout the year with little seasonal or yearly variations. Adult populations establish high immunity and the disease affects mainly young children. In unstable malaria, the transmission is seasonal with wide yearly variations with a tendency for the occurrence of malaria epidemics. The disease affects all age groups.

Pathogenesis

The symptoms and pathology are caused by the asexual erythrocytic stage of the malaria parasite. Fever and the associated symptoms of muscular pain, headache, nausea and vomiting occur when mature schizont-infected red blood cells rupture, releasing merozoites invasive to other red cells. It is presumed that endogenous pyrogens (probably interleukin-1) and other toxins are released from the ruptured schizont, but none has been identified yet.

Haemolysis of infected red cells both intravascular and extravascular (in the reticuloendothelial system) causes anaemia. Stimulation of the reticuloendothelial system (lympho-macrophage system) is shown by the enlargement of the spleen and liver.

In *P. falciparum* infection, reduced blood flow to the tissues is an important factor in the pathogenesis of clinical manifestations of severe infection (e.g. cerebral malaria, renal failure). Obstruction of microcirculation by growing trophozoite- and schizont-infected red cells may be related to reduced deformability of the red cells and to 'knob'-like protrusions from the red cell surfaces and their tendency to adhere selectively to vascular endothelium of certain internal organs. Increased vascular permeability, vasoconstriction due to hyperactivity of the sympathetic nervous system, high blood viscosity and intravascular coagulation may also be contributing factors in the development of tissue anoxia in severe falciparum malaria.

Pathology

The pathology of severe falciparum malaria consists of mainly circulatory changes. The small blood vessels of internal organs, especially brain, are congested with parasitized red blood cells. Oedema and petechial haemorrhages are often present in the brain at autopsy, probably the result of agonal cerebral anoxia. The liver is congested and enlarged with hypertrophied Kupffer cells containing malarial pigment. The spleen is enlarged and congested, with a large number of phagocytic cells containing erythrocytes and malarial pigment. In most patients dying of falciparum malaria, the lungs are oedematous and pulmonary capillaries are packed with parasitized red blood cells and white blood cells. In patients dying with acute renal failure, acute tubular necrosis is the main abnormality with numerous parasitized red blood cells in glomerular capillaries. In the intestine, the mucosa is congested and capillaries of the lamina propria are filled with parasitized red blood cells. In the placenta, intervillous spaces contain a large number of parasitized red blood cells and monocytes containing malarial pigment associated with focal syncytial necrosis, loss of syncytial microvilli and proliferation of cytotrophoblastic cells.

Acquired immunity

Immunity is gradually acquired after repeated malaria infection in endemic areas (but see also p. 845). The first evidence of immunity is a reduction of clinical symptoms and signs for a given level of parasitaemia. Subsequently the density of parasitaemia falls, gametocytes preceding asexual erythrocytic parasites. The low-level asymptomatic parasitaemia is associated with resistance to superinfection (premunition). The acquired immunity is associated with high levels of all components of immunoglobulins, IgG, IgM and IgA. Acquired immunity to malaria is very complex, affecting various stages of the malaria parasites namely, sporozoites, pre-erythrocytic stages in the liver, the erythrocytic stages of both asexual and sexual forms, and involving both humoral and cellular immune responses.

For sporozoites, antibody to circumsporozoite protein can interfere with invasion of sporozoites into liver cells. For the asexual erythrocytic stage, protective antibody may have its effect by inhibiting merozoite reinvasion, or promoting merozoite phagocytosis, or may involve opsonization of infected red blood cells. The process is primarily T-cell dependent but antibody mediated. Antigametocyte antibody can interfere with the development of sporogony in the mosquito vectors.

Malaria in pregnancy

Malaria is a major cause of abortion, stillbirth, premature delivery, low birth weight and maternal death in tropical countries (see p. 209). In areas of unstable malaria, malaria mortality rate in pregnant women is higher than that in non-pregnant women. In hyperendemic areas both clinical symptoms and parasitaemia are worse in primiparous women than in multiparous women. Placental malaria is also more frequent in primiparae than in multiparae. Birth weights of the neonates born to women with malaria are lower than controls and the differences are highest among the first-born infants and diminish progressively with increase in maternal parity.

Severe anaemia and hypoglycaemia are important complications of malaria in pregnancy. Pulmonary oedema precipitated by fluid overload or by the sudden increase in peripheral resistance, or autotransfusion of blood from the placenta, may occur just after the delivery.

Congenital malaria

Intrauterine transmission from mother to fetus can occur but the mechanism of the transplacental passage of the parasites is not fully understood. Although malaria parasites concentrate in the maternal blood spaces of the placenta, the incidence of congenital malaria is very low. Malaria parasites have been reported to be present in liver and spleen of some rare cases of stillbirths. The rarity of congenital malaria does not appear to result from the failure of parasitized erythrocyte crossing to the fetal circulation, for transmission of maternal erythrocytes across the placenta is known to occur during normal pregnancy. The incidence of parasitaemia in the newborn varies, depending on whether the cord blood or peripheral blood is examined. Examination of cord blood gives a higher incidence of parasitaemia than does peripheral blood examination. The mechanism underlying relative resistance to malaria at birth and in early life is not fully understood. The retarded growth of parasites in red blood cells containing HbF might be of advantage to newborn infants. The age of erythrocytes is suggested as another potential malariostatic factor, since old red cells containing HbF do not support growth of *P. falciparum*. The progressive ageing of red cell populations containing HbF which occurs in early post natal life may thus confer some protection against *P. falciparum* malaria.

Congenital malaria can be caused by any of the four plasmodial species which infect man. The incidence depends on the relative frequency of the different species in the area. The onset of clinical illness with detectable parasitaemia in peripheral blood may be up to two months after birth and is usually more delayed in cases of vivax or malariae than in falciparum malaria.

In endemic areas where mosquito transmission cannot be excluded, congenital malaria is diagnosed only when the parasites have been identified in the newborn within seven days of birth. If the parasites are detected during 7–28 days after birth, it is called 'neonatal malaria', implying that infection by mosquito bite cannot be ruled out. In malaria endemic areas, neonatal malaria should be included in the differential diagnosis of every case of neonatal sepsis or any acute febrile illness.

Clinical courses

Vivax and ovale malaria

Ovale malaria is clinically milder than vivax, otherwise the symptoms are similar. The incubation period is 10–20 days in vivax and 11–16 days in ovale malaria. The incubation period in some strains of *P. vivax*, especially those from temperate regions, may be prolonged up to 8–14 months. Vivax and ovale malaria often begin with the prodromal symptoms. The child may appear restless or drowsy and refuse food, while an older child may complain of headache and nausea.

Fever in the first few days is irregular remittent, going on to quotidian (daily) and then tertian intermittent (alternate day), but the clear-cut febrile paroxysms of a cold stage and a definite rigor are uncommon in infants and children. During the febrile period, the child usually feels cold and may have short episodes of shivering. The fever occurs more commonly by day than at night and usually develops in the afternoon. Convulsions are not uncommon in association with high fever in children aged six months to five years.

A classical febrile paroxysm consists of three stages: cold stage (rigor and chill), hot stage (high fever) and sweating stage. The cold stage begins with a chilly feeling followed by shiver and rigor with a rise in temperature. The patient may have headache, nausea and vomiting. This stage lasts from 15 minutes to one hour. The hot stage succeeds the cold when the rigor ceases and the patient feels hot with warm and dry skin. The hot stage lasts longer than the cold, usually two hours or more. The sweating stage begins when the temperature falls. Sweating appears first at the temples and rapidly becomes generalized and copious. The temperature falls to normal or subnormal in an hour or so. The patient feels relieved but very fatigued.

The liver usually enlarges and becomes palpable by the end of the first week. The spleen invariably increases in size during the attack and is usually palpable in the second week.

Anaemia is less pronounced in vivax and ovale than in falciparum malaria.

Parasitaemia is rarely heavy and usually less than two per cent of erythrocytes are infected. All stages of the asexual erythrocyte cycle occur in the peripheral blood at some time during the attack. Gametocytes usually appear after a week of the clinical course. The serum total bilirubin may be slightly increased but clinical jaundice is uncommon.

Relapses occur in untreated cases in which the attack spontaneously subsides and also in cases treated with blood schizontocides only. The relapse occurs after a period of clinical quiescence for some weeks or months. The relapse usually begins with fever characterized by the periodicity of the primary attack. The relapse is usually less severe and of shorter duration.

Malariae malaria

The incubation period of malariae malaria is usually longer than that of vivax malaria. It may be as long as 30–40 days and in some cases several months. The clinical picture is basically similar to that of vivax malaria except for quartan periodicity of the fever. The periodic fevers are more regularly spaced and the paroxysms are more definite. Usually less than one per cent of red blood cells are infected. All stages of the asexual parasites are usually present at any one time.

Gametocytes appear after a few weeks of the onset of the clinical attack.

Quartan malaria nephrotic syndrome

Nephrotic syndrome has been particularly reported in Guyana, East and West Africa, where malariae malaria is relatively common (see p. 797). A causal relationship between nephrotic syndrome in children and malariae malaria has been demonstrated. Malariae infection may cause nephrosis owing to granular immune complexes deposited in the renal glomeruli. The antibody in the complexes is specific for *P. malariae*. Histological changes consist of capillary wall thickening and segmental glomerular sclerosis leading to progressive glomerular damage and secondary tubular atrophy. Immunofluorescence microscopy shows globulin deposits in the basement membrane in granular, mixed or diffuse patterns.

Peak incidence is at age 4–5 years. The children present with severe generalized oedema, persistent heavy proteinuria and severe hypoproteinaemia, and most show ascites, usually without azotaemia or hypertension.

Cases with mild histological changes and a granular pattern of fluorescence are more frequently associated with response to treatment with corticosteriods or other immunosuppressants than with a mixed pattern, while a diffuse pattern is invariably associated with poor response to treatment. In cases with more severe histological changes, response to treatment is uniformly poor irrespective of fluorescence patterns. Symptomatic and supportive treatment consists of diuretics and high protein diet. A five-year study of 115 children with quartan malaria nephrotic syndrome in Uganda showed a complete remission rate of 26 per cent and an overall mortality rate of 24 per cent.

Falciparum malaria

The incubation period for falciparum malaria varies from 8 to 15 days. The child at first becomes lethargic, drowsy or irritable. He/she may refuse food and if old enough may complain of headache and nausea. Fever is usually (but not invariably) present. Where it occurs it tends to be irregular at first and in most cases remains irregularly remittent or intermittent and periodic paroxysms do not develop. Anorexia, nausea and vomiting are common. Abdominal pain and diarrhoea may occur but are not common.

Liver enlargement is a common finding in children with falciparum malaria. In an acute primary attack, liver enlargement is usually detected earlier (by the end of the first week) and more frequently than spleen enlargement. The enlarged liver is usually soft and tender and continues to enlarge as the disease progresses.

The spleen enlarges and is often palpable in the second week and enlargement progresses as the disease continues. In children who have had many attacks, the spleen may be very large and firm in consistency.

Anaemia is an important consequence of falciparum malaria in children. In acute infections, the severity of anaemia appears to be related to the degree of parasitaemia. In certain malaria endemic areas, most of the children are already affected by anaemia from other causes such as hookworm infection and malnutrition. When these children are infected with falciparum malaria, anaemia progresses rapidly and they may become severely anaemic. Children with severe anaemia (Hb less than 5 g/dl) present with tachycardia and dyspnoea or frank congestive heart failure.

In the peripheral blood, the ring form of the parasite is dominant and the more mature stages are rarely seen, except in very heavy infections and severely ill children. As the infection progresses the parasite density increases stepwise until 15–20 per cent or more of the erythrocytes are infected. Gametocytes usually appear in the peripheral blood after the second week of the disease, increase in number for a fortnight or so and then subside.

Liver function in children with falciparum malaria is less commonly disturbed than in adults. Jaundice has been observed in some children but this is mainly attributable to haemolysis, and transaminases increase slightly and transiently.

Severe manifestations of falciparum malaria

Cerebral malaria   Convulsions are common in children aged six months to five years who have high fever and it is difficult to differentiate clinically convulsions caused by malaria from those caused by other febrile illnesses. Cerebral malaria should be diagnosed if coma persists more than half an hour after convulsions in a child with falciparum malaria. In West Africa, it has been noted that convulsions are less commonly associated with malaria in malnourished children than in well-nourished ones; the frequency of convulsions increase as the parasites density rises. In cerebral malaria, the child becomes increasingly drowsy, passing into a light coma which soon deepens. The common neurological signs are those of symmetrical upper motor neurone and brainstem disturbances including dysconjugate

gaze and decerebrate and decorticate postures. Neck rigidity does not occur but mild neck stiffness is not uncommon. There are no signs of increased intracranial pressure. Retinal haemorrhages and exudate have been observed in some children with cerebral malaria. Examination of the cerebrospinal fluid usually reveals normal findings but in some cases there is a slight increase in initial pressure, leucocyte count (mostly lymphocytes up to 50 cells/dl) and protein (rarely exceeding 150 mg/dl). A rising level of lactate in the CSF (>2.5 mmol/l; normal 1.1–2.2 mmol/l) has been found to indicate a poor prognosis in cerebral malaria.

Children with cerebral malaria may show some other severe manifestations or complication of the disease (Fig. 4.12.2).

Renal dysfunction   Renal failure is relatively unusual in infants and small children. Initial oliguria is uncommon but may occur in older children. However, a slight increase in blood urea nitrogen sometimes occurs, usually due to dehydration, and returns to normal with rehydration.

Slight proteinuria (trace or one plus) is not uncommon in children with falciparum malaria. Mild and transient acute glomerulonephritis may occur but is rare.

Bleeding tendencies and spontaneous bleedings   Bleeding tendencies with prolonged coagulation time, thrombocytopaenia and decreased coagulation factors may occur in some children with severe falciparum malaria. Spontaneous haemorrhage from the gastro-intestinal tract has been observed in children with cerebral malaria.

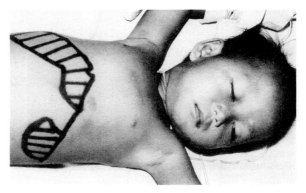

Fig. 4.12.2   Cerebral malaria with hepatosplenomegaly, severe anaemia and jaundice.

Pulmonary oedema Acute pulmonary oedema may occur in infants and children with cerebral malaria, severe anaemia or with high parasitaemia. In some cases, pulmonary oedema is due to fluid overload. Others develop pulmonary oedema with normal or negative fluid balance. Increase in respiration rate is an important early-warning sign, usually preceding the development of rhonchi and crepitations in the lungs. Acute pulmonary oedema may cause confusion with bronchopneumonia.

Haemoglobinuria Massive intravascular haemolysis with haemoglobinuria is a rare complication in children with malaria. Most, but not all, cases of haemoglobinuria in malaria are associated with G6PD deficiency and the administration of antimalarial drugs, especially primaquine. The degree of haemolysis differs among those with different variants of G6PD deficiency. Haemolysis is usually self-limiting in cases with African type in which the deficiency is only manifested in the older erythrocytes. Haemolysis can be severe and life-threatening in cases with the Mediterranean type in which the deficiency involves the entire erythrocyte population. In Thai children with the Mahidol variant of G6PD deficiency, haemolysis is self-limiting (Fig. 4.12.3).

Hypoglycaemia Severe hypoglycaemia may occur in children with severe falciparum malaria but the incidence may be lower than in adults. It results from hyperinsulinaemia induced by malaria and quinine, impaired liver function and lactic acidosis. Hypoglycaemia may present with convulsions, impaired or deteriorating consciousness, or with milder symptoms such as sweating and irregular breathing.

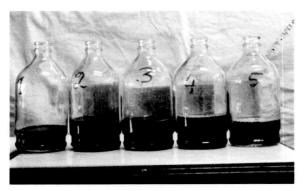

Fig. 4.12.3 Haemoglobinuria in a six-year-old boy with G6PD deficiency and falciparum malaria after antimalarial treatment. The fifth eight-hour urine collection was less dark.

Hypotension (Algid malaria) Severe hypotension occasionally occurs in patients with pulmonary oedema, metabolic acidosis, Gram-negative bacteraemias and massive gastro-intestinal haemorrhage. It is usually attributable to vasodilation and relative hypovolaemia.

Diagnosis

A definite diagnosis of malaria is made by the identification of the parasite in the blood. The presence of the asexual form must be established. The discovery of the gametocytes of *P. falciparum* only is not sufficient to confirm the diagnosis of active malaria, since they may be found in the peripheral blood for weeks after the overt attack has subsided or been cured.

In endemic areas, malaria must be suspected in all children with fever. In infants and young children, the clinical picture of malaria is less characteristic than in adults. The early symptoms of malaria are vague and can simulate other conditions. Failure to find parasites in one blood examination cannot exclude malaria, for which at least three samples, taken at 6–12 hour intervals, must be examined. However, the delay in diagnosis and treatment of falciparum malaria increases the risk of the patient. Tentative antimalarial treatment for suspected falciparum infection may be necessary in cases with negative blood examinations or in areas where facilities for blood examination are not available. Failure to control the fever within three days after administration of adequate doses of an effective antimalarial tends to exclude malaria as the cause of the disease.

Clinical judgement is needed in the diagnosis of malaria. The detection of the parasites in a blood film does not prove that the patient is suffering from malaria because parasitaemia may be entirely asymptomatic in semi-immune indigenous children. On the other hand, the chance of detecting malaria parasites in the blood is reduced in the patient who has been taking suppressive chemoprophylaxis or has been given antimalarial drugs several hours before the blood examination.

Species identification of the malaria parasite is needed in the diagnosis of malaria, since management is related to the parasite species. Tissue schizontocide (primaquine) is required for the radical treatment of vivax and ovale malaria. In areas with chloroquine-resistant *P. falciparum*, other appropriate effective antimalarials must be given in the treatment of falciparum malaria (see later).

Blood films

For diagnosis of the presence of parasites the examination of a thick blood film is sufficient. The species of the parasites can usually be identified in the thick blood film but should be confirmed by examination of a thin film which shows the undistorted parasites within the red cells. The thick blood film, in which red cells are piled upon each other, and lysed and stained at the same time, allows more red cells to be examined at a time, but the parasites liberated from the lysed red cells are distorted (see p. 979).

For the thick film, a large drop of fresh blood on a cleaned slide is spread evenly with a corner of another slide to form a round smear about 2 cm in diameter. The film is allowed to dry thoroughly before staining with Field's stain or Giemsa stain. The thin blood film is prepared in the ordinary way and stained with Wright's stain or Giemsa stain.

Once malaria parasites are identified on the blood film, it is necessary to determine whether the patient has *P. falciparum* infection, especially in an area with a chloroquine-resistant strain. All other malarial species are initially treated with chloroquine. Criteria suggestive of *P. falciparum* include prominent non-pigmented ring forms, double chromatin, multiple infection, applique form, and the diagnostic crescent-shaped gametocytes. The infected red cells are not enlarged and without pink stippling (Schuffner dots). Pigmented trophozoites and schizonts are seen only in heavy infection.

The detailed diagnostic character of human malaria parasites in both thick and thin blood films will be found in textbooks of parasitology and in handbooks mentioned elsewhere.

In falciparum malaria, parasites should be counted in relation to erythrocytes (on thin blood films) or to the white cell count (on thick films). There is a strong correlation between the level of parasitaemia and severity. The mortality is approximately one per cent with parasitaemia below $100\,000/\mu l$ increasing to more than 50 per cent where counts exceed $500\,000/\mu l$. The level of parasitaemia is also used in the clinical grading of drug resistance (S, RI, RII and RIII).

Immunological and other diagnostic techniques

Serological techniques for detecting malarial antibodies have been used in epidemiological surveys and for screening potential blood donors. The methods widely used are the immunofluorescent assay (IFA) and enzyme-linked immunosorbent assay (ELISA).

Detection of malaria parasites by radio-immunological (RIA) techniques or by DNA probes are being developed in many laboratories. One RIA can detect 0.0001 per cent parasitaemia and one DNA probe can detect as little as 0.01 ng of parasite DNA. These techniques would be very useful in processing large numbers of blood samples in screening blood donors or in malaria survey or surveillance.

Treatment

Treatment of malaria is aimed at control or eradication of the parasite, dealing with clinical manifestations and in endemic areas rendering the patient non-infective to mosquitoes.

Clinical effects of malaria result from the presence of the asexual parasite in the erythrocyte. Control of the attack is achieved by eliminating these parasites from the blood. Drugs which destroy the asexual erythrocytic forms are called *schizontocides* (blood schizontocides). Relapses of vivax and ovale malaria can be controlled by giving *tissue schizontocides* to eliminate the dormant parasites in the liver. *Gametocytocidal drugs* (gametocytocides) destroy the sexual erythrocytic forms while *sporontocidal drugs* inhibit the development of the parasite in the mosquitoes.

Available antimalarial drugs

There are eight groups of antimalarial drugs in current use:

- Cinchona alkaloids (quinine, quinidine, cinchonine)
- 4-Amino-quinolines (chloroquine, amodiaquine)
- 8-Amino-quinolines (primaquine, pamaquine)
- Biguanides (proguanil, chlorproguanil)
- Diaminopyrimidines (pyrimethamine)
- Sulphonamides and sulphones
- Antibiotics (tetracycline, erythromycin)
- Quinoline methanol (mefloquine)

The action of antimalarial drugs on different phases of the development of the malaria parasite is shown in Table 4.12.1

Quinine is the most important compound of cinchona alkaloids. Quinine has a fast action on the asexual erythrocytic stages of all species. Quinine is mainly used for the treatment of very severe infection or chloroquine-resistant falciparum malaria.

Quinidine alone and *cinchonine* in combination with

Table 4.12.1. Action of antimalarial drugs

| Drug | Sporozoites | Tissue phase | Erythrocytic phase | | Development of gametocytes in mosquito |
			Asexual forms	Sexual forms (gametocytes)	
Chloroquine Quinine Mefloquine	No action	No action	Fast action	Active against *P. vivax, P. ovale, P. malariae*; no action on *P. falciparum*	No action
Proguanil Pyrimethamine	No action	Active mainly against *P. falciparum*	Slow action	No action	Active
Sulphonamides Sulphone	No action	No action	Moderate action when given alone but active in association with pyrimethamine	No action	No significant action
Primaquine	No action	Active against *P. falciparum* and *P. vivax*	Active only in toxic dose	Fast action in all species	Active
Tetracycline	Unknown	Active against *P. falciparum*, other species unknown	Active but relatively slow against *P. falciparum*, other species unknown	No action against *P. falciparum*, other species unknown	Unknown

quinine and quinidine have been shown recently to be more effective than quinine alone in the treatment of multidrug-resistant falciparum malaria in Thailand.

Chloroquine is a very active antimalarial with low toxicity. It is the drug of choice in the treatment of chloroquine-sensitive falciparum malaria and all other species but will not prevent relapses of vivax and ovale malaria.

Amodiaquine is slightly more effective than chloroquine against falciparum malaria with low resistance to chloroquine. However, the use of amodiaquine is not encouraged after the reports of agranulocytosis related to the drug (see later).

Primaquine is used for radical cure of vivax and ovale malaria and for destroying gametocytes of *P. falciparum*.

Proguanil and *chlorproguanil* are used for prophylaxis.

Pyrimethamine is used alone for prophylaxis and in combination with *sulphonamides* or *sulphones* for treatment of chloroquine-resistant falciparum malaria. The combination has potentiating effect against asexual blood forms of *P. falciparum*.

Tetracycline is used as an adjunct to quinine for the treatment of chloroquine and quinine-resistant falciparum malaria. Its slow action precludes its use alone in treatment of malaria. *Erythromycin* may be used as an alternative to tetracycline in children less than seven years old to avoid the staining of teeth with tetracycline.

Mefloquine is very effective in the treatment of chloroquine and quinine-resistant falciparum malaria. Mefloquine has been combined with sulfadoxine and pyrimethamine with an aim to delay the development of resistance of *P. falciparum* to the drug. However, this combination has the disadvantage of adding the side-effects of sulphadoxine and pyrimethamine.

New antimalarial drugs

Qinghausu (artemisinine) is a sesquiterpene lactone peroxide extracted from the herb *Artemisia annua*, which has been used for the treatment of malaria in China for over a 1000 years. Qinghausu and two of its derivatives, artemether and artesunate, have been shown to have high efficacy against chloroquine and multidrug-resistant *P. falciparum*. It has only just become available for testing outside China.

Halofantrine, a phenanthrenemethanol, is another recently developed, synthetic antimalarial drug effective against chloroquine-resistant *P. falciparum*.

Drug resistance

Resistance of *P. falciparum* to chloroquine was first reported from South America and South-east Asia in the early 1960s. The resistance has now spread to more than 50 countries in Asia, Central and South America and Africa (Table 4.12.2 and Fig. 4.12.4). In certain areas, the parasite has also developed resistance against the combination of sulphadoxine and pyrimethamine (Fansidar), quinine or mefloquine.

Drug resistance in malaria has been defined as the 'ability of a parasite strain to survive and/or multiply despite the administration and absorption of a drug given in doses equal to or higher than those usually recommended but within the limits of tolerance of the subject'. Grading of resistance of asexual parasites of *P. falciparum* to normally recommended doses of chloroquine has been proposed *in vivo* with 28 days observation (D_{28}) after the first day of treatment (D_0) (Table 4.12.3). It may be applicable also to other blood schizontocides. Evidence of RIII observed at 48 hours after the treament has begun indicates the alternate treatment with a more effective drug.

Treatment of a simple attack

Antimalarials are usually given orally. Parenteral administration should be used only in severe cases of falciparum malaria and should be replaced by the oral route as soon as possible. Some antimalarials such as chloroquine and quinine are bitter in taste. In small children such antimalarial tablets should be given orally on a spoon after being crushed and mixed with syrup or sweetened condensed milk. In children with high fever, oral administration of antimalarial should be done after reducing the fever by tepid sponging or other effective measures to avoid vomiting.

The dosage of antimalarials should be calculated from an adult dose, adjusted to the body surface area. However, for parenteral administration of drugs, dosage should be calculated according to body weight as in Table 4.12.4.

Quinoline antimalarial drugs (chloroquine, amodiaquine, quinine, quinidine, mefloquine and primaquine) should be prescribed as amounts of base. Conversions of salt and anhydrous base are given in Table 4.12.5

Vivax, ovale and malariae malaria

Acute attacks of vivax, ovale and malariae malaria should be treated with chloroquine. The dosage of drug is adjusted to the body surface from an adult dose of 1500 mg base (25 mg base/kg) given over three days as follows:

Days of treatment	Chloroquine base
Day 1	300 mg 3 times
Day 2	300 mg
Day 3	300 mg

To reduce side-effects, especially for weak and malnourished children, the dose proportional to an adult dose of 300 mg base (6 mg base/kg) may be given three times in the first day.

To prevent relapses of *P. vivax* and *P. ovale* infection, after completion of chloroquine treatment, a 14-day course of primaquine proportional to the adult dose of 15 mg base (0.3 mg base/kg) per day is given. Some strains of *P. vivax* in the South-west Pacific and South-

Table 4.12.2. Countries where *P. falciparum* malaria resistant to chloroquine has been detected

Africa	Tanzania	Uganda	Angola
	Madagascar	Kenya	South Africa
	Zaire	Gabon	Congo
	Burundi	Malawi	Senegal
	Namibia	Zambia	Cameroons
	Mozambique	Sudan	Rwanda
	Burkina Faso	Comoros	Zimbabwe
	Benin	Ghana	Ethiopia
	Equ.-Guinea		
Americas	Bolivia	Surinam	Guyana
	Colombia	Brazil	Peru
	French Guiana	Ecuador	Venezuela
	Panama		
Asia	Bangladesh	Vanuatu	Papua New Guinea
	India	Sri Lanka	Solomon Islands
	Thailand	Burma	Vietnam
	Kampuchea	People's Republic of China	Nepal
	Malaysia	Laos	Bhutan
	Philippines		
Eastern Mediterranean	Pakistan	Iran	

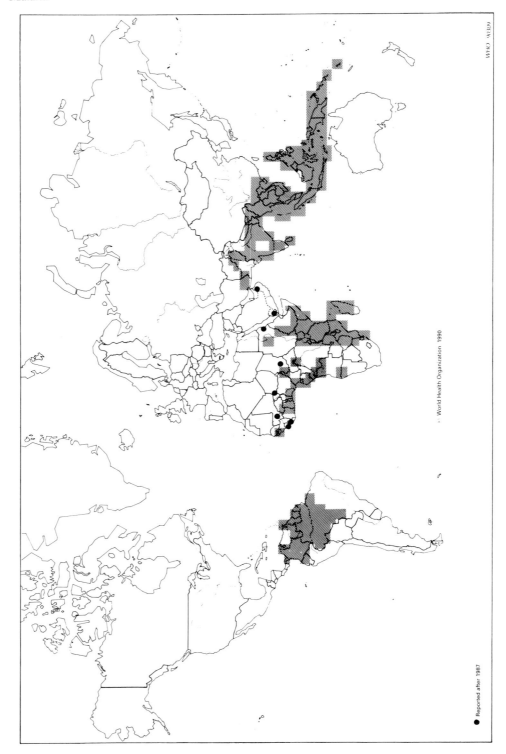

WHO 90/8191

● World Health Organization 1990

● Reported after 1987

Fig. 4.12.4　Areas where chloroquine-resistant *Plasmodium falciparum* has been reported. (Reproduced with permission from the WHO from World malaria situation, 1988. *World Health Statistics Quarterly*, 1990; **43(2)**: 68–79.)

Table 4.12.3. Grading of resistance of asexual parasites (*P. falciparum*) to schizontocidal drugs (4-amino quinoline)

Response	Recommended symbol	Evidence
Sensitivity	S	Asexual parasites disappear by D$_6$, no recrudescence by D$_{28}$
Resistance	RI	Asexual parasites disappear by D$_6$ but reappear by D$_{28}$
	RII	Asexual parasitaemia is reduced to 25 per cent or less of original level during the first 48 hours of treatment, but no clearance
	RIII	Asexual parasitaemia is reduced by less than 75 per cent during the first 48 hours of treatment or it continues to rise.

Table 4.12.4. Calculation of dosages of antimalarial drugs for children

Approx. age	Approx. weight (kg)	Fraction of adult dose
2 weeks	3.2	1/8
4 months	6.5	1/5
1 year	10.0	1/4
3 years	15.0	1/3
7 years	23.0	1/2
12 years	40.0	3/4

For the first 2 weeks of life, the dosage is divided by half, i.e. 1/16 of adult dose.

Table 4.12.5. Salt and anhydrous base equivalents of common quinoline antimalarials

	Salt (mg)	Anhydrous base (mg)
Chloroquine sulphate	204	150
Chloroquine phosphate	242	150
Chloroquine dihydrochloride	246	200
Amodiaquine hydrochloride	261	200
Primaquine phosphate	26	15
Quinine sulphate	301	250
Quinine dihydrochloride	612	500

east Asia, require an adult dose of 22.5–30 mg base (0.45–0.6 mg base/kg) for 14 days or weekly dosage of 45 mg base (0.9 mg base/kg) primaquine and 600 mg base (12 mg base/kg) chloroquine over a period of eight weeks.

In cases with G6PD deficiency, primaquine may induce haemolysis of old red blood cells and the haemolysis is usually mild. In these cases, the weekly dose of 45 mg base primaquine and 600 mg base chloroquine has been shown to produce less haemolysis than the 14-day course of primaquine 15 mg base per day.

Vivax and ovale infection acquired congenitally or by blood transfusion can be radically treated with chloroquine alone, since there are no hepatic forms. In malariae malaria, there is no need to give primaquine since hepatic forms do not occur.

Falciparum malaria

Owing to the development of resistance of *P. falciparum* to various antimalarials in many areas of the world, chemotherapy of falciparum malaria should be given according to the status of drug resistance in the areas where the infection was contracted as follows:

- areas of chloroquine sensitivity;
- areas of chloroquine resistance;
- areas of chloroquine, sulphonamide/pyrimethamine resistance.

Areas of chloroquine sensitivity Chloroquine proportional to the adult dose of 1500 mg base of chloroquine should be given over three days, as in vivax and other infections.

Areas of chloroquine resistance Acute uncomplicated falciparum malaria should be treated with a single dose of combinations of long-acting sulphonamide and pyrimethamine proportional to an adult dose of:

- Sulphadoxine 1500 mg (30 mg/kg) and pyrimethamine 75 mg (2.5 mg/kg) (one Fansidar tablet contains 500 mg sulphadoxine and 25 mg pyrimethamine).
- Sulphalene 1500 mg (30 mg/kg) and pyrimethamine 75 mg (2.5 mg/kg) (one Metakelfin tablet contains 500 mg sulphalene and 25 mg pyrimethamine).

In areas where sulphadoxine or sulphalene are not available, sulphisoxazole or sulphadiazine proportional to the adult dose of 2.0 g (40 mg/kg) initially and then 0.5 g (10 mg/kg) six hourly for five days and pyrimethamine proportional to the adult dose of 25 mg (0.5 mg/kg) once daily for three days may be given. Amodiaquine is still in common use as a second-line drug to chloroquine in parts of Africa where the differential sensitivities of falciparum parasites to the two drugs seem to be sufficient. The danger of agranulocytosis following the drug as used in treatment has not yet appeared to contradict its use.

Areas of chloroquine, sulphonamide/pyrimethamine resistance In these areas, the following regimens may be given.

1. For children older than seven years, a 5–7 day course of quinine plus a seven-day course of tetracycline given concurrently. The drug dosages are adjusted proportional to the adult dose of 500 mg base quinine (10 mg base/kg) three times per day and 250 mg tetracycline (5 mg/kg) three or four times per day.

2. For children under seven years of age to whom tetracycline should not be given, an eight-day course of quinine should be prescribed. For the first four days, quinine is given proportional to the adult dose of 500 mg base (10 mg base/kg) three times per day and for the following four days quinine is given at a 50 per cent increased dose, proportional to the adult dose of 750 mg base (15 mg base/kg) three times per day. An alternative is a 5–7 day course of standard-dose quinine plus a seven day course of erythromycin 500 mg (10 mg/kg) three times per day given concurrently.

3. A single dose of mefloquine alone or in combination with sulphadoxine and pyrimethamine. The drugs are given proportional to adult doses of 750 mg base (15 mg base/kg) mefloquine, 1500 mg (30 mg/kg) sulphadoxine and 75 mg (1.5 mg/kg) pyrimethamine. One Fansimef tablet contains 250 mg base mefloquine, 500 mg sulphadoxine and 25 mg pyrimethamine.

Gametocytocidal drugs In areas under malaria eradication or control programmes where interruption of transmission has been achieved or is close to being achieved, primaquine proportional to the adult dose of 30 mg base (0.6 mg base/kg) should be given with the last dose of schizontocidal drug to destroy the gametocytes of *P. falciparum*.

Supportive treatment

Children in many malaria endemic areas may suffer from some degree of iron-deficiency anaemia with reduced mean corpuscular haemoglobin concentration, microcytosis and hypochromia in the peripheral blood. In such cases, iron supplements may promote a rapid recovery from severe anaemia after repeated malaria attacks.

Management of severe falciparum malaria

Delay in diagnosis and treatment is the most important factor leading to the development of severe falciparum

malaria. Parasitaemia over two per cent in young children is dangerous and parasitaemia over five per cent should always be treated as severe disease. Children with high parasitaemia or with cerebral malaria or with other severe manifestations should be managed as a medical emergency.

A brief initial physical examination should be carried out to detect dehydration, pulmonary oedema, hypoglycaemia, and other conditions which may require immediate treatment. A thorough examination should be performed after the treatment has begun. Fluid intake and output should be recorded hourly with monitoring of the vital signs.

Antimalarials

In severe falciparum malaria, the aims of chemotherapy are to achieve therapeutic concentrations of antimalarial in the plasma as quickly but as safely as possible, and to maintain these throughout the treatment. The first dose of antimalarials should be given by intravenous infusion and the same route should be used for subsequent doses in cases with cerebral malaria, other severe manifestations or severe vomiting or diarrhoea. Dosages of parenteral drugs should be calculated according to body weight. Oral administration of the drug should replace parenteral therapy as soon as possible.

Areas of chloroquine sensitivity Chloroquine should be given at a dose of 5 mg base/kg diluted with normal saline or five per cent dextrose (20–30 ml/kg infused intravenously over 2–4 hours). The dose may be repeated every 12 hours to attain the total dose of 25 mg base/kg. The rate of infusion must be carefully controlled. Blood pressure should be checked frequently and the infusion rate slowed if blood pressure falls.

In areas with facilities for intramuscular injection only, the child should be treated with intramuscular chloroquine (2.5 mg base/kg then one hour later another 2.5 mg base/kg). This should be repeated every 12 hours to attain the total dose of 25 mg base/kg.

Areas of chloroquine resistance Intravenous infusion of quinine is the treatment of choice. In certain areas of chloroquine-resistant falciparum malaria, the minimum inhibitory concentration (MIC) of quinine is high. In these areas, the first dose of quinine should be given as a loading dose (20 mg base/kg) in normal saline or five per cent dextrose solution, infused over four hours. If the child has taken quinine within the previous two days, the conventional dose (10 mg base/kg) should be given. Thereafter, this dose (10 mg base/kg) is infused every eight hours.

Some children with severe falciparum malaria have a protracted course, remaining seriously ill for many days. To avoid cumulative toxicity in such cases, the dose of quinine should be reduced by one third or one half after the third day until clinical conditions improve.

In areas with facilities for intramuscular injection only, quinine dihydrochloride should be given intramuscularly at a dose of 10 mg base/kg eight-hourly with strict aseptic technique.

Supplementary doses of tetracycline or erythromycin should be started when the clinical conditions improve and the patient can take the drug orally.

Cerebral malaria

Other causes of encephalopathy should be excluded by examining the cerebrospinal fluid in all comatose children. Convulsion must be brought under control with intravenous diazepam (0.5–1.0 mg/kg) or intramuscular paraldehyde (0.1 ml/kg in a glass syringe). Comatose children should be kept on their side or in a semiprone position and should be turned frequently, to reduce the incidence of aspiration and bedsores. When coma is prolonged, naso-gastric feeding should be instituted as soon as the acute conditions and, in particular, convulsions subside.

Children with cerebral malaria usually also suffer from severe anaemia. Correction of severe anaemia with fresh blood transfusion is an important aspect of the management of cerebral malaria.

Corticosteroids are contra-indicated in cerebral malaria. Dexamethasone prolongs coma and increases the incidence of complications including pneumonia and gastro-intestinal bleedings. The use of heparin, low-molecular-weight dextran and mannitol is not recommended.

Severe anaemia

In children with high parasitaemia, there is a continued fall in haemoglobin in the few days following effective antimalarial therapy. The haemoglobin should be kept over 4.4 mmol/l (above 7.1 g/l) by slow infusion of 5–10 ml per kg body weight packed red cells or 10–20 ml per kg whole blood. Fresh blood is preferable to stored blood. Children with severe anaemia may present with tachycardia and dyspnoea. In these cases, frusemide (1–2 mg per kg) may be given in addition to blood transfusion. The first dose of antimalarial should be given with a smaller volume of intravenous fluid (10 ml/kg) over four hours.

Renal failure

Older children with falciparum malaria may present with oliguria and dehydration. Urine examination usually reveals a high specific gravity, low urinary sodium and a normal urinary sediment indicating simple dehydration and hypovolaemia. To correct this, the first dose of quinine or chloroquine is diluted in normal saline solution (20 ml/kg body weight) and infused over two hours. In most cases, urine will begin to flow. If less than 4 ml/kg of urine is produced during the first eight hours after starting the intravenous fluid, then frusemide can be tried initially at 2 mg/kg then double at hourly intervals to a maximum of 8 mg/kg (given over 15 minutes). If there is still no output of urine, dopamine (2.5 to 5 μg/kg per minute) can be infused through a central venous catheter or a large free-flowing peripheral vein. The child who fails to produce more than 4 ml/kg body weight of urine at the end of 16 hours, should be placed on a strict fluid balance and transferred to the nearest hospital with dialysis facilities (see pp. 798–800).

Pulmonary oedema

To prevent or reduce the chance of developing pulmonary oedema in children with severe malaria, the patients should be propped up at 45° and their fluid intake strictly regulated according to central venous pressure or jugular venous pressure measurement and careful observation of fluid balance.

Early detection of pulmonary oedema is very important. Once pulmonary oedema has developed, the patient should be propped upright and given a high concentration of oxygen. Intravenous frusemide should be given initially but, if the diuretics fail, venesection (10 ml/kg) should be tried.

Hypoglycaemia

Intravenous injection of 50 per cent glucose (up to 1.0 ml/kg) should be given first and followed by intravenous infusion of 10 per cent glucose. Recurrent hypoglycaemia may occur during the intravenous infusion of 10 per cent glucose and should be treated with intravenous injection of 50 per cent glucose.

Bleeding tendencies and spontaneous bleeding

Bleeding tendency and spontaneous bleeding from the gastro-intestinal tract is usually improved after the transfusion of fresh whole blood. The use of heparin in these cases is not recommended.

Hyperparasitaemia

If the parasite count exceeds 10 per cent the prognosis is bad. Exchange transfusion should be considered in these children, especially those who show severe clinical manifestations.

Malaria in pregnancy

Malaria in pregnancy must be regarded seriously, especially in the last trimester and with *P. falciparum* infections. Both mother and fetus are vulnerable to the combined effects of the parasitaemia, toxaemia, fever, anaemia, placental infarction, hypoglycaemia and the effects of overdosage, particularly of quinine in chloroquine-resistant falciparum infection. Fortunately the use of chloroquine and quinine intravenously in therapeutic doses rarely appears to cause fetal damage or to induce abortion or premature labour.

In severe falciparum infections sensitive to chloroquine, the drug should be given in full adult dose 200–300 mg (base) in 4–5 per cent glucose saline intravenously up to three times in the first 24 hours and continued daily until oral therapy can commence. In less severe infections, intramuscular chloroquine in the same dosage has almost as rapid and effective an action.

In chloroquine-resistant infections, quinine should be given, if possible intravenously, in a dose of 10 mg (base)/kg to a maximum of 500 mg (base) in 10 ml/kg in 0.9 per cent sodium chloride (normal saline) to a maximum of 500 ml over four hours. This should be repeated every 8–12 hours until considerable improvement has occurred. Maternal temperature, blood pressure, uterine contractions and fetal heart rate need to be monitored frequently during the treatment regimen. Quinine is less satisfactorily given deeply intramuscularly in single doses of 16 mg/kg base (equivalent to 20 mg/kg quinine dihydrochloride) not exceeding 1000 mg in one dose and a total dosage of 2000 mg in 24 hours.

Blood glucose levels should be checked for hypoglycaemia which above all may be responsible for fetal loss. Intravenous glucose may be necessary, initially as a bolus and then as a continuous infusion of a 10 per cent solution to maintain normal blood glucose levels.

In severe anaemia, blood transfusion may be necessary as a life-saving measure. Caesarean section may be necessary to save the fetus from further hypoxia and to remove a large reservoir of parasitized cells sequestered in the placenta.

Prophylaxis and prevention of malaria

Mass prophylaxis for children under five years living in endemic areas is not recommended. This is considered to have four disadvantages; firstly it is not feasible to achieve continuous suppression on a wide scale, secondly it may interfere with the development of protective immunity, thirdly it may accelerate the development of drug resistance, and fourthly there is a risk of accumulative toxicity. However, in endemic areas, full prophylactic protection is indicated in pregnant women, especially primigravidae, throughout pregnancy.

Prophylaxis should be given to expatriate children living temporarily in endemic areas. The prophylaxis may be continuous or only seasonal, according to the patterns of malaria transmission in the areas.

Areas with chloroquine-sensitive *P. falciparum*

Chloroquine should be given proportional to the adult dose of 300 mg base weekly. The first dose should be repeated on the second day of prophylaxis, which should be continued weekly for 4–6 weeks after leaving the endemic areas. Chloroquine should not be given for continuous prophylaxis for longer than six years.

For long-term residents, proguanil should be given proportional to the adult dose of 200 mg daily.

Areas with chloroquine-resistant *P. falciparum*

Proguanil should be given proportional to the adult dose of 200 mg daily combined, some would advise, with chloroquine 300 mg once a week.

An alternative regimen using sulphadoxine/pyrimethamine (Fansidar) can be given, proportional to an adult dose of 500 mg (10 mg/kg) sulphadoxine and 25 mg (0.5 mg/kg) pyrimethamine once a week and continued for 4–6 weeks after leaving the endemic areas. Continuous prophylaxis with sulphadoxine/pyrimethamine should not be given for longer than two years and leucocyte differential counts should be carried out at six-months intervals.

In areas with highly chloroquine-resistant *P. falciparum*, the parasites may also be resistant to sulphadoxine/pyrimethamine (Fansidar) and break through may occur under the prophylaxis with the drug combination.

Mefloquine if available, may be given proportional to an adult dose of 250 mg base once a week. However, the drug should only be used for short-term residence in malarious areas. For children exposed to *P. vivax* or *P. ovale* infection, radical treatment with 14 days of primaquine should be undertaken during the last two weeks of the prophylaxis. If the stay in the endemic area is long, the continuous use of chemoprophylaxis may become more detrimental to health than early diagnosis and immediate treatment of attacks of malaria. In these cases it will be preferable to rely on methods of avoiding infection and on effective standby drugs that can be given if an infection occurs.

In addition to the drug prophylaxis, measures of vector avoidance should be encouraged. Bed nets should be used. Houses should be screened. Avoiding exposure to mosquito bites in the evening and early morning, protective clothes and mosquito repellents will also help. Recently it has been shown that insecticide-impregnated bed nets and curtains are effective in preventing malaria. Community based health care programmes are adopting these methods of vector avoidance in many endemic malarial areas.

Malaria control

Malaria control can be approached by mosquito control, chemoprophylaxis, intermittent chemotherapy, and measures to prevent mosquitoes from biting people. In the 1950s and 1960s, malaria eradication programmes based mainly on interruption of transmission by DDT residual spraying were successful in Europe and the United States, while in many countries there was a marked reduction in malaria incidence. However, by the 1970s malaria eradication programmes in most countries had deteriorated because of the emergence of DDT resistance of the mosquito vector, drug resistance of *P. falciparum* and rising cost of operation. Now the early control methods based on mosquito control combined with measures to prevent mosquitoes biting man are becoming of practical importance again.

A malaria control programme should be developed within the strategy of primary health care, according to the local epidemiological situation including parasitological, entomological, socio-economic and other factors.

It is feasible to train lay persons in the recognition and management of malaria. Diagnosis and treatment with appropriate antimalarials by community-based workers (including volunteers) can be carried out with oral rehydration therapy and contraceptive distribution.

In countries or areas where malaria is a serious problem but where the health infrastructure is very deficient and there is no organized antimalarial service, the antimalarial strategy should concentrate initially on providing the sick with treatment. It is necessary to establish a network of diagnosis and treatment facilities at the community level that will provide full courses of an appropriate curative drug to all patients suffering from malaria as well as courses of chemoprophylaxis during pregnancy. This network of facilities may be considered as an entry point to primary health care.

In countries or areas where the primary health care system is comparatively highly developed, malaria control activities should be implemented as an integral part of the overall activities of the health system. In countries or areas where organized antimalarial services have preceded the development of primary health care at the periphery, the antimalarial service may form the basis for the development of primary health care. Paediatricians in malaria endemic areas should play an important role in rendering health education to the community whose participation is the core of primary health care.

Further reading

Bruce-Chwatt LJ. *Essential Malaria*. London, William Heinemann Medical Books, 1980.

Bruce-Chwatt LJ, Black RH, Canfield CJ *et al.* Chemotherapy of malaria, 2nd edn. *Monograph Ser. WHO*, No. 27, 1981.

Chongsuphajaisiddhi T, Sabchareon A, Attanath P. *In vivo* and *in vitro* sensitivity of falciparum malaria to quinine in Thai children. *Annals of Tropical Paediatrics*. 1981; **1**: 21-6.

Chongsuphajaisiddhi T, Sabchareon A, Attanath P. Treatment of quinine resistant falciparum malaria in Thai children. *Southeast Asian Journal of Tropical Medicine and Public Health*. 1983; **14**: 357-62.

Cook GC. Prevention and treatment of malaria. *Lancet* 1988; **1**: 32-7.

Looareesuwan S, Phillips RE, White NJ *et al.* Quinine and severe falciparum malaria in late pregnancy. *Lancet*. 1985; **2**: 4-8.

Shute PG, Maryon ME. *Laboratory Technique for Study of Malaria*, 2nd edn. London, Churchill Livingstone, 1966.

Stanfield JP. Malaria. In: Black JA (ed.) *Paediatric Emergencies*, 2nd edn. London, Butterworths, 1987: 569-77.

Warrell DA, Looareesuwan S, Warrell MJ *et al.* Dexamethasone proves deleterious in cerebral malaria: a double blind trial in 100 comatose patients. *New England Journal of Medicine*. 1982; **306**: 313-19.

White NJ, Looareesuwan S, Warrell DA *et al.* Quinine loading dose in cerebral malaria. *American Journal of Tropical Medicine and Hygiene*. 1983; **32**: 1-5.

White NJ, Warrell DA, Chantavanich P *et al.* Severe hypoglycemia and hyperinsulinemia in falciparum malaria. *New England Journal of Medicine.* 1983; **309**: 61-6.

WHO. Advances in malaria chemotherapy. *Tech. Rep. Ser. WHO*, No. 711, 1984.

WHO. WHO Expert Committee on Malaria, 18th Report. *Tech. Rep. Ser. WHO*, No. 735, 1986.

WHO, Malaria Action Programme. Severe and complicated malaria. *Transactions of the Royal Society of Tropical Medicine and Hygiene.* 1986; **80** (Suppl.): 1-50.

CHAPTER 13

Other vector-borne parasitic infections

TRYPANOSOMIASIS
H. Taelman

Trypanosomiases are parasitic diseases caused by protozoan haemoflagellates belonging to the genus *Trypanosoma* of which the subspecies *Trypanosoma brucei gambiense* and *T. b. rhodesiense* are responsible for African trypanosomiasis while the single species *Trypanosoma cruzi* produces American trypanosomiasis or Chagas' disease.

African trypanosomiasis

African trypanosomiasis (also called sleeping sickness) classically includes two main clinical varieties: the chronic, Western or Gambian form caused by the subspecies *Trypanosoma brucei gambiense* located mainly in West and Central Africa, from Senegal to southern Sudan in the north, to Angola and Zaïre in the south, and the acute, Eastern or Rhodesian form caused by the subspecies *Trypanosoma brucei rhodesiense* found in East Africa at the Sudan–Ethiopia border, in Uganda, Kenya, Rwanda, Tanzania, Zambia, Zimbabwe, Botswana, Malawi and Mozambique. Both forms coexist in Uganda and southern Sudan. Thirty-six African countries are currently endemic for the disease. It has been estimated that 50 million people are at risk of infection and that the annual incidence is 20 000 new cases, the majority being reported from Zaire.[1]

Epidemiology

Transmission of trypanosomes from man or animal to man requires a development cycle of the parasites in blood-sucking flies of the genus *Glossina*, the tsetse flies. After being sucked from peripheral blood of an infected man or animal, the trypanosomes undergo several morphological and biochemical changes.

In the mid-gut of the fly the parasites differentiate into multiplicative forms called epimastigotes, characterized by the presence of an active mitochondrion at the posterior part of the parasite. These epimastigotes eventually migrate to the salivary glands. There they ultimately differentiate into trypomastigotes which are non-multiplicative metacyclic forms living free in the lumen of the salivary glands. The subsequent step of their cycle takes place in man or animal.

Humans become infected through the bite of a tsetse fly harbouring infective trypanosomes. According to the species, tsetse flies require to variable degrees, high temperature, shade, high humidity and blood for their development. The epidemiology of trypanosomiasis results from complex interactions between man, parasite, vector, vertebrate hosts and the ecological characteristics of the environment.

The West African trypanosomiasis epidemiology is characterized by strict man–fly–man transmission. Of major epidemiological importance is the chronic course of the disease with minor incapacitation for the patient, allowing infected individuals to remain capable of working and to form mobile reservoirs upon which the flies may feed. Occasional chronic asymptomatic carriers of trypanosomes detected by serological tests have been reported. Vectors are the riverine species *Glossina palpalis*, *G. fuscipes* and *G. tachinoides*. They are usually found in hot areas with darkness and moisture where people tend to congregate, i.e. river crossings, washing and watering places, and in forest galleries along rivers.

Recent studies have shown that domestic animals (pigs, dogs, cattle, sheep) can become infected with *T. b. gambiense* but their role as reservoirs remains speculative.

Transmission of endemic East African trypanosomiasis to man usually involves game animals and the savannah group of tsetse flies. However, man–fly–man or domestic animals–fly–man cycles predominate in epidemic Rhodesian trypanosomiasis. As the clinical course of the Eastern variety is acute, infected patients are very sick and do not usually circulate. The true reservoir is not man but wild game animals, principally the bushbuck.

The main vectors are *Glossina morsitans*, *G. pallidipes* and *G. swynnertoni*. The less fastidious biological requirements of these flies explain why they are found in the savannah. Exposed people are hunters, fishermen, honey and fuelwood gatherers and occasionally safari tourists. Under normal circumstances, because of the lower exposure of children to risk, the incidence of the disease among them is much lower than in adults, but in epidemic situations the incidences according to ages tend to become similar.

Transplacental transmission as well as transmission through non-tsetse biting insects, accidental injection of contaminated material and blood transfusion have also been reported.[1, 2, 3]

Pathogenesis

Antigenic variation of the outer glycoprotein layer of the trypanosome is considered as the basic mechanism of the pathogenesis of sleeping sickness. The antigenic variation explains the cyclic appearance of new waves of trypanosomes more or less every 15 days, each new wave being destroyed by the corresponding lytic antibodies it has induced. So, the host is exposed to a variety of parasite components that induce a cascade of reactions. This mechanism also accounts for the fluctuations of the parasitaemia and the temperature, and for the continuous production of immunoglobulins, mainly of the IgM class, and of circulating immune complexes (see p. 845). These activate vasoactive peptides (kallikrein, kinine), the complement and blood coagulation systems, which in turn elicit destructive inflammatory responses and tissue damage.[4]

Clinical manifestations

Classically the course of the disease is arbitrarily subdivided into two stages: the early or haemolymphatic stage and the advanced or late or meningoencephalitic stage. However, every gradation can be encountered in both varieties of the disease. Although in adolescents and adults the Western and Eastern varieties have similar manifestations, they differ distinctly in duration of evolution. Gambian sleeping sickness is a chronic disease with a course extending over a few years while the Eastern disease is acute, lasting a few weeks or months.

After the patient has been bitten by an infective tsetse fly, a reddish tender swelling 2–5 cm in diameter – the trypanosome chancre – may develop within 5–10 days at the site of the bite but it seldom occurs in Africans affected with the Gambian form. The early stage starts with the invasion of blood and lymph nodes by the trypanosomes 7–14 days after the bite and lasts an average of one year in the Western form. It is dominated by irregular fever and persistent headache. Enlarged posterior cervical lymph nodes – Winterbottom's sign – are a frequent finding in the West African form while in the Eastern variety lymph gland enlargement is usually generalized. The glands reach a diameter of ± 1 cm, have a child testicle consistency and become smaller with time. Tachycardia and/or ECG signs of myocarditis are often found in the Rhodesian form. The patient begins to lose weight and is usually asthenic. In some paler skinned patients, an erythematous rash, called trypanides, breaks out seven to eight weeks after the onset. It is usually seen on the chest and back and is composed of several ring-shaped patches 7–10 cm in diameter, overlapping each other, giving the lesion a polycyclic aspect. Although uncommon, facial oedema is another possible early manifestation of sleeping sickness. Splenomegaly is often present but may be due to other concurrent tropical diseases.

Early neurological manifestations with normal CSF include mental dullness, modification of behaviour, insomnia, aimless gaze, tremor of tongue and eyelids, deep hyperaesthesia such as pain on locking doors – the key sign of Kerandel – or by pressure on the muscles, and generalized pruritus.

Primitive cutaneous reflexes, i.e. hand–chin (stimulation of the hand induces contraction of the muscles of the chin) or perioral (percussion of the face on the midline or touching the upper lip induces contraction of the muscles of the chin and the lips) reflexes can sometimes be evoked.

The late stage is related to the involvement of CNS by trypanosomes and is characterized by alterations of the CSF components. Trypanosomes are present in some cases but by far the most usual findings are an increased number of lymphocytes, and an elevated protein level. Morular cells – the Mott cells – which are plasmocytes distended by accumulated immunoglobulins and IgM are sometimes found. Signs and symptoms of the later stage are those of a diffuse meningoencephalitis with involvement of the extrapyramidal system. Prominent clinical features include: tremor and muscle fasciculations at various sites of the body, increase in muscle rigidity and cerebellar ataxia. However, the most impressive sign is the daytime somnolence. In the final stage, somnolence d pens to stupor and ultimately to coma. The patient if not treated, dies from intercurrent infection or undernourishment.

A feature of sleeping sickness in young children is the overlapping of the signs related to the two phases of the disease and the high frequency of neurological signs due to early involvement of the CNS in both varieties of the disease.

Trypanosomiasis in pregnancy, if untreated, results in abortion, premature labour or maternal death; successful treatment is now being reported. Only a few cases of congenital trypanosomiasis have been reported.[2, 3, 6] The affected babies may present with fever, failure of breast-feeding, weight loss, lethargy, cyanosis, dyspnoea, jaundice, hepatosplenomegaly, anaemia, cardiomegaly. In *T. b. gambiense* infection the disease may also have a protracted course and, if diagnosed late, may manifest as a neurological illness with permanent sequelae. An unusual presentation of encephalitis and mental retardation due to trypanosomiasis was recently reported by Woodruff *et al.*[5] in a child, aged two, born to an asymptomatic carrier.

Diagnosis

The clinical diagnosis of African trypanosomiasis should be considered in any person who has stayed or lived in an endemic area for this disease and who presents with one or several of the following signs: prolonged irregular fever, persistent headache, lymphadenopathy, unexplained tachycardia and neurological manifestations. Although unspecific, anaemia, increased sedimentation rate, and high IgM levels are constant biological findings in trypanosomiasis that may help in diagnosis. But definite diagnosis relies on the demonstration of the parasite.

Direct examination of a chancre or a lymph node aspirate or of CSF sediment and/or blood film may reveal long, slender ($25-30 \times 1.5-2 \mu$m) or short stumpy ($14-22 \times 4-5 \mu$m) trypanosomes. More sensitive methods are the examination of a Giemsa-stained thick blood film or, better, of the buffy coat collected from centrifuged heparinized blood. By far the most sensitive method is the diethylaminoethyl (DEAE) cellulose anion exchange centrifugation technique, by which the trypanosomes are selectively eluted and recovered on membrane filtration. A practical design* of a method for field use has been developed and allows the detection of as few as five parasites per millilitre of blood.

Because of the cyclic fluctuation of the parasitaemia, repeated blood examinations over several days are sometimes necessary to detect trypanosomes. If all these methods have failed, trypanosomes can sometimes be found in stained bone marrow smear or by animal (rat, mouse) inoculation.

Once trypanosomes are detected in peripheral blood, CSF must be examined for trypanosomes, Mott cells, WBC count, total protein and IgM level to allow the staging of the disease. Most authors consider a WBC exceeding $3-5/$ mm^3 and a total protein level higher than 25 mg/dl with the Sicard–Cantaloube albuminometer or 45 mg/dl with the sulphsalicyclic acid method or 37 mg/dl with the dye-binding protein assay† as the criteria indicative of the meningoencephalitic stage of the disease. Serological tests are of considerable diagnostic aid because they are reliable and very sensitive. They allow the selection of suspected cases in mass screening as well as in clinical individual medical care. Serological techniques such as indirect immunofluorescence and ELISA have been found very useful for surveillance. Recently, the indirect haemagglutination and card agglutination techniques have been developed as diagnostic tests for mass screening in the field.[7]‡

Treatment

Three drugs are classically used in the treatment of African trypanosomiasis: suramin, pentamidine and

---

*A m-AECT (mini-anion exchange centrifugation technique) device has been designed under the trade mark TRYVIA by International Diagnostic Laboratories (IDL) Jerusalem, Israel.
†Bio-Rad Protein Assay Kit I, Bio-Rad Laboratories, Richmond, California.
‡Teststrip IHA and Teststrip CATT Smith Kline-RIT Laboratories, Rixensart, Belgium.

melarsoprol. The first two do not cross the blood–brain barrier; therefore their use is restricted to the first stage of the disease. Melarsoprol diffuses into the brain and is thus the drug of choice for the meningoencephalitic form. The choice of the drug depends on the stage and on the variety of trypanosomiasis. It is therefore of paramount importance to determine in each case the degree of CNS involvement by CSF analysis and to specify the geographical origin of the disease.

Suramin (Bayer 205, Moranyl, Antrypol, Nathuride) is very active in the early phase of both varieties of trypanosomiasis. It is administered intravenously. After an initial dose of 2 mg/kg to test idiosyncrasy, the drug is given at a dose of 20 mg/kg (max. 1 g) on days 1,3,7,14,21. Adverse effects of this drug include febrile reactions, proteinuria, casts in urine sediment, skin rash, pain in palms and soles and desquamation of skin. Mild albuminuria is not an indication for drug withdrawal.

Pentamidine isethionate or methane sulphonate (Lomidine) is an effective drug in the alternative treatment of the early phase of Gambian and Rhodesian trypanosomiasis. It is given intramuscularly at a daily dose of 3–4 mg/kg pentamidine base for 7–10 consecutive or alternate days. The patient should be in supine position when receiving the drug because hypotension, tachycardia, tachypnoea, nausea and vomiting may occur. Other side-effects are renal insufficiency, hypoglycaemia and onset of diabetes.

Melarsoprol (Mel B, Arsobal) is an arsenical effective in each stage of either form of trypanosomiasis but its use is restricted to the second stage because of its associated high toxicity. The drug, provided in 3.6 per cent solution of propylene glycol, is administered strictly intravenously. The recommended dose schedule is 3.6 mg/kg per day for three of four consecutive days. This series should be repeated one to three times, each time after an interruption of 7–10 days. The number of series is based on the CSF findings. According to the dosage scheme proposed by Neujean, patients with 5–20 cells/mm^3 in the CSF should receive one series of four daily injections of 3.6 mg/kg; with 21–100 cells/mm^3 two series; with > 100 cells/mm^3 three series. Some authors consider this dosage regimen too high and prefer a milder schedule with slowly increasing doses mainly in severely ill patients and in children, for instance a first series of daily injections of melarsoprol at doses of 1.8–2.2–2.56 mg/kg respectively from day 1 through day 3, a second series with 2.56–2.9–3.26 mg/kg respectively from day 10 through day 12 and a third series from day 19 through day 21 at doses of 3.6 mg/kg per day.

The major toxic effect of melarsoprol is an encephalopathy which occurs in 1–5 per cent of the patients and is associated with a high mortality rate. Some authors have reported the protective effect of corticosteroids (prednisolone, dexamethasone) at doses of 0.75 mg/kg per day against this complication.

A curative course of chloroquine and a few injections of suramin before melarsoprol administration followed by prophylactic proguanil seems to improve the outcome of children treated with melarsoprol. Recent experience indicates that concurrent infection, particularly malaria and high loads of trypanosomes in the blood, increases the toxicity of melarsoprol. Recently, difluoromethylornithine (DFMO, eflornithine)* an experimental drug which penetrates the CSF and has only minor side-effects, and nifurtimox (Lampit) in use in Chagas' disease, have proven effective in the early as well as in the late stage of *T. b. gambiense* trypanosomiasis, even in cases refractory to melarsoprol.

The toxicity in pregnancy to the fetus and the excretion in breast-milk of these trypanosomicidal agents have not been determined.

Each case of trypanosomiasis must be followed up for at least two years before being declared cured. Patients in the advanced stage should undergo examination of the CSF every six months.[1, 8, 9, 10]

Control

There are three main strategies for control of African trypanosomiasis:

- Surveillance and treatment of infected individuals. Case detection can be carried out passively in health centres and/or actively by mobile teams trained to diagnose trypanosomiasis, the most sensitive and specific techniques being the serological tests, e.g. the card agglutination test for trypanosomiasis. Each case found positive should undergo clinical, biochemical and parasitological investigations. If the results of these are consistent with active trypanosomiasis, a specific treatment must be started according to the variety and the stage of the disease.

- Chemoprophylaxis. Pentamidine one i.m. injection every six months may prove successful in the prevention of *T. b. gambiense* disease, particularly in epidemic situations, but its widespread use may mask the involvement of the CNS.

- Vector control. This aims at reducing man–fly contact and hence the transmission of the disease. Approaches to vector control include game destruction, selective vegetation clearing, use of residual

*Not in trade, produced by Merrell Dow Research Centre Strasbourg, France.

insecticides by ground or aerial application, trapping using traps or screens impregnated with insecticides and tsetse fly attractants. (Traps may be obtained at ORSTOM, Brazzaville, Rep. of Congo)

The specific approach for control in a particular area should rely on extensive ecological surveys.

Individual protection may be obtained by wearing adequate light-coloured clothes covering the body when travelling in infected areas, by avoiding crossing rivers during daytime and by using insect repellents.[11]

References

1. WHO Expert Committee. Epidemiology and control of African trypanosomiasis. *Technical Report Series 739.* Geneva, World Health Organization, 1986, pp. 127.
2. Mulligan H.W. (ed.) *The African Trypanosomiases.* London, Georges Allen & Unwin, 1970, pp. 950.
3. Buyst H. Sleeping sickness in children. *Annales de la Société Belge de Médecine Tropicale.* 1977; **57**: 201–11.
4. Wery M, Mulumba PM, Lambert PH, Kazyumba L. Hematologic manifestations, diagnosis and immuno-pathology of African trypanosomiasis. *Seminars in Hematology.* 1982; **19**: 83–92.
5. Woodruff AW, Evans DA, Owino NO. A 'healthy' carrier of African trypanosomiasis. *Journal of Infection.* 1982; **5**: 89–92.
6. Triolo N, Trova P, Fusco C, Le Bras J. Bilan de 17 années d'étude de la trypanosomiase humaine africaine à T. gambiense chez les enfants de 0 à 6 ans. A propos de 227 cas. *Médecine Tropicale.* 1985; **45**: 251–7.
7. Van Meirvenne N, Le Ray D. Trypanosomiasis: diagnosis of African and American trypanosomiasis. *British Medical Bulletin.* 1985; **41**: 156–61.
8. Apted FIC. Present status of chemotherapy and chemoprophylaxis of human trypanosomiasis in the eastern hemisphere. *Pharmacology and Therapy.* 1980; **11**: 398–413.
9. Taelman H, Schechter PJ, Marcelis *et al.* Difluoromethylornithine, an effective new treatment of gambiense trypanosomiasis: results in five patients. *American Journal of Medicine.* 1987; **82**: 607–14.
10. Moens F, De Wilde M, Kola Ngato. Essai de traitement au nifurtimox de la trypanosomiase humaine africaine. *Annales de la Société Belge de Médecine Tropicale.* 1984; **63**: 37–43.
11. Molyneux DH. Selective primary health care: strategies for control of disease in the developing world. VIII. African trypanosomiasis. *Reviews of Infectious Diseases.* 1983; **5**: 945–56.

American trypanosomiasis (Chagas' disease)

American trypanosomiasis, also called Chagas' disease, is an anthropozoonosis caused by *Trypanosoma cruzi* and transmitted by haematophagous bugs, extending from Mexico to Argentina and Chile. With an estimated 16–18 million infected people and 90 million individuals at risk, Chagas' disease constitutes a major health problem in Latin America by causing severe heart disease and chronic gastro-intestinal pathology.[1]

Epidemiology

Transmission of *T. cruzi* infection from man or animal to man involves a developmental cycle in blood-sucking triatomine reduviid bugs, also known popularly as kissing bugs (barbeiros, vinchucas, chipos). Among these, the genera *Triatoma*, *Rhodnius* and *Panstrongylus* are the best adapted to human dwellings where they live in cracks of wooden or dry mud walls and grass or fibre roofs. Known reservoirs for the parasite are wild and domestic (dogs, cats) animals as well as the infected man. Bugs become infected by sucking infected blood from man or animal. Once in the gut, trypanosomes undergo several morphological and biological changes. They become infective (metacyclic trypomastigotes) in the hind-gut and are eventually eliminated with the faeces near the site of the bite during subsequent blood meals. The mechanism of transmission is contaminative, not inoculative.

Man becomes infected by contamination of the biting site of the bug or of mucous membranes by the infected faeces of the bug, through transfusion of contaminated blood, transplacentally (transmission rates up to 10 per cent in highly endemic areas) or possibly via breast-milk from infected mother to infant, accidentally in laboratories by handling the parasite or infected bugs, or by ingestion of contaminated food.

Chagas' disease is principally a problem of remote rural areas and low socio-economic groups.[2, 3, 4]

Pathogenesis

After having penetrated the skin or a mucous membrane, trypanosomes invade surrounding cells, transform into rounded parasites (amastigotes), multiply, form pseudocysts, and differentiate into trypomastigotes which are eventually released into the bloodstream. The lesion produced at the portal of entry is called a 'chagoma' and is made of parasites and inflammatory cells. Following their dissemination throughout the body, the parasites may penetrate any organ but preferentially invade the reticuloendothelial system, the myocardium and the nervous system where they differentiate into amastigotes. As a consequence of this infection, myocarditis, meningoencephalitis and hepatosplenomegaly may ensue. In the chronic phase of the disease, severe alterations of the myocardium and the conductive system of the heart are often found. These alterations result from parasitism itself as well as from cell-mediated immunity or autoimmune reactions and neuronal destruction occurring during the acute stage of the disease (see p. 845). The invasion followed by the destruction by *T. cruzi* of the ganglion cells of the myenteric plexus of the digestive tract lead to mega-oesophagus and megacolon.[2, 5]

In a recent study from Brazil, the risk of abortion in *T. cruzi* serologically positive pregnancies was twice that of seronegative pregnancies, with increased incidences of polyhydramnios and leg varicosities in the seropositive group. Stillborn fetuses show widespread dissemination of parasites with inflammatory changes, and sometimes an appearance resembling hydrops fetalis. Transmission appears maximal between the 26th and 37th week of pregnancy. The placentae show a high parasitaemia and granulomatous reactions to the parasites which may be intra- or extracellular and lie within the stroma or free in the villi, and sometimes form pseudocysts.[6]

Clinical manifestations

Seroepidemiological studies show that only 20–30 per cent of infected individuals develop overt disease. Three clinical stages are commonly recognized in Chagas' disease: an acute stage involving mostly infants and young children over five years of age, followed by an indeterminate latent stage, and finally a chronic stage usually affecting adults.

The acute stage starts after an incubation period ranging from 7 to 14 days, but in children aged less than six months this can be reduced to two days. The initial manifestation may be a painful erythematous swelling of the skin, called 'chagoma', which may reach a diameter of several centimetres or a painless bipalpebral unilateral oedema associated with a satellite retro-auricular lymph node – Romaña's sign (Fig. 4.13.1). These primary lesions (which subside after one to four months) are highly suggestive of early acute Chagas' disease but are present in only 25–30 per cent of patients. More often the early manifestations are non-specific and include fever, dyspnoea, cough, cyanosis, pallor, irritability, insomnia and refusal of feeding. A

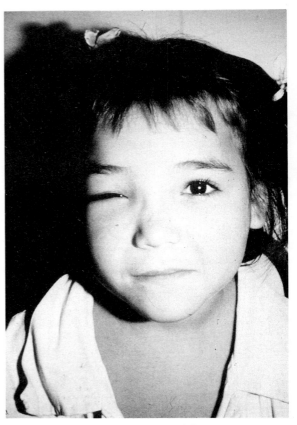

Fig. 4.13.1 Romaña's sign in Chagas' disease.

constant or remittent fever is an early and frequent symptom that may persist for one or two months. Generalized lymphadenopathy, mild hepatosplenomegaly and oedema involving lower limbs and the face are common observations.

Other manifestations are related to the systems involved:

- skin: maculo-papular or morbilliform eruption, urticaria;
- central nervous system: meningoencephalitis with focal to generalized seizures, often responsible for death of young infants;
- heart: myocarditis manifesting as tachycardia, dysrhythmias, non-specific ECG changes or congestive failure with a mortality rate of 5–10 per cent.

The manifestations of congenital Chagas' disease in its acute stage are similar to those of the acute acquired disease. They may appear at birth or a few months later. They include hepatosplenomegaly, anaemia, jaundice, oedema, petechiae, tremor and convulsions.

Occasionally gastro-intestinal involvement with development of megaoesophagus is seen.

Intrauterine deaths, prematurity and perinatal deaths are seen at a higher rate among chagasic mothers as compared with non-chagasic mothers. Acute congenital Chagas' disease must be differentiated from infectious diseases such as cytomegalovirus and herpes simplex virus infection, toxoplasmosis, and erythroblastosis fetalis. Biological abnormalities of the acute stage include presence of trypanosomes in peripheral blood, hyperleucocytosis with lymphocytosis, elevated sedimentation rate and hyperglobulinaemia. Signs and symptoms resolve gradually over 8–12 weeks and the patient enters into the asymptomatic indeterminate stage of the disease. Of the asymptomatic individuals 20–30 per cent will eventually enter the chronic stage of the disease. Chronic Chagas' disease usually strikes adults aged 20–40 years but children who survive the acute stage may also be affected.

Two major complications of the chronic stage are chronic cardiopathy and megaorgans of the digestive tract. Congestive heart failure, more commonly right-sided, is frequently the first sign of Chagas' heart disease. Other cardiac signs are premature ventricular beats, right bundle branch block and varying degrees of A–V block. Embolism of a thrombus may also supervene. Digestive manifestations are related to megaoesophagus and/or megacolon and include dysphagia, odinophagia, night regurgitation, chronic constipation, food impaction, and volvulus. ECG, echocardiography and X-ray examination may be helpful in determining the degree of involvement of the heart and/or digestive tract. Involvement of the CNS or the adrenals has also occasionally been described.

Less than 10 per cent of patients with symptoms in the chronic phase develop major complications. Death of patients usually results from intractable heart failure, arrhythmia and thromboembolism.[2, 3, 6, 7]

Diagnosis

Clinical diagnosis of Chagas' disease rests on a history of living or travelling in an endemic region and the presence of one or more of the manifestations described above. Definitive diagnosis of Chagas' disease is based on the demonstration of the parasite in blood or tissues.

The examination of peripheral blood for trypomastigotes is useful only during the acute phase of the disease. Parasites may be searched for in a wet blood smear but the sensitivity of this method is restricted to parasitaemias of 1×10^5–1×10^6/ml thereby excluding patients in the advanced stages of the disease. Giemsa-stained thin and thick blood smears are of limited value because of the destruction of *T. cruzi* by the smearing. Blood concentration techniques such as Strout's concentration test (serum from 5 cc clotted retracted blood is centrifuged and the sediment examined for trypanosomes) on clotted blood, and the microhaematocrit concentration test of Woo (a capillary tube for haematocrit filled with heparinized blood is centrifuged and the interface red blood cells–plasma (buffy coat) is examined for trypanosomes) initially used for parasitological diagnosis of African trypanosomiasis, are more sensitive methods. This latter technique is strongly recommended for the diagnosis of congenital Chagas' disease in the newborn because of its simplicity, moderate price and ease of application.

Animal inoculation or culture on suitable media are tools for isolation of parasites in suspected cases when attempts to demonstrate parasites by concentration methods have been unsuccessful. There is general agreement that the most sensitive parasitological method is xenodiagnosis. This method detects acute disease in its earliest phases and 67 per cent of those in the chronic phase. The test consists in feeding laboratory-reared reduviid bugs on patient's blood and screening the insect faeces for trypanosomes once a month for three months.

Several serological tests (complement fixation, indirect immunofluorescence, gel precipitation, indirect haemagglutination) have been developed to detect antibodies to *T. cruzi*. Serodiagnosis is of great value in selecting the patients who are infected and are thus at risk of developing chronic disease, but is of limited usefulness in the diagnosis of the acute disease. It may also corroborate a clinical diagnosis of chronic Chagas' disease.[2, 8]

Treatment

Effective treatment is based on an early diagnosis of the disease because the curative chemotherapy is limited to the acute phase of the disease. The two drugs that have proven effective and even curative in acute Chagas' disease are nifurtimox and benznidazole.

Nifurtimox, a 5-nitrofuran derivative (Lampit) is given by mouth in a daily dose of 15–20 mg/kg in children (8–10 mg/kg in adults) in four divided doses for up to 120 days. There is a geographical variation in effectiveness of the drug which is more successful in Argentina and Chile than in Brazil. Adverse side-effects include nausea, vomiting, abdominal pain, weight loss, disorientation, sensory polyneuropathy and seizures. They subside with reduction or discontinuation of therapy.

Benznidazole is a 2-nitroimidazole (Radanil, Rochagan, Ragonil) administered orally in a daily dose of 10 mg/kg for 60 days. Serious side-effects include peripheral polyneuropathy and bone marrow depression. Besides specific chemotherapy, patients with acute Chagas' myocarditis or meningoencephalitis also require supportive treatment. The treatment of patients with chronic Chagas' disease is essentially supportive. Patients with megaoesopagus and/or megacolon do sometimes derive benefit from surgery.[9]

Control and prevention

Chagas' disease is associated with disadvantage and poverty and cannot be solved without the political will of the authorities of the countries concerned. General prevention is largely based on control of transmission and includes mainly vector control by spraying of households with suitable insecticides, suppression of infected domestic animals, and improvement in housing. An insecticide fumigant canister for indoor use may be obtainable from UNDP/World Bank/ WHO Special Programme for Research and Training in Tropical Diseases, 1211 Geneva, 27 Switzerland.)

Transmission of *T. cruzi* through blood transfusion may be prevented by a careful screening of blood donors and/or treating blood with gentian violet solution in a final concentration of 1 in 4000. Laboratory personnel should take appropriate precautions when handling *T. cruzi* and infected bugs. Travellers to endemic areas should sleep in stone-built houses.[10]

References

1. Maurice JM, Pearce AM (eds). *Tropical Disease Research: A Global Partnership*. Geneva, WHO, 1987; pp. 191.
2. Brener Z, Andrade ZA (eds). *Trypanosoma cruzi e Doença de Chagas*. Rio de Janeiro, Guanabera Kaogan, 1979, pp. 463.
3. Le Ray D, Recacoechea M (eds). Chagas' disease. *Annales de la Société Belge de Médecine Tropicale*. 1985; **65** (suppl. 1): 1–232.
4. Miles MA. *Trypanosoma cruzi*: epidemiology. In: Baker JR (ed.) *Perspectives in Trypanosomiasis Research*. New York, J.Wiley Research Studies press, 1982. pp. 1–15.
5. Köberle F. Pathogenesis of Chagas' disease. In: *Trypanosomiasis and Leishmaniasis with Special References to Chagas' disease*. Ciba Foundation Symposium 20 (new series). New York, North Holland, Elsevier, 1974. pp. 137–52.
6. Bittencourt AL, Freitas LAR, Aranjo MOG *et al.* Pneumonitis in congenital Chagas' disease: a study of 10 cases. *American Journal of Tropical Medicine and Hygiene*. 1981; **30**: 38–42.
7. Bittencourt AL. Congenital Chagas' disease. *American Journal of Diseases of Children*. 1976: 97–103.
8. Van Meirvenne N, Le Ray D. Trypanosomiasis: diagnosis of African and American trypanosomiasis. *British Medical Bulletin*. 1985; **41**: 156–61.
9. Gutridge W. Trypanosomiasis: existing chemotherapy and its limitations. *British Medical Bulletin*. 1985; **41**: 162–8.
10. Marsden PD. *Reviews of Infectious Diseases*. 1984; **6**: 855–65.
11. Pepin J *et al. Lancet*. 1987; **ii**: 1431–3.
12. Doua F *et al. American Journal of Tropical Medicine and Hygiene*. 1987; **37**: 525–33.

LEISHMANIASIS
Philippe Lepage

Leishmaniasis is a group of diseases caused by parasites of the genus *Leishmania*. These organisms, originally parasites of rodents, have become adapted to canines and humans. Classically, three major clinical forms of leishmaniasis are described: visceral leishmaniasis caused by *L. donovani*; cutaneous leishmaniasis caused by *L. tropica*; and muco-cutaneous leishmaniasis caused by *L. braziliensis*.

The parasites are transmitted by sandflies (*Phlebotomus* or *Lutzomyia*). In visceral leishmaniasis, mother-to-infant transmission may occur and infections through contaminated blood transfusions have been described.[1] However, transmission other than through sandflies is rare.

The Leishmania life-cycle commences when the sandfly takes up amastigotes as it bites a human or an animal suffering from leishmaniasis. The amastigotes develop and increase in number by a process of division in the stomach of the sandfly. They become elongated (promastigotes) and move to the pharynx. The sandfly injects the promastigotes into a new host (man or animal) when it attempts to feed. The whole cycle in the sandfly takes about 10 days.[1]

Recent estimates suggest about 10 million infections in humans and 400 000 cases of visceral leishmaniasis a year.[2]

Visceral leishmaniasis (Kala-azar, Ponos)

Epidemiology

Kala-azar (which means 'black disease' in Indian language) is caused by *L. donovani* and is found from the Mediterranean coast, through the Middle East and India to the coast of China. In Africa, kala-azar occurs mainly in Sudan and East Africa; elsewhere the infection is sporadic. In the Western Hemisphere, it is found in Central America, Columbia, Venezuela, Brazil, Northern Argentina and Paraguay. At least three different epidemiological forms exist:[1, 2]

- A Mediterranean form with a canine reservoir (dogs, foxes and jackals). Children one to four years of age are mostly affected ('ponos' means infantile kala-azar).
- An Indian form with a human reservoir. The disease predominates in children older than five years. Humans are the only reservoir.
- An African form with a rodent reservoir (rats and gerbils). It especially affects subjects 10 to 20 years of age.

Clinical aspects

The incubation period usually varies from six weeks to 10 months but may be as short as 10 days or as long as 10 years. A primary skin nodule is infrequently seen, except in African leishmaniasis.

In infantile leishmaniasis, the disease may begin suddenly with fever and vomiting or insidiously with low-grade fever, weight loss, pallor and asthenia. When present, double daily spikes of fever are a characteristic sign. The spleen enlarges gradually; if the patient is not treated, the spleen can be palpated into the pelvis. Sometimes diarrhoea or dysentery are observed. Bleeding disorders become evident shortly before death. If untreated, death usually occurs after several months but the clinical course may be more protracted (one or two years).

In older children the course of the disease is frequently more chronic. Severe emaciation and brittle hair are common signs. In cases of Indian kala-azar, the skin may acquire an earth-grey color. Jaundice can be observed in 10 per cent of patients. Massive splenomegaly is found and lymphadenopathy is especially common in the African form. Untreated kala-azar has a fatality rate greater than 75 per cent.[3]

Death results from intercurrent infectious illnesses in more than 90 per cent of cases (pneumonia, amoebiasis, malaria, etc). More than 85 per cent of cases can be cured if early treatment is initiated.

Post-kala-azar dermal leishmanoid can be observed, after treatment, if all parasites are not eradicated. In the Indian form, up to 20 per cent of patients may be affected; it appears several years after therapy and may last some years. In the African form it affects about 2 per cent of the patients, appears during therapy and heals spontaneously. Post-kala-azar leishmanoid is apparently absent in the Mediterranean form. The skin is hypopigmented, erythematous and nodular lesions may be seen. It seems to represent a modified form of *L. donovani* infection in which the parasites no longer are able to invade the viscera and are localized to the skin.[1, 2, 3]

Biological findings

Anaemia is found in every case and is often severe. It is caused by haemolysis (probably due to an immune process) and by sequestration of red cells in the spleen. Leucopaenia is usually considerable with a relative increase in lymphocytes and decrease in eosinophils. The pathogenesis of neutropaenia is obscure (see also p. 845). Thrombocytopaenia is also frequently noted, responsible for the bleeding diathesis. In chronic cases, anaemia, leucopaenia and thrombocytopaenia can be reversed by splenectomy.

There is an early polyclonal rise in IgG. To a lesser extent, IgM and IgA are also elevated. This increase in IgG may exceed 5 g/dl; they are mostly non-specific and non-protective antibodies. Specific antibodies produced during active disease have diagnostic significance and are detected by indirect immunofluorescence, indirect haemagglutination and complement-fixation tests (see later). Renal, hepatic and splenic amyloidosis may occur and disappear with treatment. The dysproteinaemia usually disappears within six months of clinical recovery.

Liver function tests show evidence of hepatocellular damage in the majority of patients during active disease.[1, 2]

Diagnosis

Splenic puncture and liver biopsy are the most useful procedures but may be hazardous in case of haemorrhages. Sternal or iliac crest puncture is safer than spleen puncture. In Indian kala-azar, the organisms are regularly found in stained smears of peripheral blood, but in African and Mediterranean forms they may be difficult to isolate by this technique. Blood and bone marrow culture on NNN medium are also very useful. The *Novy, McNeal and Nicolle* (NNN) medium for *Leishmania* species and *Trypanosoma cruzi* is as follows:

> Agar 7 g
> Sodium chloride 3 g
> Distilled water 450 ml
> Defibrinated rabbit blood 150 ml

Mix agar, NaCl and water and bring to boiling to dissolve agar and salt. Autoclave at 121°C for 15 minutes. Cool to 52°C and add rabbit blood. Dispense 5 ml portions into sterile 13 mm × 100 mm screw-capped tubes, and slant the tubes in the refrigerator. If there is little moisture, a few drops of sterile water may be added with the inoculum. Medium should be tested for sterility by incubating a sample slant at 35°C for 48 hours.

Non-specific tests (such as the *formol gel test*) reflecting the elevation of serum globulins have proved useful in the diagnosis of kala-azar in field conditions. Briefly, 1 or 2 ml of clear serum of the patient is placed in a tube to which one drop of formaldehyde is added. The serum is shaken and allowed to stand at room temperature. The test is positive if the serum solidifies and becomes opaque within 20 minutes.

The indirect immunofluorescence test has a good sensitivity and specificity, as have the indirect haemagglutinin test, microenzyme-linked immunoabsorbent assay and counter-immunoelectrophoresis. The complement-fixation test is less sensitive and less specific than the above-mentioned tests due to cross-reactions with Chagas' disease and sometimes with tuberculosis and leprosy.

If leishmania are very scanty, they can be demonstrated by intraperitoneal inoculation of material (liver, spleen, bone marrow, etc.) into a hamster.

The *leishmanin test* or *Montenegro reaction* is a measure of delayed hypersensitivity to leishmanin antigen. The test is performed like the tuberculin skin test: 0.1 ml is injected intradermally and skin induration is measured after 48 to 72 hours. It becomes positive only 6 to 8 weeks after development of the active infection and remains positive for life. The change from a negative to a positive leishmanin test is the sign that the patient has developed protective cell-mediated immunity. Positive Montenegro reaction may occur among subjects with no history of kala-azar and indicates a subclinical infection with immunity to the organism.[1, 3, 4]

Treatment

Pentavalent antimonial compounds such as sodium stibogluconate are the treatment of choice of visceral leishmaniasis. The paediatric dose of sodium stibogluconate recently recommended by the World Health Organization is 20 mg/kg daily i.v. or i.m. for at least 20 days.[4] Longer treatment schedules are required for the African form than for the Indian form. Side-effects include nausea, vomiting, urticaria, bradycardia and ECG changes. If improvement is slow or incomplete, the therapy can be repeated.

If resistance to antimony is present, pentamidine (4 mg/kg i.m. three times a week for at least 5 to 25 weeks) or amphotericin B (1.5 mg/kg on alternate days by slow i.v. drip in glucose; total adult dose = 1 to 3 g) can be given.[4, 6]

After therapy, patients should be followed up every six months for at least two years. Fluorescent antibody tests should be negative after one year.

Prevention

In Europe and Asia, good control of peridomiciliary vectors of kala-azar has been achieved following control of malaria with DDT.[2] Spraying should coincide with the maximum population of sandflies. DDT application in houses has been successful in the control of the Brazilian vector of kala-azar.[2] In contrast, aerial fogging of forests is impracticable and did not reduce sandflies in Sudan.[2]

Sandfly bed nets exist, but may be intolerable in a warm climate. Mosquito nets impregnated with insecticide offer some protection. Repellents and protective clothing have been used as prophylactic measures in jungle training.

Destruction of animal reservoirs is another method of prevention. Dogs are an important domestic reservoir of kala-azar in many areas of the world. However, destruction of infected dogs is not always possible.

Antimonial treatment of dogs in quarantine has been used successfully.[2] On the other hand, the control of wild canines (foxes, etc.) is virtually impossible. Other wild animals that are important reservoirs are also difficult to control. Effective control of desert rodents has been achieved in USSR.[5]

Limited field trials of vaccines against kala-azar have, until now, proved disappointing.

Cutaneous or Old World leishmaniasis

Old World cutaneous leishmaniasis (or 'oriental sore') is caused by *L. tropica*. It is found in the Mediterranean basin, Middle and South-western Asia, and in Western and Eastern Africa.

Two types exist: rural leishmaniasis caused by *L. tropica major* with rodents (gerbils) as the natural reservoir of infection, and urban leishmaniasis caused by *L. tropica minor* with dogs as the natural reservoir.

Clinical aspects

A red, pruritic, vesicular papule appears weeks or months after the bite of a sandfly. The papule enlarges to 1 or 2 cm in diameter and then dries, presenting as an ulcer usually with sharp indurated margins. Healing occurs after 3 to 18 months, leaving a hypo- or hyperpigmented scar. Without secondary infection, there are no usual complications.[1, 3]

Diagnosis

The parasites are found by staining (with Giemsa or Wright) non-necrotic tissue of the ulcer. Culture on NNN medium is also helpful.

Treatment

The lesion tends to heal spontaneously if the patient is removed from the endemic area.

Drug therapy consists of pentavalent antimonials as in kala-azar. Other drugs (such as metronidazole, glucantine, rifampicin, levamisole, etc.) have also been used. Local injections of mepacrine in 15 per cent solution into the base of the ulcer are curative when few lesions are present. Oral and intralesional steroids have also proved useful.[1, 3, 4]

Prevention

Residual spraying for malaria control has eliminated cutaneous leishmaniasis from many countries, but with the end of many malaria eradication campaigns, leishmaniasis has returned to the Middle East.

Gerbils have been eradicated from many villages in Central Asia by poisoning their burrows. Destruction of infected dogs may also be realized.

Using live, cultured promastigotes, vaccination campaigns have been successful in USSR and Israel. Infection with *L. tropica major* protects against infection from *L. tropica minor*, but protection in the reverse direction is incomplete.[2] The development of a positive Montenegro reaction following immunization is of uncertain significance regarding protection. A significant diminution of cases following an immunization campaign is the best criterion of success.[2]

American leishmaniasis

In contrast to Old World leishmaniasis, American leishmaniasis is a rural disease common in people living in forest, or on the border of forest, of South and Central American. There are various forms of leishmaniasis in Central and South America, and muco-cutaneous leishmaniasis ('espundia') is but one of them. Each variety has its own clinical, epidemiological and pathological feature.[1, 3, 6] However, two main groups of parasites exist: the *L. mexicana* complex and the *L. braziliensis* complex. Various species of rodent represent the animal reservoir.

Leishmania mexicana complex

L. mexicana causes a simple lesion which does not metastasize. It occurs commonly on the face, on the external ear and sometimes on the upper limbs. The disease is often self-limited, but a chronic destroying lesion of the external ear ('chicle ulcer') may occur.

L. mexicana is principally found in Mexico, Guatemala and Belize. Chicle ulcer is principally an occupational disease affecting gum ('chicle') collectors. Any age may be attacked.

Leishmania braziliensis complex

L. braziliensis braziliensis causes the most severe form of American leishmaniasis, known as muco-cutaneous leishmaniasis or 'espundia'. Lesions of the mucous membranes of the nasopharynx often arise several years after healing of a cutaneous ulcer (usually of the leg) with ulceration and perforation of the nasal septum, mouth, palate and larynx. Death is frequently caused by aspiration pneumonia or intercurrent sepsis.

The disease is mainly found in Brazil, Peru, Bolivia, Ecuador, Paraguay and northern Argentina.

Diagnosis

L. mexicana grows quickly and *L. braziliensis* slowly on NNN medium and in hamsters.

Treatment

As in other forms of leishmaniasis, pentavalent antimonials are the drugs of choice in the treatment of American leishmaniasis. However, in the case of 'espundia' with mucosal lesions, therapy with pentavalent antimonials is disappointing and amphotericin B is the best treatment.

Locally applied heat can be very effective in non-metastasizing cutaneous lesions. The temperature in the lesion must be raised to between 37 and 43°C for periods of 12 hours.[1, 3, 4]

Prevention

Prevention of American leishmaniasis is extremely difficult since it is a forest zoonosis. Sleeping in tents under fine mesh netting and employing insect repellents are recommended.[1, 2, 4]

References

1. Leishmaniasis. In: Manson-Bahr PEC, Apted FIC eds *Manson's Tropical Diseases*, 18th edn. London, Baillere Tindall, 1982: 93–115.
2. Marsden PD. Selective primary health care: strategies for control of diseases in the developing world. XIV. Leishmaniasis. *Review of Infectious Diseases*. 1984; **6**: 736–44.
3. Wittner M. Leishmaniasis. In: Feigin RD, Cherry JD eds. *Textbook of Pediatric Infectious Diseases*, 2nd edition. London, WB Saunders, 1990. pp. 1562–8.
4. WHO Expert Committee. *The Leishmaniasis*. Technical Report Series No. 701. Geneva, WHO, 1984.
5. Marinkelle CJ. The control of leishmaniasis. *Bulletin of the World Health Organization*. 1980; **58**: 807–18.
6. Hart DT (ed.) *Life Sciences*. 1989; **163A**: 1–1041.

FILARIASIS
H. Taelman

Filariasis is caused by thread-like round worms of the superfamily Filarioidea. Among the hundreds of filariae existing in nature only eight infect man. *Wuchereria bancrofti*, *Brugia malayi* and *B. timori*, the lymphatic-dwelling filariae producing elephantiasis, are transmitted by mosquitoes. *Onchocerca volvulus*, the causal agent of river blindness, is transmitted by blackflies; *Loa loa*, the West African eyeworm causing Calabar swellings, is transmitted by tabanid flies; *Dipetalonema perstans*, *D. streptocerca*, *Mansonella ozzardi*, considered to be non- or weakly pathogenic for man, are transmitted by midges (also by blackflies for *M. ozzardi*). All eight filariae have some characteristics in common.

Man is infected by the bite of an insect vector carrying infective larvae. These forms, according to the species to which they belong subsequently migrate either to the subcutaneous tissues or to the lymphatics where they develop over a 3 to 12 month period into male and female adult worms (40–600 mm × 0.6 mm) called macrofilariae.

The offspring of the female adults – the microfilariae – (150–360 μm × 10 μm) live either in the blood or in the skin. The next step of the cycle takes place in the insect which becomes infected by the ingestion of microfilariae. These larvae subsequently grow through several larval stages before becoming infective larvae in the mouth parts of the insect.

Because potent infection requires intensive and repeated exposure to the parasites, most of the manifestations of the various filariae usually do not appear before the second decade of life.

As a result of the socio-economic impact of the complications associated with the filariases, such as blindness, chronic dermatitis and elephantiasis, filarial infections constitute a major public health problem in some countries of Africa and Latin America.

Onchocerciasis

Onchocerciasis, also called river blindness, is caused by *Onchocerca volvulus*. In Africa it is found in the rain forest belt and the savannahs extending from Senegal to Ethiopia in the north to Angola to Tanzania in the south. In America, the disease is found in Central and South America. In Asias, the disease is restricted to Yemen. World-wide, onchocerciasis is endemic in 34 countries with a population of 85 million at risk of infection, of whom 17.6 million are actually infected and nearly 336 000 are blind.

Epidemiology

Man is the only reservoir of the parasite and is infected by the bite of the female blackflies of the genus *Simulium* harbouring infective larvae. The focal distribution of the disease is related to the ecological requirements of the vectors. *Simulium* tend to breed in fast-running streams and rivers in Africa and in small streams in America. The various epidemiological and clinical patterns of infection result from differences in parasite strains, vectors and host responses within the endemic areas. In the rain forest, transmission takes place throughout the year and is mainly associated with skin lesions, whereas in the savannah transmission is seasonal and the eye lesions are more prevalent. In Africa, the flies bite usually on the lower parts of the body while in America they bite on the upper parts; these biting preferences might explain the different location of lesions in the African and the American disease.[1]

Clinical manifestations

Most symptoms and signs result from reactions to microfilariae in the subcutaneous tissue and the eye. The incubation period varies from one person to another but is usually not less than 12 months. Whereas most indigenous people with a light infection are asymptomatic, lightly infected expatriates usually

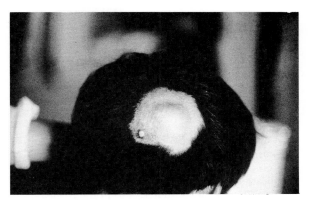

Fig. 4.13.2   *Onchocerca volvulus* nodule on the head.

exhibit complaints. Because the complications of onchocerciasis result from heavy parasitic loads, a consequence of repeated infections, the severe disease is more often found in adults than in children, who usually do not develop manifestations before the end of the first decade of life. Transplacental transmission of the infection has been recorded.

Usual manifestations of the disease are:

- Subcutaneous nodules. These are firm and non-tender. They range from several millimeters to a few centimeters in diameter and contain adult worms which may have a life span of 15 years. They are usually located over pelvis, chest wall, scapulas, spine, and head (Fig. 4.13.2).
- Dermatitis. The early lesions consist of a papular, itching rash frequently localized on the buttocks but severe itching and scratching lesions may be present all over the body. Later on a leathery thickening of the skin followed by atrophy, loss of elasticity and depigmentation may develop. The hanging groin, a pendulous skin sac containing inguinal and femoral lymph nodes, is seen in the advanced disease and may reach crippling and disfiguring proportions.
- Eye lesions. The earliest and most common eye lesion is punctate keratitis, readily distinguishable on slit-lamp examination. Pannus formation may follow this. Other lesions include iridocyclitis and chorioretinitis.
- Blindness. This is the result of corneal fibrosis, glaucoma and/or optic atrophy.
- Growth retardation and kyphoscoliosis. These were reported in some parts of Africa in earlier literature; the so-called 'Nakalanga' syndrome. The cause was obscure and could have been unrelated to the onchocercal infection always associated with identified cases. No recent reports have been seen.[1]

Diagnosis

Onchocerciasis must be considered in any patient residing or having travelled in an endemic area and presenting with one or several of the manifestations just described.

Non-specific laboratory tests such as hypereosinophilia or elevated IgE level are indications of an helminthic infection. Serological tests, because of their lack of specificity, are of limited value. Definitive diagnosis is brought by the demonstration of parasites. Microfilariae can be found in the tissue fluid of skin scarifications or in snips performed over iliac crests, buttocks, thighs and scapulas; also in the cornea or in the anterior chamber by slit-lamp examination. Macrofilariae can be displayed in nodules.

If parasites are not found despite strong suggestion of disease, a Mazzotti test is recommended. It consists in the administration of a single oral dose of 1 mg/kg of diethylcarbamazine (DEC: Banocide, Hetrazan, Notezine; max. 50 mg). If an intense papular rash ensues within a few hours, onchocerciasis is likely.[1]

Treatment

Until recently the sole available drug was DEC. This drug is active on microfilariae but not on adult worms. As DEC therapy may induce severe adverse reactions including papular rash (a Mazzotti-type reaction (Fig. 4.13.3)), fever, myalgia, exacerbation and worsening of eye lesions, it should be administered by building up within four to five days the full daily dosage of 6 mg/kg. This dose should then be continued for 21 days. Severe side-effects or worsening of keratitis may be alleviated by combining corticosteroids with DEC therapy. To avoid relapses, several courses of DEC are often required. If repeated courses have failed to eradicate the parasite, or if eye lesions are present, suramin should be used to kill the adult worms. Its usual dosage is 20 mg/kg (max 1g) once weekly for six weeks after an initial dose of 2 mg/kg (max. 100 mg) to detect idiosyncrasy. Nodules, particularly when located over the head, should be removed. Surgery is also required for larger hypertrophied skin folds such as occur in the groins.

Recently, Ivermectin (Mectizan), an avermectin derivative in a single oral dose of 100–200 µg/kg has proved very effective with only a mild Mazzotti-type reaction in some patients and without ocular worsening. The drug slowly suppresses the microfilariae and seems to damage the uterine contents of the female macrofilariae. Toxicity of the antifilarial

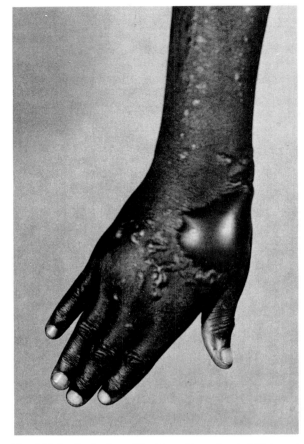

Fig. 4.13.3 Onchodermatitis. Mazzotti reaction to initial treatment with diethylcarbamazine.

drugs in pregnant women and in the embryo is not known.[3]

Control and prevention

There are two major points of attack for the control of onchocerciasis:

- Vector control by using widespread larvicides along rivers and streams – the habitats of vectors' larvae. In 1975, a massive campaign called the Onchocerciasis Control Programme, extending over the whole Volta River Basin of Africa was started by WHO. It consisted in aerial spraying of the larvicide *'temephos'* along the waterways. Although this programme has achieved considerable success in the control of *Simulium* flies, problems such as vector resistance and re-invasion of flies have arisen. Moreover, the costs of such a programme were enormous and estimated at more than several million US dollars per year.

- Mass treatment of the infected people. Because of the side-effects of DEC or suramin, this approach has given disappointing results. However, chemotherapy on a large scale might become feasible with drugs that are well tolerated, effective and easy to administer, e.g. Ivermectin.

Individual prevention is based on avoiding exposure to blackflies by use of protective clothing or repellents.[4, 5]

Loiasis

Loiasis is a filarial infection caused by *Loa loa*. Its area of distribution is irregular and restricted to the rain forest belt of Western and Central Africa and equatorial Sudan. About 2–3 million people are estimated infected with *Loa loa*. In some areas it is a major cause of morbidity and work absenteeism.

Epidemiology

The disease is transmitted to man by female tabanid flies of the genus *Chrysops*, which become infected by sucking blood from people harbouring microfilariae. These undergo a developmental cycle of two weeks in the thoracic muscles of the fly before migrating to and becoming infective in the proboscis. Man is the sole reservoir of epidemiological importance. *Loa loa* microfilariae live in the pulmonary vessels at night but appear in peripheral blood during the day with a peak at noon. Macrofilariae live in the subcutaneous tissues and occasionally appear under the conjunctivae (Fig. 4.13.4). The main vectors, *Chrysops silacea* and *C. dimidiata*, are day-biting flies usually living in the canopy of the rain forest. They are attracted by woodsmoke and by movement. Workers in rubber plantations are particularly at risk.[1, 2, 7]

Clinical manifestations

The first manifestations occur, at the earliest, 12 months after the infective bite. The morbidity rate of loiasis is greatly variable. Whereas in one area a substantial number of infected people remain asymptomatic, in another region the morbidity rate may reach 100 per cent. Children are infected as frequently as adults.

Disease syndromes are produced by macrofilariae migrating in the tissues. There are two different types of manifestation:

- Calabar swellings. These are transient, erratic, localized areas of non-erythematous subcutaneous oedema, 10–20 cm in diameter. They are slightly itchy, and last a few days. They are usually seen on the hands, wrists, forearms and legs, but may develop anywhere. They are considered an allergic reaction to the intermittent laying of microfilariae by the female macrofilariae. (Fig. 4.13.5.)
- Eye and skin troubles. Severe erythematous conjunctivitis may occur when an adult worm migrates under the conjunctiva. Occasionally the migrating worms produce a creeping worm-like eruption.[1, 2, 7]

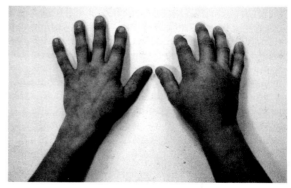

Fig. 4.13.5   Calabar swelling in loiasis.

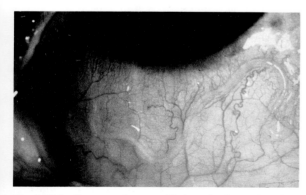

Fig. 4.13.4   Passage of a macrofilaria under the conjunctiva in loiasis.

Diagnosis

Loiasis should be suspected in any patient coming from an endemic area and presenting with skin swellings and/or eye troubles. Eosinophilia and high IgE level are non-specific biological abnormalities often present. Definitive diagnosis is established by the demonstration of the characteristic sheathed microfilariae in peripheral blood during the daytime. These can be found in the Giemsa-stained thick film or by concentration methods such as the Knott procedure. By this technique the erythrocytes are haemolysed and leucocytes and microfilariae are concentrated. Peripheral blood (5 ml) is mixed with 45 ml of 2 per cent formalin. After centrifugation of the mixture, the sediment is spread on slides, stained with Giemsa and examined for microfilariae.

The microfilarial load in the blood should be determined in each case before treatment. However, even in hyperendemic areas, microfilariae are found in no more than 35 per cent of people presenting with suggestive signs of loiasis. Serological tests, although they lack specificity may be of some help in the diagnosis, for instance in the absence of microfilaraemia.[1]

Treatment

Diethylcarbamazine is effective on microfilariae as well as on macrofilariae. DEC should be administered cautiously as for onchocerciasis. Fever, headache, malaise, vomiting, increased swellings and itching are common side-effects that sometimes necessitate the withdrawal of the drug or the use of corticosteroids. But the major drawback of DEC in the treatment of loiasis is post-therapeutic encephalitis. This is to be expected in patients with microfilaraemia $\geq$ 50 000/ml (roughly 800–1000 in a thick blood film). In this event, the microfilarial load can be lowered by apheresis and allow subsequent treatment with DEC. By this method withdrawn blood is sedimented into layers consisting of red cells, white cells, blood platelets, microfilariae and plasma. The layers of the platelets and microfilariae are extracted and the remaining components of the blood are returned to the patient. Some 1×10^7 microfilariae can be extracted by centrifugation of 3 litres of blood.[1, 2, 7, 8] Ivermectin is capable of decreasing microfilarial load without side effects.[10]

Control and prevention

Control is mainly based on:

- the destruction of the vector by the spraying of insecticides in breeding places;
- chemoprophylaxis with DEC at a dose of 5 mg/kg per day for three days each month.

Individual prevention relies on the wearing of protective clothing and the use of insect repellents.

Other Filariases

Dipetalonema perstans

D. perstans is found in West, Central and East Africa, in the Caribbean and in a few countries of Central and South America. It is regarded by many as a non-pathogenic commensal. However, an association of *D. perstans* infection with a variety of symptoms including Calabar swellings, pruritus, fever, headache, arthralgia and neurological and psychological symptoms has been reported.

D. perstans infection is diagnosed by the finding of typical unsheathed microfilariae throughout both day and night in peripheral blood. *D. perstans* is usually resistant to DEC. Mebendazole combined with levamisole seems to be more effective.

Mansonella ozzardi

M. ozzardi is confined to the Caribbean and Central and South America and is also considered as a non-pathogenic filaria. In one report, *M. ozzardi* infection has been implicated in painful arm–shoulder syndrome.

Diagnosis of the infection is based on the demonstration during day or night of unsheathed microfilariae in peripheral blood. DEC has usually no effect on the parasite.

Dipetalonema streptocerca

The geographical distribution of *D. streptocerca* is limited to the tropical rain forests of West and Central Africa. Most of the infected individuals remain asymptomatic. In some cases, *D. streptocerca* infection has been associated with dermal and lymphatic pathology. The major clinical manifestations of streptocerciasis include skin eruption and altered pigmentation, mild pruritus, inguinal lymphadenopathy and lymphoedema.

The aetiological diagnosis is based on the demonstration of unsheathed microfilariae in the skin, morphologically distinguishable from *O. volvulus* microfilariae.

DEC is an effective micro- and macrofilaricide in streptocerciasis but may produce side-effects similar to the Mazzotti reaction.[1, 2]

References

1. Janssens PG. Filariasis. In: Woodruff AW, Wright SG eds *Medicine in the Tropics*. Edinburgh, Churchill Livingstone, 1984.

2. Ottensen EA. Filariasis and tropical eosinophilia. In: Warren KS, Mahmoud AAF eds *Tropical and Geographical Medicine*. New York, McGraw-Hill, 1984.

3. Goodwin LG, Ottensen EA, Southgate BA. Recent advances in research on filariasis. *Transactions of the Royal Society of Tropical Medicine and Hygiene*. 1984; **78** (suppl.): 1–28.

4. Azziz MA. Chemotherapeutic approach to control of onchocerciasis. *Reviews of Infectious Diseases*. 1986; **8**: 500–5.

5. Greene BM. Selective primary health care: strategies for control of disease in the developing world. VI.

6. Onchocerciasis. *Reviews of Infectious Diseases*. 1983; **5**: 781–9.

6. Ogumba EO. Loiasis in Ijebu Division, West Nigeria. *Tropical and Geographical Medicine*. 1971; **23**: 194–200.

7. Fain A. Epidemiologie et pathologie de la loase. *Annales de la Société Belge de Médecine Tropicale*. 1981; **61**: 277–85.

8. Muylle L, Taelman H, Moldenhauer R *et al*. Usefulness of apheresis to extract microfilariae in management of loiasis. *British Medical Journal*. 1983; **287**: 519–20.

9. Taylor HR, Greene BM. *American Journal of Tropical Medicine and Hygiene*. 1989; **41**: 460–66.

10. Richard-Lenoble D. *et al*. *Bulletin de la Sociéte de Pathologie Exotique*. 1989; **82**: 65–7.

FILARIASIS IN CHILDREN IN ASIA

J.W.Mak

Epidemiology	Management
Community perceptions	Prognosis
Aetiology and pathogenesis	Prevention and control
Clinical manifestations	Future
Complications	References
Diagnosis	

Filariasis, a disease caused by the developing and adult forms of the nematode parasites, *Wuchereria bancrofti*, *Brugia malayi* and *B. timori*, is mainly seen in tropical and subtropical regions of the world. Of the estimated 90.2 million persons infected, 61.4 million are in the Asian region.[1] Most infections are due to *W. bancrofti* (90 per cent of all infections); *B. malayi* infection is seen mainly in Asia and *B. timori* infection is only found in certain islands of Indonesia.

The infection is non-fatal and in most endemic areas a high proportion of infected individuals may be asymptomatic. As such, the disease may easily be missed, except in those with gross deformity of the limbs.

Epidemiology

Lymphatic filariasis is seen in both urban and rural areas. Urban bancroftian filariasis is associated with poor sanitation in overcrowded slums where the principal vector mosquito, *Culex qinquifasciatus* breeds in profusion. Brugian filariasis and the rural forms of bancroftian filariasis found in various parts of Southeast Asia, are seen mainly in agricultural and estate populations and are transmitted by various *Mansonia* spp. and *Anopheles* spp. mosquitoes. The former mosquitoes breed on water plants in open swamps and

swamp forests. *Anopheles* spp. vectors (e.g. *A. barbirostris* and *A. campestris*) breed in rice fields and in some endemic areas, transmit both malaria and filariasis.

Various forms of *B. malayi*, which differ in their range of animal reservoir hosts, mosquito vectors and ecotypes, are found in endemic areas.[2] Traditionally, these parasites have been classified on the basis of their microfilarial periodicity, into periodic and subperiodic forms. This rhythmic variation in microfilarial density in the peripheral blood over the 24-hour cycle, is most marked in the periodic form. Peak microfilarial density is at night. The lowest density occurs in the day and is usually less than 5 per cent of the peak density in the periodic form but more than 10 per cent in the subperiodic form. The most highly evolved variant is the periodic form of *B. malayi* which is essentially a human parasite without any animal reservoir. *Anopheles* spp. are the principal vectors while *Mansonia* spp. serve as secondary vectors. There is at the other extreme, the subperiodic *B. malayi* variant which is zoonotically transmitted from wild (leaf monkeys) and domestic animals (cats) to man. Between these two extremes are intermediate variants with shared epidemiological features. There is no evidence that the periodic forms of *B. malayi*, *B. timori* and *W. bancrofti* can be zoonotically transmitted in nature.

Although all age groups can be infected, most infections and clinical disease are seen in young adults. This is closely associated with prolonged exposure to infective mosquitoes. However, *B. malayi* microfilaraemia has been reported even in three-month-old infants and chronic lymphoedema due to lymphatic filariasis can occur in older children. There is no vertical (placental) transmission of the disease.

Community perceptions

In some isolated communities the disease sequelae like elephantiasis have been attributed to a variety of causes, some of which include stepping on elephant dung, and being due to 'wind' in the affected limb. Whatever the attributed cause, the majority of such communities regard these afflictions with distaste. Subjects are ashamed of their deformities and conceal them from the public. There has, however, been an increasing demand for medical and surgical treatment for these lesions.

Aetiology and pathogenesis

Man is infected when an infective mosquito (those with infective larvae, L3) feeds on him. During the probing process before skin penetration by the proboscis, L3 are deposited near the puncture wound (Fig. 4.13.6). The L3 migrate into the puncture wound, reach the lymphatics and are lodged in the afferent lymphatics and the subcapsular sinus of the involved lymph nodes. Growth and development occur, the parasite moulting to the fourth stage (L4) at 10 days and after a final moult, to the fifth stage (L5) at four weeks after infection. The lymphatics and lymph nodes of the lower

limbs are usually involved, although the upper limbs can be affected as in bancroftian filariasis. In experimental studies in non-human primates, a large proportion of the worms may also be found in the thoracic duct and sacral lymph nodes and this may also be true in human infections.

The parasites reach sexual maturity in 8–12 months for *W. bancrofti* and three to four months for *B. malayi* and *B. timori* infections. Microfilariae, believed to be produced in batches, reach the circulation and are then available for further transmission. Microfilariae (Figs 4.13.7–4.13.9) taken up by a competent vector, penetrate the mid-gut and migrate to the thoracic muscles of the mosquito where they become the first-stage larvae (L1). They moult and develop into the second-stage larvae (L2) by the fifth day. A further

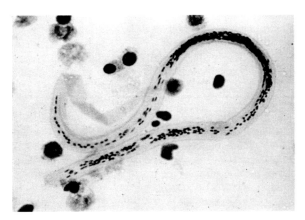

Fig. 4.13.7   *Wuchereria bancrofti* microfilaria.

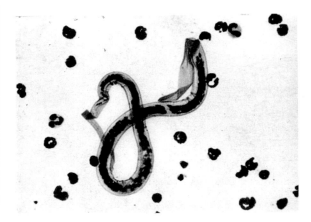

Fig. 4.13.8   *Brugia malayi* microfilaria.

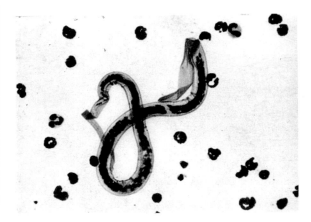

Fig. 4.13.6   Infective larvae (L3) of *Brugia malayi* emerging from the proboscis of a mosquito.

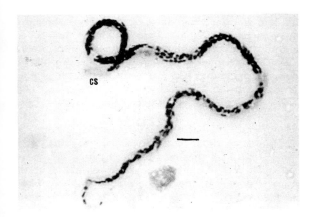

Fig. 4.13.9 *Brugia timori* microfilaria. Microfilaria exsheathed. Note long cephalic space at anterior end differentiating it from *Brugia malayi*. Scale bar = 10 μm: CS = cephalic space.

moult occurs by the 10th to 14th day and the larvae growing into the infective stage (L3). These L3 migrate to the proboscis of the mosquito to await transmission to another mammalian host.

The developing parasites will sensitize the host with moulting fluid, cuticular casts, secretions and excretions, while the adult parasites produce a variety of antigenic substances. These evoke cellular and immune responses in man and the range and intensity of such immunological responses are believed to contribute to the wide spectrum of clinical manifestation among endemic populations.

The living parasite evokes minimal pathological changes in the lymphatics, dilatation of the lymphatics being most commonly seen. At periodic intervals, believed to coincide with production of batches of microfilariae, antigens released may result in lymphangitis and lymphadenitis. Adult worms can survive for at least three to five years and microfilariae can remain viable for months in circulation. The ability of the parasite to evade the immune and other defence responses of the host is believed to be due to various mechanisms. Microfilaraemics respond poorly to filarial antigens and this is explained by the development of immune tolerance or specific immune suppression to microfilarial antigens in these patients.[3] A variety of worm products capable of acting as suppressor factors have also been identified.

Prenatal and neonatal exposure to soluble parasitic antigens (excretory–secretory antigens and other worm products), through the transplacental route and through breast-milk of infected mothers to offsprings,

may induce specific immune tolerance to filarial parasites and modify the outcome of subsequent infection. Transplacental infection does not occur as the development from microfilaria to the infective stage (L3) occurs only in the mosquito.

Clinical manifestations

There is a wide spectrum of clinical manifestation of the infection. It is, however, important to remember that infected persons may not have clinical evidence of the disease while those with signs and symptoms may not have demonstrable microfilaraemia. The recognized groups are microfilaraemia, chronic manifestations and occult filariasis.

Microfilaraemia, with or without evidence of acute disease

This represents the majority of infected individuals. In most studies there is a progressive increase in microfilarial rate with age in endemic areas. This is related to duration of exposure to infective mosquitoes. Although there is a slight preponderance of males over females, the difference is not statistically significant. Microfilaraemia has been detected in infants as young as 3–3.5 months in brugian filariasis. In *B. malayi* endemic areas with total microfilarial rates of 7.0–10.2 per cent, the rate in the age group 0–9 years was 3.4–5.4 per cent. In a highly endemic area for bancroftian filariasis in Irian Jaya, Indonesia, with a microfilarial rate of 29.9 per cent, the corresponding rate in the age group 0–9 years was 7.3 per cent.[4] In both bancroftian and brugian filariasis areas, rates increase from early infancy to reach a maximum in the age group 30–39 years after which the rates tend to plateau.

Many microfilaraemic children, as well as adults, are normally asymptomatic. In some, episodic attacks of lymphadenitis of the superficial lymph nodes usually at the inguinal region, together with retrograde lymphangitis, may also occur. There is associated fever, the affected limb may be inflamed and acute lymphoedema may occur, usually starting in the feet and ankles. The affected limb feels hot and tender. Cord-like thickening of the lymphatics may occur after a number of attacks. The lymphadenitis is aggravated by activity and sometimes the attack may be so severe as to confine the patient to bed. Such attacks come at variable intervals of once a month to once in three or four months. Each attack lasts for three or four days to a week. Children appear to have less frequent attacks. The acute lymphoedema usually resolves at the end of the attack with occasional peeling off of the skin of the affected limb. In bancroftian filariasis, genital involvement with acute orchitis, epidydimitis and funiculitis may occur. This is more commonly seen in adults and rarely in children. Attacks can be preceded by lower abdominal pain corresponding probably to lymphangitis and lymphadenitis of deep abdominal nodes and lymphatics. After the acute attacks, the affected part usually regresses to normal. With frequent attacks over time, the lesions (especially lymphoedema), become persistent and may progress to the next stage. Occasionally, affected lymph nodes may suppurate and ulcer formation develop.

Chronic manifestations

Chronic lymphoedema may occur after a number of acute attacks. There is thickening of the skin of the leg;

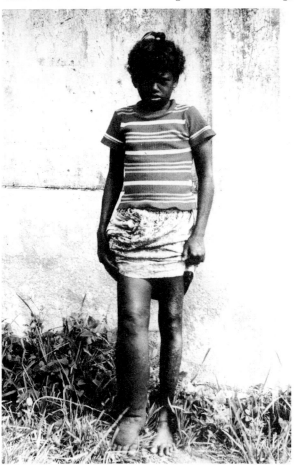

Fig. 4.13.10   Elephantiasis of the lower limb.

the lymphoedema becomes non-pitting and, in time, gross elephantiasis may occur. Chronic lesions like chronic lymphoedema and elephantiasis are less often seen in children than in adults and this is probably because progressive damage to the lymphatics may be necessary before chronic lesions can develop. Full-blown elephantiasis of the limbs has, however, been seen in children aged 10–12 years (Fig. 4.13.10). Equivalent chronic genital lesions consist of hydrocoeles and elephantiasis of the penis and scrotal sac. These are uncommon in children. Chyluria, probably due to obstruction or dysfunction of the thoracic duct and other abdominal lymphatics, is rare in children and may occur in bancroftian filariasis. Microfilariae may be detected in the chylous urine.

At the stage of elephantiasis, microfilaria are usually not detectable in the peripheral circulation.

Occult filariasis

This term is used to describe a group of filarial infections where, although microfilariae are produced, they are destroyed at various sites in the body (mainly in the lungs and spleen) through intense host immunological responses. Thus few, if any, microfilariae are demonstrable in the peripheral circulation. Within this group of patients are those that present with the syndrome known as tropical pulmonary eosinophilia. These patients have classically raised levels of eosinophils (20->50 per cent), periodic episodes of dyspnoea associated with persistent cough (usually worse at night), increased lung markings or with miliary consolidations in chest radiographs (see p. 721). Immunoglobulin levels (especially IgE) are increased. Antibody levels against homologous filarial parasites, especially against microfilarial antigens, are raised. The condition can be mistaken for bronchial asthma. Treatment with antifilarial drugs is extremely effective. Although more cases are seen in adults than in children, it is not uncommon in children.

Other forms of occult filariasis include splenomegaly with or without enlarged lymph nodes. Histologically, pools of eosinophils surrounding remnants of microfilariae in acidophilic hyaline masses can be demonstrated in the lymph nodes and other organs. These are known as Meyers–Kouwenaar bodies.

Complications

No study has been made of the adverse effect, if any, of maternal filarial infection on fetal growth and development. Lymphatic filariasis is non-fatal but infected patients, if untreated, may develop chronic lesions like elephantiasis. However, many untreated microfilarae-mics without evidence of clinical lesions do not seem to develop chronic lesions even when followed up for years. Although it appears that prolonged exposure and probably multiple infections may be necessary to induce chronic lymphoedema and elephantiasis, the role of genetic predisposition cannot be ruled out. Thus in a study of 62 elephantiasis patients and 128 controls in Sri Lanka, Singapore and Malaysia, a higher frequency of HLA-B15 was found in patients with elephantiasis.[5]

Secondary bacterial infection leading to ulcer formation is fairly common in elephantiasis. Genital elephantiasis may prevent marriage and/or inter-course. During pregnancy the lymphatic oedema may increase and vulval elephantiasis may cause problems at delivery.

In tropical pulmonary eosinophilia, failure to diagnose the condition correctly can result in undue suffering and may lead to emphysema in long-standing cases.

Diagnosis

Diagnosis of asymptomatic infection can normally be made if one is aware of the possibility of filariasis. A knowledge of where the patient comes from will indicate the possibility of filariasis. A 60 μl thick blood film should be taken for microfilaria detection after staining with Giemsa. The blood film should be obtained at night (any time after 7.00 pm) as there is a higher chance of detecting microfilariae due to the tendency of the microfilariae to peak nocturnally. If night examina-tion is not possible, DEC stimulation can be used in the day time; 100 mg DEC for those 12 years and above, and 50 mg DEC for those below 12 years should be given 30–40 minutes before blood examination in the daytime. This will stimulate the microfilariae to come out from the internal organs to the peripheral circulation.

Sometimes low-grade microfilaraemia can only be detected using concentration techniques. The Nucle-pore® membrane filtration of 1 ml of whole blood can effectively screen and detect microfilaraemia efficiently. The polycarbonate membrane (5 μm pore size, 25 mm diameter) is transparent and after filtration of the heparinized, diluted blood, can be stained and examined for parasites.

In those patients without microfilaraemia and in whom filariasis infection is suspected, serological tests to detect antibodies, like the indirect fluorescent antibody assay with sonicated microfilariae (microfila-riae broken up into tiny pieces through ultrasonic disruption), papainized microfilariae (treated with papain to expose antigenic sites) or frozen sections of adult worms of homologous parasites can be used. Titres of $\geq 1:8$ using adult worm antigen or $\geq 1:40$ using microfilaria antigens show infection. Patients with elephantiasis or occult filariasis but with active infection will have positive titres.[6]

There may be placental transfer of antibodies to the fetus.

Management

Patients with microfilaraemia should be treated with diethylcarbamazine citrate (DEC) at an oral dose of 6 mg/kg body weight daily in three divided doses for at least 14 days for *Brugia* infections and the same daily dose for 21 days for bancroftian filariasis. Reaction to the first dose can be severe in patients with high microfilaraemia. This occurs 10–12 hours after the first dose and consists of fever, nausea, joint and body aches, and rashes. These have been attributed to allergic reactions to the release of toxic-antigenic products through the destruction of microfilariae by DEC. Side-reactions can be so severe as to confine the patient to bed and normally last for 2–3 days. Few adverse reactions occur to subsequent doses of the drug. The side-reactions can be alleviated to some extent by antipyretics and antihistamines.

In some cases, inflamed nodules about 1 cm or more in diameter may occur over the site of lymph nodes or the course of the lymphatics about 7–10 days after the start of treatment. This is believed to be caused by death of adult worms. Antibiotic coverage and incision and drainage may be needed if abscess formation occurs.

It may be necessary to give more than one course (3–4 courses) of DEC to clear the microfilaraemia.

Tropical pulmonary eosinophilia should be treated with DEC at the daily oral dose of 6 mg/kg for 21 days. Patients respond very well to the drug and signs and symptoms disappear within a week. Serological monitoring of the patient would help.

Patients with acute lymphoedema and even those with elephantiasis who still have periodic episodes of adenolymphangitis should be treated with full courses of DEC. Multiple courses have to be given as it may be difficult for the drug to reach the sites of adult worms. Multiple doses given over prolonged periods at intervals of 2–3 months may bring early lymphoedema completely back to normal. Even in fairly advanced lymphoedema, multiple courses of DEC will help resolve the size of the limb and prevent further attacks of lymphangitis and lymphadenitis. Surgical interven-tion will be needed in long-standing elephantiasis to improve lymph drainage and remove excessive fibrotic tissues.

Prognosis

In patients with microfilaraemia and early signs of disease, adequate treatment with DEC will usually cure the patient and prevent the development of sequelae. DEC kills the microfilariae and all stages of the parasites in the host. More than one course may be needed. Tropical pulmonary eosinophilia can usually be cured with adequate DEC therapy. DEC therapy is not contra-indicated during pregnancy, but in view of the severe reactions which may follow DEC administration it is advisable to postpone treatment until after delivery. Side-effects can be modified by commencing treatment with fractions of the maximal dose increasing to full dosage over five to seven days and using antihistamines or corticosteroids if necessary.

Prevention and control

Protection from mosquito bites through screening of houses, use of repellants and wearing of protective clothing can minimize exposure to infection in those who visit endemic areas.

DEC at monthly doses of 5 mg/kg body weight daily for seven days kills developing parasites but may not be very practical for long-term prophylaxis.

Prevention of development of chronic sequelae is through regular examination of exposed people, followed by adequate treatment if found positive for microfilaraemia. Control programmes rely heavily on chemotherapy with DEC and to a lesser extent on vector control. DEC can be administered to endemic populations by mass chemotherapy at daily, weekly or monthly intervals or as a medicated salt. It is immaterial to the final outcome if a total dose of 36 mg/kg is given for the control of *Brugia* infection or 72 mg/kg for *W. bancrofti* infections. The objective of chemotherapy is to reduce or eliminate the source of infection for mosquitoes. Theoretically, *W. bancrofti* and periodic *B. malayi* transmission can be reduced to extremely low levels or even interrupted completely through a combination of drug administration and vector control as there are no animal reservoirs for these parasites. In contrast, in areas of subperiodic *B. malayi*, where sizeable animal reservoir hosts (leaf monkeys) exist, the control programme can only hope to reduce transmission and prevent new cases of clinical diseases.

Environmental management including provision of proper sanitation in urban areas and filling of swamps in rural areas can reduce vector breeding and contribute to effective control.

Future

A vaccine against filariasis is not feasible in the near future nor is there any work towards that end at present. A drug which is easier to administer (e.g. single dose), with less side-effects than DEC and if possible, with chemoprophylactic properties, will overcome many of the present problems in the chemotherapy and control of filariasis. A number of centres are working in collaboration with the World Health Organization towards that end.

References

1. WHO. *Lymphatic filariasis*. Fourth Report of the WHO Expert Committee on Filariasis, Technical Report Series 702. Geneva, WHO, 1984.
2. Mak JW Epidemiology of lymphatic filariasis. In: *Filariasis*. CIBA Foundation Symposium No. 127. 1987. pp. 5–14.
3. Piessiens WF, Wadee AA, Kurniawan L. Regulations of immune responses in lymphatic filariasis. In: *Filariasis*. CIBA Foundation Symposium No. 127. 1987. pp. 164–29.
4. Joesoef A, Cross JH. Distribution and prevalence of cases of microfilaraemia in Indonesia. *Southeast Asian Journal of Tropical Medicine and Public Health*. 1978; **9**: 480–8.
5. Chan SH, Dissanayake S, Mak JW *et al*. HIA and filariasis in Sri Lankans and Indians. *Southern Asian Journal of Tropical Medicine and Public Health*. 1984; **15**: 281–6.
6. Mak JW. Filariasis: diagnosis and treatment. In: Mak JW ed. *Filariasis Bulletin No. 19. Kuala Lumpur, Malaysia, Institute for Medical Research 1983*. pp. 73–81.

SECTION 5

Diseases of the Systems

Martin Brueton

CHAPTER 1

History-taking and examination

Wong Hock Boon

History-taking in paediatric patients is totally different from that in adult patients. The disease patterns are not the same, and even similar diseases seen in adults are different in children because the child is constantly developing and changing. However, the main difference is that the history is always obtained second-hand; the baby cannot talk and the young child is unable to communicate ailments accurately. Therefore, we have to rely on the parent, usually the mother. The doctor, while talking to the mother, must assess the following:

- Her general intelligence, and hence the reliability of her observations and ability to communicate them.
- Her capability as a mother and whether her history is hearsay from someone else who is closer to the baby or child, e.g. servant or foster mother. The history can therefore be third-hand rather than second-hand.
- Her psychological make-up: is she over-anxious, phlegmatic, down-to-earth, overbearing towards the child, or timid?. Only then can the credibility of the history be accurately assessed, and parental influences on the child's illness quantified.
- Her cultural and educational background, as this will 'colour' her story and attempts at self-medication, positively or negatively.
- Family size, income level and the father's occupation, since all these will have an effect on the mother's ability to take care of the child.

- The number of children she has had previously as the mother of a first child is relatively inexperienced in observation and care. Looking after too many children may also be stressful. The age of the mother is also important in this respect.

It is not difficult for the experienced doctor to 'size up' the historian, and to pick out certain aspects of the history as important, irrelevant or exaggerated, or requiring further probing.

All this can never be achieved if a rapport between the doctor and mother is not established. Most mothers are anxious when their child is ill, and therefore they need reassurance, kindness and understanding. The doctor must analyse any psychological problems which the mother may have and must talk and behave towards the mother in an appropriate manner – only then will she give a useful history. It is true that achieving rapport with people is an art. Much is dependent on the natural abilities and the upbringing of the interviewer and the interviewee, but a lot can and must be learned and practised by the doctor. The doctor's demeanour and words, should convey to the mother understanding and sympathy, and that the doctor is trying to help her because this is what she came for.

History of the present complaint

It is important to get the true sequence of events, and not what the mother considers as important. Listen to all that the mother has to say for she may have rehearsed it for hours, and cutting her off abruptly endangers rapport. Having assessed the credibility or otherwise of portions of the history, the doctor must ask leading questions. This is inevitable because the mother herself is not suffering from the illness. It is crucial to establish exactly what was observed – for example, if the mother says that the infant has had a fit, further enquiry as to its nature may reveal something totally different from a convulsion. Asking questions is an art that has to be acquired because parents frequently fail to mention certain things, e.g. knocks and falls, or bowel and bladder symptoms because they may think that they are irrelevant. The opportunity should be taken here by the doctor to 'fill in gaps' in the history. The most common 'gap' is that the mother gives the time or day of onset of an illness when the most dramatic event occurred and not necessarily the first event in a long illness. For example, the mother might say that the child had a fit at 8.00 am and was perfectly well before. Ask what the child was like at 7.00 am, the night before, the day before, several days, weeks, months before, and gradually it might transpire that the child has been drowsy on and off, with occasional vomiting for two weeks previously – a history which changes the disease-complex entirely.

History of past illness

The present problem may only be another episode of the previous illness or unconnected to any previous illness. Unless the patient is a young infant, beware of the mother who says that the child has never been ill before, which is improbable. This gives one an idea of the credibility or involvement of the historian in the child's life. Eighty per cent of all infections in children are primarily viral, and there are many viruses. Hence, there is ample opportunity for febrile episodes. Of these, pay particular attention to measles. A child is often erroneously said to contract measles five to six times because allergic rashes, German measles, exanthema subitum, exanthema infectiosum, Coxsackie virus infections, adenovirus and parainfluenza virus infection, all cause fever with rash which may be superficially indistinguishable from the rash of measles.

History of pregnancy and birth

In adults, birth has occurred a long time previously. On the other hand, the infant and child may still show the after-effects of birth, the most traumatic experience in his life so far. The following should be asked:

- Where and when was the baby born – government hospital, private hospital or home delivery? This may have a bearing on the child's condition.
- What was the baby like at birth – did he cry, was he resuscitated, was there any instrumentation, was any oxygen given, how many days did he stay in hospital, and was this on his own account or because of the mother?
- What type of birth presentation, was it – vertex, breech, Caesarean section?
- What was the pregnancy like? Ask about drugs, bleeding, toxaemia, and infection. Do not accept without question the history of the mother who says that she took no drugs during her pregnancy – many drugs and herbs may be interpreted by her as 'food'.
- What was the gestation period, and the birth weight – full-term, preterm or small-for-dates?
- What are the parity and age of mother?
- What were the amount and colour, of meconium and the day of life when passed?
- What were the first few feeds like? Was there vomiting or poor sucking?
- Was there jaundice (seen by doctor or not), and what was done – was the baby kept in hospital, given phototherapy or given exchange transfusion? Is there a family history of jaundice? What is the glucose-6-phosphate dehydrogenase (G6PD) status?
- What has the mother been told by medical and paramedical personnel?

Feeding history

Has the child been given breast-milk or fed artificially since birth? If the latter, what is the reason? The answer gives some idea of the mother's motivation and care of the baby. If artificially fed, was the baby underfed or overfed? When were solids introduced and how?

What is the child eating now? A 24-hour dietary recall from the time of history-taking is helpful. Often parents do not wish to give the impression of poverty when actually there is insufficient food to go round. Conversely, those in the higher socio-economic groups give the opposite story, that the child does not eat anything – notwithstanding this the growth is adequate. In therapeutic terms, no drug treatment is needed because often the child is obese or genetically small but healthy. So-called appetite-stimulating drugs may do harm.

Immunization history

Parents of all children attending maternal and child health clinics are given a booklet in which immunization and other health data are recorded (see p. 274). Ask for it, and you will obtain good retrospective data.

The immunization history is important because it not only indicates which infections the child is protected against but also gives an idea of the mother's own view on immunization procedures and her compliance. The history of immunization may be extended back to the mother's pregnancy. Was she immunized against tetanus and how many times? This will also suggest the care given during the antenatal period.

Family history

Construct a family diagram (see Fig. 5.1.1), as it fixes in the mind, who is who, and suffering from what, and is a reminder that many diseases have a genetic component. The arrow in the figure refers to the propositus, i.e. the child who is ill. Arabic numerals refer to every member of each generation. In this way, all relevant family members are clearly identified for the doctor and also for others. Consanguinity is easily seen. If similar symptoms, especially if suggestive of a genetic disorder, have occurred in other family members they can be marked in on the family tree.

The paediatrician should not only treat the proposi-

tus but should use the consultation to advise other members of the family.

One must recognize that some parents try to suppress information. Thus, the doctor must be tactful in eliciting the relevant information, e.g. whether the child is adopted or not, or whether there is consanguinity, as cousin–cousin, uncle–niece marriages are not uncommon amongst the certain ethnic groups.

Social history

This is very important and not only in terms of income and occupation – there are many other factors which have a bearing on the child:

- Whether both parents are with the child.
- The psychological 'make-up' of the husband and wife.
- Who has a dominant role in decision making and in the upbringing of the child, providing income and psychological stability.
- Servants and foster parent's role in the upbringing of the child. The amount of time, and what is more important, the amount of relevant involvement of the father and mother in the child's development.
- Ideas about rearing children, bearing in mind the relevance of this to disease processes in the child.
- In-laws and the part played by them in the social setting of the child.
- The amount and degree of husband/wife involvement in their careers relative to their involvement in the child's upbringing.
- Any strained relations between the husband and wife, whether with regard to child-rearing, or beyond that. Often these sensitive matters only reveal themselves after several consultations.
- Are the parents separated or divorced and what have been the effects on the child?
- The views of the parents on diseases and their attitudes towards medicines.
- The educational and cultural background will clearly have a major influence on their behaviour.
- If the child is older, how does the child 'fit' in socially? In psychological problems, it is often revealing to ask for the child's views of the whole situation.

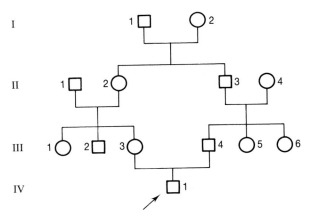

Fig. 5.1.1   A family or pedigree diagram is extremely useful in assessing genetic and environmental influences on the illness of the child (the propositus marked by the arrow). I–IV refer to generations; 1–4, etc. refer to members in each generation. Squares = males; circles = females.

Clinical examination

The clinical examination of an infant or child is much more difficult than that conducted on a cooperative adult. Hence, the doctor will have to modify the method and philosophy of clinical examination extensively.

When the parent brings the baby or child to the doctor, the doctor will have to observe the child's behaviour carefully, noting whether there is stranger anxiety or not, the relationships between parents and child, whether the child clings to the parent, and the behaviour of parent to child.

The next aspect of the examination is to assess the weight, height (length) and circumference of the skull – measurements which should have been taken before the clinical examination itself. These measurements are evaluated by local growth charts to see whether each parameter is too small or too large, e.g. the child may have a problem of poor weight gain, or short stature, hydrocephalus or microcephaly.

The next stage is a more detailed inspection of the patient. This is a much more important aspect of the clinical examination in paediatric patients than in adults and the child may be carried in the mother's arms or if cooperative, may actually lie on the couch for the examination. All the systems of the body are subjected to this inspection routine. For example, is the child in distress; is he breathless and if so, is the respiration shallow or deep; is he cyanosed, pale, or jaundiced? In dark-skinned children pallor is best seen in the tongue, inside the lips and on the gums; jaundice is readily noticed in the sclera. Is the skin normal, hyperpigmented or hypopigmented, or are there some blemishes and if so what is the type (white achromic patches, café-au-lait spots, rough ichthyotic areas, psoriatic scales, or 'flaky paint' appearance); is there excess or inadequate hair, is it brittle or hypochromic; what is the colour of the eyes, is there any heterochromia of the iris, any squint or pupillary abnormalities; are there other dysmorphic features affecting the facies, ears, mouth, lips, chin or head shape? The motor movements of the limbs are observed closely for generalized or localized weakness, wasting or incoordination, noting whether there are abnormalities in the bones, joints, hands and feet, or limb length. Abdominal movements with respiration are also observed, noting whether the abdomen is distended or not, and whether there are umbilical anomalies such as a hernia, exomphalos, secretions or bleeding. The genitalia must also be inspected.

Thus, the stage is reached when information from the history and inspection may often suggest the organ system which is involved. It is best to commence the examination of this system first and when this is completed the other systems are examined. It must be realized that the body systems are never isolated from each other. Thus, the clinical examination is not complete until the whole body is examined. It is at this

moment, that the doctor realizes that often the success or failure of the examination depends on an ability to elicit rapport with the child. It is seldom that a child is not terrified by a visit to a doctor. Such fears are natural, as a result of stranger anxiety or stressful memories of injections, operations, investigations, or separation from parents. Establishment of rapport is a learned art and takes many years of practice to achieve. Certainly, rattles, dolls and toys do help, but it is more the way the doctor speaks to the parent and speaks to the child, and the doctor's reaction to the reactions of the parent and the child which most affect cooperation. Patience and understanding of human nature of both adults (the parents) and children are essential in achieving rapport. All examination manoeuvres should be carried out painlessly and with understanding so that manoeuvres needing stressful reactions like examination of the throat with a spatula or elicitation of deep reflexes with a hammer or fundoscopy, can be performed last, lest cooperation of the child is lost early in the examination process. With practice, it is possible to inspect the throat of a crying infant or cooperative child without resorting to the use of a spatula.

The next stage is the clinical examination of the different sites and systems.

Cardiovascular system

After initial inspection, the peripheral pulses are examined. In infants, the brachial arteries are more easily felt than the radial arteries. The femoral pulses should also be palpated and if they cannot be felt or if there is femoral–radial delay, the possibility of coarctation of the aorta should be considered. With practice a bounding pulse in an infant with a patent ductus arteriosus is easily recognized.

The neck is examined for presence or absence of Corrigan's pulse, raised jugular venous pressure, or a goitre. The neck is palpated for thrills in the various areas and auscultated for murmurs. Although the presence of systolic murmurs in the neck may indicate the possibility of aortic stenosis, in infants and children, even a ventricular septal defect and pulmonary stenosis can produce systolic murmurs over the carotid arteries.

The precordium is examined in a systematic manner. It is inspected for shape and if there is a precordial bulge, there may by right ventricular hypertrophy. However, before this is concluded, it is important to exclude thoracic skeletal deformities or scoliosis. The apex beat and cardiac impulse in the precordial and epigastric areas are inspected and palpated. Thrills, the nature of any pulsations, diastolic shock in the pulmonary area or a loud first heart sound in the mitral area can all be elicited by palpation. The medical student and doctor should always analyse the cardiac findings and hazard a probable diagnosis on the basis of history, inspection and palpation before auscultation. This exercise will sharpen the doctor's clinical skills and teach him to evaluate auscultatory findings more effectively.

Finally, assessment of cardiac failure should specifically include pulmonary findings, raised jugular venous pressure, hepatomegaly, cardiac enlargement and the presence of oedema. The blood pressure should be measured using a correctly sized cuff covering two-thirds of the upper arm.

Respiratory system

In infants and children, one of the most common causes of death in the developed world or developing world is lung infection. Many of the causative organisms are viruses. Hence, examination of the respiratory tract and the lungs are important and more so in areas of the world where radiological facilities are absent or minimal. Inspection will reveal dyspnoea, cyanosis, abnormal shape of the thorax, unequal respiratory excursions; a retraction of the intercostal spaces and suprasternal area. The ears, nose and throat must also be examined carefully. In newborns, especially the preterm, chest retractions and grunting may point to respiratory distress syndrome, diaphragmatic hernia, choanal atresia or problems arising from congenital cardiac lesions.

Palpation for tracheal position, lung expansion and vocal fremitus are useful. Because of the thin chest wall, mediated percussion is usually too forceful and too insensitive to detect changes in percussion note. Direct percussion with the fingers using finger pad or using the whole index finger propped on to the third finger and flicking the index finger on to the chest wall, are sensitive methods of direct percussion. With practice, the doctor can assess the sound as well as the resistance the finger meets with the chest wall in determining different grades of impairment to direct percussion.

Auscultation in infants and children is not as rewarding as in adults who can breathe deeply on demand. However, the infant or child who is crying may also provide useful information on auscultation and with practice, the doctor can separate the crying sound from the breath sounds. Of course, crying is an added advantage for the detection of increased vocal fremitus or stridor or other voice changes, from upper respiratory tract pathology.

Finally, in areas where radiology is not easily available, in infants with a pneumothorax or pleural effusion, the diagnosis can be confirmed by using a strong torch for transillumination of the chest wall.

Abdomen

The newborn infant has a more prominent abdomen than the older child because of the large liver. Hence, the size of the abdomen varies in relation to the body, depending on the age of the infant or child. A scaphoid small abdomen in the newborn may indicate the presence of a diaphragmatic hernia or postmaturity with passage of meconium. Therefore, inspection of the abdomen can yield a lot of information; masses can be seen, gaseous distension due to malabsorption, or aerophagy noted, or fullness in the flanks suggesting ascites. Inflammation, especially of the appendix, changes the movement of the abdominal wall during breathing.

Palpation of the abdomen in an infant or uncooperative child is an art which must be learned by practice. The infant or uncooperative child invariably cries on abdominal palpation, and this crying must be accompanied by abdominal wall excursions due to diaphragmatic contraction and relaxation. The doctor will thus have to vary the depth and force of the palpating hand to coincide with these excursions. For example, if the doctor is palpating for a possible enlarged spleen, he places his hand over the left hypochondrium and when the child takes a breath before the next cry, reduces the pressure of his hand which will then be poised to feel the spleen. The liver and the kidneys can also be palpated in this way. Right iliac fossa palpation for possible appendicitis in an anxious and fearful child can be effectively done by sitting beside the child and the hand placed over the left iliac fossa and then over the right iliac fossa. No pressure is exerted by the examiner's hand but with the cooperative child's breathing or with an uncooperative child's crying, the abdominal wall 'hits' the palpating hand, which then compares the rigidity of the two sides. These are some of the ways whereby the doctor can examine the abdomen without any cooperation from the child. When examining the liver, the distance of the edge of the liver from the thoracic cage is not necessarily an accurate assessment of liver size because the liver can be pushed down by the diaphragm. Hence, percussion of the upper border of the liver will give a better idea of liver size by assessing the liver span. Inspection by stooping down and observing the anterior surface of the liver tangentially will also tell the observer whether the liver is indeed enlarged in an antero-posterior direction.

Especially useful is percussion of the left lower thorax

for the spleen, as the spleen may be enlarged and yet not palpable. Impairment of percussion note in that area may indicate that the spleen is enlarged. Similarly, percussion is useful in delineating liver size, presence or absence of a distended bladder in the suprapubic area, and so on.

Examination of the abdomen should include examination of the umbilicus whether it is wet, whether there is bleeding, its shape, as well as examination of the hernial orifices, lymph nodes and external genitalia. The latter must always be examined carefully in infants and children to exclude possible intersex states, labial adhesions, hypospadias, hydrocoele, cryptorchidism, and signs of puberty. Auscultation to note the presence and character of the bowel sounds should not be forgotten. Inspection of the anus may show fissures, skin tags or excoriation, insertion of the finger tip will reveal stenosis and abnormalities of muscle tone.

Nervous system

Much information can be gleaned about the nervous system by observation of the infant or child, noting the state of consciousness, the degree of responsiveness or rapport appropriate for the age, and the level of social and motor skills attained. Motor power is assessed by movements of the face in crying and of the limbs in clinging to the parent, walking or running. Tone can be assessed by the posture of the limbs when lying supine.

Many of the cranial nerves can be examined by inspection with few manoeuvres. Cranial nerves II, III, IV and VI can be assessed by examining the eyelids (ptosis), pupils (size, shape, reaction to light), and eye movements. The Vth nerve can be examined by blowing on the cornea and observing mouth movements. The integrity of the VIIth nerve can be tested by observing eye closure, the length of eyelashes when eyes are closed and the naso-labial grooves when crying. Nerve VIII can be assessed roughly by response to sound. Nerves IX and X can be assessed by looking into the palate of a crying infant or child. Nerve XII can be tested by inspection of tongue movements.

The tendon and superficial reflexes can be tested in the usual manner, but sensation should be tested last, as elicitation of pain responses invariably produces a crying response.

Examination of the fundus can often be achieved but in some situations a comprehensive view will require the child to be sedated, the pupils dilated with mydriatics and the procedure carried out in a darkened room.

There are other specific signs of neurological disease which can be observed or tested for, such as fits, neck stiffness and other meningeal signs, ataxia, nystagmus and the presence of clonus or involuntary movements.

Conclusion

History-taking in the real situation of much Third World practice has to be adapted to fit into the available time. With careful practical experience, the judicious, use of leading questions, 'programmed' assessment of the witness as the history-taking proceeds, consideration of the present illness in the context of previous illnesses, the birth history, feeding, immunization, family and social history can all be compacted into a very short time. If this proves impossible, it is often necessary to postpone a particularly difficult child to the end of the clinic or some other special time, especially if there is a considerable social or emotional element in the case. Whatever the problem, at the completion of the history the doctor must be able to put forward one clinical diagnosis or a few differential diagnoses (Fig. 5.1.2).

The next step is to score the differential diagnoses as possible probabilities. A maximum score of 5 is used for a definite diagnosis, with the others in descending order. During the learning stage, this is essential for practice and discipline, and later, all this may be automatically 'programmed' in the mind.

The importance of this exercise is that:

- It alerts the doctor to pay particular attention to certain aspects of the clinical and physical examina-

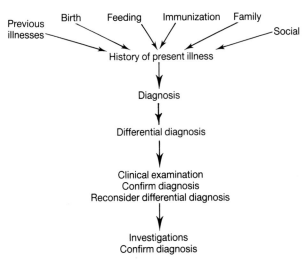

Fig. 5.1.2 Analysis of the process of diagnostic decision making.

tion, which may otherwise be missed, e.g. if tuberous sclerosis is one of the differential diagnoses, it alerts the doctor to look at the fundi for phakomas and the skin for achromic spots, even if both fundi and skin are examined as part of a full clinical examination – 'What you do not expect, you will miss'.

- As a result of the full and 'directed' physical examination, the next stage in diagnosis is reached, when the differential diagnosis is re-scored, confirmed, and new differential diagnoses brought in.

When developed fully as a complete art, the history probably plays an 80–90 per cent part in obtaining the correct diagnosis; physical examination and investigations form 10–20 per cent.

The third stage in diagnostic decision making is the selection of those investigations which are:

- Simple and can be carried out at dispensary and health centre level, e.g. urine testing, a peripheral blood film, stool examination, simple skin and mucosal scraping for microscope examination, bacterial staining and examination of relevant biological fluids, sputum examination, and blood films for malaria parasites (see pp. 974–84).
- Inexpensive but which can only be done at hospital level, such as X-rays and electrolytes.
- Relevant. This can be decided only if the doctor has gone through the process of history-taking and analysis, physical examination and re-analysis. The lazy habit of doing a whole series of 'routine' investigations is like throwing a net and seeing what fish (if any) are landed. After some time, this process 'atrophies' the brain.
- Non-invasive. This is simple to decide, by considering that if the doctor is put into the patient's place, but with his specialized knowledge, would he want the contemplated test to be carried out on himself under the circumstances? If the answer is 'No', surely, it is the same answer for the patient. This is the principle of role reversal which all doctors should practise.

CHAPTER 2

Diseases of the respiratory system

J.K.G. Webb

Acute infections of the respiratory tract (ARI) are the most common form of disease in children throughout the world. Most are mild and self-limiting, but in developing countries the minority which are serious and life-threatening constitute the third most important cause of deaths in children, after malnutrition and diarrhoea. In a 1986 review of available data, Leowski estimated the annual deaths from ARI in children under five years to be about 4 million.[1] This appalling wastage has been recognized by WHO and increasingly by individual countries as a challenge calling for a concerted strategy, with the integration of management at all levels of health services.

These considerations have dictated the organization of material in this chapter on respiratory disease. ARI have been described in much greater detail than other respiratory disorders. One section of the chapter focuses on the management of ARI in the context of primary health care.

Acute respiratory infections (ARI)

Some general considerations

Respiratory disease is marked by a limited range of symptoms and signs, most of which can occur with many different disorders. Cough, for example, is a prominent symptom in upper respiratory tract infections (URTI), allergic rhinitis and asthma, laryngitis (croup), bronchitis, bronchiolitis and pneumonia, bronchiectasis and parasitic infections. Cough is thus an important symptom of respiratory disease, but is of no great value in differential diagnosis. Nevertheless, by careful attention to all signs and symptoms through a history taken from the mother (or older children) and by meticulous observation of the patient, a working diagnosis can be made in most cases, even before more specialized investigation. Certainly history and observation are far more informative than the stethoscope.

Important symptoms and signs

- Cough – character, timing, associated factors, provoking factors, and whether productive or non-productive of sputum.
- Sputum – quantity, character, mucoid, purulent, or blood-stained.
- Stertor – a 'snoring' sound produced in both inspiration and expiration from the posterior pharynx.
- Stridor – a harsh, crowing vocal sound produced in the region of the larynx or trachea during inspiration. It may also occur in expiration when there is external compression of the airways.
- Wheeze – a long musical sound produced in the chest during expiration which may be prolonged and accompanied by unusual effort.
- Tachypnoea – quick breathing. The normal respiration rate at rest is about 30 per minute in infancy, decreasing through childhood to 20 per minute in the adult.
- Recession – indrawing of the intercostal spaces, supraclavicular fossae and the lower chest wall along the line of insertion of the diaphragm during inspiration.
- Cyanosis – a dusky bluish colour replacing the normal pink or red seen in the cheeks, lips, conjunctivae, tongue, buccal mucosa and palms of the hands. It is recognizable when the reduced (unoxygenated) haemoglobin in the blood exceeds 5 g/dl. It is therefore less readily apparent in the presence of anaemia.

All the above signs and symptoms can be recognized by health auxiliaries and careful training should enable them to understand their significance.

Other signs which are important but more difficult to recognize include:

- asymmetry of the chest, and of chest movements;
- deviation of the trachea from the mid-line;
- displacement of apex beat, and cardiac dullness as evidence of mediastinal shift;

and the whole range of more subtle signs which may be elicited by percussion and auscultation.

Classification of ARI

The respiratory tract is a continuous mucosal surface comprising:

- nose and paranasal sinuses, mouth, tonsils and pharynx, eustachian tubes and middle ear; these together comprise the upper respiratory tract (URT);
- larynx, with adjacent supraglottic region, including the epiglottis;
- trachea and bronchi;
- bronchioles;
- alveoli and lung parenchyma.

This mucosal surface is constantly exposed to invasion, or colonization, by a large range of viruses or bacteria, any one of which is capable of producing inflammation and disease at any level. Because there is no sharp line of demarcation or barrier between different levels of the tract, disease is not necessarily restricted to a single level. Nevertheless, infections tend to conform to consistent patterns which favour a classification of diseases on the broad anatomical basis indicated above.

ARI: Hospital presentation

In this section the various disease categories are described as they present, and can be investigated and treated in a well-equipped hospital.

Aetiology

During the past 30 years the aetiology of ARI in children has been intensively investigated in developed countries. These investigations have focussed on hospital patients and community populations, and have included cross-sectional, longitudinal and cohort studies. Bacteriological techniques have identified *Streptococcus pneumoniae* and *Haemophilus influenzae* as the main bacterial pathogens, with *Staphylococcus aureus*, haemolytic streptococci and enteric bacilli as less frequently involved. These bacteria are frequently carried in the nose or throat: their presence, in contrast with viruses, does not necessarily imply a pathogenic role. Virus isolation techniques using primary and continuous epithelial and fibroblast cell cultures, the identification of viruses in naso-pharyngeal secretions by immunofluorescence, and various serological techniques including the enzyme-linked immunosorbent assay (ELISA), have clarified the predominant role of viruses in childhood ARI in developed countries. The viruses mainly involved are the respiratory syncytial virus (RSV), adenoviruses, the influenza A and B viruses, parainfluenza viruses, rhinoviruses and coronaviruses. *Mycoplasma pneumoniae* is also important. Most of these viruses are associated with all categories of ARI, from URTI to pneumonia. However, certain agents are particularly associated with certain categories, examples being RSV with seasonal epidemics of infantile bronchiolitis, and the parainfluenza viruses with croup. Although bacteria remain an important cause of childhood pneumonia in developed countries, most pneumonias are caused by a virus. Evidence is accumulating that bacteria are a relatively more important cause of pneumonia in developing countries. Recent studies suggest that *Pneumocystis carinii* and *Chlamydia trachomatis* may also be important.

Upper respiratory tract infections

URTI include the common cold, otitis media, pharyngitis and tonsillitis. These together constitute the most common forms of childhood illnesses. Limited data from longitudinal community studies indicate an incidence in urban populations in both developed and developing countries of five to eight episodes of URTI annually. In rural populations the incidence is lower, averaging one to three episodes a year.

The common cold (coryza)

This presents with nasal irritation, sneezing, nasal discharge which is mucoid at first, later muco-purulent, nasal obstruction, and to a variable extent sore throat with redness and swelling of the fauces, tonsils and pharynx. Systemic upset ranges from negligible to moderate malaise, irritability and fever. In the vast majority of cases, symptoms subside spontaneously over 7–10 days; however, occasionally they may be the prodrome of a number of infections, such as whooping cough, measles and bronchiolitis. Causative agents include the whole range of respiratory viruses, many enteroviruses, and *Herpes virus hominis*. Except for haemolytic streptococci which can cause coryza in infants, the role of bacteria is probably always secondary, pneumococci and *H. influenzae* particularly contributing to the purulent nasal discharge present in the later stages of the infection.

Treatment is unnecessary in most cases. If fever and irritability are a problem, paracetamol (60–120 mg for infants; 120–250 mg for 1–5 years; 250–500 mg for > 5 years, repeated 4–6 hourly) can be helpful. If nasal obstruction in an infant is causing feeding difficulty, the nose should be cleared before feeds, by suction, or with twists of cotton wool, or cloth twisted into a wick. The usefulness of decongestant nasal drops (e.g. 0.5 per cent ephedrine in normal saline) is uncertain; they are not recommended by WHO. Antibiotics make no contribution to recovery in the vast majority of cases. However, in a minority, purulent discharge may persist,

suggesting secondary bacterial infection, with possible involvement of paranasal sinuses. Treatment with an antibiotic may then be indicated; procaine penicillin, ampicillin, amoxycillin or cotrimoxazole are likely to be appropriate but if bacteriology is available this can be confirmed by culture and sensitivities.

Otitis media

A mild infection of the middle ear requiring no specific management occurs in the course of many upper respiratory virus infections. More serious infections may develop in the course of a coryza, or as an isolated process.

Such middle ear infections are extremely common, and in developing countries tend to be overlooked. One survey of rural school-age children in India found 13–20 per cent suppurative otitis media (OM). Impaired hearing was found in 5–8 per cent of schoolchildren, nearly half of the deafness being secondary to OM.[2]

Pain is the main symptom described by the older child. But in infants, the age group most prone to OM, symptoms are non-specific. Irritability, restlessness, bouts of screaming, anorexia, vomiting, fever, occasionally with convulsions, are all characteristic features. Rarely, OM presents as unexplained fever with no pain or local symptoms.

Diagnosis depends on seeing and recognizing the changes in the ear drums. Visualization of the drums is thus an essential part of the examination of all sick children. The changes are, progressively, loss of light reflex, diffuse redness, bulging with disappearance of bony landmarks, and perforation with muco-purulent discharge.

Frank OM must be assumed to be bacterial in origin. *Strep. pneumoniae* and *H. influenzae* are the most common pathogens, and treatment with an appropriate antibiotic is currently favoured. Procaine penicillin, ampicillin, amoxycillin or cotrimoxazole are all likely to be effective, and should be given for five to ten days. If discharge occurs, the external auditory meatus (EAM) must be kept clear, and as far as possible dry, by suction and/or careful mopping with dry cotton swabs. A sodden EAM is liable to secondary infection with *Pseudomonas aeruginosa* and other bacteria, and healing becomes more difficult.

This conventional view of management has been questioned. A large trial in general practice in Europe found that more than 90 per cent of frank OM in children aged 2–12 years resolved completely within two weeks without antibiotic, only analgesics and ear drops being used.[3] If it can be shown that antibiotics contribute only marginally to the resolution of OM, this would allow the lower cost management important to Third World health budgets. However, until the long-term effects of withholding antibiotics have been established, particularly on hearing and the incidence of recurrent or chronic discharge, treatment of OM with antibiotics is to be preferred.

Pharyngitis and tonsillitis

In the most common form of tonsillo-pharyngitis, sore throat and dysphagia are the main symptoms. The usual signs are diffuse redness and slight swelling of palate, fauces and tonsils; tonsillar exudate and swelling and tenderness of tonsillar and upper cervical lymph nodes may or may not be present. Tonsillo-pharyngitis may occur on its own, or as part of a diffuse URTI along with coryza and cough.

This clinical picture may be caused by many of the respiratory viruses or the respiratory bacterial pathogens, particularly Group A streptococci. Bacterial and viral infections cannot be certainly differentiated on clinical grounds, although a fiery red mucosa with tonsillar exudate, lymphadenopathy and fever would favour a streptococcal infection. Some hospital studies suggest a streptococcal aetiology in 10–20 per cent of cases of acute pharyngitis. A point prevalence of 4 per cent for streptococcal pharyngitis was found in one study of schoolchildren in rural communities in South India, with an annual incidence of acute rheumatic fever of 1.6–1.7 per 1000, and a prevalence of 5 per 1000.[2] In the urban environment of Kampala, Uganda, 40 per cent of 82 infants had ASO titres of greater than 1 in 200 with 16 per cent greater than 1 in 400.[4]

Tonsillo-pharyngitis usually resolves spontaneously in the course of about a week. Rare complications are peritonsillar cellulitis (quinsy) and, in older children particularly, the late sequelae of streptococcal infection, glomerulo-nephritis and acute rheumatism. By the time infection with a nephritogenic strain of streptococcus can be recognized, the stage is set and treatment probably does not prevent the development of nephritis. However, to reduce the risk of the other complications, and also the period of infectivity, antibiotic treatment of streptococcal infections is recommended. The difficulty is to differentiate the streptococcal from the more frequent viral infections. Microbiological studies can help in individual cases and in epidemics, but most often management must be decided on clinical grounds.

A reasonable plan is to treat most cases supportively, e.g. with paracetamol, reserving penicillin for children under five years who have pharyngeal exudate and lymphadenopathy, and older children with lympha-denopathy with or without exudate. To eradicate a streptococcal infection, penicillin needs to be given as one intramuscular injection of benzathine penicillin, or ten days of procaine penicillin or penicillin V.

Other forms of pharyngitis occur less commonly. Shallow pale-based ulcers 2–4 mm in diameter with surrounding erythema scattered over the fauces, palate and buccal mucosa are characteristic of infection with Coxsackie A virus (herpangina); this usually causes significant systemic upset with fever and malaise lasting several days, but is self-limiting.

Similar shallow ulcers may be caused by infection with Herpes simplex. In a primary herpetic infection, ulceration may be extensive over the buccal mucosa and gums, causing local pain and dysphagia with regional lymphadenopathy, and accompanied by fever and malaise. In a secondary infection, ulceration is more localized with relatively little systemic upset. Resolution occurs spontaneously in 7–10 days; treatment is symptomatic. Topical treatment with one of the antiviral agents, idoxuridine or acyclovir may help resolution, but these are expensive and of only marginal value.

Buccal ulceration may also be due to Vincent's infection. In this, there is typically a gingivitis with erosion of gum margins, the ulcers are deeper and contain grey slough, and there is a characteristic sour foetor oris. Diagnosis can be readily confirmed by identification of the bacilli *Fusiformis fusiformis* in a Gram-stained film. This infection responds readily to penicillin but in the malnourished child it can progress with frightening rapidity to local gangrene and potentially extensive tissue destruction (noma; cancrum oris). In such cases, the immediate correction of anaemia by transfusion and of malnutrition is essential.

Ulcerative and exudative tonsillo-pharyngitis must be very carefully differentiated from membranous infections. Membrane is likely to be more firmly adherent to the underlying tissue; it may be localized to one or both tonsils, extend from a tonsil on to the fauces, or be confined to the fauces, palate or pharynx. Membrane signifies diphtheria and ordinarily requires immediate treatment with antitoxin. The anginose form of infectious mononucleosis is characterized by membrane clinically indistinguishable from diphtheritic, but diagnosis is possible on the basis of other clinical and haematological criteria.

Croup

Croup is the term used for acute inflammation in the region of the larynx or trachea. This causes upper airway obstruction, of which the characteristic signs are inspiratory stridor and a hoarse resonating sound heard with coughing or crying. Croup occurs most frequently between 18 months and 4 years of age. It embraces a spectrum of conditions which can be conveniently considered in three categories: laryngitis, laryngo-tracheo-bronchitis, and acute epiglottitis.

Laryngitis

The majority of children who present with inspiratory stridor are experiencing an acute non-suppurative infection in the region of the larynx. This produces inflammatory swelling of the true cords, and of the subglottic and less frequently the supraglottic regions. It is caused by one of the respiratory viruses, especially one of the parainfluenza group (see also p. 618). The illness usually begins as a typical URTI with coryza, the characteristic laryngeal signs appearing after a day or two. Less often, inspiratory laryngeal stridor is the first sign of illness. Fever and systemic upset are usually modest and it is the degree of respiratory obstruction that determines the severity of the illness. The loudness of the stridor is no guide to severity; dramatic respiratory noises may be tolerated by some children with nonchalance. When laryngeal obstruction is significant, breathing becomes progressively more arduous, the accessory respiratory muscles are called into play, and striking supraclavicular, intercostal and lower costal recession occur with every inspiration. The severity of inspiratory recession is the critical sign to watch. If inspiratory effort fails to match demand, hypoxia develops, the child becomes increasingly restless and anxious, and finally cyanosis appears. Signs in the lungs are usually limited to the stridor and some diminution of air entry. A chest radiograph is usually normal.

In the great majority of cases, the process resolves spontaneously over a period ranging from a few days to two weeks.

Laryngo-tracheo-bronchitis

The term laryngo-tracheo-bronchitis is reserved for those cases of croup in which the inflammatory process involves the trachea and bronchi as well as the larynx, and where bronchial secretions or exudate are the major cause of respiratory obstruction. Most cases are probably initiated by one of the respiratory viruses, measles being important in some countries. Bacteria, particularly *Strep. pneumoniae* and *Staph. aureus*, appear to play a more important role in developing countries than in developed.

Children with laryngo-tracheo-bronchitis tend to be more seriously ill than those with laryngitis. High fever, and prostration commonly develop, with marked signs of respiratory obstruction and persistent cough which is ineffective in clearing secretions. Clinical and radiological signs of segmental collapse and consolidation related to bronchial occlusion are usual. The course is prolonged, the restoration of normal bronchial mucosa being likely to take several weeks.

Acute epiglottitis

This relatively uncommon form of croup is a fulminating cellulitis involving the supraglottic region and epiglottis caused by an *H. influenzae* type b. The clinical picture is distinctive. Onset is abrupt with high fever, sore throat, hoarseness and cough, increasing respiratory obstruction and prostration, all developing over a few hours. The child characteristically sits silent and anxious, leaning forward, with mouth open, saliva drooling, and straining to breathe.

Because the inflammatory swelling is so severe and progresses so rapidly, throat examination at any stage may exacerbate the respiratory obstruction, even fatally. The diagnosis must be suspected on the basis of history and general observation. Local examination must be delayed until preparations for tracheal intubation or tracheostomy have been made.

Diagnosis can be confirmed by direct laryngoscopy which will reveal the bright red swollen epiglottis and supraglottic oedema and by laryngeal swab and blood cultures which are likely to be positive for *H. influenzae* type b, and by a polymorph leucocytosis. All these tests should be undertaken only during the anaesthesia required to establish the airway. A lateral radiograph of the neck will demonstrate obliteration of the airway but the marginal contribution this makes to diagnosis does not justify the disturbance involved for the child.

Differential diagnosis

The differential diagnosis of the three categories of croup depends essentially on careful clinical observation of the particular features already described. Bacteriology is helpful in epiglottitis, but only retrospectively. Virology is helpful to understanding, but relevant to management only if rapid diagnosis by the direct fluorescent antibody technique is available.

Other conditions which may cause laryngeal stridor of sudden onset include laryngeal diphtheria, the laryngospasm of tetany, a foreign body in the larynx or trachea, and a retro-pharyngeal abscess. All these can be recognized by careful attention to the history and mode of onset and the associated clinical findings and

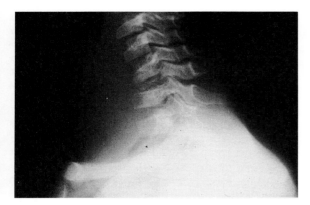

Fig. 5.2.1 Retropharyngeal abscess causing anterior displacement and narrowing of the trachea.

local signs, supported by bacteriology (for diphtheria), blood chemistry (a low serum calcium in tetany) and radiographs of epiphyses for rickets and a lateral of the neck for retro-pharyngeal abscess (Fig. 5.2.1).

Management

In all forms of croup, the primary concern in management is the maintenance of a clear airway. However, the rapidity with which life-threatening respiratory obstruction may develop varies between the three categories and broad management guide-lines differ accordingly.

In simple viral croup, an adequate airway is usually maintained without intervention. Supportive therapy includes quiet reassurance to calm anxiety, nursing in a comfortable upright position, humidifying the inspired air (by humidifier, or steam-kettle), and encouraging drinking to maintain hydration. While stridor is present, regular responsible observation must be maintained so that increasing respiratory difficulty and chest recession will be recognized early and endotracheal intubation performed as early as may be necessary.

In laryngo-tracheo-bronchitis, once respiratory difficulty develops, tracheostomy is likely to be necessary to allow the efficient clearing of bronchial secretions and exudate by regular aspiration. If the secretions are purulent, a bacterial role should be assumed. The choice of antibiotic can be determined by culture of secretions with sensitivities, but treatment should be started without delay with an antibiotic effective against *Strep. pneumoniae*, *H. influenzae* and *Staph. aureas*, e.g. cotrimoxazole, amoxycillin or chloramphenicol.

If epiglottitis is suspected then intubation or tra-

cheostomy are almost certain to be necessary; and the sooner this is performed the better. This is a difficult procedure and should be undertaken by the most skilled operator available, ideally a paediatric anaesthetist. Under anaesthetic, the necessary examination and tests can be carried out and endotracheal intubation performed. Infection with *H. influenzae* should be assumed while awaiting bacteriological confirmation, and treatment started at once with chloramphenicol intravenously or intramuscularly 100 mg/kg in 24 hours, divided into four doses.

Children with a tracheostomy or endotracheal tube are best nursed, initially at least, in a special unit where all staff are thoroughly familiar with the techniques of maintenance and the management of extubation. Apart from this, no special measures are required beyond good general nursing and the maintenance of hydration either intravenously or by naso-gastric tube if drinking is difficult. Recovery from epiglottitis can be expected within a few days, but is likely to be slower in tracheobronchitis.

Acute bronchitis

Within the spectrum of ARI of childhood, cases occur in which there is evidence of involvement of the bronchi but not of the larynx, bronchioles or lung parenchyma. Such cases fall into the diagnostic category of acute bronchitis but they are a heterogeneous group lacking the distinct clinical profile of croup or bronchiolitis. The cause may be any of the respiratory viruses, with a variable secondary role by bacteria.

The most prominent symptom of bronchitis is a harsh barking cough. This may be the first symptom of illness, or may develop in what begins as typical URTI. Systemic upset and fever vary from mild to severe. The course is variable. The cough may become loose with the production of sputum which may become purulent. Lung signs will be restricted to rhonchi and crepitations, with no evidence of air-trapping or consolidation. A chest radiograph may show signs of bronchial thickening but none of consolidation or collapse.

This clinical picture is relatively uncommon in healthy children but more likely to occur in those who are debilitated by anaemia, malnutrition or other chronic diseases. In typhoid, a bronchitic cough may develop during the second week of a gradually escalating fever. In the basically healthy child, the illness is likely to resolve spontaneously; a simple linctus or a mixture based on ammonium chloride may be good for morale. If cough with purulent sputum persists, possible complicating factors should be considered (see pp. 719–20). A chronic bacterial infection may be res-

chronic bacterial infection may be responsible. If several sputum cultures are positive with the same predominant organisms consistently present, a prolonged course of antibiotic chosen to match the sensitivities of the organisms cultured may be of value. Physiotherapy with postural coughing may be helpful. Other conditions which may contribute to the continuation of infection include protein–energy malnutrition, anaemia, and various chronic debilitating diseases. Correction of these if present may be more important than treatment aimed specifically at the bronchial infection.

Acute bronchiolitis

Acute bronchiolitis is a disease of infancy caused by infection with a respiratory virus, and distinguished by an inflammatory reaction in the walls of the bronchioles and the peribronchiolar tissues, the alveolar walls and spaces being spared. Plugging of the lumen of bronchioles by inflammatory exudate gives rise to obstruction of the lower airways which is responsible for the distinctive features of the illness.

Aetiology

Although almost all the respiratory viruses may cause bronchiolitis, the winter epidemics which occur annually in the conurbations of Europe and North America are chiefly caused by the respiratory syncytial virus (RSV) (see p. 618). Epidemics of RSV bronchiolitis have not yet been described in developing countries but may well occur. Most cases occur between the ages of six weeks and ten months; the typical clinical picture is never seen in the newborn period and it becomes increasingly rare after one year of age. Breast-feeding affords some protection against RSV bronchiolitis.

Clinical features

The illness characteristically begins as an URTI; the infant appears slightly unwell, with low-grade fever, a blocked nose with some minor discharge, cough and feeding difficulty. Within 24–48 hours the signs of lower airways obstruction appear. Breathing becomes more difficult, lower costal and intercostal recession develop and sibilant rhonchi and fine crepitations may be heard in the lungs. The chest tends to become distended with an increase in antero-posterior diameter. The respiration rate increases, commonly to 60 (even to 80) per minute; heart rate also rises to above 150 per minute. Severe cases may become cyanosed. The chest remains

hyper-resonant with obliteration of cardiac dullness and medium crepitations as well as rhonchi are heard on auscultation.

This picture of acute respiratory distress may develop rapidly over a few hours or more gradually. It may last for 24 hours or several days. In most cases, respiratory obstruction resolves spontaneously within 24 to 48 hours. Breathing becomes easier and less rapid and all the abnormal signs gradually disappear over a few days, lower costal recession tending to persist the longest. In a minority of cases, respiratory obstruction persists to a point where the infant becomes exhausted by the effort of breathing. Respirations become more laboured, slower, and less effective, cyanosis deepens and without aided respiration the infant will die.

Diagnosis

Diagnosis is based on the clinical signs already described supported by a good quality chest radiograph. The classical radiological signs of bronchiolitis are air-trapping with depression and flattening of the diaphragm, and an increase of the translucent space anterior to the heart shadow as seen in a lateral view. Peribronchial thickening is typically seen as increased linear markings but rarely as double parallel lines, and occasional opacities caused by small subsegmental areas of collapse may also be seen.

Diagnosis is based primarily on the clinical signs. In practice, the importance of the chest radiograph is to exclude pneumonia. The white cell count is slightly or moderately raised and is therefore of little value in differentiating bronchiolitis from pneumonia. Rapid virus diagnosis by the direct fluorescent antibody technique or by ELISA, applied to naso-pharyngeal secretions, can be of great value in establishing the presence of a likely causative agent.

Management

Ribavirin, given by aerosol, is moderately helpful if RSV is the cause, but careful attention to points of detail in supportive therapy can critically affect outcome. The infant should be nursed in a position which makes breathing as easy as possible. This can be conveniently achieved on a frame inclined at approximately 40° from the horizontal. The infant needs to be securely supported on this so that he cannot fall forwards or sideways. This can be achieved by means of a suitably designed sling which fits snugly around buttocks, hips and perineum, with holes for the thighs and leaving chest and arms completely free. The long ends of the sling should be wide enough not to create easily and should pass behind the shoulders and over the top of the frame. In this position the infant can rest comfortably and the pressure of the abdominal contents on the diaphragm is reduced so that breathing is unimpeded. This position is also convenient for giving feeds and for clinical examination of the chest.

Oxygen is of accepted value and absolutely essential if cyanosis develops. Humidity is of accepted value. Both oxygen and humidity can be satisfactorily provided in a tent with a mechanical humidifier. In a hot climate, oxygen may be administered best by means of a nasal catheter (see below). The maintenance of hydration is essential. While the infant is unable to suck, feeds may be given by a fine naso-gastric tube. Occasionally, intravenous fluids may be preferable; in this case it is important to ensure against fluid overload.

Corticosteroids are of no value. Antibiotics have no action against the causative virus so their only value can be against secondary bacterial infection. When pneumonia can be excluded by a negative chest radiograph, bronchiolitis can safely be treated without antibiotics, their use being reserved for the later stages in the small minority of cases where secondary bacterial infection delays resolution.

The great majority of cases recover spontaneously but in a small minority the burden of breathing becomes excessive and they will die without mechanical ventilation. When the resources for ventilation are available, the difficult judgement of when to intervene has to be made. Blood-gas analysis can supplement clinical criteria, but does not eliminate the need for clinical judgement. Some infants may require ventilation with a PCO_2 of 60 mmHg, whereas others may manage on their own with a PCO_2 level of above 100 mmHg. There is no doubt that intubation and intermittent positive pressure or some other form of mechanical ventilation sustained over a few days can be life saving. The pathological changes in the lung, even in the very severe cases, are reversible and complete recovery can occur.

Second attacks of typical bronchiolitis occasionally occur within a few weeks of the first illness; RSV may be responsible on both occasions. Infants who have had a very severe illness may have a number of lower respiratory infections in rapid succession, but whether the bronchiolitis has rendered them unduly vulnerable, or whether the infections are an expression of a predetermined vulnerability is unclear.

Pneumonia

The term pneumonia means inflammation of the lung parenchyma, that is the alveolar walls and spaces, and the interstitial tissues. Pneumonia may be caused by a wide range of respiratory viruses and bacteria. The histopathological changes vary, being largely interstitial in viral infections, and in the alveolar walls and spaces in bacterial. However, in both there is consolidation of lung with the obliteration of air spaces which interferes with gaseous exchange, and gives rise to the characteristic clinical and radiological features.

Aetiology

In developed countries, pneumonia is for the most part a precise diagnosis based on clinical features supported by radiography. The aetiology has been extensively and intensively studied. It is clear that in primary pneumonia developing in healthy infants and children, viruses are largely responsible. All the respiratory viruses are capable of causing pneumonia but the RSV, influenza A and B, and adenoviruses are particularly important (see pp. 604, 618). *M. pneumoniae, Strep. pneumoniae* and *H. influenzae* cause a number of pneumonias in older children; *Staph. aureus* may cause pneumonia as part of a septicaemia in infants and young children.

In the developing world, no such complete picture of the aetiology is available. Present understanding depends on fragmentary data, which are being added to all the time: from these a provisional picture has to be constructed.

A number of studies have shown that the same respiratory viruses are as active in the developing as in the developed world, but the extent to which these may be the sole pathogen in pneumonia is not clear. Considerable efforts have been made to determine the role of bacteria. Because bacteria may be carried in the upper respiratory tract and yet not be involved as a pathogen in the lung, and because blood culture understates lung involvement, the only really dependable evidence is provided by the culture of aspirates from consolidated lung in children not already treated with antibiotics.

The procedure carries some risk so is not used routinely. Good lung aspirate data are therefore scanty. Such data as are available are concordant, about 60 per cent of aspirates being positive for pathogenic bacteria.[5] Shann's findings in Papua New Guinea[6] are representative: bacteria were isolated from lung, blood or both from 79 of 83 children with radiological consolidation, *H. influenzae* from 33 (40 per cent) *Strep. pneumoniae* from 28 (34 per cent) and both organisms from 18 (22 per cent). This contrasts with 11.1 per cent positive bacterial cultures in a comparable study of children with pneumonia in Newark, USA. The figure of 60 per cent is likely to be understating the true role of bacteria because culture techniques can never be infallible.

While the importance of bacteria is therefore clear, the relative importance of other agents, and of various possible modifying factors, still needs to be clarified. In a study from Papua New Guinea,[7] Shann has shown how complex the true picture is. Paired sera from 94 children aged 1–24 months admitted to hospital with pneumonia showed evidence of recent infection with RSV in 22, *P. carinii* in 23, *C. trachomatis* in five, *M. pneumoniae* in five, and cytomegalovirus in one (but 86 showed CMV antibody). They conclude that all these organisms may be important causes of pneumonia in young children in developing countries, in addition of course to the bacteria whose role had been earlier defined in the same hospital.

In the light of present information it seems reasonable to conclude that in developing countries bacteria are playing a major pathogenic role in about two-thirds of the pneumonias of children. The respiratory viruses and a number of other organisms are also involved. The factors which may be responsible for the difference in relative importance of bacteria between developed and developing countries merit continuing study in relation to the formulation of appropriate treatment plans.

Clinical features

Pneumonia occurs at all ages but is most common and most severe in the first year of life.

Pneumonia in an infant may develop during an illness which starts as URTI, or may begin without evidence of involvement of the upper respiratory tract. Fever, cough, tachypnoea, dyspnoea with grunting expiration and active alae nasi, intercostal and lower costal recession, abnormal signs in the lungs, and progressive systemic upset with inability to suck or feed are the characteristic features. Lung signs are variable; they may be no more than fine crepitations in one or more zones, or there may be evidence of more extensive consolidation with diminished air entry, impaired percussion note, and bronchial or tubular breath sounds. Cyanosis may develop. Where pneumonia develops during septicaemia, the infant deteriorates very rapidly, becoming toxic and collapsed within a few hours. In a staphylococcal infection, localized signs of consolidation appear early, and because of rapid tissue necrosis, a check-valve mechanism may develop in a feeding bronchus with the formation of pneumatocoeles which may rupture into the pleura leading to pneumothorax and empyema. If the check valve continues to operate, a tension pneumothorax develops with progressive displacement of mediastinum causing circulatory collapse from interference with right heart filling.

In older children, pneumonia is more likely to develop as a primary process without preceding upper respiratory infection. Presenting symptoms will be fever, cough, pleural pain, tachypnoea and dyspnoea, and signs of lobar consolidation are more likely to be found than in infants. Apical pneumonia may present with meningism, and requires special care in clinical and radiological examination to identify what may initially be a very localized consolidation.

M. pneumoniae commonly occurs in older children. Radiological changes tend to be more marked than clinical signs suggest; consolidation varies from patchy broncho-pneumonic to larger single foci which may correspond to a broncho-pulmonary segment. The diagnosis is made more likely by the presence of a skin rash, often of the erythema multiforme type, or of a bullous myringitis.

The clinical picture is usually fairly clear-cut, but, as in infants, if the child is debilitated by malnutrition, tuberculosis, chronic diarrhoea or other long-standing disease, fever, cough and dyspnoea may be inconspicuous, even in the presence of extensive consolidation. In children with severe anaemia from whatever cause, pneumonia may precipitate congestive cardiac failure, producing a complex clinical picture in which the pneumonic contribution is difficult to define.

Aspiration pneumonia frequently develops in children who are comatose as a result of meningitis, encephalitis, malaria, toxaemia as in typhoid, or dehydration and dyselectrolytaemia, and also in children with any form of respiratory paralysis, as in poliomyelitis. In all such cases, pneumonia developing in a hypostatic lung may be missed unless specifically looked for; if missed and therefore untreated, consolidation may progress to suppuration and abscess formation.

Although pneumonia, both viral and bacterial, may resolve spontaneously and completely, it is always a serious illness carrying a significant mortality. The initial septicaemic or viraemic phase may be overwhelming; if consolidation is extensive the heart may fail from a combination of hypoxia and exhaustion; consolidation may proceed to suppuration with the formation of a lung abscess or empyema. The presence of concomitant chronic disease or malnutrition worsens the prognosis.

Diagnosis

Although the diagnosis of pneumonia can often be made confidently on the basis of clinical features alone, and although in very early cases radiological changes may be minimal, recognition of pneumonic consolidation relies critically on radiological appearances (Figs 5.2.2–5.2.5). Radiography will establish the presence,

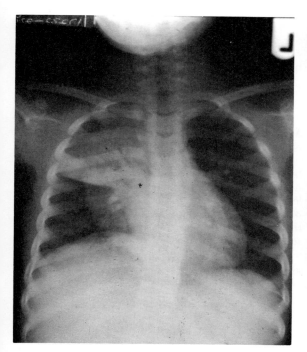

Fig. 5.2.2   Right upper lobe pneumonia in a 6 year old child. The shadowing had entirely resolved after one week.

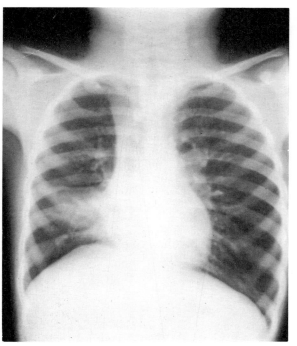

Fig. 5.2.4   Right middle lobe consolidation in a 7 year old with pneumonia.

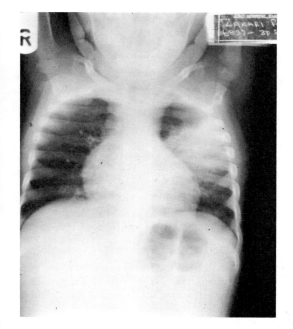

Fig. 5.2.3   Left upper lobe pneumonia in a 3 year old child.

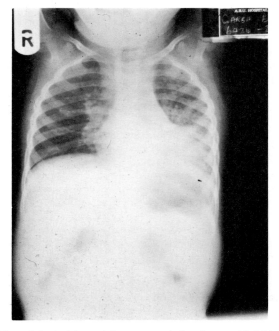

Fig. 5.2.5   Left lower lobe pneumonia in a 2 year old child.

type and extent of consolidation, the presence of pleural thickening or fluid, and the development of lung abscesses or pneumatocoeles or pneumothorax. Serial films to monitor the course of the disease and to confirm resolution, are essential in all but the most straightforward cases (see also pp. 1019–24).

Bacteriology can help both in diagnosis and management. Blood culture in the early stages of the illness, or culture of a largyngeal cough swab, or sputum if available, may all help to identify a lung pathogen, and its antibiotic sensitivities. Culture of lung aspirate is valuable for research and in difficult cases, but should not be a routine diagnostic procedure.

Rapid virus diagnosis by direct antigen detection techniques applied to naso-pharyngeal secretions is very helpful if a particular virus is suspected, but available only in selected centres. Virus identification by tissue culture or serology is a valuable research tool but because of the time lag is rarely helpful to management.

Treatment

Although some cases of pneumonia are caused by viruses, all cases should be treated as though bacterial in origin. The radiological appearances of consolidation caused by the alveolar exudate of a bacterial infection and the interstital pneumonia of a virus infection cannot be distinguished. Moreover, even if a virus can be identified in naso-pharyngeal secretions, bacteria may also be involved in the pneumonic process. All cases of pneumonia must therefore receive antibiotics.

The antibiotic selected must be effective against *Strep. pneumoniae* and *H. influenzae* as the most likely bacteria to be involved. Choices include:

Benzylpenicillin	10–30 mg/kg daily in 2–4 doses, i.m.
Procaine penicillin	300 mg once daily, i.m.
Cotrimoxazole (by mouth)	120 mg twice daily, 6 weeks–5 months
	240 mg twice daily, 6 months–5 years
	480 mg twice daily, 6–12 years
	960 mg twice daily, >12 years
Amoxycillin (by mouth)	125 mg 8-hourly, up to 10 years
	250 mg 8-hourly, >10 years
Pivampicillin (by mouth)	500 mg 12-hourly

Of the above, cotrimoxazole has the advantage of being active against *Staph. aureus* and also against *P. carinii* and *C. trachomatis*, and this may prove to be important. If *Staph. aureus* is the pathogen involved, or strongly suspected to be, a penicillinase-resistant penicillin should be used as first choice, e.g.

Flucloxacillin	125 mg 6-hourly, by mouth
	or 125 mg 6-hourly, i.m.
	or 250 mg 6-hourly, slow i.v.

Mild or moderately severe infections will respond to oral therapy. In severe infections, or where retention of oral medication is in doubt, a parenteral route should be used. If the resources are available, the safest and most effective route of administration and probably the least disturbing for the child is by continuous intravenous infusion. A strong case can be made for starting treatment in this way in all cases, but particularly for a staphylococcal infection.

If infection with *M. pneumoniae* is proved or suspected, erythromycin should be given by mouth, 125–250 mg every six hours.

In very severe cases where the organism is unknown, and the quickest possible response is essential, parenteral chloramphenicol 50–100 mg/kg per day divided into four 6-hourly doses by i.m. or i.v. infusion may be used, or flucloxacillin combined with an aminoglycoside like gentamicin (3 mg/kg every 12 hours for child up to two weeks of age, and 2 mg/kg every 8 hours from two weeks to 12 years, i.m. or slow i.v.). Treatment should ordinarily be continued for about 10 days but may have to be for longer for complete resolution in severe cases.

Supportive therapy

Fluids. If an infant is on the breast and able to suck, breast-feeding should be continued. Older children should be encouraged to drink sufficient to meet daily requirements. If this is not possible hydration must be maintained by naso-gastric tube or intravenous infusion. Inappropriate secretion of antidiuretic hormone may occur in pneumonia, so it is especially important to avoid fluid overload which can lead to pulmonary oedema.

Posture. As in bronchiolitis, the child should be supported in a semi-upright position. An infant may rest most comfortably if held in his mother's arms.

Oxygen. Oxygen should be given to all children who are cyanosed, or seriously ill with marked dyspnoea and recession. This may be by means of a tent. Where supplies of oxygen are limited or cost is a factor, the most economical route of administration is by nasal catheter, at a rate of one litre per minute using a low flow-meter to achieve this. The oxygen should be humidified.

Clearing the nose as already described is important in infants.

A neutral thermal environment is desirable; over-heating or chilling add to a child's burdens, the former carrying a risk of convulsions. If the child's temperature rises above 39°C, paracetamol should be given.

Where pneumonia complicates or is complicated by protein–energy or other nutritional deficiency, this needs to be corrected as rapidly as possible. This may mean early administration of high calorie and protein feeds by naso-gastric tube, and if felt necessary intramuscular vitamin A. Severe anaemia is a partic-ular hazard, and may call for a small slow transfusion of packed red cells, repeated if necessary; if heart failure is also present, a careful exchange transfusion covered by digoxin and frusemide may be life saving. In HbS anaemia, pulmonary sicklings can have complications caused by pneumonia or Gram-negative organisms (see pp. 828–30). Such children require high concentrations of oxygen, if possible hyperbaric or by positive pressure ventilation. If clinical or radiological signs of pleural fluid develop, or of pneumothorax, the diagnosis should be established immediately by pleural aspiration and the appropriate treatment instituted.

Pneumonia, if severe, may cause weight loss and debility, which will require supervised nutritional rehabilitation during convalescence.

ARI: A community health problem

Epidemiology

ARI have long been recognized as the most common form of illness in children throughout the world, with pneumonia the third major cause of deaths in develop-ing countries after malnutrition and diarrhoea. During the last 20 years, a clearer picture of morbidity and mortality from ARI in the developing world has been taking shape. Some of the details contributing to this picture have been reviewed by Pio *et al.*[5]

A number of community-based longitudinal studies have shown that children in urban areas have five to eight ARI annually during the first five years of life. In rural areas the incidence of ARI is lower, one to three episodes per year. This overall incidence is much the same in developed and developing countries, unlike diarrhoea where the incidence is very much higher in developing countries. The duration of episodes of ARI is also similar in developed and developing countries. However, the difference in annual incidence of pneu-monia is striking, 30–40 per 1000 children under five years of age in urban areas in the USA, compared for

Table 5.2.1 Deaths from pneumonia and influenza as underlying cause per 100 000 children 1–4 years of age in four countries, 1979–81.

Country	Year	No. per 100 000
France	1980	0.7
Netherlands	1981	1.1
Egypt	1979	173.6
Guatemala	1979	251.0

Adapted from WHO, *World Health Statistics Annual*, Geneva, WHO, 1983. Cited by Pio *et al.*, in *Acute Respiratory Infections in Childhood*, University of Adelaide, 1985.

example with 94.1 per 1000 in one Indian study, and 256 per 1000 in the first year of life, and 62 per 1000 in children aged one to four years in one district of Papua New Guinea. The differences in ARI-related mortality rates are even more striking (see Table 5.2.1). More-over, the rate of decline in mortality rates is faster in many developed countries than developing, so the gap is widening.

A number of risk factors have been shown to contribute to high mortality from ARI. These include low birth weight, malnutrition, and anaemia, and poor accessibility to adequate treatment facilities including supplies of antibiotics and other drugs. The incidence of low birth weight (< 2500 g) is 5–7 per cent in developed countries against 15–30 per cent in developing: the contrast in the incidence of malnutrition is even greater. Indoor air pollution has been identified as a risk factor for respiratory infection, but not as having an effect on ARI-related mortality.

On the positive side, a protective effect against ARI has been demonstrated for breast-feeding. In a case-control study in Newcastle-upon-Tyne, UK, breast-feeding was shown to halve the risk of admission to hospital with RSV infection in children 0–5 months of age.[8]

Attempts have been made to quantify the contribu-tion of vaccine-preventable diseases to ARI-related mortality in children. Without immunization, all chil-dren can be expected to develop measles and pertussis before they reach the age of five years. Both these dis-eases carry a definite mortality. In both, pneumonia or laryngo-tracheo-bronchitis is a common complication, especially in the presence of malnutrition. Estimated deaths from these two diseases are shown in Table 5.2.2.

The relative importance of viruses and bacteria in the aetiology of severe ARI is of critical importance in any consideration of community health. Limited commu-nity studies of carrier rates for pathogenic bacteria in the upper respiratory tract suggest these may be higher

Table 5.2.2   Estimated deaths from measles and pertussis in developing countries (excluding China), 1983.

	Measles[a]	Pertussis[b]
Survey data from 25 countries	2 088 000	608 000
All other developing countries	401 000	127 000
Total	2 489 000	735 000

[a] Based on immunization coverage data, assuming vaccine efficacy of 95 per cent and that 95 per cent of unimmunized children will get measles.
[b] Based on immunization coverage data, assuming vaccine efficacy of 80 per cent and that 80 per cent of unimmunized children will get pertussis.
Data reproduced from Pio *et al*., in *Acute Respiratory Infections in Childhood*, University of Adelaide, 1985.

in developing countries. For example, in Goroka, Papua New Guinea, weekly cultures of nasal secretions in 22 infants showed that by the third month of life, all had acquired at least one strain of both *Strep. pneumoniae* and *H. influenzae*.[5] The evidence for a major role for pathogenic bacteria in about two-thirds of childhood pneumonias has already been presented in the section on pneumonia (see pp. 713–14).

These community data reveal the scale of the burden imposed by ARI on children in developing countries. While some of the factors contributing to this burden are amenable only to long-term measures, others can clearly be tackled with resources that could be made available immediately. A decision for immediate action was taken by the World Health Assembly in 1982 when it approved a comprehensive ARI programme of services and research, within the WHO Seventh General Programme of Work, 1984–89.

A strategy for control

A Technical Advisory Group (TAG) was established. The reports prepared by this TAG and other publications the TAG has generated provide comprehensive reviews of the relevant scientific data, and detailed guidelines for the development of ARI control programmes and the integrated management of ARI through primary health care and hospital services.[9, 10]

The essential argument for the strategy now advocated is as follows. A very large number of infants and young children in developing countries are at present dying from pneumonia. Most of these children never reach hospital, so die without benefit of modern medicine. Many of those who reach hospital arrive too late for treatment to be effective. Many of the pneumonias are initiated by measles or pertussis which could be prevented by immunization. In perhaps two-thirds of all pneumonia deaths *Strep. pneumoniae* or *H. influenzae* play

a major role, so many might be prevented by early treatment with an antibiotic. Early treatment with antibiotics could never be made available on the required scale if their use is restricted to doctors. Antibiotic treatment must therefore be made available through village-level health workers (VHWs). This could result in wasteful misuse of antibiotics on a potentially gigantic scale. Misuse can be prevented if health workers are suitably supervised, and if they can be taught first how to distinguish between children with ARI who do not require antibiotic treatment and those who do; and secondly, precisely what action to take for children in each of these categories. Guide-lines for such action are now referred to as 'Standard Management Plans'. Training health workers for such a role is clearly a massive undertaking but equally clearly forms a logical component of the training for primary health care to which virtually all developing countries are already firmly committed.

The strategy which has been developed in response to the above reasoning is made up of three elements: an expansion of the programme of immunization (EPI), training of health workers and communities in the recognition of serious ARI and in the understanding of the treatments available, and the development of standard treatment plans which are agreed, approved and followed at all levels of health care. These three elements, EPI, training and standard treatments, are logical and uncontroversial provided the goal of the health services is clearly perceived as the health of all children in the community served. Already in pilot projects in a number of different countries, the strategy is being successfully implemented.

Primary health care of ARI

Implementation of this strategy for the control and management of ARI must be the responsibility of the primary health care (PHC) team. The first element of the strategy, the expanded programme of immunization (EPI) is already an integral part of PHC. The particular emphasis on immunization against pertussis and measles is therefore no more than a reinforcement of established practice. The second and third elements, training and the adoption of standard treatments, are innovative and involve enhanced responsibilities for VHWs.

The essential point in this development is the realization that childhood pneumonia requires treatment with an antibiotic given on the spot by a VHW in exactly the same way as a child with diarrhoea requires immediate oral rehydration therapy. Once this is accepted, it becomes clear that the VHW needs to be trained first of all to recognize the child with pneumonia among the scores, perhaps hundreds, of children he/she will see with simple URTIs. Secondly, the VHW needs to know the standard treatments for URTI and for pneumonia which have been worked out, accepted, and are being followed by the whole PHC team.

VHWs cannot be trained to use stethoscopes – in fact there is no need. Shann[11] in Papua New Guinea has evaluated the different signs and symptoms of respiratory disease as discriminators for pneumonia, and has found rapid breathing (defined as more than 50 per minute) to be both sensitive and specific. Leventhal[12] correlated respiratory signs and symptoms with radiological consolidation and found tachypnoea to be the best discriminator. Shann has shown it is possible to train VHWs to recognize rapid breathing reliably. They are taught to examine the child when resting quietly, preferably lying on the mother's lap. If they have a watch, they count the breaths in a minute. However, Shann found this was not necessary; they were able to recognize rapid breathing as abnormal when breathing was specifically assessed, even without timing.

Shann found in the same way that recession, with indrawing of intercostal spaces and the lower chest wall, was the most reliable discriminator for severe pneumonia. He found VHWs could also be trained to recognize this sign.

These observations, already confirmed by others, are the basis for the standard treatments currently recommended by WHO.[10]

- ARI with cough and normal breathing: treat supportively.
- ARI with cough and rapid breathing but without recession: treat with antibiotic at home.
- ARI with cough, rapid breathing and recession: refer to hospital.

Supportive treatment includes guidance on feeding, fluids, thermal environment, cleaning the nose and posture, as already described (see p. 716).

The choice of antibiotic needs to take account of the likely bacteria, their sensitivities, the relative costs of alternative antibiotics, and their side-effects. Cotrimoxazole is effective against *Strep. pneumoniae*, *H. influenzae* and *Staph. aureus* (as well as *P. carinii* and *C. trachomatis*). It is cheap, needs to be given only twice a day, and has few side-effects. Cotrimoxazole is therefore the first-choice antibiotic to be given by a VHW for the home treatment of pneumonia (dosage as given on p. 716).

This description of a standard treatment for pneumonia illustrates a way in which it is possible to make modern medicine accessible to remote populations.

Clearly, the extent to which this approach can be developed will depend on many variables, including particularly the level of ability of the VHWs and the quality of training and supervision they receive. As the PHC infrastructure becomes securely established, it will be possible to introduce more elaborate standard treatments.

Judgement on what is possible in this regard must in the end be the responsibility of the local PHC managers who are themselves responsible for training and supervision. However, optimal management of ARI in communities will be achieved when standard treatments are developed as an integrated exercise, all the relevant experts including paediatricians and microbiologists at regional level sharing the responsibility.

This collaboration between professionals in the endeavour to manage ARI efficiently in the community, and to reduce childhood deaths from pneumonia, is desirable for several reasons. As already indicated it will help to ensure that standard treatments are the best possible in the light of present knowledge. It will also help to ensure that concordant guide-lines are followed at all levels of health care, in the community, at first-referral health centres and in hospital. And finally it will help those working in hospitals to see their role as providing support to PHC and to contribute positively from their experience to the improvement of standard treatments and training programmes.

Suppurative lung disease

Cough with the production of purulent sputum indicates pulmonary suppuration. This is occasionally an acute process, or, more commonly, a subacute or chronic condition.

Acute suppuration: lung abscess

Acute pulmonary suppuration occurs most often in the course of a septicaemia, *Staph. aureus* being commonly responsible. In such cases, lesions are usually multiple, taking the form of pneumatocoeles (see p. 714). Initially, septicaemia dominates the clinical picture with fever, possibly convulsions, and peripheral circulatory collapse, lung signs being relatively inconspicuous. Gradually the lung signs dominate with tachypnoea, dyspnoea, cough, evidence of consolidation and possibly of mediastinal shift from pleural fluid or pneumothorax. Later there may be expectoration of frank pus. Most cases will resolve on intravenous antibiotics, flucloxacillin and gentamicin being an appropriate starting combination, until the infecting pathogen and its sensitivities have been identified from blood or sputum culture. Empyema, pneumothorax or other possible complications will require appropriate management.

Lung abscess may develop in the course of any pneumonia, especially if this is inadequately treated, or occurs in a malnourished, debilitated or anaemic child. It may also arise from secondary infection of a hydatid cyst, from infection in a lobe, or broncho-pulmonary segment collapse following bronchial obstruction by an inhaled foreign body, or by extension from an extrapulmonary focus such as a subphrenic or hepatic abscess. In such cases surgical intervention is likely to be necessary.

Chronic suppuration: bronchiectasis

A child presenting with chronic cough and purulent sputum with recurrent exacerbations accompanied by fever is likely to have some form of bronchiectasis. This is the common end-stage of a number of different pathways and is characterized by chronic inflammation of bronchial walls and adjacent interstitia, with irreversible dilatation of affected bronchi. Bronchiectasis may be focal or diffuse; possible causative mechanisms are listed in Table 5.2.3.

Table 5.2.3   Bronchiectasis: types and causes.

Focal
Arising through infection in a lobe or broncho-pulmonary segment collapsed by bronchial occlusion from:

- pneumonia, particularly in measles or pertussis
- an inhaled foreign body
- compression or stenosis, e.g. from a tuberculous hilar lymph node.

Diffuse
Lung previously normal, damage occurring from:

- recurrent bronchitis (or bronchiolitis)
- severe pneumonia, either bacterial or viral, particularly certain adenoviruses

Lung abnormality present as in:

- cystic fibrosis
- immotile-cilia syndrome
- bronchomalacia

Cystic fibrosis

Cystic fibrosis is a genetically determined disorder characterized by undue vulnerability of the lower respiratory tract to recurrent and continuing infection, by deficient or absent pancreatic exocrine secretion and consequent malabsorption, and by an abnormally high concentration of sodium and chloride in the sweat. The essential metabolic defect is still not known. The mode of inheritance is autosomal recessive. The gene frequency is 1 in 20–25 in Caucasian populations, giving a disease incidence of about 1 in 2000. The gene is rare in non-Caucasians, so the disease is excessively rare in developing countries. In developed countries it is the most common cause of chronic suppurative lung disease.

Immotile-cilia syndrome

The genetically determined association of dextrocardia or situs inversus, chronic sinusitis and bronchiectasis has been known since it was first described by Kartagener in 1933. More recently a basic defect in muco-ciliary transport associated with ultrastructural abnormalities of the cilia has been identified.[13] Since this ciliary abnormality appears to be constant, and the other features of the syndrome are variable, 'immotile-cilia syndrome' is the favoured designation. The ciliary defect accounts for the most characteristic feature of the syndrome, which is vulnerability to recurrent and persistent infection of both the upper and lower respiratory tracts.

Bronchomalacia

This uncommon disorder is characterized by abnormally compliant bronchi due to extensive deficiency of bronchial cartilage. It is uncertain whether the cartilage deficiency is congenital or acquired.[14]

Management

While some of these predisposing conditions or causative mechanisms are amenable to specific therapy, e.g. tuberculosis, foreign body, and the malabsorption of cystic fibrosis, the management of the bronchiectasis is common to all, and is primarily medical not surgical. The object of treatment is to keep the bronchi clear of muco-purulent secretions by chest percussion and postural drainage, and to prevent or control infection by appropriate antibiotic therapy. In mild focal bronchiectasis this may involve no more than a slightly prolonged course of antibiotic in higher than normal dosage during episodes of infection. In severe established bronchiectasis, regular drainage twice a day and continuous antibiotic prophylaxis will be required. Careful tailoring of the antibiotic regimen to the individual is essential.

Parasitic infections of the lung

Many species of parasite pass through the lungs at one stage in their life-cycles and some cause the following diseases: ascariasis, schistosomiasis, and strongyloidiasis. If the infective load is modest, this lung passage may be relatively symptom-free. If the load is heavy, respiratory symptoms may be marked, with cough, haemoptysis, wheeze, fever, eosinophilia, and transient patchy consolidation in chest radiographs. However, even where the prevalence of such parasites is high, this clinical picture seems to be rare, or unrecognized. In addition, there are at least two parasitic infections where respiratory symptoms persist over long periods.

Tropical pulmonary eosinophilia

This is a relatively common disease in India, Sri Lanka and Malaysia; it has been described infrequently in other East Asian countries, and in parts of Africa and the Caribbean.

Aetiology

The disease is caused by a filarial infection, in which, unlike bancroftian filariasis where microfilariae circulate freely, the microfilariae become trapped and killed in the capillaries of affected tissues where they produce granulomatous lesions.[15] (See p. 694.) The reason for these differing tissue responses has not been finally established. That the microfilariae are morphologically indistinguishable from those of *Wuchereria bancrofti* does not completely exclude an explanation based on the hypothesis that the infection in tropical pulmonary eosinophilia (TPE) is zoonotic. However, the finding of higher levels of reaginic antibody of the IgE class to filarial antigen in patients with TPE, than in patients with typical filariasis, and the fact that the levels were higher against human filarial antigen than against the dog parasite *Dirofilaria immitis*, makes it seem more likely that the explanation lies in a differing host response to the same parasite, characterized in TPE by hypersensitivity.[16]

Clinical features

All age groups are affected. The main symptoms are cough and wheeze which are worse at night. In young children particularly, lymph nodes and liver may be enlarged, and there may be weight loss and failure to thrive. If untreated, symptoms persist for months. There is always a massive eosinophilia in the peripheral blood, eosinophil counts of 40 000–50 000 per mm^3 being common. The chest radiograph is almost always abnormal, changes ranging from generally increased lung markings to diffuse coarse mottling.

Diagnosis

The combination of persistent wheeze and cough, massive eosinophilia and compatible changes in the chest radiograph, occurring in a region where TPE is prevalent, is diagnostic. Confirmation would be provided by finding a raised titre of complement-fixing antibody in the serum to filaria antigen, or more simply by a therapeutic trial with diethylcarbamazine.

Treatment

A five-day course of diethylcarbamazine, (10 mg/kg per day, divided into two or three doses) usually effects complete cure, with rapid relief of symptoms. If symptoms persist after two to three weeks, diethylcarbamazine should be repeated in a dose of 20 mg/kg per day. If symptoms still persist the diagnosis should be reviewed.

Paragonimiasis

This disease was at one time not uncommon in East Asia, and has been reported in India, West Africa, and parts of Central and South America. It is now becoming rarer.[17] (See p. 643.)

Aetiology

The disease is caused by infection with a lung fluke, of the genus *Paragonimus*. The life-cycle of this fluke includes a stage in a fresh-water snail, and another in crayfish and crabs. Human infection occurs through eating these crustacea uncooked. In man, the lung is the main target organ, but other tissues including pleura, muscle, intestinal wall and brain may be involved. In the lung, the fluke provokes a fibrous reaction, becoming encysted, but continuing to release eggs into the bronchi.

Clinical features

The onset is usually insidious and the course chronic, with cough, occasionally productive, the main symptom.

Control

Infection can of course be avoided by not eating uncooked shellfish, and by care in their preparation.

Treatment

Bithionol (20–50 mg/kg per day) given by mouth at a total of 10–15 doses on alternate days appears to be the most satisfactory treatment.

Pleural effusion, empyema and pneumothorax

There are many possible causes of a pleural effusion in a child (see Table 5.2.4). Whenever pleural fluid is suspected, it should be aspirated for diagnostic purposes, further action being dictated by the findings (see p. 1013). In practice, the most common finding will be a serous or purulent exudate which has collected in the course of a pneumonia, most often staphylococcal. In such a case, the essential treatment is the antibiotic regime appropriate for the pneumonia. But as much of the pleural fluid as possible should be withdrawn. If fluid recollects, it should be aspirated again, and an intercostal catheter inserted with underwater drainage. If thick pus is found, thoracotomy with removal of pus, resection of a piece of rib and underwater drainage may be necessary.

Table 5.2.4   Possible causes of pleural effusion.

Neoplasm	Primary mesothelioma
Infection from adjacent structures	Secondary to leukaemia, neuroblastoma, lymphoma
Lung	Pneumonia, tuberculosis
Chest wall	Osteitis of rib
Diaphragm	Subphrenic or hepatic abscess
Systemic diseases	
Septicaemia	Empyema

Empyema secondary to a staphylococcal pneumonia may be complicated by a pneumothorax, in which there may be mounting positive pressure. If the pneumothorax is under tension with pressure on the mediastinum interfering with right heart filling, circulatory collapse develops rapidly. Needling the chest to release pressure can be life-saving. In any case, the correct treatment for the pyopneumothorax is to maintain underwater drainage of the pleural cavity until infection has been controlled by antibiotics, and resolution occurs.

Asthma

Asthma is now understood to be 'a disease characterized by an increased responsiveness of the trachea and bronchi to various stimuli and manifested by widespread narrowing of the airways that changes in severity either spontaneously or as a result of therapy' (American Thoracic Society).

Mechanisms and prevalence

The essential defect in asthma is a hyper-reactivity of the bronchi which respond to a variety of triggers by constriction and by increased secretion of mucus. Both contribute to the airways obstruction which is the cause of symptoms. The diagnosis of asthma in children used to be reserved for severe and persistent wheezing in older children, the 'wheezy bronchitis' of a younger age-group being regarded as a distinct entity. Long-term community studies suggest that all wheezing, apart from bronchiolitis in early infancy, is due to this common defect of bronchial hyper-reactivity.[18] This defect is probably determined genetically, though the exact mode of inheritance is still not clear. Atopy, which may be defined as an abnormal tendency to produce IgE antibodies in response to normal exposure to environmental allergens, is present in most but not all subjects with bronchial hyper-reactivity. Hay fever and eczema are therefore common, though not constant, associations.

Known triggers which provoke broncho-constriction are:

- exposure to an allergen to which previous sensitization has occurred;
- viral respiratory infections;
- vigorous exertion, which is linked to tracheal cooling;
- emotional stress.

The degree of broncho-constriction provoked in an individual by any of these triggers may vary from time to time, but the essential hyper-reactivity seems to persist.

The presence of bronchial hyper-reactivity can be demonstrated in up to 90 per cent of symptomatic asthmatics by formal testing. The simplest method is by exercise; running for six minutes fast enough to raise the heart rate to 180 per minute will cause broncho-constriction which can be measured with a peak flow meter, a reduction of peak flow rate of over 20 per cent being regarded as abnormal. A second method is by histamine challenge, in which increasing concentrations of histamine are inhaled from a nebulizer under standardized conditions.

Community studies of wheezing in developed countries suggest a prevalence of 12–20 per cent.[18] This includes the whole spectrum of severity, some children having only a few episodes of wheezing in early child-hood, with only a small proportion remaining sympto-matic into adult life. There is some evidence that the prevalence in developed countries is increasing.[19] Pre-valence in developing countries is not well documented, but is certainly very much lower.

Clinical features

Wheezing is the dominant symptom. This is most marked in expiration which is prolonged. Depend-ing on the severity of airways obstruction, breath-ing requires increasing effort marked by intercostal recession.

The pattern of attacks varies markedly from child to child, and from time to time in the individual child. In general, respiratory infections are the most important trigger in early childhood, the other triggers operating increasingly and in combination if symptoms continue into later childhood.

Any child with asthma can experience a severe, even life-threatening, attack at any time. In mild or moderate asthma, there may be no abnormal findings between attacks. In severe persistent asthma, the chest becomes deformed with elevation of the shoulders, increased antero-posterior diameter, and prominent Harrison's sulci. Eczema or hay fever may or may not be present.

Diagnosis

Diagnosis depends essentially on the history, except during an attack, when rhonchi, prolonged expiration, and costal recession may all be present. A chest radiograph is not essential. Most of the time it will be normal, though segmental or even lobar collapse can develop during severe attacks. Rapidly reversible airways obstruction is really compatible only with a diagnosis of asthma, but in some countries other causes of wheezing may be important, e.g. tropical pulmonary eosinophilia.

Management

The most important aspect of management is explain-ing the disorder to the family and to the child when old enough, enabling them as far as possible to be self-suffi-cient in managing the problem (see also p. 972).

Three categories of drug are useful in treatment. Salbutamol is an effective selective bronchodilator. It can be given by mouth (0.15 mg/kg 6-hourly), by inhalation as a dry powder, a rotacap, or by metered aerosol (200 μg, 4–6 hourly), by nebulizer using a respirator solution containing 2.5–10 mg, repeated up to 4-hourly, or by slow intravenous injection, 250 μg. Of the xanthine bronchodilators, intravenous amino-phylline (5 mg/kg, over 15 minutes) is useful in very severe asthmatic attacks, and slow-release tablets by mouth (225–450 mg) are helpful in controlling night symptoms. Finally, corticosteroids are valuable both in prophylaxis, and in the treatment of acute severe asthma. Beclomethasone dipropionate by metered aerosol or inhaled in powder form (100–200 μg 2–4 times daily) affords valuable protection: hydrocortisone (3–4 mg/kg every 3–4 hours) is useful in the treatment of acute severe asthma.

Quick symptomatic relief of episodic wheezing is conveniently provided by salbutamol by metered aerosol. Children below six to eight years of age can usually not handle an aerosol efficiently; they may manage the rotacaps, or administration by nebulizer may be necessary. Bronchodilators alone may suffice; if not, additional relief may be obtained with prophylactic beclomethasone, which is associated with absolutely minimal side-effects. The aim should be to find the the-rapeutic regimen which enables the child to lead as full and normal a life as possible.

Any child with asthma may experience a very severe, even life-threatening, attack at any time. Parents should be warned of this, taught to recognize signs of severity and told what to do. Ordinarily this means immediate admission to a hospital. Life-threatening asthma should be treated with nebulized salbutamol, intravenous hydrocortisone and aminophylline, and oxygen, together with support measures as described for pneumonia (see p. 716).

Inhaled foreign body

Inhalation of a foreign body is relatively common in the toddler age group. Any object small enough to go in the mouth may be inhaled, but seeds, grains, nuts, grams (legumes) are most commonly involved. At the time of inhalation, there is likely to be a sudden bout of violent and sustained coughing. If inhalation is suspected immediate referral to a hospital with facilities for bronchoscopy is essential.

In hospital, if the child is seen early with a history of possible inhalation, perhaps with a newly acquired wheeze and with supporting clinical and radiological signs of segmental or lobar collapse or of localized emphysema, the diagnosis is straightforward. If, how-ever, the child is seen only after some days, the history of inhalation may not be available and the clinical pic-ture, particularly with a vegetable foreign body, will be one of spreading pneumonia, with cough, fever, dyspnoea and evidence of lung consolidation or collapse. In such cases, the diagnosis is likely to be missed unless the possibility is in mind, and the relevant questions are asked specifically.

To make the correct diagnosis is of the greatest practical importance because without bronchoscopy and removal of the foreign material, resolution of the pneumonia or collapse will at best be slow and the risk of permanent lung damage will be considerable. Bronchoscopy should always be performed without delay if a foreign body is suspected; successful removal usually leads to rapid recovery.

References

1. Leowski J. Mortality from acute respiratory infections in children under 5 years of age: global estimates. *World Health Statistics Quarterly*. 1986; **39**: 138–44.
2. Steinhoff MC, John TJ. Acute respiratory infections of children in India. *Pediatric Research*. 1983; **17**: 1032–3.
3. Van Buchem FL, Peeters MF, van't Hof MA. Acute otitis media: a new strategy. *British Medical Journal*. 1985; **290**: 1033–7.
4. Stanfield JP, Bracken PM. Antistreptolysin O titres in the childhood population in rural and semi-rural Buganda. *East African Medical Journal*. 1973; **50**: 153–8.
5. Pio A, Leowski J, ten Dam HG. The magnitude of the problem of acute respiratory infections. In: Douglas RM, Kerby-Eaton E, eds. *Acute Respiratory Infections in Childhood*. Adelaide, University of Adelaide, Department of Community Medicine, 1985. pp. 3–16.
6. Shann F, Gratten M, Germer S *et al.* Aetiology of pneumonia in children in Goroka Hospital, Papua New Guinea. *Lancet*. 1984; **2**: 537–41.
7. Shann F, Walters S, Pifer LL *et al.* Pneumonia associated with infection with pneumocystis, respiratory syncytial virus, chlamydia, mycoplasma, and cytomegalovirus in children in Papua New Guinea. *British Medical Journal*. 1986; **292**: 314–27.
8. Pullan CR, Toms GL, Martin AJ *et al.* Breast-feeding and respiratory syncytial virus infection. *British Medical Journal*. 1980; *281*: 1034–6.
9. *Programme of acute respiratory infections.* WHO Technical advisory group on acute respiratory infections. 1983 Report of first meeting, Geneva WHO/TRI/ARI. TAG. I/83.3. 1985 Report of second meeting. Geneva WHO/RSD/85.18.
10. *Respiratory infections in children: management at small hospitals.* Background notes and manual for doctors. 1986: WHO/RSD/86.26.
11. Shann F, Hart K, Thomas D. Acute lower respiratory tract infections in children: possible criteria for selection of patients for antibiotic therapy and hospital admission. *Bulletin of World Health Organisation* 1984; **62**: 749–53 (Reprint No. 4453).
12. Leventhal JM. Clinical predictors of pneumonia as a guide to ordering chest roentgenograms. *Clinical Pediatrics*. 1982, **21**: 730–4.
13. Eliasson R, Mossberg B, Camner P *et al.* The immotile cilia syndrome. *New England Journal of Medicine*. 1977; **297**: 1–6.
14. Williams HE, Landau LI, Phelan PD. Generalized bronchiectasis due to extensive deficiency of bronchial cartilage. *Archives of Disease in Childhood*. 1972; **47**: 423–8.
15. Webb JKG, Job CK, Gault EW. Tropical eosinophilia: demonstration of microfilariae in lung, liver and lymph-nodes. *Lancet*. 1960; **I**: 835–42.
16. Ottesen EA, Neva FA, Paranjape RS *et al.* Specific allergic sensitization to filarial antigens in tropical eosinophilia syndrome. *Lancet*. 1979; **I**: 1158–61.
17. Malek EA. Public health importance of helminthic disease and basic principles for their control. V. Helminthiasis transmitted by snail intermediate hosts. WHO *Document/Helminths/2*. 1961.
18. McNicol KN, Williams HE. Spectrum of asthma in children: I. Clinical and physiological components. II. Allergic components. III. Psychological and social components. *British Medical Journal*. 1973; **4**: 7–20.
19. Editorial. Bronchial asthma and the environment. *Lancet*. 1986; **ii**: 786–7.

CHAPTER 3

Diseases of the gastro-intestinal tract

Martin Brueton

Gastro-intestinal infections causing diarrhoea, vomiting and abdominal pain currently overshadow most of the other alimentary disorders which occur in children in the tropics and subtropics. These symptoms can be non-specific, and frequently occur in infections and other diseases which do not primarily affect the gut. It is therefore essential to carry out a full general examination and to elicit a clear history. Gastroenteritis and other causes of acute and chronic diarrhoea are discussed on pp. 455–495. Parasitic infections of the gut other than those due to protozoa are discussed on pp. 633–656. Surgical causes of acute abdominal symptoms arising from intestinal obstruction, perforation or appendicitis are discussed on pp. 894–7, which also describe the management of congenital abnormalities of the gastro-intestinal tract (see pp. 889–93). This chapter covers other causes of intestinal and hepatic disorders, initially following a symptom-based approach to diagnosis.

Vomiting

Some of the important causes of vomiting are shown in Table 5.3.1. The timing, frequency and amount of vomitus should all be noted, together with the presence or absence of blood or bile. Projectile vomiting should be distinguished from regurgitation.

Gastroesophageal reflux and hiatus hernia

Effortless regurgitation of stomach contents due to gastroesophageal reflux is often seen in healthy babies in the first few months of life. Most of them have a normally placed gastroesophageal junction and yet have a tendency to reflux, probably due to an immaturity of the integration of the various factors which effect lower oesophageal closure. This usually causes no distress, except to the parents. Weight gain is generally satisfactory, and in the majority of infants the symptoms have resolved by the age of six months to one year.

Table 5.3.1 Causes of vomiting in infants.

Feeding problems
Infections
  Enteral
    oral candidiasis
    gastroenteritis
  Parenteral
    respiratory tract
    otitis media
    urinary
    central nervous system
    septicaemia
Gastroesophageal reflux
  hiatus hernia
Intestinal obstruction
  congenital malformations
  pyloric stenosis
  intussusception
Malabsorption
  coeliac disease
  cow's milk protein intolerance
  lactose intolerance
Cerebral
  birth trauma
  hydrocephalus
  meningoencephalitis
  intracranial space-occupying lesions
Metabolic disorders
  galactosaemia
  idiopathic hypercalcaemia
  aminoacidaemias
Endocrine
  adrenogenital syndrome
Renal
  renal tubular acidosis
  uraemia

Table 5.3.2 Causes of vomiting in the older child.

Infections
Acute appendicitis
Drug ingestion
Cyclical vomiting
Diabetic ketoacidosis
Migraine
Motion sickness
Peptic ulceration
Intestinal obstruction
Dietary indiscretion

Simple management measures include posturing the baby in a semiprone position with the head raised, and thickening the feeds. More severe reflux may be associated with a hiatus hernia or a partial thoracic stomach. Oesophagitis is then more likely to develop, causing blood to be seen in the vomit, failure to thrive and in some cases stricture formation; aspiration may also occur. If any of these features are seen, further investigations are required. The presence of significant reflux, a hiatus hernia or oesophagitis on barium studies indicates treatment such as reducing the volumes and increasing the frequency of individual feeds, and the use of antacid therapy, H_2 blockers and prokinetic drugs.

Vomiting in older children

Some of the main causes of vomiting in older children are shown in Table 5.3.2.

Haematemesis

Common sources of bleeding in childhood include the oesophagus, where mucosal tears may follow prolonged retching, and the naso-pharynx where a history of epistaxis and swallowed blood is relevant. More serious causes include oesophagitis, oesophageal varices, coagulation disorders, gastritis, duodenal ulceration, and acute poisoning.

Diarrhoea

Definitions, pathogenesis and classification are presented on pp. 456–7. Chronic diarrhoea is usually associated with infections and malnutrition. Hidden within these patient populations, there are undoubtably a few children with primary underlying mucosal transport disorders. The possible diagnoses include congenital disaccharidase deficiencies (lactase, sucrase, isomaltase), glucose–galactose malabsorption, and chloride-losing diarrhoea. Other rare causes of small bowel malabsorption include lymphangiectasia, abetalipoproteinaemia, acrodermatitis enteropathica and congenital microvillus atrophy. The more common conditions described here are lactose malabsorption, colitis and *Clostridium perfringens* infection.

Lactose malabsorption

Malabsorption of lactose occurs when there is a reduction of lactase activity in the microvillus brush border of the enterocytes. Unabsorbed lactose passes on to be metabolized in the caecum by the normal gut flora, the stools becoming fluid, acidic and containing glucose (see pp. 465–6). The most common cause of lactase deficiency is the damage to the enterocyte brush border which occurs in many small bowel enteropathies. This secondary impairment will resolve with the enteropathy. Congenital lactase deficiency is an extremely rare autosomal recessive disorder in which there is probably a defect in the protein synthesis of lactase. Adult lactase deficiency occurs in 50–90 per cent of non-Caucasians but only 2–30 per cent of Caucasians. Lactase activity appears *in utero* at 28 weeks per cent of gestation and is therefore low in some preterm infants; the levels are highest in infancy. Children with lactase deficiency develop explosive, watery diarrhoea from the initial introduction of milk feeds – they will tolerate monosaccharides.

Adaptive, demographic and genetic theories have been propounded to explain the adult variations which are seen; genetic theories are currently favoured.

Clinical features and management

The passage of watery stools with pH < 5.5 and containing reducing substances as demonstrated by Clinitest tablets is suggestive of lactose malabsorption. The patient also experiences colicky abdominal pain, abdominal distention and increased flatus. The relation of clinical symptoms to lactose ingestion is quantitative and is dependent upon the length of small bowel which is deficient in lactase and the efficiency of colonic water reabsorption. Thus, many people who are malabsorbing lactose are nevertheless able to ingest limited amounts of milk and milk products without producing diarrhoea. In childhood their symptoms are mild, but maybe brought to light by gastroenteritis, malnutrition or other causes of mucosal damage.

Lactose malabsorption is confirmed if the exclusion of lactose from the diet relieves the symptoms and subsequent challenge using lactose, 2 g/kg body weight in a 10 per cent solution, causes a recurrence, with acidic stools positive for the presence of reducing substances. Normal lactose absorption may be confirmed by demonstrating a rise in blood glucose after an oral lactose load. However, absence of a rise may reflect inadequate ingestion or variation in the rate of gastric emptying rather than malabsorption. If lactose has reached the colon and been metabolized by bacteria, hydrogen will be produced and may be measured in expired air after a lactose challenge. Lactase may be measured directly in a mucosal biopsy specimen which may also be examined histologically to demonstrate an enteropathy.

Treatment with a lactose-free milk in infants will control symptoms. It is unusual to have to exclude all dairy products in older children. When lactose malabsorption is secondary to acute gastroenteritis, it is usually possible to reintroduce cow's milk after two to four weeks. In some infants gastroenteritis results in mucosal damage, and sensitization to cow's milk and other dietary proteins may occur. The consequent disruption of the enterocyte brush border maintains lactase deficiency, and it may not be possible to reintroduce cow's milk for several months.

Colitis

The cardinal symptoms of colitis are rectal bleeding, diarrhoea, the passage of mucus and abdominal pain. Infections are the most common cause, particularly *Shigella*, *Salmonella*, *Campylobacter* and *Entamoeba histolytica* (see pp. 459–90). Inflammatory bowel disease is rare, but well recognized to occur in childhood. The aetiological diagnoses include ulcerative colitis, Crohn's disease and hypersensitivity to cow's milk protein.

Ulcerative colitis

Ulcerative colitis is characterized by diffuse inflammation and ulceration of the mucosa of the rectum and colon proximal to it. The peak incidence periods are the first year of life and between eight and nine years of age. The aetiology is unknown but probably reflects an interaction between infective, genetic and immunological factors. In addition to the above symptoms, most children present with weight loss, nausea, lack of energy and low-grade fever. Abdominal examination generally reveals non-specific tenderness. Extra-intestinal manifestations include erythema nodosum, arthritis, mouth ulcers and pyoderma gangrenosum. Occasionally, life-threatening fulminating toxic dilatation of the colon occurs.

Investigation and management Infections must first be excluded. A double-contrast barium enema shows proctitis and an abnormal colonic mucosal pattern with loss of haustration, pseudopolyp formation and disordered motility. Mucosal biopsies should be taken at sigmoidoscopy or colonoscopy to confirm the diagnosis.

Fluid and electrolyte disturbances and anaemia must be recognized and corrected, and the diet must contain adequate protein and calories. Specific therapy includes oral prednisolone 60 mg/kg per day (or 0.25–0.75 mg/kg per day in a single morning dose and sulphasalazine 50–100 mg per day in four divided doses). Topical rectal corticosteroids are also useful. Prednisolone should be gradually withdrawn to leave the patient on maintainance sulphasalazine (20–30 mg/kg per day in two divided doses). Opiates and anticholinergic drugs should be avoided since they predispose to the development of toxic megacolon.

The clinical course is chronic with relapses and remissions. Surgery is indicated if acute symptoms do not respond to intensive medical care, if perforation occurs, or if persisting disease activity leads to chronic ill health and developmental delay. There is an increased incidence of malignancy which is related to the duration and extent of the disease; it is of the order of 3.5 and 4.5 per cent between 10 and 20 years from the onset of disease.

Crohn's disease

Crohn's disease causes chronic inflammation of the whole thickness of the bowel wall. Its aetiology is obscure. Histologically, granuloma and fissure formation also occur. The terminal ileum and the colon are particularly affected, although any part of the alimentary tract may be involved with normal bowel in between and with sparing of the rectum.

The symptoms are non-specific and their significance is frequently not appreciated. Useful clues are the presence of painless perianal fissures, or a right iliac fossa mass in the presence of finger clubbing. Nutritional deficiencies are common and are caused by malabsorption and loss of protein and blood into the gut. Extra-intestinal lesions are less common than in ulcerative colitis. An important differential diagnosis is tuberculosis.

Investigation and management   Barium studies of both the small and large bowels are necessary. Oedema, spasm and fibrosis cause narrowing (string sign), patchy involvement is seen (skip lesions), fistulae may be demonstrable, and in the colon, eccentric lesions with rose thorn (spikey) ulcers are seen. Ideally, histological confirmation of a diagnosis should be achieved. Steroids and sulphasalazine are effective in inducing a remission, but are not curative and do not prevent relapse. Attention should be paid to supportive measures and the maintainance of a good nutritional state – the latter is correlated with prolonged remissions. Surgical resections of affected bowel are palliative since the recurrence rate is high. Acute indications for surgery include perforation, haemorrhage and obstruction. Chronic indications include growth retardation, delayed puberty, subacute obstruction and fistulae.

Clostridium perfringens

Clostridium perfringens causes several types of diarrhoeal illness, including food poisoning and necrotizing jejunitis. It is a Gram-positive bacillus with aerotolerant spores, and it produces a variety of toxins. *C. perfrin-* *gens* type A food poisoning presents as watery diarrhoea, with abdominal pain but not vomiting, after an incubation period of 8–20 hours. Signs of systemic illness do not occur and these symptoms usually resolve after 24 hours. In contrast, necrotizing enteritis is a much more serious disease accompanied by vomiting, severe abdominal pain, bloody diarrhoea and ultimately shock. The mortality rate is high. Differential diagnoses include acute shigellosis, acute ulcerative colitis, and other food poisoning syndromes. Treatment is supportive, however, when necrotizing jejunitis occurs surgical resection of the involved bowel must be considered when signs of toxaemia and complications appear.

Constipation

Constipation defined as difficulty or delay in the passage of stools frequently has its origin in factors related to toilet training, diet and behavioural problems. Congenital causes such as Hirschsprung's disease are rare (see p. 899). Intestinal obstruction is discussed on pp. 890-2 and hypothyroidism on pp. 806-7. Acute constipation may occur during a febrile illness or period of anorexia. If the subsequent passage of a hard stool causes a rectal mucosal abrasion or fissure, blood may be seen on the stool and defaecation may become painful and infrequent. Most acute episodes improve spontaneously, but some children continue to retain stools and subsequently have great difficulty in straining to open their bowels. Abdominal distention develops and remarkable faecal masses may accumulate and become readily palpable. Parental anxiety tends to exacerbate the situation, faecal soiling or spurious diarrhoea may occur, and the psychodynamics of the family may need to be taken into account when undertaking management. Physical examination should exclude obvious anal and spinal abnormalities. Rectal examination reveals a ballooned rectum with the stool close to the anal verge. A regular bowel habit should be established by combining a diet of sufficient bulk with the use of a stimulant laxative such as senna. Since many patients are anorexic at this stage, a bulk purgative such as lactulose is useful initially. Laxatives should not be commenced if enormous, rocky faecal masses are present – the lower bowel should first be emptied using an enema which it should not be necessary to repeat. Relapses are common, and laxatives may be required for several months after a normal pattern of defaecation has been regained to cover the period during which the dilated lower bowel with its diminished sensation is returning to normal.

Abdominal pain

Recurrent abdominal pain is common yet notoriously difficult to evaluate in children. Most of the large series reported reflect experience in Europe and North America where it is unusual to make an organic diagnosis in an otherwise healthy child of school age. In the tropics, colic frequently accompanies gastro-intestinal infections, but there are numerous other possible causes arising from the gut and other intra-abdominal organs as well as referred pain from surrounding structures (Table 5.3.3). A large group of healthy children remain in whom emotional causes need to be evaluated.

Acute abdominal pain always requires careful assessment, particularly for infants in whom it must never be immediately assumed that the source of their discomfort is gastro-intestinal. An account of the surgical differential diagnosis and management of acute abdominal pain is given on pp. 894–7. In colicky infants in whom no precise cause may be found, attention should be paid to feeding practices and the possibility that their behaviour may be reflecting parental anxiety or depression.

Table 5.3.3 Causes of recurrent abdominal pain in childhood.

Gastro-intestinal
  Gastroenteritis
  Helminth infections
  Tuberculosis
  Mesenteric adenitis
  Malabsorption syndromes
  Hepatitis
  Gallstones
  Pancreatitis
  Peptic ulcer/gastritis (*Helicobacter* infection)
  Subacute obstruction
  Inflammatory bowel disease
Extragastro-intestinal
  Renal infections
  Renal calculi
  Pneumonia
  Diabetes mellitus
  Sickle cell disease
  Epilepsy
  Migraine
  Lead poisoning
  Metabolic disorders (porphyria)
  Referred pain from spine, gonads
  Pyomyositis
  Gynaecological disorders

Rectal bleeding

Rectal bleeding is most commonly due to local lesions or infections. Pathogens include *Salmonella*, *Shigella*, *Campylobacter* and *Entamoeba histolytica*. Fissures may be associated with constipation. There is a great diversity of other causes, including chronic inflammatory bowel disease, a Meckel's diverticulum, colonic polyps, (usually benign), vascular malformations, Henoch Schönlein purpura and haemorrhagic disorders. An intussusception may also present with rectal bleeding, as may massive upper gastro-intestinal bleeding. When taking the history it must be established whether or not the blood is coming from the rectum or the genito-urinary tract. It is also important to distinguish between bright red or dark red blood mixed with the stools and streaks of blood on the outside of a stool, as would occur with a lesion in the rectal ampulla or anal canal. In the neonate, rectal bleeding may also be caused by necrotizing enterocolitis. In infants, in the absence of a local lesion or infection, the cause often remains obscure and spontaneous resolution occurs.

Mucosal immunity

The gastro-intestinal tract is continually exposed to a bewildering variety of microbiological, dietary and environmental antigens. There is therefore often a requirement to confine immune responses to the mucosa. This contrasts with the effect of parenteral antigens which have long been recognized to induce active systemic humoral and cellular immunity. Oral exposure to antigen characteristically generates a protective local mucosal IgA and cell-mediated immune response, and simultaneously a systemic tolerance or hyporesponsiveness which suppresses subsequent antigen-specific IgG and IgM antibody and cell-mediated activity. This dichotomy is dependent on the immunoregulatory functions of the mucosal-associated lymphoid tissue (MALT).

The MALT forms a substantial lymphoid organ within the body. Lymphocytes are distributed in considerable numbers throughout the lamina propria and in lesser numbers in the epithelium. The lamina propria also contains many isolated lymphoid follicles with larger aggregates in the Peyer's patches, appendix and tonsils. In the epithelium, the predominant cells are T lymphocytes. The lamina propria contains a heterogeneous group of cells including B and T lymphocytes, macrophages, monocytes, and large numbers of plasma cells secreting immunoglobulin, particularly IgA. Antigen entry occurs preferentially through the Peyer's patch epithelium. The importance of antigen access at other mucosal sites is not clearly defined in man but there is evidence that it occurs in the immature infant and situations where the mucosa has been damaged, resulting in altered permeability. Following sensitization in the Peyer's patches, lymphocytes migrate within the lymphatics to the bloodstream from which they preferentially 'home' to the intestinal mucosa as predominantly IgA-producing cells. The major function of intestinal antibodies is immune exclusion at the mucosal surface. IgA is well placed to inhibit absorption of food antigens by complexing with them and promoting their degradation. IgA also reduces bacterial adhesion and toxin binding to enterocytes and is involved with antibody-dependent, cell-mediated cytotoxicity. Although it is difficult to study T lymphocyte function within the mucosa, it is clear that various aspects of cellular responses fulfil a crucial role. Recognition of the importance of mucosal immunity will lead in due course to the development of oral immunization programmes.

The regulation of mucosal immune responses is complex and may be modified in various situations. These include the presence or absence of damage to the mucosa, factors such as infection and adjuvants, and the maturity, state of nutrition and genetic potential of the individual. In man there are three particular situations in which dietary protein intolerance appears to be more common: in infancy, in children born to atopic parents, and after gastroenteritis. In the neonatal period it is likely that some aspects of mucosal immune function are immature, and thus the protection afforded by the mother's milk assumes greater importance. Human milk contains many non-specific immune factors such as macrophages, lysozyme, lactoferrin and the C3 and C4 components of complement. Specific immunity is provided by IgA, which includes antibodies in milk directed against enteric antigens.

The interaction between gastroenteritis and malnutrition, particularly around the weaning period is a crucial factor affecting morbidity and mortality in the non-industrialized world. There is no doubt that the impact of both these factors and their secondary effects has important implications for the regulation and effectiveness of mucosal immune responses.

Opportunist infections

Opportunist infections of the gut are common in AIDS (see pp. 600–4). Bacterial diarrhoeas occur with the usual infecting organisms (such as *Shigella*, *Campylobacter* and *Salmonella*) but the illnesses may be devastating. *Giardia lamblia*, *Entamoeba histolytica* and *Cryptosporidium*

are also encountered, together with cytomegalovirus infections and *Mycobacterium avium intracellulare*.

Protozoal infections

The protozoal pathogens which commonly infect man are *Giardia*, *Cryptosporidium* and *Isospora* (see pp. 459–95).

Cryptosporidiasis

Cryptosporidium was discovered in 1907 in mice – however, the first human infection was not reported until 1976. Since 1982, reports of cryptosporidiasis have increased dramatically, in parallel with the incidence of AIDS. Schizogony and gametogony take place in epithelial cells of the small intestinal tract, oocysts are produced and shed in the faeces, and transmission occurs by the faeco-oral route from person to person or via contaminated food.

In immunocompetent patients, typical symptoms include the passage of four to six watery or mucoid motions a day for up to two weeks, with anorexia, vomiting and abdominal pain. The disease is self-limiting and may mimic giardiasis or other intestinal infections. Asymptomatic infections and the carrier state have often been reported. In immunocompromised hosts cryptosporidiasis causes a severe and chronic diarrhoeal illness, with profuse watery diarrhoea, dehydration and malabsorption.

The diagnosis may be made by demonstrating oocysts in faecal, duodenal or biopsy material, and occasionally in sputum. Special techniques applied to identify oocysts in the faeces include formalin concentration and staining with modified acid-fast stain, Giemsa, safranin, trichrome or auramine. A serological immunofluorescent antibody test is also available.

The only antimicrobial agent which currently appears to be effective in treatment is the macrolide antibiotic spiramycin.

Coccidiasis

Isospora and *Sarcocystis* are intracellular coccidian protozoa related to *Crytosporidium*. After ingestion of oocysts, asexual and sexual reproduction of *Isospora belli* takes place in enterocytes in the small intestinal tract. Oocysts are later excreted in the faeces, however, some sporulate in the intestinal tract leading to internal auto-infection and long-term maintenance of isosporiasis.

Sarcocystis alternates between intermediate hosts such as cattle or pigs. Reproduction of encysted parasites which have been ingested takes place in the small intestine, resulting in the excretion of oocysts or sporocysts.

The true prevalence of isosporiasis is difficult to assess since the coccidia may be difficult to identify in stools. It is more often diagnosed in patients with AIDS. The infection causes acute diarrhoeal disease which can lead to severe dehydration. Occasionally, diarrhoea becomes chronic and may persist for years. In sarcocystiasis, the symptoms may mimic food poisoning after the ingestion of contaminated meats.

The diagnosis of coccidiasis relies upon demonstration of the parasite in faeces or duodenal aspirates. Treatment with antiprotozoal drugs has been unsatisfactory. In chronic or severe cases, tinidazole, furazolidone, and combinations of pyrimethamine and sulphadiazine, trimethoprim and ampicillin have been used.

Diseases of the mouth

Lips

Congenital malformations such as cleft lip and haemangiomata pose special problems. Both may cause long-term disfigurement, particularly in areas where there are no facilities for plastic surgery. Intensive home visiting by an experienced nurse who understands the culture of the community will not only assist the family to solve feeding problems, but will also inspire confidence in the parents of the child.

Cheilosis with raw, red, sore lips can result from sensitization to certain fruit rinds, such as the skins of mangoes and cashew nuts. It can also arise from vitamin deficiency, such as acute ariboflavinosis. This can be responsible for angular cheilosis, which may be exacerbated by constant exposure to the sun and dry winds. Deeper, often relatively painless fissures (rhagades) may occur in congenital syphilis.

Mouth

On examination, inflammation, pigmentation, and gingival and dental abnormalities should all be noted. Ulceration is the most common lesion of the oral mucosa. Acute ulcers can be caused by trauma and infection. Recurrent aphthous ulcers are shallow with a yellow/white base and a surrounding rim of erythema. They may be multiple and involve the gums, tongue and palate. Their aetiology is unknown and their appearance is non-specific. They may occur in nutritional deficiency and in association with inflammatory bowel disease and various systemic gastro-intestinal

and dermatological diseases. Curative treatment is unsatisfactory: antiseptics give symptomatic relief; topical steroids may be of benefit if used early in the prodromal phase of localized burning and pain before the ulcers appear. Oral hygiene must be maintained. Tube feeding or drinking through a straw may be necessary to maintain fluid balance.

Viral infections

Herpes simplex virus type I causes vesiculo-erosive lesions which can extend into a severe gingivo-stomatitis (see p. 615). The onset is with a fever and sore throat with cervical lymphadenopathy. The child later becomes systemically unwell with the pyrexia subsiding over one to two weeks. The patients are infectious and undernourished children are particularly at risk. Specific treatment is with acyclovir. Herpes labialis (cold sores) is a less severe infection with the type I Herpes simplex virus. It causes vesicular eruptions around the lips and occurs in all age groups. It is precipitated by multiple factors, such as a cold, exposure to sunlight, and meningococal and pneumococcal infections.

Herpangina is caused by several types of Coxsackie A viruses (see p. 606). After an abrupt onset of fever, pharyngitis and dysphagia, small papules or vesicles with a red areola develop into superficial ulcers on the anterior faucial pillars and the structures posterior to them. Cervical lymphadenitis is uncommon.

Coxsackie A infections, especially A16, also cause the hand, foot, mouth syndrome in which vesicles progressing to ulcers occur in any part of the mouth and are associated with vesiculo-pustular lesions on the hands and feet which later desquamate.

Fungal infections

Candida albicans (monilia, thrush) causes creamy white patches with superficial mucosal ulceration (see p. 628). Individual lesions resemble milk curds but are adherent with surrounding intensely red inflammation. They may become confluent, extending widely over the oral and pharyngeal mucosa and down into the oesophagus. Infections occur when hygiene is poor, in malnourished children and after courses of antibiotics. Treatment is with nystatin suspension (100 000 units) after feeds or with imidazoles, e.g. miconazole.

Tongue

The traditional place that inspection of the tongue holds in even a cursory examination of any patient is a measure of the numerous, albeit non-specific changes that have been described. Glossitis is an important feature of nutritional deficiencies (riboflavin, niacin, folic acid and vitamin B_{12}). A geographic tongue showing a map-like appearance of normal epithelium and denuded pink areas is of no pathological significance.

Teeth

The time of eruption of teeth appears to be one of the few developmental indices which are relatively unaffected by factors which delay the development of other physical characteristics. Thus, the stage of eruption of teeth is very helpful in assessing the age range in a community. Nonetheless, in some ethnic groups (such as the Bantu of South Africa) the permanent teeth erupt early. In general, the range for eruption of primary or deciduous teeth is 5–30 months, and for shedding is 6–13 years. The mandibular teeth erupt before the maxillary in the order of central then lateral incisors, first molars, canines, and finally second molars. Natal teeth may cause nursing difficulties and should be removed, as should supernumerary teeth which occasionally appear. In some normal individuals, one or more permanent teeth can fail to erupt.

In traditional societies, dental caries is rare in children in the tropics. Many of the dental problems encountered arise from disorders which affect the gum. This picture is, however, rapidly changing. The great increase in the consumption of refined sugars, over-milled flours and sweets among the population of developing countries has caused an alarming increase in the incidence of dental caries. Instruction in good oral hygiene and eating habits will reduce its incidence and also the simple forms of gingivitis. Local practices which promote healthy teeth must be encouraged. The teeth should be cleaned twice a day. If a chewing stick is used as the local toothbrush it must not be employed so vigorously that the gingival margins become traumatized. The consumption of fruits such as oranges and mangoes at bedtime is useful in cleaning the teeth. Ingestion of concentrated sugars and sweets between meals should be kept to a minimum. Small children should not be allowed to fall asleep with a bottle of milk or to hold one in the mouth for prolonged periods. Fluoridation of water supplies to prevent dental caries is beginning to be used in some subtropical and tropical countries.

Cleft palate

When this occurs in children in tropical areas it poses serious social and feeding problems. Support and encouragement for the family is essential, and mothers must be taught to feed their children with cup and spoon until the child is old enough to speak.

Uvula

Uvulectomy is a practice carried out by native surgeons, particularly in northern Nigeria. The uvula, observed to be pointing downwards towards the throat is regarded as a symbol of doom and therefore has to be removed. A severe illness may follow as cellulitis of the surrounding tissues causes respiratory obstruction or septicaemia.

Cancrum oris

This condition involves a rapidly progressive erosive gangrenous lesion of the gums, the neighbouring bones, and the buccal mucosa of the cheeks. It arises in malnourished children, and may follow an attack of measles or herpetic gingivitis, during which local trauma allows access for *Borrelia vincenti* and *Fusiformis fusiformis* which initially cause necrotic ulcerative gingivitis. Eventually the cheeks may be perforated and the teeth fall out. There is a characteristic fetid odour and the regional lymph nodes are enlarged. The disfigurement produced by these lesions (Fig. 5.3.1) gives rise to enormous social handicaps for the children. Vigorous treatment with penicillin usually halts the progress of the disease. If, however, the damage produced is already great, difficult plastic surgery will be necessary.

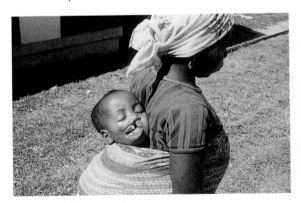

Fig. 5.3.1 Cancrum oris.

Parotid glands

Parotid swelling occurs in kwashiorkor, Chagas' disease, HIV infection, calcific pancreatitis, and when local calculi are present. It is also caused by mumps, Coxsackie and other viruses. Bacterial infections causing suppurative parotitis require treatment with antibiotics and sometimes surgical drainage.

The pancreas

Pancreatitis

The most important feature of acute pancreatitis is abdominal pain. This is usually sudden in onset and of great severity. The pain is maximal in the upper abdomen and characteristically, but by no means always radiates centrally through to the back. Vomiting may also be a prominent symptom. Physical examination will reveal varying degrees of shock, fever, and localized abdominal guarding or rigidity. The patient is usually quiet and lies on his side with legs slightly bent. In the most severe form, acute haemorrhagic pancreatitis, haemorrhagic ascites develops and a bluish discoloration of the flanks or around the umbilicus may be seen. The presence of a palpable mass in the upper abdomen may indicate that a pseudocyst has developed. The most important laboratory test is the level of serum amylase – a fourfold increase above the normal value being consistent with the diagnosis.

Viral infections are the most important cause of acute pancreatitis in childhood; trauma and drug-induced inflammation are less common. Viruses which have been implicated include mumps, Coxsackie B5, influenza, Epstein–Barr virus and hepatitis B. Pancreatitis may be induced by penetrating injuries, however, it is more frequently associated with blunt abdominal trauma. Drug-induced pancreatitis is well described after exposure to corticosteroids or sodium valproate. Various metabolic disorders are associated with pancreatitis, including hyperlipidaemia, hyperparathyroidism and hypercalcaemia. Associated hepatobiliary disorders are probably less important factors in paediatric compared with adult practice. An important congenital anomaly which is now shown to increase the incidence of pancreatitis in some children is a malfusion of the ventral and dorsal pancreatic anlage. It is more common than annular pancreas with an incidence of up to 5 per cent. This pancreas division malformation results in two independent duct systems: the ventral system communicating with the common bile duct and a separate dorsal system which may have a narrow orifice opening in the accessory ampulla. Dilatation of the pancreatic duct system may then be found.

Treatment has two main aims: to restore fluid and electrolyte balance and to provide adequate analgesia. Morphine is contra-indicated since it causes spasm of the sphincter of Oddi; pethidine is usually recommended. Pancreatic secretion is decreased by nasa-gastric decompression of the stomach and drainage of gastric secretions. Antibiotics are only of use if a pancreatic abscess develops or when blood cultures or other signs indicate sepsis.

Pancreatic insufficiency

Chronic severe protein malnutrition may result in pancreatic insufficiency, and atrophy of the pancreas was described soon after the recognition of kwashiorkor. A calcific form of chronic pancreatitis has also been associated with malnutrition and is almost endemic in the Indian subcontinent, particularly in the state of Kerala. It appears that this syndrome differs from the reversible pancreatic atrophy seen in kwashiorkor. It is well known that the susceptibility of the pancreas to toxic agents in increased in malnutrition, thus the aetiology may be a multifactorial combination of poor nutritional status, toxins and infection. These forms of chronic pancreatitis are associated with steatorrhoea and, in many cases, the onset of diabetes mellitus.

In Caucasian populations the most common cause of pancreatic exocrine insufficiency is cystic fibrosis; however, this is excessively rare in other ethnic groups. Various rare congenital abnormalities of pancreatic secretion have also been recognized, such as enterokinase and colipase deficiency.

Indirect evaluation of pancreatic function includes an estimation of faecal fat excretion and investigation of the stools for tryptic activity. Direct pancreatic function tests involve duodenal intubation and stimulation of secretion using a standard test meal or intravenous secretin and cholecystokinin. The activities of lipase, trypsin, and amylase are measured in duodenal juice together with the bicarbonate concentration and the volume secreted. Various preparations of pancreatic extracts are available for replacement therapy. The dose required to control steatorrhoea varies from patient to patient.

The liver

Hepatic disorders commonly occur in tropical countries because of the constant bombardment of stimuli which the liver receives as viruses, bacteria, ova, adult parasites, enteric endotoxins and other antigens pass through it via the portal vein. Numerically the most common severe liver diseases are those associated with B, non-A and non-B hepatitis viruses which cause acute hepatitis (see pp. 610–14) and chronic hepatitis,

Table 5.3.4 Pathological mechanisms and parasitic diseases of the liver.

Reticuloendothelial hyperplasia
Malaria
Kala-azar
Acute toxoplasmosis
Trypanosomiasis
Schistosomiasis
Necrosis
Amoebic abscess
Cyst formation
Echinococcus
Granuloma formation
Schistosomiasis
Visceral larva migrans
Bile duct obstruction
Liver flukes

cirrhosis and hepatoma. Many parasitic infections affect the liver. Some of the major pathological processes are listed in relation to the pathogens involved in Table 5.3.4. Hepatic involvement is often present in patients with systemic bacterial infections, e.g. pneumococcal lobar pneumonia. In addition there are disorders which are specific for certain localities, such as Indian childhood cirrhosis and veno-occlusive disease.

Cirrhosis

Cirrhosis is the end-stage of many forms of injury to the liver. It is defined pathologically as a replacement of the normal hepatic architecture by regenerative nodules which are surrounded by marked fibrosis. This proliferation of connective tissue and distortion of the structure of the liver disrupts the intralobular circulation and precipitates portal hypertension. There are many classifications of cirrhosis, according to the aetiology, the pathological appearances of micro- or macro-nodules, and the extent of fibrosis and hepatocellular necrosis. A further major division is into patients with postnecrotic cirrhosis following any form of hepatocellular damage, and those with biliary cirrhosis in which the primary abnormality is in the biliary tree, the hepatic parenchyma being relatively unchanged initially. The clinical course of cirrhosis may be divided into compensated and decompensated stages.

Aetiology

The liver is capable of phenomenal regrowth following severe injury. However, in some patients this return to normality fails to occur. The factors controlling

hepatic regeneration are obscure. One common feature appears to be that when hepatocellular necrosis occurs near the portal tracts abnormal amounts of collagen are more likely to accumulate and the stage is then set for the continuing distortion of lobular architecture described above.

There are numerous causes of cirrhosis which occur in temperate as well as tropical regions. These include viral hepatitis, congenital abnormalities of the biliary tract, and various familial metabolic disorders such as Wilson's hepato-lenticular degeneration, Gaucher's and Niemann–Pick diseases and galactosaemia. Each region of the tropics has its own spectrum of chronic liver disease. Cirrhosis can be peculiar to specific regions, for example Indian childhood cirrhosis, cirrhosis following veno-occlusive disease, malnutrition and parasitic diseases, haemosiderosis due to iron overload, and oriental cholangiohepatitis. Some of these conditions are discussed here following a general account of clinical aspects of cirrhosis. *Schistosoma mansoni* infection is discussed on p. 652.

Clinical features

The characteristic clinical features arise from chronic hepatocellular failure and portal hypertension. In compensated cirrhosis, the principal features will be those of the underlying cause. The onset of anorexia and malabsorption leads to malnutrition and failure to thrive. Portal hypertension is associated with a reduction in effective hepatic blood flow and the development of collateral vessels such as oesophageal varices which bypass the liver. The abdomen becomes prominent as hepatosplenomegaly and ascites develop and dilated superficial abdominal vessels appear, radiating from the umbilicus towards the systemic circulation. The liver edge feels firm and sharply defined but as the disease progresses it shrinks in size and the area of hepatic dullness is reduced. The most prominent change in the peripheral circulation is the presence of vascular spider naevi, in the drainage area of the superior vena cava. These lesions contain a central arteriole with numerous fine vessels radiating from it – pressure on the centre of the lesion causes complete blanching. Palmar erythema is a feature with clubbing and white nails. As decompensation occurs, peripheral oedema and ascites are seen. The onset of encephalopathy is accompanied by a characteristic fetor hepaticus, a sweetish, slightly faecal smell on the breath. The appearance of jaundice, spontaneous bruising and epistaxis are all grave signs; septicaemia is often a terminal event.

Investigations

Routine laboratory investigations of liver function may be normal in the presence of cirrhosis. The disturbances which often occur are an increase in serum transaminases and a fall in serum albumin. Alkaline phosphatase concentrations are elevated, especially in biliary cirrhosis, and the prothrombin time is frequently prolonged. The serum bilirubin is commonly normal until decompensation occurs. The most sensitive and easily available test of liver function is the bromsulphalein clearance test which normally shows less than 5 per cent retention of an injected dose 45 minutes after its intravenous administration. A peripheral blood count will often show a modest reduction in total white cell count and haemoglobin with acanthocytosis (burr cells) in advanced disease.

A barium meal may show varices in the oesophagus, stomach or duodenum; occasionally peptic ulcers are evident. Ultrasound, scintiscans and endoscopy are all useful. Liver biopsy is the definitive investigation which confirms the diagnosis of cirrhosis. However, it may well not provide an indication of aetiology.

Management

The aims of management are first to control the underlying cause of the liver disease whenever possible, and secondly to prevent or treat complications. The complications are similar to those which occur in adults but the impact of nutritional deficiency is greater in the growing child. Malnutrition arises from anorexia and malabsorption of fat and the fat-soluble vitamins; specific supplements of vitamins A, D and K must be given in the diet. Hypoalbuminaemia due to reduced albumin synthesis leads to oedema and ascites as portal hypertension develops. An additional factor in the redistribution of fluid in the body is an increase in the total body water associated with a rise in aldosterone production and increased renal sodium reabsorption. Although ascites can cause numerous complications it may be present for long periods or recurrently without causing problems. If treatment is decided upon, the key-stone of management is sodium restriction. Very low sodium diets are unpalatable, thus restriction to 10–20 mmol/day or a no-added salt regimen is more practical. The diuretic of choice is an aldosterone antagonist (spironolactone) which has the additional advantage of countering the potassium depletion which is encountered in cirrhotic patients. Frusemide may be added later, and close biochemical monitoring will be required. Therapeutic paracentesis is not advised unless gross acute symptoms arise from raised intra-abdominal pressure. Diagnostic paracentesis is, however, essential in the presence of unexplained fever, diarrhoea, abdominal pain or encephalopathy.

Bleeding from varices or associated peptic ulceration is a major complication. Following stabilization of the patient's condition, the site of bleeding should ideally be identified if facilities are available. If the bleeding is not profuse, bedrest, mild sedation, antacids and H2 blockers (ranitidine) are useful. If bleeding continues pitressin may be used as an emergency measure, infusing 20 U/100 ml of 5 per cent dextrose over 2–40 minutes. Oral propranolol 1 mg/kg/day may also be used. In a referral unit balloon tamponade is carried out using a Sengstaken–Blakemore tube, followed by surgical procedures such as injection of the varices with sclerosants, or proceeding to a porto-systemic shunt. Since the presence of blood in the bowel will precipitate encephalopathy, the patient should be given purgatives and neomycin (see later).

Hepatic encephalopathy

Hepatic encephalopathy is characterized by intellectual impairment and clouding of consciousness, progressing to personality changes, stupor and coma. A flapping tremor of the hands occurs, the tendon reflexes are initially increased but later decreased, and varying neurological signs develop indicating organic brain disease. An acute severe form occurs in fulminant hepatitis. A chronic encephalopathy may be exacerbated by gastro-intestinal haemorrhage, dehydration, infection or renal failure. The pathogenesis of this syndrome is complex; it is thought that ammonia, methionine, toxins, short-chain fatty acids and biogenic amines may all have a role to play in it. Reye's syndrome is an important cause of encephalopathy and coma which is discussed on pp. 744–5. The basic aims of treatment are to improve liver function and prevent ammonia accumulation. The latter is achieved by dietary protein restriction, and the use of neomycin to reduce the bowel flora and thus the bacterial production of urea within the gut. Lactulose produces an osmotic diarrhoea, the acid pH further reducing colonic ammonia reabsorption. Attention must also be paid to electrolyte balance and the treatment of any precipitating causes.

Indian childhood cirrhosis

Indian childhood cirrhosis (ICC) is a micronodular cirrhosis in which the hepatocytes contain large amounts of copper and copper-binding protein and Mallory's hyaline. It presents late in the course of the disease, there is no accepted treatment, and the mortality is high. It is seen almost exclusively among children in India, Burma, Pakistan and Sri Lanka. Although the peak incidence is between one and three years of age, it can affect children between two weeks and ten years of age. It occurs in all classes and is seen more often in the villages than in the urban centres of India.

The aetiology is unknown. The high incidence of consanguinuity, the familial occurrence and the recognized association with the C3F gene support a multifactorial inheritance. The association with copper-contaminated milk and excessive copper levels in many organs supports the importance of environmental factors. Immunological dysfunction has been demonstrated, while the role of infections and inborn errors of metabolism continues to be investigated.

Clinical features

Most children are asymptomatic during the early stages of the disease. A low-grade fever, anorexia and irritability are associated with abdominal distension with an enlarged smooth liver with a sharp 'leaf-like' edge readily palpable below the right costal margin. Progression to cirrhosis takes from one to eight months, splenomegaly is constant, the liver becomes harder, ascites and jaundice develop and progression to decompensation occurs. The cause of death is almost exclusively hepatocellular failure, often precipitated by gastro-intestinal bleeding or infection. A palpable gall-bladder is an especially bad prognostic sign.

The classic histopathology on liver biopsy (see earlier) enables the diagnosis to be confirmed. The hepatic concentration of copper has been reported to be as high as 6 600 μg/g dry weight (normal less than 50 μg/g). Wilson's disease is distinguished by a presentation later on in life, the presence of Kayser–Fleischer rings, and hypercaeruloplasminaemia. Treatment of ICC with D-penicillamine has so far been disappointing.

Hepatic veno-occlusive disease

Veno-occlusive disease of the liver refers to post-sinusoidal obstruction involving the small hepatic veins. It is the result of a toxic liver injury produced by pyrrolizidine alkaloids amongst other agents. It was initially recognized in Jamaican children and found to be the result of the ingestion of medicinal 'bush tea' made from *Crotelaria* plants.

Initially the disease was thought to be limited in distribution to the Caribbean countries and South America. However, similar outbreaks have been described caused by pyrrolizidine alkaloids from contaminated bread in South Africa, wheat in Afghanistan, cereals in Northern India and herbal tea in Britain. Epidemics have been reported in times of drought where staple foods have become contaminated with toxic plants. There is also some evidence that malnutrition increases susceptibility to poisoning from such toxins.

Histopathologically the findings are of centrilobular congestion with haemorrhagic necrosis of the parenchymal cells arising from fibrous obliteration of central and sublobular veins. Recovery from an acute episode is accompanied by recanalization of the small veins. Chronic ingestion leads to centrilobular fibrosis progressing to a micronodular cirrhosis.

Clinical features

The initial acute phase of veno-occlusive disease is marked by the sudden onset of epigastric pain, hepatomegaly and ascites without significant jaundice. Recovery usually takes four to six weeks but it may be incomplete leading to a subacute stage characterized by recurrent ascites and firm hepatomegaly. If a collateral circulation develops the disease may resolve completely during the early stages. However, progression to cirrhosis (see earlier) with prominent portal hypertension and intractable ascites occurs in the chronic form of the disease.

Differential diagnosis and treatment

The differential diagnosis is that of portal hypertension. Once centrilobular hepatic congestion has been recognized on a liver biopsy, the Budd–Chiari syndrome must be excluded. This condition involves occlusion of the hepatic vein. Thus, on liver biopsy the majority of central vein branches are patent, in contrast to veno-occlusive disease where there is fibrous occlusion of the central veins.

An early diagnosis can often reverse the course of disease; thus, ingestion of alkaloids or other toxic drugs must be stopped. The general management of portal hypertension and cirrhosis was discussed on p. 735.

Liver fluke infections

The liver flukes are trematode worms which in man inhabit the bile ducts (see pp. 736–8). The important human parasites are *Clonorchis sinensis* and *Opisthorchis viverrini* of the superfamily Opisthorchioidae which occur mainly in the Far East, and *Fasciola hepatica* which is widely reported from Africa, Asia, South and Central

America and Europe. Adult worms of *C. sinensis* and *O. viverrini* shed their eggs into the biliary system and they are then voided in the faeces. The first intermediate hosts are snails in which ciliated miracidia hatch and develop further into sporocytes, rediae and cercariae. These are released and enter the second intermediate hosts which are various species of fresh-water fish and crayfish, where they develop into metacercariae. When man or another mammal eats raw or improperly cooked fish, the parasites excyst in the duodenum and migrate into the biliary ducts where they mature into adult worms. Infection is highly endemic in some areas of Thailand and Laos. The main factors responsible are: the habit of consuming raw fish food, which is also given to young children; poor hygiene resulting in pollution of water supplies; and the prevalence of *Bithynia* snails and fresh-water fish.

F. hepatica requires the snail genus *Lymnaea* and water plants to which the metacercariae attach. Human infestation is found in people of lower socio-economic standing who are associated with livestock or who eat uncooked water plants (especially watercress) or drink contaminated unboiled water containing viable metacercariae.

Pathology

The presence of the adult liver flukes in the distal biliary ducts provokes adenomatous hyperplasia of the biliary epithelium with thickening of the walls and crypt formation. When the duration of infection is prolonged, periductal inflammation with portal fibrosis occurs, the bile ducts dilate and the liver hypertrophies. In severe infections, necrosis and atrophy of hepatocytes occurs with the formation of multiple biliary cysts. Secondary bacterial infection causes further damage as a result of cholangitis, cholecystitis and stone formation. There is a high association between liver fluke disease and cholangiocarcinoma.

Clinical features

The clinical manifestations of infection depend upon the number of worms, the duration of infection, the degree of liver damage and nutritional status. In mild to moderate infection the patients are usually symptomless – some may complain of anorexia, flatulence, indigestion and intermittent right upper quadrant discomfort; others may show intermittent diarrhoea and mild obstructive jaundice. In more severe infestations the three features of dyspepsia, right hypochondrial pain and diarrhoea become more prominent but are rather non-specific complaints in themselves. Heavy infestations produce features of localized biliary obstruction with jaundice and the attendant complications of stones, cholangitis and abscesses. Oedema and ascites may be observed with the advance of malnutrition and cirrhosis.

The signs and symptoms of fascioliasis are in general more drastic and acute than those of the Opisthorchiida. During the acute phase of migration of the young parasites to the liver, abdominal pain with shock may be seen due to intra-abdominal haemorrhages from the liver capsule. A peripheral eosinophilia may be present and ectopic sites of fluke migration may catch the unwary, presenting as subcutaneous masses which may be up to 6 cm in diameter, itchy and painful, with inflammatory features.

Diagnosis and treatment

The most pertinent test is finding the ova in the stools of the patient, or in fluid obtained from duodenal intubation or aspiration from liver cysts. The eggs require about five months from the initial infection to appear in the stool; thus duodenal aspiration may enable their recovery earlier. A variety of complement-fixation and intradermal tests have been described but these are not generally available.

Liver function tests may be useful to detect obstructive jaundice. A polymorphonuclear leucocytosis is often seen in children with cholangitis and abscess. Although an eosinophilia is common it may be caused by a variety of helminthic diseases. The biliary tract may be investigated in more detail radiologically.

The differential diagnosis is extensive and includes intestinal parasitic infections, amoebic hepatitis and liver abscess, hydatid cysts, viral hepatitis, cirrhosis and carcinoma of the liver. Specific chemotherapy for liver fluke infections is so far unsatisfactory. Most of the drugs employed have been either ineffective or produced unacceptable toxicity. Some of the drugs which have been used include chloroquine phosphate (5 mg/kg per day for six weeks), dehydroemetine (2.5 mg/kg per day on alternative days for 12–15 doses) and niclosamide (1–2 mg/kg for two or three days).

Hetol (hexachloroparaxylene) has been used in China and Japan but has multiple side-effects, including sensitization. It is contra-indicated in those with a history of contact dermatitis using the drug. A more recent promising medication is praziquantel (Biltricide). (See p. 646.)

Most patients presenting with acute cholangitis respond to conservative treatment with intravenous fluids and antibiotics, usually in the form of aminoglycosides and/or cephalosporins. Emergency surgery is indicated when there are signs of general peritonitis or empyema of the gall-bladder.

In theory, these diseases can be prevented by not eating raw fish. However, changing cultural practices is difficult. Extermination of snails by molluscicides is impractical. Control by biological means and changes in the environment have been tried.

Hydatid disease (echinococcosis)

Infection with cestodes of the genus *Echinococcus* causes solitary (*E. granulosus*) or multiple (*E. multilocularis*) cysts in the liver (see also p. 643). The adult parasites live in the intestine of dogs, jackals and other carnivores. The larval stage causes the disease in the intermediate hosts which are various herbivores such as sheep, cattle, camels and buffaloes, and occasionally man. Children usually become infected by accidentally ingesting the faeces of dogs. Oncospheres emerged from ingested eggs, penetrate the intestinal mucosa and in most cases reach the liver. However, they can also be distributed to the lungs as well as to many other anatomical sites (see p. 643). Larval development produces fluid-filled cysts (Fig. 5.3.2) which grow slowly by concentric enlargement (1–5 cm per year) but are well tolerated until they become large enough to cause pain or dysfunction by compression. They are surrounded by a connective tissue adventitial reaction of variable intensity. The disease is endemic world-wide, wherever there is major livestock rearing activity.

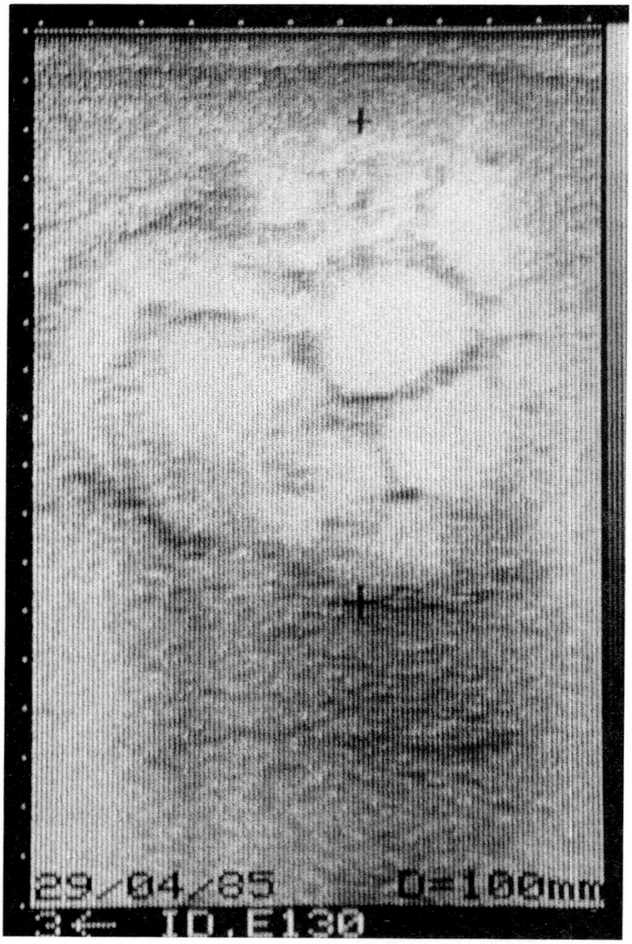

Fig. 5.3.2   Ultrasound showing hydatid cyst. (Courtesy of the Hydatid Unit, AMREF, Kenya.) See also Figs. 4.10.6 and 4.10.7.

Clinical features and diagnosis

The symptomatology is extremely variable and never pathognomonic. The liver is enlarged (see p. 643). A live cyst will destroy surrounding structures by compression rather than infiltration, and, depending on its location, this may or may not produce symptoms. Secondary bacterial infection can cause a liver abscess. Rupture with sudden release of hydatid fluid produces allergic reactions such as urticaria, wheezing and oedema or even anaphylactoid shock. Secondary larvae (protoscolices) may be released locally or transported via the bloodstream to give rise to new cysts in distant sites. Diagnostic puncture of a suspected cyst should never be performed because of the dangers of allergic reactions, infection and secondary hydatidosis.

The Casoni intradermal test has been used for many years; it relies on immediate and delayed responses to an antigen prepared from hydatid fluid. It is non-specific and gives variable positivity rates. The complement-fixation and latex agglutination tests give reliable results but a negative finding does not rule out the diagnosis since antibodies may be absent or masked in an immune complex. Immunoelectrophoresis techniques are more specific. Ultrasonography and other scanning techniques are of value in localizing the cysts and differentiating them from other space-occupying lesions.

Treatment

Surgery remains the treatment of choice when sophisticated facilities are available, but there is a significant morbidity and mortality. Formalin and cetrimide have been injected into the cyst to kill the protoscolices before enucleation. Chemotherapy remains unsatisfactory, although various benzimidazole derivatives such as mebendazole, flubendazole and albendazole have given promising results. The limiting factor is penetrability of the cyst wall by the therapeutic agent. Thus, high dosages are required and ideally the plasma levels need to be monitored because of extreme individual variations in intestinal absorption. Albendazole (200–400 mg daily for 28 days in repeated courses) is appearing to revolutionize the treatment of hydatid disease. Surgical removal is now being limited to the occasional very large or resistant cysts and is performed at the end of a course of Albendazole. Prevention through health education aimed at disposing of infected offal and treatment and reduction of the dog population is the best approach to control.

Amoebic liver abscess

The liver is the most frequent extragastro-intestinal location of amoebiasis caused by *Entamoeba histolytica*. Amoebiasis is ubiquitous in tropical countries, particularly in conditions of overcrowding and low socio-economic status. The majority of infected people become healthy cyst carriers. Amoebic liver abscess (ALA) occurs in less than 4 per cent of infected individuals when trophozoites in the caecum and ascending colon embolize to the liver via the portal vein from thrombosed venules of the gut wall. An amoebic liver abscess is a well-defined area in which the liver parenchyma is completely replaced by necrotic material, surrounded by a ring of congested liver tissue. It may vary in size from a pin-point lesion to an extremely large mass, particularly affecting the right lobe of the liver. Complications may arise from local compression or rupture into the peritoneal cavity.

Clinical features and diagnosis

Liver abscess classically presents with intermittent fever, weakness, night sweats and tenderness over the right hypochondrium. There may be right shoulder pain and many children have signs at the base of the right lung. Laboratory investigations may be normal but usually reveal a leucocytosis, a rapidly rising erythrocyte sedimentation rate and a moderate anaemia. Elevated levels of alkaline phosphatase and direct bilirubin are often found but can be absent even when large amounts of liver parenchyma have been destroyed. Radiological screening shows an elevation and hypomotility of the right hemidiaphragm. Ultrasound and other scanning techniques may detect filling defects in the liver but cannot identify the aetiology. Serodiagnosis is of enormous value, using the immuno-fluorescent antibody technique, counter-current immunoelectrophoresis or enzyme-linked immunosorbent assays. They may give negative results in the early phases of the disease or in immunosuppressed individuals. Stool examination does not contribute to the diagnosis since intestinal amoebiasis may be concomitant or absent (see p. 477). Exploratory liver puncture should only be undertaken in experienced hands, if the differentiation from a pyogenic abscess has proved difficult and when the possibility of liver echinococcosis has been eliminated. The classic anchovy paste appearance of the aspirated material from ALA is typical but not constant, *E. histolytica* may be found on Giemsa staining or culture of the terminal portion of the aspirate.

Treatment

Treatment was revolutionized by the discovery of the nitroimidazole derivatives, metronizadole, tinidazole and ornidazole. Metronidazole (Flagyl) should be given in a dose of 25–40 mg/kg per day for ten days (see p. 487). Antibiotics should be given if a secondary bacterial infection is suspected. Surgical intervention is now only required for some secondary bacterial complications. Subsequent treatment with an active contact amoebicide (e.g. diloxanide furoate) has been recommended to eradicate cysts in the bowel lumen and avoid relapses.

African haemosiderosis

Haemosiderosis is characterized by an increase in total body iron and usually results from exogenous iron introduced via the gastro-intestinal tract or parenterally. It has been well described in African populations. Initially this siderosis was thought to be secondary to a metabolic defect. However, it was soon discovered that the iron content of the diet was high as a result of the use of rusty cooking pots. Haemosiderosis also occurs in children with chronic haemolytic anaemias, the intravascular haemolysis releasing large amounts of haemoglobin iron which is taken up by the hepatocytes. Normally iron absorption from the gastro-intestinal tract would be decreased but because of the ineffective haematopoiesis and chronic haemolysis this does not happen and iron absorption actually increases. The liver becomes enlarged and pathologically it appears rusty brown with histological changes showing a micronodular cirrhosis and excess stainable iron in the hepatocytes, Kupffer cells and portal tracts. Some patients with siderosis do not develop cirrhosis; this supports the possibility that the hepatic changes arise from a multifactorial aetiology. There is experimental evidence that the siderotic liver is more vulnerable to hepatotoxins, viruses and nutritional deficiency.

Clinical features and diagnosis

Iron overload without significant tissue damage is usually asymptomatic. As childhood progresses, firm hepatomegaly and splenomegaly develop. Serum iron levels are usually elevated as is the serum ferritin. Various secondary features may arise from associated abnormal ascorbic acid metabolism, osteoporosis, and pancreatic fibrosis. The diagnosis of iron overload depends on liver biopsy. There is no specific treatment for established haemosiderosis. The ideal approach is prevention, either by reducing the dietary intake of iron or, in the case of thalassaemia major, by treating with chelating agents such as desferrioxamine (p. 832).

Further reading

Anderson CM, Burke V, Gracey M. *Paediatric Gastroenterology*, 2nd Edn. London, Blackwell Scientific, 1987.

Bhagwat AG, Walia BNS. Indian childhood cirrhosis: a commentary. *Indian Journal of Pediatrics*. 1980; **48**: 433–7.

Bhave SA, Pandit NA, Pradham AM. Liver disease in India. *Archives of Disease in Childhood*. 1982; **57**: 922–8.

Craig PS, Zeyhle E, Romig T. Hydatid disease: research and control in Turkana. II. The role of immunological techniques for the diagnosis of hydatid diseases. *Transactions of the Royal Society of Tropical Medicine and Hygiene*. 1986; **80**: 183–92.

Degremont A. Parasite diseases of the liver. *Balliere's Clinical Gastroenterology*. 1987; **1**: 251–72.

Martinez–Palomo A ed. *Amoebiasis, Human Parasite Diseases*. Amsterdam, Elsevier, 1986.

Mowat AP. *Liver Disorders in Childhood*: 2nd Edn. London, Butterworths, 1987.

Tanner MS, Bhave SA, Kantarjian AH *et al.* Early introduction of copper-contaminated milk feeds as a possible cause of Indian childhood cirrhosis. *Lancet*. 1983; **ii**: 992–5.

Thompson JE, Forlenza S, Verma R. Amoebic liver abscess: therapeutic approach. *Reviews of Infectious Diseases*. 1985; **7**: 171–9.

Walker–Smith JA. *Diseases of the Small Intestine in Childhood*. London, Butterworths, 1988.

CHAPTER 4

Disease of the central nervous system

Suresh Rao Aroor

Children with neurological disorders comprise a significant proportion of paediatric practice. Approximately 30 per cent of all children admitted to an active teaching hospital and 40–60 per cent of patients admitted to tertiary paediatric care have neurological diseases which are primary or secondary to other systemic conditions. The higher incidence of neurological disease in the paediatric age group in recent years, is probably more apparent than real, and it results from our increasing ability to detect disturbances within the nervous system.

Neurological diagnosis is dependent on the evaluation of the history, the performance of a careful and detailed neurological examination, and the utilization of appropriate ancillary procedures.

Coma

Coma is a state of unconsciousness that differs from syncope, in being sustained, and from sleep in being less easily reversed. A normal level of consciousness (wakefulness) depends upon activation of the cerebral hemispheres by groups of neurones located in the brainstem and known as the reticular activating system (RAS). This is a highly complex polysynaptic region in the very core of the upper pons and the mid-brain, which bifurcates into both thalamic regions and ultimately becomes widespread within the hemispheres. Both the cerebral hemispheres, the RAS, and the connections between them must be preserved for normal consciousness. The principal causes of coma are, therefore bilateral hemispheric damage or a brain-stem lesion that damages the RAS.

The pharmacological or biochemical vulnerability of the RAS is reflected in the appearance of coma in nearly every variety of severe metabolic disturbance and the fact that the RAS is the major site of action of numerous pharmacological and toxic agents.

Differential diagnosis

One of the initial diagnostic decisions is whether the alteration in consciousness is due to a process which is primarily intra or extracranial. The intracranial processes are subdivided into those in which focal signs are likely and those in which no focal signs may be anticipated. The major categories of intracranial processes with focal brain dysfunction include trauma, haemorrhage, tumours, certain forms of infection, and brain infarction. The intracranial processes causing coma without focal signs include meningitis, encephalitis, cerebral malaria, and subarachnoid haemorrhage.

The extracranial processes which cause coma can be divided into those encephalopathies arising as a result of endogenous metabolic derangements, and those due to exogenous toxins. All major dysfunctions of the body's vital organ systems result in endogenous metabolic derangements, which ultimately lead to coma.

Infectious causes

Infections of the central nervous system (CNS) and its coverings should be suspected in every comatose child. A lumbar puncture, the single most valuable diagnostic test, should be performed if there is no papilloedema. Infections of the CNS could be of bacterial, viral, protozoal (cysticercosis, amoebiasis and malaria) or fungal aetiology. The other infectious causes of coma include postinfectious and parainfectious encephalomyelitis, acute haemorrhagic leucoencephalopathy, and severe systemic infections (bacterial pneumonia, pyelonephritis, soft tissue abscesses and enteric fever). Neuro-infections are discussed in detail elsewhere (see pp. 745–56).

Metabolic causes

Numerous systemic metabolic disorders lead to coma (Table 5.4.1). Usually the loss of consciousness occurs slowly or over a matter of several days and the underlying metabolic state is suspected on other clinical grounds.

Disorders of electrolytes are frequently accompanied by coma. Hyponatraemia may be due to adrenal

Table 5.4.1   Metabolic and vascular causes of coma.

Metabolic causes	Vascular causes
Hypoglycaemia	Hypertensive
Hypoxia	encephalopathy
Hepatic failure	Hypotension
Acidosis	Haemorrhage
Alkalosis	intracerebral
Hypercapnia	subarachnoid
Hyper- and hypocalcaemia/	subdural
magnesaemia	Thrombosis
Osmotic abnormalities	Vasculitis
Diabetes	Embolization
Hyperosmolar states	Bleeding diatheses
Injudicious intravenous therapy	Aortic stenosis
Hypertonic dehydration	Asystole
Diabetes insipidus	
Gastroenteritis	
Hypotonic states	
Inappropriate ADH secretion	
Excess water intake	
Uraemia	
Porphyria	
Vitamin deficiency/dependency	
states	

insufficiency or acute water intoxication. Hypertonic dehydration is accompanied by loss of water from the brain to the vascular compartment. The brain actually shrinks away from the inner table of the skull and bridging veins may be torn, leading to a subdural haematoma.

Hypoglycaemia of any aetiology may lead to coma. This condition is rather infrequent, but is an important cause of deep coma, episodic confusion, and convulsions. The essential biochemical abnormality is a blood sugar level of less than 1.4–1.9 mmol/l (lower in infants) lasting for about 90 minutes and leading to exhaustion of the stores of cerebral glucose and glycogen. The most common causes of hypoglycaemic coma are endocrine dysfunction, ketotic hypoglycaemia, drugs, toxins, malnutrition, insulinoma, Reye's syndrome, and glycogen-storage disease. The diagnosis depends largely upon the history and the documentation of a reduced blood sugar during an attack.

Uraemia is a common cause of metabolic coma at all ages, including the newborn. The exact pathophysiology of coma in renal failure is poorly understood. A multifactorial cause is likely, including increased permeability of the blood–brain barrier to toxic substances (such as organic acids) and an increase in brain calcium or cerebrospinal fluid (CSF) phosphate content. Signs are usually focal.

Hypoxia may occur as a result of many causes. Severe hypoxic episodes with coma may occur in children with cyanotic congenital heart disease. Hypercapnia, the accumulation of carbon dioxide in the blood, may be seen in severe pulmonary disease. It can also be seen in association with massive obesity.

Hepatic failure may lead to coma associated with an elevated blood ammonia.

Vitamin deficiencies have been associated with alterations of consciousness. Of particular importance in children are pyridoxine deficiency and dependency. Abnormalities of intermediary carbohydrate metabolism from vitamin deficiency (pellagra, beriberi) may lead to coma.

Alterations in magnesium and calcium ion concentrations may lead to coma. Acidosis/alkalosis of a metabolic and/or respiratory nature may also be associated with coma.

Vascular causes

Vascular disease is much less common in the paediatric age group than in adults. Often it is related to systemic vasculitis (collagen vascular disease, polyarteritis nodosa, lupus erythematosus and granulomatous angiitis). Failure to perfuse the brain adequately may be caused by abnormalities of the intracranial vasculature, abnormalities of the blood (methaemoglobinaemia or acute haemolysis), or decreased cardiac output (severe congestive heart failure or haemorrhagic shock). Hypotensive or hypertensive episodes often lead to loss of consciousness (Table 5.4.1).

Subdural haemorrhage may follow trauma. Subarachnoid haemorrhage in the child, as in the adult, is usually due to trauma or rupture of an aneurysm. Diagnosis is established by the finding of grossly bloody spinal fluid or by CT scan.

Venous thrombosis is more common than arterial thrombosis in young children. Sickle cell anaemia is an important predisposing cause. Thrombosis of the cerebral veins, and especially the dural sinuses, is seen following severe dehydration or pyogenic infection of the paranasal sinuses, middle ear, or mastoid. The spinal fluid usually contains red blood cells during the course of the disorder, but it is rarely frankly bloody.

Intracerebral and intraventricular haemorrhages are rarely seen in the older child in the absence of a disorder of the clotting mechanism or inflammation of vessels.

Miscellaneous causes

Common endocrinological causes of coma are diabetes mellitus, Addison's disease, Cushing's syndrome, phaeochromocytoma, thyrotoxicosis, and hypothyroidism.

Other important causes of coma include trauma, toxins, lead and other poisonings, drugs, degenerative diseases, and seizure disorders.

Increased intracranial pressure

Space-occupying lesions such as haematomas, abscesses, neoplasms, tuberculomas, and hydatid cysts may cause raised intracranial pressure. This may be exacerbated by the onset of acute obstructive hydrocephalus. Of childhood brain tumours, 65 per cent are subtentorial; thus, in contrast to adults, increased intracranial pressure and coma are more common presentations. Metastatic tumours are less common in children than in adults; Wilm's and Ewing's tumours occasionally metastasize to the brain. Diffuse infiltration of the meninges may complicate acute leukaemia.

Early management of the comatose child

In assessing and managing a comatose patient, it is first necessary to detect and treat any immediate life-threatening condition: haemorrhage is stopped, the airway is protected with intubation whenever necessary (including the prevention of aspiration in a patient who is vomiting), and the circulation is supported. If the diagnosis is unknown blood is drawn for investigations, after which 50 per cent dextrose is given intravenously. A simple way of keeping these entities in mind is to recall the essential requirements for brain metabolism: adequate oxygen, optimum circulation to get oxygen to the brain, and glucose as substrate. If trauma is suspected, damage to internal organs and fracture of the neck should be taken into consideration until radiographs determine otherwise.

Examination of the comatose child

The next step is to ascertain the site and cause of the lesion. The history should be obtained from whoever accompanies the patient. Examination should include the following: the skin, nails and mucous membranes for pallor, cyanosis, jaundice, sweating, hypo or hyperpigmentation, petechiae, dehydration or signs of trauma: the breath for acetone or fetor hepaticus; and the fundi for papilloedema, or subhyaloid haemorrhages. Fever may imply infection; hypothermia may occur with hypothyroid states, hypoglycaemia, sepsis in premature infants, or infrequently with a primary brain lesion. Urinary or faecal incontinence may signify an unwitnessed seizure. The ears and nose are examined for blood or CSF. Resistance to passive neck flexion suggests meningitis, or subarachnoid haemorrhage, but it may be absent in patients who are deeply comatose.

The neurological examination of the comatose child is quite different from routine neurological examinations. In the most common conditions associated with coma there tends to be a rostral–caudal deterioration in nervous system functions as the process worsens. Rostral–caudal deterioration refers to the sequential loss of certain functions beginning with the cerebral cortex, then the upper brainstem, mid-brain, pons, and finally the medulla. A rapid assessment of the anatomical level in a given patient can be made by examination of the state of consciousness, pupils, eye movements, respiration, and remaining motor functions.

Objective assessment of the level of consciousness is essential. The Glasgow scale is an example of this, scoring 1–15 in three areas of responsiveness. These are:

1	The best motor response	–	6 obeying	3 abnormal flexing
			5 localizes	2 extensor response
			4 withdraws	1 none
2	The best verbal response	–	5 orientated	
			4 confused conversation	
			3 inappropriate words	
			2 incomprehensible sounds	
			1 none	
3	Eye opening	–	4 spontaneous	2 to pain
			3 to speech	1 none

These scores, together with pupillary reactions to light and vital signs, should be recorded on a head chart at least hourly intervals.

The state of extra-ocular movements is another valuable way of establishing the level of remaining nervous system functions. If cervical injury has been ruled out, oculocephalic testing (the doll's eye manoeuvre) is performed by passively turning the head from side to side. With an intact reflex arc, the eyes move conjugately in the opposite direction. A more vigorous stimulus is produced by irrigating each ear with ice water; a normal, awake person has nystagmus with the fast component in the opposite direction to the ear stimulated. In the mesencephalic stage of deterioration, the eyes no longer move easily with the doll's eye manoeuvre. Once the pons and medulla have been involved there is no response in the eye movements to doll's eye manoeuvre or ice water caloric stimulation.

The respiratory pattern is another useful marker relating to the severity of brain damage. Postural changes are often instructive in the comatose patient; these include decerebrate rigidity and flaccidity.

Laboratory investigations

If the history and immediate physical examination do not point to a probable cause for loss of consciousness then further investigations are indicated. Immediate blood studies should include a haemoglobin level, haematocrit, and estimation of total and differential leucocyte counts. Measurements of serum electrolytes, including calcium and magnesium, serum ammonia, blood glucose, and urea, and liver function tests should be carried out.

An electroencephalogram (EEG) can be useful in a comatose patient. It can distinguish coma from psychic unresponsiveness. In metabolic coma, the EEG is always abnormal, and it may reveal asymmetries or evidence of clinically unsuspected seizure activity. If there is evidence of raised intracranial pressure, a lumbar puncture and examination of the spinal fluid should not be undertaken.

Reye's syndrome

Reye's syndrome is a severe disorder characterized by fatty infiltration of the liver and an acute non-inflammatory encephalopathy without evidence of meningeal involvement. Recent epidemiological data suggest that this syndrome is one of the most common neurological complications of viral infections in childhood. Most paediatricians now consider Reye's syndrome as the possible diagnosis when a young child presents with recurrent vomiting and an altered state of consciousness several days after a viral- or influenza-like illness. They also believe that early recognition of this syndrome, coupled with prompt supportive care, can interrupt the possible sequence of events that may culminate in coma.

The syndrome is mostly seen in children during the first decade of life. Both sexes are equally affected. The precise aetiology of this syndrome remains obscure. However, there is clearly an important association with the antecedent viral illness. Several viruses have been implicated, especially influenza viruses and varicella. Salicylates have also been implicated. Thus, the disorder may be the consequence of a synergistic effect between an infective agent and drugs.

Children usually present with copious and protracted vomiting within a few hours; they either become lethargic or go into a hyperexcitable state. In mild cases, recovery occurs uneventfully from this stage. However, in the majority of cases disturbances in level of consciousness develop, with progresssion to a comatose state. The peak of illness may develop over three to four hours or over a period of one to two days. The more rapid the progression, the worse the prognosis. When death occurs, it is most often within 24 hours and usually within three days of the onset of symptoms. If the child survives, rapid recovery to a virtually normal state occurs.

The fundoscopic examination usually shows evidence of raised intracranial pressure due to cerebral oedema. Investigations reveal abnormalities in liver function – chiefly high levels of serum transaminases and ammonia – and the prothrombin time is usually prolonged. Jaundice is most unusual but hypoglycaemia is frequently present, especially in children less than four years old. An important negative finding is the lack of a significant pleocytosis in the CSF. In addition, there are several other metabolic disturbances, none of which are pathognomonic. Fatty accumulation is present in most tissues, particularly the liver, kidney and heart. This is noticeably absent in the brain. The liver biopsy shows characteristic microvesicular fat in every liver cell. There is no displacement of the nucleus of the hepatocyte and no inflammatory cell response. Reversible mitochondrial swelling is seen in both the liver and the brain. The differential diagnosis includes viral encephalitis, bacterial meningitis, and toxic and metabolic encephalopathies.

Management

Since no specific aetiology for Reye's syndrome has been determined, management largely consists of supportive care, with particular attention to the control of increased intracranial pressure. Continuous infusion of 10–20 per cent glucose is advocated to prevent hypoglycaemia.

Extraordinary attention must be given to the development and control of cerebral oedema. Intracranial pressure monitors have been used to aid management. Cerebral oedema may be controlled as discussed above.

Other therapeutic considerations have included exchange transfusion, peritoneal dialysis, hepatic coma regimen, and the administration of various metabolites and chemicals. The total experience with each of these procedures is either limited or discouraging.

Neuro-infections

These infections are among the most dramatic and potentially devastating illnesses that attack infants and children. Effective treatment is dependent upon the early recognition of the disease, identification of the organism responsible, and prompt provision of effective, specific and supportive therapy.

Bacterial meningitis

The first year of life is a time of special risk, not only because of the greater frequency of meningitis at this time but also because the signs of meningeal inflammation may be less distinct and sequelae more frequent when bacterial agents attack the immature brain. Virtually any bacterium is capable of causing meningitis but different age groups within the paediatric population are predisposed to meningitis caused by certain organisms (Table 5.4.2). A variety of Gram-negative and Gram-positive organisms, can produce either single or recurrent episodes of meningitis in children with dermal sinuses communicating with the subarachnoid space (see also pp. 577–9).

Table 5.4.2 Most common causes of bacterial meningitis at various ages.

Birth to 4 weeks
Group B streptococcus
Escherichia coli
4 weeks to 12 weeks
Streptococcus pneumoniae
Group B streptococcus
Salmonella sp.
Listeria monocytogenes
3 months to 3 years
Haemophilus influenzae
Streptococcus pneumoniae
Neisseria meningitidis
Mycobacterium tuberculosis
Over 3 years
Streptococcus pneumoniae
Neisseria meningitidis
Mycobacterium tuberculosis

Meningitis caused by *Mycobacterium tuberculosis* continues to be a problem in the tropics and subtropics, and hence will be dealt with separately (pp. 536–8).

The most frequent route of infection is via the bloodstream. Traumatic rupture of the anatomical defences or direct spread from infections in contiguous tissues, such as the ears and sinuses may also occur. Chronic suppurative otitis media is a common problem in the paediatric population and is an important source of bacterial meningitis.

Symptoms and signs

The clinical presentation and signs depend on a number of factors, the most important of which are the age of the child, the duration of illness, and the aetiology. In meningococcal infections, a generalized purpuric rash may occur. Neonates respond to meningeal infections in many different ways, and few of them suggest CNS disease. The signs are usually those of infection in general. Fever is the most common, hypothermia occurs less often. Irritability, lethargy, vomiting, lack of appetite, and seizures are common, but signs of meningeal irritation are late features.

Beyond four months, infants with meningitis usually manifest febrile responses, signs of meningeal irritation in the form of neck rigidity. Kernig's and Brudzinski's signs, and tenseness of the anterior fontanelle, progressing if untreated to opisthotonus (Fig. 5.4.1).

Older children, usually present with fever, headache, vomiting, mental confusion, lethargy, and seizures.

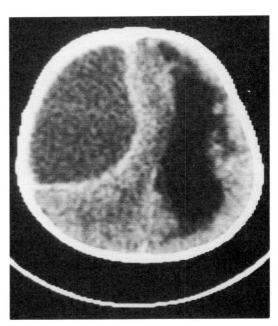

Fig. 5.4.2 Subdural effusion. CT scan showing compression of the ipsilateral ventricle with dilatation of the opposite ventricle.

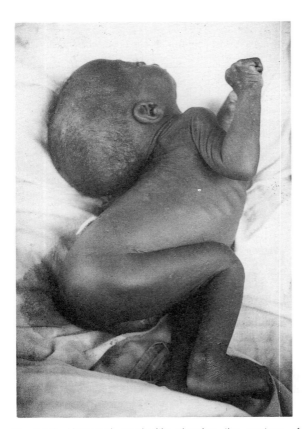

Fig. 5.4.1 Untreated meningitis showing the posture of opisthotonus.

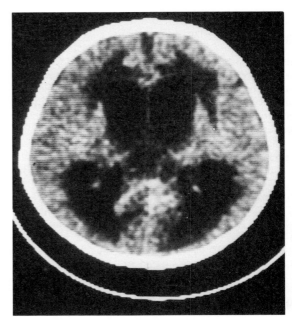

Fig. 5.4.3 Hydrocephalus. CT scan showing dilatation of both lateral ventricles.

This is followed by a progressive decline in sensorium within 24–36 hours. An occasional child will present following a generalized convulsion; this can erroneously be assumed to represent a febrile convulsion unless the CSF is examined. Convulsions can occur in up to 35 per cent of children with acute meningitis during the course of the illness.

Focal neurological deficits are generally not seen in acute meningitis, but occur in meningitis of tuberculous or fungal aetiology and in viral meningoencephalitis.

The presence of papilloedema within the first few days after the onset is unusual in acute meningitis, and the diagnosis should be questioned. Other possible considerations under these circumstances include brain abscess, extradural and subdural collections of pus (Fig 5.4.2.), and tuberculous or fungal meningitis. In neonatal meningitis the mortality and morbidity rates can be high. The most notable severe residual deficits include hydrocephalus (Fig. 5.4.3), seizures, mental retardation, deafness, hyperactive behaviour and cranial nerve or long tract signs.

Diagnostic studies

Studies that should be performed include blood count, urine analysis, serum glucose, electrolytes and urea, tuberculin skin test, skull and chest radiographs, blood, urine and CSF cultures and analysis. Additional tests may have to be considered under special circumstances. In children with recurrent meningitis, serum immunoglobulins should be measured and sinus and mastoid radiographs should be obtained. Additional procedures not to be overlooked include transillumination of the skull of the infant, if subdural effusions are considered, over the last few years, ultrasonography has assumed considerable importance in the evaluation of neuro-infections in the neonate and infant.

CSF examination

The examination of CSF is an essential and often critical tool in the evaluation and management of patients with neuro-infection (see pp. 980–1, 1011).

Classically in cases of pyogenic meningitis the CSF is turbid with a polymorphonuclear pleocytosis. The cell count ranges between 100 and 10 000 per mm^3, with a protein level above 0.4 g/l and sugar less than 2.5 mmol/l (less than 40 per cent of a simultaneous blood sugar level). Occasionally one may see a normal CSF or a predominantly lymphocytic pleocytosis early in the course of illness, or when the patient has received antimicrobial therapy. A repeat lumbar puncture carried out 8–24 hours later might show the classical picture of pyogenic meningitis. A predominance of polymorphonuclear cells early in the clinical course of viral meningitis or during the course of tuberculous meningitis is quite common.

Examination of stained smears of CSF is currently the most widely used laboratory test for rapid diagnosis of bacterial meningitis. It is positive in about 50–70 per cent of cases. Culture is important in diagnosis and it provides information regarding antibiotic sensitivity. Newer techniques for detection of microbial antigens, such as countercurrent immunoelectrophoresis, ELISA and also nucleic acid hybridization probes, are becoming available for the detection of bacterial antigens.

Therapy

The preferred antimicrobial therapy for the neonate differs from that recommended for older children, as Gram-negative organisms and group B streptococci are those most frequently encountered. Previously, a combination of either penicillin or ampicillin with an aminoglycoside (usually gentamicin) was used. Newer cephalosporins may be effectively substituted for aminoglycoside therapy but must be combined with ampicillin.

Intraventricular instillation of aminoglycosides may be considered in selected patients with ventriculitis which has been confirmed by ventricular tap.

The maximal daily doses and routes of administration of antibiotics used in neonates and infants are shown in Tables 5.4.3 and 5.4.4. They should be continued for two weeks. In meningitis caused by group B streptococci, pneumococci and meningococci, penicillin alone is used. For the therapy of *H. influenzae* meningitis, a combination of ampicillin and chloramphenicol is employed until the sensitivity pattern of the isolate becomes available. If the organism is sensitive to ampicillin, chloramphenicol is discontinued.

Table 5.4.3 Drug dosages for bacterial meningitis in neonates.

Drug	Dose/day
Ampicillin	
Premature	50 mg/kg, i.v.
Full-term	150 mg/kg, i.v.
Gentamicin	5–7.5 mg/kg, i.m.
Chloramphenicol	
Premature	25 mg/kg, i.v.
Full-term	50 mg/kg, i.v.
Methicillin	50–100 mg/kg, i.v.
Penicillin	50 000–100 000 units/kg, i.v.

Table 5.4.4 Maximal daily dose and route of administration of antibiotics used in bacterial infections of the CNS, in infants over two months old.

Antibiotics	Dose/day	Interval (h)/route
Penicillin G	200 000 U/kg	4 or 6 i.v.
Ampicillin	300–400 mg/kg	4 or 6 i.v.
Carbenicillin	400–600 mg/kg	4 or 6 i.v.
Chloramphenicol (4 g max.)	100 mg/kg	6 i.v. or orally
Gentamicin	5 mg/kg	8 i.v. or i.m.
Methicillin	200–300 mg/kg	6 i.v.
Oxacillin	200 mg/kg	6 i.v.
Amikacin	15 mg/kg	8 i.v. or i.m.
Cefotaxime (14 g max.)	200 mg/kg	6–8 i.v.
Metronidazole (4 g max.)	30 mg/kg	6 i.v.

When examination of Gram-stained spinal fluid shows no organisms, a combination of ampicillin and an aminoglycoside is recommended for the initial treatment of infants less than two months old, ampicillin and chloramphenicol for children from three months to five years old, and aqueous pencillin G and chloramphenicol for older children. Cephalosporins show good activity against *Haemophilus*, meningococcal and pneumococcal organisms. Subdural effusions are seen most frequently with *Haemophilus* meningitis. The indications for subdural taps in infants include the development of a tense, bulging anterior fontanelle after two to three days of therapy with other evidence of improvement, and the onset of focal seizures or hemiparesis.

Supportive therapy

Good nursing care, prevention of aspiration, and monitoring of vital signs are all critical aspects of management. Attention must be paid to fluid balance; intravenous fluid are often essential. Fluid overload arising from the presence of inappropriate antidiuretic hormone secretion will necessitate fluid restriction.

The control of cerebral oedema secondary to infection is difficult. Mannitol has a rapid effect and is given intravenously in a dose of 2 g/kg over 30 minutes. Dexamethasone at a dose of 0.5 mg/kg per 24 hours is also very effective but is probably better in preventing cerebral oedema than in treating an established case. Corticosteroids may also reduce the inflammatory exudate and excessive fibrin deposition.

Convulsive disorders are common and primarily

occur during the first 12–48 hours of illness, probably as a result of cerebral irritation or ischaemia.

Intracranial abscess

Intracranial suppuration may occur in several sites: between the skull and dura (extradural), between the dura and arachnoid (subdural), or any site within the substance of the brain (Fig. 5.4.4). Abscesses within the brain can be solitary or multiple and may be associated with an extracranial suppurative focus. The infections can arise from an extension from adjacent sites such as the middle ear, mastoid, paranasal sinuses, and midline congenital dermal sinus, or following penetrating injuries to the skull; or they can arise from the bloodstream owing to pulmonary infection, and from shunting in cyanotic congenital heart disease.

Streptococci, staphylococci and pneumococci are the organisms most frequently recovered. Anaerobic bacteria of many types have also been identified. Gram-negative bacilli are often found in cerebral abscesses in infants.

The most common early symptoms in children are headache, vomiting followed by lethargy, fever and seizures. This is followed by deterioration in level of sensorium and the onset of focal neurological signs.

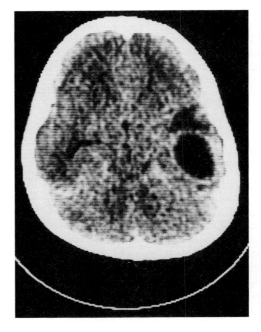

Fig. 5.4.4 Cerebral abscess. CT scan showing translucent area in the right temporal lobe.

Papilloedema is present in many, but not all, children and abducens weakness with diplopia frequently develops as a false localizing sign. An abscess within the cerebellar hemispheres presents with progressive cerebellar dysfunction in conjunction with manifestations of increased pressure.

Diagnostic studies

Fever and blood leucocytosis are suggestive of an infectious process. Skull X-rays are of little definitive help, except for the evidence of increased pressure manifested by suture spread. Sinus and mastoid films may reveal a potential source of infection. Electroencephalography is a valuable tool for localizing a cerebral abscess; it may reveal a focus of high voltage, delta-wave focus activity.

If a cerebral abscess is strongly suspected, lumbar puncture should be avoided and is contra-indicated if papilloedema is present.

Treatment

Treatment is based on surgical drainage or aspiration and the use of appropriate antimicrobial agents. Pending the results of sensitivity tests, penicillin and chloramphenicol are given intravenously; consideration may be given to the addition of metronidazole. Antibiotics should continue to be administered in a similar manner and on a similar basis as in bacterial meningitis.

Tuberculosis

For a discussion of tuberculosis of the CNS see pp. 536–8.

Viral diseases

Viruses may reach the CNS through a number of routes following their entry into the body. Of these, the haematogenous route is by far the most important. During the stage of viraemia, viruses invade the CNS via the cerebral capillaries and the choroid plexus. Another pathway of infection is along the peripheral nerves; centripetal movement of viruses is accomplished by retrograde axoplasmic spread. Experimentally it has been shown that viruses may spread to the CNS by penetrating the olfactory mucosa, but the role of this pathway in human infection is not certain.

Viruses which have invaded the nervous system, have diverse clinical and pathological effects (Table 5.4.5). (See also pp. 600–23) Thus, some infections

Table 5.4.5 Neurological disorders associated with viral infections.

Acute illnesses
  Aseptic meningitis
  Encephalitis
  Acute transverse myelitis
  Poliomyelitis, polio-like myelitis
  Postinfectious, postvaccination encephalomyelitis
Chronic illnesses
  Subacute sclerosing panencephalitis
  Progressive rubella panencephalitis
  Progressive multifocal leucoencephalopathy
  Kuru
  Creutzfeldt–Jakob disease
Intrauterine — neonatal illnesses
Viral-related disorders
  Reye's syndrome
  Acute cerebellar ataxia
  Guillain–Barré syndrome
  Opsoclonus–polymyoclonus
  Bell's palsy
  Benign sixth-nerve palsy of childhood

confined to the meningeal cells, give rise to a benign aseptic meningitis and others involve parenchymal cells and lead to the more serious disorder of encephalitis. In some viral infections the susceptibility of particular cell groups is even more specific, e.g. polio and rabies. Some viruses cause chronic infections of the CNS in man, producing progressive brain disease, e.g. subacute sclerosing panencephalitis.

Viral infections of the CNS occur in epidemics in different parts of the world (see p. 605). Periodicity and seasonal prevalence are characteristic features, for example of arbovirus, measles and poliovirus. However, some viral diseases of the CNS, such as Herpes simplex encephalitis, occur sporadically.

Diagnosis

The CSF findings in meningitis, encephalitis, or meningoencephalitis may be similar, consisting of an increase in pressure, pleocytosis of varying degree, a moderate protein content elevation, and a normal glucose content. The diagnosis in non-fatal cases can be made by a combination of serological tests and by the inoculation of blood, naso-pharyngeal washings, faeces, or CSF into susceptible animals or cell culture systems.

Enteroviruses

Enteroviruses, including polioviruses, Coxsackie viruses and echoviruses, are known to involve human beings. These viruses include four newly recognized members of the enterovirus group (see p. 606).

Acute anterior poliomyelitis

Poliomyelitis is an acute infectious disease, characterized by preferential involvement of the motor neurones of the spinal cord and brain. It results in an asymmetric flaccid paralysis of the voluntary muscles.

The poliovirus is an enterovirus. There are three antigenically distinct types, and infection with one does not protect against the others. Type I virus is generally more virulent than types II and III. Type I has been the most frequent cause of endemic and epidemic paralytic disease and type II is the least paralytogenic strain. Acute anterior poliomyelitis is world-wide in distribution, and due to vaccination, has almost disappeared from industrialized countries. It may occur in sporadic, endemic, or epidemic form. Infants under the age of one year are rarely attacked. In a country where hygiene is poor, most sufferers are between the ages of two and four years. After the age of five years, most individuals are immune, and after 25 years the disease is rare. The incubation period varies from 6 to 20 days and can be somewhat shorter or more prolonged in certain cases. Spread is from individual to individual by the faecal–oral route. The virus multiplies in the pharynx and ileum, probably in lymphoid tissue of the tonsils and Peyer's patches. The virus then spreads to cervical and mesenteric lymph nodes and can be detected in the blood shortly thereafter. Infection of the nervous system by way of viraemia is likely. Transmission of poliovirus along the peripheral nerve fibre pathway is a possibility under certain circumstances.

Pathology

In the acute stage, the spinal cord is congested, soft and oedematous, and minute haemorrhages may be visible in the grey matter. One of the striking features of the pathology of this disease is the selectivity of distribution of the lesions and the almost consistent sparing of other parts of the CNS. In the spinal cord, the most severe grey matter lesions are in the anterior columns. The degree of damage varies from one level to another but is often most intense at the cervical or lumbar enlargements of the cord. The inflammatory reaction can also involve the intermediate and posterior horns, but not to the extent of the involvement of the anterior horns. Within the brainstem, cellular infiltration can be seen in many of the cranial nerve motor nuclei, but is most apparent in the region of the vestibular nuclei and the

reticular formation. Unlike most other types of viral encephalitis, the cerebral cortex is characteristically spared.

The microscopic pathology of paralytic polio varies, depending on the duration of the illness at the time of death. The earliest visible changes in the spinal cord in the acute stage consist of infiltration with lymphocytes and polymorphonuclear leucocytes in the anterior horns, in addition to chromatolysis of nerve cells in the region. Congestion of vessels and petechial haemorrhages may also be observed when the inflammatory reaction is intense. The spinal meninges commonly exhibit inflammatory cell infiltration of variable degree, while the cerebral meninges may be entirely spared. With the passage of time beyond the acute insult, the cellular infiltration becomes less dense, but neurones that are irreversibly damaged undergo necrosis and neuronophagia. This is followed by atrophy of the anterior roots due to loss of myelinated nerve fibres, and denervation atrophy of the muscles involved. In the chronic stages, severely damaged anterior horns contain few or no viable neuronal elements, and may assume a cavitied or cystic appearance to gross observation.

Clinical manifestations

The clinical picture of poliomyelitis ranges from a non-specific mild febrile illness to a severe and potentially fatal paralytic disease. Infections caused by the polioviruses have been classified as asymptomatic, abortive, non-paralytic, and paralytic. Types of paralytic polio include spinal, bulbar, and bulbo-spinal. Polioencephalitis is much less common than either the spinal or the medullary form of the disease. Of the different neurological syndromes that can occur in polio, approximately 45 to 50 per cent of cases are predominantly spinal, 10–15 per cent are bulbar, 15 per cent are bulbo-spinal, and 1–5 per cent have 'encephalitic' features, reflecting extensive damage within the brainstem and diencephalon.

Poliomyelitis is a mild disease of short duration in most patients. It has been estimated that for every paralytic case there are 100 to 1000 infected individuals who are not paralyzed. Exposure to the virus may lead to the development of immunity without any symptoms of illness – asymptomatic cases. Abortive poliomyelitis, also termed the 'minor illness', is a non-specific illness lasting for hours to a few days, characterized by fever, headache, malaise, sore throat, nausea, vomiting, and abdominal pain. One or several of these symptoms may be present in various combinations. There are no signs of CNS involvement and the CSF is normal. However, the protein of the CSF may be found to be elevated two or three weeks later, indicating that inflammatory changes may have occurred sub-clinically. This phase, the 'minor illness', is followed by temporary improvement with remission of fever for 48 hours, or may merge into the second phase, 'major illness', in which headache is more severe and is associated with pain in the back and limbs, sometimes with muscle tenderness. The symptoms closely resemble those of other forms of viral meningitis. In non-paralytic cases, the patient recovers after exhibiting, in mild or more severe form, either or both of the phases of the preparalytic stage. The spinal fluid usually contains an increase in cells and protein.

The illness of greatest consequence is paralytic poliomyelitis. Following the initial prodromal illness, and a few days of apparent well-being, there will be recurrence of the febrile illness with meningeal signs. Limb pain or painful muscle spasms may be the first evidence of parenchymal neurological involvement, but more often the rapid evolution of flaccid muscle weakness is observed within one or two days after the onset of the meningeal signs. Weakness or paralysis develops quickly, and, once begun, it achieves its maximal severity within 48 hours in most cases. The pattern of muscle weakness in paralytic polio varies a great deal from patient to patient but asymmetry of limb involvement is a notable, though not invariable, feature. Certain muscle groups of one arm or leg are selectively affected in some cases, but in others flaccid paraplegia or quadriplegia will occur. Upper cervical or thoracic cord involvement results in diaphragm and intercostal muscle weakness manifested by a shallow, rapid, but regular respiratory pattern. Physical examination may reveal loss of neck control and muscle tenderness, and in sitting posture the patient will place the arms behind the back for support (tripod sign). The deep tendon reflexes are normal early in the disease, but become diminished as weakness progresses.

Bulbar polio may occur with or without spinal cord disease and is manifested by dysfunction of lower cranial nerves, often in asymmetric fashion. The most life-threatening aspect of bulbar polio results from inflammation of certain nuclear groups of the medullary reticular formation, the so-called vaso-motor 'centres'. The respiratory pattern in such cases is characterized by its irregularity, punctuated by episodes of apnoea, in addition to hypertension and abnormalities of the rate and rhythm of the pulse. Peripheral vascular collapse or the sudden development of pulmonary oedema are common terminal events in such cases. Facial paralysis has been observed in some patients, while external ophthalmoplegia is infrequent.

The unusual neurological manifestations, that have been described with poliovirus are acute cerebellar ataxia, association with Reye's syndrome, and the onset of progressive anterior horn cell degeneration in adults who have experienced paralytic polio in childhood.

Laboratory studies

The blood picture is usually normal, although a mild leucopenia may be found in the early stage of the illness. The CSF usually reveals a pleocytosis which initially may be largely polymorphonuclear but rapidly becomes lymphocytic in nature. The cell count ranges from 50 to 200/mm^3 in most cases, but can be greater or less in some others. By two or three weeks after onset, the cell count decreases to normal or near normal. The protein content is normal in the early stages of the illness, and may be slightly elevated during the second or third week after the onset of paralysis.

Neutralizing antibodies and complement fixation tests on serial specimens are the most valuable laboratory diagnostic aids for poliovirus infections, in addition to techniques to isolate and type the virus from stool and naso-pharyngeal specimens. Unlike other enteroviruses, the poliovirus can rarely be isolated from the CSF in patients with neurological infection. Complement fixation tests are less specific than neutralizing antibody tests.

Prognosis

The prognosis for non-paralytic poliomyelitis is good. The prognosis in paralytic infection varies with the site and severity of paralysis. In bulbar poliomyelitis the mortality rate is approximately 10 per cent, whereas in paralysis due to spinal cord involvement the mortality rate is approximately 1 per cent. Respiratory failure is responsible for most of the deaths. Recovery from paralysis usually begins within one week. The rate of recovery is most rapid during the first three months. Muscles that remain completely paralysed after an interval of three months usually do not show return of function. Weakened muscles continue to improve for a period up to one year.

Differential diagnosis

The non-paralytic phase must be differentiated from other types of aseptic meningitis. The paralytic phase must be differentiated from the Guillain–Barré syndrome and other cases of polyneuritis. The presenting symptom of infectious polyneuritis is symmetric paralysis, which usually progresses for more than one week and is not accompanied by fever, and physical examination reveals generalized hypo- or a reflexia. The absence of CSF pleocytosis and a marked rise in protein in the presence of a progressive paralysis also suggests polyneuritis.

Treatment

No specific treatment is available. Therapy is supportive and symptomatic. Medical management is directed towards making the child comfortable, minimizing skeletal deformation and anticipating complications. Since physical activity in the preparalytic stage increases the risk of severe paralysis during the acute illness, bed rest is indicated. Relief of muscle pain can be accomplished by periodic application of hot moist packs. A neutral position with the feet at a right angle, knees slightly flexed and hips and spine straight, is achieved by use of boards, sandbags, and occasionally light splint shells. Active and passive movements are indicated as soon as the pain has disappeared.

Respiratory failure is treated with respiratory assistance. Bladder paralysis usually lasts only a few days and can be managed temporarily by parasympathetic stimulants, such as bethanechol, and manual compression of the bladder. If catheterization must be performed the strictest asepsis is essential.

Treatment of the convalescent stage involves physiotherapy, application of appropriate corrective appliances, muscle re-education, and orthopaedic measures (see pp. 914–16).

Prevention

Control of poliomyelitis has been achieved by the use of orally administered live attenuated virus vaccine (Sabin). This has largely replaced the formalin-inactivated preparation (Salk) (see p. 82).

Coxsackie viruses

An increasing number of Coxsackie virus strains have been reported as causing infections of the human nervous system (see p. 606). The clinical pictures produced by the various strains are indistinguishable. Most commonly affected are children between five and nine years of age, although no age group is immune.

The Coxsackie viruses are classified into group A with 24 types and group B with six types. Both strains are known to involve the nervous system.

Clinical syndromes caused by Coxsackie viruses vary. The most common CNS manifestation is an asep-

tic meningitis, and infrequently encephalitis. There is an initial prodromal phase lasting two to seven days with malaise, loss of appetite, nausea, and fever. Group A infections may be associated with herpangina, skin rash, and rarely parotitis. Group B infections may produce myalgia or pleurodynia and infrequently myocarditis in the newborn.

The prodromal phase is followed by headache, vomiting, neck pain and drowsiness. Physical examination may reveal signs of meningeal irritation and a variable level of sensorium. Occasionally, paralysis simulating poliomyelitis, acute cerebellar ataxia or encephalitic signs may be predominant. The course of the illness is characteristically benign with complete recovery.

There is no specific treatment. Therapy is largely supportive and symptomatic.

Echoviruses

This group of viruses is the most frequent cause of enterovirus infection of the nervous system. The clinical manifestations are variable, but the most common is an aseptic meningitis. A total of 34 types of echovirus are currently recognized; so far 24 of these have been demonstrated to produce aseptic meningitis in man, with or without skin rash.

The symptomatology and course of the illness are similar to those described in cases of meningitis caused by Coxsackie virus. The initial systemic illness may be followed by fever, headache, vomiting, neck pain and photophobia. The illness usually terminates in seven to ten days. Minor symptomatology may persist for several months.

Seizures, coma, or other signs of cerebral dysfunction indicating an encephalitis have been reported. Acute ascending polyradiculomyelitis and acute cerebellar ataxia of short duration have also have described.

No specific treatment is known. Therapy is supportive and symptomatic.

Lymphocytic choriomeningitis

Lymphocytic choriomeningitis is a benign viral infection of the meninges caused by an arenavirus (see p. 609). This name is derived from the striking lymphocytic infiltration in the choroid plexus seen with infections in susceptible animals. The reservoir for the virus is the grey house mouse. Infection may be transferred to man by indirect contact with infected mice.

The most frequent clinical form of the disease is a mild lymphocytic meningitis. This presents with symptoms and signs of meningeal involvement. These symptoms persist for about two weeks and are usually followed by complete recovery. In a few children, the encephalitic picture predominates.

Medical management consists of supportive therapy.

Arboviruses

The CNS infection caused by arboviruses is usually an encephalitis. Sometimes clinical manifestations of an aseptic meningitis are also produced.

Like other viruses, arboviruses present with different clinical pictures, from the subclinical to the most fulminant with rapid progression to death within 24–48 hours after the onset of illness (see pp. 604–6).

Of great significance in India is Japanese B encephalitis. The other arboviruses most frequently affecting the nervous system and resulting in encephalitis are Western, Eastern, and Venezuelan equine encephalitis, St Louis, Murray Valley, and California encephalitis, and tick-borne arbovirus encephalitis.

The onset of illness is usually sudden, with fever, headache, vomiting, neck pain, and sometimes followed by focal or generalized convulsions, drowsiness, stupor, or coma. Symptoms usually persist for about 10 days, then gradually subside. In fatal cases, the course is rapidly downhill.

In any patient with suspected viral encephalitis it is important to exclude the possibility of a postinfectious or postvaccination encephalitis.

In the acute phase the condition has to be differentiated from bacterial infections, Reye's syndrome, cerebral malaria, and febrile convulsions. A prolonged period of unconsciousness, focal neurological deficits, or cytochemical alterations in CSF should raise doubts about the diagnosis of arbovirus encephalitis. The treatment is symptomatic.

Japanese encephalitis

Japanese encephalitis (JE) virus is an RNA virus and belongs to group B arboviruses (flaviviruses) (see p. 605). It is a difficult virus to culture, however, culture can be achieved on primary cell lines from monkey kidney or chick embryo fibroblasts, and recently in arthropod tissue culture systems. The hosts or reservoirs of infection are pigs and birds. The mosquito is the main vector; *Culex tritaeniorhynchus* being the most commonly implicated species. The natural cycle of JE virus is bird–mosquito–bird and pig–mosquito–pig. Man becomes a host only when the population of infected mosquitoes increases in an endemic area.

Japanese encephalitis is seen in an area extending from India to Japan. Several large epidemics have occurred in Japan, Korea, and India, where the majority of cases were children younger than 15 years of age.

Pathology

Cerebral oedema is a prominent feature in most of the cases and mainly affects the grey matter. Haemorrhages and focal necrotic lesions are observed predominantly in the cerebral cortex, thalamic nuclei, corpus striatum, and brainstem. Perivascular mononuclear infiltration is seen. The clinical picture is indistinguishable from other types of arbovirus encephalitis, characterized by a brief history of fever, headache, neck pain, and vomiting, followed by an altered sensorium, convulsions, and motor paralysis. Weight loss is quite marked. Alteration of sensorium is present in 85–90 per cent of cases. It may vary from mild drowsiness to coma. In fulminant cases a totally unresponsive state may result, and may finally terminate in death. After a period varying from a few days to a few weeks of the encephalitic phase, in those who survive, either steady improvement occurs or the neurological deficit stabilizes. In those who develop neurological deficit at the onset, the chances of complete recovery are 80 per cent.

The cerebrospinal fluid reveals mild to moderate lymphocytic pleocytosis, usually less than 200 cells/mm^3 and the proteins are normal or mildly elevated with normal sugar content. The definitive diagnosis is established by virological studies. Diagnosis can also be established in the absence of virus isolation by demonstrating at least a fourfold rise in antibody titre in the convalescent serum.

The overall experiences indicate that roughly one-third of the cases fully recover, one-third are left with residual neurological deficits, and the rest prove to be fatal. A significant proportion (approximately 50 per cent) of those who recover are left with deficits in the form of intellectual impairment, behavioural changes, disorders of tone, and motor paralysis.

There is no specific treatment, but adequate general and supportive measures considerably influence the mortality and morbidity.

Killed vaccine prepared from mouse brain inoculated with the Nakayama JE strain has been widely used for immunization. After two doses, adequate levels of antibody titre are attained and offer good protection.

Encephalitis can occur with common childhood viral illnesses like measles, mumps, chickenpox, and rubella. The spectrum of clinical symptomatology of CNS involvement includes encephalitis, aseptic meningitis, and encephalomyelitis. Although children are more susceptible, young adults may also acquire the disease.

In the pathogenesis, two major hypotheses have been proposed: direct viral invasion of the CNS; and an autoimmune reaction against neural tissue or tissue–viral complex.

Measles (rubeola) encephalitis

Encephalitis occurs in 1 to 2 per 1000 children with measles and usually develops 7–10 days after the onset of the rash. However, it may develop during the prodromal period or up to two weeks after the onset of the rash (see p. 500). Recurrence of the fever, headache, vomiting, neck pain, and seizures may herald the onset; coma may ensue. Recovery may be rapid or may take up to a month. The mortality is high (10–15 per cent) and permanent sequelae occur in approximately 20 per cent of survivors.

Aseptic meningitis, acute cerebellar ataxia, optic neuritis, and transverse myelitis are other CNS complications of measles.

The diagnosis is usually made on available clinical information aided by a history of measles, exposure to contact, or presence of the measles rash. In unusual cases isolation of the virus from tissues other than brain tissue may be helpful. Therapy is supportive and symptomatic. The attenuated measles vaccine reliably induces active immunity.

Mumps meningoencephalitis

The incidence of aseptic meningitis associated with mumps varies with different epidemics, in the range 1–10 per cent (see p. 514). The nervous system involvement occurs several days to two weeks after the onset of the parotitis. However, nervous system involvement may precede the parotitis or parotitis may not develop at all. The onset is abrupt with symptoms and signs of meningeal involvement. These symptoms usually subside, along with the parotid swelling within one week. The case fatality rate of mumps meningoencephalitis is about one per cent. The most common residual complication is deafness.

On occasion, myelitis, optic neuritis, cerebellar ataxia, Guillain–Barré syndrome, or other cranial nerve palsies have been reported. The diagnosis is obvious clinically, when a child develops aseptic meningitis in association with acute parotitis. To establish the diagnosis it is necessary to isolate the virus or demonstrate a rise in antibodies to mumps virus. Treatment is symptomatic. The live attenuated mumps virus vaccine reliably produces adequate antibodies and protects against natural mumps in vaccinated individuals.

Chickenpox (varicella) encephalitis and Herpes zoster

The incidence of chickenpox encephalitis is not precisely known. An incidence of 7–55.8 per 100 000 cases has been reported in the USA and those at great risk are adults and children below five years of age. The most common neurological complication of chickenpox consists of encephalitis (see p. 517). This generally occurs in the post-eruptive period but can occur in the pre-eruptive period also. Cerebellar ataxia, myelitis, aseptic meningitis, and optic neuritis may occur. Estimates of mortality rates in varicella encephalitis vary from 5 to 25 per cent.

Herpes zoster infection reflects reactivation of a latent virus. The disease is most often seen in adults but may be seen in children with malignancy, especially lymphoma and leukaemia. Crops of clustered vesicles are distributed unilaterally along one or adjacent sensory nerves.

The diagnosis of CNS involvement by the varicella-zoster virus depends on the clinical history and manifestations.

Treatment is symptomatic. Antiviral therapy for the neurological complications of varicella-zoster virus infection is less effective than in herpes simplex infection. Acyclovir prevents complications in the immunocompromised and in the neonate if started within five days of onset of the disease (see Table 4.8.2 p. 616).

Herpes simplex encephalitis

Herpes simplex virus (HSV) occurs in two distinct serological and biological types. Involvement of the nervous system in infants and children beyond the newborn age group is by the HSV type 1. The most frequent portal of entry is the naso-pharyngeal passages. The virus finds its way to the nervous system either through a haematogenous or neurogenic pathway. HSV type 2 is frequently the agent causing a primary generalized herpetic infection in the neonatal period. The infection is acquired during birth (see pp. 615–16).

The clinical manifestation in older children consists of an initial prodromal illness lasting for a week. This is followed by neurological involvement, including aseptic meningitis and encephalitis of a diffuse or focal nature. Aseptic meningitis is seen in about 20 per cent of cases. This is relatively benign and patients recover in a week. More frequently, herpes is associated with encephalitis. This could be a diffuse encephalitis presenting as fever, papilloedema, meningeal irritation and global confusion, or a focal encephalitis, usually of the orbital or temporal regions of the brain, causing anosmia, memory loss, disordered behaviour, and olfactory or gustatory hallucinations. Localizing signs are found in about 75 per cent of patients – mostly focal seizures and paralyses. The EEG is most sensitive and focal abnormalities are found in 80 per cent of proved cases. Angiography suggests the presence of a mass lesion, often localized to the temporal lobes. The CT scan shows an area of low attenuation involving one or both temporal lobes and is abnormal in 59 per cent of biopsy proven cases. The mortality from herpes encephalitis ranges from 37 to 70 per cent if untreated. Approximately half of the survivors have major residual deficits.

The diagnosis of a Herpes simplex infection of the brain depends on the isolation of the virus from the nervous system or the demonstration of the intrathecal production of virus specific antibodies. Attempts to isolate the virus from the CSF have not been successful. Isolation of the virus from brain biopsy, and more rapid diagnostic adjuncts, including light microscopy, electron microscopy, and immunofluorescent staining, have met with a higher degree of success. However, considering the low toxicity and the high efficacy of acyclovir, and the possible complications of brain biopsy, this procedure is no longer recommended.

Treatment

General supportive measures and therapy for increased intracranial pressure and seizures are indicated. While specific chemotherapeutic agents such as idoxuridine and cytosine arabinoside have been utilized in treatment of Herpes simplex encephalitis, there has been no demonstration of effectiveness in controlled studies. More recently, vidarabine and acyclovir have been shown conclusively to reduce both the mortality and the morbidity in this disease. Owing to the toxicity of vidarabine, acyclovir has become the drug of first choice. It should be started immediately on presumptive diagnosis of HSV encephalitis (see p. 616).

Chronic viral infections

The vast majority of viral infections involving the nervous system consist of an acute process but there are

a few in which the infection is chronic. These slowly progressive diseases are called slow virus diseases. They include subacute sclerosing panencephalitis (SSPE), progressive multifocal leucoencephalopathy (PML), and HIV encephalopathy (see p. 602), Creutzfeldt-Jakob disease, kuru, and rubella subacute panencephalitis. Of these, the first and the last primarily affect children.

Subacute sclerosing panencephalitis

SSPE is the most common of the chronic virus infections to affect children. The onset has been most often between 5 and 15 years. The disease is most common in males by a ratio of 3:1. The observation of an early measles infection, in 50 per cent before two years of age and in 80 per cent by four years of age, is probably related to some pathogenetic factor in the disease (see p. 500). The period from the known measles infection to the development of encephalitis is usually between three and nine years.

Clinical features

Four stages of the disease are described for both diagnostic and therapeutic purposes. The first stage, usually of several months duration, is marked by an insidious deterioration in behaviour and intellectual performance, but the exact time of onset may be difficult to determine. This stage usually blends into stage two. In stage two, mental deterioration becomes progressively more obvious and the characteristic periodic abnormal movements develop; these are described as myoclonus. These spasms start abruptly, but cease gradually and last at least one second. They are usually bilateral and symmetrical but may be unilateral or asymmetrical and may affect the whole limb or parts of the limbs; they are repetitive and stereotyped and result in clumsiness and frequent falls. Apart from the periodic spasms, seizures of more conventional types may also occur. Mild focal neurological deficits may appear. The ophthalmic manifestations include cortical blindness, focal chorioretinitis, nystagmus, and optic atrophy. Stage two lasts for one to four months, and the duration varies from one month to one year.

In the third stage of the disease there is evidence of extrapyramidal and/or pyramidal dysfunction. Dementia is severe and the child becomes bedridden. The spasms and convulsions continue. The fourth stage with decerebrate rigidity and coma is reached one or more years from the onset and may last for a few months to a few years. The tempo of the illness is variable. Rarely, spontaneous arrest of the disease in the second stage, lasting for a few months to a few years has been reported.

The clinical diagnosis of SSPE is confirmed by several studies. One finding is the characteristic EEG pattern of recurrent stereotyped periodic complexes of high voltage slow waves. In stages three and four there is in addition a slowing of background rhythm.

Serum and CSF studies reflect the hyperimmune response, with an elevation of the measles antibody titres. In those cases with atypical clinical and laboratory features, brain biopsy for fluorescent antibody studies, light and electron microscopy, and viral cultures for isolation of measles (rubeola) virus can be useful in establishing the diagnosis.

The variable natural history of SSPE with occasional prolonged remissions makes assessment of the results of treatment difficult. Numerous agents, including steroids, amantadine, cytosine arabinoside, isoprinosine, interferon, and transfer factor, have not altered the course of the disease. Anticonvulsants have only been effective in controlling the seizures.

Epilepsy in infancy and childhood

A seizure may be defined as a sudden transient disturbance of body movement or mental function, while epilepsy may be defined as a series of such stereotyped seizures. Epilepsy is not a specific disease; it is a symptom or sign of brain malfunction, the aetiology of which can be static or progressive.

Clinical types

Grand mal (major motor)

These are generalized tonic–clonic convulsions, often not preceded by an aura. The attack begins with loss of consciousness. A tonic phase in which the trunk and limbs are held rigid for a few seconds is followed by a clonic phase involving repetitive flexion and extension movements. Respiration is laboured, cyanosis, salivation and urination may occur, and in the postictal period the child may be stuporous, confused and ataxic.

Focal seizures begin in one limb. In these attacks the eyes and head turn away from the side of the lesion and the ipsilateral limb extends. Sometimes there is a definite progression to jerking in the hand, arm and face with loss of consciousness when the contralateral side is involved – the Jacksonian attack.

Petit mal

This is a form of generalized seizure in which there is a brief absence or arrest of consciousness lasting 5–10 seconds. During this period there is retention of posture but a lack of all other motor activity; thus speech, walking and other limb movements cease and the child stares vacantly in front of him and is unaware of what is said or of what is taking place around him. After a few seconds his face may flush and his eyelids twitch and he continues the activity in which he was previously engaged. Many attacks may occur during the day; the first indication of the disorder may be a deterioration in school performance.

Psychomotor seizures (temporal lobe epilepsy)

Foci of temporal lobe activity lead to a variety of sensory disturbances – anxiety, visceral sensations, feelings of 'déjà vu', and olfactory hallucinations. Minor motor activity may occur simultaneously, such as lip-smacking, chewing and fumbling movements. This may be followed by drowsiness or inappropriate automatisms.

Myoclonus

This is a form of generalized seizure consisting of a single brief jerk, or sometimes a series of jerks, usually of a limb but sometimes of the whole body, which may result in the child suddenly falling to the ground. Infantile spasms are a serious form of myoclonus occurring in the first year of life and associated with EEG appearances of hypsarrhythmia.

Status epilepticus

This is a condition in which there is a continuous prolonged seizure or several epileptic seizures in succession without recovery of consciousness in-between.

Causes

The poorer the environment, and the more disadvantaged the community, the more likely it is that convulsions in childhood are secondary to CNS pathology, such as meningitis, encephalitis, fever, trauma, metabolic and electrolyte disturbances, or vascular accidents (see Table 5.4.6). The better the environment, the more likely the convulsions are to be primary, that is idiopathic. Febrile convulsions and infantile spasms are discussed below; neonatal convulsions are discussed elsewhere (pp. 234–5).

Table 5.4.6　Causes of epilepsy.

Non-structural brain damage
　Idiopathic
　Febrile convulsions
　Perinatal anoxia
　Meningitis/encephalitis
　Metabolic disorders
　　e.g. hypoglycaemia
　　　　hypocalcaemia
　　　　hypomagnesaemia
　　　　hypernatraemia
　　　　phenylketonuria
　Poisoning, drug ingestion
　Pyridoxine deficiency
Structural brain damage
　Head injury
　Congenital malformations
　Brain abscess
　Chronic infections
　　e.g. cysticercosis
　　　　toxoplasmosis
　Tumours
　Neurocutaneous syndromes
　　e.g. tuberose sclerosis
　　　　neurofibromatosis
　Degenerative disorders
　　e.g. leucodystrophies

Conditions simulating convulsions

Syncope

These vaso-vagal attacks are most common in adolescent girls (see also pp. 402–8). They usually follow standing, especially in a hot environment. Sometimes they are preceded by fatigue and emotional stress.

Breath-holding attacks

These occur in young children and are precipitated by crying, arising because of pain, anger, fear, or frustration. There may be cyanosis or pallor, followed by limpness and occasionally by twitching.

Hysteria

In this situation there is no aura and consciousness is not truly lost. Movements are more or less coordinated and often clonic; there is no definite sequence and micturition and tongue-biting are rarely seen. The attack terminates suddenly and the child then resumes normal activity.

Tics

Tics are repetitive movements which can be voluntarily controlled.

Investigation

A full clinical history and examination is essential, taking into account features in the other systems of the body as well as the central nervous system. This assessment will determine whether more detailed investigation is necessary. Useful clinical pointers for common conditions must be recognized. For instance, unconsciousness in association with convulsions might suggest meningoencephalitis, cerebral malaria, or hypoglycaemia; a child with diarrhoea and vomiting who then convulses is likely to be dehydrated with electrolyte imbalance, while a young child with high fever and no localizing signs may have bacterial meningitis and require an early lumbar puncture. An EEG may help to confirm a clinical diagnosis of epilepsy, but it is not unusual for an EEG to be normal in a child with unequivocal epilepsy, and to be abnormal in a child who has never had a seizure. In petit mal epilepsy the EEG shows typical regular (three per second) spike and wave discharges. In infantile spasms the EEG appearance of hypsarrhythmia is diagnostic. If metabolic disorders or infections are suspected, the appropriate clinical, pathological and microbiological investigations should be carried out. Skull X-rays may reveal asymmetry or intracranial calcification. CT brain scans are rarely justified.

Treatment

Before treatment, the physician must decide whether or not there is an underlying precipitating disorder which can be treated or removed. Having reached a diagnosis and controlled the seizures, the measures needed to prevent recurrence may need to be considered. It is best to become thoroughly familiar with a few anticonvulsant drugs (Table 5.4.7) suitable for the different types of epilepsy (see also p. 972). The smallest dose which successfully produces control should be used. Treatment is introduced with one drug alone, continuing with a starting dosage for three to four weeks. The dose is then increased if necessary until the seizures are controlled or side-effects appear. If adding a second drug proves to be effective, the first one is gradually withdrawn. In some children, particularly brain-damaged infants, it has to be accepted that adequate control cannot be achieved without undue drowsiness. If several drugs are introduced one should

Table 5.4.7 Drugs used in the treatment of epilepsy.

Drug	Type of epilepsy	Starting dose (mg/kg per 24 h)	Side-effects		Therapeutic range (µg/ml)
			Minor (often dose related)	Major (usually uncommon)	
Phenobarbitone	Grand mal Neonatal	3–6	Sedation, hyperactivity, irritability	Learning impairment, nausea, headaches	15–30
Carbamazepine	Temporal lobe Grand mal	10–20	Lethargy, dizziness (increase dose slowly), dry mouth, nausea, diplopia	Purpura, blood dyscrasias	4–10
Sodium valproate	Grand mal Petit mal Myoclonic	20–50	GI disturbances, transient hair loss, tremor	Thrombocytopaenia, liver dysfunction	50–100
Phenytoin	Grand mal	5–10	Skin rashes, gum hypertrophy, ataxia, hirsutism, acne, GI disturbances	Nystagmus, blood dyscrasias	5–20
Ethosuximide	Petit mal	20–50	Sedation, ataxia, GI disturbance	Blood dyscrasias	40–100
Diazepam	Status	0.1–0.2 intravenous as required	Drowsiness, respiratory depression	Bronchial hypersecretion	
Nitrazepam	Infantile spasms	0.5–1.0	Sedation, drooling	Bronchial hypersecretion	

Paraldehyde is given for status epilepticus — i.m. 0.1 ml/kg in a glass syringe.
ACTH is used in infantile spasms — 40–80 units daily.
GI = gastro-intestinal.

be aware of their interactions, e.g. phenobarbitone reduces the effective blood level of phenytoin. In general, therapy should be continued for three years after the last convulsion; thereafter the dose can be gradually reduced over a period of a few months; sudden cessation of therapy may lead to status epilepticus.

In status epilepticus the immediate care of the child is that of any unconscious person: the airway should be preserved by placing the child prone on his side. The drug of choice to stop seizures is intravenous diazepam: 5–10 mg is often sufficient in the smaller child but 20 mg or more may be needed in others. This drug is unreliable intramuscularly or orally, but can be given rectally if necessary. Alternative drugs are intramuscular paraldehyde and intravenous phenytoin. Failure to respond to these measures suggests that marked cerebral oedema has occurred. This may be treated with intravenous dexamethasone (0.5 mg per kg); frusemide or intravenous mannitol are alternatives. If all these measures fail, general anaesthesia may be required for several hours.

Unfortunately social problems are common in children with epilepsy. It is a disorder which is often regarded with fear and suspicion by the lay person. Thus, it is most important to educate the family and the community to accept the child and his condition by explaining carefully why such bizarre manifestations occur, otherwise there is a danger that the child will be rejected both at home and at school.

Infantile spasms

This condition can be diagnosed in the presence of the triad of flexion spasms (salaam attacks), developmental regression/retardation and hypsarrhythmia – the EEG finding of continuous, random, generalized sharp and slow wave discharges of high voltage. The onset is often in the first few months of life. In some 40 per cent of patients the aetiology is unknown; in the remaining 60 per cent, the predisposing factors may be prenatal (congenital defects, intrauterine infection), perinatal (anoxia), or postnatal (neuro-infections, metabolic disorders, tuberose sclerosis, or trauma). There is a high subsequent incidence of mental retardation and neurological abnormalities. The cardinal features of the syndrome are repetitive short muscular contractions that lead to trunk flexion and occasionally extension; sometimes the attacks occur in clusters of 30–40 spasms, often preceded by a cry.

Many patients respond to ACTH (40–80 units per day), if commenced early in the course of the disease, and nitrazepam (0.5–1.0 mg/kg per day). Despite treatment there is developmental retardation of varying degree in approximately 90 per cent of cases.

Febrile convulsions

A febrile convulsion is defined as a seizure occurring in a child aged between six months and five years, associated with fever but without any evidence of intra-cranial infection or pre-existing neurological abnor-mality. These convulsions occur in 2–5 per cent of young children; the peak incidence is 13–15 months in girls and 15–18 months in boys. There is an increased incidence in some families. The most common causes of fever are upper respiratory tract infections, but almost any disorder which causes a rise in temperature can precipitate a fit in susceptible children. In addition to various viral infections, shigella gastroenteritis and malaria are particularly likely to cause convulsions in these children. Overall, one-third of the children who have a febrile convulsion are likely to have one or more recurrences when febrile.

Most attacks are short-lived; longer-lasting convul-sions should be terminated using diazepam (see earlier). Any site of infection should be identified; in young infants in whom underlying meningitis is difficult to exclude with certainty, a lumbar puncture should always be done. A thick blood film should be examined for malarial parasites. Pyrexia should be reduced by tepid sponging, fanning, maintaining fluid intake and giving antipyretic drugs such as paracetamol (120 mg) six-hourly.

Recurrence is more likely in young children, particularly boys with a positive family history. Advice should be given on reducing fever and malarial prophylaxis in endemic regions. Intermittent adminis-tration of anticonvulsants is preferred, although some patients with recurrent convulsions require prophylac-tic treatment (see earlier). The overall prognosis is excellent; however, in patients in whom convulsions precipitated by fever are prolonged, temporal lobe damage can occur (see also p. 972).

Disorders of the spinal cord

Sudden or gradual development of symptoms arising from diseases of the spinal cord is an important problem

Table 5.4.8   Differential diagnosis of paraplegia.

Abscess, extradural
Trauma
Discitis (pyogenic)
Transverse myelitis
Schistosomiasis
Tuberculosis
Hydatid disease
Syphilis
Tumours
leukaemia
neuroblastoma
Burkitt's lymphoma
Anterior spinal artery occlusion
Nutritional myelopathy
Lathyrism
Spinal dysraphism
Myelomeningocele

in the tropics. The causes of paraplegia are shown in Table 5.4.8. In acute transverse myelitis the child complains of back pain, followed by weakness of the legs and then development of a flaccid paralysis, often with a sensory level at or below T10 with loss of sphincter control. The cause is frequently not identi-fied. Arachnoiditis may result from infection or follow intrathecal drugs or trauma. Tuberculosis of the spine and paraplegia are discussed on pp. 539–52, 916–20.

Lathyrism occurs in central India as an endemic or occasionally epidemic condition. It starts with muscle cramps, weakness and stiffness; the onset of paraplegia is often acute. It is caused by ingestion of *Lathyrus sativus* (legume) seeds, usually eaten in greater amounts during food shortages. The chemical agent causing it, beta-*N*-oxalylaminoalanine can be destroyed by boiling in a large volume of water before cooking.

Myelomeningoceles are associated with a spina bifida in which there is a laminal defect with herniation of the spinal cord and its membranes to form a sac. The nerve supply beyond is compromised; hydrocephalus is present in 70–90 per cent of cases. Spinal dysraphism describes a spectrum of disorders in which the spinal canal may be narrowed or broadened or obstructed with central spurs of fibrous tissue, cartilage or bone which may tether the spinal cord. The presence of an underlying abnormality may be indicated by growth of hair over the lumbo-sacral region, a postanal dimple, or a pigmented naevus or subcutaneous lipoma overlying the lower back. Although many of these spinal disorders may occur at any level, the most common are in the cervical and lumbo-sacral regions.

Investigation

Investigations should include screening for acute and chronic infections, and radiology of the spine and chest. A lumbar puncture may be carried out in some cases, after careful consideration. Myelography should clearly define the subarachnoid space throughout the region of clinical interest.

Ataxia

Some of the causes of ataxia are listed in Table 5.4.9. In acute cerebellar ataxia following a viral infection truncal ataxia, tremor and nystagmus may be seen. A mild pleocytosis may be present in the CSF with some elevation of the protein level. There is no specific treatment; about two-thirds of cases recover completely.

Table 5.4.9 Causes of ataxia.

Acute cerebellar ataxia
  e.g. varicella
     measles
     polio
Raised intracranial pressure
  e.g. posterior fossa tumours
     abscess
     neuroblastoma
Nutritional recovery syndrome
Acute labyrinthitis
Drug or toxin ingestion
Uncontrolled epilepsy
Kuru
Congenital syndromes
  e.g. metabolic disorders
     Friedreich's ataxia
     ataxia telangiectasia

In children recovering from kwashiorkor, a syndrome of coarse tremors, postural abnormalities, exaggerated tendon jerks and cog-wheel rigidity of the limbs has been described. There have been reports from various parts of the world of young children with tremors, anaemia and malnutrition; specific aetiological and nutritional deficiencies have not been identified.

Kuru is a disease which occurs exclusively in the Fore people living in a small region of Papua New Guinea. The disease occurs in children of both sexes after the age of four years and in adult women after the age of 20 years, adult males being infrequently affected. The disease runs an inexorable course to death within one year of its onset with a fine irregular tremor, locomotor ataxia and emotional lability. The symptoms rapidly progress to inability to walk and the superimposition of coarse tremors and choreiform movements. Soon the patients are unable to sit or swallow, death following from inanition or bronchopneumonia. The cause has been confirmed to be a slow virus infection transmitted by ingestion during ritual cannibalism.

Neuropathies

A rapidly evolving flaccid paralysis suggests the following clinical possibilities: paralytic spinal poliomyelitis and encephalomyelitis, Guillain–Barré syndrome (acute idiopathic polyneuritis), tick-bite paralysis, and various secondary acute myelopathies and polyneuropathies. Bacterial exotoxins in diphtheria and botulism are well recognized to cause paralyses. Chronic poisoning with metals such as lead, arsenic and mercury can lead to neuropathies. Certain ixodid ticks cause paralysis when attached to the skin. This has been attributed to a toxin injected from the salivary glands of the female tick. An ascending flaccid paralysis progresses rapidly, often accompanied by pain and parasthesiae; respiratory failure occurs unless the entire tick (including the mouth parts) is removed.

Guillain–Barré syndrome is thought to be an autosensitivity phenomenon following infections with mycoplasma or viruses including the Epstein–Barr virus. One to two weeks following non-specific respiratory or gastro-intestinal symptoms, symmetric weakness of the lower extremities develops which may ascend rapidly to the arms, trunk and face. Muscle tenderness and spinal root pains are frequent; fever is uncommon; facial weakness may occur early. On examination, the symmetrical flaccid weakness is usually greater proximally; bulbar involvement may occur. CSF examination shows a raised protein with normal glucose and cell counts. Electromyography shows a marked reduction in nerve conduction velocities with denervation after 10–21 days. The clinical course is progressive over a few days to two weeks, the major complications being respiratory failure and superinfection. The management is supportive, although some authorities advise corticosteroids; the majority of cases recover completely.

Further reading

Dekker, PA. *Epilepsy; A manual for Medical and Clinical Officers in Kenya*. Kenya Association for the Welfare of Epileptics, PO

Box 44599, Nairobi, Kenya, 1990.

Delgado-Escuada AV, Wasterlain CG, Treiman DM. Current concepts in neurology: management of status epilepticus. *New England Journal of Medicine*. 1982; **306**: 1337-40.

Del Rio M, Chrane D, Shelton S *et al*. Ceftriaxone versus Ampicillin – Chloramphenicol for treatment of bacterial meningitis in children. *Lancet*. 1983; **1**: 1241-4.

Emerson R, D'Souza BJ, Vining EP *et al*. Stopping medication in children with epilepsy: predictors of outcome. *New England Journal of Medicine*. 1981; **304**: 1125-9.

Feigin RD. Bacterial meningitis beyond the neonatal period. In: Feigin RD, Cherry JO eds. *Textbook of Paediatric Infectious Diseases*. Philadelphia, USA, WB Saunders, 1981: 293-308.

Molevi A, Le Frock JC. Infections of the central nervous system. *Medical Clinics of North America*. 1985: **69**: 1-434.

Nelson KB, Ellenberg JH. Prognosis in children with febrile seizures. *Pediatrics*. 1978; **61**: 720-7.

O'Donohue NV. *Epilepsies of Childhood*. London, Butterworths, 1985.

Rose FC, ed. *Paediatric Neurology*. London, Blackwell Scientific Publications, 1979.

Shaywitz BA, Rothstein MD, Venes JL. Monitoring and management of increased intracranial pressure in Reye syndrome: results in 29 children. *Pediatrics*. 1980; **66**: 198-204.

CHAPTER 5

Cardiovascular disease

F. Jaiyesimi

Cardiovascular diseases of children in the technically developed temperate countries comprise, almost entirely, congenital heart disease. In Canada, for instance, cardiac malformations account for over 90 per cent of childhood heart disease.[1] In the developing countries of the tropics and subtropics the spectrum is widened by a considerable prevalence of infections-related acquired heart disease[2] (Table 5.5.1). The common types and major manifestations of heart disease in childhood are described in this chapter.

Major manifestations of heart disease

Heart disease may manifest with cyanosis, heart murmurs, abnormal electrocardiogram, cardiomegaly, or heart failure, depending on its nature and severity.

Brief descriptions of these manifestations are given here; congestive heart failure is discussed in more detail because of its immense clinical significance.

Heart failure

Congestive cardiac failure is often the ultimate sign of severe cardiac stress. The causes are numerous and vary from one paediatric age group to another (Table 5.5.2). However, the haemodynamic consequences are similar, since they are mainly the effects of inadequate stroke output and increased central venous pressure.

Manifestations

Cough, breathlessness, inability to feed well, vomiting and failure to thrive are the most prominent manifestations. Swelling of the body is an uncommon symptom

Table 5.5.1 Patterns of heart disease in a tropical developing country (Nigeria) and an industrialized nation (Canada).

Disease	Relative frequency (%)	
	Nigeria[2]	Canada[1]
Congenital heart disease	71	92
Rheumatic heart disease	11	6
Cardiomyopathies	9	–
Infective pericarditis	8	1
Others	1	1

Data from 1, Keith JD, in *Heart Disease in Infancy and Childhood*, New York, Macmillan, 1978.
2. Antia *et al.*, in *Paediatric Cardiology* vol. 4, Edinburgh, Churchill Livingstone, 1982.

Table 5.5.2 Important causes of heart failure in children.

Age group	Causes
Newborn period	Birth asphyxia
	Septicaemia
	Congenital heart disease (persistent ductus arteriosus in preterms, transposition of the great arteries, tricuspid atresia)
1 month–5 years	Congenital heart disease (persistent ductus arteriosus, ventricular septal defect, transposition of the great arteries, tricuspid atresia)
	Anaemia
	Bronchopneumonia
	Septicaemia
	Pericarditis
	Cardiomyopathy
Above 5 years	Rheumatic heart disease
	Cardiomyopathy
	Pericarditis

in infants and young children. Assessing the jugular venous pressure in infants is a difficult, if not futile, assignment. Furthermore, the jugular venous pressure may be spuriously elevated in a restless, crying child. Consequently this sign is of value only in the older child who can be quietened during physical examination. The more reliable signs are: tachycardia, which may be associated with gallop rhythm; tachypnoea with or without fine crepitations at the lung bases; an enlarged, soft and tender liver; and cardiac enlargement. In severe heart failure the peripheral pulses are thready, the skin is cold, and the patient may be restless and his sensorium clouded as a result of cerebral hypoxia.

Management

The principal objectives of management are to reduce cardiac workload and improve myocardial perfor-

mance. These often require treating the cause of the heart failure whenever possible, bed rest in a sitting position, and administration of diuretics and digoxin (Table 5.5.3). Whenever potassium-wasting diuretics are prescribed it is essential to check the serum potassium level regularly and give supplemental potassium if necessary. This may be in the form of potassium chloride or fresh fruit juices.

Oral administration of digoxin is to be preferred: it is convenient, safe, and adequate for most occasions. Where persistent vomiting renders oral digoxin unsuitable, an intramuscular preparation is the next choice. Intravenous digoxin is best reserved for critically ill patients. Similarly, 'digitalizing' doses are hardly ever necessary; and patients receiving such large doses must be carefully observed for signs of digoxin toxicity. These include vomiting, bradycardia and cardiac arrhythmias. If any of these signs are observed, digoxin should be discontinued promptly and hypokalaemia corrected, if present. After 48–72 hours, and provided urine production is adequate, most of the digoxin would have been excreted. The drug can then be re-commenced, using a reduced dose.

Children with heart failure are often anorexic, and do not willingly accept salt-free diets. Besides, the hot tropical climate promotes considerable sweating and induces thirst. For these reasons the practice in many centres is to restrict salt and fluid intake only if maximal safe doses of digoxin and diuretics fail to control the heart failure.

Severely breathless infants may need to be fed via a naso-gastric tube; oxygen given via a tent, face mask, or nasal tube often has a salutary effect on patients who show signs of cerebral hypoxia. Assisted ventilation, coupled with intravenous frusemide (1 mg/kg), usually provides prompt relief for patients with pulmonary oedema. It is particularly essential in young infants who tend to get easily overwhelmed by the high ventilatory workload imposed by pulmonary oedema.

Aggressive management modalities, such as the use of glucagon, other inotropic agents and systemic vasodilators, are hardly ever indicated in children.

Cardiomegaly

Increased cardiac workload may induce one or more of three compensatory phenomena: tachycardia, cardiac dilatation, and cardiac hypertrophy. The nature of the workload determines whether dilatation or hypertrophy will predominate. For instance, increased pressure load on the left ventricle, such as that imposed by aortic valve stenosis, induces more hypertrophy than dilatation, whereas in chronic anaemia left ventricular

Table 5.5.3   Drugs commonly used in the treatment of cardiovascular disorders.

Drug	Dosage	Usual route	Side-effects/precautions
Anticongestive			
Digoxin (neonates)	0.01 mg/kg	oral	Vomiting, bradycardia
(1 month–2 years)	0.02 mg/kg	oral	arrhythmias
(above 2 years)	0.01 mg/kg	oral	i.m./i.v. dose = 75% oral dose
Chlorothiazide	20–40 mg/kg per day	oral	Hypokalaemia
Hydrochlorothiazide	2–5 mg/kg per day	oral	Hypokalaemia
Hydroflumethiazide	2–5 mg/kg per day	oral	Hypokalaemia
Frusemide	1.0 mg/kg stat	i.v.	Hypokalaemia
	1–4 mg/kg per day	oral	Hypokalaemia, hyponatraemia
Spironolactone	2–4 mg/kg per day	oral	
Potassium chloride	62.5–500 mg/day	oral	
Anti-arrhythmic			
Propranolol	0.1 mg/kg stat	i.v.	
Verapamil	1.0 mg/kg per day	oral	These drugs are myocardial depressants
Diphenylhydantoin	2–5 mg/kg stat	i.v.	
Lignocaine	2–3 mg/kg 8-hourly	oral	
Procainamide	2–5 mg/kg stat	i.v.	
	10–15 mg/kg 6 hourly	oral	
Antihypertensive			
Diazoxide (Trimetaphan)	5 mg/kg	i.v. fast	Hyperglycaemia
Hydralazine	0.10–0.25 mg/kg stat	oral	Hypotension, skin flushing
	0.60 mg/kg per day	i.m./i.v.	
Methyldopa	5.0–10.0 mg/kg stat	i.v.	
	10–15 mg/kg per day	oral	Hypotension, haemolytic anaemia
Reserpine	0.02–0.05 mg/kg stat (max. 2.5 mg)	i.m.	Nasal congestion, flushing of the skin, drowsiness
	0.025 mg/kg per day	oral	
Others			
10% Calcium gluconate	0.50–1.0 ml/kg stat	i.v., slowly or via drip	Fast injections can precipitate cardiac arrest
Noradrenaline	4 mg in 1000 ml i.v. fluid	i.v. drip	Rate of infusion depends on response
Aminophylline	5 mg/kg stat	i.v., slowly	Cardiovascular collapse may occur with fast injections
Atropine sulphate	0.01–0.02 mg/kg dose (maximal 6 mg/dose)	oral, subcutaneous or i.v.	Dry mouth, increased intraocular pressure, arrhythmias

dilatation is more prominent than hypertrophy. When the heart fails, there is progressive cardiac dilatation. Nonetheless, cardiac enlargement, defined as a cardio-thoracic ratio greater than 0.5, is not always a sign of cardiac disease: it may occur in children with narrow thoracic cavities. Conversely, the heart size may be normal if the heart disease is trivial, and even in some types of severe heart disease, such as constrictive pericarditis and Fallot's tetralogy.

Cyanosis

Cyanosis may be central or peripheral. In peripheral cyanosis the tongue and buccal mucosa are pink but the extremities, especially fingers and toes, are bluish and cold. The usual underlying cause is impaired venous drainage resulting from either venous obstruction or severe heart failure. It is an entirely venous pheno-menon; and the arterial oxygen saturation is normal. It is therefore not quite as ominous as central cyanosis, in which the arterial oxygen saturation is usually reduced to below 70 per cent, and the tongue, buccal mucosa, lips and nail beds are bluish. Birth asphyxia, respiratory distress syndrome and cyanotic congenital heart disease are the most common causes of central cyanosis in neonates. Beyond the newborn period cyanotic congenital heart disease is the main cause.

Heart murmurs

Most structural cardiovascular defects cause turbulent blood flow and are therefore associated with heart murmurs. These may be systolic or diastolic, and either soft or harsh depending on the underlying defect. Systolic murmurs are often loud and therefore easily audible: and they are sometimes sufficiently loud as to be palpable as thrills. Diastolic murmurs, on the other hand, are usually soft and are particularly difficult to appreciate in a child who is crying or has a tachycardia.

Serious heart disease may exist without appreciable murmur. This is especially true of myopericardial disorders. Conversely, not all murmurs denote heart disease. Indeed, about 40 per cent of healthy children have innocent murmurs. These are commonly ejection systolic in timing, soft and, as a rule, are never associated with a thrill. They are most frequently heard over the pulmonary area. Very occasionally, innocent diastolic murmurs are heard, especially in children with sickle cell anaemia. A venous hum, another common type of innocent murmur, begins in systole and continues into diastole, just like the murmur of persistent ductus arteriosus (p. 766), but unlike the latter, it is usually confined to or loudest at the upper right sternal border; it can be abolished by turning the head in various directions, or by pressing on the jugular vein, and it is not associated with bouncy pulses.

Abnormal electrocardiogram

In rhythm or conduction disorders ECG abnormalities may be the only signs of heart disease. In addition, electrocardiography provides a simple, non-invasive and fairly reliable means of assessing myocardial mass, unlike chest radiographs which assess heart size. Caution needs to be exercised in interpreting ECGs obtained from children because normal patterns vary from one paediatric age group to another, and within the same age group in different races. In this regard, doctors in tropical Africa will do well to remember that tall R-waves, elevated ST segments, and T-wave changes in left precordial leads are seen in up to 20 per cent of healthy black children.[3] In addition sinus arrhythmia and occasional premature ventricular contractions are common in healthy children.

Congenital heart disease

Owing to the inadequacy of health resources in most developing countries congenital cardiac defects are detected late and corrective surgery is feasible in very few centres. Consequently, the morbidity and case fatality rates are higher than in the technically developed countries. The incidence is, however, similar – between 3.5 and 7.0 per 1000 births. So also is the relative prevalence of the various types, except that obstructive aortic lesions are relatively uncommon in negroes. The possibility that associated abnormalities may be present in other systems must not be forgotten. Table 5.5.4, which shows the relative frequency of the various cardiac defects in Nigeria, typifies the general pattern in most developing countries. The main features of these defects are summarized below. They are broadly divided into cyanotic and non-cyanotic types. By convention, patients with right-to-left shunts fall into the cyanotic category, while patients who do not have right-to-left shunts are regarded as non-cyanotic even if they are cyanotic for other reasons, such as a low cardiac output.

Non-cyanotic heart disease

Pulmonary valve stenosis

Stenosis of the pulmonary valve causes hypertrophy of and increased pressure within the right ventricle. A pressure gradient exists across the pulmonary valve and, quite often, the pulmonary blood flow is reduced. Heart failure may occur in severe cases; and patients who have associated patent foramen ovale or septal defect may develop right-to-left shunt across such communications.

Symptoms are uncommon in mild cases, but severe stenosis may manifest with dyspnoea on exertion, effort

Table 5.5.4 Relative prevalence of the main types of cardiac malformation in 635 Nigerian children.

Simple defects (76%)		Complex defects (24%)	
Obstructive lesions (12%)	Left-to-right shunts (64%)		
Pulmonary valve stenosis (9%)	Ventricular septal defect (35%)	Fallot's tetralogy	10%
Coarctation of aorta (2%)	Patent ductus arteriosus (22%)	Transposition of the great arteries	5%
Aortic valve stenosis (1%)	Atrial septal defect (7%)	Others	9%

angina, or heart failure. In such cases the peripheral pulse volume is reduced, there is a prominent left parasternal heave, and a systolic thrill may be palpable over the pulmonary area, the same location where the characteristic rough systolic ejection murmur is usually loudest. In the absence of heart failure the chest radiograph may be normal, but the ECG often reveals varying degrees of right ventricular hypertrophy.

Pulmonary valve stenosis, aortic valve stenosis and coarctation of the aorta may, especially in infants, be mistaken for one another. In such cases, cardiac catheterization or echocardiography is often required to ascertain the correct diagnosis. Definitive treatment consists of pulmonary valve repair or replacement.

Coarctation of the aorta

This lesion is usually located distal to the left subclavian artery, around the insertion of the ductus arteriosus. Since it creates an impediment to blood flow, the blood pressure is elevated proximal to the lesion (e.g. in the arms) and reduced in areas distal to it. For the same reason, the upper limb pulses are full whereas lower limb pulses are either barely palpable or completely absent. These features may, however, be masked by a coexisting patent ductus arteriosus. Infants with severe coarctation may present in heart failure, and systemic hypertension is a common complication in older children. Other features include a suprasternal pulsation and thrill, coupled with a systolic murmur which is best heard at the upper sternal borders. On chest X-ray, the heart is usually slightly enlarged, and erosion of the inferior surfaces of the ribs may be seen in older children. ECG obtained from infants with coarctation may show right ventricular hypertrophy; but beyond infancy left ventricular hypertrophy is the usual finding.

The main measures in treatment include the control of heart failure, administration of antihypertensive agents which reduce the afterload (such as propranolol), and surgical resection of the coarctation.

Aortic valve stenosis

In this disease, ejection of blood from the left ventricle is impeded; the systolic pressure within the ventricle rises while that in the aorta remains low–normal. The increased pressure load on the ventricle results in hypertrophy, and may eventually cause heart failure.

Most of the patients are asymptomatic before onset of heart failure, but a few may present with exercise intolerance, effort angina and, rarely, syncopal attacks. The principal signs include a forceful apex beat, suprasternal pulsation, a systolic thrill in the upper right sternal border, and an ejection systolic murmur which is best heard over the aortic area. The presence of small-volume peripheral pulses and other signs of heart failure usually denotes severe stenosis. In compensated aortic stenosis the cardiac size on chest radiograph may be normal, but ECG reveals varying degrees of left ventricular hypertrophy in all but the mildest cases. Further proof of the diagnosis may be obtained at cardiac catheterization or echocardiography.

Aortic valve repair or replacement is the mainstay of treatment.

Left-to-right shunts

The malformations that make up this subgroup are atrial septal defect, ventricular septal defect, and patent ductus arteriosus. They produce varying degrees of cardiac volume overload, increased pulmonary blood flow and, ultimately, pulmonary hypertension. Very rarely the pulmonary hypertension may become so severe as to reverse the intracardiac shunt, thus causing cyanosis. Fast breathing, frequent chest infections, inability to feed well, and failure to thrive are common manifestations of both ventricular septal defect and patent ductus arteriosus. So is heart failure. Atrial septal defect, however, produces minimal symptoms and is frequently an incidental discovery.

Each of these three defects has its own fairly characteristic physical signs. In atrial septal defect these comprise a soft systolic murmur in the pulmonary area and wide, fixed splitting of the second heart sound. Ventricular septal defect produces a pansystolic murmur which is loudest at the mid or lower left sternal border and is often palpable as a thrill. Patent ductus arteriosus is characterized by bouncy pulses, a wide pulse pressure, and a continuous murmur over the pulmonary area. This murmur, too, is often palpable as a thrill. The distinguishing features of all three defects are shown in Fig. 5.5.1. In a preterm neonate the clinical course of respiratory distress syndrome may be complicated by opening of the ductus arteriosus. This may be difficult to detect clinically since a murmur may be absent or very soft. Early signs of a significant left-to-right shunt are increasing congestive cardiac failure, and an increasing oxygen dependence and ventilatory insufficiency.

Management of children with left-to-right shunts often entails prevention or prompt treatment of intercurrent chest infections, control of heart failure, maintenance of adequate nutrition, and surgical closure of the defect.

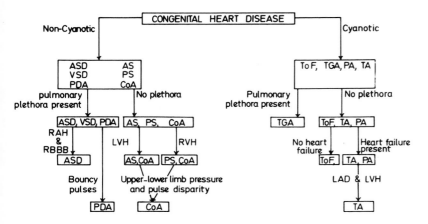

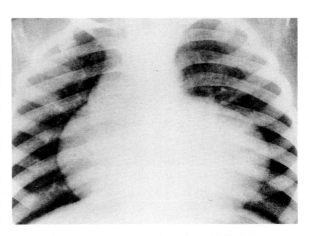

Fig. 5.5.1 Schematic approach to the diagnosis of the major cardiac malformations.

Cyanotic heart disease

Fallot's tetralogy

This is the most common cyanotic heart disease in children aged more than one year; and it is encountered so frequently that every general practitioner or paediatrician must expect to meet some cases at one time or another. It has four main components: obstruction at the outflow path of the right ventricle, right ventricular hypertrophy, a high ventricular septal defect, and a large aorta which straddles the interventricular septum. This combination results in increased right ventricular pressure, reduced pulmonary blood flow (pulmonary oligaemia) and, ultimately, shunting of blood from the right ventricle through the ventricular septal defect into the aorta.

The manifestations include growth retardation, reduced exercise tolerance, squatting, clubbing, and central cyanosis which, during hypercyanotic spells, may be so intense as to cause convulsions and coma. The cyanosis usually becomes manifest during the second half of the first year of life, or later. In typical cases, the peripheral pulses are of small volume, there is a prominent left parasternal heave, and auscultation reveals a single second heart sound and a systolic murmur which is loudest at the mid-left sternal edge. Heart failure rarely complicates Fallot's tetralogy, and this marks it out from the other common cyanotic malformations. Pulmonary oligaemia and a boot-shaped heart (Fig. 5.5.2) are the most common radiographic features; and the ECG usually shows right ventricular hypertrophy.

There are important medical aspects to the treatment of children with Fallot's tetralogy. During a hypercyanotic spell the child should be huddled into a

Fig. 5.5.2 Chest radiograph of a patient with Fallot's tetralogy. Note the boot-shaped heart.

knee–chest position in bed, and given oxygen. Next, propranolol (0.1 mg/kg body weight) or morphine sulphate (0.2 mg/kg) is administered intravenously to relax the outflow path of the right ventricle. It is usually necessary to correct concurrent metabolic acidosis by administering a base, such as 8.4 per cent sodium bicarbonate (1–2 ml/kg). If a child has frequent cyanotic spells it is wise to keep him on oral propranolol (1.0 mg/kg per day) and to expedite arrangements for surgical treatment. Erythropheresis may need to be performed in patients whose haematocrit levels exceed 65 per cent.

Surgery for Fallot's tetralogy may be in the form of a palliative shunt, such as an anastomosis between the subclavian and pulmonary arteries, or total correction of the defects.

Transposition of the great arteries

This complex malformation is the most common cyanotic cardiac defect in young infants. In the most common variant, the aorta arises from the right ventricle and the pulmonary artery from the left ventricle. The systemic and pulmonary circulations are parallel. Hence some form of communication, be it patent ductus arteriosus or a septal defect, is obligatory; as is bidirectional shunting of blood. Central cyanosis is noticeable shortly after birth and heart failure is the rule rather than the exception. These features, together with the radiographic signs which comprise an egg-shaped heart and pulmonary plethora (Fig. 5.5.3), distinguish transposition of the great arteries from the tetralogy of Fallot.

Treatment often entails the control of heart failure and alleviation of cyanosis through the creation of a large interatrial communication. Total correction is feasible in well-equipped centres.

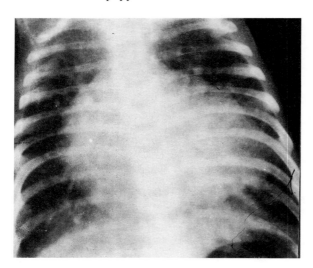

Fig. 5.5.3 Chest radiograph in transposition of the great arteries. The heart is egg-shaped and the lung fields are plethoric.

Tricuspid atresia and pulmonary atresia

These two cyanotic defects are encountered occasionally in infancy, and may be differentiated from transposition of the great arteries and Fallot's tetralogy on the basis of features outlined in Fig. 5.5.1. It must be noted, though, that precise diagnosis and definition of cardiac anatomy in children with congenital heart disease often requires special investigations, such as cardiac catheterization, angiocardiography, and echocardiography.

Pericardial diseases

Pericardial diseases are often caused by infections: acute pericarditis by pus-forming organisms and chronic pericarditis by the tubercle bacilli. Either of these can result in pericardial constriction. Viral pericarditis probably occurs more frequently than is recognized, but it is not an important cause of ill-health; neither is involvement of the pericardium by collagen disorders or intrathoracic tumours. In this section the important causes of pericardial effusion will be highlighted, but only purulent pericarditis and constrictive pericarditis will be considered in any detail.

Pericardial effusion

Important causes of pericardial effusion in childhood include:

- purulent pericarditis;
- rheumatic heart disease;
- endomyocardial fibrosis;
- chronic congestive heart failure;
- nephrotic syndrome;
- liver cirrhosis;
- tuberculous pericarditis;
- juvenile rheumatoid arthritis.

The effusion in acute rheumatic carditis, infective pericarditis, endomyocardial fibrosis, and juvenile rheumatoid arthritis is an exudate. It is therefore very cellular and the protein content is usually about 30–40 g/l. By contrast, the pericardial fluid in hypoproteinaemic states (e.g. nephrotic syndrome and liver cirrhosis) and in chronic congestive heart failure, including chronic rheumatic heart disease, is a transudate; it is relatively acellular and the protein content rarely exceeds 10 g/l. Spontaneous haemorrhagic pericardial effusion usually denotes a malignancy, but may occasionally be due to tuberculosis.

Purulent pericarditis

This is the most common form of pericardial disease encountered in paediatric practice in the tropics. It occurs equally in both sexes and throughout the paediatric age group, but the peak incidence is in the first five years of life.

Aetiology

The disease seldom occurs alone. It is usually associated with a septicaemia or other intrathoracic infections, notably postmeasles bronchopneumonia, empyema thoracis, and lung abscess. Between 20 and 40 per cent of the cases are attributable to *Staphylococcus aureus* septicaemia, and in most of such cases other foci of infection, including pyoderma, pyomyositis, septic arthritis, and empyema thoracis, are usually evident. Other organisms that may cause purulent pericarditis are *Pneumococcus* spp., *Pseudomonas aeroginosa*, *Klebsiella* spp. and, especially in infants, *Escherichia coli*.

Clinical features

The usual history is that the child has been unwell for many days, or since an attack of measles. Anorexia, fever, cough, and dyspnoea are the most prominent symptoms. Very observant parents might have noticed an exacerbation of the symptoms, coupled with some puffiness of the face, a few days before presentation. About a quarter of the older patients may complain of retrosternal chest pain.

The patients look quite ill (temperatures are likely to be in the range 38–40°C) and more than half of them will have other signs of systemic infection, such as anaemia, splenomegaly and hepatomegaly. The cardiac signs depend largely on the volume of the pericardial exudate. If this is minimal, tachycardia and a scratchy pericardial rub may be all that can be detected. But if the pericardial exudate is copious, the peripheral pulses will be fast and thready; the pulse pressure will be small, due to a reduction in systolic and elevation of diastolic pressure; and the apex beat might be impalpable. The jugular venous pressure will be elevated, and will rise further during inspiration (Kussmaul's sign). In about a third of the patients, the heart sounds are muffled and signs of heart failure are prominent. Murmurs are not heard.

Investigations

Leucocytosis and moderate anaemia are common haematological findings. If the pericardial effusion is considerable, the cardiac silhouette on X-ray is likely to be enlarged and globular (Fig. 5.5.4) while the ECG might show low-amplitude QRS deflections with flat or inverted T-waves. Rapid evolution of these signs makes the diagnosis more certain. Echocardiography can also demonstrate the presence of pericardial effusion.

Pericardiocentesis enables the clinician to ascertain the nature of the pericardial fluid. Besides its diagnostic

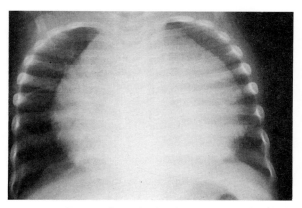

Fig. 5.5.4 Chest radiograph showing an enlarged globular cardiac silhouette in a patient with purulent pericarditis. (Courtesy of Professor WP Cockshott.)

importance pericardiocentesis can be therapeutic, and indeed life-saving in situations where pericardial evacuation is required and appropriate surgical facilities are unavailable. The procedure is relatively safe, provided appropriate precautions are taken (see p. 1014). First, premedication with morphine sulphate (0.10–0.20 mg/kg) or pethidine (1.0–2.0 mg/kg) is essential in order to minimize the patient's anxiety and restlessness during the procedure. Secondly, ECG monitoring is helpful but not compulsory. Thirdly, the elected site should be generously infiltrated with a local anaesthetic. We have found it best to attempt the tap via the xiphisternal angle, with the patient propped up in bed and the needle pointing towards the left axilla. It is advisable to use a fine venepuncture needle as a 'sound' to determine the distance of the pericardium from the skin. Having done that a big-bored needle is next used to aspirate the pericardial exudate, specimens of which are sent for bacteriological studies. The infecting organism can be isolated from the pericardial aspirate or blood culture in 50–75 per cent of cases.

Differential diagnosis

Cardiomyopathies and severe viral myocarditis can also produce a globular, murmurless heart. However, in these two conditions signs of septicaemia are absent, there is no pus within the pericardial sac, and echocardiography shows mainly dilated and hypocontractile ventricles. Other causes of pericardial effusion should also be considered in the differential diagnosis.

Treatment and prognosis

Treatment of purulent pericarditis entails a three-pronged approach: administration of effective doses of appropriate antibiotics (based on culture report or a knowledge of the spectrum of bacterial infections in the locality), complete drainage of the pus within the pericardial space (see p. 1014) and antifailure measures in appropriate cases. Supportive measures include the correction of anaemia and maintenance of adequate nutrition. Where treatment is delayed or ineffective, purulent pericarditis may be complicated by pericardial constriction or fatal myocardial damage.

Constrictive pericarditis

Constrictive pericarditis is a form of restrictive heart disease where a rigid, densely fibrosed and sometimes calcified pericardium acts as a splint which impairs both diastolic relaxation and systolic contraction of the heart. The constriction may involve all or part of the pericardium, but it generally tends to be more marked over the right heart chambers. It is almost always a complication of tuberculous or pyogenic pericarditis.

Clinical features

The disease is often difficult to recognize clinically because the symptoms are vague and frequently tend to suggest an abdominal rather than cardiac pathology: anorexia, lassitude and abdominal swelling are more prominent symptoms than cough and dyspnoea. But the physical signs are fairly distinctive in advanced cases. The precordium is usually quiet. The jugular venous pressure is elevated, the arterial pulses are fast, and the pulse pressure is low (usually less than 30 mmHg); and prolonged inspiration further accentuates these signs. The heart sounds are muffled in about half of the patients. Occasionally an extra sound – a pericardial 'knock' – may be heard in early diastole; when present this 'knock' is virtually diagnostic of pericardial constriction. The liver is enlarged in almost all cases; ascites and pedal oedema are also common signs.

Investigations

Pericardial calcification, a diagnostic radiographic sign which is best demonstrated on a lateral or oblique view, is present in about a third of the patients. The cardiac size remains normal in up to 60 per cent of the patients, but the pulmonary veins are almost always congested. Bifid P-waves, low-amplitude QRS complexes, and flat or inverted T-waves are the main ECG findings. Where the chest X-ray and ECG do not provide adequate clues

to the diagnosis, demonstration of a thickened pericardium on echocardiography, or at cardiac catheterization, will be essential for a definite diagnosis.

Differential diagnosis

Most of the physical signs of pericardial constriction can be produced by endomyocardial fibrosis of the right ventricle, and by severe myocardial damage complicating purulent pericarditis. However, tricuspid regurgitation is invariable in endomyocardial fibrosis, common in severe myocardial damage but extremely uncommon in constrictive pericarditis. Chest radiographs in endomyocardial fibrosis show pulmonary oligaemia, whereas in the other two conditions the lungs are congested. Where these signs are inconspicuous, distinguishing these conditions will require echocardiography or cardiac catheterization. Considerable ascites occurs commonly in constrictive pericarditis, liver cirrhosis and nephrotic syndrome; but in the last two conditions the chest radiographs and ECG are usually normal.

Treatment and prognosis

Treatment consists of administration of antifailure and antituberculous drugs, in appropriate cases, followed by pericardiectomy. If effective treatment is delayed, constrictive pericarditis can lead to myocardial atrophy and progressive hepatic fibrosis. Hence, it is important to prevent the disease by preventing tuberculosis, and by treating purulent pericarditis promptly and effectively.

Myocardial diseases

Acute myocarditis

Aetiology

The causes of acute myocarditis are many and diverse. Most prominent among them are viral infections (especially those due to Coxsackie B, measles, polio and mumps viruses), septicaemic states such as meningococcaemia, typhoid and staphylococcal septicaemia, rheumatic fever, American trypanosomiasis (Chagas' disease), and diphtheria. Less common causes include neonatal rubella, cytomegalovirus infection, and toxoplasmosis. Emetine, being rarely used now, has ceased to be an important cause of myocarditis, but its place is being slowly taken by daunorubicin and doxorubicin (Adriamycin), both anti-neoplastic agents.

Clinical features

Chagas' disease and diphtheritic myocarditis are considered separately (below) while rheumatic myocarditis is described elsewhere in this chapter.

Most cases of viral myocarditis are subclinical and self-limiting. For instance, 29 per cent of Nigerian children studied during an attack of measles had ECG features suggestive of myocarditis; but none of them had clinical evidence of heart disease.[4] Reports of autopsy studies also confirm the relative infrequency of overt myocarditis: only 32 cases were seen in the University College Hospital, Ibadan over an eight-year period during which there were 884 autopsies.[5] Fifteen of the 32 cases were in patients aged 10 years or less.

Where symptoms occur at all, they are commonly those of an associated upper respiratory tract infection: fever, malaise, headaches, and nasal discharge. Clinical signs are also usually unimpressive, consisting mainly of tachycardia, gallop rhythm, atrioventricular conduction defect, or premature ventricular contractions. Features of severe myocarditis include muffled heart sounds, cardiac arrhythmias, and congestive cardiac failure. In cases where myocarditis complicates a septicaemia, clinical features of this latter condition predominate, coupled with heart failure.

Investigations

Tests aimed at ascertaining the aetiology should include virus isolation studies, for which throat swab, rectal swab, or stool specimens are required. Serological studies on paired sera taken four to six weeks apart or during the acute and convalescent phases of the illness are of immense value in the diagnosis of toxoplasmosis and viral infections. If a septicaemia is suspected, blood cultures are mandatory. Depending on the severity of the myocardial damage, the ECG may be normal or reveal prolonged P–R intervals, bizarre QRS configurations, and flat or inverted T-waves. Where heart failure has occurred an enlarged globular heart and pulmonary venous congestion will be visible on chest radiograph.

Treatment and prognosis

The main ingredients of management are bed rest, diuretics, and digoxin. But the cardiac glycoside needs to be administered cautiously because patients with acute myocarditis are prone to digoxin toxicity. Specific antimicrobials should also be given in appropriate cases. Response to treatment is generally satisfactory but varying degrees of cardiac enlargement may persist

for a long time. Such cases may progress to dilated cardiomyopathy (p. 772).

Chagas' disease

This is a distinct form of parasitic myocarditis caused by *Trypanosoma cruzi* (see pp. 679–82). It is endemic in, and virtually confined to, Central and South America where it affects mainly socially disadvantaged people who live in poor houses with thatched roofs and cracked walls that provide refuge for the vector reduviid bug. Children seem to be particularly susceptible to American trypanosomiasis, and in a study by Blandon and his colleagues 75 per cent of the trypanosome-positive subjects were younger than 15 years.[6]

Clinical features

There are two main forms of cardiac involvement in Chagas' disease: an acute myocarditis occurs at the time of infection, followed some 10 or more years later by a chronic myocardial disease. The acute form, which is the more common variant in children, is usually part of a generalized illness characterized by inoculation chagoma (an indurated skin swelling) or Romana's sign (see p. 680) (unilateral conjunctivitis with palpebral oedema), fever, lymphadenopathy, splenomegaly, heart disease and meningoencephalitis. Acute myocarditis occurs in about 70 per cent of the cases and manifests with tachycardia, conduction defects and heart failure.

In chronic Chagas' disease the heart is heavy, the chambers are dilated, but the left ventricle is thinned out and its apex is often aneurysmal. Atrioventricular valve regurgitation, cardiac failure, conduction defects and rhythm disorders are the usual manifestations at this stage of the disease.

Investigations

Aetiological diagnosis in the acute phase depends on xenodiagnosis or demonstration of the trypanosomes in blood films; but in the chronic form it requires echocardiographic or angiocardiographic demonstration of the characteristic cardiac features, coupled with positive complement fixation or other serological tests.

Treatment and prognosis

The results of drug treatment for the acute phase of American trypanosomiasis have improved following the introduction of nitroimidazole derivatives (e.g. benznidazole). These compounds suppress parasitaemia in up to 90 per cent of the patients. Nonetheless between 5 and 10 per cent of the patients succumb to heart failure during this phase of the disease; and there is no clear evidence that drug treatment halts the progression of the cardiac disease. Similarly, the myocardial dysfunction associated with the chronic phase of Chagas' disease responds poorly to drug treatment. Efforts aimed at preventing the disease should therefore be intensified.

Diphtheritic myocarditis

Peripheral circulatory failure occasionally occurs early in the course of diphtheria as a result of toxic damage to the splanchnic parasympathetic nerves. However, the more serious cardiovascular complication is the toxic myocarditis which occurs in about 20 per cent of the patients. It commonly develops in the second week of the illness, and in unimmunized children.

In fatal cases the heart is large, pale and flabby; and histology usually reveals fatty degeneration of the myocardium, scanty mononuclear cell infiltration, and necrosis of the specialized conductive tissues.

The clinical manifestations comprise tachycardia, muffled heart sounds, atrioventricular and intraventricular conduction defects, and heart failure.

Treatment and prognosis

Bed rest, diuretics and digoxin are the main ingredients of medical treatment of diphtheritic myocarditis. Corticosteroids (e.g. prednisolone 1–2 mg/kg body weight) are also commonly prescribed. Administration of antibiotics and the specific antitoxin are standard measures in the treatment of diphtheria, but antitoxin therapy does not influence the outcome of diphtheritic myocarditis. The mortality rate varies from 5 to 50 per cent, and is highest in unimmunized patients.

Dilated cardiomyopathy

Dilated cardiomyopathy, by which is meant heart muscle disease of unknown aetiology, occurs in all age groups but is more common in adults.

Aetiology

A history suggestive of recent viral respiratory infection is common, histological evidence of viral myocarditis is, however, usually lacking. This has prompted the suggestion that the disease may be the result of an immune reaction triggered off by a viral infection. Protein–energy malnutrition is not a cause of dilated cardiomyopathy.

Pathology

The heart is pale and flabby. Varying degrees of hypertrophy and dilation are noticeable in all the cardiac chambers, but the changes are usually most prominent in the left ventricle. In that chamber the trabeculae carneae are arranged in a fine lace pattern and the mitral valve leaflets are rendered incompetent by dilation of the valve ring. Patchy endocardial scarring is a common feature; and mural thrombi are seen in some cases.

Clinical features

About 20 per cent of the patients are asymptomatic. In such cases, the cardiomyopathy is usually an incidental finding during chest radiography. Where symptoms are present they usually consist of cough and effort dyspnoea. A poor left ventricular impulse is a fairly constant physical sign; a ventricular gallop is also common and a soft mitral regurgitation murmur is audible in 30 to 50 per cent of the patients. Features of heart failure may or may not be present, depending on the severity of the disease. The blood pressure is usually normal.

Investigations

Leucocytosis is a common finding. The chest radiograph shows an enlarged and rather globular heart, but pulmonary venous congestion is evident only in patients with heart failure. ECG features consist of tall R-waves and flat or inverted T-waves in leads V4–V6. Echocardiography or left ventricular angiocardiography will in most cases confirm the presence of a dilated, hypertrophied but poorly contractile left ventricle.

Differential diagnosis

Other causes of mitral regurgitation, such as rheumatic heart disease and endomyocardial fibrosis, must be considered in the differential diagnosis. These two conditions are described elsewhere in this chapter. On occasions when constrictive pericarditis manifests with a large, globular heart it may simulate dilated cardiomyopathy, but a careful analysis of the ECG will usually reveal the correct diagnosis.

Treatment and prognosis

Patients who present in heart failure should be managed in the standard fashion. Fortunately, the response to treatment is usually satisfactory, though varying degrees of cardiomegaly may persist for a long time. The long-term prognosis is uncertain.

Tropical left ventricular aneurysms

Left ventricular aneurysms have been reported in children and young adults from most countries in tropical Africa. They are, however, uncommon. In Nigeria, for instance, such aneurysms account for less than 0.5 per cent of heart disease in children.

Aetiology

The aetiology is uncertain. None of the usual causes of ventricular aneurysms, namely, myocardial ischaemia, trauma, and collagen disorders, have been implicated. Rather it does appear, from clinicopathologic studies, that infection-induced damage to parts of the left ventricle may be a prerequisite for the development of the aneurysms.

Pathology

The aneurysms are often located beneath the aortic or mitral valve ring, from where they may burrow through the ventricular septum, the posterior wall of the left ventricle, or the left atrial wall. Less commonly, the aneurysm is located at the apex of the left ventricle. Subaortic aneurysms may be 3–5 cm in diameter, while those located in the submitral region could be much larger, up to 10 cm. Such aneurysms weaken the related valve rings and render the valves incompetent. In addition, large submitral aneurysms may stretch the circumflex branch of the left coronary artery and thereby precipitate myocardial ischaemia.

Clinical features

About a third of the patients are asymptomatic. The rest may present with fever, precordial pain, palpitations and symptoms of left ventricular failure. A double apical impulse is the most characteristic physical sign, but it is detected in less than 50 per cent of the patients. Other features include an apical third heart sound, signs of heart failure, and the murmur of aortic or mitral regurgitation, depending on which valve is affected.

Investigations

Submitral aneurysms can be recognized fairly easily on plain chest radiographs because they often produce visible bulging of the left heart border. Fluoroscopy may reveal paradoxical pulsation and specks of calcification, but the precise location and size of the aneurysm is best determined at angiocardiography. Low-voltage QRS deflections, flat or inverted T-waves, and pathological Q-waves in left ventricular leads are the main ECG findings.

Differential diagnosis

Subaortic and small submitral aneurysms which do not produce a visible bulge on the heart border may be indistinguishable clinically from other causes of incompetence of the affected valve. Precise diagnosis in such cases requires angiocardiography.

Treatment and prognosis

Treatment consists of control of heart failure and excision of the aneurysm during cardiac bypass surgery. Where surgery is not feasible, death may occur from heart failure, ventricular arrhythmia, or rupture of the aneurysm. Infective endocarditis and systemic thrombo-embolic events may also complicate the disease.

Endomyocardial fibrosis

Endomyocardial fibrosis (EMF) occurs world-wide but is most prevalent in the hot and humid parts of tropical Africa and, to a lesser extent, in Brazil and southern parts of India. It is, by and large, a disease of children and young adults, with about 70 per cent of the patients aged between five and 20 years. Both sexes are equally affected.

Aetiology

The aetiology of EMF is still incompletely understood but substantial advances in knowledge have occurred since those days when the disease was erroneously attributed to malnutrition, excessive plantain consumption and, later, a 'tropical immunological syndrome'. There now exists considerable evidence that hypereosinophilia (or the hypersensitivity reaction it denotes) may, in susceptible individuals, initiate the cardiac damage which ultimately results in EMF. In Nigeria, eosinophilia caused by helminthic infections has been identified as a precipitating factor.[7] But not all

EMF patients have eosinophilia, and there have been instances where dilated cardiomyopathy preceded or coexisted with EMF. It therefore seems that EMF may have more than one cause.

Pathology

The disease may affect one or both sides of the heart. All three layers of the heart are involved, but the dominant lesions are in the endocardium and the subendocardial myocardium. Pericardial effusion is present in about a quarter of the cases; and in some cases of right ventricular EMF the apex of the right ventricle is visibly retracted, creating a notch between it and the left ventricle. The gross anatomy of the interior of the heart is remarkable: the endocardium is replaced by a meshwork of fibrous tissue which begins at the apex and spreads through the free wall of the ventricle to the recesses of the atrioventricular valve (Fig. 5.5.5). In the process, the ventricular cavity is reduced and the papillary muscles bound down, thus rendering the related valve incompetent. The resultant regurgitation of blood from the ventricle causes dilatation of the corresponding atrium. Curiously enough, the outflow tracts of the ventricles are usually unaffected.

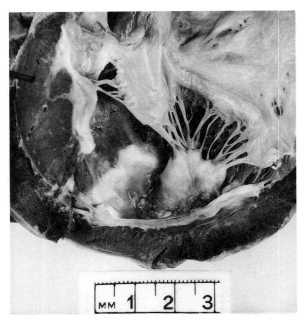

Fig. 5.5.5 Gross pathology of the heart in right ventricular EMF. (Courtesy of Dr DH Connor.)

Haemodynamics

The fibrosis results in impaired ventricular contractility during systole and restricted relaxation in diastole. The former causes a reduction in stroke output and tissue perfusion, while the latter leads to elevated central venous pressure and either systemic or pulmonary venous congestion, depending on whether the disease affects the left or right ventricle.

Clinical features

EMF of the left ventricle is manifested clinically with symptoms and signs of mitral regurgitation, pulmonary hypertension and heart failure. When the right ventricle is affected the features are more striking. Abdominal swelling and cough are the principal symptoms, but facial swelling and effort dyspnoea are also common. In advanced cases, the jugular veins are distended and show a large systolic pulsation, indicating tricuspid regurgitation; the peripheral pulses are feeble, the heart sounds are distant and, in most cases, no murmur is audible. Atrial fibrillation occurs in about a quarter of the patients. Ascites, a large, firm but pulsatile liver, and growth retardation are fairly constant features. The ascites is often massive, presumably because it is produced through three mechanisms: elevated central venous pressure, hepatocellular dysfunction with hypoalbuminaemia and reduced serum oncotic pressure, and a low-grade peritoneal reaction. Pleural effusion is commonly present. Proptosis and central cyanosis are present in about a half of the patients, and close to a third of them have clubbing of the digits. Less common features include periorbital hyperpigmentation and enlargement of the parotid glands. Ankle oedema is remarkably minimal.

Investigations

Chest X-ray findings in patients with left ventricular EMF are non-specific and comprise moderate cardiomegaly with pulmonary venous congestion. In right ventricular disease, however, the appearances are very characteristic. The heart has a globular shape, the size is markedly enlarged (due to a combination of pericardial effusion and an enormously dilated right atrium), but the lung fields are oligaemic (Fig. 5.5.6). In a few patients, specks of calcification are visible in the outflow path of the right ventricle.

The ECG facilitates the clinical recognition of EMF considerably. The P-waves are tall and peaked in right ventricular EMF but bifid or broad in left ventricular disease; and in both situations the QRS complexes are

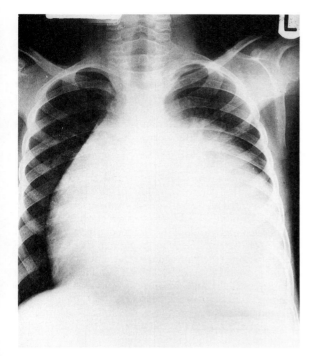

Fig. 5.5.6 Chest radiograph in right ventricular EMF. The cardiac silhouette is enormous and the lung fields are oligaemic.

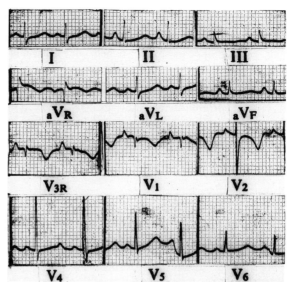

Fig. 5.5.7 ECG obtained from a seven-year-old boy with right ventricular EMF. Note the low voltages, and the virtually diagnostic qr pattern in leads V3R and V1.

of low amplitude while the T-waves are either flat or inverted. All these are non-specific changes, though. The most useful sign is a qr pattern over leads V3R, V1 or V2 (Fig. 5.5.7). This pattern is present in between 60 and 90 per cent of children with EMF but is rare in any other acquired heart disease in childhood.[8]

Echocardiographic assessment of the affected ventricle may reveal dense endocardial echoes, atrioventricular valve prolapse, reduced ventricular contractility, sudden obliteration of the cavity and, in patients with right ventricular EMF, dilated infundibulum.[9] The pathological anatomy of the heart and the deranged haemodynamics can also be demonstrated by cardiac catheterization and angiocardiography.

Differential diagnosis

A mitral regurgitation murmur induced by left ventricular EMF may be mistaken for that of rheumatic heart disease or dilated cardiomyopathy. In these two other conditions, however, the ECG show tall R-waves in the left ventricular leads, and no qr pattern is seen. The echocardiographic and angiocardiographic features are also different.[2] The clinical features of non-calcific constrictive pericarditis may closely resemble those of right ventricular EMF. In such cases, a precise diagnosis may be impossible without echocardiography and other sophisticated cardiac investigations. Very occasionally tuberculous pericarditis may cause a massive pericardial effusion and thus mimic right ventricular EMF; but the absence of tricuspid regurgitation and pulmonary oligaemia in such cases facilitates the differential diagnosis.

Treatment and prognosis

Administration of diuretics in large doses is the mainstay of medical treatment. Digoxin is of limited value, except in patients who have atrial fibrillation, but may be administered all the same in the hope that it will improve contractility of the unfibrosed myocardium. Even then low doses are prescribed because the heart rate in EMF patients is often relatively slow for the degree of cardiac disease. Abdominal paracentesis is a safe and effective means of providing relief for patients with massive ascites. The ascites usually recurs, though, and paracentesis may need to be repeated at frequent intervals. If the main problem is pericardial effusion, rather than ascites, partial pericardiectomy or a valved pericardio–peritoneal shunt will decompress the heart and facilitate improved myocardial performance. Definitive surgery, consisting of endocardiectomy with or without valve replacement, appears to be beneficial in carefully selected cases.[10]

In most medically treated patients the course of EMF is characterized by progressive cardiac failure, hepatic fibrosis, recurrent ascites, and growth retardation. Heart failure is the most common mode of death.

Endocardial diseases

Rheumatic fever

Prevalence

Acute rheumatic fever and chronic rheumatic heart disease still constitute a major health problem in the developing countries. In West Africa and the West Indies the prevalence of rheumatic heart disease is about 1.0 per 1000 children; in India the rates range from about 5 per 1000 in Vellore to 11 per 1000 in Delhi;[11] and rates of 9 and 15 per 1000 have been reported from South and North Africa, respectively.[12, 13]

Rheumatic fever affects even the very young, beginning from about the age of three years, but the peak incidence occurs between six and ten years and first attacks are uncommon after adolescence. It is slightly more common in girls than in boys. Clustering of cases within a family occurs occasionally, thus raising the possibility of a familial, probably genetic, predisposition.

Aetiology

The disease is usually a sequel to group A β–haemolytic streptococcal pharyngitis (see p. 515). The risk to an individual child is small, though, since less than 5 per cent of children with this form of pharyngitis are likely to develop rheumatic fever. Generally, whether or not a child will develop rheumatic fever after an episode of streptococcal pharyngitis depends on individual susceptibility, the promptness or otherwise with which effective treatment is given, and the rheumatogenicity of the infecting streptococci.

Pathology

Rheumatic fever causes proliferative and exudative inflammatory reactions in several connective tissues, but notably those in joints, heart and brain. Effusions into joint capsules, pericardial or pleural spaces result from exudative reactions, while the proliferative process is typified by the Aschoff nodules which are generally most abundant in the left atrial myocardium.

The cardiac lesions comprise fibrinous pericarditis, myocarditis and endocarditis, the last being most conspicuous in the left ventricle, and on the mitral valve which becomes roughened and oedematous. Varying degrees of cardiac enlargement may occur at this acute stage; and mitral regurgitation is common. Later on, as healing progresses, the pericarditis resolves virtually completely, the myocardium may be scarred, and the valve edges become thickened and rolled up. The papillary muscles become stout and shortened, thus preventing full approximation of the valve leaflets during ventricular systole. Commissural adhesions may subsequently lead on to valve stenosis.

These changes are not the results of direct invasion of the heart by streptococci; but beyond that not much else is certain about the pathogenesis of rheumatic fever and rheumatic heart disease. Antigenic similarities between the human heart and group A streptococci have been demonstrated by many workers, and it is widely believed that the cardiac damage is sequel to an immune reaction between heart tissues and antibodies produced by the body against the streptococci.

Clinical features

The diagnosis of acute rheumatic fever is traditionally based on the revised Jones criteria (Table 5.5.5), according to which the diagnosis may be made if there are two major manifestations, or if there is a combination of one major and two minor manifestations, plus evidence of streptococcal infection. The relative

Table 5.5.5 Revised Jones criteria for the diagnosis of rheumatic fever.

Major manifestations	Minor manifestations	Evidence of streptococcal infection
Carditis	Arthralgia History of rheumatic fever	Raised ASO titre (or increased titre of other specific antistreptococcal antibodies)

Polyarthritis
Sydenham's
  chorea
Erythema
  marginatum
Subcutaneous
  nodules
	Fever
	Increased P–R
	  interval
	Raised ESR
	
	Increased C-
	  reactive protein
		Positive throat culture

Table 5.5.6 Frequency of major manifestations of rheumatic fever in four developing countries.

Manifestation	Frequency (%)			
	Cameroons[14]	Egypt[15]	Nigeria	India*
Arthritis	80	59	59	53
Carditis	100	50	90	60
Chorea	20	12	5	4
Erythema marginatum	10	Not stated	2	2
Subcutaneous nodules	10	Not stated	1	2

* Compiled from data quoted by Sanyal *et al. Circulation*, 1974; **49**: 7–12.

frequencies of the major manifestations in four countries are shown in Table 5.5.6.

As stated earlier, rheumatic fever causes a *pancarditis*. The pericardial inflammation may manifest initially as a pericardial friction rub and, later, as an exudate. The myocarditis is evidenced by tachycardia, conduction and rhythm disorders or, in severe cases, soft heart sounds and heart failure. But endocarditis with valve damage, and hence cardiac murmur, is the most serious lesion because it frequently leads to chronic heart disease. Rheumatic *arthritis* is typically polyarticular, fleeting and not symmetrical. The large joints, such as the ankles, knees, elbows and wrists are the favourite sites. *Chorea* is seen mostly in peripubertal female patients; and is seldom concurrent with other rheumatic manifestations. *Erythema marginatum*, an evanescent erythematous skin rash with an irregular edge, is confined to the trunk. This centripetal distribution, coupled with the fact that it causes no itching, makes it very easy to miss the rash. *Rheumatic nodules* are best sought for near bony prominences, joint capsules or muscle tendons, especially over the elbows, occiput and spine. The *minor manifestations* are common clinical phenomena and therefore need not be described here. It is sufficient to state that, generally, the child with rheumatic fever looks quite sick; he lies in bed with his limbs flexed, apparently trying to minimize the joint pains.

Investigations

Laboratory tests are relevant only in so far as they confirm the presence or absence of the manifestations of rheumatic fever. But two points need be stressed. First, throat swab culture for β-haemolytic streptococci is positive only in about a third of patients with rheumatic fever. Secondly, the ASO titre can be considered significantly elevated only if it exceeds 200 i.u.

Differential diagnosis

The following should be considered in the differential diagnosis of rheumatic fever.

- Sickle cell disease.
- Septicaemia with infective endocarditis.
- Juvenile rheumatoid arthritis.

The first two diseases are discussed elsewhere in this chapter. Juvenile rheumatoid arthritis may, at its early stages, be mistaken for rheumatic fever but as the disease progresses the chronicity of the joint lesions and the usual absence of heart murmurs facilitate the differential diagnosis.

Treatment and prognosis

Treatment should aim to eradicate any streptococci that the patient may still be harbouring, suppress the inflammatory reactions, and reduce cardiac workload. These objectives can be achieved through bed rest, the administration of a course of penicillin (e.g. procaine penicillin 0.3–0.6 mega units daily for ten days, or a single injection of 0.6–1.2 mega units of benzathine penicillin) and salicylate therapy, using aspirin in a dose of 80–100 mg/kg body weight per day. Oral prednisolone (1.0–2.0 mg/kg body weight per day), or any equivalent corticosteroid, is indicated in patients who show signs of severe carditis, namely, extreme tachycardia, copious pericardial exudate, rapidly progressive valve damage, or heart failure. The steroid may be administered concurrently with the salicylate until signs of severe carditis have subsided. When that happens the steroid is withdrawn gradually; but the salicylate should be continued and the patient's physical activity curtailed until all signs of rheumatic activity have regressed and the ESR is normal. The usual antifailure measures are also applied until heart failure is controlled.

Death in the acute phase is uncommon but may occur in patients with severe carditis. In some other patients, the disease runs a subacute course, with incapacitating valve disease developing within one year. Altogether, about 75 per cent of children with acute rheumatic fever subsequently develop chronic rheumatic heart disease.

Prevention

The prevention of rheumatic fever and rheumatic heart disease are interwoven; both will therefore be considered together here.

Primary prevention This aims at preventing a first attack of rheumatic fever. It can be achieved through: (i) prevention of overcrowding; (ii) improved nutrition, so that the children will be better able to resist infections; (iii) health education and provision of essential health facilities in both urban and rural areas; and most important of all (iv) prompt and effective treatment of streptococcal infections. This last objective can be achieved by a 7–10 days course of either oral penicillin (250–500 mg four times a day) or procaine penicillin 0.3–0.6 mega units daily, i.m.). A single dose of benzathine penicillin (0.6–1.2 mega units) will achieve the same result.

Secondary prevention   The aim here is to prevent a recurrence of acute rheumatic fever in a child who has already suffered one attack, or who already has rheumatic heart disease. The main thrust is the prevention of streptococcal infections by long-term antibiotic prophylaxis, such as the administration of benzathine penicillin every three to four weeks or oral penicillin 250 000 units twice daily. If the child is allergic to penicillin, oral sulphadiazine (250–500 mg twice daily) or erythromycin (250 mg twice daily) can be substituted. The prophylaxis can be discontinued five years after the last attack of rheumatic fever or when the patient reaches the age of 18 years, whichever is later. Close surveillance is usually necessary to ensure compliance.

Chronic rheumatic heart disease

Pattern of valve involvement

The mitral valve is involved in practically every child who has chronic rheumatic heart disease: 64 per cent of the patients studied in our unit had pure mitral regurgitation, 17 per cent had combined mitral regurgitation and stenosis, and pure mitral stenosis was present in only 3 per cent of the patients. Mitral valve disease was associated with aortic valve disease in 8 per cent and with tricuspid regurgitation in 6 per cent of the patients. The mean age of the patients at presentation was nine years, but a few of them already had mitral stenosis at the age of five years. Similar instances of juvenile mitral stenosis have also been reported from other tropical developing countries.[17] It is believed to result from repeated attacks of acute rheumatic fever and the associated intense host reactions.

Clinical features

A few patients are brought to hospital on account of excessive precordial activity, but the majority present with symptoms of congestive cardiac failure.

The signs are those of the underlying valve defect, plus heart failure if such a complication exists. In mitral regurgitation the apex beat is diffuse and heaving, and a systolic thrill is frequently palpable there. Auscultation usually reveals a long, blowing systolic murmur which is loudest at the apex or towards the left axilla. The mitral stenosis murmur is also best heard at the apex, but because it is soft and occurs in diastole it is easily missed. Turning the patient to his left side often makes the murmur louder. Aortic regurgitation is characterized by bouncy pulses, a wide pulse pressure, suprasternal pulsation, and a soft early diastolic murmur which is best heard between the apex and the aortic area, and in held expiration. The auscultatory findings in congenital and acquired aortic stenosis are similar, but rheumatic aortic stenosis rarely occurs alone; some other valve lesion is usually present.

Investigations

Chest X-ray signs in mitral valve disease include cardiomegaly, a convex contour to the left heart border, and pulmonary venous congestion. The aorta is often dilated in patients with aortic valve disease. ECG signs of left ventricular hypertrophy are commonly seen in aortic valve disease and in mitral regurgitation; but in mitral stenosis the ECG shows right ventricular hypertrophy and biatrial dilatation. Further definition of the nature and extent of rheumatic valve damage usually requires sophisticated cardiac investigations.

Differential diagnosis

Other important causes of mitral regurgitation include endomyocardial fibrosis, dilated cardiomyopathy, sickle cell disease, and mitral valve prolapse. They are described elsewhere in this chapter.

Atrial myxoma and constrictive pericarditis may, rarely, simulate mitral stenosis. But for all practical purposes mitral stenosis in the tropics should be ascribed to rheumatic carditis until otherwise proven. The presence of another valve lesion makes the diagnosis fairly certain. A patent ductus arteriosus (p. 766) is about the only common condition that needs be considered in the differential diagnosis of rheumatic aortic regurgitation.

Treatment and prognosis

The definitive treatment of rheumatic valve disease is surgical. If heart failure is present it should be treated in the usual manner. Infective endocarditis and recurrences of acute rheumatic fever worsen the prognosis in rheumatic heart disease. Both complications should therefore be prevented by applying measures outlined elsewhere in this chapter. Pulmonary hypertension and atrial fibrillation also affect the prognosis adversely. Severe heart failure is the most common cause of death.

Infective endocarditis

Available reports indicate that infective endocarditis is relatively uncommon in children. It accounts for less than 1.0 per cent of cardiac diseases seen in the paediatric cardiology service in the University College Hospital, Ibadan. Brockington and Edington[5] identified 64 cases over an eight-year period; only one was in a patient aged below 10 years.

Aetiology

Acute bacterial endocarditis is often due to *Staphylococcus aureus* septicaemia, but may occasionally be secondary to infections by *Pseudomonas aeruginosa, Klebsiella sp., Escherichia coli, Streptococcus viridans* and *Streptococcus pneumoniae*. Mostly, however, these other organisms invade previously damaged valves or sites of congenital cardiac defects and cause a subacute illness. Fungal and rickettsial endocarditis seem to be rare in tropical paediatric practice.

Clinical features

These are attributable to septicaemia, cardiac damage, and thrombo-embolic episodes. In *acute endocarditis* features of septicaemia predominate. There is often a history of skin sepis, abrasion or trauma, followed days later by an acute illness characterized by high fever, chills, cough and dyspnoea. The child looks quite toxic and pale, and the temperature may persist at above 39°C. Evidence of valve incompetence is discernible if carefully sought; so also are signs of rapidly progressive heart failure. In the *subacute disease* toxaemia is less pronounced and anaemia is moderate. The main features are the persistent fever, the murmur of valve incompetence, and signs of heart failure. Splenomegaly is common, but clubbing of the digits occurs in less than a third of the patients. Osler's nodes, skin petechiae and splinter haemorrhages are distinctly rare.

Investigations

The common laboratory findings include microscopic haematuria (in 30–50 per cent of cases), normocytic anaemia, leucocytosis with toxic granules, and raised erythrocyte sedimentation rate. Blood cultures are positive in up to 80 per cent of patients not previously treated with antibiotics. Echocardiography is also very useful: it can detect valve vegetations in up to 80 per cent of cases.

Differential diagnosis

Acute malaria in a child with an innocent murmur may be mistaken for infective endocarditis. However, the fever of malaria subsides one to two days after administration of effective antimalaria drugs, unlike the persistent fever of endocarditis. Many of the signs associated with bacterial endocarditis are also seen in acute rheumatic carditis, and in sickle cell disease. These conditions are described elsewhere. In general, if blood cultures are positive in any child who has a significant cardiac murmur it is wise to assume that he has endocarditis and to treat accordingly. The subsequent course of the illness, especially the promptness or otherwise of the response to antibiotic therapy, will usually indicate the correct diagnosis.

Treatment

Medical treatment, aimed at eradicating the infection, controlling heart failure and providing general support, must commence as soon as the necessary blood samples have been sent for bacteriological studies. The initial choice of antibiotics will depend on the clinical suspicion with regards to the probable pathogen or a knowledge of the common pathogens in the community. In any case the regimen should be a combination of antibiotics that are effective against both Gram-positive and Gram-negative organisms. Cloxacillin (100 mg/kg per 24 h, i.v.) plus gentamicin (5.0–7.5 mg/kg per 24 h slow i.v. or i.m.) is one such combination. Appropriate changes are made subsequently, depending on the results of bacteriological studies and the response to treatment. Antibiotic therapy should continue until repeated blood cultures are sterile and the child has been afebrile for at least two weeks.

Other measures in the management include the correction of anaemia and administration of antifailure drugs in appropriate cases. Very occasionally the affected valve may need to be excised to eradicate the infection.

Prognosis

Bacterial endocarditis is a severe illness with a case fatality rate of between 25 and 50 per cent. This poor prognosis is often due to misdiagnosis and delays in starting effective treatment.

Prevention

The prevention of infective endocarditis revolves around the prompt investigation and effective treatment of bacterial infections in children. Besides, cardiac patients should receive antibiotic prophylaxis before any procedure that may cause a bacteraemia. These include dental surgery, colonic or bladder instrumentation, and cardiac catheterization. The prophylaxis could be in the form of penicillin and streptomycin, given intramuscularly 45–30 minutes before the procedure and continued for two or three days after; ampicillin may also be used.

Mitral valve prolapse

Mitral valve prolapse (floppy mitral valve, billowing mitral valve, click-murmur syndrome) is believed to be common beyond infancy. It occurs in association with congenital cardiac malformations (notably septal defects), thoracic wall deformities, and cardiomyopathies, as well as with rheumatic heart disease and Marfan's syndrome. A familial tendency has also been observed in some cases. However, no aetiological factor is discernible in about 60 per cent of cases.

Clinical features

The associated mitral regurgitation is usually trivial. Quite often the first hint of the disease comes from cardiac auscultation and comprises an apical mid- or late-systolic click, with or without a systolic murmur. Postural changes alter the intensity of these abnormal sounds: they are accentuated by standing, held expiration, and by lying in a left lateral position while squatting and vasoconstriction tend to reduce their intensity.

Investigations

ECG and chest radiographs are of little value in diagnosis. Left ventricular angiocardiograms may demonstrate the prolapse and regurgitation, but the diagnosis can be ascertained much more rapidly and safely by echocardiographic demonstration of the characteristic posterior movement of the posterior mitral valve leaflet in late systole.

Treatment and prognosis

No specific treatment is required because the disease hardly ever poses any significant haemodynamic problem and the prognosis is good.

Miscellaneous heart disorders

Anaemia

The cardiovascular sequelae of acute anaemia include tachycardia and a reduction in pulse volume. In severe cases these initial signs are followed by progressive hypotension and heart failure, all culminating in complete cardiovascular collapse. These signs are largely the results of hypovolaemia and tissue hypoxia. In chronic anaemia, on the other hand, the pathophysiology is a composite of tissue hypoxia and hypervolaemia. This is true of all haemoglobinopathies, but more so of sickle cell disease and thalassaemia major, in which conditions anaemia is often severe. Furthermore, the abnormal shape of the erythrocytes in sickle cell disease leads to hyperviscosity, which in turn imposes more strain on the heart. The account that follows below relates to the cardiovascular features of sickle cell disease (see pp. 828–31).

Cardiac dilatation and tachycardia are fairly regular findings. The tissue hypoxia causes a reduction of the peripheral resistance, hence the peripheral pulses are bounding and the pulse pressure increased. The circulation is hyperdynamic, the heart sounds are loud, and an innocent murmur is a common feature. With time the increased cardiac workload leads to ventricular hypertrophy. Myocardial ischaemia may result from hypoxaemia, or from thrombotic occlusion of a coronary artery by sickled erythrocytes; but it is a very rare complication. Repeated pulmonary infarctions may, in the older sickler, lead to pulmonary hypertension and cor pulmonale. But this, too, is an uncommon event. A sudden exacerbation of the anaemia can, of course, precipitate heart failure. This tends to occur when the haematocrit drops to below 15 per cent.

Treatment

This consists of correction of anaemia, control of heart failure, treatment of any concurrent illness, and adoption of the usual measures for the routine management of children with sickle cell haemoglobinopathy. In patients with severe anaemia, heart failure may be averted by administering a fast diuretic (e.g. frusemide 1–2 mg/kg, i.v.) 30 minutes before transfusing packed red blood cells (15 ml/kg body weight), or by undertaking an exchange blood transfusion. The latter, however, is more tedious and is hardly feasible in a busy paediatric unit.

Cor pulmonale

Cor pulmonale, otherwise known as pulmonary hypertensive heart disease, may complicate any respiratory disorder which causes significant hypoxaemia, increases the pulmonary vascular resistance, or in some other way increases the ventilatory workload. Acute cor pulmonale is common in children, the main causes being acute laryngo-tracheo-bronchitis, bronchiolitis and acute bronchopneumonia. Of these three causes, bronchopneumonia is the most common, and it tends to cause heart failure, especially in infants and very young children. Chronic cor pulmonale, on the other hand, often results from pulmonary tuberculosis, lung abscess, bronchiectasis or, in Egypt, pulmonary schistosomiasis. Bronchial asthma rarely causes cor pulmonale in children.

Clinical features

The common features are those of the underlying lung disease, coupled with signs of right heart failure. The very young patients may, however, have signs of biventricular failure. In chronic cor pulmonale especially there is a prominent parasternal heave and the pulmonary closure sound is accentuated. ST segment depression and flat or inverted T-waves are the principal ECG findings in acute cor pulmonale. In chronic cases there usually is, in addition, ECG evidence of right atrial and right ventricular hypertrophy. Chest radiographs commonly show signs of the primary pulmonary disorder, cardiac enlargement and, in chronic cor pulmonale, prominent main pulmonary arteries.

Treatment

This consists of the institution of anti-failure measures, oxygen therapy, and treatment for the underlying pulmonary disease.

Malnutrition: Kwashiorkor

Pathology

Cardiac involvement in protein–energy malnutrition has been widely reported, though more of the reports have emanated from necropsy than from clinical studies. In kwashiorkor the heart is pale, flabby and atrophic; and depletion of the epicardial layer of fat is a striking feature. On microscopy there is diffuse myocardial atrophy and necrosis, and in about 50 per cent of the cases these degenerative changes are also evident in the conductive tissues (see p. 342).

Clinical features

Four main patterns of clinical manifestations are recognized. The first consists of ECG changes only, notably diminished QRS complexes and flat or inverted T-waves. Secondly, there may be features of a low output state, with a small pulse pressure but no other signs of heart failure. Chest radiographs from patients who present this way often show a small heart. Less commonly, the cardiac involvement manifests as congestive cardiac failure. This may be precipitated in the acute phase of kwashiorkor by myocardial atrophy, anaemia, electrolyte and trace metal imbalance (particularly deficiency of potassium, calcium, magnesium, or zinc), and by intercurrent chest infection or septicaemia. More often, though, heart failure occurs during nutritional rehabilitation. At this phase an increase in serum protein and oncotic pressure, coupled with increased sodium intake in patients who receive milk supplements, may expand the plasma volume to an extent that the compromised myocardium is unable to sustain, thus causing heart failure. Sudden death caused by cardiac arrhythmias represents the fourth and most serious form of cardiac manifestation of malnutrition.

Treatment

Treatment consists of nutritional rehabilitation, administration of anti-failure drugs, careful control of fluid and salt intake, and the prompt eradication of any other source of cardiac stress. The prevention and management of protein–energy malnutrition are described elsewhere.

Beriberi

Beriberi, a nutritional disease caused by thiamine (vitamin B_1) deficiency, is still encountered with considerable frequency in parts of South-east Asia (see pp. 373–4). Two fairly distinct forms are recognized in children: infantile beriberi in young infants who are wholly dependent on breast-milk obtained from thiamine-deficient mothers; and juvenile beriberi in older children fed mainly polished rice.

The salient cardiac features of infantile ('wet') beriberi include cyanosis, dyspnoea, tachycardia and acute cardiac failure with pulmonary crepitations, hepatomegaly and generalized oedema. In juvenile ('dry') beriberi cardiac features are less prominent and may be no more than a wide pulse pressure or an accentuated pulmonary valve closure sound. Very rarely, older children may present with a severe form of beriberi ('shoshin') characterized by biventricular failure, shock and coma.

A diagnosis of beriberi may be confirmed either by a determination of erythrocyte transketolase activity or by a therapeutic trial of parenteral thiamine (25 mg i.v. or 50–100 mg i.m. stat). In patients with infantile beriberi parenteral thiamine induces diuresis and clinical improvement within 24 hours. Once this diagnostic response is observed thiamine (25 mg, i.m.) is given for three days, after which the oral preparation can be administered in a dose of 10 mg twice daily until full recovery occurs. The response in 'dry' beriberi is generally less impressive; and it is often necessary to administer other B vitamins and institute general supportive measures.

Systemic hypertension

Prevalence

Population studies of blood pressures in children from different backgrounds and countries have led to the delineation of normal blood pressure levels in various paediatric age groups. From such studies, for instance, it has been established that the systolic pressure in both sexes increases from about 92 mmHg at the age of four years to about 110 mmHg at 12 years, while the diastolic rises from about 60 to 70 mmHg.[18, 19] Two such population studies have also revealed that about 5 per cent of West African children have high blood pressures.[20]

Aetiology

Renal diseases are the most commonly identified causes in hospital-based studies. Less common causes include coarctation of the aorta, prolonged corticosteroid therapy, and neuroblastoma. However, results of population studies suggest that most children with hypertension have no discernible cause.

Clinical features

Most of the patients do not have signs that are directly referrable to the elevated blood pressure, but if the disease is longstanding and severe there may be signs of target organ damage, namely, heart failure, renal failure, or hypertensive retinopathy with visual impairment. A large and sudden increase in blood pressure, such as may occur in acute glomerulonephritis, could precipitate a hypertensive encephalopathy. The main features of this are headaches, confusion, convulsion, and coma.

Investigation

Every case must be thoroughly investigated with a view to identifying any underlying cause. The investigation should begin with tests designed to identify renal disease (see pp. 784–805). Where aortic or renal artery obstructions are suspected arrangements should be made for selective angiography.

Treatment and prognosis

The blood pressure must be lowered promptly if there is hypertensive encephalopathy or if the diastolic pressure exceeds 120 mmHg. In such an emergency, a combination of intravenous hydralazine (0.15 mg/kg six-hourly) and diazoxide (5 mg/kg when needed) is suitable, the diazoxide being given everytime the diastolic pressure equals or exceeds 120 mmHg. Where the hypertension is less critical it can be controlled gradually, using any of several oral antihypertensive agents (Table 5.5.3). The addition of a diuretic agent often enhances control of hypertension, especially in patients who have renal disease; and where a treatable cause is found the appropriate treatment should be given. The prognosis is best in such cases; and worst in cases associated with chronic bilateral renal disease.

References

1. Keith JD. Prevalence of heart disease. In: Keith JD, Rowe RD, Vlad P eds. *Heart Disease in Infancy and Childhood*. New York, Macmillan 1978.
2. Antia AU, Jaiyesimi F. Heart disease in African children and adolescents. In: Godman M ed. *Paediatric Cardiology, Vol. 4.* Edinburgh, Churchill Livingstone, 1982. pp. 656–66.
3. Bertrand E, Charles D, Ravinet L *et al.* Electrocardiograms in subjects free from cardiovascular disease. *Tropical Cardiology.* 1982; **8**: 149–56.
4. Jaiyesimi F. Electrocardiographic abnormalities during measles. *Nigerian Medical Journal.* 1976; **6**: 267–73.
5. Brockington IF, Edington GM. Adult heart disease in Western Nigeria. *American Heart Journal.* 1972; **83**: 27–40.

6. Blandon R, Johnson CM, Leandro I *et al.* Chagas' disease in children. In: Godman M. ed. *Paediatric Cardiology, Vol. 4.* Edinburgh, Churchill Livingstone, 1982. pp. 614–9.

7. Jaiyesimi F. Controversies and advances in endomyocardial fibrosis. *African Journal of Medicine and Medical Science.* 1982; **11**: 37–46.

8. Jaiyesimi F. Scalar electrocardiograms in children with endomyocardial fibrosis. *Tropical Cardiology.* 1981; **7**: 117–25.

9. Puigbo JJ, Combelas I, Acquatella H *et al.* Endomyocardial disease in South America. *Postgraduate Medical Journal.* 1983; **59**: 162–8.

10. Metras D, Coulibaly AO, Quattara K *et al.* La chirurgie cardiaque à L'Institut de Cardiologie d'Abidjan 1978–1983. *Tropical Cardiology.* 1984; Special No., 81–7.

11. Koshi G, Benjamin V, Cherian G. Rheumatic fever and rheumatic heart disease in rural South Indian children. *Bulletin of the World Health Organization.* 1981; **59**: 599–603.

12. McLaren MJ, Hawkins DM, Koornhof HJ *et al.* Epidemiology of rheumatic heart disease in black school children of Soweto, Johannesburg. *British Medical Journal.* 1975; **3**: 474–8.

13. Strasser T, Rotta J. The control of rheumatic fever and rheumatic heart disease. *WHO Chronicle.* 1973; **27**: 49–55.

14. Muna WFT, Nko'o S, Din-Dzietham R *et al.* Acute rheumatic fever and carditis: an echocardiographic study. *Tropical Cardiology.* 1985; **11**: 179–84.

15. Kassem AS, Badr-El-Din MK, Ibrahim FY *et al.* The pattern of rheumatic fever in Alexandria. *Abstracts of Pan African Congress of Cardiology*, Lagos, 1981, No. 34.

16. Sanyal SK, Thapar MK, Ahmed SH *et al.* The initial attack of acute rheumatic fever during childhood in north India. *Circulation.* 1974; **49**: 7–12.

17. Tandon R. Rheumatic fever today. In: Godman M. ed. *Paediatric Cardiology*, Vol. 4. Edinburgh, Churchill Livingstone, 1982. pp. 606–13.

18. Akinkugbe OO, Akinkugbe FM, Ayeni O *et al.* Biracial study of arterial blood pressures in the first and second decades of life. *British Medical Journal.* 1977; **1**: 1132–4.

19. Blankson J, Larbi EB, Pobee JOM *et al.* Blood pressure levels of African children. *Journal of Chronic Disease.* 1977; **30**: 735–43.

20. Muna WFT, Kingue S, Nko'o S. Left ventricular wall thickness in children with hypertension. *Tropical Cardiology.* 1986; **12**: 9–13.

CHAPTER 6

Disorders of the kidney and urinary tract

Yap Hui Kim

Disorders of the kidney and urinary tract are frequently seen by paediatricians in most urban centres. The pattern of renal disease seen in the tropics is influenced by geographical, socio-economic, as well as cultural factors such as the use of skin lightening creams and herbal medicines.[1] Infections are common and are easily overlooked in young children.

Glomerulonephritis accounts for a large proportion of the renal disorders seen in hospitalized children. Poststreptococcal nephritis is still a major problem in the tropics, in view of the high prevalence of skin infection complicating scabies.[1] Other infectious agents such as *Plasmodium malariae*,[2] *Schistosoma mansoni* and *S. haematobium*,[3] and hepatitis B,[4] also have a significant role in the pathogenesis of immune-complex nephritis.

On the other hand, the importance of renal malformations and genetic disorders is relatively unknown except in urban centres, due to the lack of sophisticated diagnostic equipment in rural regions.

This chapter will address some of the common practical problems facing the primary care practitioner.

Methods of investigation

A brief outline of easily applied techniques is given below, with more detailed discussion in subsequent sections. (See pp. 974–84, 1010–11).

Abnormal urinary elements

Cells

Small numbers of red and white blood cells as well as tubular epithelial cells are excreted in normal health. Pyuria can be most usefully defined as > 10 white blood cells/mm^3 of uncentrifuged urine using a modified Fuchs–Rosenthal counting chamber. Note that urinary tract infections should not be diagnosed on the basis of pyuria alone.

Girls may have 50–100 white blood cells per millilitre without any evidence of bacteriuria. 'Sterile' pyuria may be caused by conditions such as renal tuberculosis, schistosomiasis, fever, urethritis, calculus disease and glomerulonephritis.

Haematuria has been defined as > 6 red cells/mm^3 in uncentrifuged urine; or > 3 red cells per high power-field on sediment from spun urine. Using the Addis count on a timed urine collection, a red cell excretion rate of $> 15\,000$/m^2 of body surface area per hour has been considered abnormal.

Casts

Red cell casts reflect glomerular bleeding. Granular casts indicate renal parenchymal inflammation, but their discovery may require repeated search of centrifuged deposits.

Protein

Tests for proteinuria are best carried out on early morning urine to minimize the effects of posture and exertion. Stick testing (e.g. albustix) has the advantages of speed and simplicity. Quantitative determination is best made on a timed overnight collection, the upper limit of normal being 4 mg/h per m^2 of body surface area. Heavy proteinura is usually defined as > 40 mg/h/m^2.

Bacteriuria

The main problem is to avoid contamination of urine samples by perineal and preputial bacteria (see pp. 1010–11). The diagnosis of infection is based on the urine culture and colony count. Significant bacteriuria is defined as the presence of a pure growth of $> 100\,000$ colonies/ml of urine from a clean-catch mid-stream specimen.

In infants, suprapubic puncture is a safe and reliable means of eliminating contamination; catheterization is not justified. A useful quick screening method is to do a Gram-stain of the urine and examine it under an oil-immersion lens ($\times 1000$). The presence of at least one bacterium per field correlates closely with 100 or more bacteria per millilitre. Dip-slide urine culture is another rapid and convenient method of diagnosing an infection in the out-patient setting; urine is voided directly on to the culture medium.

Renal function

Glomerular filtration rate (GFR)

Measurement of the GFR is one of the most useful means of assessing disease severity and of monitoring the response to treatment. It is determined by measuring the volume of plasma completely cleared per minute of a substance which is filtered through the glomeruli and neither excreted nor reabsorbed by the tubules. Endogenous creatinine clearance is the most popular method but it requires an accurately timed urine collection. Measurement of isolated serum urea and creatinine concentrations is of limited value, since they can be normal in the presence of a moderately impaired GFR. Serial measurement of creatinine can be helpful in monitoring the response of severe renal disease to treatment. An estimate of the GFR can be obtained using the formula of Schwartz *et al.* where

$$\text{GFR ml/min per } 1.73 \text{ m}^2 = \frac{\text{height(cm)} \times 40}{\text{p creatinine } (\mu \text{ mol/l})}$$

Urine concentration and dilution tests

These tests of tubular function should be carried out separately. They involve fluid deprivation when studying the capacity of tubules to excrete solutes while conserving water, and a high water load when testing tubular excretion capacity. In advanced renal failure, progressive nephron destruction causes the urine specific gravity to be fixed around 1.010.

Renal structure

Imaging

Plain abdominal radiographs may reveal the renal outlines. Intravenous pyelography detects structural abnormalities. Micturating cystourethrograms will show vesico-uretic reflux and posterior urethral obstruction due to urethral valves. When available, ultrasound and isotope scanning studies give valuable information (see Urinary tract infection, below). If satisfactory visualization is not obtained, cystoscopy and retrograde pyelography may be advisable.

Renal biopsy

Percutaneous needle biopsy is of great value in the management of some cases of nephrotic syndrome and persistent glomerulonephritis. Its use should be confined to centres with facilities for processing and interpreting the material obtained.

Urinary tract infection

Urinary tract infection (UTI) is a common cause of hospitalization and morbidity in children. Its incidence varies with age and sex. Surveys of children attending out-patient services have reported frequencies of UTI ranging from 0.4 to 5 per cent.[5] In neonates, there is a male predominance with a female to male ratio of 0.4:1. There is a progressive increase in this ratio to 1.5:1 at two to six months, and 10:1 after two years of life.

In the tropics, there is an increased frequency of UTI in malnourished children, ranging from 10 to 30 per cent.[6] In some regions there also appears to be an association between bacteriuria and schistosomal infection.

Microbiology

The intestinal flora has been recognized as the major source of urinary pathogens. The majority of uncomplicated urinary tract infections are caused by *Escherichia coli*. Other organisms include *Proteus* in older boys, *Klebsiella* in neonates, and coagulase-negative *Staphylococcus* in pubertal children. Where an underlying structural abnormality is present, *Pseudomonas enterococcus* and even *Candida albicans* may be the invading organisms.

Approach to the child with urinary tract infection

The clinical significance of diagnosing the presence of UTI in an infant or a child lies in its role as a possible indicator of an underlying structural or functional abnormality, which may require specific therapy to prevent progressive renal damage. Early diagnosis and treatment is therefore of utmost importance. However, such efforts may be frustrated by the lack of specific symptoms and signs. Hence, it behoves every paediatrician to have a high index of suspicion when presented with a sick child, and especially in malnutrition which is not responding to a full protein and calorie intake.

Clinical features

The symptoms of urinary tract infection are influenced by the following factors: the age and sex of the patient, the presence of complications, the site of the infection (i.e. whether it is a cystitis or pyelonephritis), the number of previous infections, and the time interval since the last infection.

Infants tend to present with a variety of non-specific symptoms, such as fever, vomiting, diarrhoea, convulsions, neonatal jaundice, failure to thrive, feeding problems, screaming attacks, and irritability. In addition, the young child may complain only of abdominal pain. The older child may have loin pain or symptoms directly related to micturition, such as frequency, urgency, dysuria, enuresis or cloudy urine.

Careful clinical examination may identify enlarged kidneys due to hydronephrosis, with or without a palpable bladder suggesting bladder outlet obstruction. Rectal examination may reveal the shelf-like protrusion of posterior urethral valves. Underlying neurological abnormalities such as spina bifida, must be excluded.

Screening tests

Urine collection, microscopy and microbiology have already been discussed. Several chemical tests using reagent strips have been developed for the detection of bacteriuria. The nitrite test (N-Multistix, Ames) correlates with formal cultures in 80 per cent of cases, and is good for detection of Gram-negative bacteria.

Uroradiological investigations

Every child who presents with the first proven urinary tract infection has to be investigated to exclude the presence of structural abnormalities which may require surgery, or vesico-ureteric reflux where antibiotic prophylaxis is necessary. Congenital abnormalities of the urinary tract are found in about 50 per cent of these children, with a slight male preponderance, especially in infancy.[7]

An intravenous urogram (IVU) or ultrasound is required to detect upper tract abnormalities such as dilatation of the pelvicalyceal system or cortical scarring (see pp. 900–1). In addition, useful information will be obtained regarding renal size, the thickness of the renal parenchyma, width of the ureters, size and shape of the bladder and the amount of residual urine. If available, the ultrasound is a less invasive technique, and is useful especially in infants less than six months of age, because the poor concentrating ability of the kidneys at this age may result in difficulty in obtaining a good renal image on the IVU.

A micturating cystourethrogram (MCU) is also recommended in children below the age of five years, to detect the presence of vesico-ureteric reflux, and assess its severity. In boys, it is important to examine the voiding images carefully to look for posterior urethral valves. As the prevalence of vesico-ureteric reflux and the likelihood of renal scarring decreases with age, the MCU is not routinely required in the older child unless there is a history of recurrent urinary infection, hypertension, impaired renal function, or evidence of bladder outlet obstruction. The MCU is usually carried out two to four weeks after antibiotic therapy.

In recent years, radionuclide renal scans, such as diethylene-triamine-penta-acetic acid (DTPA), have been used to study differential renal function, differentiate between mechanical and functional obstruction, and follow the progression of reflux by isotope cystography. The dimercaptosuccinic acid (DMSA) scan has been found to be useful in identifying early renal parenchymal scars, not picked up by the other imaging techniques.

Management

Early and aggressive treatment of the first urinary tract infection is important, especially in infancy, in order to prevent renal scarring. The overall plan of management of urinary tract infection in childhood is outlined in Fig. 5.6.1.

Treatment of symptomatic infection

Therapeutic doses of antibiotics are usually recommended for 7 to 10 days, although infection should be eradicated within 48 hours in most instances.[8, 9] Short-course therapy, ranging from a single dose to four days, has been used in the treatment of uncomplicated urinary tract infections. However, it is often difficult to define this entity in the child presenting for the first time.

The common antibiotics used are listed in Table 5.6.1. As the most frequent organism isolated is *E. coli*, ampicillin is the drug of choice. However, resistance to this antibiotic has been on the increase, especially in recurrent infections. Co-trimoxazole is a highly effective oral antibiotic against *E. coli*, *Klebsiella pneumoniae*, and *Proteus mirabilis*. Nitrofurantoin also has a greater than 90 per cent efficacy against *E. coli*. Cephalexin is another useful alternative.

When upper tract involvement is suspected in the sick child, parenteral antibiotics, such as gentamicin, should be used. The aminoglycosides are very effective;

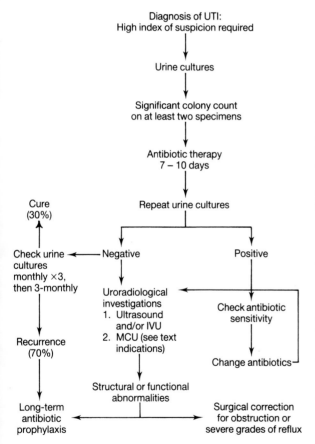

Fig. 5.6.1 Management of urinary tract infections (UTI) in children. IVU = intravenous urogram; MCU = micturating cystourethrogram.

Table 5.6.1 Common antibiotics used in the treatment of urinary tract infection in children.[a]

Antibiotic	Therapeutic dosage (mg/kg per day)	Prophylactic dosage (mg/kg per day)
Co-trimoxazole[b]		
trimethoprim	8	1–2
sulphamethoxazole	40	5–10
Trimethoprim	8	1–2
Ampicillin	50–100	
Amoxycillin	30–50	
Cephalexin	25–100	
Nitrofurantoin[b]	5–7	1–2
Nalidixic acid[b]	50	20
Gentamicin[c]	3–5	

[a] Modified from Yap HK, *Medical Progress*, 1986, 25–31.
[b] Check G6PD status of child before administration.
[c] Only given parenterally.

however, if renal impairment is present, the dosages have to be adjusted. Here, use of the third-generation cephalosporins which have less nephrotoxic side-effects, may be safer.

Within 48–72 hours after instituting the appropriate antibiotic therapy, most children should respond with resolution of clinical symptoms. A repeat urine culture should be done at this time. Persistence of infection could be due to resistant organisms, inadequate drug dosage, or the presence of an obstructed urinary system. Ideally monthly repeat urine cultures should be carried out for several months after an infection.

Recurrent urinary tract infection

Recurrent infection is seen in at least 70 per cent of children after initial treatment. A large proportion of these are related to the presence of an underlying structural defect. Local non-anatomical factors involved in recurrence include poor perineal hygiene, chronic constipation, tight-fitting clothing resulting in moisture accumulating in the perineum and colonization of the prepuce in boys.

The overall management of the child with recurrent infections must include procedures that promote bladder emptying. Correction of mechanical causes of obstruction may be required to prevent recurrences. Where functional bladder emptying is a problem, manoeuvres such as bladder training, use of autonomic drugs or intermittent catheterization may be necessary to reduce the residual urine. Children in whom no anatomical defect is demonstrated, should be encouraged to drink plenty of fluids, and empty their bladder regularly. Constipation has to be relieved.

Prophylactic antibiotic therapy

Low-dose prophylactic antibiotics are indicated in children with underlying structural defects, or vesico-ureteric reflux. Children with recurrent symptomatic infections may also benefit from prophylaxis for a six to 12 month period.

Co-trimoxazole, trimethoprim and nitrofurantoin are suitable prophylactic agents used as a single nightly dose (see Table 5.6.1). Nalidixic acid is also useful, but is usually given twice a day. A rise in intracranial pressure has been described in infants and children with its use, and it is contra-indicated in neonates.

Vesico-ureteric reflux

Vesico-ureteric reflux (VUR) is a condition in which there is a backward flow of urine from bladder to the

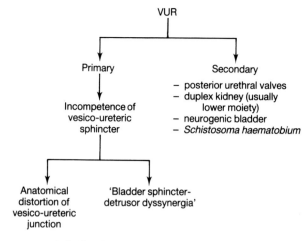

Fig. 5.6.2 Causes of vesico-ureteric reflux (VUR) in childhood.

ureter. It occurs when the pressure in the bladder exceeds that provided by the sphincteric mechanism of the vesico-ureteric junction. It is associated with atrophic pyelonephritis; scarring occurs more commonly in the upper and lower poles of the kidney, where intrarenal reflux has been seen previously on the MCU. The aetiology of VUR is depicted in Fig. 5.6.2.

It has been increasingly recognized in the majority of children with primary VUR that no anatomical defect can be identified. Owing to the dynamic interrelationships of the bladder sphincter and detrusor contractions during voiding, the pressures impinging on the immature vesico-ureteric sphincter may result in varying degrees of reflux. There is a familial occurrence of VUR, with a multifactorial mode of inheritance, the risk in first-degree relatives being 10–12 per cent.

Management

At least 30 per cent of children with VUR have associated renal scarring. If urinary infection is prevented, renal growth, even in scarred kidneys, may be normal.[8] The natural history of primary VUR is that of spontaneous resolution in about 80 per cent of undilated ureters, and 40 per cent of dilated ureters. This is related to 'maturation' of the sphincteric mechanism due to lengthening of the intramural segment of the ureter as it passes more obliquely through the bladder wall, with increasing age of the child.

There has been much controversy surrounding the management of primary VUR. Controlled trials of medical treatment versus surgical reimplantation of the ureters have yet to demonstrate an advantage of any one modality of treatment.[10] The child should be maintained on low-dose antimicrobial prophylaxis until the reflux has resolved, or he is postpubertal and infection-free for at least a year. Urine cultures should be done every three months, or whenever he is febrile or symptomatic.

Surgical treatment is recommended for those children with gross VUR associated with anatomical malformations, or if there are repeated 'breakthrough' infections. Another indication for early ureteric reimplantation is in those children living in regions where close follow-up is not possible, and compliance with antibiotic prophylaxis is doubtful.

Haematuria

Incidence and causes

Haematuria is a common urinary abnormality seen in children. The most frequent causes are listed in Table 5.6.2. In communities where infection by *S. haematobium* is endemic, screening for haematuria and proteinuria is a useful indicator of the morbidity pattern and intensity of infection. Poststreptococcal glomerulonephritis is still a frequent cause of renal disease in tropical countries, and haematuria may be the sole presenting feature. Cystitis is a common cause of haematuria. In children, culture-negative cystitis is usually due to a viral aetiology. Adenoviruses 11 and 21, influenza virus, and a papova-like virus have been implicated. Rarely, tuberculosis has to be excluded.

Sickle cell trait and sickle cell–haemoglobin C disease are associated with episodic gross urinary bleeding. It is less commonly seen in homozygote sickle cell disease. IgA nephropathy is a common cause of recurrent gross haematuria in children, especially in some Asian communities. The patient frequently develops gross haematuria concurrent with an infection, usually upper respiratory. The entity of benign recurrent haematuria, familial (inherited in an autosomal dominant fashion) and non-familial, is associated with thinning of the glomerular basement membrane, seen only on electron microscopy. In Alport's syndrome, the glomerular basement membrane is attenuated with a characteristic 'basket weave' appearance. This disease has a more progressive course, especially in boys.

Table 5.6.2   Common causes of haematuria in children.

Glomerular disorders
  Postinfectious glomerulonephritis*
  Other types of primary glomerulonephritis, e.g. membrano-
    proliferative*, membranous, Henoch–Schönlein nephritis*
  Systemic lupus erythematosus*
  IgA nephropathy (Berger's disease)*
  Hereditary nephritis (Alport's syndrome)*
  Thin membrane disease (benign recurrent haematuria,
    familial and non-familial)*
  Haemolytic-uraemic syndrome
Non-glomerular disorders
  Prerenal causes
    Coagulopathies, e.g. haemophilia*, disseminated
      intravascular coagulopathy
    Sickle cell anaemia*
    Drugs, e.g. aspirin
  Postrenal causes
    Urinary tract infection
    Trauma
    S. haematobium infection
    Cystitis
    Urethritis
    Renal tuberculosis
    Hydronephrosis
    Renal tumour, e.g. Wilms's tumour
    Bladder tumor, e.g. rhabdomyosarcoma*
    Urolithiasis*
    Hypercalciuria*
    Foreign bodies
    Renal vein thrombosis
    Polycystic kidney disease
    Arterio-venous malformations

* These disorders may present with the syndrome of recurrent gross haematuria.

Haematuria occurs in about 15 per cent of patients with hydronephrosis. With relatively minor trauma, asymptomatic gross haematuria may result. In recent years, hypercalciuria has been increasingly recognized as a cause of asymptomatic haematuria in children.

Approach to the child with haematuria

Haematuria is usually first suspected in a child who presents with 'red' or 'smoky' urine, or who had a routine dipstick test which was 'positive for blood'. Other causes of 'red' urine, such as urate crystals on the diaper, or red dyes found in certain foods, should be excluded.

Microscopic examination of a fresh specimen of urine will readily establish the presence of haematuria. Haemoglobinuria, which occurs commonly in African and Chinese children with glucose-6-phosphate dehydrogenase (G6PD) deficiency, can hence be differentiated.

Clinical assessment

The presence of dysuria, frequency, urgency and other lower urinary tract symptoms may point towards a urinary infection or foreign body. Associated loin pain may suggest urolithiasis. A concurrent or recent respiratory infection may suggest IgA disease or poststreptococcal nephritis respectively. The past medical history should focus on any bleeding diathesis and any recent drug therapy. It is important to obtain a family history or a history of trauma or bruising suggestive of a bleeding tendency.

On physical examination, features of chronic renal disease such as growth retardation and rickets, should be looked for. Hypertension and oedema may indicate an underlying glomerulonephritis. Rashes, arthritis and other features of a vasculitic process should be excluded. Abdominal masses should be palpated for. Local examination of the perineum may exclude obvious causes such as vulvitis in girls or meatal ulceration in boys.

Laboratory investigations

As the incidence of a significant glomerular lesion is low in children with asymptomatic microscopic haematuria, we have to identify those children where more invasive tests, such as renal biopsy, are likely to yield a significant abnormality. In addition, it is important to diagnose those disorders where some form of definitive therapy can be offered, such as tumours or calculus disease.

The next step in this approach would be to differentiate between the glomerular and non-glomerular causes of bleeding. Table 5.6.3 lists the initial laboratory tests which may be helpful in identifying those children who require further evaluation. The presence of red cell casts on urine microscopy indicates an underlying glomerulonephritis. It is important that this is performed on a fresh urine sample. Phase contrast microscopic examination of the urine is also useful, as the presence of dysmorphic red cells would indicate a glomerular bleed, while isomorphic cells point towards a non-glomerular aetiology. The Wright's stain has also been used to demonstrate red cell morphology, and it has the advantage of not requiring a phase contrast microscope. In regions endemic for *S. haematobium* infection, the urine should be examined for ova.

In those children where a glomerular lesion is implicated, other tests such as antinuclear antibody titre may be performed if the appropriate clinical setting is present. The indications for a renal biopsy are:

Table 5.6.3   Initial laboratory work-up in a child with haematuria.

Laboratory findings	Glomerular haematuria	Non-glomerular haematuria
1. Red cell casts on urine microscopy	+	–
2. Red cell morphology on phase contrast microscopy or Wright's stain	Dysmorphic	Isomorphic
3. Proteinuria	Significant if >1 +	– (1 + if gross haematuria)
4. Urine culture	–	+ in urine infection
5. Urine for ova (in regions endemic for schistosomiasis)	–	+ in *S. haematobium* infection
6. Urine for TB culture (in endemic regions)	–	+ in renal TB
7. Urine calcium excretion or urine calcium/ creatinine ratio	N	>0.1 mmol/kg per day or >0.7 mmol/mmol indicate hypercalciuria
8. Antistreptolysin O titre or anti-DNase B titre	+ in PSGN	–
9. C3 levels	Low in PSGN, MPGN, lupus nephritis	N
10. Sickle cell test	–	+ in sickle cell anaemia and trait
11. Urinalyses for family members	+ in familial benign haematuria	–

N = normal; PSGN = poststreptococcal nephritis; MPGN = membrano-proliferative glomerulonephritis.

significant proteinuria, development of hypertension or renal impairment, persistently low C3 levels, or family history suggestive of Alport's syndrome.

Where a non-glomerular aetiology is indicated from the initial work-up, a renal ultrasound should be done to exclude hydronephrosis and Wilms's tumour.

A micturating cystourethrogram and cystoscopy are indicated if the child has repeated episodes of gross haematuria, with red cells which are isomorphic in character.

Urinary schistosomiasis

S. haematobium infection is endemic in certain regions of the tropics (see pp. 650–6). It presents as haematuria, proteinuria, pyuria and the presence of the character-istic ova in the urine. In affected areas, a high propor-tion of patients with *S. haematobium* infection develop renal damage following obstructive lesions, and also probably by immunological mechanisms. Screening for infection in children is hence important in endemic regions, so that early chemotherapy may be instituted to achieve reversal of most of the lower tract abnormali-ties. Dipstick examination of the urine for haematuria and proteinuria is not only useful in identifying possible infection, but it also correlates with the urinary egg-count, which is an indicator of the intensity of infection.

Radiological, cystoscopic and pathological changes in the urinary tract are related to the intensity of infection. Radiographic abnormalities have been demonstrated in at least 50 per cent of infected children.[3] In the bladder, nodular filling defects are commonly seen. Calcification and fibrosis resulting in a small capacity bladder are late consequences. The ureters, especially in their lower third, may also be affected, resulting in filling defects or a beaded appearance. Fibrosis may result, with narrowing at the vesico-ureteric junction, causing stasis and dilatation of the upper ureters. Ureteral calcification, including stones, is also common. The kidney may become hydronephrotic secondary to obstruction in the lower urinary tract. Cystoscopic findings include mucosal inflammation, schistosomal tubercules and nodules, and abnormal ureteric orifices due to erosion by granulation tissue, followed by fibrosis.

Sickle cell nephropathy

Gross haematuria is one of the most dramatic manifestations of sickle cell anaemia (see pp. 828–31). It is usually secondary to microthrombi formation with infarction, following sickling in the vasa recta. Another important consequence of this is impairment of the counter-current mechanism, resulting in abnormalities in renal water conservation and hyposthenuria.[11] Renal hydrogen excretion is also impaired, with development of an incomplete form of distal tubular acidosis.

Glomerular injury has also been described in sickle cell disease, presenting clinically as the nephrotic syndrome in children. The occurrence of focal and segmental glomerulosclerosis can be explained by the hyperfiltration theory, as increase in glomerular filtra-tion rate has been demonstrated. Another histological entity seen in association with the disease is membrano-proliferative glomerulonephritis, giving rise to the possibility of immune-complex mediated injury.

Acute nephritic syndrome

Approach to the child with acute nephritic syndrome

The acute nephritic syndrome is classically diagnosed when the child presents with oedema, oliguria, haema-turia and hypertension. The various causes of this disease are listed in Table 5.6.4. Poststreptococcal nephritis is still predominant in the tropics due to the frequent occurrence of skin infections and scabies.[1] In addition, other infectious agents such as *Staphylococcus aureus* or *epidermidis* may be involved in the genesis of immune complexes. Hence, in evaluating the child with acute nephritis, it is important to ask about any previous infective episode, or any predisposing factors, such as the presence of ventriculo-atrial shunts or cardiac prostheses. The child should also be examined

Table 5.6.4 Causes of the acute nephritic syndrome.

Postinfectious glomerulonephritis
  Bacterial
    Group-A β-haemolytic streptococci
    Streptococcus viridans
    Staphylococcus aureus
    Leptospirosis
    Salmonella typhi
    Syphilis
  Viral
    Hepatitis B
    Cytomegalovirus
    Epstein–Barr virus
    Measles
    Mumps
    Varicella
  Parasitic
    Malaria
    Toxoplasmosis
    Trypanosomiasis
    Filariasis
  Rickettsial
    Scrub typhus
  Fungal
    Coccidioides immitis
Glomerulonephritis secondary to systemic disease
  Lupus nephritis
  Henoch–Schönlein nephritis
  IgA nephropathy
Drugs and toxins
  Antivenom
  Antitoxin
  Postvaccination
  Organic and inorganic mercurials
  Sulphonamides
Hereditary nephritis
Membrano-proliferative glomerulonephritis

for signs of an underlying vasculitic disorder, such as rash or arthritis.

Laboratory investigations

The initial laboratory work-up, shown in Table 5.6.5, includes microscopic examination of a fresh specimen of urine. The urinary sediment frequently contains dysmorphic red cells, white cells, and casts – granular, hyaline and more specifically, red cell casts. Proteinuria is usually present, and may reach the nephrotic range, even in poststreptococcal nephritis. The serum albumin may be reduced slightly, due to dilution and urinary protein loss. The glomerular filtration rate is usually reduced, with elevations in the blood urea nitrogen and serum creatinine.

Table 5.6.5 Initial diagnostic work-up in the child with acute nephritic syndrome.

Demonstration of glomerular injury
  Urinalysis
  Renal function assessment — blood urea nitrogen serum
           creatinine
Acute-phase reactants
  Erythrocyte sedimentation rate
  Complement levels — total haemolytic complement activity
          C3, C4
Serological studies
  Antibodies to streptococcal products
  — antistreptolysin O (ASO)
  — antideoxyribonuclease-B (ADNase-B)
  — antihyaluronidase (AHase)
  Antinuclear antibody
  Hepatitis B surface antigen
Cultures
  Throat swab
  Swab from skin lesions

The erythrocyte sedimentation rate is usually elevated, and may be very high in patients with lupus nephritis. Decreases in total haemolytic complement activity and C3 levels are seen in postinfectious nephritis, lupus nephritis, and membrano-proliferative glomerulonephritis. In addition, in lupus nephritis where there is involvement of the classical complement pathway, C4 levels are also decreased.

Anaemia is usually present, due to a haemodilutional effect. If there is evidence of associated haemolysis, then lupus nephritis must be considered (Coomb's positive haemolytic anaemia). A differential diagnosis of haemolytic–uraemic syndrome must also be excluded.

Evidence of previous streptococcal infection is provided by positive throat or skin cultures, or by serological markers. The ASO (antistreptolysin O) titre

can be detected 10 to 14 days after a streptococcal pharyngitis. However, this is often not elevated in pyoderma, due to binding of streptolysin O by lipids in the skin. The ADNase-B titre is raised in more than 95 per cent of pyoderma-associated poststreptococcal nephritis. Positive culture for group A streptococcus is found in only 20 per cent of patients.

In regions endemic for hepatitis B infection, the hepatitis B surface antigen should be looked for.

Problems

The clinical problems seen in the acute nephritic syndrome are a result of the decreased glomerular filtration rate, and consequent hypervolaemia due to salt and water retention. It is important to identify them early, to prevent significant morbidity and even mortality.

Circulatory congestion. This is manifested clinically as oedema, ascites, raised jugular venous pressure, tense enlarged liver, cardiomegaly, and (in the more severe cases), pulmonary oedema. The chest roentgenogram frequently shows an enlarged cardiac silhouette, with evidence of pulmonary vascular congestion, and occasional pleural effusion.

Hypertension with or without encephalopathy. Blood pressure elevation is often directly related to the volume expansion, and the plasma renin and aldosterone levels are usually suppressed. The child may develop severe headaches, vomiting, somnolence, confusion, seizures and coma. Visual disturbances, including occipital blindness, are occasional manifestations. Encephalopathy is most often associated with an acute rise in blood pressure; however, serious neurological manifestations have been described without severe hypertension.

Acute renal failure. Oliguria is common; however, anuria is rare and usually indicates an underlying crescentic glomerulonephritis. The child may develop symptoms of uraemia, necessitating dialysis.

Hyperkalaemia. The serum potassium levels have to be monitored closely, as hyperkalaemia is one of the major contributors to mortality.

Therapeutic interventions have to be instituted early to prevent serious sequelae. Management of these complications will be discussed in the section on acute renal failure.

Post-streptococcal glomerulonephritis

Acute post-streptococcal glomerulonephritis follows infection of the skin or throat by nephritogenic strains of group A haemolytic streptococci (see p. 515).

Epidemiology

In tropical and subtropical regions, post-streptococcal glomerulonephritis tends to occur in epidemics, and is usually associated with impetigo.[12] On the other hand, sporadic post-streptococcal nephritis is commonly associated with pharyngitis. It is more prevalent in school-age children with a mean age of onset of five to seven years. Subclinical disease is common, and has been described both in epidemics as well as in family contacts. The attack rate in families has been estimated to range from 20 to 38 per cent.

Several studies have looked into the association of post-streptococcal nephritis with HLA antigens. An increased incidence of HLA-DW5 and DR3 has been described in affected siblings, while the frequency of HLA-DRW4 is increased in unrelated patients. Further studies, however, are required to establish a possible relation to susceptibility to disease.

Pathogenesis

Several strains of streptococci have been described in association with nephritis. These 'nephritogenic' strains include types 1, 3, 4, 6, 12, 25 and 49 found in pharyngeal infections and types 2, 49, 55, 57 and 60 associated with pyoderma.

In recent years, attention has been directed at determining the nature of the nephritogenic antigen. Immunofluorescent studies have demonstrated the presence of streptococcal antigens in the glomeruli.

The common lesion seen on light microscopy is an endocapillary proliferative glomerulonephritis. Crescents occur in less than 0.5 per cent of cases. IgG and C3 are usually deposited in a granular fashion along the basement membrane in the peripheral capillary loops, and in the mesangium. Electron microscopy shows the characteristic 'humps' in the subepithelial regions.

Clinical features

Post-streptococcal glomerulonephritis usually occurs after a latent period of 10 to 14 days following a streptococcal pharyngitis, and 14 to 21 days after a skin infection. The classical features of the acute nephritic syndrome are only seen in about 40 per cent of children with post-streptococcal nephritis.[12] Oedema is the most common finding, seen in 85 per cent of children, with anasarca occurring in 36 per cent of children below six years of age. Gross haematuria, usually described as 'smoky reddish-brown urine', is present in 30 to 70 per cent. Hypertension is common, and may be the initial manifestation. Circulatory congestion is present in the majority of children, but true cardiac failure is rare. The nephrotic syndrome occurs in less than 4 per cent of patients, while a rapidly progressive course with acute renal failure occurs in less than 0.5 per cent of sporadic post-streptococcal nephritis, and is even rarer in the epidemic form.

Management

Therapy is directed at the complications of the acute nephritic syndrome. Bed rest is recommended only for those children with problems such as severe hypertension. A no-added-salt, 1–2 g sodium diet may be useful in those with oedema and hypertension. Judicious use of diuretics, especially frusemide, may be helpful.

Antibiotic therapy is useful to eradicate any concurrent streptococcal infection, but has no influence on the course of the disease. Routine penicillin prophylaxis is not recommended.

Renal biopsy should be considered in the following situations:

- 'Atypical' presentation such as anuria or nephrotic syndrome.
- Delayed 'resolution' with persistent low serum complement levels, significant hypertension, azotaemia, and macroscopic haematuria after four to six weeks.

Prognosis

The long-term prognosis in acute post-streptococcal glomerulonephritis is controversial. In large studies in children following the epidemic form of the disease,[13] the outcome after 10 to 12 years was excellent, with chronic renal failure developing in less than one per cent. Persistent abnormalities, such as haematuria and proteinuria, were found in about 10 per cent.

In general, the prognosis appears to be favourable in young children, and in the nephritis associated with epidemics.

Henoch–Schönlein nephritis

Henoch–Schönlein purpura is a generalized vasculitis characterized by a purpuric urticarial rash on the extensor surfaces of the lower legs, buttocks and occasionally, the arms. In addition, arthritis or arthralgia, gastro-intestinal manifestations such as pain, haemorrhage and intussusception, and uncommonly, neurological symptoms may be seen. It commonly occurs in children between the ages of two and

11 years, with a male to female ratio of 1.15 to 2.0. A history of preceding infection is often obtained; however, no specific aetiological agent has been identified, although β-haemolytic streptococci, mycoplasma, drugs, food allergens, insect bites and vaccinations have been variously implicated.

Renal involvement has been reported to range from 22 to 92 per cent. The most common renal manifestation is haematuria with or without proteinuria. In a review of childhood Henoch–Schönlein nephritis, Meadow *et al.* noted the presence of haematuria in almost all the patients, and this was complicated by a nephritic–nephrotic picture in about 40 per cent.[14] The renal pathology ranges from a minimal lesion to severe crescentic glomerulonephritis, with focal segmental proliferative glomerulonephritis being the most common. Immunofluorescence studies show the presence of mesangial deposits of IgA and C3, with IgG as a frequent accompaniment. In addition, skin biopsies usually reveal granular deposits of IgA along the dermal vessels of both the purpuric and unaffected skin.

In general, the prognosis in patients presenting with haematuria alone tends to be favourable. Those with nephrotic syndrome complicated by hypertension, azotaemia, oliguria, and/or hypoproteinemia are at increased risk of active renal disease, with progression to renal failure occurring in about 50 per cent. The presence of crescents on renal biopsy is also associated with a poorer outcome. It has yet to be demonstrated that any form of therapy can influence the outcome in Henoch–Schönlein nephritis. Corticosteroids appear to affect favourably soft tissue swelling, joint and gastrointestinal manifestations. The results of immunosuppressive therapy for the nephritis appear to be equivocal.

Lupus nephritis

Systemic lupus erythematosus is a multisystem disorder which is more common and severe in patients of Asian or African origin. One of the major causes of mortality is renal failure. The clinical presentation of lupus nephritis ranges from asymptomatic urinary abnormalities (such as haematuria and proteinuria) to nephrotic syndrome, and rarely rapidly progressive renal failure. Evidence of other system involvement, such as malar rash, oral ulceration, arthritis or serositis, may be present. In addition, the patient may have a positive lupus erythematosus (LE) cell preparation, elevated antinuclear antibody, or anti-double-stranded DNA antibody titres. With active renal involvement, the serum complement levels are usually low.[15]

The most common histological finding in lupus nephritis is diffuse proliferative glomerulonephritis with the classical 'wire-loop' appearance. Active lesions show the presence of mesangial and endothelial cell proliferation with karyorrhexis, fibrinoid necrosis, disruption of capillary walls, polymorphonuclear leucocytic infiltration, cellular crescents, and fibrin thrombi. With progression to chronicity, segmental sclerotic lesions and tubulo-interstitial fibrosis may be seen. Electron-dense deposits may be seen in the mesangial, subendothelial or subepithelial regions. Immunoglobulins and complement are deposited in a granular pattern. Other histological types, such as mesangial, focal proliferative and membranous glomerulonephritis, may occur, and are usually associated with a less severe clinical course.

The treatment of lupus nephritis is controversial, and is aimed at preventing renal deterioration. Steroid therapy is indicated in those with active renal disease, such as nephrotic syndrome. In addition, immunosuppressive agents such as cyclophosphamide and azathioprine, and even plasmapheresis have been advocated for patients with severe disease. The survival rate in children with lupus nephritis has been reported to range from 45 to 75 per cent at 10 years.

Nephrotic syndrome

Nephrotic syndrome is a common renal disorder seen in childhood. In the West, the incidence is approximately 2 per 100 000. However, in African and Indian children, the incidence appears to be higher, ranging from 11 to 16 per 100 000.

Definition

The nephrotic syndrome is characterized by oedema, massive proteinuria, hypoalbuminaemia, and hyperlipidaemia. Massive proteinuria can be defined as a protein excretion rate of at least 40 mg/m^2 per hour or an excretion of greater than 50 mg/kg per day or 4 + albumin on dipstick examination of the urine for at least three consecutive days.[16] The serum albumin is usually 2.5 g/dl or less. There is elevation of the plasma cholesterol early, with increase in the triglycerides when the serum albumin falls to about 1 g/dl.

In developing countries in the tropics, the clinical recognition of nephrotic syndrome may be rendered difficult by endemic problems such as nutritional oedema. The detection of ascites is useful, as it differentiates nephrotic syndrome from kwashiorkor, where ascites is a rare finding.

Approach to the child with nephrotic syndrome

Once the diagnosis of nephrotic syndrome has been established, the next step is to determine its aetiology. In children, approximately 90 per cent result from a primary glomerulopathy, with only 10 per cent being secondary to a systemic disease. The various causes are listed in Table 5.6.6. The most common is minimal change disease. Classically in this condition, the glomeruli appear normal on light microscopy, however, there is fusion of foot processes on electron microscopy. In some children, there is an association between steroid-responsive nephrotic syndrome and the presence of atopic disorders, as well as certain HLA

Table 5.6.6 Causes of nephrotic syndrome and the relative frequency in children and adults.

	Frequency (%)	
	Children*	Adults
Primary glomerulopathies		
Minimal change disease	76	16
Membrano-proliferative glomerulonephritis	8	4
Focal and segmental glomerulosclerosis	7	6
Focal and global glomerulosclerosis	2	
Mesangial proliferative glomerulonephritis	2	2
Proliferative glomerulonephritis	2	23
Membranous nephropathy	2	25
Chronic glomerulonephritis	1	
Congenital nephrotic syndrome	<1	
Secondary causes		
Infections — Malaria		
Hepatitis B		
Schistosomiasis		
Syphilis		
Vasculitis — Lupus nephritis		
Henoch–Schönlein nephritis		
Polyarteritis nodosa		
Allergies — Food allergens		
Hay fever		
Bee-stings		
Drugs and Toxins — Heavy metals (gold, mercury)		
Trimethadione		
Penicillamine		
Cardiovascular — Renal vein thrombosis		
Haemolytic–uraemic syndrome		
Sickle cell anaemia		
Malignancies — Lymphoma		
Leukaemia		
Hereditary — Alport's syndrome		

* Adapted from *Kidney International*, 1978; **13**.

markers. In the tropics, infections, such as hepatitis B, malaria and schistosomiasis, appear to be important in the genesis of the disease in children.[18] Membranous nephropathy occurs more commonly, in about 12 to 30 per cent of nephrotic children. In certain communities, heavy metal poisoning has to be considered as an aetiological factor, such as following the use of mercurial skin lightening creams.

After excluding a secondary cause for the nephrotic syndrome, it is important to differentiate minimal change disease from other causes of the primary nephrotic syndrome, as this has implications for both therapy and prognosis. In general, the criteria associated with minimal change nephrotic syndrome are an age of onset between one and six years, absence of hypertension, haematuria and renal failure, normal serum complement levels and highly selective proteinuria. In areas where quartan malarial nephropathy is prevalent, poorly selective proteinuria, as determined by a ratio of clearance of IgG to transferrin that is

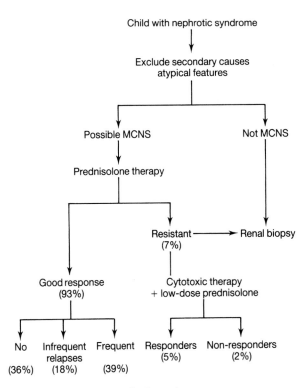

MCNS=minimal change nephrotic syndrome.

Fig. 5.6.3 Approach to the child with nephrotic syndrome. (Modified from Barnett *et al*, in *Pediatric Kidney Disease*, 1978, Little Brown & Co., Boston.)

greater than 0.1, is commonly indicative of this aetiology. The most accurate and non-invasive discriminator for minimal change disease is the response to steroid therapy.[19] It has been shown that 92 per cent of children with this form of nephrotic syndrome responded to an initial eight week course of prednisolone with complete loss of proteinuria.

Renal biopsy is indicated in those children who present with atypical features of the nephrotic syndrome and in those with frequent relapses and severe steroid toxicity where cytotoxic therapy is considered. Fig. 5.6.3 outlines the management plan for the child with nephrotic syndrome.

Management

There are two important considerations in managing a child with the nephrotic syndrome.[20] First, minimal change disease is the most common cause in childhood, and secondly, this disease has an excellent long-term prognosis, with a mortality rate of less than 4 per cent resulting from complications of the disease rather than renal failure. Hence, it is essential to look for complications and institute therapy early.

Supportive care

There is no necessity to restrict the child's activity unless he is symptomatic from massive oedema. Salt restriction has not been shown to lessen oedema, but excessive salt intake probably results in increased water retention. Fluid restriction is also unnecessary unless the child is in renal failure.

The major complication of nephrotic syndrome is hypovolaemia. These children present with symptoms of nausea, dizziness, vomiting and abdominal pain. On examination they appear sweaty with cold extremities, the pulse is weak, and rapid and orthostatic hypotension is present. Therapy consists of infusion with intravenous salt-poor albumin 0.5 to 1.0 g/kg over four to six hours, followed by intravenous frusemide 1 g/kg to induce a diuresis. It is important to monitor these children for hypertension and pulmonary oedema resulting from mobilization of the extracellular fluid.

The use of diuretics to treat oedema should be limited to those in whom there is gross oedema resulting in problems of skin breakdown, respiratory distress or hypertension. Usually only the loop diuretics, such as frusemide, are effective. However, they should be used judiciously as they may aggravate any existing hypovolaemia, and may lead to electrolyte imbalance, especially hypokalaemia.

There is an increased incidence of infections in nephrotic patients. The common pathogen found is *Strep. pneumoniae*, resulting in septicaemia, cellulitis, and peritonitis. Immunizations with live-attenuated vaccines should be avoided during the nephrotic episode, and while the child is on steroid therapy.

Another consequence of the nephrotic syndrome is a hypercoagulability state, probably related to low levels of antithrombin III. This may result in various thrombo-embolic phenomena, including renal vein thrombosis leading to an increase in proteinuria.

Initial therapy

In the child with uncomplicated nephrotic syndrome, initial therapy is with prednisolone, at 60 mg/m^2 per day (2 mg/kg per day) in divided doses, until the urine is protein free for at least three consecutive days. The patient is then given 40 mg/m^2 (1 mg/kg per day) on alternate days for four more weeks before tapering the prednisolone dose. Remission is generally seen within two weeks, with 94 per cent of the steroid-responders doing so within a month.

Treatment of relapses

Over 50 per cent of children who respond to initial steroid therapy will relapse. Recurrent proteinuria is commonly precipitated by upper respiratory infections, and may clear spontaneously once the infection resolves. 'Frequent relapsers' are defined as having two relapses within six months of initial therapy, while 'steroid dependence' is defined as recurrence of significant proteinuria as the steroid dose is being tapered. In both groups of children, a long-term alternate day maintenance dose of steroids is recommended, and is aimed at using the lowest steroid dose that will keep the child protein free. In this way, long-term adverse effects of steroid therapy, may be minimized.

Therapy with cytotoxic agents such as cyclophosphamide or chlorambucil, is generally reserved for those children with frequent relapses or who are steroid dependent, and have significant steroid toxicity. Cyclophosphamide is usually given in a dose of 2 to 2.5 mg/kg per day for eight weeks, in conjunction with a tapering steroid dose. It has been shown that the gonadal toxicity is related to a cumulative dose of greater than 250 mg/kg or exposure to the drug for more than 60 days. Leucopaenia, haemorrhagic cystitis, alopecia, oral ulceration and susceptibility to infections are other side-effects of the drug. Chlorambucil at a dose of 0.2 mg/kg per day for eight weeks has also been used. This is generally associated with fewer toxic effects; however, seizures have been a therapeutic problem.

Management of steroid-resistant nephrotic syndrome

A renal biopsy is important in this group of nephrotic children to differentiate the 7 per cent of minimal change disease which falls into this category from other causes of nephrotic syndrome such as focal and segmental glomerulosclerosis. Remission may be induced in those children with minimal change disease using cytotoxic drugs. Even in the group with focal and segmental glomerulosclerosis, 17 per cent will lose their proteinuria with prednisolone therapy, although they may develop late non-response. Another 11 per cent may respond to cytotoxic therapy.[16]

Hepatitis B-associated nephrotic syndrome

In Asian and African children where there is a high carrier rate for hepatitis B surface antigen, there is also a disproportionately high incidence of membranous nephropathy.[21] (See pp. 611–13.) The common histological types of glomerulopathies associated with hepatitis B virus are membranous nephropathy and membrano-proliferative glomerulonephritis. Demonstration of the hepatitis B surface antigen in the affected glomeruli has been variably reported. On the other hand, the hepatitis B e antigen, which is a smaller molecule, is postulated to be capable of inducing immune-complex glomerulonephritis.

The natural history of hepatitis B virus-associated membranous nephropathy is one of slow resolution over several years.

Quartan malarial nephropathy

The association between *Plasmodium malariae* infection and the nephrotic syndrome was first recognized by Atkinson in 1884. It has a peak incidence at about five years of age, and is rare in the first two years of life (see p. 662). It occurs more frequently in malnourished children. The onset of oedema is usually insidious, but most patients have fever early in the course of the illness, which may be of the characteristic quartan pattern with spikes every 72 hours.[2] Hypertension is unusual, except in those with renal impairment. There is associated hepatosplenomegaly in 50 per cent of patients, as well as anaemia.

The main histological abnormality seen is thickening of the glomerular capillary walls, which may be segmental in the early stages. With progression of the lesion, there is segmental sclerosis, tubular atrophy, and interstitial inflammation. Occasional small fibro-epithelial crescents may occur. On electron microscopic examination, the basement membrane is irregularly thickened. Immunofluorescence studies reveal IgG, IgM, and occasional C3 deposited in a granular or diffuse pattern along the capillary walls. The *P. malariae* antigen is detected in about one-third of patients.

The natural history of this disease is one of persistent proteinuria, with slow progression to renal failure. The majority of children have poorly selective proteinuria, and are resistant to steroid therapy, which is usually associated with a high risk of complications. Cyclophosphamide therapy has occasionally resulted in a remission, but its use has been complicated by adverse effects, especially serious infections. Hence it is probably indicated only in children with mild histological lesions, where remissions have been reported. Antimalarial agents have not been shown to have any benefit.

Acute renal failure

Definition

Acute renal failure denotes any abrupt and severe deterioration of renal function. There are essentially two clinical types, oliguric renal failure where the urine output is less than 1 ml/kg per hour or 300 ml/m^2 per day, and non-oliguric renal failure where the glomerular filtration rate ranges from 5 to 15 ml/min per 1.73 m^2. This degree of renal function is insufficient to handle the increased load of metabolic end-products resulting from the hypercatabolic state.

Causes

The cause of renal failure in childhood varies in different centres, depending not only on the diseases endemic in that region, but also on the patterns of referral. In Europe and North America, renal failure is predominantly a consequence of renal hypoperfusion, haemolytic–uraemic syndrome, and congenital urinary tract anomalies. In the tropics, infections are an important cause of renal failure in childhood. *Plasmodium falciparum* malaria is endemic in some regions in Africa and South–East Asia, and infection has been associated with intravascular haemolysis and renal failure, a condition which has been termed 'blackwater fever'.[22] (See p. 671.) G6PD deficiency may also be a cause of renal failure consequent upon intravascular haemolysis triggered by drugs such as antimalarials, or infections such as typhoid fever.

The haemolytic–uraemic syndrome is an important cause of childhood renal failure in South America and

Table 5.6.7 Causes of acute renal failure in childhood.

Prerenal
  Functional renal failure
    Severe volume depletion
    Shock
    Sepsis
    Severe cardiac failure
    Intravascular haemolysis
    Trauma
  Nephrotoxins
    Antibiotics, e.g. aminoglycosides
    Heavy metals, e.g. mercury, lead
    Toxins, e.g. shake venom
  Hepato-renal syndrome
Renal
  Glomerulonephritis
    Postinfectious glomerulonephritis
    Lupus nephritis
    Henoch–Schönlein nephritis
    Wegener's granulomatosis
  Vascular and thrombotic
    Haemolytic–uraemic syndrome
    Renal vein thrombosis
  Interstitial disease
    Allergic, postinfectious, interstitial nephritis
    Papillary necrosis
    Fulminating pyelonephritis
Postrenal
  Obstructive uropathy
    Posterior urethral valve
    Neurogenic/non-neurogenic bladder
  Uric acid crystallization
    Treatment of myelo-proliferative disorders

South India, where it usually follows bacillary dysentery.[23] In addition, severe dehydration due to infectious diarrhoea is still a significant prerenal factor leading to acute tubular necrosis. Snake venom poisoning also accounts for some cases of renal failure in the tropics.

The aetiology of acute renal failure can be conveniently approached by considering the various disorders under prerenal, renal, and postrenal causes (see Table 5.6.7).

Approach to the child with acute renal failure

The symptoms and signs of acute renal failure are non-specific, and are usually related to the accumulation of metabolic end-products. The child may present with anorexia, nausea, vomiting, diarrhoea, drowsiness, convulsions and coma. Renal failure should be suspected when there is accompanying oliguria or anuria, hyperventilation due to acidosis, or hypertension.

In most instances, careful clinical evaluation will suggest the underlying cause. The initial laboratory work-up should include a complete blood count and peripheral smear to look for fragmented red cells and thrombocytopaenia which are present in the haemolytic–uraemic syndrome. Urinalysis and cultures should be done.

It is important to recognize the prerenal causes early so that definitive therapy can be instituted to prevent progression to established acute renal failure. The postrenal causes must also be excluded, as surgical intervention in the obstructive uropathies may be necessary for maximum recovery of renal function.

Differentiation between prerenal, renal and postrenal causes

Urinary sediment. Microscopic examination of the urinary sediment may be helpful in elucidating the underlying aetiology. The presence of dysmorphic red cells and red cell casts would suggest a glomerulonephritis. Eosinophils may be seen in acute interstitial nephritis, especially that secondary to drugs. Renal tubular epithelial cells, cell debris, and tubular cell casts may be present in acute tubular necrosis. Specific crystals, e.g. of uric acid can be identified if tubular obstruction due to crystal deposition is suspected.

Diagnostic indices. Tests which are useful in differentiating reversible prerenal from established acute renal failure include urine osmolality, urine to plasma osmolality ratio, urine to plasma urea ratio, urine to plasma creatinine ratio, urinary sodium concentration, fractional excretion of sodium (FeNa), and renal failure index (RFI). Both these indices can be calculated readily from plasma (P) and urine (U) measurements of sodium (Na) and creatinine (Cr).

$$RFI = U_{Na}/U_{Cr} \times P_{Cr}$$

$$FeNa = U_{Na}/U_{Cr} \times P_{Cr}/P_{Na} \times 100$$

Table 5.6.8 outlines the use of these indices in the evaluation of the child with renal failure.

Therapeutic trial of volume expansion. If the child is not oedematous and an obstructive cause has been excluded, a fluid challenge is given to determine if the oliguria is prerenal in origin: 20 ml/kg of normal saline or plasma (if the patient is in shock) is infused intravenously over half to one hour. If oliguria still persists after extracellular volume has been restored, intravenous frusemide (2 mg/kg) is administered. Mannitol (0.5 mg/kg) may be given as a 20–30 minute infusion; however, failure to respond with a diuresis may result in a hyperosmolar state with its attendant neurological and cardiovascular complications. If no increase in urine output occurs following these

Table 5.6.8 Diagnostic indices in acute renal failure (RF).

	Prerenal		Established RF	
1. Urine osmolality (mOsm/kg water)	>500		<350	
2. Urine sodium (mEq/l)	<20		>40	
3. U/P urea	>8		<3	
4. U/P osmolality	>1.15		<1.1	
5. U/P creatinine	>40		<20	
6. RFI	<1	(<3*)	>1	(>3*)
7. FeNa	<1	(<2.5*)	>1	(>2.5*)

Data from Miller TR *et al.*, *Annals of Internal medicine*, 1978; **89**: 47–50. U = urine, P = plasma, RFI = renal failure index, FeNa = fractional excretion of sodium.
* Criteria used in neonates (adapted from *Pediatrics*; **65**: 57 © 1980).

manoeuvres, then established acute renal failure has to be suspected, and fluid administration correspondingly reduced.

Detection of postrenal causes. The clinical examination is important to exclude enlargement of the kidneys or a palpable bladder. Rectal examination may reveal the presence of posterior urethral valves. In renal failure, the most useful tests to demonstrate the cause of obstruction are ultrasonography and MCU. The IVU is generally contra-indicated because of the osmotic load of the contrast agents. In addition, there is poor visualization of the kidneys in renal failure.

Role of renal biopsy. Renal biopsy should be considered where a rapidly progressive form of glomerulonephritis or allergic interstitial nephritis is suspected from the clinical evaluation and examination of the urinary sediment. Diagnosis is important as some type of definitive therapy may be offered, such as plasmapheresis for Goodpasture's syndrome. A renal ultrasound should be done before biopsy to establish that the kidney is normal in size or enlarged, rather than shrunken due to chronic disease.

Management

Prompt recognition of prerenal failure and its treatment with volume expanders may prevent the development of established renal failure. Once renal failure is established, there is no treatment modality that will enhance recovery of renal function. The goal of therapy in this instance is to maintain normal body composition while awaiting spontaneous improvement. The oliguric phase usually lasts from 5 to 11 days.

Management of the problems encountered is now discussed.

Fluid overload. Daily fluid intake is restricted to insensible losses, calculated either on the basis of surface area at 300 ml/m^2, or on the basis of caloric intake at 30 ml/100 cal, plus any additional losses such as urinary output, faecal losses or sweating in the tropics. The aim is to achieve a loss of 0.5 to 1.0 per cent of the body weight daily.

Increased nitrogenous waste products. Optimal caloric and protein intake will aid in decreasing catabolism, hence alleviating the uraemic state. A protein intake of 1 g/kg per day is recommended. Because of the fluid restriction, the caloric intake may be inadequate unless high caloric feeds such as Polycose are included. For those patients who are unable to take orally, total parenteral nutrition should be considered.

Hyponatraemia. This is usually dilutional due to volume expansion. Hence both salt and fluid restriction are necessary to prevent complications such as hypertension.

Hyperkalaemia. Hyperkalaemia must be treated aggressively to prevent sudden death. If the serum potassium is greater than 7 mol/l, or ECG changes, or arrhythmias are present, the following intravenous medications should be given immediately – 2.5 mol/kg of sodium bicarbonate, 0.5 ml/kg of 10 per cent calcium gluconate over 5 to 10 minutes, and 0.5 g/kg of 50 per cent glucose. If the hyperkalaemia persists, insulin at a dose of 1 unit for every 5 g of glucose may be given, and preparation for dialysis should be undertaken. If the serum potassium is 5.5–7 mol/l, an ion-exchange resin such as Kayexylate 1 g/kg may be used.

Hypocalcaemia. Calcium supplementation at 50–100 mg/kg per day may be required to treat hypocalcaemic tetany. In addition, the serum phosphorus levels may have to be controlled with phosphate binders.

Hypertension. Diuretics, such as frusemide (2–5 mg/kg per dose), may be useful in acute nephritis when the child is still able to respond with a diuresis. For the treatment of hypertensive crisis, in addition to diuretics, drugs such as diazoxide (5 mg/kg per dose), sodium nitroprusside (0.5–0.8 g/kg per min infusion) or hydralazine (0.15–0.5 mg/kg per dose) may be given intravenously for immediate action. Recently, sublingual nifedipine has been found to be useful in the management of hypertensive emergencies without the potential problem of hypotension seen with diazoxide. For long-term control of blood pressure, agents such as propranolol, hydralazine, methyldopa or captopril may be used.

Acidosis. Sodium bicarbonate at 1–3 mol/kg per dose may be used to correct the acidosis. However, this will increase the sodium load to the body, and dialysis may be required if treatment is difficult.

Convulsions. In acute renal failure, this may be due to

several causes such as hypertensive encephalopathy, hypocalcaemia, hyponatraemia, severe azotaemia, and intracranial haemorrhage especially in neonates. Anticonvulsants may be used, but correction of any underlying metabolic derangement is essential.

Anaemia. Severe anaemia must be treated cautiously with transfusions, in view of the volume-expanded state. In neonates, exchange transfusion may be performed.

Infection. This is an important cause of death in acute renal failure. Nephrotoxic antibiotics, such as aminoglycosides, should be avoided if possible, but if their use is imperative, then dosage adjustments are necessary, with proper monitoring of the serum antibiotic levels.

Indications for dialysis

When conservative measures fail, dialysis should be considered. In children, peritoneal dialysis is generally the most convenient and technically easiest form of dialysis to perform.[26] The indications for dialysis include severe hyperkalaemia, unresponsive to medical treatment, intractable acidosis, severe fluid overload with uncontrolled hypertension or congestive cardiac failure, progressive uraemia, and deterioration of the general condition. There is evidence that early and judicious use of dialysis, before deterioration of the patient, has been effective in decreasing mortality due to acute renal failure.

Haemolytic–uraemic syndrome

The haemolytic–uraemic syndrome is characterized by a triad of microangiopathic haemolytic anaemia, thrombocytopenia, and acute renal failure. It is a well-documented cause of acute renal failure in childhood in certain regions.[23] It is often preceded by gastroenteritis and upper respiratory infection. Infectious agents linked to the disease include *Shigella, Salmonella*, Coxsackie, echoviruses and adenoviruses. A familial tendency has also been reported, and both autosomal dominant and recessive modes of inheritance have been suggested.

Glomerular capillary endothelial cell injury is the most common finding on histology. The capillary lumen is markedly reduced by swollen and detached endothelial cells, fibrin thrombi and platelets. Patchy or diffuse cortical necrosis may be seen. There may be thrombosis of the small arterioles.

Therapy is mainly supportive, with early dialysis preferred. The use of heparin, streptokinase or antiplatelet agents does not appear to have any additional benefit.[27] Poor prognostic factors include a non-diarrhoeal prodrome, familial involvement, progressive reduction in renal function, persistent or recurrent thrombocytopaenia, severe neurological involvement, and histological evidence of predominant arteriolar changes or acute diffuse cortical necrosis. Mildly affected patients tend to do well, but at least 20 per cent of those with severe disease may develop long-term sequelae, such as hypertension, proteinuria, and progressive renal failure.

Chronic renal failure

Chronic renal failure is usually diagnosed when a raised serum creatinine level is found either incidentally in the work-up of a child with some general problem such as short stature or pallor, or in the course of an evaluation of symptomatology related to the urinary tract. The symptom complex of uraemia is generally absent until the glomerular filtration rate has decreased to less than 15 ml/min per 1.73 m^2, as the remnant nephrons are capable of regulating body homoeostasis through adaptive alterations in tubular function.

Approach to the child with chronic renal failure

When an elevation of the serum creatinine is detected, the first step is to determine if the reduction in renal function is acute or chronic in origin.

Features of chronicity

A history of polyuria, polydipsia and enuresis occurring after bladder control has been attained, may suggest a concentrating defect seen in chronic renal dysfunction. The past history may reveal a previous acute glomerulonephritis, surgical procedures for a congenital urinary tract abnormality or urinary tract infection in infancy. Enquiry into the family history is also important, in order to exclude hereditary disorders such as Alport's syndrome, cystinosis, juvenile nephronophthisis and infantile polycystic disease of the kidney, which lead to chronic renal failure.

On physical examination, assessment of growth is important, as those children with long-standing renal impairment, such as that seen with congenital maldevelopment of the urinary tract, usually show evidence of retarded growth. In contrast, those with acquired lesions (such as glomerulonephritis) which tend to occur later in childhood, have lesser disturbance in growth. Other features which suggest chronicity include a sallow discoloration, pallor, dystrophic finger nails, chronic hypertensive retinopathy, and evidence of rickets.

Establish the cause

Chronic glomerulopathies constitute the most common cause of chronic renal failure in childhood, especially in the older child.[28] Renal dysplasia, chronic pyelo-nephritis associated with severe vesico-ureteric reflux, and obstructive uropathies such as posterior urethral valves in boys, are significant causes of renal failure, which usually develops within 5 to 15 years of diagnosis. Renal dysplasia is often suggested by the concomitant presence of other congenital abnormalities, such as imperforate anus, congenital heart disease, and spina bifida.

Examination of the urine may be helpful in indicating an underlying glomerulonephritis if red cell casts are present. Some proteinuria is invariably present in chronic renal disease, with the possible exception of juvenile nephronophthisis in its early stages. However, heavy proteinuria is often seen in glomerulopathies or reflux nephropathy.

The renal size frequently gives an important clue to the underlying aetiology (see Fig. 5.6.4). A plain abdominal X-ray or ultrasound of the kidneys are useful non-invasive tests, and they have the additional advantage of not being dependent on renal function, as is required by the IVU. Large kidneys suggest an underlying obstruction, polycystic disease (usually the autosomal recessive variety in children), or cystic dysplasia. Small and unequal-sized kidneys with irregular contour are seen in severe vesico-ureteric reflux with scarring. Glomerulopathies and tubulo-interstitial disease generally result in symmetrically contracted kidneys.

Management

The aims in the management of the child with chronic renal failure are to:

- improve or stabilize renal function, promoting the maintenance of normal body homoeostasis;
- promote as much growth in the child as possible;
- permit the child to lead as active and normal a life as possible.

Fig. 5.6.5 outlines the management plan in these children.

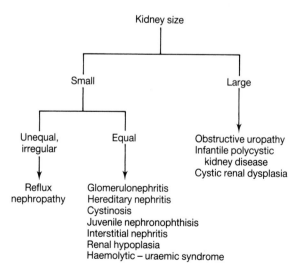

Fig. 5.6.4 Classification of causes of chronic renal failure according to renal size.

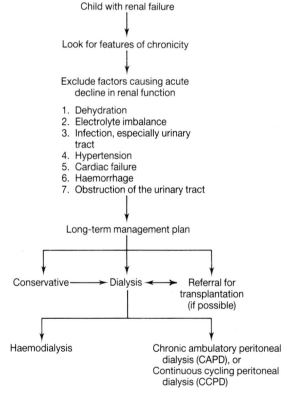

Fig. 5.6.5 Outline of management of the child with chronic renal failure.

Factors causing deterioration in renal function

Many children with chronic renal failure remain at a stable level of decreased glomerular filtration rate for many years. Hence, when there is a deterioration in renal function, it is imperative to exclude any acute reversible factors.

Children with tubular disorders, either primary or associated with obstruction, may have problems of 'salt-wasting', acidosis or concentration defects. They may develop dehydration, and electrolyte and acid–base imbalance, especially during episodes of urinary tract infections or intercurrent illnesses. Hypertension may be a problem in some forms of glomerulonephritis, reno-vascular disease, or reflux nephropathy, and may lead to further deterioration in renal function if not controlled. Other acute factors include cardiac failure and haemorrhage.

Persistent obstruction of the urinary tract must be excluded, as surgical correction may be necessary. Following the ultrasonographic evaluation, an MCU may be required to assess the bladder outlet, bladder morphology, and the presence of any vesico-ureteric reflux.

Conservative management

In many developing countries, the resources for dialytic therapy for children with end-stage renal disease are limited. Therefore, conservative measures are of increased importance.

Nutrition Anorexia is often seen in children with chronic renal failure, thus making it difficult to provide sufficient calories and protein for growth. Protein restriction of 1.5–2 g/kg body weight is recommended when the glomerular filtration rate is below 25 ml/min per 1.73 m^2. This should be in the form of proteins with high biological value, such as egg, milk and fish. Further restriction may be necessary when the renal function decreases to less than 10 per cent of normal, to minimize the uraemic symptoms. These children usually require caloric supplementation to achieve an intake close to the recommended daily allowance, and to prevent protein catabolism.

Acidosis Children with chronic renal failure usually develop acidosis, as the remnant nephrons are unable to excrete the daily acid load of 2–3 mol/kg per day. In addition, there may be a renal tubular defect resulting in bicarbonaturia. Hence, they require 2–3 mol/kg per day of sodium bicarbonate or sodium citrate (Shohl's solution) to maintain a normal acid–base status.

Fluid and electrolytes Fluid restriction is usually unnecessary and may be detrimental, unless there is evidence of oedema, as may be seen in the child with end-stage disease. The thirst mechanism is a good regulator of the amount of fluid intake in most instances. Sodium intake may be limited to 40–90 mol/day, that is 'no added salt', so as to avoid the development of hypertension. Where renal sodium loss is a problem, a free sodium intake, or even supplementary salt tablets may be required. Potassium intake has to be adjusted according to the serum potassium levels, as both hyperkalaemia and hypokalaemia may be problems, depending on the type of renal lesion.

Renal osteodystrophy One of the major problems of chronic renal failure is a disturbance in calcium and vitamin D metabolism resulting in defective bone mineralization. Biochemically, this is reflected by the presence of hyperphosphataemia, hypocalcaemia, and elevated serum alkaline phosphatase levels. Control of hyperphosphataemia is achieved both by dietary restriction and the use of oral phosphate binders, such as aluminium hydroxide or calcium carbonate, taken with meals. Aluminium hydroxide should be used with caution due to the danger of aluminium bone disease and aluminium encephalopathy. Once control of the serum phosphate level is achieved, calcium supplementation may be required, and use of a vitamin D metabolite, such as dihydrotachysterol (dose 15 μg/kg per day) or calcitriol (dose 14 ng/kg per day), to improve intestinal calcium absorption is usually necessary. The serum calcium and phosphate levels, and the urinary calcium–creatinine ratio should be monitored closely to avoid problems of metastatic calcification.

Dialysis and transplantation

Careful medical management of children with chronic renal failure can prevent rapid deterioration of the already compromised kidney function, and also lead to an improvement in the quality of life. However, ultimately, dialysis or transplantation is required to maintain life. In developed countries, haemodialysis and more recently, chronic peritoneal dialysis are acceptable modalities for end-stage care.[26] Rehabilitation following successful renal transplantation is also possible in these children. Unfortunately, in many developing countries, such tertiary medical care is extremely costly and, especially where there are more pressing problems in other areas of primary health, these facilities will at present be limited. The paediatrician's role in these regions will hence include counselling of parents to prepare them for the management of the dying child, and also genetic advice where indicated.

Miscellaneous problems

Congenital abnormalities of the urinary tract

Developmental abnormalities of the kidney can affect either the renal parenchyma or the collecting system. Disordered renal morphogenesis can result in renal dysplasia where there is abnormal differentiation with formation of primitive glomeruli and tubules with associated cystic dilatation and cartilaginous metaplasia, or renal hypoplasia or agenesis where there is diminution in renal tissue mass. Abnormal development of the collecting system may result in such conditions as hydronephrosis, partial or complete duplications, and posterior urethral valves.

To the paediatrician, the clinical significance of congenital renal abnormalities is that many of these disorders are severe, and associated with progressive renal failure. Early detection and surgical intervention in the various forms of obstructive uropathies may minimize the renal damage (see pp. 900–1); this is especially important in infancy and early childhood where the potential for renal growth is greatest.

Renal tubular acidosis

Renal tubular acidosis (RTA) is a syndrome characterized by hyperchloraemic acidosis associated with an inappropriately alkaline urine, in the presence of normal or slightly reduced glomerular function. Four types of RTA have been described, all of which occur in childhood.[29]

Type 1 or classic distal RTA

In this form of RTA a defect in the distal tubule is present, resulting in an inability to generate a hydrogen ion gradient between the tubular fluid and blood. The urine pH remains high (>6.2), even in the face of severe metabolic acidosis. In infants and children, this is commonly associated with bicarbonaturia, and has been termed type 3 RTA. Failure to thrive is the most common presentation. Other manifestations include dehydration, vomiting, polyuria, and constipation. Acute hypokalaemic paralysis may occur in 25 per cent of children. Hypercalciuria and nephrocalcinosis are frequent complications.

Type 1 RTA may be inherited as an autosomal dominant disorder, and can be associated with other genetic disorders like Ehlers–Danlos syndrome and Marfan's syndrome. It may occur secondary to nephro-calcinosis, drugs such as amphotericin-B, autoimmune disorders, sickle cell nephropathy, and in the transplant kidney.

Diagnosis is confirmed by an ammonium chloride loading test, where there is an inability to acidify the urine (<6.2) with decreased excretion of titratable acid and ammonium ion. Therapy consists of sodium bicarbonate or citrate 1–3 mol/kg per day.

Type 2 or proximal RTA

This form of RTA is characterized by a defect in proximal tubular reabsorption of bicarbonate. It may occur as an isolated defect, but is commonly associated with other transport defects as seen in Fanconi's syndrome, such as glycosuria, aminoaciduria, phosphaturia, and uricosuria. In infants, it may occur as a transient disorder, or may be associated with metabolic diseases such as cystinosis.

These patients are able to acidify the urine to less than pH 5.5. Growth retardation and rickets are common findings. Nephrocalcinosis is absent. Urinary potassium loss is a problem. Children with this type of RTA require large doses of bicarbonate, 10–15 mol/kg per day. In addition, potassium supplementation is necessary. Hypophosphataemia and rickets are treated with Vitamin D analogues and phosphate solutions.

Type 4 or hyperkalaemic RTA

Type 4 RTA is the most common type of RTA in children, and is characterized by hyperchloraemic acidosis, hyperkalaemia and the ability to acidify the urine to less than pH 5.5. It is due to a deficiency of aldosterone or decreased tubular responsiveness to the hormone, and has been classified into five subtypes on the basis of the pathophysiological mechanism. Hyperkalaemic RTA may occur in association with obstructive uropathy. Treatment consists of alkali therapy, 4–20 mol/kg per day, and diuretics for the hyperkalaemia.

Urolithiasis

Calculus disease of the urinary tract in children is common in some regions of the tropics and subtropics. In Pakistan, northern Thailand and in the Nile Delta region of Egypt, there is a high frequency of bladder stones, especially in boys of preschool age.[30] The disease tends to occur in rural regions, and is associated with malnutrition and recurrent episodes of gastroenteritis.

Renal stone formation in childhood is often due to metabolic disorders, such as distal renal tubular acidosis, cystinuria, or primary hyperoxaluria. Idiopathic hypercalciuria is the most common metabolic abnormality encountered. Other factors include a high oxalate diet seen in some regions, enteric diseases, total parenteral nutrition, primary hyperparathyroidism, infantile hypercalcaemia, vitamin D intoxication, obstructive uropathies with or without infection, and prolonged immobilization.

Common presenting symptoms of renal stones are gross haematuria, abdominal or loin pain and renal colic. Occasionally, calculi are detected radiologically in the investigation of a child with urinary tract infection. Disturbances of micturition, such as frequency, urgency and dysuria, occur in patients with bladder stones. Investigations should be aimed not only at the detection of urological complications, but also at determining the underlying aetiology, so that the risk of recurrence may be minimized.

Medical management of renal stones consists of encouraging a high fluid intake, especially important in the hot climate of the tropics. Thiazide diuretics have been used in the treatment of renal hypercalciuria. In addition, potassium citrate has been found to be useful in increasing the urinary citrate and pH, thus inhibiting crystallization of calcium oxalate and phosphate which leads to stone formation.

References

1. Hendrickse RG. Epidemiology and prevention of kidney disease in Africa. *Transactions of the Royal Society of Tropical Medicine and Hygiene*. 1980; **74**: 8–16.
2. Hendrickse RG, Adeniyi A. Quartan malarial nephrotic syndrome in children. *Kidney International*. 1979; **16**: 64–74.
3. Oyediran ABOO. Renal disease due to schistosomiasis of the lower urinary tract. *Kidney International*. 1979; **16**: 15–22.
4. Hsu HC, Lin GH, Chang MH *et al*. Association of hepatitis B surface (HBs) antigenemia and membranous nephropathy in children in Taiwan. *Clinical Nephrology*. 1983; **20**: 121–9.
5. Marr TS, Traisman HS. Detection of bacteriuria in paediatric out-patients. *American Diseases of Children*. 1975; **129**: 940–3.
6. Morton RE, Lawande R. II. Frequency and clinical features of urinary tract infection in paediatric out-patients in Nigeria. *Annals of Tropical Paediatrics*. 1982; **2**: 113–17.
7. Smellie JM, Normand ICS. Urinary tract infection. Clinical aspects. In: Williams DI, Johnson JH eds. *Paediatric Urology*. London, Butterworths, 1982. pp. 95–111.
8. Smellie JM, Normand ICS. Urinary infections in children 1985. *Postgraduate Medical Journal*. 1985; **61**: 895–905.
9. Yap HK. Treatment of urinary tract infections in children. *Medical Progress*. 1986. pp. 25–31.
10. Birmingham Reflux Study Group. Prospective trial of operative versus non-operative treatment of severe vesicoureteric reflux: two years' observation in 96 children. *British Medical Journal*. 1983; **287**: 171–4.
11. De Jong PE, van Eps LWS. Sickle cell nephropathy: new insights into its pathophysiology. *Kidney International*. 1985; **27**: 711–17.
12. Rodriguez-Iturbe B. Epidemic poststreptococcal glomerulonephritis. *Kidney International*. 1984; **25**: 129–36.
13. Potter EV, Lipschultz SA, Abidh S *et al*. Twelve to seventeen-year follow-up of patients with post-streptococcal acute glomerulonephritis in Trinidad. *New England Journal of Medicine*. 1982; **307**: 725–9.
14. Meadow SR, Glasgow EF, White RHR *et al*. Schönlein–Henoch nephritis. *Quarterly Journal of Medicine*. 1972; **41**: 241–58.
15. Tan EM, Cohen AS, Fries JF *et al*. The 1982 revised criteria for the classification of systemic lupus erythematosus. *Arthritis and Rheumatism*. 1982; **25**: 1271–7.
16. McEnery PT, Strife CF. Nephrotic syndrome in childhood: management and treatment in patients with minimal change disease, mesangial proliferation, or focal glomerulosclerosis. *Pediatric Clinics of North America*. 1982; **89**: 875–94.
17. International study of kidney disease in children. *Kidney International*. 1978; **13**: 159–65.
18. Abdurrahman MB. The role of infectious agents in the aetiology and pathogenesis of childhood nephrotic syndrome in Africa. *Journal of Infectious Diseases*. 1984; **8**: 100–9.
19. International Study of Kidney Disease in Children: the primary nephrotic syndrome in children. Identification of patients with minimal change nephrotic syndrome from initial response to prednisone. *Journal of Pediatrics*. 1981; **98**: 561–4.
20. Barnett HL, Schoeneman M, Bernstein J *et al*. Minimal change nephrotic syndrome. In: Edelmann CM Jr ed. *Pediatric Kidney Disease*. Boston, Little, Brown and Company, 1978. pp. 704.
21. Seggie J, Nathoo K, Davies PG. Association of hepatitis B (HBs) antigenaemia and membranous glomerulonephritis in Zimbabwean children. *Nephron*. 1984; **38**: 115–19.
22. Adu D, Anim-Addo Y, Foli AK *et al*. Acute renal failure in tropical Africa. *British Medical Journal*. 1976; **1**: 890–2.
23. Raghupathy P, Date A, Shastry JCM *et al*. Acute renal failure in south Indian children: a ten-year experience. *Annals of Tropical Paediatrics*. 1981; **1**: 39–44.
24. Miller TR, Anderson RJ, Linas SL *et al*. Urinary diagnostic indices in acute renal failure. A prospective study. *Annals of Internal Medicine*. 1978; **89**: 47–50.
25. Mathew OP, Jones AS, James E *et al*. Neonatal renal

failure. Usefulness of diagnostic indices. *Pediatrics*. 1980; **65**: 57–60.

26. Fine RN. Peritoneal dialysis update. *Journal of Pediatrics*. 1982; **100**: 1–7.

27. Fong JSC, de Chadarevian JP, Kaplan BS. Hemolytic–uremic syndrome. Current concepts and management. *Pediatric Clinics of North America*. 1982; **29**: 835–56.

28. Potter DE, Holliday MA, Piel CF *et al.* Treatment of end-stage renal disease in children – a 15 year experience.

Kidney International. 1980; **18**: 103–9.

29. McSherry E. Renal tubular acidosis in childhood. *Kidney International*. 1981; **20**: 799–809.

30. Naqvi SA, Risvi SA, Shahjehan S. Bladder stone disease in children; clinical studies. *Journal of the Pakistan Medical Association*. 1984; **34**: 94–101.

31. Taylor CM and Chapman S (eds.) *Handbook of Renal Investigations in Children*. Guildford, Butterworths, 1989; pp. 25–34.

CHAPTER 7

Endocrine and metabolic disorders

Wong Hock Boon

Endocrine disorders in the tropics are similar to those occurring in temperate lands, except that some diseases are more commonly seen in particular ethnic groups. The most common endocrine gland affected by disease is the thyroid. Diabetes mellitus, hypoparathyroidism, disorders of the sex organs, congenital adrenal hyperplasia and pituitary diseases, amongst others, are also encountered.

Thyroid disorders

Hypothyroidism

Two groups of causes are important: endemic goitre and congenital hypothyroidism. In recent years the term iodine deficiency disorders (IDD) has been adopted to include goitre, endemic cretinism and hypothyroidism so as to emphasize the very serious effect that iodine deficiency has on the development and function of the nervous system.[11]

Endemic goitre

Most cases of endemic goitre arise in areas lacking in iodine, notably those far from the sea, such as in the Himalayan mountains, South-east Asian countries, the South American Andes, New Guinea, the Philippines and Indonesia.[1] The thyroid gland compensates for a lack of iodine by increased activity producing hyperplastic tissue which may culminate in goitres of immense size (Fig. 5.7.1). Lack of adequate compensation may result in hypothyroidism. However, in some areas, the genes for dyshormonogenetic hypothyroidism may also be present so that deaf-mutism may be encountered. Endemic goitre potentially can take a large toll, and 30 years ago it was estimated that 200 million people were affected. Yet its prevention is relatively simple and cost-effective – addition of iodine to salt or injection of iodized oil.

Congenital hypothyroidism

The incidence of congenital hypothyroidism or cretinism varies in different ethnic groups but is approximately 1 in 3000 to 1 in 6000 livebirths. In the past it usually had a poor prognosis because of delays in diagnosis. As a result, screening for hypothyroidism in the neonatal period has been established. This is usually carried out by estimating thyroid-stimulating hormone (TSH) and T_4 in cord blood or T_4 in blood on filter paper in the first two weeks of life. Estimation of these hormones is fairly expensive. Low levels sometimes give rise to a false positive diagnosis so that recall hormone estimations add further to the cost. Yet, in communities which can afford it, this screening strategy is now routine and follow-up studies have shown that

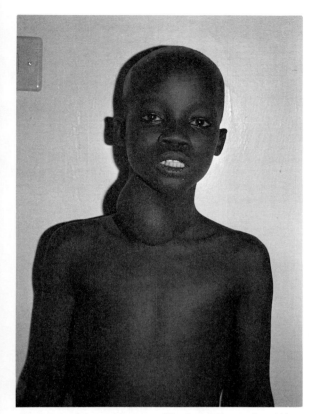

Fig. 5.7.1 A large adenoma of the thyroid in a euthyroid boy.

Table 5.7.1 Neonatal hypothyroid index.

Clinical features		Scores
Typical facies		3
Dry skin		1.5
Open posterior fontanelle (>0.5 cm)		1.5
Feeding problems		1
Constipation		1
Inactivity		1
Hypotonia		1
Umbilical hernia	(>0.5 cm)	1
Enlarged tongue		1
Skin mottling		1
Total		13

babies diagnosed and treated so early in life have an improved developmental status.[2]

Hypothyroid screening has made it possible to evaluate the so-called diagnostic clinical signs of congenital hypothyroidism. A scoring system can be used in those communities that are unable to afford routine hypothyroidism screening procedures (Table 5.7.1). A score of greater than three should select babies that need to have TSH and T_4 hormone levels estimated as well as an X-ray for bone age. Prolonged jaundice, distended abdomen, hoarse cry, slow deep tendon reflexes and hypothermia are features that were shown not to be significantly different from normal controls. It is worth mentioning two points in the clinical diagnosis of congenital hypothyroidism: some ethnic groups show abnormal facies which may resemble those of congenital hypothyroidism; and Beckwith's syndrome may also be wrongly diagnosed as congenital hypothyroidism. Treatment for hypothyroidism with thyroid hormones is for life; the dose of levothyroxine in the new born is 0.025 mg per day, gradually increasing to 0.1 mg/m² per day. Sometimes there is sufficient

thyroid tissue to prevent overt cretinism and keep the child euthyroid until the later demands of growth and activity outgrow thyroid production and juvenile myxoedema develops (Fig. 5.7.2).

Hyperthyroidism

Hyperthyroidism in the child occurs at any age: about 10 per cent before five years, 20 per cent from 5 to 10 years, and 70 per cent after 10 years. Although hyperthyroidism in childhood comprises only about 1 per cent of cases at all ages, it accounts for 15 per cent of all paediatric thyroid diseases. The most common variety of hyperthyroidism is Graves's disease, but like paediatric hypothyroidism congenital hyperthyroidism is occasionally seen. This occurs in mothers who had or are having hyperthyroidism during pregnancy, whether they are treated or not, and is due to possible transmission of thyroid-stimulating immunoglobins (TSIg) from mother to fetus. Hence, in the majority of cases, the condition is transient as the antibodies disappear in the baby after birth; however, cases have been described where the hyperthyroidism is more 'permanent'.[3] It is probably best to treat all cases of congenital hyperthyroidism with antithyroid drugs because there is evidence that excess thyroid hormones in the newborn period causes premature craniostenosis and possible mental retardation in later life. The signs and symptoms are similar to hyperthyroidism in children but confined to the period of the neonate. Thus, there is a visible goitre in 70 per cent of cases with hyperactivity, excess perspiration, tremulousness, tachycardia, and exophthalmos with a voracious milk intake but with poor weight gain. Besides antithyroid drugs, propanolol may be necessary. Withdrawal of drugs depends on the progress: if there is no recurrence then it is the usual transient variety but if signs and symptoms recur treatment will have to be continued.

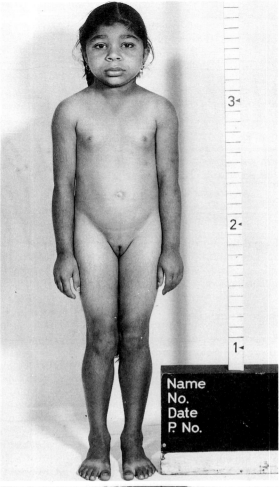

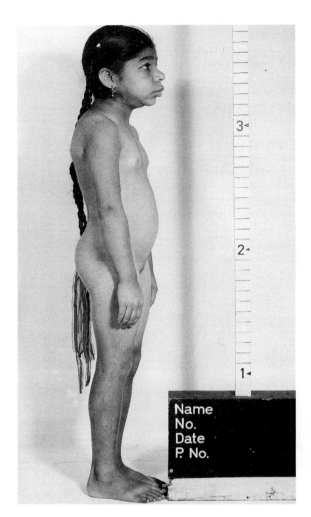

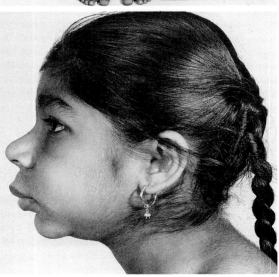

Fig. 5.7.2 Juvenile myxoedema in a 12-year-old Indian girl.

Childhood hyperthyroidism is typically of Graves's disease variety and the signs and symptoms are similar to those seen in adults. The toxicity is gradual in onset, and the signs and symptoms which may differ from those seen in adults include the following:

- Behavioural problems; these are often the initial presenting symptoms.
- School performance; this often deteriorates with shortened attention span, deteriorating handwriting, and hyperactivity.
- Increase in both water and food intake; some cases may actually put on weight; some are referred because of polyuria and polydipsia.
- Inordinate height velocity; this may precede the usual classical signs and symptoms.
- Tremors are less common.

Diagnosis is confirmed by thyroid hormone estimation with raised T_3 and T_4 and low TSH.

Treatment essentially comprises the use of anti-thyroid drugs such as carbimazole (20–40 mg/day) or propylthiouracil (6–7 mg/day). Propanolol may be necessary initially if hyperactive signs and symptoms are excessive. Dosage changes will depend on the clinical features and thyroid hormone levels. Usually, treatment will have to be continued for two years. Relapses occur in half the cases. These may receive further courses of antithyroid drugs, but if compliance is poor surgery is recommended. Although there are proponents for the wider use of radioactive iodine in the treatment of childhood hyperthyroidism, the possible late complications of thyroid carcinoma still deter many from using this form of treatment.

Thyroiditis

Thyroiditis is not uncommon in children and can be acute, subacute or chronic.

The acute variety can occur as a result of bacterial or viral infection but the most common is bacterial with the presence of pus, i.e. an acute suppurative thyroiditis. There are no significant thyroid hormone changes and the treatment is as for any bacterial suppuration.

Subacute or de Quervain's thyroiditis is considered to be an adult disease and is rarely seen in children.

Chronic thyroiditis is not uncommon, and in most cases is an autoimmune type (Hashimoto's thyroiditis). It often starts as a visible goitre and histology shows a lymphocytic thyroiditis. Females are affected more than males with a peak age incidence of around 10 years. Initially, patients are euthyroid but some show mild signs of hyperthyroidism, which are usually transient. There may be concomitant signs of other autoimmune disorders, and some thyroid antibodies are often present in high titre. Some remain euthyroid but many finally become hypothyroid. If the diagnosis is in doubt, biopsy should be carried out. Treatment comprises giving T_4 (thyroxine) for about two years, after which it is withdrawn. One-third of patients remain euthyroid but the rest will show signs and symptoms of hypothyroidism so that thyroxine treatment will have to be continued.

Thyroid carcinoma

Thyroid carcinoma is rare in childhood and usually presents as a thyroid nodule. There may or may not be enlarged lymph nodes. With thyroid scanning, these usually present as 'cold' nodules but there are other 'cold' nodules which are not carcinomatous. Invariably, nodules in the thyroid in the paediatric age group should be followed up with biopsy to confirm or exclude the diagnosis of thyroid carcinoma. The prognosis with surgery is good if carried out early, as the tumour is slow-growing and spread is initially slow.

Diabetes mellitus

Nearly all cases of childhood diabetes mellitus are type I often also referred to as insulin-dependent diabetes mellitus (IDDM). Besides IDDM, in the tropics, there is a peculiar form of pancreatic diabetes[4] called J diabetes, as it was described in Jamaica. It is associated with chronic malnutrition but is rare in children, with onset between ages 15–40 years. In spite of severe hyperglycaemia, ketosis is uncommon, and there is relative resistance to insulin. Some show pancreatic calcification while others do not. It is uncertain whether the rarity of ketosis is due to malnutrition with little fat distribution or whether it is a maturity onset diabetes (NIDDM) with malnutrition.

IDDM is a multifactorially inherited disease,[5] dependent on both polygenes and the environment. Environmental triggers include virus infection, e.g. Coxsackie viruses, as well as psychological factors. Polygenes involve to some extent the HLA genes but these certainly are not the only ones involved. Among Caucasians HLA-DR3 and DR4 predispose to IDDM. DR2 seems protective but this is not absolute, i.e. there are individuals with DR3 and DR4 who do not suffer from IDDM and individuals without DR3 and DR4 who suffer from IDDM. For example, the significant HLA haplotypes seen in IDDM among Chinese in Singapore and Chinese in Shanghai are not identical.

Since inheritance is multifactorial, it is uncommon for more than one member of the family to suffer from IDDM, compared with the high incidence of affected family members in NIDDM (non-insulin dependent diabetes mellitus or type II). The risk of an offspring of a patient with IDDM also being affected is 5 per cent. In IDDM, there is evidence of autoimmunity against the pancreas with insulitis and a gradual fall in insulin production.

The clinical presentation of IDDM can be acute or gradual. In the acute type of presentation, it is often preceded by a virus infection and severe ketosis. Those with gradual onset present with polyuria, polydipsia, loss in weight, and lethargy, which may also culminate in diabetic ketoacidosis (DKA).

Diagnosis is confirmed by testing the urine for glucose (glycosuria) with ketones and hyperglycaemia. Such cases do not need a glucose tolerance test (GTT) for confirmation, although less obvious cases will do so. Criteria for the different states of intolerance to glucose

Table 5.7.2 Glucose tolerance test (GTT).

	Glucose concentration (mmol/l (mg/dl))			
	Whole blood		Plasma	
	Venous	Capillary	Venous	Capillary
Fasting value	≧6.7 (≧120)	≧6.7 (≧120)	≧7.8 (≧140)	≧7.8 (≧140)
2 hr value	≧10 (≧180)	≧11.1 (≧200)	≧11.1 (≧200)	≧12.2 (≧200)

1.75 g per kg up to 75 g for the GTT are shown in Table 5.7.2.

The differential diagnosis of polyuria is usually simple for the more common causes – diabetes mellitus, central or nephrogenic diabetes insipidus (DI), chronic renal failure, and psychogenic polydipsia. The following sequence of tests is used:

- Confirm polyuria and polydipsia by observation for 24 hours. Patients with polyuria usually pass 2.5 litres of urine in 24 hours.
- Test the urine for glucose and ketones. If positive, diabetes mellitus is the diagnosis.
- If negative for sugar, test for blood urea and creatinine. If levels of both are raised, chronic renal failure is confirmed. This leaves central or nephrogenic diabetes insipidus and psychogenic polydipsia.
- With free access to fluids the early morning urine osmolality is estimated. If the urine osmolality is more than 150 mosmol/kg, psychogenic polydipsia is the cause.
- Finally, central DI is confirmed by giving ADH (pitressin) and observing disappearance of the polyuria. With nephrogenic DI, ADH will have no effect since this disease is not due to lack of ADH but to absent receptors in the renal tubular cells.

The main problem of IDDM is that in spite of insulin, morbidity due to microvascular and macrovascular complications are still significant; 7 per cent die after 20 years of the disease and 60 per cent die after 40 years. With increasing life span in many countries, this is unacceptable. When one adds the morbidity before premature death, previous modes of therapy are relatively ineffectual. Therefore, the parents and the child must be educated about the disease – how diabetic complications arise and how close blood glucose control can be achieved with home monitoring. Treatment of the IDDM child consists *not only* of insulin injections. Other aspects of the disease, such as diet, exercise, life-style, psychological attitudes, genetic counselling, and hypoglycaemic episodes, must be considered also.

Treatment

Ketoacidosis Diabetic ketoacidosis requires urgent treatment. The condition is recognized by the presence of significant dehydration, vomiting, acidotic respiration, hyperglycaemia, heavy ketonuria, and glycosuria with an impaired level of consciousness. The body weight must be recorded and accurate fluid balance records kept. Whenever possible, blood glucose, electrolytes and acid–base studies should be carried out before treatment and at four-hourly intervals thereafter. An infection screen should also be arranged. Emergency management involves intravenous fluids, calculating the initial 24 hour requirement by assuming 10 per cent dehydration plus maintenance according to age and body weight. The rate of infusion should be one-third of the 24 hour requirement in the first four hours, one-third over the next eight hours, and the balance over the succeeding 12 hours. If the patient is severely hyperosmolar these volumes must be reduced. Saline 0.9 per cent is given initially; when the blood glucose has fallen below 15 mmol/l, 4.3 per cent dextrose and 0.18 per cent saline should be used. Soluble insulin at 0.05 units/kg body weight intramuscularly should be given on presentation. Provided blood glucose monitoring is available this dose may be repeated one to two-hourly until the blood glucose level has fallen below 15 mmol/1, the rate of fall should not exceed 4–5 mmol/h otherwise there is a danger of cerebral oedema. Potassium should not be given until urine flow has been established. The metabolic acidosis will usually resolve without specific correction with bicarbonate in all but the most severe cases. Oral feeding can usually begin some 12 hours after admission with small quantities hourly. The fluid should include glucose at 20 g three-hourly and potassium supplements or fruit juices. Further subcutaneous soluble insulin should be given according to the blood sugar level or the amount of glycosuria and ketonuria. These doses may be given four-hourly followed by six-hourly, and then three times daily before meals.

Hyperglycaemia without severe acidosis or dehydration Soluble insulin in a dose of approximately 0.5 units/kg is given subcutaneously three times daily at the start of each main meal. Four-hourly blood and urine glucose monitoring is useful. When ketonuria has disappeared and moderate stabilization has been achieved, a change to a once or twice daily insulin regimen may be made, using initially about three-quarters of the total daily soluble dose. The choice of insulin preparation is often a matter of personal preference. In general, it is better to use a twice daily regimen of a short-acting insulin than to attempt a once daily regimen of intermediate or long-acting types. This is particularly so where the meals or injection may be somewhat irregular in timing; the simple rule of not having the injection until just before the meal makes late hypoglycaemic states less likely.

Much has been written about the dietary control of carbohydrate intake. Counsels of dietary perfection must be tempered with such practical matters as the availability of a trained dietician or nutritionist with local food and language experience and the educational attainment of the parents. As a general guide, 1000 kcal/day are necessary at one year, increasing by approximately 100 kcal/day each year until puberty. The carbohydrate intake should be spread over the day. There is no evidence that the overall approach to management is any different from that prescribed in Europe or North America. In general, there is no place for oral hypoglycaemic therapy in children.

Hypoglycaemia

Hypoglycaemia in the paediatric age group is not uncommon, and if prolonged and severe, its effects on the developing brain can be devastating. The level of blood glucose which causes signs and symptoms of hypoglycaemia is dependent not only on the blood level but also on the passage of glucose across the blood–brain barrier, which varies in different individuals because of genetic variation. Hence, it is neuroglycopenia which is important rather than the blood glucose level. Yet, a 'working level' of blood glucose is necessary for practical purposes, and it is usually assumed that hypoglycaemia occurs when the blood glucose is below 1.1 mmol/l (20 mg/dl) during the first three days of life in preterm and small-for-dates infants; below 1.7 mmol/l (30 mg/dl) for full-term infants; and below 2.2 mmol/l (40 mg/dl) for all age groups beyond the immediate neonatal period; others claim that the lowest acceptable limit should be 2.2 mmol/l (40 mg/dl).

Prompt diagnosis of hypoglycaemia is an emergency. Patients with conditions (see later) known to produce hypoglycaemia should have their blood glucose deter-

mined and certain neuroglycopenic signs and symptoms looked for (Table 5.7.3).

Hence, when hypoglycaemia is suspected and after blood is taken for blood glucose determination, intravenous glucose should be given immediately followed by oral glucose. The cause of the hypoglycaemia is then investigated. At the outset it is necessary to test the urine for ketones. A simple classification of the aetiology of hypoglycaemia is to divide the causes into two main groups: the ketotic and the non-ketotic. The non-ketotic variety occur with excess insulin, i.e. when there is hyperinsulinism, while the ketotic variety have normal appropriate levels of plasma insulin for the degree of hypoglycaemia. Insulin prevents lipolysis of the adipose cells so there will be no excess of fatty acids to produce ketones; thus, non-ketotic hypoglycaemia is associated with hyperinsulinaemic hypoglycaemia. If there is no hyperinsulinism, hypoglycaemia will evoke lipolysis to produce fatty

Table 5.7.3   Symptoms of neuroglycopenia.

Newborn: often non-specific	
Fits	Coma
Floppiness	Abnormal cry
Dyspnoea or apnoea	Pallor
Tremors	Feeding difficulties
Hyperactivity	Cyanosis
Infant and child	
Pallor/sweating	Abnormal behaviour
Fits	Headache
Drowsiness/coma	Syncope
Lethargy	Nausea/vomiting

Table 5.7.4   Causes of hypoglycaemia.

Transient neonatal
Non-ketotic: hyperinsulinism
        Infant of diabetic mother
        Erythroblastosis
        Beckwith's syndrome
Ketotic: Birth hypoxia
        Small-for-dates baby
Persistent neonatal/infancy
Non-ketotic: hyperinsulinism
        Nesidioblastosis (islet cell hyperplasia, adenoma)
        Beckwith's syndrome
Ketotic: (a) Enzyme deficiency
        Glycogen storage disease
        Pyruvate enzyme deficiencies
        Fructose 1–6-diphosphatase deficiency
        Galactosaemia
        Fructose intolerance
        Maple syrup urine disease
     (b) Hormone deficiency
        Growth hormone deficiency
        Hypothyroidism
        Glucocorticoid deficiency
        Glucagon deficiency
Children
Non-ketotic: hyperinsulinism
        Islet cell adenoma
        Insulin administration
        Oral hypoglycaemics
Ketotic: Islet cell adenoma
        Insulin administration
        Oral hypoglycaemics
        Fulminant hepatitis
        Reye's syndrome
        Starvation
        Salicylates
        Alcohol

acids so that ketosis will be produced as an alternative source of fuel. The causes of hypoglycaemia are given in Table 5.7.4.

Adrenal disorders

The most common adrenal disorder is the autosomal recessive condition, congenital adrenal hyperplasia (CAH). In females, the most obvious presentation is ambiguous external genitalia. Here we consider the problem of ambiguous external genitalia due to CAH as well as other causes.

Ambiguous external genitalia

The problems of ambiguous external genitalia (AEG) should be recognized and dealt with at birth, not later. It is a medical emergency to assign sex and explain to the parents how to bring the child up in the male or female gender with minimal psychological and physical problems on the part of the child. In general, the paediatrician should assign the correct sex as early as possible so that the legal sex on the birth certificate, the name, the mode of upbringing and clothing, all reflect the sex assigned.

The first step is to establish whether the baby with AEG is 46 XX and hence Barr body positive (chromatin positive) or 46 XY and Barr body negative (chromatin negative). If chromosome culture facilities are unavailable, simple staining with 1 per cent orcein of buccal epithelium obtained by scraping the inside of the cheek, will be sufficient to decide whether the baby is chromatin positive or negative. The chromatin negative cases with a Y chromosome can also be confirmed by staining the lymphocytes with quinacrine sulphate

Table 5.7.5 Ambiguous external genitalia

Chromatin positive
  Congenital adrenal hyperplasia
  Drugs in pregnancy
  Maternal arrhenoblastoma
  True hermaphroditism
  Others
Chromatin negative
  True hermaphroditism
  Testosterone synthesis defect
  Deficient androgenic action
    (a) Partial syndrome of testicular feminization
    (b) 5 α-reductase deficiency
  Leydig cell agenesis
  Anorchia
  Fetal pituitary and hypothalamic disturbances
  Others

and finding the Y fluorescence. Thus, there is usually no problem in assigning a baby with AEG to one of these two subgroups.

Next, is the problem of sex assignment. A simple rule is that all chromatin-positive babies with AEG should be assigned the female sex role because in spite of the AEG, most chromatin-positive cases have female internal genitalia (uterus, tubes and vagina) as well as female gonads (ovaries). With surgical treatment of the external genitalia, many such cases will grow up and function as normal physical and psychological females and bear children.

The causes of AEG in chromatin-positive and chromatin-negative patients are listed in Table 5.7.5.

Chromatin-positive patients

One of the most common causes of chromatin-positive AEG is congenital adrenal hyperplasia. This is due to deficiency of one of the enzymes involved in the metabolism of the adrenocortical hormones. Fig. 5.7.3 depicts the three limbs of the adrenocortical hormones – the aldosterone limb, the cortisol limb and the sex hormone limb.

The most common enzyme deficiency is 21-hydroxylase deficiency. This causes deficiency of cortisol and, by negative feedback on the pituitary, ACTH production is increased. The block at the 21-hydroxylase level causes testosterone to be over-produced so that virilization of the external genitalia of the female occurs with consequent ambiguous external genitalia. If the 21-hydroxylase in the aldosterone limb is affected severely, there will also be symptoms and signs of adrenal crises – the patient will be a salt-loser and death can occur if diagnosis is delayed and adequate treatment not given. Diagnosis of 21-hydroxylase deficiency and 11-hydroxylase deficiency causing congenital adrenal hyperplasia is made by finding raised levels of 17-hydroxyprogesterone in the plasma and raised 17-ketosteroids in the urine. Since the condition is inherited in an autosomal recessive manner, other siblings may be affected and there may be parental consanguinity. Treatment is by giving hydrocortisone for life, which will reduce ACTH and hence testosterone production with reduction in virilization. If there are salt-losing signs and symptoms, fludrohydrocortisone with or without sodium chloride is also given. Patients brought up as females can marry and produce children. Short stature may occur due to the effect of androgen on early bony fusion. The 21-hydroxylase gene is closely linked with the HLA genes on chromosome 6, so that prenatal diagnosis is

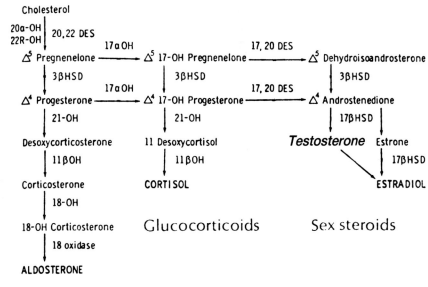

Fig. 5.7.3 Simplified scheme showing the three metabolic limbs of the adrenal cortex. The most common cause of congenital adrenal hyperplasia is deficiency of the enzyme 21-hydroxylase. Key: OH = hydroxylase; DES = desmolase; 3β-HSD = 3β-hydroxysteroid dehydrogenase; 17β-HSD = 17β-hydroxysteroid dehydrogenase. (Reproduced from Wong HB, *Journal of the Singapore Paediatric Society*, 1983; **25**: 44–51.)

possible if the HLA haplotypes are determined for the affected child and the parents.

The other chromatin-positive AEG patients do not show continuing virilization. Thus, plastic operations on the external genitalia are all that is needed for treatment and prognosis is usually much better.

Chromatin-negative patients

In contrast to chromatin-positive patients who should be brought up as females, chromatin-negative patients may be brought up as males or females, depending on the cause and the appearance of the external genitalia and the structure of the genitalia ducts. If the sex assignation of a chromatin-negative true hemaphrodite is female, then testicular tissue should be removed. Otherwise, plastic operations should be carried out to fit the child for the male or the female role, depending on the decision for sex assignation.

Acute adrenal insufficiency

As already mentioned, acute adrenal insufficiency can occur in congenital adrenal hyperplasia of the salt-losing, 21-hydroxylase deficiency type. Addisonian crisis, from whatever cause, is an emergency – its recognition is important and the deficient hormones should be given immediately. Clinically, children with acute adrenal insufficiency complain of abdominal pain and anorexia, with vomiting and diarrhoea. These prodromal symptoms are soon followed by a fall in blood pressure, dehydration and collapse, ending in death. There is hyponatraemia and a hyperkalaemia with excessive loss of sodium in the urine.

Besides congenital adrenal hyperplasia and hypoplasia, infections such as meningococcaemia (Waterhouse–Friderichsen syndrome), adrenal haemorrhage, and treatment with long-term corticosteroids can also cause Addisonian crises.

Adrenal hypercorticism

Hypercorticism, the opposite of adrenal insufficiency, can result iatrogenically by treatment of various diseases with exogenous corticosteroids. Cushing's syndrome encompasses all varieties of hypercorticism, while Cushing's disease is hypercorticism due to excess ACTH production from the hypothalamic–pituitary unit. The main feature of Cushing's syndrome is easily recognized as it resembles the iatrogenic Cushingoid appearance. Obesity, hirsutes, buffalo-hump, seborrhoea and acne, hypertension and poor carbohydrate tolerance are usually found. The greatest difficulty is distinguishing Cushing's syndrome from ordinary obesity: in the former there is retardation in height while in the latter there is increased height.

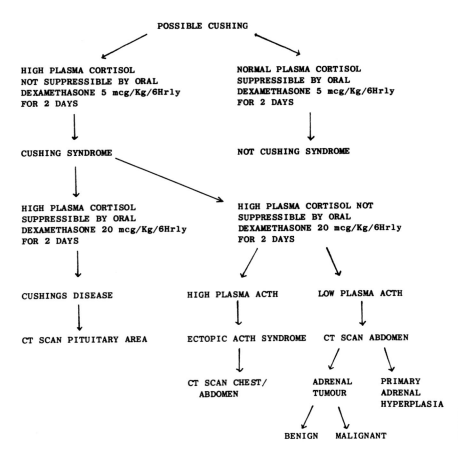

Fig. 5.7.4 Scheme for diagnosis of a possible case of Cushing's syndrome.

No single pathognomonic test can distinguish Cushing's syndrome from Cushing's disease but a simple diagnostic regimen[6] is shown in Fig. 5.7.4.

Treatment of Cushing's syndrome secondary to an adrenal tumour or an ectopic ACTH-secreting tumour is surgical removal. However, treatment of Cushing's disease is not so straightforward and less than ideal. The aim is to restore normal cortisol production. Cortisol production may be decreased by adrenalectomy or by using metyrapone which blocks the conversion of 11-desoxycortisol to cortisol. The alternatives are pituitary surgery, irradiating the pituitary, or using drugs which influence the release of ACTH from the pituitary.

Bilateral adrenalectomy may be total or subtotal[7]. Recurrence is about 10 per cent due to inadequate removal of adrenal tissue or the non-recognition of ectopic adrenal tissue. Life-long cortisol replacement is necessary for those with total adrenalectomy. Trans-

sphenoidal surgery on the pituitary has advanced considerably in safety and efficacy, and in expert hands, 90–95 per cent remission rates have been achieved. Radiotherapy to the pituitary gland utilizing 3500–5000 rads has some degree of success.

Drug treatment using cyproheptadine, serotonin antagonists and bromocryptine, a dopamine agonist, have had some degree of success. Cyproheptadine inhibits the release of corticotrophin-releasing factor (CRF) at the hypothalamic level and at the same time increases the cortisol action on CRF release. It also inhibits the release of ACTH at the pituitary level; side-effects include increased appetite with weight gain, depression of the CNS, and vision problems. Bromo-cryptine inhibits the stress-induced release of CRF and also directly suppresses ACTH secretion at the pituitary level. However, long-term treatment with this drug has been rather disappointing.

Hypogonadism

Most of the problems in hypogonadism appear during puberty, especially in females. However, in males, the appearance of the external genitalia long before puberty may suggest male hypogonadism obvious at birth, e.g. the presence of a micropenis, or in boys with bilateral undescended testes. Thus, the paediatrician is more likely to be consulted for male hypogonadism, while the endocrinologist and the obstetrician will be consulted for female hypogonadism.

Both male and female hypogonadism may be primarily gonadal or primarily hypothalamic–pituitary. The former is usually referred to as hypergonadotrophic hypogonadism while the latter is hypogonadotrophic hypogonadism. Because of primary affection of the gonads, there may be increased gonadotrophic hormones via the negative feedback mechanisms – hypergonadotrophic. If the hypothalamic–pituitary unit is involved, there is a decrease of the gonadotrophic hormones – hypogonadotrophic hypogonadism.

Male hypogonadism can be caused by a wide variety of abnormalities, as Fig. 5.7.5 shows. A scheme for the investigation of male hypogonadism is shown in Fig. 5.7.6. The most common variety of delayed puberty in boys is constitutional delay. The time of onset of puberty is highly variable; some boys achieve puberty much later than others in terms of chronological age. Their growth and development are compatible with the bone age rather than their chronological age, which clearly highlights the unreliability of the latter as far as maturity is concerned. Boys with constitutional delay are 'slow-growers' and thus their bone age, height and puberty are all delayed in terms of chronological age. Since the cause is polygenic, delay could also have affected the father and siblings. Testicular stimulation tests utilizing human chorionic gonadotrophic or luteinizing hormone-releasing hormone will show a rise in testosterone in these boys. Reassurance is important for the boy and his parents and in time, pubertal changes will occur. The treatment of other varieties of male hypogonadism depends on the cause.

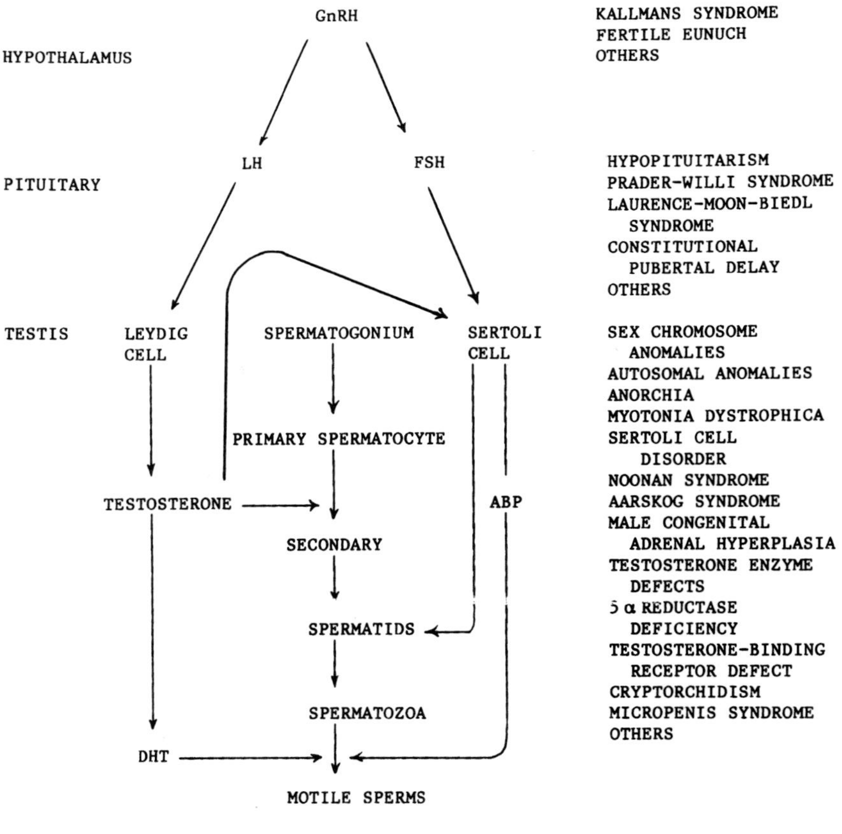

Fig. 5.7.5 Outline of possible causes of male hypogonadism in children. The left-hand diagram shows the different levels where the relevant causes (on the right side) may operate. Key: GnRH = Gonadotrophin releasing hormone; LH = Luteinizing hormone; FSH = Follicle stimulating hormone; ABP = Androgen binding protein; DHT = dihydrotestosterone.

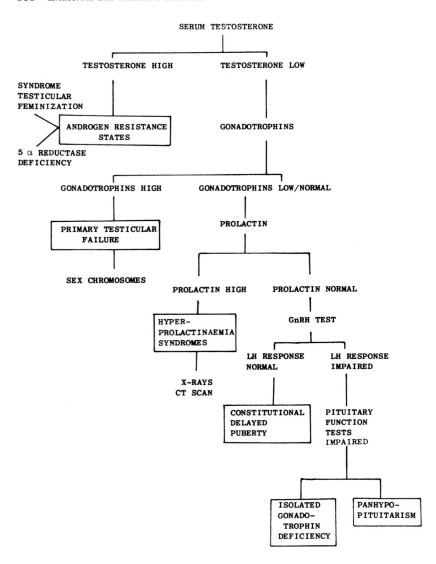

SERUM TESTOSTERONE

TESTOSTERONE HIGH   TESTOSTERONE LOW

SYNDROME
TESTICULAR
FEMINIZATION
                  ANDROGEN RESISTANCE   GONADOTROPHINS
                       STATES

5 α REDUCTASE
DEFICIENCY

GONADOTROPHINS HIGH   GONADOTROPHINS LOW/NORMAL

                                    PROLACTIN

              PRIMARY TESTICULAR
                   FAILURE

       SEX CHROMOSOMES

                        PROLACTIN HIGH   PROLACTIN NORMAL

                                                 GnRH TEST
              HYPER-
              PROLACTINAEMIA
              SYNDROMES
                                    LH RESPONSE   LH RESPONSE
                                    NORMAL   IMPAIRED
                        X-RAYS
                        CT SCAN
                                    CONSTITUTIONAL   PITUITARY
                                    DELAYED   FUNCTION
                                    PUBERTY   TESTS
                                                     IMPAIRED

                                         ISOLATED   PANHYPO-
                                         GONADO-   PITUITARISM
                                         TROPHIN
                                         DEFICIENCY

Fig. 5.7.6 Simplified scheme for investigating the cause of male hypogonadism.

Pubertal delay may also be caused by environmental factors such as systemic disease and chronic malnutrition. Studies of the long-term effects of malnutrition show that whereas height and bone age are retarded, bone age which closely correlates with the maturation of secondary sexual characteristics is not so severely affected as growth (height). The net result is that growth, though it may have longer to continue, ceases before optimal (genetic) height is attained. The secular trend as health and nutrition improves is towards increasing growth velocity, earlier maturity and puberty, and increasing ultimate adult height.

The most common variety of female hypogonadism is Turner's syndrome, a condition which can often be diagnosed at birth because of the associated somatic features. Many of these babies have lower birth weights and show a low hair line with webbing of the neck, a flat shield-shaped chest, cubitus valgus, nevi, or lymphoedema of the dorsum of the feet and hands. There may be associated cardiac anomalies, especially coarctation of the aorta. As the child grows, shortness of stature becomes obvious. Confirmation of the diagnosis is simple as most cases lack Barr bodies (chromatin negative) in spite of an unequivocal female appearance.

Sex chromosomes studies will show that the majority are 45 X0. However, chromatin-positive cases of Turner's syndrome do occur, e.g. isochromosome of the long arm of X, deletion of the short arm of X, mosaics of XX/X0 and so on. Nearly all cases of Turner's syndrome (like Klinefelter's syndrome, XXY) are not inherited in the strict sense and it is extremely rare to see more than one case of Turner's or Klinefelter's syndrome in a single family. The cause is usually non-disjunction at meiosis of the sex chromosomes of one of the parental gametes or non-disjunction of the sex chromosomes of the zygote. This is important to bear in mind when giving genetic advice.

Calcium and phosphate metabolism

Although permanent diseases of the parathyroids do occur in the paediatric age group, hyperparathyroidism is rare. Hypoparathyroidism occurs as a transient phenomenon in newborns, as part of the di George syndrome and in idiopathic hypoparathyroidism and pseudohypoparathyroidism. However, two common conditions involving calcium and phosphate metabolism occur in the paediatric age group: hypocalcaemia and rickets.

Vitamin D_3 or cholecalciferol is taken in food. In addition, its precursors in the skin can be converted to cholecalciferol by sunlight; hence, rickets is more common in pigmented races living in temperate lands. However, cholecalciferol has minimal activity, being a prohormone. It has to undergo two other changes before it shows optimal activity. It is hydroxylated at the carbon-25 position to form 25-hydroxycalciferol in the liver. Then, in the kidney, it is hydroxylated a second time at the carbon-1 position to form the potent vitamin D, i.e. 1,25-dihydroxycalciferol. Hence, lack of vitamin D occurs because of poor diet, malabsorption, and lack of sunlight, and also as a result of liver and kidney diseases.

Figure 5.7.7 summarizes the important factors that determine serum calcium and phosphate levels.

There is a tendency for hypocalcaemia to occur at birth in all newborns. The exact cause is still uncertain, but, many agree that it occurs as follows. Maternal calcium and phosphate are transferred maximally to the fetus in the third trimester to build up the bones in the fetus. As a result, during this late period of fetal life, fetal parathormone (PTH) is low and fetal calcitonin (CT) is high, so as to deposit calcium in the bones. When the cord is severed at birth, low fetal PTH and high fetal CT would produce hypocalcaemia. It is at this time that the parathyroid glands will normally increase

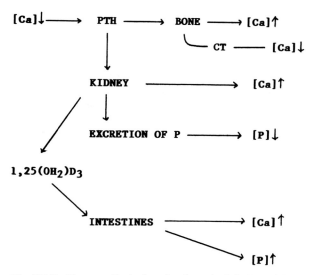

Fig. 5.7.7 Diagram illustrating the important factors determining serum calcium and phosphate levels. (PTH = Parathormone, CT = Calcitonin).

the production of PTH to offset the hypocalcaemia, so that early neonatal hypocalcaemia does not take place. This explains why hypocalcaemia is more likely to occur in preterm infants. Stress at birth, e.g. by asphyxia, also tends to increase CT production.

Hypocalcaemia

Hypocalcaemia is most common in infancy, although it can occur in later life (Table 5.7.6). (See also p. 380). Hypocalcaemia in the neonatal period may present differently from hypocalcaemia in later life when tetany is seen. In the neonatal period, hypocalcaemia may produce seizures, jitteriness, hyperreflexia, hypertonus, clonus and hyperalertness.[8] The pathogenesis of

Table 5.7.6 Pediatric hypocalcaemia.

Neonatal
  Early
    Hypocalcaemia of premature infants
    Hypocalcaemia in infants of diabetic mothers (IDM)
  Late
    Transient hypoparathyroidism
    Di George syndrome
    Hypomagnesaemia
Postneonatal
  Hypoparathyroidism
  Pseudohypoparathyroidism
  Rickets
  Renal failure

---

the hypocalcaemia in the infants of diabetic mothers is also uncertain but possibly the increased fetal size of these infants may be responsible for increased calcium needs. Early neonatal hypocalcaemia occurs during the first three days of life when the parathyroids finally increase PTH production and alleviate the hypocalcaemia. Late neonatal hypocalcaemia occurs in those infants where the parathyroids take longer to compensate but finally do so and hypocalcaemia disappears. Di George syndrome occurs as a result of poor development of the third and fourth pharyngeal pouches and branchial arches. Besides other structures, the thymus and the parathyroids are derived from these arches so that the facies is abnormal with hypoparathyroidism and immunodeficiency. There may also be congenital heart disease. The usual initial presenting symptoms and signs are those of hypocalcaemia. Hypomagnesaemia may impair parathyroid function so that hypocalcaemia supervenes and this it achieves by inhibiting PTH secretion and blunting end-organ responses to PTH. Hypocalcaemia due to magnesium deficiency can be eliminated by giving magnesium (0.5–1.0 ml of 5 per cent magnesium sulphate intramuscularly). (See also p. 381).

Postneonatal hypocalcaemia can be seen when there is idiopathic hypoparathyroidism, pseudohypothyroidism, rickets and renal failure. Idiopathic hypoparathyroidism is rare in children. It can be familial or isolated or can occur as a result of autoimmunity to the parathyroid and other endocrine glands and to other tissues, e.g. pernicious anaemia or adrenal insufficiency. Patients with hypoparathyroidism may present with fits, calcification of the basal ganglia and other organ disorders. Treatment with vitamin D and calcium ameliorates the condition. Patients with pseudohypoparathyroidism also show signs and symptoms due to hypocalcaemia but the PTH levels are normal or even higher than normal. This is not due to deficiency of PTH or to hypoparathyroidism but to end-organ failure to respond to PTH. The signs and symptoms are similar to those of hypoparathyroidism but mental retardation and short stature are common.[9] In addition, there is brachydactyly of the metacarpals and metatarsals, especially fourth and fifth. The facies is round with calcification in the lens and subcutaneous tissues.

Rickets

Rickets is osteomalacia in growing bones. Osteomalacia is due to failure of calcification of bone matrix, while osteoporosis is caused by rarification of bones due to a poor protein matrix (Fig. 5.7.8). The most common

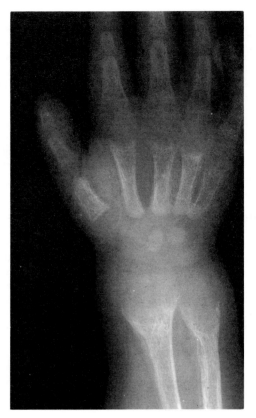

Fig. 5.7.8 Classical cupping of the metaphyses of the radius and ulna with osteoporosis and delayed epiphyseal growth in a four-year-old child.

cause of rickets is lack of vitamin D (see also pp. 376–9). Causes in the paediatric age group are shown in Table 5.7.7.

Nutritional rickets can occur in the tropics but is not common, mainly because of adequate sunlight. However, in extreme malnutrition or following the cultural habits of swaddling infants or women wearing excess clothing, rickets can occur. Rickets is not uncommon in tropical ethnic groups who migrate to temperate lands, as a result of lack of sunlight and poor nutrition.

The infant with nutritional rickets is irritable. The skull is soft (craniotabes) with frontal bossing and late closure of the anterior fontanelle. There is bowing of the arms and legs with delay in sitting, crawling and walking. There is bending of the ribs, and enlargement of the bone ends of the arm and legs. Funnel chest (pectus excavatum), pigeon chest (pectus carinatum) and Harrison's sulci are seen (Table 5.7.8). X-ray features are pathognomonic (Fig. 5.7.8). Management

Table 5.7.7 Causes of rickets.

Nutritional
  Lack of vitamin D in diet
  Malabsorption
  Lack of sunlight
Rickets of infancy
  Osteopenia in low-birth-weight babies
  Obstructive jaundice syndrome in infancy
Metabolic rickets
  Calciopenic rickets
  Phosphopenic rickets
  Fanconi's syndrome

Table 5.7.9 Childhood rickets.

Mendelian
  Sex-linked hypophosphataemic rickets (XLH)
  Autosomal dominant hypophosphataemic rickets (HBD)
  Autosomal recessive vitamin D-dependent rickets
    (VDD type I)
  Autosomal recessive vitamin D-dependent rickets
    (VDD type II)
Fanconi's syndrome
  Autosomal recessive
  Acquired forms

Table 5.7.8 Clinical and biochemical features of preterm osteopaenia.

Clinical features	Biochemical
Craniotabes	Serum calcium: low to low–normal
Bony expansion of wrist	Serum phosphate: low to low–normal
Costochondral bending	Serum alkaline phosphatase: raised
Rib fractures	Serum parathormone: raised
Respiratory distress	Urine amino acids: non-specific increase
Convulsions	$1,25(OH)_2D_3$: low
Radiological signs	

is through prevention by good health habits, and giving vitamin D to those pregnant women and newborns who are predisposed to nutritional rickets.

The most common form of rickets in infancy is seen in developed countries. Increasing numbers of neonates of low, very low, and extremely low birth weight are surviving because of intensive perinatal care. As a result of failure of calcium passage from mother to fetus, these babies lack both calcium and phosphate from birth.

The management of osteopenia of prematurity is to anticipate it in preterms and to offer adequate calcium, phosphate, or vitamin D, or all three; milk formulas containing 1200 mg/l of calcium, 600 mg/l of phosphate, and 800–1200 mg i.v. vitamin D may be needed to prevent and treat rickets when it has occurred.[10]

Rickets is also associated with prolonged cholestasis (conjugated hyperbilirubinaemia) in infancy due to biliary atresia or severe hepatitis. There is raised conjugated bilirubin; jaundice usually starts at one month of age with hepatosplenomegaly, the presence of bile in the urine and absence of constitutional signs and symptoms in most cases. The cause of the rickets is an inability to absorb the fat-soluble vitamin D because of

reduction or absence of bile in the intestine as a result of cholestasis or biliary obstruction. Treatment is the treatment of the cause, together with the use of vitamin D. The diagnostic strategy in neonatal cholestasis is shown in Fig. 5.7.9.

Childhood rickets is often due to Mendelian inherited disorders (Table 5.7.9).

Acquired renal osteodystrophy

Acquired renal osteodystrophy is due to chronic renal failure and is the only form of rickets where the serum phosphate is raised, i.e. it is a hyperphosphataemic rickets. All other forms of rickets are hypophosphataemic. Sex-linked hypophosphataemic rickets (XLH) is due to a genetic defect in the proximal renal tubule so that there is a defect in phosphate reabsorption giving rise to rickets. Clinically, a male hemizygote will be more seriously affected than a female. Bow legs are usually detected when the child begins to walk at 12–18 months of age. Premature sagittal synostosis may be seen. The serum calcium is normal but the serum phosphate is low and hence it is a hypophosphataemic form of Mendelian rickets. X-rays show typical features of rickets. Autosomal dominant hypophosphataemic rickets (HBD) also shows normal serum calcium but with a low serum phosphate: males and females are equally affected. Treatment of both XLH and HBD consists of giving vitamin D in a dose of 10 000–50 000 i.v. of calciferol and a phosphate solution to counteract the loss of phosphate in the urine in the form of Joulie's solution in a dose of 5–15 ml five times a day. Joulie's solution is made up of dibasic sodium phosphate (136 g per volume) and phosphoric acid (85 per cent, 58.8 g per volume) in one litre of tap water. The pH is 4.9 with an osmolality of 1725 mosmol and provides 30.4 mg of organic phosphates per ml. With the above dose, the serum phosphate should be kept above 3 mg/dl. Surgical osteotomy may be resorted to if the bone deformities are severe.

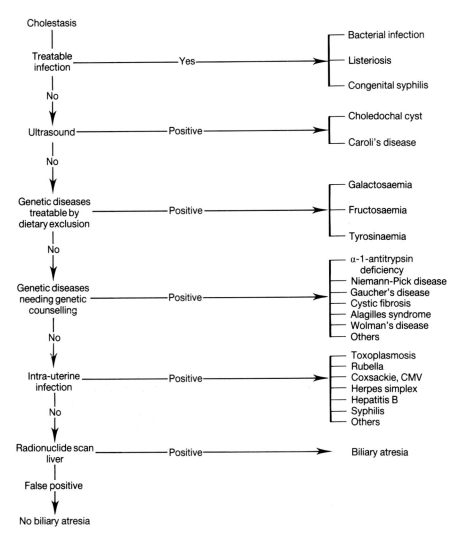

Fig. 5.7.9 Diagnostic strategy for identifying causes of direct hyperbilirubinaemia of infancy.

In the vitamin D-dependent rickets (VDD) serum phosphate is low but, unlike the hypophosphataemic rickets (XLH and HBD), serum calcium is also low. VDD are referred to as calciopenic rickets. The mode of inheritance is also different in that they are autosomal recessive. In type I VDD rickets, there is a failure of renal conversion of $25(OH)D_3$ to $1,25(OH)_2D_3$, i.e. a deficiency of D-1 α-hydroxylase in the kidney. Therefore, there is a marked decrease in serum $1,25(OH)_2D_3$. In type II VDD rickets, the serum $1,25(OH)_2D_3$ is normal or high but there is an end-organ failure to respond to $1,25(OH)_2D_3$. The clinical features of rickets are similar to the hypophosphataemic rickets, and treatment of VDD type I rickets consists of the use of $1,25(OH)_2D_3$. It is more difficult to treat VDD type II but larger doses of $1,25(OH)_2D_3$ may be needed.

Fanconi's syndrome causing rickets usually results in failure of renal tubular reabsorption of phosphates as well as other renal tubular defects. The syndrome can be idiopathic or occur in various disorders such as cystinosis and galactosaemia. It can also be acquired, as in tetracycline poisoning. Treatment consists of phosphate supplements and $1,25(OH)_2D_3$ with additions e.g. of potassium, water, bicarbonate, etc., depending on the number of substances which are not reabsorbed in addition to the phosphates.

References

1 Stanbury JB, Kroc RC. *Human development and the thyroid gland and relation to endemic cretinism*. New York, Plenum, 1972.

2 Glorieux J, La Vecchio FA. Psychological and neurological development in congenital hypothyroidism. In: Dussaulf JH, Walker P eds. *Congenital Hypothyroidism*. London, Butterworths, 1983. pp. 411-30.

3 Fisher DA. Pathogenesis and therapy of neonatal Grave's disease. *American Journal of Diseases of Children*. 1976; **130**: 133-4.

4 West KM. Diabetes in the tropics: some lessons for western diabetology. In: Podolsky S, Viswarathan M eds. *Secondary diabetes*. New York, Raven Press. 1980. pp. 249-55.

5 Wong HB. Insulin-dependent diabetes mellitus: strategy for prevention and management. *Annals of the Academy of Medicine, Singapore*. 1985; **14**: 334-42.

6 Lie WK, Wong HB. An approach to the diagnosis and treatment of Cushing's Syndrome in children. *Journal of the Singapore Paediatric Society*. 1985; **27**: 69-73.

7 Gold EM. The Cushing Syndrome: changing views in diagnosis and treatment. *Annals of Internal Medicine*. 1979; **90**: 829-44.

8 Wong HB. Some endocrine and metabolism emergencies in infants and children. *Journal of the Singapore Paediatric Society*. 1983; **25**: 44-51.

9 Lewin IG, Papapoulos SE, Tomlinson S *et al*. Studies of hypoparathyroidism and pseudohypoparathyroidism. *Quarterly Journal of Medicine*. 1978; **47**: 533-48.

10 Steichen JJ, Gratton TC, Tsang RC. Osteopenia of prematurity; the cause and possible treatment. *Journal of Pediatrics*. 1980; **96**: 528-34.

11 Hetzel BS. *The Story of Iodine Deficiency: an International Challenge in Nutrition*. Oxford, Oxford University Press, 1989. pp. xii, 236.

Haematological disorders

C. Chintu

The bone marrow manufactures at least three cellular components of the blood: erythrocytes, platelets and granulocytes. All these cells arise from a pluripotential stem cell which produces, after appropriate stimuli, three types of committed stem cells. These three types produce, respectively, the erythroid series, the megakaryocytic series and the granulocytic series. The range of haemotological disorders encountered is illustrated in Table 5.8.1. Erythroid disorders are discussed first.

Table 5.8.1 Epidemiology of blood diseases in children in the tropics.

Nutritional anaemias	
Parasitic diseases	— hookworm
	— malaria
	— kala-azar (visceral leishmaniasis)
Genetic anaemias	— haemoglobinopathies
	— thalassaemias
	— G6PD deficiency with haemolysis
Eosinophilia	— intestinal helminths
	— filariasis
	— allergy (asthma, eczema)
Purpura	— meningococcal septicaemia
	— dengue haemorrhagic fever
	— Brazilian purpuric fever
Leukaemia	— acute lymphoblastic leukaemia
Lymphomas	— Burkitt's lymphoma
	— Hodgkin's disease
	— lymphosarcoma

Anaemia

Anaemia is defined as a haemoglobin concentration or packed cell volume below the normal range for age and sex. Anaemia is not a disease in itself but a sign of many disorders. Common causes are shown in Table 5.8.2.

Table 5.8.2 Common causes of childhood anaemia in the tropics.

Low birth weight
Nutritional deficiencies of iron, folate, cyanocobalamin
Infections that interfere with food intake and intestinal
  absorption — diarrhoea, respiratory infections, measles
Parasites — hookworm, *Trichuris* (whipworm), malaria,
  leishmaniasis, schistosomiasis
Genetic anaemias — haemoglobinopathies (HbS, HbE),
  thalassaemias
Loss of intact red blood cells

In many children, more than one of the listed causes contributes to the anaemia.

Symptoms and signs

General symptoms of anaemia include lethargy, fatigue, sleeplessness, impaired memory, poor concentration, palpitations, throbbing headache, anorexia, and shortness of breath on slight exertion. Other symptoms relate to the cause of anaemia, for example chills and fever in malaria. Atrophic changes in the stomach may lead to dysphagia and the Plummer–Vinson syndrome.

The signs of anaemia include pallor, tachycardia, a collapsing pulse in severe anaemia, pedal oedema, and atrophic glossitis (see also p. 780). Other signs relate to the specific cause of anaemia, for example jaundice and splenomegaly in haemolytic disorders. In iron-deficiency anaemia the nails break and splinter haemorrhages may be seen; the concave appearance of the nails is referred to as koilonychia. Cracking of and soreness of the mouth as well as corners of the mouth (angular stomatitis) are often associated, although these changes may also occur in other deficiencies such as of vitamin B_{12} and other B group vitamins.

Investigation

The nutritional history, episodes of bleeding and chronic ill health have a major bearing on the choice of investigative procedures (see p. 982). The history, coupled with physical examination will lead one to the most appropriate laboratory tests, listed in Fig 5.8.1 (see also p. 975). To these may be added a thick film for malaria parasites, stool microbiology and a serum bilirubin. Anaemia can be objectively diagnosed by measuring the haemoglobin concentration and haematocrit. The haematocrit is roughly three times the haemoglobin concentration. These two indices may provide values of mean corpuscular haemoglobin concentration (MCHC). The relationship is shown in the following equation (Hb = haemoglobin; PCV = packed cell volume).

$$\underset{\text{(g/dl)}}{\text{MCHC}} = \frac{\text{Hb (g/dl)}}{\text{PCV}}$$

The normal MCHC value = 31–35 g/dl. This range cannot be exceeded, as the red blood cells are normally filled with haemoglobin. However, low values (below this range) are found in iron deficiency, thalassaemia, and other microcytic anaemias.

The red cell count (RBC) and PCV are useful in the

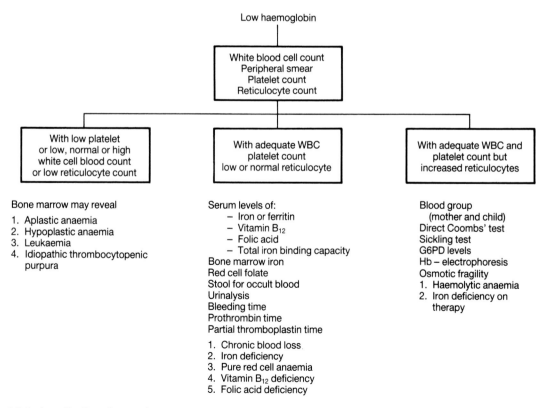

Fig. 5.8.1 Investigation of anaemia.

calculation of mean corpuscular volume (MCV) and mean haemoglobin concentration (MCH).

$$MCV \text{ (fl)} = \frac{PCV}{RBC/l} \times 10^{15}$$

Normal MCV value = 78–85 fl

$$MCH \text{ (pg)} = \frac{Hb \text{ (g/l)}}{RBC/l} \times 10^{12}$$

Normal MCH value = 24–34 pg
(pg = picogram; fl = femtolitre)

Estimates of the 'normal' haematological values in the tropics and subtropics are scanty and vary from region to region; they depend upon environmental, economic, geographical, and perhaps genetic factors. The newborn has high haemoglobin concentrations in the range of 160–180 g/l. Thereafter the haemoglobin concentration begins to drop as erythropoiesis decreases. In a normal, nutritionally well-fed infant the haemoglobin concentration begins to rise after three months of age to levels above 110 g/l. From 6 to 14 years the haemoglobin concentration rises to 120 g/l and may reach adult levels thereafter (Fig. 5.8.2).

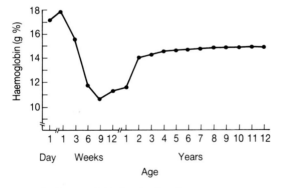

Fig. 5.8.2 Haemoglobin levels at various ages.

The peripheral blood examination will enable abnormalities of the shape, size and haemoglobinization of the red blood cells to be identified (Table 5.8.3). Examination of the peripheral smear will reveal the morphology of the white cells and give an indication of the numbers. Very immature cells indicative of leukaemia will be evident on a peripheral smear. In the tropics, eosinophilia would be indicative of parasitic infestation. Platelet counts would reveal thrombocytopenia which sometimes may accompany immune thrombocytopenic purpura, aplastic anaemia or leukaemia. A peripheral

Table 5.8.3   Red blood cell morphological abnormalities.

RBC morphology	Commonly seen
Microcytosis with hypochromia	Iron-deficiency anaemia Thalassaemia Pyridoxine deficiency
Macrocytosis	Folic acid deficiency Vitamin B_{12} deficiency Thiamine deficiency
Microcytes and macrocytes	Multiple nutritional deficiency as in kwashiorkor and marasmus
Microspherocytes	Congenital hereditary spherocytosis ABO haemolytic disease
Reticulocytosis and normoblasts	Active erythropoiesis (as in haemolytic anaemia and in iron deficiency on iron therapy)
Target cells (increased)	Thalassaemia, haemoglobinopathy, and liver disease
Heinz bodies	Postsplenectomy, functional asplenia, e.g. sickle cell anaemia, congenital asplenia Certain drugs
Parasite in RBC	Malaria
Distorted RBC Acanthocytes	Liver disease, rare congenital haemolytic anaemia
Burr cells	Microangiopathic haemolytic anaemia and renal disease

smear may sometimes be used to estimate the adequacy of platelets in the peripheral blood if other methods of platelet count are not available.

The serum ferritin and serum iron are both low in iron-deficiency anaemia. Although the former is more sensitive, ferritin is an acute-phase protein and is high during acute infections, even when iron deficiency is present. The sensitivity of serum ferritin is therefore decreased in the tropics where infections are common. Absence of stainable bone marrow iron may indicate depletion of iron stores, but not necessarily anaemia. Total iron binding capacity is quite high in iron deficiency and like serum ferritin or serum iron is useful in following therapy.

Serum or red folate levels are low in macrocytic anaemia due to folic acid deficiency. Since vitamin B_{12} may produce the same peripheral blood and bone marrow smear, it is prudent to measure both folate and vitamin B_{12} if possible. However, folic acid deficiency is more common in children than vitamin B_{12} deficiency, particularly in severe protein–energy malnutrition and chronic haemolytic anaemias.

Reticulocyte counts are low in untreated iron deficiency, in leukaemia, and in hypoplastic or aplastic anaemia due to any cause. The white blood cell count is low in hypoplastic or aplastic anaemia, although in the early stages the count may be at the lower limit of normal. In the black African there is relative leucopenia. Where doubts exist, a bone marrow aspiration may resolve the issue. In a few cases, the bone marrow aspiration may be normal initially because of patchy hypoplastic or aplastic sites in various areas of the bone marrow.

Bone marrow aspiration (see p. 1011) may yield information leading to the diagnosis of infiltrative lesions, such as leukaemia, neuroblastoma, myelofibrosis, and lipid storage diseases such as Gaucher's disease. It may also reveal features of hypoplasia or aplasia. Special stains may show ringed sideroblasts and an absence of stainable iron. Evidence of parasites (e.g. malaria and trypanosomes) may also be seen.

Iron deficiency anaemia

Iron deficiency is the most common cause of anaemia in children in the subtropics and tropics, and indeed in the whole world. A committee on nutrition of the American Academy of Pediatrics recommended that all infants receive iron-fortified formula until at least 12 months of age.

The growing fetus is an efficient parasite and draws its iron requirement from its mother against a concentration gradient. The fetus may thus become iron replete at the expense of the mother. In the newborn, most of the iron is in the circulating red blood cell, followed by the liver, tissue and bone marrow. The haemoglobin concentration is reduced during the first few weeks of an infant's life, being lowest at about two to three months of age. This is because of the reduced life span of the fetal red cell and the decreased erythropoiesis due to an initial polycythemic state. The released iron is stored in the bone marrow for future use.

At about four months of age erythropoiesis becomes active and the iron stores are mobilized in the formation of haemoglobin, myoglobin, and other tissue enzymes such as the cytochrome group of enzymes. If no exogenous supply of iron is given to the infant the iron stores will be depleted. It is estimated that among 12–18 month old infants of economically deprived families in America, the incidence of iron deficiency is approximately 40 per cent. The incidence is higher in African countries where the peak of protein–energy malnutrition is between 12 and 18 months.

Iron deficiency is not synonymous with iron-deficiency anaemia; one can be iron deficient without being anaemic. About 10 per cent of the naturally occurring iron in cereals, in green and yellow vegetables, strained meat, fortified milk formulas and fruits is absorbed by a full-term infant. Cow's milk is a poor source of iron and breast-milk has 0.3 mg of iron per litre (half of this is absorbed by the intestine). Iron absorption from vegetables may be enhanced by the addition of meat, fish or foods containing vitamin C, such as citrus fruits. Preterm infants do not absorb iron as efficiently as full-term newborns.

The total body iron of an adult is about 5 g, whereas that of infant is about 0.5 g. To make up the deficit which goes to production of haemoglobin, myoglobin and other enzymes, the infant should take in approximately 0.8 mg of iron per day. Additional iron is required to replace the ongoing losses in the gastro-intestinal tract and sweat, so that daily requirements of 0.8–1.5 mg are required during infancy, childhood and early adolescence. Since only 10 per cent of iron is absorbed, a daily intake of 10–15 mg iron must be ingested, for growth, protein and haemoglobin synthesis (see also p. 384).

Causes of iron deficiency

The causes of iron deficiency are many and there is often interaction between causative agents or factors. The causes are as follows:

Inadequate supply of iron

- Prematurity, twins and low-birth-weight babies.
- Fetal blood loss at or before delivery in conditions such as abruptio placenta, placenta praevia, twin-to-twin transfusion, bleeding from an unclamped cord.

Inadequate intake of iron

- Lack of adequate iron in diet.
- Prolonged milk feeding without supplementary cereals or semi-solids.

Impaired absorption

- Chronic diarrhoea in protein–energy malnutrition.
- Malabsorption.
- Gastro-intestinal abnormality.
- Milk allergy.

Blood loss

- Acute haemorrhage – concealed or external.
- Parasitic infection – hookworm, amoebiasis, schistosomiasis.

Laboratory investigation

The haemoglobin will be less than 10 g/dl. The MCV is also decreased to less than 24 pg, the MCH to less than 78 fl, and the MCHC to less than 30 g/dl. The peripheral blood smears show microcytosis and hypochromia. The reticulocyte count is low, although after haemorrhage it may be as high as 3–6 per cent. Thrombocytopenia may be present; the white cell count is normal. Stool examination should be done to exclude hookworm or *Trichuris trichuria* or gastro-intestinal bleeding. Urinalysis is important to exclude *Schistosoma haematobium* as cause of loss of blood in the urine. The platelet counts may be low in immune thrombocytopenica purpura, aplastic and hypoplastic anaemia; they are also low in hypersplenism. The bone marrow may show absence of stainable iron. The serum iron is reduced and transferrin saturation is also low, below 120 μg. In the absence of this test, a low haemoglobin alone should be an indication for iron therapy.

Treatment

A definite diagnosis should be made wherever possible before giving iron. The most common preparation and cheapest form of iron is ferrous sulphate which contains 20 per cent elemental iron by weight, whereas ferrous gluconate contains 10–12 per cent by weight. A total of 6 mg/kg of elemental iron in three divided doses for three or four weeks is recommended and provides adequate treatment. The iron must be given between meals, as some foods interfere with its absorption.

In rare cases where oral iron cannot be taken, parenteral iron may be used; the indications include:

- intolerance of oral iron;
- poor absorption in small bowel malabsorption syndromes;
- frequent blood loss;
- when the patient is unreliable in taking oral iron, e.g. mentally disturbed patients.

The dose required to raise the Hb above 10 g/dl (normally to 12.5 g/dl) can be calculated from the following formula:

$$\text{Blood volume} \times \frac{12.5 - \text{Hb}}{100} \times 3.4 = \text{Dose (mg)}$$

The blood volume of children is approximately 70–80 ml/kg body weight.

Iron dextran complex and iron sorbital citric acid complex are available; however, these may cause anaphylactic reactions, urticaria, oedema, arthralgia and fever. Infants in tropical countries such as Papua New Guinea who received intramuscular injections of iron dextran have been found to suffer increased attacks of *P. falciparum* malaria and respiratory infections. In the newborn an increase in Gram-negative bacterial meningitis has been reported.

The response to parenteral therapy is no different from oral therapy and a reticulocytosis is expected within three to four days. Blood transfusion is reserved for those who are:

- acutely bleeding;
- in cardiac failure;
- severely anaemic in association with infection, particularly respiratory.

If there are no facilities for testing donor blood for HIV infection, transfusion should only be done as a last resort. Transfusion in the presence of severe cardiac failure must be approached with great caution. Very often the symptoms and signs of cardiac failure due to severe anaemia will abate when the child is propped up in bed at rest. If blood transfusion is decided upon, it should be given as packed cells, slowly and combined with a diuretic. The venous pressure in neck veins and liver and signs of pulmonary congestion must be oberved. Sometimes a modified exchange transfusion will save a child in extremis.

Hypoplastic and aplastic anaemias

Hypoplastic anaemias represent a heterogenous group of disorders in which the production of red blood cells and their precursors is depressed. Acquired hypoplastic anaemia is uncommon. Chronic hypofunction of erythropoiesis may be congenital or secondary to systemic disorders such as renal disease, collagen diseases, chronic infection and certain endocrine deficiencies. In all these conditions, the basic and underlying cause must be treated before the anaemia can be expected to improve.

Acute aplastic anaemia

Idiopathic erythroblastopenia is a transient condition occurring in infants and young children. The aetiology is unknown but it is sometimes preceded by a respiratory illness suggesting an infectious cause. The previously normal haemoglobin can drop to as low as 8 g/dl with a reticulocyte count in the range of 0–0.2 per cent. The serum iron is elevated and evidence for haemolysis is lacking.

The peripheral blood smear is normocytic and normochromic. The white cells and platelets are normal. Most patients recover in about a year's time, or sooner with the use of prednisone.

Hypoplastic anaemia can be induced by radiation, chemical agents (e.g. benzene, lead, insecticide), and drugs (e.g. chloramphenicol, gold-containing drugs, sulphonamides). The resulting pancytopenia is associated with infections and bleeding episodes, as well as the signs and symptoms of anaemia. A careful history of drug ingestion and exposure to chemicals is therefore very important in investigating selective depression of red blood cell precursors. Withdrawal of the offending drug or toxic substance often leads to cure or the arrest of the progression of the disease. Prednisone in doses of 1–2 mg per kg body weight per day may be useful. Supportive blood transfusions may help to relieve the symptoms. Blood transfusion must be weighed against the development of iron overload and infections such as hepatitis B and acquired immune deficiency syndrome (AIDS).

Replacement of bone marrow with infiltration of abnormal tissue should be considered in some cases of aplastic anaemia. This may occur in leukaemia, neuroblastomas and lipid storage diseases.

Pure red cell aplasia may occur in protein–energy malnutrition. A good number of these patients respond to riboflavine administration orally or intramuscularly. The red cell aplasia in protein–energy malnutrition is independent of folic acid and vitamin B_{12} deficiencies. In any haemolytic anaemia, depression of the regeneration of the red blood cell may lead to decompensation in a patient with a chronic haemolytic process as occurs in sickle cell disease, congenital spherocytosis and thalassaemia.

Congenital aplastic anaemia (Blackfan–Diamond syndrome)

This was described by Blackfan and Diamond and is a primary defect resulting in selective depression of red blood cell production. It has been reported in families, although a few cases are sporadic. Abnormalities in tryptophan metabolism have been implicated but the cause of the condition is unknown. It is associated with congenital malformations such as skeletal or renal abnormalities, mental retardation, and congenital heart disease. It presents in early infancy with symptoms of anaemia.

Treatment

The mainstay of treatment is steroids. Prednisone in doses of 20–30 mg/day produces normalization of the haemoglobin and reticulocytes. The stunting of growth is serious and the minimal dose required to maintain near-normal levels of haemoglobin must be used. The steroids probably work by interfering with the erythroid inhibitors. Supportive blood transfusion should be given carefully to avoid iron overload. About 50 per cent of patients respond to this therapy.

Haemolytic anaemias

This group includes a variety of disorders which are characterized by a reduction in the life span of red blood cells. The most common causes are shown in Table 5.8.4.

Table 5.8.4 Causes of haemolytic anaemias.

With minor splenomegaly
  G6PD deficiency
  Autoimmune haemolytic anaemia
  Haemolytic–uraemic syndrome
  β-thalassaemia minor (heterozygous)
  HbH thalassaemia
  HbE thalassaemia
  Acute infections such as malaria
  Sickle cell anaemia in older children
With marked splenomegaly
  Sickle cell disease
  β-thalassaemia major
  HbE β-thalassaemia
  Hereditary spherocytosis
  Malaria in tropical splenomegaly syndrome
  Visceral leishmaniasis (kala-azar)

In the full-term newborn, blood group incompatibility, glucose-6-phosphate dehydrogenase (G6PD) deficiency and infection are the most common causes (see pp. 222–8, 440). The rhesus blood group is rare in tropical Africa. As rhesus disease becomes less in other parts of the tropics and subtropics, through passive immunization during pregnancy and immediately after delivery, ABO haemolytic disease and G6PD will become the major causes of anaemia and neonatal jaundice. It should be emphasized that haemolytic anaemia in the newborn, from whatever cause, is usually accompanied by jaundice. Haemolytic anaemias associated with both jaundice and tea-coloured urine are due to intravascular haemolysis; the urine colour is due to haemoglobinuria which can be detected in the urine spectroscopically. Of course haematuria and bile must be excluded.

Intravascular haemolysis can occur in G6PD-deficient people if predisposing factors such as ingestion of oxidant drugs, fava beans and infections are present. The inheritance of G6PD deficiency is most commonly sex-linked, thus affecting males. In autoimmune haemolysis the Coomb's test is positive; it is negative in G6PD deficiency.

Therapy depends upon the cause of the anaemia. Very often treating the cause, such as treatment of malaria, or removal of oxidant drugs in a G6PD-deficient person, will stop further haemolysis. Supportive management, such as exchange transfusion in the newborn with severe anaemia and jaundice, is life saving. Simple blood transfusion is also indicated when the anaemia is acute or is causing incapacitating symptoms. Splenectomy improves anaemia in spherocytosis but does not cure the disease. In all chronic haemolytic anaemia, folic acid is indicated because of very active erythropoiesis.

Haemoglobinopathies

In early fetal life there are two types of haemoglobin: Gower 1 and Gower 2. Gower 1 consists of four E chains whereas Gower 2 consists of α_2 and ϵ_2 chains. These are replaced late in fetal life by fetal haemoglobin (HbF) of $\alpha_2 \gamma_2$ chains, HbA_2 of $\alpha_2 \delta_2$ chains and HbA of $\alpha_2 \beta_2$ chains. After birth the production of γ chains is switched off, so that in adult life the only normal haemoglobin of significance is HbA; HbF and HbA_2 may persist in late childhood in a smaller percentage than at birth.

Haemoglobinopathies are disorders which result from the production of abnormal haemoglobin chains because of the substitution of an amino acid in one of the globin chains due to the alteration of a single base in a codon (triple-base code) in a gene. Inadequate synthesis of normal haemoglobin occurs in thalassaemia syndromes.

Sickle cell diseases

Sickle cell diseases are characterized by the inheritance of two abnormal genes responsible for the formation of haemoglobin. One of the two abnormal genes is responsible for the formation of haemoglobin S (HbS). Examples of sickle cell diseases are HbSS, HbSC and HbS – Thalassaemia.

Sickle cell haemoglobin (HbS) is the product of the substitution of valine for glutamic acid in position 6 of the β chain and the mutant gene is inherited in an autosomal recessive manner. HbC results from a replacement of glutamic acid by lysine in position 6 of the β chain. In the homozygous (sickle cell anaemia) state, haemolytic anaemia is induced when the haemoglobin is deoxygenated leading to sickling (polymerization of HbS molecules into filaments) of the erythrocyte.

The sickle cell gene is widespread throughout Africa where its incidence ranges from 5 to 40 per cent. It is also found in South America, the West Indies, the United States, Greece, Cyprus, the Middle East and India.

Both the heterozygous state (HbAS) and homozygous state (HbSS) can be demonstrated by the sickling test, but only the homozygous state shows anaemia. The homozygous state, or sickle cell anaemia, has about 60–90 per cent haemoglobin S with the remainder being fetal haemoglobin; no normal haemoglobin (HbA) is produced. Heterozygous carriers (HbAS) have some protection from infection with *P. falciparum* malaria, and this accounts for the selection and perpetuation of the gene for sickle haemoglobin.

Clinical features The clinical course of sickle cell anaemia (HbSS) tends to be more severe in Africans than in Saudi Arabs because the latter possess some

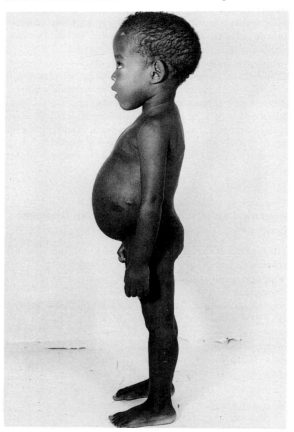

Fig. 5.8.3 Bossing of the skull and hepatosplenomegaly in sickle-cell anaemia.

fetal haemoglobin (HbF) that protects red cells from sickling at low oxygen tension. Homozygous (HbSS) individuals may become symptomatic after the third month of life when production of fetal haemoglobin decreases naturally. One-third of patients develop symptoms by their first birthday and two-thirds by their second birthday. Extramedullary haematopoiesis may result in hepatosplenomegaly and skull bossing (Fig 5.8.3). The increased diploë can be seen radiologically as a 'hair on end' appearance (Fig 5.8.4a). Features of sickle cell anaemia during the first two years include: *dactylitis* – painful swelling of fingers or toes (hand–foot syndrome) due to vascular occlusion with sickled cells of capillaries supplying the digits (Fig 5.8.5); *pneumococcal infection* involving the lungs and meninges or presenting as septicaemia; *acute splenic sequestration* with acute enlargement of the spleen trapping a significant volume of red cells and causing a sudden fall in haemoglobin concentration and the risk of death from circulatory failure. This last complication is often preceded by a minor illness such as an upper respiratory tract infection. Recurrence of acute splenic sequestration is common but may be prevented by splenectomy. Prompt transfusion to maintain the peripheral circulation is needed during episodes of acute splenic sequestration. Both the tendency to acute splenic sequestration and susceptibility to pneumococcal infections reflect impaired functioning of the spleen in early childhood. Enlargement of the spleen may no longer be palpable by the age of eight years because of repeated infarcts and subsequent fibrosis.

As the child grows older, the typical facies and body morphology of sickle cell disease becomes apparent (Fig. 5.8.3). Bossing of the head, hyperplasia of the maxillae disproportionately long arms and legs as compared to the trunk, abdominal protrusion and mild icterus develop. Children beyond the preschool age suffer *painful vaso-occlusive crises* with acute attacks of bone pain in the arms, legs, joints, back or chest, or of abdominal pain with nausea and vomiting (see p. 897). The pain may last from hours to days. Infection, particularly malaria, is often a cause of these crises when

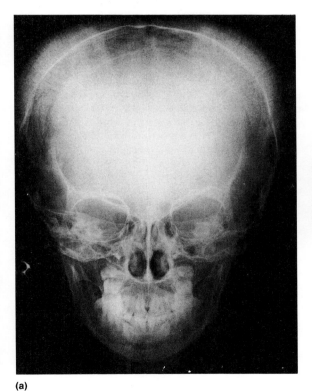

(a)

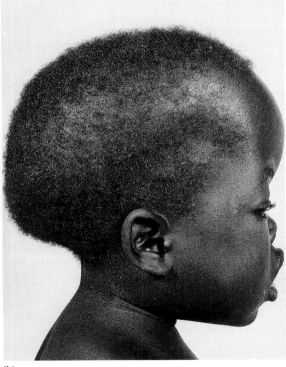

(b)

Fig. 5.8.4 a) X-ray of skull in sickle-cell anaemia, showing 'hair on end' appearance and loss of medulla. b) External appearance.

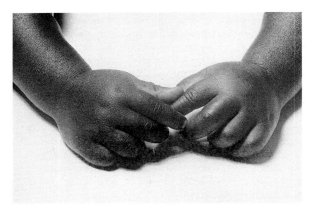

Fig. 5.8.5   Sickle-cell anaemia hand–foot syndrome.

patients have fever, dehydration and a rapid pulse rate. Avascular necrosis of bones, e.g. femoral head and humeral head, may lead to joint deformity. Osteomyelitis is another complication of sickle cell disease and the pathogens are *Salmonella* and *Staphylococcus* in more than half the cases.

Sickle cell nephropathy with haematuria and glomerular damage is described on p. 791.

Aplastic crises with depression of red cell precursors in the bone marrow and severe anaemia of rapid onset are usually associated with parvovirus infection. Epidemics of aplastic crises all related to recent parvovirus infection have been reported in Jamaica during the decade 1975–85.

In adolescence, retardation of physical and sexual development creates special problems. Advice on contraception is needed on attainment of sexual maturity, although with proper management, risks during pregnancy are small. Chronic leg ulceration develops most frequently during adolescence.

Sickle cell disease in Saudi Arabia is common in oasis areas where 1 in 250 are born with HbSS. These Arabs with HbSS tend to have a milder disease because of high levels of fetal haemoglobin and a high prevalence of α thalassaemia. Fetal haemoglobin prevents sickling of deoxygenated HbS molecules. Anaemia is mild (Hb 8–10 g/dl). Painful vaso-occlusive crises are the most frequent reason for medical attention and these tend to occur in the winter months. Splenic function is lost more slowly than in Africans, but there is still an increased risk of pneumococcal infection.

Diagnosis   This depends on the presence of sickled red cells on microscopy of blood mixed with one drop of 2 per cent sodium metabisulphite solution (sickling test). Haemoglobin electrophoresis shows the presence of HbS (which moves more slowly than adult haemoglobin), and the absence of HbA.

Management   General measures, such as nutrition, prophylaxis against infection, and prompt diagnosis and therapy of infections, are important in children with sickle cell disease. The avoidance of extremes of temperature, maintenance of hydration, and education of patient and family about the disease are also recommended. *Folic acid* supplements are required, particularly in Africa. Zinc supplementation improves healing of leg ulcers. Iron supplementation should be avoided, except in the presence of marked iron deficiency.

All children with sickle cell disease should be given a full course of *immunization* against diphtheria, tetanus, whooping cough, poliomyelitis, measles and tuberculosis. Protection against pneumococcal infection is recommended, using prophylactic penicillin from the age of six months. Pneumococcal immunization with polyvalent vaccine may be delayed until two years of age and revaccination done at four years before termination of penicillin prophylaxis. Protection against malaria must be given until adulthood. The antimalarial drug prescribed depends on geography, e.g. pyrimethamine 25 mg weekly for West Africa and chloroquine 150 mg weekly in other countries (see pp. 672–3).

Infections should be treated promptly with appropriate parenteral antibiotics and hydration because dehydration and haemoconcentration precipitate painful crises.

Blood transfusion is indicated in acute splenic sequestration when there is a precipitate fall in haemoglobin, and during aplastic crises when patients become severely anaemic (see also p. 780). Patients requiring anaesthesia and surgery are given a blood transfusion to dilute the concentration of circulating red cells with HbS in order to avoid vaso-occlusive complications. The number of blood transfusions received by a patient should be monitored to avoid iron overload.

The ultimate therapy in sickle cell disease would be the administration of therapeutic agents that would inhibit sickling. However, there is no single effective agent currently available.

Prognosis   The survival and quality of life enjoyed by these children has improved with the control of malaria by chemoprophylaxis, with prompt treatment of infections, and through better nutrition. However, homozygous HbS individuals still have a mortality rate in excess of 10 per cent in Jamaica in the first two years of life, in spite of the absence of malaria. Most deaths occur during the first five years of life. The principal causes of death are acute splenic sequestration, pneumococcal pneumonia, septicaemia and meningitis.

As the child grows older, symptoms tend to decrease and health improves. Unfortunately some children suffer cerebral infarction, sometimes repeated, which may leave them handicapped (as in cerebral palsy) to a greater or lesser extent for the rest of their lives.

Thalassaemias

Thalassaemia is an inherited disorder of haemoglobin production in which there is a reduction in the rate of synthesis of one globin chain resulting in anaemia. There are two main types: one affecting the synthesis of α chains of haemoglobin (α-thalassaemia) and the other affecting the synthesis of β chains (β-thalassaemia).

Thalassaemia was originally described in people of Mediterranean origin, thus gaining its name from the Greek word *thalassa*, the sea. However, this condition has since been found to be widespread in the Middle East, India, and South-east Asia. The severe form of anaemia, β-thalassaemia, presents early in life and is associated with splenomegaly and bone changes.

The α-thalassaemias are prevalent in Saudi Arabia, Thailand and other parts of South-east Asia, Greece, Italy and Africa. The deficiency of α-chains leads to an excess of γ-chains in the fetus and β-chains in the adult. These globin chains are unstable and form tetramers, HbBart's ($\gamma 4$) and HbH ($\beta 4$) that are unable to delivery adequate oxygen to the tissues because of their oxygen affinity. The clinical presentation of α-thalassaemia can vary from lethal hydrops fetalis to mild anaemia.

β-thalassaemia

This is a condition in which there is a deficiency of β chain production with a consequent net excess of α chains produced in normal amounts. This imbalance in globin chains leads to precipitation of the α chains in the bone marrow and in erythrocytes, resulting in ineffective erythropoiesis, a shortened red cell life span and anaemia. Two main types of β-thalassaemia are recognized on the basis of β chain synthesis: β-thalassaemia$^+$ and β-thalassaemia^0 in which there is partial or total deficiency of β chain production respectively. Clinical features of these two types of β-thalassaemia are similar and the conditions can only be diagnosed on haemoglobin electrophoresis. β-thalassaemia^0 occurs in Greece, Northern Italy, parts of the Middle East, Indian subcontinent, and South-east Asia. β-thalassaemia$^+$ is found in other parts of Italy and is the usual form in Negroes. A less common type of β-thalassaemia, $\delta \beta$-thalassaemia, results from suppression of both β and δ chain synthesis. Interaction occurs between β-thalassaemia and β chain variants; for

example, in HbS producing sickle cell thalassaemia the severity of the condition depends upon the possession of the β-thalassaemia^0 gene.

The usual form of β-thalassaemia is inherited in an autosomal recessive manner, the affected child having both parents heterozygous for the abnormal gene. There is a high incidence of the β-thalassaemia gene (1–15 per cent) in Mediterranean, Middle Eastern and South-east Asian countries.

Homozygous β-thalassaemia, a condition of severe anaemia, was first described in 1925 by Thomas Cooley and Lee, in children who died unless frequent blood transfusions were given.

Clinical features Although affected infants are normal at birth, anaemia of insidious onset is obvious by the third month of life and becomes progressively severe. The infant fails to thrive and may have intermittent fever, poor feeding and non-specific symptoms of ill-health. Parents usually seek medical help during the first six months when the infant has pallor with splenomegaly. There is stunting of growth in children, who also show skeletal changes due to hyperplasia of the bone marrow in the skull (bossing of the frontal bones) and of maxillary bones resulting in a characteristic appearance – the thalassaemic facies. Radiological findings associated with these skeletal changes include the 'hair on end' appearance in the skull and widening of the cortex of bones in the hands and feet. Moderate to marked hepatosplenomegaly is present and skin pigmentation is increased. Puberty is delayed and secondary sex characteristics undeveloped.

Most children with homozygous β-thalassaemia require regular blood transfusions. General health is poor from chronic haemolytic anaemia complicated by recurrent infections and folic acid deficiency. As the spleen enlarges, secondary hypersplenism with thrombocytopenia and leucopenia may develop and increase the tendency to bleeding and infection.

Repeated blood transfusions and increased intestinal absorption of iron, resulting from ineffective erythropoiesis and chronic anaemia, lead to haemosiderosis and death in the second and third decades from cardiac failure as a result of iron deposition in the myocardium. Pancreatic haemosiderosis may cause diabetes mellitus and iron deposition in the liver results in nodular cirrhosis.

Haematological findings The blood picture resembles that of severe iron-deficiency anaemia. Anaemia is usually severe with haemoglobin levels of 2–5 g/dl. Examination of a stained peripheral blood film shows marked anisocytosis (variation in size) and poikilocytosis (varied cell shape) of the erythrocytes.

Microcytosis predominates, hypochromia is striking, target cells are prominent, and tear-drop cells and cell fragments are often seen before splenectomy. The reticulocyte count is elevated and some nucleated red cells are usually present. Granular cytoplasmic inclusion bodies, representing aggregates of α chains, may be demonstrated by the staining with methyl violet of normoblasts and reticulocytes of splenectomized patients. The bone marrow shows marked erythroid hyperplasia, basophilic stippling of the erythroblasts and increased iron deposition. Haemoglobin electrophoresis in homozygous β-thalassaemia invariably shows an increase in fetal haemoglobin HbF (10–90 per cent). Adult haemoglobin HbA is absent in β-thalassaemia^0 while variable amounts are found in β-thalassaemia$^+$. HbA$_2$ may be reduced, normal or occasionally elevated. Small amounts of free α chains can be demonstrated on starch gel electrophoresis.

Red cell survival studies have nearly always shown a reduced ^{51}Cr survival time and two cell populations: one with normal survival containing HbF and the other with much shorter survival. The osmotic fragility test reveals an increased resistance to haemolysis. Serum bilirubin is usually slightly raised but insufficient to produce clinical jaundice. Serum iron is invariably elevated and the iron-binding protein completely saturated.

Pathophysiology of the anaemia   The anaemia of homozygous β-thalassaemia is the result of intramedullary red cell destruction, shortened red cell life span, secondary impairment of haem synthesis and peripheral circulatory haemodilution. The deficiency of β chain synthesis leads to a large excess of α chains. In some red cells, γ chains produced in relatively large amounts, combine with the α chains to form HbF and ensure a normal life span. In other cells where γ chain production is insufficient, the excess α chains rapidly precipitate. Cells with large α chain precipitates are destroyed within the bone marrow causing ineffective erythropoiesis. The less affected cells are released into the circulation and removed during passage through the spleen. These processes result in anaemia requiring blood transfusion which together with increased intestinal iron absorption produces haemosiderosis. Fetal haemoglobin has a high affinity for oxygen and releases less oxygen to the tissues than HbA. This factor compounds the tissue hypoxia caused by the anaemia and increases the production of erythopoietin which leads to bone marrow expansion and extramedullary haemopoiesis with skeletal and organ changes.

Management   There is no specific treatment for β-thalassaemia but non-specific measures of blood transfusion, folic acid, ascorbic acid and iron-chelating agents have been used with promising results. The basis of treatment is the correction of the anaemia without inducing iron overload and siderosis of vital organs. To achieve this, diagnosis should ideally be established in infancy. The haemoglobin concentration should be raised to the normal range and maintained at this level by blood transfusions. In 1964, Wolman reported that if a patient's haemoglobin was kept in the normal range by increasing transfusions to raise the haemoglobin from 9 g/dl to 14 g/dl the patient could live a normal life without shortening survival. Children exclusively treated from infancy with six-weekly blood transfusions that aim to raise the haemoglobin level from 9 g/dl to 14 g/dl are virtually normal until they are 12 years old when they start showing symptoms due to iron overload.

It is, therefore, necessary to use iron chelating agents to treat the fatal iron loading. Desferrioxamine is the drug that has been used since the mid-1960s. It has to be administered by subcutaneous or intravenous injection and its action is enhanced when ascorbic acid is given to correct deficiency of this vitamin associated with iron overload. Iron is excreted in urine and stool and about 200 mg of iron is removed in the urine during a 24-hour continuous infusion of desferrioxamine. In many cases, 12-hour overnight subcutaneous infusions given with a small syringe pump into the anterior abdominal wall may be as effective as 24-hour continuous infusions and interfere less with daily routine. These 12-hour subcutaneous infusions at doses as low as 0.5 g can produce negative iron balance in young children with previous transfusion iron loads of less than 10 g, so that iron toxicity may prove to be preventable. Infusions may be inconvenient for the patient but are superior to bolus injections in leaching iron. The dose of desferrioxamine required varies from 20 to 40 mg/kg per day. Desferrioxamine infusions should be given for six days per week together with ascorbic acid. Splenectomy would be required when hypersplenism is present. The recent advance in treatment by the use of an oral preparation, 1, 2-dimethyl-3-hydroxypyrid-4-one, which is an effective chelator of iron, gives hope to thalassaemic patients world-wide.

The policy of maintaining the patient's haemoglobin above 10 g/dl has reduced the need to resort to splenectomy for massive splenomegaly during early childhood when there is a major risk of life-threatening infection in splenectomized children. Splenectomy may be required in late adolescence when there is a progressive shortening of the interval between transfusions.

Heterozygous β-thalassaemia The carrier of the β-thalassaemia gene is usually asymptomatic until the stress of pregnancy or infection induces anaemia which does not respond to iron therapy. Clinical examination reveals little apart from a palpable spleen. The haemoglobin concentration is rarely less than 10 g/dl, the mean cell volume (MCV) and mean cell haemoglobin (MCH) are low but the mean cell haemoglobin concentration (MCHC) is often within the normal range. The blood film shows anisocytosis, microcytosis or moderate degree of hypochromia, basophilic stippling and a variable number of target cells. A reticulocyte count of 5 per cent is usual. The red cell osmotic fragility test shows an increased resistance to haemolysis. Haemoglobin electrophoresis shows an increase in HbA_2 (3.5–6.5 per cent) in most cases, and an HbF level seldom above 3 per cent. The main problem in diagnosis is the differentiation of this condition from iron deficiency. When iron deficiency develops in an individual with heterozygous β-thalassaemia the HbA_2 level may fall but is restored to its previous level when iron stores are replenished. If the HbA_2 and HbF levels are normal and the patient is not iron deficient, the possibility of α-thalassaemia should be considered in Middle Eastern and South-east Asian peoples. No treatment is required for heterozygous β-thalassaemia patients unless they develop symptomatic anaemia during pregnancy or infection, when folic acid supplements should be given. Iron is neither necessary nor helpful.

Prevention Recent interest has centred on the antenatal diagnosis of homozygous β-thalassaemia between 12 and 18 weeks and on the possible termination of affected pregnancies. *In vitro* globin chain synthesis techniques applied to pure fetal blood or to mixed maternal–fetal blood samples are capable of diagnosing homozygous β-thalassaemia^0 and β-thalassaemia$^+$. Analysis of chorion villus tissue may be a better method of prenatal diagnosis. It will be many years before antenatal diagnosis will be fully available in countries where thalassaemia is a common disorder.

α-thalassaemias

The α-thalassaemias are disorders in which there is defective synthesis of chains leading to an excess of γ chains in the fetus and β chains in the adult. There is a depression of all haemoglobins containing α chains, that is HbA, HbA_2 and HbF. The γ and β chains being unstable, precipitate to form tetramers, HbBart's (γ4) and HbH(β4), haemoglobins that have a high oxygen affinity and are unable to deliver adequate oxygen to the tissues. The level of HbBart's in the newborn (0.5 per cent and above) has been used as an indicator of the presence of the α-thalassaemia gene in population studies. Using this criterion, the incidence of α-thalassaemia in Saudi Arabia is more than 50 per cent and in Thailand 20 per cent. The levels of HbBart's in Saudi Arabian newborn infants ranged from 0.5 to 16 per cent of the total haemoglobin, but hydrops fetalis and HbH disease were rarely recorded. This disorder also occurs in other parts of South-east Asia, Mediterranean countries and Africa.

Haemoglobin H disease This form of α-thalassaemia is common in South-east Asia and is seen in some Mediterranean countries and in the Middle East. It is the result of interaction between the α-thalassaemia 1 gene and the α-thalassaemia 2 gene. The disorder shows great clinical variability but most patients have a moderate anaemia (Hb 8–9 g/dl), splenomegaly and a normal life expectancy. Anaemia may be severe during infection, pregnancy, or from haemolysis induced by the ingestion of oxidant drugs (such as sulphonamides). Gallstones occur in adults.

Morphological changes in red cells include hypochromia, microcytosis, red cell fragmentation, target cells and basophilic stippling. The MCV and MCH are low. On incubation of the red cells with brilliant cresyl blue for 30 minutes numerous HbH inclusion bodies are visible. The bone marrow shows marked erythroid hyperplasia and some inclusion bodies are detectable in red cell precursors on incubation with methyl violet. The haemoglobin pattern consists of HbH (5–25 per cent), HbA, HbA_2, HbF and small amounts of HbBart's in some cases. Neonates have about 25 per cent of HbBart's and small amounts of HbH but the proportions are reversed by the end of the first year. In South-east Asia, 40 per cent of patients with HbH disease have small amounts of an α chain variant, Hb Constant Spring, a haemoglobin which migrates slowly between the origin and HbA_2 at pH 8.6 on starch gel or cellulose acetate electrophoresis. Haemoglobin Constant Spring has an elongated α chain in which there are 31 extra residues attached to the C-terminus in addition to the normal 141 amino acid residues.

HbH tends to precipitate in the cell as the erythrocytes age, so older cells contain single large inclusion bodies (Heinz bodies). These cells are subjected to mechanical trauma and have a shortened life span.

Haemoglobin H disease results from the inheritance of both α-thalassaemia 1 and 2 genes or the heterozygous state of an α-thalassaemia 1 gene with the Hb Constant Spring gene.

Most patients with HbH disease do not require therapy, except for folic acid during pregnancy. Prompt treatment of infections is advisable and oxidant drugs should be avoided.

Haemoglobin Bart's hydrops fetalis   This is the most severe manifestation of α-thalassaemia (homozygous state of α-thalassaemia 1 gene) common in South-east Asia but rare in other parts of the world. There is total suppression of α chain synthesis with gross excess of γ chains that form tetramer $\gamma 4$, HbBart's, a high oxygen affinity haemoglobin. Clinical features are similar to those of hydrops fetalis due to severe rhesus haemolytic disease. Affected infants are either stillborn at about 34 weeks gestation, or if liveborn survive only a few minutes. They are pale and grossly oedematous with marked hepatosplenomegaly. The placenta is grossly enlarged. Severe anaemia is present (Hb < 6 g/dl). Blood film shows many nucleated red cells, anisocytosis, poikilocytosis, hypochromia, basophilic stippling and target cells. The reticulocyte count is high and the serum bilirubin raised. Haemoglobin electrophoresis reveals HbBart's (95 per cent) and small amounts of HbH, but no HbF or HbA.

The risk of recurrence of HbBart's hydrops fetalis is one in four for every pregnancy.

Glucose-6-phosphate dehydrogenase deficiency (G6PD)

Glucose-6-phosphate dehydrogenase (G6PD) is an essential enzyme in the pentose phosphate pathway of glucose metabolism. G6PD is activated by NADP and inhibited by NADPH. In the absence of G6PD the generation of NADPH is produced in very little quantity to meet the metabolic demand in the pentose phosphate pathway (see also pp. 222–8, 440).

G6PD deficiency is genetically determined and is located on the X chromosome, affecting male offspring of mothers who are heterozygous. The disorder occurs in about 18 per cent of black Americans. In black Africans it ranges from 5.7 to 21.6 per cent, depending upon the tribe sampled. The disorder is found amongst the Mediterranean Littoral, that is the Sardinians, Greeks, Sephardic Jews and orientals.

There are several variants of G6PD. The well-known ones are G6PDA$^+$ and its deficiency is as designated as G6PD^{A-}. This is common in blacks who show haemolysis in 10–15 per cent. The second variant is G6PD^B which is found amongst Caucasians in whom haemolysis is not so common. G6PD Mediterranean is an even more severe condition than G6PD^{A-} found in blacks. The oriental variants of deficiency may be severe.

The global incidence of G6PD deficiency parallels

Table 5.8.5   Agents causing haemolysis in G6PD deficiency.

Drugs and chemicals	
Chloroquine	Primaquine
Diaphenylsulphone (Dapsone)	Pamaquine
Salicylates	Pentaquine
Probenecid	Nalidixic acid
Quinidine	Nitrofurantoin
Sulphanilamide	Niridazole
Sulphacetamide	Phenylhydrazine
Sulphamethoxazole	Methylene blue
	Naphthalene

Other agents
Fava beans and pollen (*Vicia faba*)
Infections (bacterial pneumonia, typhoid, viral hepatitis)
Diabetic ketoacidosis
Uraemia

the area covered by malaria, particularly falciparum malaria. This leads to the suggestion that G6PD deficiency may offer some protection against malaria.

Diagnosis   The diagnosis of G6PD deficiency depends largely on recognizing predisposing factors such as drugs, metabolic acidosis and infections (see Table 5.8.5). The deficiency is confirmed by assay of G6PD activity. However, in the presence of high reticulocyte counts the G6PD activity may be normal. Methylene blue and tetrazoline reagent are used in the diagnosis.

Bleeding disorders

The various abnormalities which present as bleeding disorders are shown in Table 5.8.6.

Diagnosis

If onset of the disorder is in the neonatal period then intrauterine infection must be considered. If, however, it occurs between three and five days of life, haemorrhagic disease of the newborn must be borne in mind. Prolonged bleeding occurring after circumcision is always suggestive of haemophilia and must be investigated. Transient thrombocytopenia may occur in a child born to a mother with idiopathic thrombocytopenic purpura. Family history is very important, as some inherited bleeding disorders (such as factors VIII and IX deficiency) are inherited as sex-linked recessive conditions. Others like Von Willebrand's disease are inherited as a dominant illness, in which case both males and females are affected equally.

The site of bleeding may give a clue as to what to exclude or include in the investigations. Bleeding into

Table 5.8.6 Epidemiology of bleeding disorders in the tropics.

Blood vessel abnormality
  Scurvy
  Septic or toxic vasculitis (meningococcal septicaemia and some viral haemorrhagic fevers e.g. yellow fever)
  Anaphylactoid purpura (Henoch–Schönlein)
Platelet abnormality
  Thrombocytopenia
    Malignancy (leukaemia, tumours)
    Viral infections (chickenpox, dengue haemorrhagic fever, Marburg, Congo/Crimean haemorrhagic fever)
    Visceral leishmaniasis (kala-azar)
    Marrow damage by drugs and chemicals
    Aplastic anaemia
    Idiopathic thrombocytopenic purpura
    Disseminated intravascular coagulation (septicaemia, severe anoxia)
  Abnormal platelet function
    Von Willebrand's disease (lack of plasma factor for platelet adhesiveness)
Abnormal coagulation
  Congenital
    Haemophilia (factor VIII deficiency)
    Christmas disease (factor IX deficiency)
  Acquired
    Haemorrhagic disease of the newborn (transient deficiencies of prothrombin, and factors VII, IX, X, corrected by vitamin K)

the joints is characteristic of haemophilias. Bleeding into the skin (purpura) is commonly seen in thrombocytopenic and in Henoch–Schönlein purpura. Bleeding from the nose is common in Von Willebrand's disease. Bleeding from the gums is often seen in scurvy.

Inquiry into associated diseases such as liver disease, malignancy, leukaemias, systemic lupus erythromatosus, and renal disease may explain the bleeding.

Drug ingestion may cause bleeding, e.g. salicylates and warfarin.

Laboratory investigations

- *Haemoglobin and peripheral blood.* The Hb will indicate how anaemic the patient is. The peripheral smear will indicate roughly the number of white blood cells, their type and degree of maturity (see p. 978).
- *Platelet count.* This is important, particularly when estimation from a peripheral smear is difficult.
- *Whole blood clotting time.* This measures the time taken for whole blood in a glass tube to clot. It is prolonged in the deficiencies of intrinsic clotting factors and in the presence of anticoagulants. It is not a very sensitive test and may be normal in factor VIII deficiency.

- *Prothrombin time (PT).* This measures the extrinsic factors. It is therefore prolonged in deficiencies of factors II, V, VII and X. It is normal in haemophilia and Christmas disease.
- *Partial thromboplastin time (PTT).* This measures factors in the intrinsic coagulation cascade. It is prolonged in deficiencies of factors XII, XI, IX, VIII and X.
- Thromboplastin generation test. This will measure the individual factors in the intrinsic system. However, it is time consuming and largely replaced by using plasmas deficient in a single factor and PTT.

Haemorrhagic disease of the newborn

Haemorrhage in the newborn may occur from a variety of causes, such as thrombocytopenia and disseminated intravascular coagulation as a result of such conditions as hypoxia and shock (see pp. 229–33). Only haemorrhage due to vitamin K deficiency and characterized by deficiency of prothrombin and factor VII will be discussed here.

The incidence of haemorrhagic disease of the newborn is unknown, although some studies have reported 0.25–0.5 per cent. This may well be because it is sometimes difficult to separate vitamin K deficiency from other causes of bleeding in the newborn. The administration of vitamin K and the introduction of early feeding have affected the incidence greatly.

Bleeding usually occurs in the second or third day of life although it has sometimes occurred as late as two weeks after birth. Bleeding may occur from the umbilical cord, nose, gastro-intestinal tract, circumcision site, skin and scalp. Prolongation of bleeding from veins or capillary puncture sites is yet another manifestation. Some newborns, particularly preterm asphyxiated neonates, may have intracranial and pulmonary haemorrhage, partly because of vitamin K deficiency.

Laboratory investigation will reveal prolongation of prothrombin time and factors II, VII, IX and X will be deficient.

Therapy

Newborns at risk and those with hypoxia should prophylactically receive vitamin K 1 to 2 mg orally or intramuscularly. The newborn with bleeding should receive the same dose, preferably intravenously as intramuscular injection may cause haematoma and anaemia. Fresh blood should be transfused if the newborn is anaemic.

Haemophilias

The signs and symptoms of factor VIII and factor IX deficiencies are very similar. The severity of haemophilia varies greatly and some cases may only be discovered after surgical procedures, such as tooth extraction. Others may develop crippling haemarthoses and contractures. The severity of the clinical presentation correlates well with the levels of factors VIII or IX in the circulation. Both are inherited as sex-linked recessive disorders although in about 25 per cent of cases of factor VIII deficiency, there is no family history – these probably represent new mutations. Factor VIII deficiency is the most common accounting for about 80 per cent of haemophilia. Newborn males may bleed from the umbilicus or bleed excessively after circumcision; bleeding from injection sites is common. As a child begins to crawl, stand or walk he begins to have bruises and haematomas. By three years of age most severe haemophiliacs have had a major bleeding episode. Haemarthosis, haematuria and bleeding into other vital organs may occur.

Laboratory investigations

The partial thromboplastin time is markedly prolonged and so is the thromboplastin generation test. The prothrombin time is normal. Factor VIII assay will show low levels.

Treatment

Part of the management should be devoted to genetic counselling after available information from history and laboratory investigation has been collected. Prevention of trauma forms an integral part of treatment; padded playpen cribs should be used. Protective knee and elbow pads should be considered, particularly when children are engaged in physical activities.

Replacement therapy with factor VIII concentrate is the treatment of choice in a patient who bleeds. The cheapest is cryoprecipitate which can be prepared in the blood bank using fresh plasma. The blood must be tested for HIV to minimize the acquisition of AIDS by these patients. One bag of cryoprecipitate per 5 kg will raise factor VIII to 40 or 50 per cent. Commercial preparations of pure factor VIII concentrate are available but expensive for the majority of countries in the subtropics. In the absence of cryoprecipitate, fresh whole blood or fresh frozen plasma can be given.

Therapy of Christmas disease

This consists of giving fresh plasma or fresh frozen plasma, 10 ml/kg every 12–24 hours, depending upon the extent of the bleeding and the response. The danger of HIV infection must always now be kept in mind.

Von Willebrand's disease

This is due to factor VIII deficiency, a capillary defect and decreased platelet adhesiveness associated with prolonged bleeding time. The most common symptoms are epistaxis and bleeding from the mouth and upon tooth extraction. In girls, excessive menstrual periods may be encountered. Clotting time, prothrombin time and platelet counts are normal. Often the thromboplastin generation test is employed to make the diagnosis. Treatment consist of administration of cryoprecipitate.

Idiopathic thrombocytopenic purpura

This is the most common platelet disorder in children. The cause is still unknown but evidence for an immunological basis is overwhelming, particularly in the chronic form. It usually follows a respiratory infection and is characterized by easy bruising and purpura. Haemorrhages into the gastro-intestinal tract do occur and if cerebral haemorrhage occurs this may lead to death. Apart from evidence of bleeding the child is normal and the spleen is not palpable. The diagnosis is made from the peripheral blood smear which shows scanty platelets; this is supported by a platelet count which is usually less than 50 000/mm^3. In every case a bone marrow test must be performed to exclude leukaemia. The bone marrow in idiopathic thrombocytopenic purpura shows normal or increased numbers of megakaryocytes.

Treatment

The disorder is self-limiting in children and about 75 per cent recover spontaneously within a few weeks. About 15 per cent recover in about six months to one year. The remainder form a chronic group, 10 per cent of whom are cured by splenectomy.

The use of corticosteroids is controversial but may probably hasten the recovery phase. Immunosuppressive drug such as vincristine and cyclophosphamide are used in cases where splenectomy has not been successful. Administration of immunoglobulin has transient benefit but could be helpful during surgical procedures.

The spleen

The large mass of reticulo-endothelial and lymphoid cells in the spleen plays an important part in the body's immune response to infection. It is also a site of extramedullary erythropoiesis. The causes of splenomegaly are numerous and are summarized in Table 5.8.7.

Table 5.8.7. Some causes of splenomegaly in children in the tropics.

Infections
    Bacterial — septicaemia, tuberculosis, typhoid, endocarditis
    Parasitic — malaria, visceral leishmaniasis (kala-azar), schistosomiasis (with cirrhosis), toxoplasmosis
    Viral — rubella, Herpes simplex, cytomegalovirus, infectious mononucleosis
    Mycotic — histoplasmosis
Blood diseases
    Haemolytic anaemias
    Haemoglobinopathies — sickle cell disease
    Thalassaemia
Congestive splenomegaly
    Secondary to portal vein obstruction — veno-occlusive disease
    Secondary to cirrhosis
    Congestive heart failure
Malignancies
    Leukaemia
    Hodgkin's disease, lymphosarcoma, Burkitt's lymphoma
Collagen diseases
    Rheumatoid arthritis
    Systemic lupus erythematosus
Others
    Haemangioma
    Lymphangioma

Tropical splenomegaly syndrome

Children and young adults in many areas of the tropics and subtropics may suffer from gross splenomegaly. In many cases this is probably ascribed correctly to a prevailing disease such as malaria or kala-azar, yet in many other cases the evidence for any specific infection is slight and the response to treatment is poor. Detailed investigations may only reveal varying degrees of hypersplenism. The condition is considered to be an abnormal immune response associated with malaria, but the pathogenesis and natural history are poorly understood. In India, children with gross splenomegaly and portal hypertension have been described with varying degrees of non-cirrhotic portal fibrosis.

Clinical features

Those most affected are children from four years of age to puberty. The patients usually present with a history of general weakness, swelling of the abdomen with a dragging abdominal pain, a progressively enlarging abdominal mass and mild recurrent episodes of fever; very occasionally children present with frank haematemesis. The history may extend over several months or years, growth may be stunted and secondary sexual characteristics delayed.

The spleen is moderately or greatly enlarged, it is firm and mobile but seldom tender. The liver is usually enlarged 2–3 cm below the costal margin, its edge being firm, uniform and non-tender. The lymph nodes are not enlarged. Anaemia, leucopenia and thrombocytopenia are common. The former has been shown to be due to the combination of an increased plasma volume diluting a normal or even raised red cell mass, pooling of red cells is the spleen, and increased red cell destruction. The bulk of the increased plasma volume has been shown to be due to overproduction of immunoglobulins. The bone marrow is usually hyperplastic. The intrasplenic pressure is raised and splenovenography may show a large dilated portal vein, usually without oesophageal varices. Liver biopsy shows varying degrees of hepatic sinusoidal lymphocytosis, these cases have a markedly raised antibody titre against malaria. The serum albumin is reduced, other liver function tests are usually normal; the IgM concentration is markedly increased.

Treatment

Prolonged therapy with antimalarial drugs is the treatment of choice for those children with hepatic sinusoidal lymphocytosis. Treatment should be continued for a year or more as the response to therapy may be very slow. Discontinuing treatment usually leads to a rapid relapse if the patient continues to live in a malarious area. Successful antimalarial therapy leads to a great reduction in spleen size and plasma volume associated with a rise in the haemoglobin concentration and a return to normal of the red cell survival.

There remains a small group of patients for whom surgical intervention may be required. The indications include severe protracted pain, and severe portal hypertension. Splenectomy carries a distinct mortality risk, there is a danger of severe bleeding from highly vascular adhesions, and over-transfusion is a risk in the presence of an expanded blood volume. Following splenectomy there is an increased incidence of overwhelming infections.

Neutrophil disorders

Recurrent infections, such as pneumonia, boils, urinary tract infections, and fever of unexplained origin, should be investigated for deficiency in numbers or function of the white cells. If there is associated anaemia and easy bruising, then investigation for bone marrow failure should be instituted.

Causes of bone marrow failure have already been discussed. Brief mention of the disordered function of white blood cell will be made here. Leucocyte numbers range between 5×10^9 and 10×10^9/l although in certain individuals leucocytes between 2×10^9 and 4×10^9/l are encountered, especially in the black Africans. A neutrophil count of less than 1.5×10^9/l constitutes neutropenia, which results in diminished phagocytosis and killing power of the neutrophils.

Drug-induced neutropenia is common and should be looked for in a patient who has infection while on drugs. Drugs such as chloramphenicol, sulphonamide, propothiouracil, carbimazole, diphenylhydantoin, amodiaquine, and many others, will cause leucopenia and neutropenia.

Cyclical neutropenia is a rare condition which is characterized by a fall in the neutrophil count at three-week intervals. Severe infections are unusual. It may be associated with pancreatic exocrine insufficiency, dwarfism and metaphyseal abnormalities in the Schwachman–Diamond syndrome.

Chronic granulomatous disease of childhood is by far the most common of the disorders of intracellular bacterial killing. This is characterized by repeated infections in the first year of life; e.g. leg ulcers, abscesses, pneumonia, tonsillitis, lymphadenitis, hepatosplenomegaly and mouth ulcers. It is inherited as an X-linked disorder. It is diagnosed by a failure of white cells to reduce nitroblue tetrazolium.

Further reading

Hardisty RM, Weatherall DJ. *Blood and its Disorders*, 2nd edn. Oxford, Blackwell, 1982.

Hinchcliffe RF, Lilleyman JS (eds). *Practical Paediatric Haematology: A Laboratory Worker's Guide*. New York, Wiley, 1987.

Nathan DG, Oski FA (eds). *Haematology of Infancy and Childhood*. New York, Saunders, 1987.

Serjeant JR. *Sickle Cell Disease*. Oxford, Oxford University Press, 1985.

Weatherall DJ (ed.). *The Thalassaemias*. Edinburgh, Churchill Livingstone, 1983.

CHAPTER 9

Immunological disorders

Badrul Alam Chowdhury and Ranjit Kumar Chandra

A wide variety of diseases in man are associated with disorders of the immune system. An effective immune system consists of antigen-specific host defence mechanisms like the T cell system of cell-mediated immunity, and the B cell system of immunoglobulins; and non-specific defences like the phagocytic system of polymorphonuclear leucocytes and mononuclear macrophages, complement system, lysozyme, interferon, and skin and mucous membranes. A breakdown of any of these barriers leads to immunodeficiency. Depending on the cause and time of onset, immunodeficiency diseases are classified as primary or secondary.

In this chapter the development of the immune system and both primary and secondary immunodeficiency diseases are discussed.

Development of the immune system

Various components of the immune system develop at different rates during fetal and early postnatal life. All immunocompetent cells such as lymphocytes, monocytes, and polymorphonuclear leucocytes are derived from undifferentiated haemopoietic stem cells, but differentiate into various cell types under the influence of different micro-environmental factors. Lymphocytes and macrophages acquire unique surface markers as differentiation proceeds, some of which are subsequently lost. These cell markers can be used to identify different cell lines that have unique functions in the generation of immune responses.

T Cells

The T cell system is responsible for a variety of host defence functions, including control of infections, particularly viral and fungal, graft rejection, graft-versus-host reactions, tumour immunity, immuno-logical tolerance, delayed skin hypersensitivity, and regulation of the immune system. Precursors of T lymphocytes arise first about the fourth week of gestation from pluripotential stem cells in the blood islets of the yolk sac, and subsequently mature under the influence of the thymus. The thymic rudiment develops at about six weeks from endoderm of the third and fourth pharyngeal pouches. The organ soon becomes seeded with blood-borne lymphoid precursor cells and it migrates caudally to the anterior mediastinum. Thymus-processed T lymphocytes enter the general circulation and migrate to function in the secondary lym-

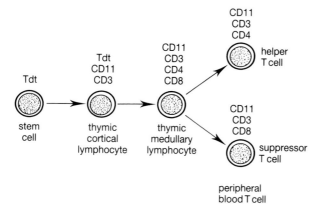

Fig. 5.9.1 Sequential acquisition of markers in different stages of T cell maturation.

phoid organs like the spleen and lymph nodes.

Various markers are present in different stages of T cell maturation within and outside the thymus (Fig. 5.9.1). The enzyme terminal deoxyribonucleotidyl transferase (Tdt) is present in stem cells and immature cortical cells, but not in the mature medullary and peripheral lymphocytes. The receptor for sheep erythrocytes (CD11), which is a classical marker for the human T cell, develops at the early stage of differentiation in thymic cortex and persists thereafter. CD3 (or Leu 4) surface glycoprotein, which is involved in antigen recognition by T cells, also appears in the thymic cortical stage but somewhat later than sheep erythrocyte receptor, and is maintained on mature T lymphocytes. CD4 (or Leu 3) and CD8 (or Leu 2) antigens, which are markers for helper and suppressor T lymphocytes, respectively, appear along with CD3, but one or the other is lost during thymic differentiation so that only one type is present in mature T cells committed to a particular function.

B Cells

B lymphocytes are responsible for antibody production and humoral immunity. Like the T cells, precursors of B cells arise from pluripotential stem cells, but their path of migration is different. In the chicken embryo, primary B cell lymphopoiesis occurs in a hindgut lymphoepithelial organ called the bursa of Fabricius. Like the thymus, the bursal rudiment develops as an outpouching of endodermal cells, becomes infiltrated by blood-borne lymphoid precursor cells which organize in the cortex and medulla, and matures in close contact with the epithelial cells. Mammals do not

have a discrete organ for B cell maturation. Like other haemopoietic cells, B lymphocytes probably develop initially in the fetal liver starting from eight to nine weeks of gestation, and later in the bone marrow where the developmental process continues into adult life.

B lymphocytes mature through various stages known as lymphoid stem cells, pre-B cells, immature B cells, mature B cells, and finally, on antigen stimulation, plasma cells (Fig. 5.9.2). During maturation the cells acquire surface immunoglobulins which act as the cell surface antigen receptor. The early stem cells proliferate and undergo immunoglobulin gene rearrangement to give rise to pre-B cells which express cytoplasmic immunoglobulin M heavy chain. Depending on size, two populations of pre-B cells are recognized. Large pre-B cells, which precede small cells, are found only in the fetal liver and bone marrow, whereas small pre-B cells also occur in the circulation and peripheral lymphoid tissues. In the next stage of development, light chains of kappa or lambda type are synthesized, and the cells acquire IgM surface immunoglobulin. These cells, now called immature B cells, also acquire C3 and IgG Fc receptors. They differentiate further into mature B cells with the expression of surface IgD. At the same time subpopulations of surface IgG and IgA expressing cells also appear. Each of the B cell lineages is committed for the rest of its life to a specific antigen-binding and antibody-producing capability dictated by the surface immunoglobulin. Given the known number of B cells in the body and the infinite number of antigens in the environment, the generation of antibody diversity is not fully understood. Immature and mature B cells respond differently to antigen exposure. Both cell types bind antigen with surface immunoglobulin which results in its loss by capping and endocytosis. In mature B cells the process is reversible with the re-expression of surface immunoglobulin, while in immature cells the process is irreversible resulting in the loss of the particular clone. This mechanism explains the removal of clones bearing antibodies to self-antigens.

After production in fetal liver and bone marrow, B cells migrate in the circulation and function in

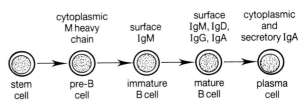

Fig. 5.9.2 Expression of immunoglobulins in different stages of B cell maturation.

secondary lymphoid tissues. On antigenic stimulation they develop into antibody-forming plasma cells. Although the human fetus is capable of forming antibody of the IgM class as early as 10 weeks of gestation, the level of circulating antibody of fetal origin is very low throughout gestation. Even at birth it constitutes only 1 to 2 per cent of the adult level. The newborn have broad lymphocyte diversity, but their antibody responses are qualitatively restricted and different from those of adults. They fail to respond to polysaccharide antigens with repeating antigenic determinants, and their response to protein antigens is slow to shift from IgM to IgG class. Maternal IgG transmitted across the placenta and secretory IgA in the breast-milk play an important role in the protection of the fetus and the newborn.

Phagocytic and antigen-presenting cells

Polymorphonuclear neutrophils and mononuclear phagocytes (blood monocytes and fixed tissue macrophages) play an important role in host defence through their ability to ingest and digest particulate pathogens. Mononuclear cells also have an antigen-presenting function which is essential for T cell activation. Development of these cells commences at about the sixth week in the fetal liver, and later in the spleen and bone marrow. After birth, bone marrow becomes the site of myelopoiesis. The phagocytic and chemotactic function of neutrophils is acquired early in fetal life, but their activity is less due to the lower opsonizing ability of fetal serum. The phagocytic function of mononuclear cells develops early during gestation, but their antigen-presenting function develops somewhat later.

Complement

The complement system is made up of at least 20 different plasma proteins. They are important mediators of antigen–antibody reactions and also provide non-specific protection against micro-organisms. The complement proteins appear during early development of the fetus and are detected about the same time as circulating immunoglobulins. Their concentration in the newborn ranges from 50 to 60 per cent of the adult level. Thus, complement components, together with phagocytic cells, are probably more important in the protection of the fetus and newborn than are antibodies.

Immune deficiency diseases

Immune deficiency diseases are a group of disorders in which there is an abnormality in one or more

parameters of host defence mechanisms due to a primary defect in the immunocompetent cells (primary immunodeficiency) or secondarily to systemic disease processes or conditions (secondary immunodeficiency). Primary immunodeficiencies are either congenital or acquired, and are classified according to whether the defect involves cell-mediated immunity (T cell function), humoral immunity (B cell function), or both.

Table 5.9.1   Immune deficiency diseases.

Primary immunodeficiency
Combined T and B cell disease
   Severe combined immunodeficiency disease (SCID)
   Immunodeficiency with thrombocytopenia and eczema
     (Wiskott–Aldrich syndrome)
   Immunodeficiency with ataxia–telangiectasia
Primary T cell disease
   Thymic hypoplasia (DiGeorge's syndrome)
Primary B cell disease
   Infantile X-linked agammaglobulinaemia
   Transient hypogammaglobulinaemia of infancy
   Selective immunoglobulin (IgA, IgM etc.) deficiency
   X-linked immunodeficiency with increased levels of IgM
   Immunodeficiency with thymoma
   Common varied immunodeficiency
Secondary immunodeficiency
Malnutrition
Infections
   Viral, e.g. human immunodeficiency virus (HIV), measles,
    Epstein–Barr virus, congenital rubella
   Bacterial, e.g. tuberculosis, lepromatous leprosy,
    septicaemia
   Spirochaetal, e.g. syphilis
   Fungal, e.g. chronic mucocutaneous candidiasis,
    coccidioidomycosis
   Parasitic, e.g. trypanosomiasis, schistosomiasis
Cancer
Immunosuppressive therapy
   Corticosteroids
   Cytotoxic drugs
   Radiation
Trauma
   Surgery
   Burns
   Accidents
Loss of immunocompetent cells or proteins
   Nephrotic syndrome
   Protein-losing enteropathy
   Intestinal lymphangiectasia
   Tricuspid regurgitation
Miscellaneous
   Sarcoidosis
   Hodgkin's disease
   Collagen disorders
   Splenectomy
   Renal failure
   Myotonic dystrophy
   Cirrhosis

Most of these diseases are rare, genetically determined, and are observed more often in children. Secondary immunodeficiencies are not caused by intrinsic abnormalities in development or function of T or B cells. The best known of these are immunodeficiency associated with malnutrition, and acquired immunodeficiency syndrome (AIDS) caused by human immunodeficiency virus (HIV) infection. The classification of immune deficiency diseases into primary and secondary, and that of T or B cell defect is somewhat arbitrary, as there is always a close cooperation between different cells of the immune system and defect in one leads to some alteration in the other. However, the classification serves the purpose of drawing rough boundaries between different clinicopathological syndromes. A working classification of immune deficiency diseases listing the main recognized types is given in Table 5.9.1. In this section the clinical features common to all immune deficiency states and evaluation of patients with immunodeficiency is described, followed by brief description of some common immunodeficiency diseases.

Common clinical features

Immunodeficiency syndromes are characterized by unusual susceptibility to infection, cancer, autoimmunity and allergy. Infection is caused by impaired host resistance. Malignancy is caused by increased susceptibility to oncogenic viruses, failure of immune surveillance to detect virus infected or early malignant cells, and inability of cytotoxic T cells to destroy such cells. Autoimmunity is caused by a failure of immunoregulatory cell function. Allergy is caused by loss of the mucosal barrier of the gastro-intestinal and respiratory tracts which allows antigens to enter the body and provoke an IgE response. In most patients with immunodeficiency the presenting feature is infections of increased frequency, duration, or severity, or infections with unusual organisms. The age of onset and type of infection provide the first clues to the nature of the immune defect. If the onset is before six months of age, the possibility of a T cell defect is high – as transplacentally acquired antibodies protect the infant up to this time; whereas after six months infections may be due to either T or B cell defects.

B cell defect

Children with defects in humoral immunity have an increased susceptibility to infection with extracellular encapsulated organisms like *Haemophilus influenzae* and *Streptococcus pneumoniae*. They suffer recurrent or chronic sinopulmonary infections, meningitis, or bacteraemia. The occurrence of unusual infections, like *H. influenzae* meningitis in older children and severe infestation with the intestinal parasite *Giardia lamblia*, warrants consideration of humoral immune deficiency. These patients also have altered responses to common viral infections like *Varicella zoster*, and rubella. The clinical course of primary infection does not differ from that of the normal host; however, long-lasting immunity may not develop. As a result, multiple recurrences of these infections may occur. Intact T cells in these patients can control the viral infections, but the B cell defect fails to generate long-lasting immunity.

T cell defect

Children with defects in cell-mediated immunity are predisposed to infection with intracellular bacteria such as *Mycobacteria, Listeria, Legionella*; fungi such as *Candida, Cryptococcus, Aspergillus*; protozoa such as *Pneumocystis carinii*; and viruses such as Herpes simplex, Varicella zoster, and cytomegalovirus. Very commonly, these patients develop disseminated viral and fungal infections, particularly mucocutaneous candidiasis, and atypical infections like *Pneumocystis carinii* pneumonia. T cell deficiency is always accompanied by abnormalities of antibody response; as a result, patients also suffer from overwhelming bacterial infections.

Combined T and B cell defect

Children with defects in both cell-mediated and humoral immunity are susceptible to the whole range of infectious agents, including those not commonly considered pathogenic. Multiple and severe infections with viruses, bacteria, fungi, and protozoa occur, often simultaneously. These patients also cannot reject foreign tissues. As a result, blood transfusions can cause fatal graft-versus-host disease due to persistance of donor lymphocytes.

Evaluation

A careful history and physical examination usually indicates the type of immunodeficiency and can guide the selection of laboratory tests. A history of normal response to childhood viral vaccination excludes severe combined immunodeficiency disease (SCID) and severe defects in cellular immunity. Absence of palpable lymph nodes or diffuse lymphoid hyperplasia suggests some underlying immunodeficiency. The laboratory tests used to evaluate immunological status range from simple office procedures to sophisticated methods requiring special technical skills. In most cases simple procedures are adequate.

Humoral immunity

Deficiency of humoral immunity is usually accompanied by low serum concentrations of one or more classes of immunoglobulin. Immunoglobulin levels must be interpreted in relation to age; wide ranges are seen in the normal population. Normal adult values of IgM (100 mg/dl) are reached by about one year, of IgG (1000 mg/dl) by five to six years, and of IgA (200 mg/dl) by puberty. This happens at younger ages in developing countries because of the frequent exposure to infection. In the presence of borderline values, the capacity to produce specific antibodies can be measured following vaccination or infection. Enumeration of B lymphocytes is of value in determining the pathogenesis of certain types of immune deficiency. B lymphocytes are identified by using monoclonal antibodies directed against membrane-bound markers like immunoglobulins, IgG Fc or C3 receptors. B lymphocyte function can be evaluated *in vivo* by Schick test or *in vitro* by pokeweed mitogen stimulation. In children who have previously received diphtheria vaccine, a negative Schick test reflects adequate antibody production.

Antibody deficiencies may be mimicked clinically by a deficiency of complement components. Thus, the estimation of C3 and total haemolytic complement is of importance. Opsonic function of plasma is another important test of host defence. The assay detects the presence of opsonins (some antibody and complement fragments) in the patient's plasma.

Cellular immunity

Enumeration of T lymphocytes and their subsets is an important test of cellular immunity. T lymphocytes are identified by their expression of surface molecules which can bind sheep erythrocytes, forming E-rosettes. The monoclonal antibody CD11 or Leu 5 can also recognize the sheep erythrocyte receptor. Other monoclonal antibodies are also available which can recognize antigens on mature T cells (CD3 or Leu 4), T helper-inducer subsets (CD4 or Leu 3), and T suppressor-cytotoxic subsets (CD8 or Leu 2). T lymphocyte function can be evaluated *in vivo* by delayed hypersensitivity skin tests using common recall antigens like tetanus toxoid, purified protein derivative, streptokinase–streptodornase, mumps, *Candida*, and *Trichophyton*. Positive skin tests in the presence of

previous exposure denote intact cell-mediated immunity. T lymphocyte function can be evaluated *in vitro* by estimating the capacity of cells to proliferate in response to antigens to which the patient is previously sensitized or to polyclonal T cell mitogens phytohaemagglutinin and concanavalin A. The ability of stimulated T cells to produce lymphokines can also be measured. Other tests of T cell function include their ability to be activated in mixed lymphocyte culture, and to lyse target cells.

Primary immunodeficiency

Severe combined immunodeficiency disease

This disease which involves both T and B cell function is inherited in an autosomal recessive or X-linked manner. In the common severe form of SCID (Swiss-type agammaglobulinaemia), the basic defect is thought to lie in the lymphoid stem cells, resulting in the absence of both types of immunocompetent cells. Increased susceptibility to infection is noted at three to six months of age, and infants rarely survive beyond two years without treatment.

The peripheral lymphocyte count is less than $2 \times 10^9/l$. Serum immunoglobulin levels are usually one per cent of normal, and antibodies do not form after vaccination or infection. Delayed cutaneous hypersensitivity to common recall antigens is negative. Lymph node biopsy shows absence of follicles, lymphocytes and plasma cells.

Treatment

Passive administration of gamma-globulin is temporarily effective. Bone marrow transplantation usually provides long-lasting reconstitution of the T and B cell systems.

Immunodeficiency with thrombocytopenia and eczema (Wiskott–Aldrich syndrome)

This is an X-linked recessive disorder characterized by eczema, thrombocytopenia, and recurrent infections. Both T and B cells are defective. Serum IgM is usually decreased, IgA and IgG are normal, and IgE increased. T cells are anergic and do not respond to antigens. Affected children rarely survive more than 10 years, dying of infection, bleeding, or lymphoreticular malignancy. Treatment by histocompatible bone marrow transplants usually corrects both the immunological and haematological abnormalities. In patients lacking suitable donors, splenectomy may improve platelet count and bleeding diathesis.

Immunodeficiency with ataxia–telangiectasia

This is an autosomal recessive disorder characterized by cerebellar ataxia from infancy and oculocutaneous telangiectasia, and variable T and B cell deficiency which starts 5 to 10 years later. Serum and secretory IgA deficiency is seen in approximately 80 per cent of the children, and a smaller number have reduced serum IgA, IgG2 and IgG4 levels. Defective T cell function, and maldevelopment of the thymus is also present. Affected individuals usually die of chronic pulmonary disease or lymphoreticular malignancy by the second or third decade. Treatment is only symptomatic.

Thymic hypoplasia (DiGeorge's syndrome)

DiGeorge's syndrome occurs due to maldevelopment of the third and fourth pharyngeal pouches resulting in aplasia of the thymus and parathyroid gland. Immunologically the syndrome represents a pure T cell deficiency. The principal manifestations of the disease are neonatal tetany and increased susceptibility to infection. Associated abnormalities may include cardiac defects, shortened philtrum, abnormal ears, and hypertelorism.

T cells are virtually absent from circulation and functional T cell assays are abnormal. Serum immunoglobulin levels are usually normal, antibody responses to antigen may be low. Serum calcium is reduced, phosphorus is elevated, and parathyroid hormone is absent.

Infantile X-linked agammaglobulinaemia

This disease with an X-linked pattern of inheritance is characterized by defects in B cell function with an intact T cell system. The basic defect is thought to be a developmental block in the differentiation of pre-B cells.

There are usually no symptoms up to the first 5 to 6 months of life due to the presence of maternal antibody. Thereafter the infant develops recurrent infection with pyogenic organisms. Some affected children also have arthritis of large joints.

B lymphocytes are virtually absent in the peripheral circulation. Serum IgG levels are less than 200 mg/dl, IgM and IgA levels are less than one per cent of normal. T cell number and functions are normal.

Gamma-globulin injection is the mainstay of treatment. The injections are usually given intramuscularly at a dose of 0.2 to 0.4 ml/kg, or intravenously at a dose of 400–800 mg/kg. Frequency of treatment is determined by monitoring the blood IgG level.

Transient hypogammaglobulinaemia of infancy

In this reversible syndrome the physiological hypogammaglobulinaemia of infancy is unusually prolonged and severe. Normally the levels of IgG drop to 300 to 400 mg/dl between 3 and 6 months of age as the maternal IgG is catabolised. The levels thereafter rise, reflecting the infant's synthetic capacity. In this condition, levels of IgM, IgG, and IgA remain low for a long period. A reduced number of helper T cells has been proposed as the underlying cause of this disorder.

Isolated deficiency of IgA

This is the most common primary immunodeficiency, occurring in approximately 1 in 600 individuals of European origin. The disease is familial, but the pattern of inheritance is unknown. Isolated cases are also reported following intrauterine infections in the newborn, e.g. rubella, and phenytoin treatment in older children and adults. Since secretory IgA is the major immunoglobulin protecting the mucous membranes, these patients suffer from recurrent respiratory and gastro-intestinal infection, and an increased incidence of atopic and autoimmune diseases. Treatment is symptomatic as IgA cannot be effectively replaced exogenously, and its use would risk the development of IgG antibodies to IgA. However, in the subgroup with combined IgA–IgG2 deficiency, gammaglobulin therapy is safe and effective. Spontaneous recovery has been reported in about one-third of affected children.

Secondary immunodeficiency

Immunodeficiency in malnutrition

In children with protein–energy malnutrition (PEM), both cell-mediated and humoral immunity are depressed (see pp. 335–58). Malnutrition during fetal life can also cause profound immunodeficiency during the postnatal period, reflecting the severe effect of nutritional deficiency on the developing immune system. Isolated deficiency of some nutrients like vitamins, minerals, and trace elements also alters immune function. Among them the effects of iron and zinc are well known. Iron deficiency lowers host resistance due to reduced activity of the enzyme myeloperoxidase required in phagocytosis, and of ribonucleotide reductase necessary for DNA synthesis. Deficiency of zinc occurs in acrodermatitis enteropathica – a rare autosomal recessive condition of zinc malabsorption, and also in total parenteral nutrition, malabsorption, and due to excess dietary phytates. Zinc is essential for the function of many enzymes, and its deficiency mainly affects cell-mediated immunity.

Clinical findings

The prevalence, severity, and duration of infection is increased in children with PEM. The pattern of pathogens isolated mimics that of other immuno-deficiency states. In addition to opportunistic infections such as *Pneumocystis carinii* pneumonia, common infections like gastroenteritis, measles, tuberculosis, amoebiasis, and hepatitis occur in malnourished children with increased frequency and severity. Infants who are small for gestational age suffer from the sequelae of decreased immune function far longer than do appropriate-for-gestational age preterm infants.

Laboratory findings

Lymphopenia is common in malnourished children (often below $0.5 \times 10^9/l$). Total T and helper T cell counts are markedly decreased, suppressor T cell counts are slightly reduced or unaltered, and the B cell count is unaltered. *In vivo* and *in vitro* T cell functions are decreased. Serum immunoglobulin levels are normal or increased due to repeated infections, while secretory IgA is decreased. The serum concentrations of almost all complement components, especially C3, are reduced, and lysozyme is decreased in serum and mucous secretions. Phagocytes are slow in chemotactic response and intracellular microbial killing is reduced. The thymus of malnourished children is markedly atrophied.

Immunodeficiency in infectious disease

In tropical countries viral, bacterial, and parasitic infections are very common. Immunodeficiency caused by malnutrition is mainly responsible for the increased incidence observed. Certain infectious diseases also depress immune function, which in turn increases the frequency and severity of infection and further complicates malnutrition. Malnutrition and infection thus go hand-in-hand, and immunodeficiency is the vital link between them.

Immunodeficiency in viral infections

Viral exanthems have profound effects on the immune system. A classical example is the loss of tuberculin test positivity during measles infection. *In vitro* assays also show suppression of T cell functions in measles. Some other viral infections, such as chickenpox, rubella and influenza, also depress cell-mediated immunity. B cells are classically affected in Epstein–Barr virus infection. These effects are due to infection of the leucocytes by virus, and secondary to the release of mediators with powerful non-specific effects (see pp. 600–23).

Immunodeficiency in bacterial infections

A number of bacterial infections are associated with impairment of immune responses. Intracellular bacteria usually depress cell-mediated immunity. Thus, in miliary tuberculosis (see p. 520) and lepromatous leprosy (see pp. 557–8), delayed skin hypersensitivity and other assays for T cell functions are altered. Pyogenic organisms depress chemotaxis and intracellular bacterial killing by phagocytes. In secondary syphilis and cholera, T cell functions are often abnormal.

Immunodeficiency in protozoal infections

Non-specific immunosuppression is a universal feature of protozoal infection, which probably explains the observation that children with protozoal infection are especially susceptible to bacterial infection and it may account for the association of Burkitt's lymphoma with malaria. Specific suppression of antibody or cellular response has also been described for some protozoans. Malaria depresses humoral immunity and in particular affects antibody production to antigens requiring T cell help. Leishmaniasis affects cell-mediated immunity, probably due to increased suppressor cell reactivity (see p. 683). In trypanosomiasis both types of response are depressed – the African trypanosomiasis mainly affects the antibody response (see p. 676), while the American trypanosomiasis mainly alters cell-mediated immunity.

Immunodeficiency in helminthic infections

In schistosomiasis a significant depression of cell-mediated immunity is observed. Delayed skin hypersensitivity is suppressed, and lymphocyte proliferation to antigens and mitogens are depressed. Larvae of *Trichinella spiralis* release lymphotoxic factors which alter antibody responses to T–dependent antigens. Immunodeficiency in other helminthic infections has not been studied adequately, but non-specific immunosuppression is believed to occur as in protozoal infection.

Acquired immunodeficiency syndrome (AIDS)

See pp. 600–604.

Further reading

Chandra RK ed. *Primary and Secondary Immunodeficiency Disorders*. Edinburgh, UK, Churchill Livingstone, 1983.

Chandra RK. Nutrition, immunity, and infection: present knowledge and future directions. *Lancet*. 1983; **i**: 688–91.

Chandra RK. Immunocompetence in undernutrition. *Journal of Pediatrics*. 1972; **81**: 1194–200.

Cohen S, Warren KS eds. *Immunopathology of Parasitic Infections*, 2nd Edn. Oxford, UK, Blackwell Scientific, 1982.

Forum on B cell ontogeny. *Annals of Immunology*. (Paris). 1984; **135** (2): 187–92.

Kaplan LD, Wofsy CB and Volberding PA. Treatment of patients with acquired immunodeficiency syndrome and associated manifestations. *Journal of the American Medical Association*. 1987; **257**: 1367–70.

LeDouarin NM, Dieterlen-Lievre F, Oliver PD. Ontogency of primary lymphoid organs and lymphoid stem cells. *American Journal of Anatomy*. 1984; **170**: 261–99.

Owen JJ, Jenkinson EJ. Early events in T lymphocyte genesis in the fetal thymus. *American Journal of Anatomy*. 1984; **170**: 301–10.

Rosen FS, Cooper MD, Wedgwood RJP. The primary immunodeficiencies. *New England Journal of Medicine*. 1984; **311**: 235–42.

Rubinstein A, Bernstein L. The epidemiology of pediatric acquired immunodeficiency syndrome. *Clinical Immunology and Immunopathology*. 1986; **40**: 115–21.

CHAPTER 10

Diseases of the skin

A.N. Okoro

INTRODUCTION

The healthy skin of the newborn child in the tropics is exposed from birth to a hazardous disease-ridden environment. This, together with the inadequate care and protection characteristic of such situations, accounts for the rapid rise in incidence of skin diseases throughout childhood. Some of the pathogenic factors in this environment are amenable to change and control, using available and affordable primary health care measures.

Consideration of skin diseases in children should therefore encompass examination of various aspects of these diseases, the mobilization of primary health care concepts for their treatment and control, and amelioration of the aetiological environmental factors by combined and coordinated governmental and international action. The care of the child's skin thus belongs to the entire health care community comprising the parents, primary health care team, non-specialist doctors, dermatologists, paediatricians and government. Mothers are potentially good 'home dermatologists' and, with adequate health education, they can become a vital link in the health care chain.

Infestations by animal parasites, bacterial, fungal and viral infections and nutritional disorders are among the diseases of underdevelopment. Their domination of the 'top ten' skin diseases suggests persistence of adverse environmental factors – these are examined here.

Major aetiological factors

The physical (geographical) environment, the disease agents and the host (man) are the dominant factors determining the pattern of these skin diseases. Man contributes to his skin diseases by his way of life – poor personal and community hygiene, disease-infested rural dwelling, overcrowding in rural or unplanned urban settings, poor nutrition and a low socio-economic level based on poor scientific and technological development.

The disease agents flourish in the environment of the home, surroundings, farms, forests, water sources, markets and work places. The temperature of the tropical and subtropical regions, the rainfall and humidity in the rain forest regions, the dust and aridity of the desert and savannah regions and the vagaries of climatic changes favour the disease agents and their vectors. Socio-political upheavals also hamper development and depress the quality of life and level of health of the affected communities.

Man's way of life has an influence over the environment and disease agents. Both factors are largely amenable to alteration by human effort; so is the pattern of skin diseases in children alterable for the better (Table 5.10.1).

Table 5.10.2 shows the rising incidence of skin diseases with age. The strikingly low incidence of neonatal dermatoses is due partly to the lack of necessary expert routine examination of the skin at birth, and partly to the sheltered environment of neonatal life.

Table 5.10.1   Primary health care measures against skin diseases.

Diseases	Primary health care measures
Onchocerciasis and other filariases	Vector control with larvicides and insecticides Prompt and adequate chemotherapy
Scabies and pediculosis	Improved personal and family hygiene Prompt and adequate treatment
Dracunculiasis	Water boiling and filtering Elimination of cyclops (water fleas) from infested ponds or wells Provision of wholesome drinking water Prompt and adequate treatment
Larva migrans, jiggers and tumbu fly	Avoidance of contact with contaminated soil or dust
Common bacterial infections	Improved personal hygiene Prompt and adequate antibiotic treatment
Leprosy	Contact tracing Surveys of risk groups Other control measures Vaccination (under trial) Prompt and adequate multidrug therapy
Fungal infections	Improved personal and family hygiene Prompt and adequate treatment
Warts and molluscum contagiosum	Improved personal and family hygiene Prompt and adequate treatment
Herpetic infections and varicella	Avoidance of contact with affected individuals
Nutritional disorders	Adequate and balanced nutrition Protein and vitamin supplements

Table 5.10.2   Rising incidence of skin diseases with age.

Age group	No. cases	%
Neonatal (1–28 days)	50	0.6
1–12 months	940	10.8
1–5 years	2100	24.2
6–10 years	2349	27.0
11–15 years	3233	37.2

Table 5.10.3 'Top ten' groups of skin diseases in children.

Disease group	No. cases	%
Infestations by animal parasites	2587	28.5
Eczema or dermatitis	1725	19.0
Bacterial infections	1184	13.0
Fungal infections	905	9.9
Viral infections	589	6.4
Papulo-squamous eruptions	464	5.1
Allergic eruptions	463	5.1
Nutritional disorders	330	3.6
Pigmentary disorders	239	2.6
Skin tumours	120	1.3

This table accounts for 94.8 per cent of skin diseases in this series (1968–85).

Table 5.10.4 Other skin diseases in children.

Disease group	No. cases	%
Keratoses	89	0.9
Acne vulgaris	74	0.8
Drug eruptions	63	0.7
Congenital conditions	44	0.5
Hair disorders	36	0.4
Sweat disorders	32	0.4
Pruritus	19	0.2
Connective tissue disorders	17	0.2
Bullous eruptions	11	0.1
Nail disorders	5	0.05
Miscellaneous (unclassified)	86	0.9
Total	465	5.2

In this table which constitutes only 5.2 per cent of the prevalent skin diseases, genetic and developmental factors tend to count more than alterable environmental factors.

Thereafter, the incidence of skin diseases rises with age and increasing exposure to adverse cultural and environmental conditions and disease agents, the developing immunological competence of the growing child notwithstanding.

The 'top ten' groups of skin diseases are shown in Table 5.10.3. These constitute nearly 95 per cent of skin diseases seen in children. The first objective of their description is to make them fairly easily recognizable by the primary health care team (including mothers), non-specialist doctors, dermatologists and paediatricians. The second is to guide the primary health care workers on what they can treat and what should be referred to the non-specialist doctor or to the dermatologist or paediatrician.

Table 5.10.4 indicates the incidence of other skin diseases in children.

INFESTATIONS BY ANIMAL PARASITES

Scabies, lice, bedbugs, jiggers and fleas may share the homes of man. The larvae of larva migrans (creeping eruption) and cutaneous myiasis (tumbu fly) can infest compounds or gardens. The vectors of dracunculiasis (guinea-worm) and schistosomiasis can infest ponds and wells and streams. The insect vectors of the filarial worms can infest farms, forests and river banks. Children growing up in such infested environments fall victim to the disease agents, and the warm closeness of families leads to easy spread of the diseases.

Scabies

The contagious disease scabies is caused by the itch mite, *Sarcoptes scabiei* which is transmitted by close personal contact. A number of children from the same family, compound or school tend to present at the same time. Itching, most pronounced at night, is the constant presenting symptom. Epidemics of scabies are frequent in refugees camps and in other depressed socio-economic situations.

The common primary lesions are isolated papules, or lines of papules (runs), while secondary lesions may include pustules, vesicles, bullae, scabs, crusts, erosions and excoriations. Cellulitis or eczematization may also result. The common sites of these lesions are the webs and sides of the fingers, the wrists, the ulnar borders of the hands and forearms, the elbows, the axillary folds, the areola of the breasts, the abdomen, the umbilicus, the external genitalia, the thighs, the buttocks, the natal cleft, the knees, ankles and feet (Fig. 5.10.1).

Confirmation of the diagnosis is by identification of the mite in blunt scrapings from broken papules or vesicles, examined on a slide using a hand lens or the low power of a microscope.

Complications of untreated or wrongly treated scabies include secondary bacterial infection leading to pyoderma, cellulitis, lymphadenitis and even septicaemia. Eczematization may be provoked by irritant topical applications. A few patients may develop acarophobia, a delusion that the infestation persists in spite of successful treatment.

Treatment　All children and other affected members of the family should be treated together. After a thorough bath with soap and sponge at night, the appropriate scabicide is rubbed firmly into the skin from the neck down to the toes. This procedure should be repeated on two or three successive nights. Benzyl

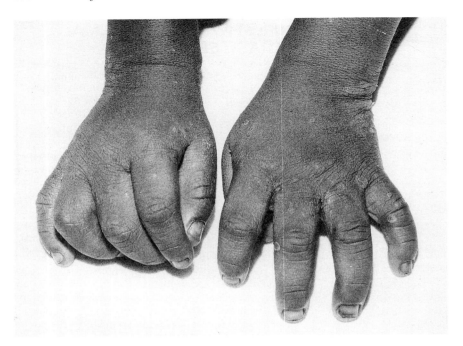

Fig. 5.10.1 Scabies: lesions in webs, sides of fingers, wrists.

benzoate emulsion (25 per cent) is the standard scabicide and the cheapest. Others include Ascabiol and Eurax (crotamiton). A soap containing 10 per cent tetraethyl thiuram monosulphide (Tetmosol) is also useful. Antihistamines should be given for the relief of itching, and appropriate antibiotics for secondary bacterial infection.

Pediculosis (lice infestation)

Pediculosis presents with itching of the affected parts and the lice and their nits (eggs) are seen easily on careful search. They are spread by close contact and the sharing of combs, brushes and clothing material.

Treatment Pediculosis capitis is treated by cutting the hair and applying a 5 per cent DDT emulsion, gamma-benzene hexachloride shampoo or 0.5 per cent malathion lotion. Pediculosis corporis is managed by treating the bedding and clothing with DDT powder or gamma-benzene hexachloride powder and then washing. The skin lesions can be treated with calamine lotion and antihistamine tablets or syrup. Pediculosis pubis is treated in the same way as pediculosis capitis.

Larva migrans (creeping eruption)

The larvae of certain worms inadvertently get into the skin and produce an itchy tortuous inflammatory reaction as they wander about in the skin aimlessly, destined to die without further development because man is not their natural host (see p. 639).

Treatment The larvae are frozen with ethyl chloride spray. Thiabendazole applied topically is also larvicidal. If infestation is extensive or visceral, thiabendazole (3–5 g orally) may be given weekly until larval activity stops.

Tumbu fly

The larvae of *Cordylobia anthropophaga* (tumbu fly) may enter the skin directly from the soil or through clothes which may have fallen on the ground. The disease presents as painful erythematous or dusky boil-like swellings. Within one to two weeks the maggots mature and push their way out of the skin, drop to the ground and pupate.

Treatment This consists of pressing out the maggots, destroying them and treating the cellulitis with antibiotics.

Jiggers

The pregnant female of *Tunga penetrans* (sand flea) attaches itself to the skin of the toe or foot, burrows into the dermis and grows rapidly. Its presence causes itching and soon a tender swelling the size of a bean or maize seed pushes to the surface. It is full of eggs which are discharged on to the ground. Cellulitis, secondary bacterial infection and even tetanus can develop from the associated dirty wound.

Treatment   The jigger should be prised out carefully and destroyed. The wound should be treated with antiseptics and systemic antibiotics may be necessary. A course of tetanus toxoid should be given.

Filarial infections

See pp. 686–96.

ECZEMA

The child's skin is the same sensitive organ in the tropics and subtropics as it is in the temperate region. The atopic diathesis has the same associations and organ involvements. Type IV hypersensitivity reaction forms the same basis for allergic contact dermatitis, and primary irritant dermatitis always depends on the concentration of the chemical agent. The high position of eczema in the 'top ten' of Table 5.10.3 is, therefore, not a surprise. It occurs in all races, social classes and ages.

Eczema is a distinctive inflammatory reaction in the skin, characterized in the acute stage by erythema or duskiness, papules, vesicles and bullae, and accompanied by itching. In the subacute stage, the vesicles and bullae break or are scratched open, and exudation, scabs, crusts and scales develop. In the chronic stage, scaling is more prominent and lichenification and hyperpigmentation may develop.

Eczema or dermatitis may be caused by exogenous factors, or by inherited or acquired factors which predispose the body to act in a hypersensitive way to substances which would not normally be antigenic.

Endogenous eczema

This is a constitutional disorder in which the precipitating causes are difficult to identify and are not reproducible by patch testing. It is more common in children than exogenous eczema or dermatitis which is more usual in adults who are more exposed at work, at home or at play to various allergens.

Forms of endogenous eczema seen in children include atopic eczema, seborrhoeic eczema, nummular eczema, nutritional eczema, and flexural infective eczema. Eczematization of scabies, onchodermatitis and other infestations are also common.

Atopic eczema

An atopic child readily develops IgE-mediated hypersensitivity reactions. This may present as infantile eczema starting in the first year of life or as atopic eczema in childhood or in adolescence.

Infantile eczema

This presents, at about three to six months, with erythema or duskiness on the cheeks and forehead associated with itching. Papules and vesicles develop later, and flexures; the neck and the elbows and knees in particular become involved. In the subacute stage, exudation and scaling occur, and secondary bacterial infection may follow. The trunk and other parts of the limbs may become affected (Fig. 5.10.2).

The condition tends to wax and wane over the years, responding positively but irregularly to appropriate treatment. The child may grow out of it in late childhood or the condition may become chronic with thick scaling, lichenification and hyperpigmentation. It is comparatively rare in rural tropical areas, possibly

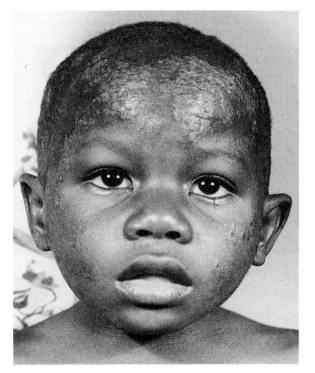

Fig. 5.10.2   Atopic eczema: scaling on forehead and cheeks.

because of prolonged breast-feeding which reduces the extent of foreign antigen exposure at an early age.

Atopic eczema starting in late childhood or adolescence presents with intensely itchy, scaly, flexural lesions studded with deep-seated papules and vesicles. Lichenification, fissuring, and hyperpigmentation follow prolonged scratching and diverse topical applications.

There is often a family history of atopic eczema or other atopic conditions, including bronchial asthma, allergic rhinitis (hay fever), urticaria and migraine. A child with atopic eczema may develop bronchial asthma or any of the other conditions while the atopic eczema is active or after it has cleared up.

Treatment   Children with atopic eczema tend to be sensitive. They should be treated with the minimum of fuss and allowed to grow up normally. Atopic eczema responds to corticosteroid lotions in the acute stage, creams in the subacute stage and ointments in the chronic stage. These should be used in the lowest possible concentration[1] and the ointments may be diluted with up to five parts of emulsifying ointment. Starting with applications thrice daily, the treatment should be tailed off weekly down to daily applications. In mild cases or when the more expensive corticosteroid preparations cannot be afforded, calamine lotion (with or without 3 per cent coal tar solution) may be used to good effect. Antihistamine syrup or tablets (e.g. chlorpheniramine, mepyramine, promethazine) may be given for the relief of itching, and sedatives may be given if itching or distress disturbs sleep. It is most important to advise against the use of irritant soaps and disinfectants, frequent baths and undue scratching.

Seborrhoeic eczema

This is the form of endogenous eczema which affects mainly the principal sebum-bearing areas of the body. It usually presents in infancy as the so-called 'cradle cap', fine yellowish or brown greasy scaling on the scalp. Also involved are the forehead, eyebrows, periauricular region, naso-labial folds, neck, axillae, presternal and interscapular regions. Later, other flexures and the whole trunk may be covered. The lesions may become erythematous or dusky and exudative but itching is not as severe as with atopic eczema. The condition does not usually persist into late childhood.

Treatment   With corticosteroid topical applications, emulsifying ointment and antihistamines, seborrhoeic eczema can be effectively managed. Scalp lesions respond to spirit shampoo, selenium sulphide shampoo, corticosteroid lotions or simple olive oil.

Other forms of endogenous eczema

Nummular or discoid eczema presents as itchy discoid or coin-shaped clusters of papules and vesicles which readily become exudative and scaly or crusted. The common sites are the dorsa of the hands or feet, arms, legs and trunk.

Flexural infective eczema presents as exudative lesions with scales and crusts and scabs with secondary bacterial infection, involving the flexures. It may be bilateral or unilateral.

These forms respond to treatment appropriate to the stage of eczema.

Exogenous eczema or dermatitis

Exogenous eczema is due to factors reaching the skin from outside. These factors are easy to demonstrate by patch testing, applying the suspected substances on the skin under occlusion and observing the reaction of the skin 48 hours later. A positive test will show erythema and vesicles.

Primary irritant dermatitis

When a strong acid, alkali, organic solvent or plant or animal product of sufficient concentration comes in contact with the skin, it produces blisters in the nature of a chemical burn within about 24 hours.

Children who play about with chemicals, plant juices or insects with vesicant (blister-producing) body fluids may produce primary irritant dermatitis on their skin. The lesions are painful rather than itchy. Unripe fruit juices, such as cashew, may produce such lesions around the lips of children. On healing, they may leave hyperpigmented circumoral macules.

Allergic contact dermatitis

This is an inflammatory skin reaction to a substance to which the skin has become sensitized by previous contact, a type IV hypersensitivity reaction, which may have taken days or weeks to develop. It is characterized by itching, erythema or duskiness and papules, vesicles and bullae. The primary lesions usually indicate the site of the original contact.

A host of allergens can produce allergic contact dermatitis in children of various ages. In infancy, napkin (diaper) dermatitis may result from a combination of contact with strong alkaline soaps or detergents with which the napkins are washed and ammonia formed from urine-soaked napkins.

Diverse baby soaps, lotions, creams, or oils of unspecified contents can provoke contact dermatitis on various parts of the body. Hair shampoos, deodorants and cosmetics, clothing materials including synthetic fibres and wool, and medicaments applied topically are among other causes of allergic contact dermatitis in children. Medicated soaps, disinfectants, sulphur ointment, penicillin ointment, tincture of iodine, sulphonamide ointments and antihistamine creams are among the causes of dermatitis medicamentosa.

Diagnosis of allergic contact dermatitis is made from a good history and confirmed by patch testing.

Treatment This begins with eliminating contact with the suspected or patch test-proved allergens. Application of the topical corticosteroid appropriate to the stage of dermatitis (see earlier) and administration of antihistamines are useful. Sedatives may be given if sleep is disturbed.

In mild cases or when corticosteroid applications are unaffordable, calamine lotion can be used to good effect. Irritant applications and soaps should be avoided.

Generalized exfoliative dermatitis

This is a widespread inflammatory reaction with scaling all over the body. It may complicate existing dermatitis or may develop on its own. In severe cases, there is generalized exudation with loss of fluid and protein and secondary bacterial infection. The condition may be life-threatening, and call for prompt and adequate fluid replacement intravenously, control of the severe reaction with systemic corticosteroids and antihistamines and combating infection with appropriate systemic antibiotics.

BACTERIAL INFECTIONS

The external environment abounds with bacteria. Many bacteria are entrapped in the extensive net of the skin. Some are killed by the acid mantle of the skin. Some survive and live as commensals, while others become pathogenic and invade the skin.

Factors which favour the establishment of skin infections in children include poorly developed immunity, severe illness, malnutrition, trauma (abrasions, scratches and cuts) and insect bites. The warm closeness of family and friends and the low standards of personal and community hygiene contribute to the easy spread of bacterial infections. Common bacterial infections include impetigo neonatorum, impetigo contagiosum, ecthyma, folliculitis, sycosis cruris, furunculosis, carbuncles, pyoderma, cellulitis and gangrene.

Impetigo neonatorum

Thin flaccid bullae may appear on the skin of the newborn within hours or days of birth and spread rapidly over the body (see pp. 233–40). This must be distinguished from congenital causes of bullous eruptions, e.g. epidermolysis bullosa.

Impetigo neonatorum which is due to *Staphyloccus aureus* infection may spread through the hands of nurses to other neonates in the same nursery; the initial infection may have been introduced by a mother, nurse, doctor, midwife or other hospital staff or by a visitor who may be a carrier of pathogenic bacteria in the skin, nose or upper respiratory tract. An epidemic may ensue with high mortality unless prompt action is taken to isolate and treat the affected neonates. Death may result from septicaemia, gastroenteritis, pneumonia, lung abscesses, glomerulonephritis, osteomyelitis or meningitis.

Treatment The infected neonate or neonates must be promptly isolated and treated with large doses of the appropriate antibiotics determined by antibiotic sensitivity tests on skin swabs and blood cultures. Massive systemic treatment with a widespectrum antibiotic, e.g. cloxacillin, must be started at once.

Impetigo contagiosum

This presents as rapidly enlarging thin-walled vesicles or bullae on erythematous or dusky bases. These quickly become pustular, rupture and spread to adjacent or distant parts of the body by contact.

The raw, broken surfaces are covered with yellowish, brown or haemorrhagic exudates which dry to form scabs and crusts. The sites commonly affected are the exposed parts – face, neck, scalp, hands and feet – but covered parts may also be affected (Fig. 5.10.3a and b).

Treatment. Antiseptics, e.g. gentian violet, locally and antibiotics systemically are used. Topical antibiotics, e.g. neomycin, bacitracin and polymyxin, are also effective. On healing, hyperpigmented macules remain for some time but there is no scarring.

Ecthyma

This variant of impetigo contagiosum may develop in malnourished or debilitated children. The bullae of impetigo break and the erosions ulcerate deeply. Treatment is with adequate doses of antibiotics given

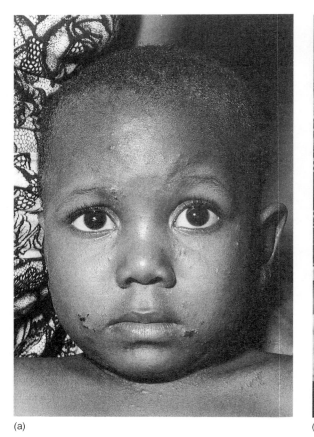

(a)

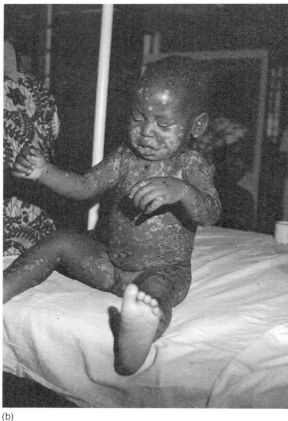

(b)

Fig. 5.10.3   Impetigo contagiosum. (a) Scabs on various parts of the face. (b) Extensive scarring of body.

systemically. On healing, deep punched-out scars remain (Fig. 5.10.4).

Hair follicle infections

The mouths of hair follicles harbour the greatest number of commensals and pathogenic bacteria. Trauma at the site or increased virulence of the bacteria will lead to infection of the hair follicles at various levels.

In folliculitis, infection is restricted to the mouths of the hair follicles. Small, yellowish pustules present on the scalp or the glabrous skin. In sycosis cruris, usually affecting the anterolateral aspect of the lower legs, infection spreads down to about the middle of the hair follicles, and tends to be recurrent or chronic. In furunculosis (boils) the roots of the hairs are infected. Round or dome-shaped nodules develop, necrose and suppurate. The common sites are the scalp, neck, large folds, buttocks, groins, perineum and trunk. The boils should be treated by incision and drainage, and appropriate antibiotics given systemically.

Treatment   Mild cases of folliculitis may be treated with gentian violet or other antiseptic applications. Other cases call for topical application of combinations of neomycin, bacitracin and polymyxin in the form of spray, cream or ointment. Gentamicin cream is also very effective. For sycosis cruris, penicillin G should be given in adequate doses while swabs are taken for culture and antibiotic sensitivity tests. The most appropriate antibiotic is then given. In furunculosis, suppurating lesions should be incised and drained.

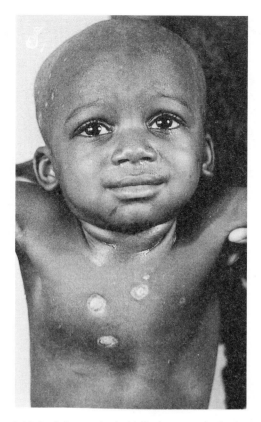

Fig. 5.10.4   Ecthyma: healed with deep punched-out scars.

Carbuncles

Caused by deep staphylococcal infection, these present as erythematous or dusky, indurated, painful and tender masses on the neck, back, waist, buttock, thigh or other site. Carbuncles may suppurate and discharge through multiple sinuses or may necrose, slough, and ulcerate. Suppurating lesions should be incised and drained. Factors which predispose to carbuncles include malnutrition, debility and prolonged corticosteroid therapy.

Pyoderma

A mixed picture of impetigo, cellulitis, folliculitis and furunculosis with ulceration and granulation may complicate simple bacterial infections or scabies, pediculosis, onchodermatitis or other infestations, or may complicate a systemic disease.

Antibiotics should be given and any underlying disease treated.

Cellulitis

Unlike the usually localized superficial or deep staphylococcal infections, streptococcal infections spread widely or in streaks (see pp. 514–16, 579). Cellulitis is usually a streptococcal infection which may be acute, subacute or chronic, affecting the skin and subcutaneous tissue. It may follow a scratch, pin or thorn prick, cut, bite, fissure, wound or ulcer, but may also develop on apparently normal skin.

Cellulitis begins as a red or dusky patch which becomes hot, indurated or oedematous and tender. It may spread in reddish or dusky streaks along the lymphatics to regional lymph nodes which become swollen and tender. There may be associated fever and malaise. Local complications may include necrosis and gangrene, and septicaemia may develop. Following recurrences or chronicity, localized lymphoedema may occur.

Diagnosis is based on the clinical picture and bacterial culture.

Treatment. Prompt and adequate treatment with penicillin G is required until antibiotic sensitivity test results indicate more specific treatment. The affected parts should be rested and any underlying systemic disease treated.

Gangrene

Necrosis or death of circumscribed parts of the skin may follow severe infectious fevers such as varicella (chickenpox), rubeola (measles), septicaemia, protein–energy malnutrition, leukaemia, or any debilitating illness. Other conditions which may be complicated by gangrene include severe pyoderma, genital ulceration, postoperative wound infection and *Pseudomonas pyocyanea* infection.

Specific treatment   This should include antibiotics and surgical excision of necrotic tissue.

Tropical ulcer

Neglect or wrong treatment of small injuries in hot, humid unhygienic settings still leads to rapidly growing, necrotic painful ulcers often with raised or undermined edges. The feet and lower legs are the common sites.

Treatment   This involves resting the affected leg, cleaning the ulcer with eusol, acriflavine, hydrogen peroxide or potassium permanganate solution, and dressing with medicated dressings. Appropriate systemic antibiotics should be given, and skin grafting may be necessary after good granulation tissue has formed.

Mycobacterial skin diseases

In children, the mycobacterial skin diseases of importance are leprosy, Buruli ulcer and tuberculosis of the skin.

Leprosy

See pp. 553–76.

Mycobacterium ulcerans infection (Buruli ulcer)

This may present as erythematous or dusky, firm, painless nodules or areas of induration. These may break down months later to form extensive shallow necrotic ulcers with undermined overhanging edges. The ulcers become chronic and heal exceedingly slowly leaving disfiguring scars (Fig. 5.10.5).

The first reported cases of Buruli ulcer were seen in Mengo, Uganda (1897) and in Barnsdale, Australia (1948) but the cluster of cases seen in the Buruli district of Uganda in the late 1950s gave the disease its name. Other cases have since been reported in other parts of Africa, Asia and the Americas.

Atypical acid-fast bacilli, *Mycobacterium ulcerans* may be demonstrated in smears from ulcers or in biopsy specimens.

Treatment   This is very difficult. Mycobactericidal drugs and co-trimoxazole have been tried with variable results. Wide excision with skin grafting may be called for.

Tuberculosis of the skin

In children, the most common manifestations of cutaneous tuberculosis include tuberculous adenitis, papulonecrotic tuberculide and papular tuberculide.

Tuberculous adenitis presents as 'cold abscesses' in the neck or other folds. These may break down to form sinuses. Bacilli may be found in biopsy material and the tuberculin test is usually positive. Investigations usually reveal visceral tuberculosis.

Papular and papulonecrotic tuberculide may be hypersensitivity reactions in the skin to occult visceral infection. The tuberculin test is usually positive but bacilli are seldom found in the lesions.

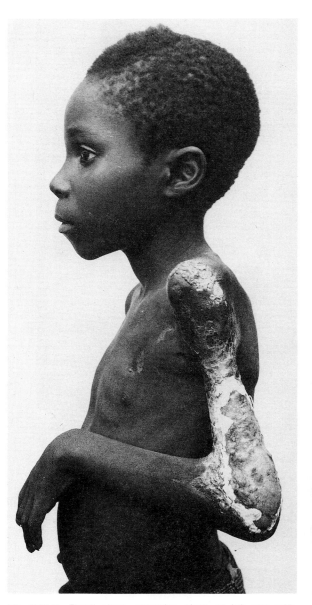

Fig. 5.10.5   Buruli ulcer: extensive ulcer on left arm with ankylosis of left elbow.

Lupus vulgaris

This is not a sensitivity reaction, but an actual infection of the skin with tubercle bacilli. It is a hypertrophic, granulating, necrotic lesion often affecting and disfiguring the face, but it can occur anywhere on the body (Fig. 5.10.6).

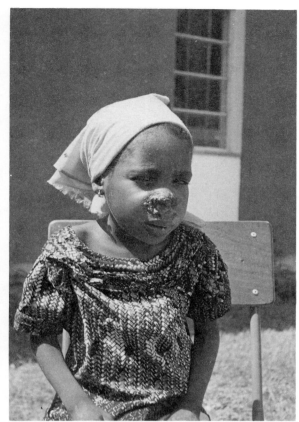

Fig. 5.10.6 Characteristic lesions of lupus vulgaris with granulomatous destruction of the skin and connective tissues.

Miscellaneous

It must be borne in mind that numerous skin rashes are associated with systemic disorders, such as Still's disease, as well as various bacterial infections. In meningococcaemia, there may be a purpuric or petechial rash and occasionally pink tender macules or papules over the trunk and extremities may develop, sometimes with haemorrhagic centres (see p. 578). In typhoid fever, pink maculopapular lesions (rose spots) are found on the trunk and chest, particularly during the second week of the disease (see pp. 584–6). In rheumatic fever, erythema marginatum is characteristic (see pp. 776–8).

FUNGAL INFECTIONS

Spores of various fungi abound in nature and, given the hot humid tropical and subtropical environment, the warm closeness of families and friends, and poor personal and community hygiene, children are readily infected with these spores.

Fungal infections may be superficial, involving the skin, mucosa, hair or nails; deep, involving subcutaneous tissues; or visceral, causing great constitutional upset.

Superficial fungal infections

Dermatophytes, which cause superficial infections, invade the top layers of the epidermis and its appendages and digest the keratin for nourishment. Superficial fungal infections can be caught by direct contact with another person (anthropophylic), an animal (zoophilic), and the soil (geophylic) or by indirect contact with clothing, combs, brushes, footwear, household furniture or farm equipment. The most common superficial fungal infections are the tineal infections and candidiasis.

Tineal infections

Tinea versicolor

Tinea versicolor presents as yellowish-brown, brown or dark-brown macules in irregular patches or confluent sheets of dry scales over the upper trunk, shoulders, neck and face (see pp. 627–8). Often the lesions are most prominent over the interscapular and sternal regions, and sometimes there is perifollicular concentration of lesions.

Tinea versicolor is mainly of cosmetic inconvenience and causes little or no itching. It is more common in later childhood and adolescence than in early childhood. It runs a chronic course, with a tendency to recurrence after apparent spontaneous regression and after inadequate treatment.

Infection is caused by *Malassezia furfur* which can be demonstrated microscopically in skin scrapings taken from the lesions, and treated on a microscope slide with potassium hydroxide solution 10–20 per cent. It shows up microscopically as short hyphal elements and clusters of spores which fluoresce under Wood's filtered ultraviolet radiation. It does not grow in Sabouraud's medium.

Treatment Topical application of effective keratolytic agents remains the best method, provided the treatment is for an adequate length of time. The older remedies readily available and affordable include Whitfield's ointment (compound ointment of benzoic acid), salicylic acid ointment, selenium sulphide suspension, tolnaftate and sodium hyposulphite solution. The imidazole derivatives are more effective but more expensive, e.g. clotrimazole, tioconazole, bifonazole.

Ringworm infection (tinea)

A variety of dermatophytes (*Microsporum*, *Trichophyton* and *Epidermophyton*) cause ringworm of the skin, hair and nails in children (see also pp. 624–7). Zoophilic infections provoke inflammatory reactions more readily than anthropophylic infections. Some fungal infections may provoke a papulo-vesicular eruption on a site away from the infection site.

Immunological factors may affect the development, spread and chronicity of fungal infections, and prolonged corticosteroid therapy may encourage the development and spread of fungal infections.

Clinical presentation of ringworm infections The pattern varies with the part of the body affected and with such factors as dryness, moistness and texture of the skin, and the species of fungi. The resulting lesions may be annular, circinate, discoid or irregular in outline. They may be dry, scaly, inflamed, exudative, boggy, hypertrophic, warty, or secondarily infected. Ringworm infections are usually itchy.

A simple classification of ringworm infections is on anatomical basis: tinea capitis (scalp), tinea corporis (glabrous skin), tinea axillaris (axillae), tinea cruris (groin), tinea manuum (hands), tinea pedis (feet), tinea unguium (nails).

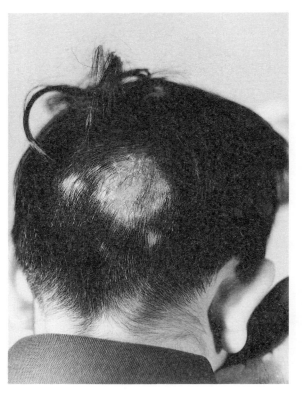

Fig. 5.10.7   Tinea capitis in three-year-old Indian boy.

Tinea capitis

Tinea of the scalp is most common in young children before adolescence. It usually presents as dry, scaly patches of hair loss, the invaded and weakened hair shafts having broken off at various levels (Fig. 5.10.7)

Tinea capitis may become inflamed if the invading fungus is zoophilic or if itching has provoked much scratching. Secondary bacterial infection of the scalp may also develop, leading to occipital or cervical lymphadenitis.

Named variants of tinea capitis include kerion, a boggy painful and tender swelling due to zoophilic or secondary bacterial infection, and favus, a crusted, moth-eaten or honey-comb picture covering most of the scalp.

The causal fungi vary from region to region, but *Microsporum* and *Trichophyta* are the most common ones. *M. audouini*, *M. canis*, *M. gypseum*, and *M. ferrugineum* are frequently isolated. Among the *Trichophyta*, *T. soudanense*, *T. violaceum*, *T. schoenleini*, *T. tonsurans* and *T. mentagrophytes* are most commonly isolated.

Tinea capitis tends to regress spontaneously with the advent of puberty and sophistication, the increased outpouring of sebum reinforcing the body's defences against fungal infection.

Tinea corporis

This refers to infection of the glabrous skin (face, neck, and limbs), and excludes axillae, groins, hands and feet which are described separately.

The characteristic lesion is annular, concentric, circinate or irregular and scaly with an active border and a tendency to clearing towards the centre. Activity at the border may include raised edges, papule or vesicle formation, inflammation, exudation or secondary bacterial infection. Large areas of the trunk or limbs may be covered by centrifugal extensions at various points of the initial lesion. Tinea corporis is usually itchy (Fig. 5.10.8.)

The causal fungi include *Trichophyton*, *Microsporum* and *Epidermophyton* of various species.

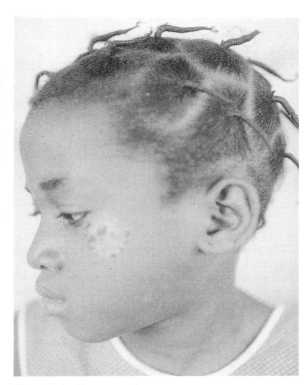

Fig. 5.10.8   Tinea corporis.

Tinea axillaris

Because of the moistness and hairiness of the axillae, infection in adolescent children may present as irregular inflammatory or scaly lesions with a tendency to secondary bacterial infection. Itching may be intense.

Trichophyton is the most common fungus but *Epidermophyton* may also be encountered.

Tinea cruris

Infection of the groin presents as scaly, circinate erythematous lesions which may spread from the groins downwards to the thighs, inwards to the scrotum or vulva, upwards to the pubic region and backwards to the buttocks. Itching is intense and scratching leads to secondary bacterial infection. *Trichophyton* predominates but *Epidermophyton* can also be encountered.

Tinea pedis and tinea manuum

These are less common in children than in adults but do occur. They may start on the dorsa or sides of the feet or hands as scaly roughly circinate lesions and spread to the soles or palms and the toe or finger webs. They may also develop on the soles or palms *de novo*, as rough scaly plaques with indistinct edges, and a tendency to papule or vesicle formation. In the toe or finger webs, they may cause maceration and become secondarily infected. The predominant fungus is *Trichophyton*.

Tinea unguium

Infection in this case usually starts at the free edge of the nail and extends to the nail plate to varying depths. The affected nails may become yellowish or brown, brittle, frayed, or ridged vertically or horizontally. They may crumble or peel off when greatly weakened.

Tinea unguium may develop as part of infection of the feet or hands or may develop on its own. It is usually chronic. *Trichophyton* is the most common fungus isolated.

Diagnosis of ringworm infections

Because of the high incidence of these infections and their variegated clinical presentations which may resemble other dermatoses, care should be taken with their clinical diagnosis, and mycological diagnosis should always be aimed at for confirmation. Some fungi may fluoresce under Wood's filtered ultraviolet lamp.

Mycological diagnosis   Skin or nail scrapings or nail or hair clippings should be placed on a microscope slide, flooded with 10–20 per cent potassium hydroxide solution, warmed over a Bunsen burner to digest the keratin, covered with a cover slip, and examined under a microscope. Mycelia and spores of various fungi can usually be demonstrated. The addition of a drop of blue ink often shows up the mycelia more clearly.

Scales, skin or nail scrapings and hair or nail clippings can be cultured on Sabouraud's medium. Fluffy, matted or creamy colonies appear within days or weeks and the coloured stains which are produced in the medium help to identify the species of fungi. *Trichophyton rubrum* produces a deep red stain. Subcultures from these colonies can be prepared in advanced mycological laboratories.

Differential diagnosis   Tinea capitis may be confused with alopecia areata, seborrhoea capitis, pyoderma, folliculitis decalvans, chronic discoid lupus erythematosus and trichotillomania. Tinea corporis may resemble tinea versicolor, seborrhoeic eczema, nummular eczema, pityriasis rosea, psoriasis, lupus vulgaris, or secondary syphilis. It must also be distinguished from tuberculoid or indeterminate leprosy in which there is loss of sensation within the lesions. Tinea axillaris and tinea cruris may be difficult to differentiate from candidiasis, intertrigo, flexural eczema, seborrhoeic eczema and erythrasma, a bacterial infection. Tinea manuum and pedis may resemble contact dermatitis, candidiasis, keratoderma, cheiropompholyx or podopompholyx. Tinea unguium may be confused with chronic paronychia, aspergillosis, psoriasis, nail dystrophy, trauma, nail biting, cosmetic staining, or nail discoloration by antibiotics or heavy metals.

Treatment of ringworm infections

When mycological diagnosis has confirmed clinical diagnosis, the choice of treatment may be made on economic grounds. The cheaper, older topical applications may be effective but call for prolonged use, one or two months or more. The more expensive newer topical applications are effective over a shorter period. The systemic antifungal agents are quickly effective but very expensive. Some have undesirable side-effects.

Topical applications   Keratolytic agents are effective against lesions which are small, few in number and not chronic. Lesions of the glabrous skin (tinea corporis, axillaris, cruris, manuum and pedis) respond better than tinea capitis or tinea unguium. These agents are in the form of ointments, creams, liquid or powder, and are applied two or three times daily according to need. Whitfield's ointment (Ung. acid benz. co) comprises 5 per cent benzoic acid, 3 per cent salicylic acid and 25 per cent soft paraffin in hydrophilic ointment. Salicylic acid ointment may be used in 5–10 per cent strength. Tolnaftate and haloprogin (Halotex) are used as cream, liquid or powder. The new imidazole derivatives, Clotrimazole (Canesten), tioconazole (Trosyd), bifonazole (Mycospor) and miconazole (Daktarin) are all very effective in liquid, cream or ointment preparations.

Systemic antifungal agents   The advent of griseofulvin in the late 1950s simplified the treatment of various ringworm infections. It should not be used when diagnosis is not made or is in doubt. It should also not be used against tinea versicolor and candidiasis which are not susceptible.

Griseofulvin is given orally, and on absorption and incorporation into keratin, inhibits the metabolism and growth of many species of fungi – *Trichophyton*, *Microsporum* and *Epidermophyton*. It is therefore effective against tinea infection of various parts of the body,

including the nails. The dose is 10–20 mg/kg per day in divided doses. The duration of treatment varies with the type and chronicity of infection, from about one month in tinea corporis up to six months in tinea unguium. The side-effects are mild, including headache, nausea and urticaria.

Imidazole derivatives are also available and effective orally. Ketoconazole (Nizoral) (200 mg orally daily) is effective against tinea versicolor, dermatophyte and yeast infections.[2] Reported side-effects include pruritus, gastro-intestinal upset and transient fever chills and hepatotoxicity.

Candidiasis (moniliasis)

Yeast-like fungi, including *Candida albicans*, *C. tropicalis* and *C. parapsilosis*, can infect the skin and mucous membranes in children (see p. 628). In infants, infection of the buccal mucosa presents as thrush. This is seen as clusters of creamy, milky or greyish spots, macules or sheets on the lips, tongue, palate or cheeks. The infection may spread down the pharynx, oesophagus or further down the gastro-intestinal tract. This spread may cause diarrhoea and constitutional upset. The anal and vaginal mucosa may also be infected. Systemic candidiasis may develop in debilitated or immunocompromised children with conditions such as AIDS.

Dusky red macerated or erosive lesions may develop in the skin folds of the neck, flexures and flanks. Fissuring or bleeding may follow scratching of these lesions, and secondary bacterial infection may develop.

Chronic paronychia occurs causing the nail folds of the fingers and toes to become swollen and tender with distortion of the nails later. Pus may be expressed between the nail fold and the nail plate.

Mycological diagnosis   Swabs from the affected parts may be smeared on a microscope slide, treated with potassium hydroxide solution, and examined under the microscope for spores. Culture of specimens on Sabouraud's medium usually grows glistening creamy colonies. Microscopic examination of specimens from these colonies reveals spores of various *Candida* species.

Treatment   Superficial lesions respond to topical applications of mycostatin and imidazole derivatives – clotrimazole, miconazole, tioconazole and bifonazole. Amphotericin B (Fungizone) and 5-fluorocytosine are also effective topically. Systemic candidiasis calls for amphotericin B intravenously. Imidazole derivatives, e.g. ketoconazole (3 mg/kg daily), can also be given orally.

Deep fungal infections

Fungal infections may involve the skin and subcutaneous tissue, fascia, fat, muscles, tendons, bones and joints. These include actinomycosis, mycetoma, histoplasmosis, sporotrichosis, chromomycosis and phycomycosis. Their incidence is low compared with dermatophytoses, but they are usually chronic and disabling and can be lethal when viscera are involved.

Actinomycosis

This presents as chronic suppurating granulomata on the abdomen, chest, neck or other sites. Microscopic examination and culture of swabs from discharging sinuses will show *Actinomyces israelii*, the causal organism.

Treatment   Procaine penicillin ($1–5 \times 10^6$ units daily) or tetracycline (1–2 g daily) should be given until the lesions clear up.

Mycetoma (Madura foot)

Mycetoma presents as nodules, granulomata or verrucose lesions of the foot and leg with general induration of the affected limb. There may be secondary bacterial infection with suppuration and the development of chronic discharging sinuses. The underlying muscles, tendons and even bone may become involved and the affected limb may become a useless burden. The full picture seldom manifests until adult life, but earlier lesions may be seen in children (see p. 630).

Confirmation of the diagnosis is by microscopic examination and culture of swabs from the discharging sinuses. The commonly isolated organisms include *Nocardia brasiliensis*, *N. asteroides*, *N. transvalensis*, *Streptomyces somaliensis*, *Madurella mycetomi*, *M. grisea* and *Leptospareria senegalensis*.

Conditions which need to be differentiated from mycetoma include osteomyelitis (bacterial); lymphoedema which is even, and does not suppurate; elephantiasis which usually extends further up the legs; actinomycosis which may affect other sites more commonly than the legs; and Kaposi's sarcoma which is more nodular, may be haemorrhagic, and is rare in children.

Treatment   There is as yet no regularly effective specific treatment. Cotrimoxazole, diaminodiphenyl sulphone, griseofulvin and the imidazoles given orally have all proved useful on occasions. A useless foot may have to be amputated.

Histoplasmosis

Various species of *Histoplasma* may invade subcutaneous or deeper tissues or the viscera (see p. 631). Infection with *Histoplasma duboisii* presents as cutaneous and subcutaneous nodules which tend to umbilicate and suppurate or ulcerate as they grow. In disseminated infections, lymph nodes and bones may be invaded and there may also be pulmonary lesions. Infection with *H. capsulatum* characteristically affects the lungs, and presents with productive cough and constitutional upset.

Confirmation of diagnosis is by microscopic examination of swab or biopsy material, sputum, blood or bone marrow.

Treatment   For visceral and non-visceral histoplasmosis, the appropriate treatment is systemic. Amphotericin B, 0.5 mg–1 mg/kg body weight in 5 per cent glucose infusion. Oral ketoconazole 200 mg daily promises good results.

Chromomycosis

Chromomycosis presents as nodules and warty plaques on the feet and legs (see p. 630). The affected limb becomes oedematous, indurated and verrucose, and the lesions may ulcerate and become secondarily infected. Chromomycosis is caused by phialophora of various species which can be isolated in culture from scrapings or biopsy material.

Treatment   This is with intravenous amphotericin B. Oral ketoconazole (200 mg daily) and 5-fluorocytosine (6–8 g daily) have also been found to be effective.

Subcutaneous phycomycoses

This presents as a slowly developing non-tender subcutaneous rubbery induration with distinct edges. The overlying skin is taut and hyperpigmented. The common sites are the thighs, buttocks and trunk (see p. 629).

Diagnosis is by biopsy and microscopy and culture which will demonstrate the causal organisms. These are phycomycetes, e.g. *Basidiobolus ranarum*.

Treatment   An old empirical remedy which is still effective in treatment is potassium iodide 10–50 drops in water or milk daily in divided doses. Ketoconazole, diaminodiphenyl sulphone and co-trimoxazole orally, and amphotericin B intravenously have been found to be effective in some cases.

VIRAL INFECTIONS

Viruses cause a wide variety of skin diseases in children of all ages. The most common infections are warts, Herpes simplex, Herpes zoster, varicella, rubeola (measles), rubella (German measles), molluscum contagiosum, Kaposi's varicelliform eruption and infectious mononucleosis. Some viruses may cause severe or lethal illness. (See also pp. 600–623.)

Most viral infections clear up spontaneously while others call for treatment, specific or non-specific. Specific antiviral agents have been developed, e.g. idoxuridine and acyclovir (see p. 616).

Warts (verrucae)

These are benign tumours which result from epithelial hyperplasia of skin or mucous membrane invaded by papilloma viruses (DNA viruses). They begin as small papules and develop various patterns, depending on the site, skin texture, moistness or dryness, and pressure on the skin.

Plane, flat or juvenile warts (verruca plana)

These present on the face, hands and fingers as small, flat, smooth skin-coloured papules which may coalesce or remain discrete. Some lesions appear flush with the skin. Many plane warts regress or resolve spontaneously.

Common warts (verruca vulgaris)

Skin-coloured, brown or greyish papules or rough verrucose plaques develop mainly on the exposed parts. They are more itchy and more chronic than plane warts but some may also regress spontaneously. Filiform and digitate warts develop in thread-like or finger-like patterns which grow more rapidly than common warts. Plantar warts and palmar warts present as hard hypertrophic nodules or calluses on the soles or palms. Because of pressure, they do not project much above the surface and they are painful and tender. Anogenital warts grow profusely into moist dusky clusters which if neglected may become secondarily infected and malodorous.

The diagnosis is based on the history and characteristic clinical picture. Papilloma virus infections can be diagnosed by the detection of specific viral DNA with hybridization techniques. These techniques are only available in specialized laboratories. Biopsy for histopathology shows acanthosis, but is also not routinely done.

Treatment. In children, spontaneous regression occurs in up to 60 per cent of cases. The remainder may require topical applications, chemical destruction, cold surgery (liquid nitrogen), diathermy, excision or 'charming'. Topical applications include 25 per cent podophyllin in alcohol; 25–40 per cent salicylic acid ointment with or without adhesive plaster; wart paste comprising trichloracetic acid 3 per cent, salicylic acid 20 per cent and glycerin 5 ml; 10 per cent benzoyl peroxide cream is effective against juvenile warts. Freshly prepared liquor arsenicalis is useful in anogenital warts. Chemical destruction with formalin, phenol, nitric acid, or glacial acetic acid is good for common warts and plantar and palmar warts after careful paring with a scalpel or razor blade. Excision, diathermy or curetting under local anaesthesia may be required for digitate, plantar and palmar warts, while sessile, filiform warts can be tied off with a black thread or suture.

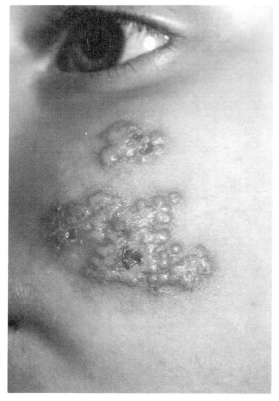

Fig. 5.10.9   Herpes simplex eruption on cheek.

Herpes simplex

Herpes simplex (labialis, febrilis) presents as burning crops of clear tense vesicles around the lips, eyes, nose, external genitalia or other parts (Fig. 5.10.9). There may be associated low-grade fever, eruptions may occur associated with pneumococcal and meningococcal infections. The condition is usually mild, clearing up a few days, but the rate of recurrence is high. Some severe cases may become erosive or ulcerative, and viraemia may lead to severe illness, notably encephalitis.

Treatment Non-specific treatment includes treatment of the underlying febrile illness, the relief of symptoms, e.g. burning, itching or pain, and a wide range of topical applications – ether, chloroform, providone iodine, levamisole. Topical treatment with antiviral products is of doubtful benefit. In severe Herpes simplex infections systemic treatment with acylovir is indicated (see pp. 615–16). Antiseptics or antibiotic creams are useful for secondary bacterial infection.

Kaposi's varicelliform eruption

This rare disease is due to Herpes simplex infection of an eczematous child. The face and limbs are studded with papules, pustules and vesicles. Acyclovir is effective; prevention of secondary bacterial infection is important.

Varicella (chickenpox)

This infectious fever of childhood, with an incubation period of 1–3 weeks, is characterized by crops of clear, tense vesicles, widespread on the body, but more profuse on the trunk than on the limbs and face, and associated with fever, malaise and itching (see p. 616). Secondary bacterial infection may lead to ulceration of broken vesicles and superficial scarring. Varicella is caused by the same virus as *Herpes zoster* (see later). Complications include pneumonia, glomerulonephritis and meningoencephalitis.

Treatment This consists of the relief of itching with calamine lotion and antihistamine, and control of bacterial infections with antibiotics.

Herpes zoster

This presents as prodromal burning sensation over a dermatome followed by erythema and clusters of tense, painful vesicles over the same area (see p. 617). These vesicles break, and superficial ulcers develop which heal with scarring. These lesions develop over the cutaneous distribution of cranial or spinal nerves. Among the cranial nerves, the trigeminal nerve is the most commonly affected, and among the spinal nerves T_2-T_{10} are the most frequently affected. The virus remains dormant in the posterior roots of these nerves after an episode of chickenpox. Complications of Herpes zoster include scarring, post-herpetic neuralgia, and keratitis in association with Herpes zoster ophthalmicus.

Treatment. Prompt and adequate control of pain with analgesics is vital. Idoxuridine and acyclovir have been used for treating keratitis although their efficacy is unproven. Antibiotics should be given if secondary bacterial infection develops. Chlorpromazine is useful in the management of post-herpetic neuralgia.

Measles

See pp. 496–502.

Molluscum contagiosum

This presents as non-itchy, discrete, glistening papules which may become globular as they enlarge in size.

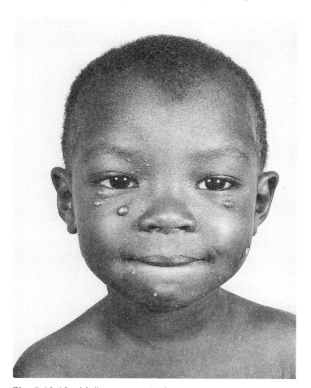

Fig. 5.10.10 Molluscum contagiosum.

Large lesions become umbilicated as the centres degenerate. Newer lesions are produced by autoinoculation of viral particles from older lesions (Fig. 5.10.10.) Some lesions regress spontaneously. Others do so after secondary bacterial infection. Apart from smallpox, which has been eradicated, molluscum contagiosum is the only strictly human poxvirus disease.

Treatment   This is by curettage of sizeable lesions. The bleeding bases are then touched with tincture of iodine or with compound tincture of benzoin. Systemic antibiotics may be required for secondary bacterial infection.

PAPULO-SQUAMOUS (SCALY) ERUPTIONS

These common skin diseases are distinguished by their characteristic patterns of scaling but their primary lesions are papular. The incidence of pityriasis rosea, lichen planus and psoriasis varies from place to place, but in most of the tropics, pityriasis rosea is the most common and psoriasis the least common.[3]

Pityriasis rosea

This disease starts with a solitary circular or ovoid erythematous papulo-vesicular eruption (the herald patch) on the trunk, upper arm or thigh. About one to two weeks later, numerous similar but smaller circular or ovoid scaly lesions appear, mainly on the trunk, neck, upper arms and thighs but possibly extending to the face, forearms and lower legs (Fig. 5.10.11).

Itching may be mild or moderate, but there is usually no fever or constitutional upset. The condition is self-limiting lasting 6–12 weeks and clearing up gradually without leaving any pigmentary changes or scars. Eczematization may follow topical application of irritant or sensitizing medicaments or soap. The aetiology of pityriasis is uncertain, but a viral aetiology is postulated.

Diagnosis is based on the distinctive history and morphological pattern. Histopathology will show mild dermatitis with superficial spongiosis.

Differential diagnosis   Tinea vesicolor is mainly on the upper trunk. *Malassezia furfur* can be demonstrated in skin scrapings. Seborrhoeic eczema is more profuse in the sebum-bearing areas and flexures. Tinea corporis is seldom as widespread and symmetrical. Psoriasis has much thicker scales and has a predilection for pressure area.

Treatment   Itching is relieved with antihistamines, e.g. chlorpheniramine syrup (5 ml) or tablets (2–4 mg

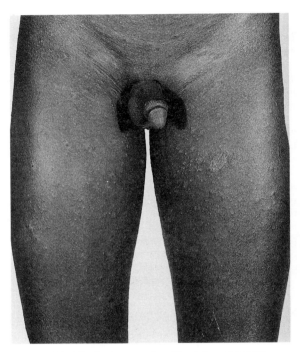

Fig. 5.10.11   Pityriasis rosea: herald patch on left thigh.

twice daily). Soothing lotions or creams, e.g. calamine, tone down the scaling and relieve the itching. More severe lesions can be treated with corticosteroid creams or ointments.

Lichen planus

This disease is characterized by shiny, flat-topped violaceous or slaty-grey papules or plaques which start around the wrists, lower trunk or lower legs and later appear in other sites. Itching is usually moderate or severe and the more the child scratches the more the lesions extend to the scratched areas (Kobner phenomenon). As the lesions age or subside, they became hyperpigmented. Variants of the condition include mucosal, nail, bullous generalized and hypertrophic lesions. Psychogenic and autoimmune factors are thought to be involved in the aetiology.

Histology reveals hyperkeratosis, hypergranulosis, acanthosis, prolongation of the rate ridges and a band of lymphocytic infiltration in the upper third of the dermis.

Differential diagnosis   Psoriasis, lichenified eczema, lichenoid drug eruptions, and secondary syphilis may be confused with lichen planus.

Treatment Itching, insomnia and stress may be controlled with antihistamines, sedatives and tranquilizers respectively. Soothing lotions and creams are also helpful. In acute widespread or bullous eruptions, systemic corticosteroids may be called for, e.g. prednisolone tablets 10 mg three times daily for two weeks and tailed off appropriately.

Psoriasis

With the strong familial and climate elements in this condition, the incidence varies with different races and climates. It is less common in the subtropics and tropics than in temperate regions. The presentation is, however, characteristic, with thick silvery or greyish lamellated scales on or around the scalp, on the elbows and knees, the extensor surfaces of the limbs and the trunk and waist. Itching is mild or moderate. The margins are sharp, and the unaffected skin appears normal. The guttate variety consists of discrete scaly papules of widespread distribution on the trunk and limbs.

Psoriasis is a chronic dyskeratotic disorder which waxes and wanes over the years, with or without treatment. The sites of healed lesions appear normal with no obvious pigmentary changes.

Histology shows hyperkeratosis, parakeratosis, acanthosis and micro-abscesses in the epidermis, and capillary dilatation and round cell infitrates in the dermis.

Differential diagnosis Scalp lesions may be mistaken for tinea capitis, seborrhoea capitis or folliculitis. Lesions on the trunk may resemble secondary syphilis but scaling is not prominent in syphilis and serological tests are positive. Seborrhoeic eczema, pityriasis rosea and tinea corporis and tinea vesicolor may also resemble psoriasis. Hypertrophic lesions of lichen planus and lichen simplex chronicus may also be confused with psoriasis. Psoriasis has been misdiagnosed as leprosy since biblical times (2nd Kings Chapter 5) and both diseases continue to be misdiagnosed to this day.

Treatment The wide range of various topical applications used indicates the non-specificity and limited efficacy of many of them. Ultraviolet radiation is the mainstay of modern treatment, the skin being pretreated with tar bath, brine as in the Dead Sea programme or psoralens orally. Other non-specific topical applications in current use include 1 per cent coal tar paste, dithranol ointment and corticosteroid ointment. Retinoic acid analogues can also be used for oral treatment but have the drawback of suspected teratogenicity.

ALLERGIC ERUPTIONS

Allergy, the altered tissue reaction to substances with which the body had had previous contact, may be considered protective, the aim of the reaction being to stop or minimize further absorption of the unacceptable antigens. Skin eruptions associated with such allergic reactions in children include urticaria, angio-oedema, erythema multiforme, erythema annulare, erythema nodosum, granuloma annulare, papular urticaria and purpura.

Urticaria

Urticaria is a very common disorder marked by the sudden or gradual appearance of itchy evanescent raised wheals of variable sizes and shapes on the skin or mucosa. The wheals may be pale, skin-coloured or erythematous. They may be circular, ovoid, annular or irregular in shape, varying from a pin-head to a geographical pattern many centimetres across, and looking like an orange skin with its multiple pitting. Some wheals may last some minutes, hours, days or weeks. Others may become chronic or recurrent. The severity of wheals varies from the mildest inconvenience of burning, through uncontrollable itching to anaphylaxis with peripheral vascular collapse and impending death.

The wheals are produced following the release of histamine or histaminoid substances from mast cells in the dermis which can be provoked by antigens, immunoglobulins or complement. Histamine, bradykinin, kallikrein, acetycholine and prostaglandins cause cutaneous vasodilatation and localized tissue oedema. This fluid accumulation stretches the skin into the familiar pattern of wheals. There is no tissue destruction and when the reaction subsides or is counteracted with antihistamines or vasoconstrictors the affected skin returns to normal.

Aetiology Causes of urticaria include allergic and non-allergic factors. Allergens may get into the body by: ingestion – food, drinks, drugs, parasites[4], micro-organisms; inhalation – chemical fumes, insecticides, sprays, deodorants; injection or inunction – insect, fish and other animal stings or bites, drugs, plant and animal bristles, e.g. bacteria, other micro-organisms and animal parasites. Chronic urticaria may be associated with systemic diseases, infections, reticuloses, autoimmune diseases and neoplasms. Non-allergic or mixed factors include mechanical pressure, heat or cold, sunlight, and familial, hormonal and psychogenic factors.

Differential diagnosis Insect bites or stings can be

traced to source. Erythema multiforme may have other elements, e.g. vesicles, bullae and mucosal lesions. Localized lymphoedema is usually more extensive, more chronic and the affected part is indurated. Localized myxoedema will show other features of thyroid disease. Oedema of renal origin is symmetrical, with puffiness of the face and eyelids, oedema of other parts and proteinuria.

Treatment   The most vital measures in the management of urticaria are identification, elimination and avoidance of the cause. Antihistamines should be given orally or parenterally, depending on the severity of the reaction. In severe cases, adrenaline (1 ml of 1/1000 solution) is given subcutaneously slowly.

Angio-oedema   Sudden or gradual gross oedema of the skin and mucosa may develop as a reaction to allergens (food or drugs). The lips, nose, eyes, tongue, pharynx and larynx swell to the point of causing dyspnoea and dysphagia. Bronchospasm, nausea, vomiting and abdominal cramps may also develop. In severe angio-oedema, adrenaline subcutaneously and intravenous hydrocortisone hemisuccinate (50–100 mg intravenously) should be given promptly.

Erythema multiforme

Erythema multiforme is marked by an acute or insidious eruption of a variety of lesions – erythema, macules, papules, vesicles, bullae, iris or target lesions, urticaria, annular lesions or purpuric spots or blotches. The most common sites are the face, peri-oral region, external genitalia, hands and feet. There may be associated fever and constitutional upset and the condition may be recurrent or cyclical.

The causes are numerous and include bacterial infections, viral infections and drugs, e.g. sulphonamides, salicylates, phenolphthalein, barbiturates, diaminodiphenyl sulphone, pyrimethamine and penicillin.

In the severe variant known as toxic erythema multiforme (Stevens–Johnson syndrome) the cutaneous lesions are accompanied by mucosal erosion of the mouth, eyes, throat and external genitalia. There is severe constitutional upset and secondary bacterial infection and exudative lesions all over the body may lead to severe fluid, electrolyte and protein loss.

Treatment   Identification, elimination and avoidance of the aetiological factor are vital. Antihistamines relieve itching and burning. Underlying infection require appropriate systemic antibiotics. In toxic erythema multiforme, systemic corticosteroids should be given first parenterally and later orally. The dosage should be tailed off over the weeks. Fluid and electrolyte loss should be corrected by intravenous infusion.

Toxic epidermal necrolysis

In this grave condition, which may be due to drugs or severe bacterial infection, large flaccid bullae develop rapidly over the child's body. They rupture and large painful denuded areas resemble those of a severe scald. It calls for heroic efforts with systemic corticosteroids and antibiotics to stave off death.

Erythema nodosum

This hypersensitivity reaction presents as tender erythematous nodules on the limbs or other parts and is associated with tuberculosis, leprosy, streptococcal infections, coccidioidomycosis, histoplasmosis and drugs, e.g. sulphonamides. It is uncommon in children.

Granuloma annulare

This presents in young children as pale, skin-coloured or erythematous, palpable, circular or circinate plaques with raised beaded margins. Some lesions are button-shaped with ringed edges and flat centres. These painless and non-itchy lesions may be solitary, few and localized or numerous and widespread. They are most common on the dorsa of hands and fingers, the wrists, forearms, ankles, feet and legs.

Granuloma annulare may last for a few months or longer; it resolves spontaneously and leaves no scars. Some cases may recur. The cause is unknown: it may be an autoimmunue reaction. Some cases have been associated with insect bites, tuberculin tests or other forms of dermal trauma.

Treatment   Many cases resolve slowly but spontaneously. Some resolve more rapidly following a partial biopsy. Intralesional injection of corticosteroids hastens the resolution of some lesions but skin atrophy or hypopigmentation may result.

Papular urticaria

This presents as a recurrent eruption of itchy erythematous, papular or vesicular eruption on the limbs and trunk, usually in infants and young children under five years old. The early urticarial elements are not prominent, and excoriations frequently lead to secondary bacterial infection, and impetiginous, pustular and pyodermic elements supervene.

The initial urticarial and papular reaction is an allergic reaction to insect bites (e.g. sandflies, mites, fleas, bedbugs). The subsequent secondary bacterial infection and the recurrent extensive eruptions are often out of proportion to the number or severity of further bites. There may be other host factors since all siblings and children of the same age range in the same family or compound do not suffer from papular urticaria, although they may all get bitten by the same insects.

Treatment The home, nursery or school environment should be investigated and the source of bites removed. Infested pets should be treated with effective insecticides. The child should be given antihistamine syrup or tablets and the skin treated with calamine lotion. For secondary bacterial infection, topical as well as systemic antibiotics should be given. To guard against further bites, the mother should dab insect repellants on the child's exposed skin.

NUTRITIONAL DISORDERS

Undernutrition and malnutrition are prevalent in the subtropics and tropics, and children suffer much more than adults with protein-deficient and vitamin-deficient diets. The skin and its appendages and the mucosa often show the outward visible signs of systemic nutritional deficiency due to inadequate intake, absorption or utilization of nutrients including vitamins.

The common manifestations of these disorders are kwashiorkor and vitamin B deficiency (see pp. 324–66, 373–5). The manifestations of the other vitamin deficiencies are uncommon.

Kwashiorkor

In severe protein–energy malnutrition seen most commonly in young children, the skin manifestations include:

- Pigmentary changes. Generalized hypopigmentation due in part to the stretching of the skin by oedema. Erythema, duskiness and hyperpigmentation in the face, flexures, pressure points and hands, feet and legs give a pellagroid picture.
- Desquamation. Scaling, peeling, blistering and rupture of the hyperpigmented areas leave erosions which are readily infested and may ulcerate.
- 'Crazy paving'. Cracking and fissuring of hyperpigmented skin on the face, trunk and limbs.
- Mucosal changes may include angular cheilitis, glossitis, magenta tongue, rhinitis, conjunctivitis and vulvovaginitis.
- Hair changes. Hair loses its texture and lustre and becomes thinned and discoloured, brown, yellowish, ginger or reddish. The dullness and lack of lustre result from the weathering of the cuticle.

Treatment This will include dietary measures such as dried skimmed milk of gradually increasing strength, multivitamin and iron supplements and Darrow's Solution and glucose to correct the electrolyte imbalance. Prompt treatment is required of intercurrent bacterial infection and helminthic infestation. Health education of the mother and community, and improvement of socio-economic standards are important.

Vitamin B deficiency

The manifestations are due to deficiency of many rather than of single fractions of vitamin B. The picture is therefore usually mixed and distinctive features are described only for riboflavine, and nicotinic acid deficiency.

Phrynoderma (follicular hyperkeratosis)

This condition may develop in early or later childhood. It is characterized by grouped spinous or papular eruptions, rough to touch, over the points of friction – elbows, knees, ulnar border of forearms, shoulders, scapular regions and buttocks. The skin of the affected areas and extensor surfaces is dry and rough. It is due to a mixed deficiency of various components of vitamin B, and there may be associated cheilitis, magenta tongue, and dyssebacia.

Treatment Replacement of the deficient vitamin by administration of vitamin B injections intramuscularly and orally is carried out until the skin eruptions clear up. The diet should be enriched with animal and vegetable proteins. Salicylic acid ointment 10 per cent is useful in dealing with the keratotic lesions.

Pellagra

Nicotinic acid and tryptophan deficiency cause dermatitis, diarrhoea and dementia. The exposed parts of the skin become erythematous and then oedematous with vesicles and bullae. The vesicles and bullae break, the affected parts desquamating and leaving sharply demarcated hyperpigmented areas. The skin changes may be exacerbated by sunlight causing burning, itching and pain.

Treatment Replacement of the deficient factors with nicotinic acid or nicotinamide (50–100 mg three times daily) is required until the condition improves. Vitamin B complex should be given orally or intramuscularly, and a high-protein diet ensured. Soothing applications and antihistamine tablets will help to control the itching and desquamation.

Riboflavine deficiency

This is characterized by cutaneous changes (dyssebacia, erythema and scrotal dermatitis) and mucosal changes (angular cheilitis and magenta tongue). Correction of the deficiency requires riboflavine (5 mg three times daily, orally), multivitamin supplements and a high-protein diet.

Hypovitaminosis-B

Deficiency of vitamin B not gross enough for the appearance of the more distinctive syndromes may result in widespread skin dryness, patchy hypopigmentation, diffuse palmo-plantar hyperkeratosis and magenta tongue. This condition can be corrected with vitamin B complex orally or intramuscularly and by improving the diet generally.

PIGMENTARY DISORDERS

The degree of melanin pigmentation of the skin distinguishes various races and what is considered normal for each race is clear. Any striking deviation from normal is usually embarrassing.

Vitiligo (leucoderma, white skin)

In this condition, common in all ages, symptomless depigmented macules of varying sizes and shapes appear on previously pigmented skin. Vitiligo may be localized or extensive, and hair in the affected areas may also be depigmented. The exposed parts are more commonly affected than the covered parts. It causes great concern because of the fear that it may be leprosy. Many cases are idiopathic and familial. Some may be associated with trauma (wounds, ulcers, burns) or with sunburn, alopecia areata, infections or endocrine disorders. The aetiology of vitiligo is unknown. Autoimmune and neurochemical factors may be responsible for making the melanocytes non-functional.

Tuberculoid leprosy is differentiated by its association with sensory and motor loss and peripheral nerve thickening. Achromic naevi are present at birth or appear a little later.

Treatment   This is very difficult, but spontaneous repigmentation does occur in some cases. Meladinine paint and tablets and 8-methoxypsoralen paint and tablets have been found useful in some cases. Psoralens and UVA therapy may be helpful.

Albinism

Albinos are seen in all races and lack melanin in their skin, hair and eyes. Albino children in the subtropics and tropics suffer from the ill effects of strong sunlight on their eyes and skin. Photophobia, nystagmus, strabismus and poor vision make life difficult for them at home, at school, at work or at play. Their skin lacks the protection against actinic radiation which melanin offers. As they grow older, these children develop sunburn, freckles, lentigines, solar keratosis, solar elastosis and skin cancer.[5] Oculocutaneous albinism is inherited as an autosomal recessive genetic defect. Both parents of an albino child must be heterozygotes (carriers of the trait) even if both are normally pigmented.

Care of the albino skin   All albino children should be registered so that care can be taken of their eyes and skin as early as possible. Protective skin lotions, creams, protective clothing and head gear should be organized on a regular basis. In teenagers, lentigines, keratosis and elastosis should be treated with 5-fluorouracil cream to guard against neoplastic changes.

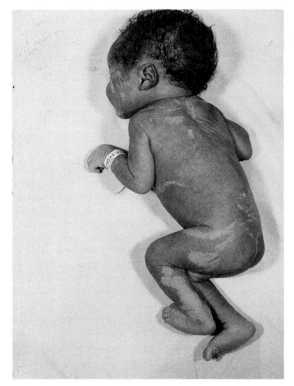

Fig. 5.10.12   Infant with marked incontinentia pigmenti.

Incontinentia pigmenti, a rare X-linked disorder, presents at birth or afterwards with linear erythemetous streaks and plaques of vesicles, particularly on the limbs (Fig. 5.10.12). There is a high incidence of other defects such as dental and ocular abnormalities, alopecia, retardation and seizures.

SKIN TUMOURS

Skin tumours of interest in children include capillary haemangioma, cavernous haemangioma, blue naevus, melanocytic naevus, granuloma telangiectaticum, lymphangioma, multiple neurofibroma, and squamous cell carcinoma.

The essence of accurate diagnosis is to differentiate from one another, the benign and harmless, the potentially dangerous, and the malignant tumours, so that appropriate action can be taken in each case, to observe, to treat or to refer to the expert.

Haemangiomata

These are developmental abnormalities of dermal blood vessels.

Capillary haemangioma

This presents at birth or within weeks as purplish or dusky stains of variables sizes and shapes on the face, neck trunk or limbs. A capillary haemangioma may increase in size with the growth of the child, and it may fade or persist. Treatment is difficult. Cosmetic firms produce special types of powder (cover mark) which can be matched with the child's complexion and used to conceal the blemish.

Cavernous haemangioma (strawberry naevus)

This presents within days or weeks of birth, as a reddish spot or as a fleshy purple or dusky soft tumour on the face, neck, trunk or limbs (Fig. 5.10.13). Cavernous haemangiomata grow larger in the first few months but spontaneous regression or disappearance occurs within the first five to seven years.

Haemangiomata may be complicated by trauma, infection, haemorrhage, thrombosis, ulceration and scarring. Lesions with mucosal involvement are more liable to these complications.

If treatment is essential, short course of systemic corticosteroids have been used; carbon dioxide snow and superficial X-rays may cause scarring.

Blue naevus

This presents as a bluish or blue-black macule or plaque on the back or buttocks. It is due to developmental

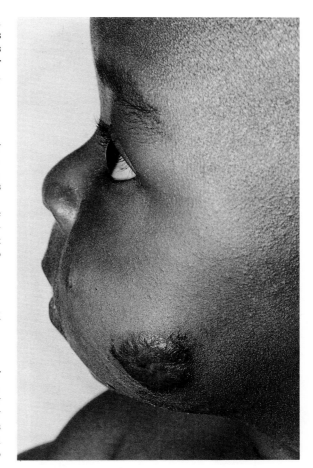

Fig. 5.10.13 Cavernous haemangioma.

arrest of melanocytes in the dermis. Only a raised or nodular lesion may call for excision. Macular lesions call for no treatment, except for reassurance.

Melanocytic naevus (mole)

This presents as a bluish or blue black lesion which may be flat, raised or hairy. Naevi may be few or numerous, erupting at intervals during childhood. Only disfiguring lesions may need to be excised. In adult life, lesions at sites where they are prone to repeated trauma may turn malignant, and call for excision.

Lymphangioma

This may present as clusters of papules or soft nodules or as soft skin-coloured tumours. Lymphangiomata are common in sites where the skin is loose. Trauma may lead to bacterial infection and sinus formation.

Granuloma telangiectaticum

This presents as a small, rapidly growing, reddish or dusky vascular tumour at the site of a minor injury such as a bite, pin-prick or scratch. Treatment is by diathermy or excision under local anaesthesia.

Multiple neurofibromata (von Recklinghausen's disease)

This presents as numerous, soft, skin-coloured papules or nodules and small fleshy tumours erupting during childhood on various parts of the body. Careful examination will reveal brown or hyperpigmented macules of varying sizes on the trunk and limbs. These are known as café au lait spots. No treatment is necessary during childhood, but large or disfiguring tumours may be excised.

Squamous cell carcinoma and basal cell carcinoma

In teenage albino children constantly exposed to strong sunlight, keratotic plaques developing on exposed parts may develop into squamous cell carcinoma (Fig. 5.10.14). These should be treated by early excision.

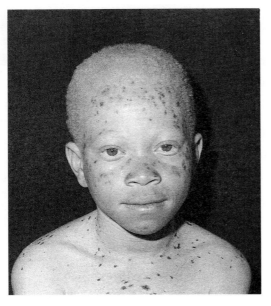

Fig. 5.10.14 Albino child with keratotic plaques on face and shoulders.

LESS COMMON SKIN DISEASES

Of the less common skin diseases which constitute about 5 per cent of the total, acne vulgaris, drug eruptions, bullous eruptions, connective tissue diseases and the keratoses will be described.

Acne vulgaris

Most adolescents are familiar with the condition acne vulgaris, pimples, as a fact of life. Pimples may start as early as the age of 9 or 10 years but may be unnoticed then. Peak incidence is earlier in girls (14–15 years) than in boys (16–17 years). Onset corresponds closely with the menarche in most girls.

The early papules on a greasy skin are commonly situated on the face, sternal region, upper back and shoulders. Interference in the form of rubbing, scratching or squeezing leads to secondary bacterial infection and cellulitis. Increased sebum production results from sebaceous gland stimulation by androgens and progesterone. Increased keratinization at the mouths of the hair follicles results from follicular wall irritation by fatty acids from sebum. These fatty acids result from the splitting of sebum by lipase produced by *Propionibacterium acnes* resident in hair follicles. Sebum thus accumulates behind the blocked hair follicles, solidifies and forms the bulk of the 'yellow heads' and 'black heads' of acne vulgaris.

Management   Reassurance of the physiological basis of acne and the generally good prognosis is essential. Aggravating factors, friction, squeezing and rich greasy foods, are best avoided. Specific treatment is aimed at controlling sebum production or accumulation, reduction of the bacterial load on the skin and controlling excessive keratinization of the hair follicles. Benzoyl peroxide controls bacterial load and sebum accumulation[6], tetracycline taken orally helps to reduce the bacterial load, and tretinoin lotion (vitamin A) reduces keratinization.

Drug eruptions

Children are as liable to drug reactions as adults, and commonly used drugs can produce these eruptions from overdose, hypersensitivity, or idiosyncrasy.

Urticarial eruptions

These may result from treatment with salicylates, penicillin, sulphonamides, antitetanus serum, laxatives, antimalarials, and barbiturates.

Fixed drug eruption

These present as bullae, erosion and residual hyper-pigmentation which tend to recur with repeated administration of the same or related drugs. Sulphonamides, phenolphthalein in laxatives, antimalarials, codeine, salicylates, diaminodiphenyl sulphone and barbiturates are the common causes.

Epidermolysis bullosa

This presents in childhood with recurrent bullae on points of friction or tension with or without trauma. The broken bullae may ulcerate and leave dystrophic scars. The condition is usually familial and has no specific treatment.

Connective tissue diseases

These autoimmune disorders characterized by fibrinoid degeneration of collagen in various tissues involves the skin and other organs.

Systemic lupus erythematosus may present in childhood as erythematous eruptions on the face, trunk and limbs. Visceral involvement (heart, kidneys, lungs) is usually insidious and may be difficult to diagnose early. Lassitude, pallor, myalgia and hepatosplenomegaly may be present. Investigations include ESR, detailed haematological investigations, demonstration of LE cells in the peripheral blood, serological examination for antinuclear factor, and detailed renal function tests. Treatment is with systemic corticosteroids, but immunosuppressive drugs, e.g. azathioprine, cyclophosphamide and 6-mercaptopurine, may be required.

Chronic discoid lupus erythematosus, the distinctive dusky, scaling and scarring connective tissue disorder is rare in children.

Scleroderma may present as morphoea, a circumscribed plaque of hardened or atrophic skin, or as more widespread oedema followed by atrophy and binding down of the skin of the face, limbs and trunk to underlying structures. The hands and feet may be cold with Raynaud's phenomenon in cold water.

Keratoses

Chronic hyperkeratosis of the palms and soles may extend to the wrists and ankles, forearms and shins, elbows and knees. The condition may start in early childhood. It is inherited as an autosomal dominant gene.

Ichthyosis vulgaris (fish skin), congenital ichthyosi-

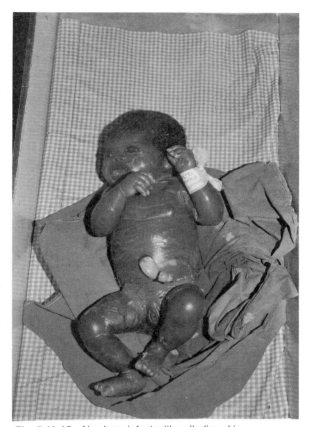

Fig. 5.10.15 Newborn infant with collodian skin.

form erythroderma, collodian skin (Fig. 5.10.15) and localized ichthyosiform hyperkeratosis are other forms of disordered keratinization.

Treatment Is difficult, but keratolytic topical applications, e.g. 2–5 per cent salicylic acid ointment, emulsifying ointment and vitamin supplements, may be found useful.

Keloid

This disfiguring condition is due to an overgrowth of collagen in the dermis. Africans are particularly prone to develop keloid scars at the site of burns or other injury, especially if infection has occurred. The overlying skin becomes firm and shiny. Surgical removal is useless, since the growth recurs, usually increased in size. Some lesions regress using carbon dioxide snow or steroid-impregnated adhesive tape; X-rays have been used.

References

1. David TJ. The practical management of atopic eczema in childhood. *Postgraduate Doctor (Africa)*. 1986; **8**(5): 156–9.
2. Heel RC. In: Levine LM ed. *Ketoconazole in the Management of Fungal Diseases*. Sydney, ADIS Press, 1982.
3. Okoro AN. Papulosquamous eruptions. In: *Pictorial Handbook of Common Skin Diseases*. London, Macmillan, 1981. pp. 85–90.
4. Pettit JHS. Urticaria. In: *Manual of Practical Dermatology. Medicine in the Tropics*. Edinburgh, Churchill Livingstone, 1983. pp. 101–3.
5. Okoro AN. Albinism in Nigeria. *British Journal of Dermatology*. 1975: **92**: 485–92.
6. Schutte E, Cunliffe WJ, Forster RA. The short-term effects of benzoyl peroxide lotion on the resolution of inflamed acne lesions. *British Journal of Dermatology*. 1982; **106**: 91–4.

CHAPTER 11

Neoplastic diseases

C.L.M. Olweny

Introduction

Third World health problems

Health problems of the Third World differ significantly from those of the industrialized, developed world in many ways. The major differences include the age structure of the population, infant mortality, overall disease pattern and the availability or non-availability of health services. The Third World population is characterized by the very large population of children. About 45 per cent of the population is under the age of 15, whereas in the developed countries only 20 per cent of the population fall into this age group. In developing countries, mortality rates are 10–20 times higher for infants and children aged one to four years than in the developed countries. Though the under-fives account for only 20 per cent of the entire population, they account for 60 per cent of all the deaths in developing countries. Against this background health planners and health workers in these countries, inundated with infectious diseases, perpetuate the myth that cancer and especially childhood cancers are rare.

Very few accurate statistical data on neoplasms are available from the tropics.[1] The latest compilation of cancer incidence in five continents has for instance, little or no information on tropical and subtropical countries.[2] Numerically, the majority of the world's cancer patients are in the developing countries. This is based on estimated cancer incidence rates of 260 and 102 per 100 000 population for developed and developing countries, respectively.[3] Given that 75 per cent of the world's 4220 million people are to be found in the developing countries, it can then be estimated that 2.84 million cancer cases occur each year in developed countries and 3.03 million cases per year in the developing countries. In many tropical areas, patients present themselves for treatment at an advanced-disease stage and some may never appear at all. This further adds to the false impression of the relative rarity of tumours. However, data produced by the World Health Organization (1977)[4] would tend to support the contention that once an individual has survived the first five years, life expectancy in the developing countries is only eight or nine years less than in the developed countries and the three leading causes of death are similar world-wide, namely cardiovascular disease, cancer and accidents.

Symptoms and signs in oncology

Oncology, the study of malignant diseases, cuts across all disciplines of medicine. The symptoms and signs observed in oncology may occur in any organ system. The general and systemic symptoms of fever, weight loss and diaphoresis are non-specific and in the tropics these may be the result of infectious or parasitic conditions, especially malaria, trypanosomiasis and leishmaniasis.

Most cancers, however, present as a swelling, hence the synonym 'tumour' often used to describe malignant and non-malignant conditions. A swelling in the jaw in a child may suggest Burkitt's lymphoma; an abdominal swelling may suggest Burkitt's lymphoma or Wilms' tumour, while scalp swelling may be due to metastatic neuroblastoma.

Cancers manifesting in the central nervous system (CNS) commonly present with the classic triad of headache, vomiting and papilloedema which are features of raised intracranial pressure. These may be seen in primary brain tumour or tumours invading the CNS secondarily, as is common in patients with leukaemia and malignant lymphoma. Cord compression syndrome (presenting as limb weakness, paraplegia and urinary and/or faecal incontinence) may be a manifestation of Burkitt's lymphoma. In Uganda, Burkitt's lymphoma is the most common cause of paraplegia in children under 15 years of age. However, tuberculosis or spinal epidural abscess from staphylococcal osteomyelitis and septicaemia must be borne in mind.

Oncological symptoms and signs referrable to the reticuloendothelial system are: weakness and pallor due to anaemia, body swelling, lymph node swelling and hepatosplenomegaly. In a tropical environment, these features are more likely to be the result of parasitic diseases, such as chronic malaria (idiopathic tropical splenomegaly syndrome), leishmaniasis and trypanosomiasis, than the result of malignancy.

Abdominal swelling due to accumulation of ascites or organ involvement by tumour is often observed. The most common organs involved in children include kidney, spleen, liver and ovary. Again, as with paraplegia, Burkitt's lymphoma is the most common cause of ovarian tumour in girls under 15 years of age in Uganda.

Haematuria, a common presenting symptom in many urological tumours, may be missed because the child may not consider it important to report. If it occurs in an environment where schistosomiasis is endemic, it may be regarded as 'developmental norm', i.e. male 'menarche', or it may not be noticed because of the use of a pit latrine.

Differences between childhood and adult cancers

Apart from leukaemias, lymphomas and brain tumours, childhood tumours tend to be rare in adults. Most childhood cancers are sarcomas while carcinomas are rare. Childhood cancers very infrequently involve epithelial tissues. They tend to be deep-seated, thus making screening impracticable as such deep-seated tumours rarely present with external bleeding and tumour cell exfoliation is uncommon. Thus, the adult screening techniques, such as mammography, chest X-rays, stool blood tests, and the pap smear, have no equivalent counterparts for the early detection of cancers in children. The diagnosis of cancer in children is often incidental and, in the majority of cases, made at an advanced stage when distant metastases have occurred.[5]

Cure for childhood cancers

A study by Miller and McKay[6] presented new evidence for the curability of childhood cancers by documenting significantly decreased death rates. The study concluded that from 1965 to 1984, there had been an 80 per cent reduction in the number of childhood cancer deaths from Hodgkin's disease; a 68 per cent reduction in deaths due to kidney cancer, primarily Wilms' tumour; 50 per cent reduction in deaths due to leukaemia and bone sarcomas: 32 per cent fewer deaths due to non-Hodgkin's lymphoma and 31 per cent fewer deaths from all other types of cancers in children.

Progress observed in the treatment of childhood cancers over the last two decades was not due to major scientific or therapeutic advances but resulted from successive clinical trials of new treatment strategies. Furthermore, the rational combination of the three important therapeutic modalities of the time – surgery, radiotherapy and chemotherapy (combined modality approach) – contributed immensely to the progress. In addition, children were almost always referred by their primary physicians to major paediatric medical centres where clinical research of management was being undertaken. Progress in these and other areas has led to the curability of a number of childhood cancers in developed countries. The curable cancers include acute leukaemias, lymphomas, Wilms' tumour, osteogenic sarcoma, Ewing's sarcoma and rhabdomyosarcoma. Unfortunately, the cure of childhood cancer continues to elude many developing countries. This is mainly because of the following:

- The perpetuated myth that cancer is rare in developing countries. Consequently, little attention is paid to cancer as a problem and minimal effort is made to provide appropriate cancer control delivery systems. Some developing countries have not even bothered to formulate national cancer policies.

- Lack of cancer management facilities. Most tropical and sub-tropical countries cannot afford the capital outlay for installation and maintenance of radiotherapy equipment, and cytotoxic drugs are expensive and often unavailable.
- Lack of trained personnel. Oncology training is often undertaken either in Europe or North America and many such foreign graduates do not return home upon completion of their courses.
- Delay in hospitalization while patients seek the opinion of traditional healers.
- Delay in making the diagnosis: At an International Congress of Paediatric Oncology held in Barcelona, Spain, in 1984, it was pointed out that in Argentina, while the average duration from first symptom to hospitalization was one month, the average duration from first medical examination to diagnosis was 12 months. This delay was attributed to lack of oncological information and lack of appropriate training given to paediatricians and general practitioners.
- Lack of support facilities like histopathology, and transfusion services.

Apart from the above, few countries can afford the luxury of separate cancer wards. It is not uncommon to find children with leukaemia/lymphoma who are severely immunosuppressed being nursed in the same ward as other children with measles, tuberculosis, chickenpox, infective diarrhoea and typhoid.

Childhood tumours in developing countries

Certain tumours occur exclusively in infancy and early childhood, for example cerebellar medulloblastoma, nasopharyngeal fibroma, malignant suprarenal neuroblastoma, Wilms' tumour and retinoblastoma. Across the tropical belt in Africa, Burkitt's lymphoma occupies a special place. Childhood tumours account for just over 10 per cent of the total malignancies seen in Uganda. Malignant lymphomas, however, constitute well over 50 per cent of all childhood tumours recorded and Burkitt's lymphoma is by far the most common, occurring more often than all the other lymphomas put together.[1] Other tumours commonly observed in children in Uganda include soft tissue and bone tumours, retinoblastoma and leukaemia (Table 5.11.1).

The situation in neighbouring Kenya is very similar. Childhood malignancies account for 10 per cent of all malignancies recorded in the Kenya Cancer Registry, and the order of frequency is similar to that in Uganda. The rest of this chapter will deal with some of the more common tumours seen in the tropics.

Table 5.11.1 Childhood tumours in Uganda.

	No.	%
Solid reticuloendothial (lymphomas)	377	49.6
Soft tissue and bone	116	15.2
Retinoblastomas	57	7.5
Nephroblastomas	56	7.4
Leukaemias	54	7.1
Sympathetic system	17	2.3
Ovary	14	1.8
Liver	12	1.6
Glioma and intracranial	10	1.3
Teratoma (extragenital)	10	1.3
Testes	6	0.7
Epithelial (nasopharynx)	6	0.7
Others	26	3.7
Total	761	100.0

Adapted from Templeton AC, *Tumours in Tropical Countries*, 1973, Berlin Springer.

Lymphoid malignancies

In 1947, Elmes and Baldwin analysed 1000 tumours collected in Lagos during 1935–44 and referred to lymphosarcoma which constituted 5.3 per cent of all tumours.[7] Their report made no mention of other tumours of the reticulorendothelial system. Subsequently, in a study involving 1038 tumours seen during 1960–63 in Ibadan, Nigeria, 233 (22.4 per cent) were tumours of the reticuloendothelial system. Of these, childhood lymphoma (presumably Burkitt's) was by far the most common constituting 28.8 per cent, followed by lymphosarcoma, reticulum cell sarcoma and Hodgkin's disease representing 19.3 per cent, 15 per cent and 12.4 per cent of reticuloendothelial tumours respectively.[8] As already indicated, the pattern in East Africa is very similar. However, this pattern is in contrast to the situation in England or the USA where Hodgkin's disease is the most common lymphoreticular tumour observed (Table 5.11.2). Because of the high frequency of Burkitt's lymphoma in tropical Africa, it will be dealt with here first.

Burkitt's lymphoma

In 1958, Dr Denis Burkitt,[9] described 28 cases of sarcoma of the jaw seen in Kampala, Uganda; the entity is now named after him. Dr Burkitt reported that 'round-cell' sarcomas seemed to occur with extraordinary frequency in the jaws of children in tropical East Africa. The distribution of the tumour within Africa, as well as the discovery of similar cases in Papua New Guinea, suggested an intriguing geographical relationship between this lymphoma and climatic

Table 5.11.2 Percentage distribution of tumours of lymphoreticular system in different countries.

Country	Histiocytic lymphoma (% of total)	Lymphocytic lymphoma (% of total)	Hodgkin's lymphoma (% of total)	Others (% of total)
UK	22	26.3	47.2	4.5
USA	16.2	32.6	49.7	1.7
Japan	64.4	14.3	16.2	5.2
Uganda (excluding Burkitt's)	38.6	31.0	30.4	0.0
Uganda (including Burkitt's)	23.7	19.2	18.5	38.6

Modified from Templeton AC, *Tumours in Tropical Countries*, 1973, Berlin Springer.

conditions such as temperature, rainfall, altitude and latitude.

Epidemiology

In Africa, Burkitt's lymphoma (BL) is distributed across a broad band south of the Sahara, between approximately 10° north and south of the equator (lymphoma belt). Within this belt there are pockets where the tumour is extremely rare and these happen to be high-altitude areas, such as the Kenyan Highlands, Rwanda, Burundi and the plateaux of Zambia and Zimbabwe. BL is restricted to those areas with an annual rainfall of over 50 cm and an average temperature in the coolest month of over 15.6°C. The distribution led to the original hypothesis that an arthropod-borne (possible mosquito) virus may be responsible. Within this lymphoma belt, the incidence of BL varies from zero to 7.6 per 100 000 population.

In Latin America, 2–5 per cent of childhood lymphomas are BL. In Brazil, BL represents 13.5 per cent of non-Hodgkin's lymphomas. Outside the endemic areas of sub-Saharan Africa and Papua New Guinea, BL occurs sporadically in the USA. Israel and Northern Europe. Other interesting epidemiological features of BL include time–space clustering, as well as time trends in incidence observed especially in the West Nile District of Uganda and in the North Mara District of Tanzania.[10]

Clinical features

BL commonly affects children with the peak age between four and seven years (Fig. 5.11.1). It is uncommon below one year of age; less than 1 per cent of children get it below two years. Less than 10 per cent of patients are diagnosed after the age of 15 years. Males are affected twice as commonly as females.

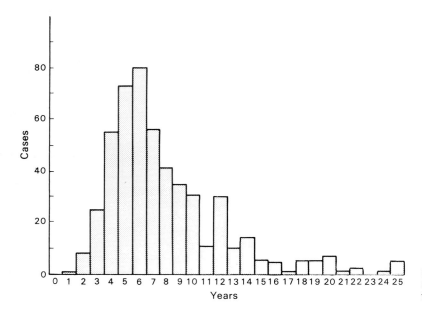

Fig. 5.11.1 Age distribution of Burkitt's lymphoma in 280 patients up to the age of 25 years (Uganda).

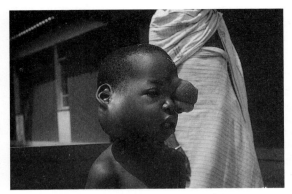

Fig. 5.11.2 Burkitt's lymphoma, presenting as tumour in all four quadrants of the jaw in a four-year-old boy (Nigeria).

BL in endemic area presents with jaw swelling in 75 per cent of cases. The maxillae are affected more frequently than the mandibles. Maxillary tumour often involves the orbit as well (Fig. 5.11.2). The first clinical evidence is often loosening of teeth. Non-jaw tumours present mainly as an abdominal mass (Fig. 5.11.3.) and virtually any organ in the abdomen (liver, kidney, ovaries, suprarenal and retroperitoneal nodes) can become involved. Abdominal presentation is seen in 60 per cent of patients. The third most common mode of presentation is with CNS involvement, which is seen in 30 per cent of patients. This often presents as cranial nerve palsy with or without malignant spinal fluid pleocytosis. Peripheral node involvement is rare in endemic cases.

In non-endemic areas of the world, e.g. USA, the most common site of presentation is with abdominal disease in 90 per cent (often ovary and ileocaecal). Peripheral node disease occurs in 20 per cent, while jaw involvement is observed in about 10 per cent of patients. CNS involvement occurs in 5 per cent and this figure doubles if the marrow is involved. It would appear that jaw tumour is the most common mode of presentation in the young children while abdominal disease increases in frequency with age.

Histology

The classic histological appearance is the uniform proliferation of immature cells 10–25 μm in diameter. They have rounded nuclei with two to five prominent nucleoli. The cytoplasm stains deeply and, because of the high content of RNA, it is strongly pyroninophilic. Interspersed within the monotonous sheets of cells are macrophages, which give the so-called 'starry-sky' appearance.

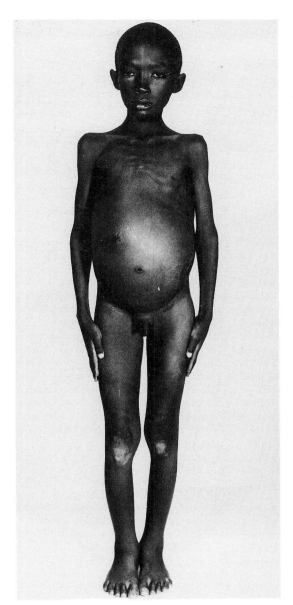

Fig. 5.11.3 Burkitt's lymphoma, presenting as abdominal swelling in an eight-year-old boy. The patient had liver and kidney involvement and malignant ascites (Uganda).

Aetiology

There is a strong association between endemic BL and Epstein–Barr Virus (EBV). The discovery of EBV in 1964 by Epstein, Achong and Barr led to a series of studies that implicated this virus as a causative factor in BL. The evidence supporting EBV as a major causative factor in endemic BL is based on the following observations:

- EBV transforms normal human B cells into continuously growing cell lines carrying EBV DNA, and these cell lines have features of malignant transformation.
- Patients with endemic BL have unusually high titre of antibodies to EBV antigens.
- All the tumour cells in 97 per cent of properly authenticated cases carry multiple copies of the EBV genome and express EBV membrane antigen as well as EBV nuclear antigen (EBNA).[11]
- The prospective sero-epidemiological study conducted in the West Nile District of Uganda identified 16 cases of BL in 42 000 children over a seven year period. In this study an unusually high titre of antibodies to virus capsid antigen was observed many months or years before clinical manifestation. The risk of developing endemic BL for those with such high antibody titres was 80 times higher than for matched controls.[12]
- In New World monkeys, EBV is experimentally oncogenic. EBV has probably fulfilled the Koch–Henle postulates of oncogenesis and is thus one of the leading contenders of human oncogenic virus. Apart from BL, EBV is known to be the cause of infectious mononucleosis and to be causally associated with nasopharyngeal carcinoma. In non-endemic areas, EBV-associated BL is observed in only 10–15 per cent of cases.

Malaria

Apart from EBV there are certainly other environmental factors involved and prominent among these is hyperendemic malaria. Malaria may be responsible for a 5–10 fold increase in BL frequency. The mechanism by which malaria could favour BL development would seem to be related to its effect on cellular immunity. Chronic severe falciparum malaria infection may lead to an intense host response with proliferation of the lymphoreticular system and particularly of the B lymphocytes. This proliferation of EBV-infected B lymphocytes provides a much higher statistical opportunity for an abnormal cell with specific chromosome abnormality to emerge. The observation that patients with sickle cell trait (AS haemoglobin) who are substantially protected from severe life-threatening falciparum malaria are also protected from BL would tend to support the role of malaria. The demonstration

that the incidence of BL falls in a population in which malaria is controlled further confirms the role of malaria.[10]

Chromosomal abnormalities

Three specific translocations t(8;14), t(8;22), and t(2;8) having in common 8q 24 band involvement are thought to be present in the majority of BL cases. The most common translocation is t(8;14) observed in 80 per cent of all translocations. Translocation t(8;22) occurs in 15 per cent of cases and t(2;8) in 5 per cent. These translocations are observed in all BL tumours, irrespective of EBV genome status and whether it is endemic or not. EBV is not by itself able to induce BL translocations as these chromosome rearrangements are not seen in infectious mononucleosis or in EBV-induced lymphoblastoid cell lines.[13] In 1979, George Klein of the Karolinska Institute postulated a three-stage pathogenetic step required for the development of endemic BL: (1) EBV transforms B cells, and immortalizes them; (2) an environmental factor, e.g. holoendemic malaria, promotes polyclonal proliferation of B cells; and (3) a cytogenetic error (i.e. 14q +) emerges and endows the cell with survival advantage.

Oncogenes

These are genes which cause cancer. The first transforming gene to be isolated was from a human bladder cancer cell line. DNA from human bladder cancer cell line was found to transform (transfect) cultured mouse 3T3 cells to a neoplastic state. Generally oncogenes are innocuous as long as they are quiescent and undisturbed, but stimulated into activity they can switch cells into cancerous growth. Oncogene activation may result from a variety of mechanisms common among which are point mutation, DNA rearrangement and chromosomal translocation. Activated *myc* (avian myelomatosis virus) oncogene has been detected in BL, promyelocytic leukaemia, small-cell cancer of the lung, neuroblastoma and retinoblastoma.

The discovery that genes for human immunoglobulin heavy chains are located on band q32 of chromosome 14, whereas the genes for the kappa and lambda light chains are on band p11 of chromosome 2 and band q11 of chromosome 22, respectively, led George Klein to predict that chromosome 8 probably carried an oncogene and the translocation, e.g. t(8;22) was transferring the oncogene close to the immunoglobulin gene. His predictions have been borne out.

The *myc* oncogene has been identified on band q24 of chromosome 8.

Clinical staging

Although BL is classified morphologically among the non-Hodgkin's lymphomas, it does not conform to the Ann Arbor staging system of non-Hodgkin's lymphomas. This is probably because in endemic areas BL is principally an extra-nodal disease. The first attempt at clinical staging was by Ziegler in 1972. Subsequently, in 1974, Ziegler and Magrath suggested another staging system which better correlated with survival[14] (Table 5.11.3). In this staging system, tumour volume appears more important than location of the tumour and CNS involvement does not necessarily place patients into a poor prognostic category. The abdomen is capable of accomodating large tumour volume before patients seek medical opinion, while jaw tumours grow to grotesque size quickly and because of the disfiguring facial appearance medical opinion is sought early.

Table 5.11.3 Staging for Burkitt's lymphoma used by investigators in Uganda and National Cancer Institute Bethesda, USA.

Stage	Criteria
A	Solitary extra-abdominal site
AR	Resected intra-abdominal tumour
B	Multiple extra-abdominal sites
C	Intra-abdominal tumour with or without facial tumour
D	Intra-abdominal tumour with sites other than facial

(Reproduced from Ziegler JL and McGrath IT, *Pathobiology Annual*, 1974; **4**: 129–42.)

Treatment of BL

The goal of treating endemic BL is cure. Every child should therefore, be given the best opportunity towards achieving this. Patients should be referred as soon as possible (once a diagnosis is suspected) to a central hospital with appropriate facilities.

BL can be treated by surgery, radiotherapy and chemotherapy. Surgical approaches include: (1) biopsy for diagnosis, (2) reduction of tumour volume (debulk operation), (3) laminectomy to relieve spinal cord compression, and (4) insertion of Ommaya reservoir for intraventricular therapy. Because BL is a rapidly growing tumour with a potential doubling time of 24 hours and growth fraction of 100 per cent, it should be regarded as a medico-surgical emergency. Any planned surgery should be performed within hours of admission. Cases of BL should not be placed at the end of the operation list – they tend to be postponed for lack of operation time and/or left to the more junior members of the surgical team.

The treatment of choice for BL is chemotherapy. Before initiation of specific chemotherapy, patients should be given fluids orally or intravenously to ensure a high urinary output of 100–150 ml/hour. A potent diuretic (e.g. frusemide) may be necessary to achieve this. Part of the fluid should be in the form of sodium bicarbonate to make the urine alkaline. This is all in anticipation of tumour lysis syndrome, a common complication of chemotherapy of BL. Because of the extreme sensitivity to cytotoxic chemotherapy, rapid lysis of tumour leads to release of intracellular elements, notably potassium, phosphates and urates. This will result in hyperkalaemia, hyperphosphataemia hyperuricaemia and secondary hypocalcaemia. This is often the cause of sudden unexpected death in apparently 'well' children within 24–48 hours of initiation of chemotherapy. Patients at great risk include those with a large abdominal tumour (stages C and D), those with high lactic acid dehydrogenase levels and those with high uric acid levels. Patients at considerable risk may benefit from prophylactic haemodialysis or peritoneal dialysis. Allopurinol (100 mg three times daily) should be be started 24–48 hours before specific therapy to prevent uric acid nephropathy.

The single most effective cytotoxic drug is cyclophosphamide, given as a bolus intravenous injection of 40 mg/kg and repeated 2–3 weeks later (Fig. 5.11.4). However, combination chemotherapy consisting of cyclophosphamide, vincristine (Oncovin) and methotrexate (COM), though similar to cyclophosphamide alone in remission induction, is superior to the single agent in preventing systemic relapse. The dose and schedule of COM combination is shown in Table 5.11.4. Treatment with single agent or with combination chemotherapy results in 80 per cent complete response rates and an overall response rate of 90 per cent (complete + partial). About 50 per cent of those achieving complete responses will relapse. Those relapsing within three months (early relapse) do badly in subsequent therapy and are unlikely to respond to previously successful chemotherapy. Those relapsing after three months (late relapse) do well and tend to respond to the initial induction regimen.

About 30 per cent of patients have CNS involvement either at presentation or on relapse. Such patients benefit from intrathecal administration of cytosine arabinoside (Ara-C), 30 mg for three days, followed by

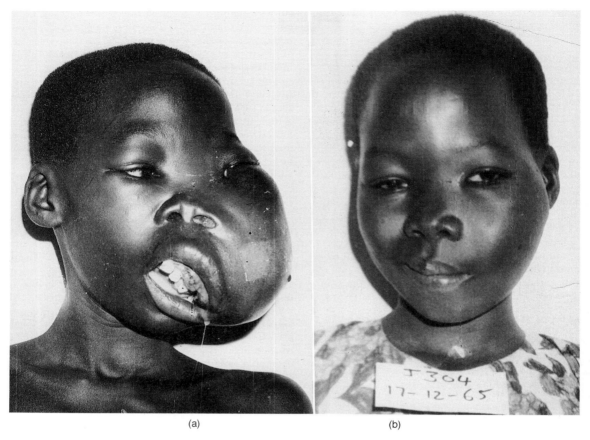

(a)   (b)

Fig. 5.11.4 (a) Burkitt's lymphoma, presenting as massive tumour of the left maxilla in a nine-year-old girl. (b) Same child 3.5 weeks after two injections of cyclophosphamide (Uganda).

Table 5.11.4 COM combination chemotherapy for Burkitt's lymphoma.

Drug	Dose	Route	Schedule
Cyclophosphamide	30 mg/kg	i.v.	Day 1
Vincristine (Oncovin)	1.4 mg/m^2	i.v.	Day 1
Methotrexate	15 mg/m^2	oral	Days 1–3

Course repeated 2–3 weeks later.

methotrexate, 15 mg on the fourth day. The finding of malignant cerebrospinal fluid pleocytosis does not necessarily augur a poor prognosis as up to 30 per cent of such patients can be salvaged.[15] Prophylactic administration of methotrexate, in addition to systemic therapy, may prevent the development of CNS relapse. Burkitt's lymphoma is a radiosensitive tumour. However, its peculiar cell kinetics call for modification of conventional radiotherapy. Each day's dose of radiotherapy is superfractionated to three treatments given four hourly. Unlike the situation in acute leukaemia, prophylactic cerebrospinal irradiation in BL does not seem to prevent CNS relapse.

Hodgkin's disease

Hodgkin's disease in the tropics has an unusual clinical and histopathological presentation. The disease shows a shift towards the young age group. Furthermore the age-specific incidence seems to be unimodal with a single peak in childhood. There is, in addition,

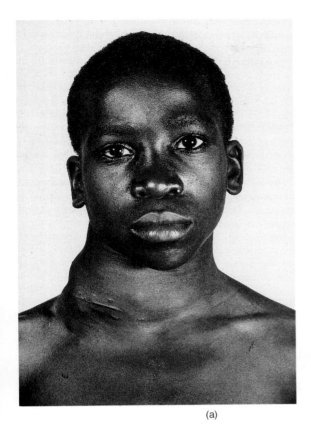
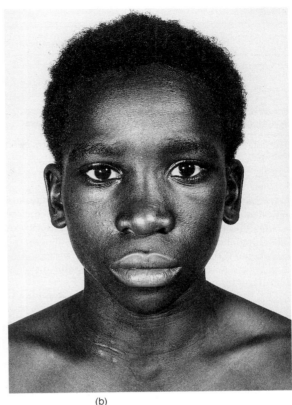

(a)   (b)

Fig. 5.11.5 (a) Hodgkin's disease, presenting as a cervical node swelling in a 12-year-old boy (Uganda). (b) Same child after six cycles of MOPP therapy.

an excess of the mixed cellularity and lymphocytic depletion types and a relative deficiency of the lymphocytic predominant and nodular sclerosis types.[16] The presenting feature of Hodgkin's disease is most often with peripheral lymphadenopathy (Fig. 5.11.5a, b). However, in most tropical countries patients present at an already-advanced disease stage, probably due to delay in reporting to hospital.

Treatment

Like BL, Hodgkin's disease is potentially curable, even at an advanced stage. Children with Hodgkin's disease should therefore, be transferred to central hospitals and offered appropriate therapy.

In general, early-stage Hodgkin's disease is best treated with radiotherapy. Many hospitals in the tropics still lack radiotherapy facilities. For this reason, and because most patients present with advanced-stage disease, chemotherapy seems to be the only reasonable and often the only available mode of treatment for all stages.

Single agents have been ineffective in inducing a high percentage of complete remissions in this disease. Drug combinations are more effective in achieving this goal.[17] The four-drug combination devised by DeVita (Table 5.11.5) has been shown to give over 75 per cent complete remission rates in several studies. In Uganda, the complete response rate in childhood Hodgkin's disease patients treated by the four-drug combination MOPP was 88 per cent and over 70 per cent of these children were disease-free five years after cessation of chemotherapy.[16] The complications of chemotherapy can be divided into acute and delayed or late complications. Acute complications include nausea, vomiting, diarrhoea, alopecia, myelosuppression and

Table 5.11.5   MOPP therapy for Hodgkin's disease.[a]

Drug	Dose (mg/m^2)	Route of administration	Schedule of administration
Nitrogen mustard	6	i.v.	On days 1 and 8
Vincristine	1.4	i.v.	On days 1 and 8
Procarbazine	100	oral	For 14 days
Prednisone[b]	40	oral	For 14 days

[a] The course is repeated every 3 weeks to complete remission when two more courses are given.
[b] Prednisone is omitted for courses 3 and 4.

metabolic effects related to steroid therapy. The late complications include Herpes zoster and gynaecomastia. This last complication appears related to germinal epithelial damage which in turn is dependent on the age when MOPP therapy is begun. Those treated after 11 years of age are more likely to develop this problem than those treated before that age.

The issue of staging laparotomy is occasionally raised. This matter is only relevant in those areas where radiotherapy facilities exist and the findings at staging laparotomy may influence decision-making as to the treatment to be given. If all stages are to be given cytotoxic chemotherapy, then staging laparotomy should not be considered. In any case, staging laparotomy and splenectomy are likely to place the child at grave risk of developing severe infections subsequently, notably cerebral malaria. Thus, unless the child can be closely followed up and is going to live in an environment where mosquito control is adequate (i.e. some cities) then staging laparotomy should be avoided.

Leukaemias

Leukaemias are neoplastic disorders characterized by an abnormal generalized purposeless and self-perpetuated proliferation of any subgroup of leucocytic series. In tropical Africa, there appears to be a low incidence of leukaemias, presumably due to underdiagnosis, high frequency of anaemia and splenomegaly, associated infections, malaria and sickle cell disease. In tropical America, although leukaemias are the most common malignant haematological disorder seen in countries like Brazil and Costa Rica, the overall incidence is still considerably lower than in the developed countries of Europe and North America.[18]

The clinico-pathologic pattern of leukaemias in the tropics is similar to that observed in the temperate climates. However, there are minor variations, such as the paucity of cases in the age group under five years. In tropical Africa, there is a higher prevalence of acute myeloid than lymphatic leukaemias.[1] In addition, there is a high frequency of chloromatous tumours in acute myeloid leukaemias in childhood and this may be mistaken for BL. This observation, initially reported from Uganda, has been confirmed by investigators working in Kenya, Nigeria, Sudan and Tanzania. By contrast, childhood acute lymphatic leukaemia (ALL) accounts for more than 80 per cent of acute leukaemias seen in tropical America.

The initial manifestations of acute leukaemia are often non-specific and may include easy fatiguability, weakness, lassitude and palpitations. These are all features of anaemia and in a tropical environment chronic blood loss from hookworm or schistosomiasis is often considered first. Some patients present with fever and infection, usually respiratory. The finding of massive hepatosplenomegaly is often thought to be the result of chronic malaria or schistosomiasis, while lymph node enlargement is regarded as tuberculous in origin. Bleeding tendency occurs more with acute myelogenous leukaemia, especially the promyelocytic type, and may be the result of disseminated intravascular coagulation. Bone pains tend to be ignored and regarded as 'growing pains'. Other possible causes in a tropical setting include osteomyelitis, sickle cell disease and rheumatic fever.

Treatment of acute leukaemias

Childhood ALL is potentially curable and, as with most childhood tumours that are curable, every effort must be made to give the child the best chance of achieving that goal. This requires referral to a central hospital where diagnosis can be confirmed and appropriate treatment instituted.

The treatment of acute leukaemias can be classified into two main categories: supportive and definitive. Supportive therapy involves correction of anaemia, control of infection and nutritional support. Definitive therapy involves the use of cytotoxic agents. Such therapy is done over three phases: induction, consolidation with CNS prophylaxis and maintenance. For ALL the induction regimen consists of vincristine and prednisone. Cooperative group studies in Argentina, Brazil, Cuba and Uruguay indicate that high remission rates (>80 per cent) can be achieved even in a tropical environment.[19] Other drugs that can be used for induction include daunomycin and L-asparaginase. Consolidation (often referred to as re-induction) uses the same drugs as for primary induction.

Maintenance therapy is usually continued for up to 24 months with methotrexate and 6-mercaptopurine. CNS leukaemia is the most frequent form of extramedullary relapse in childhood ALL. CNS prophylaxis clearly reduces the incidence of this complication. Cranial irradiation with intrathecal methotrexate is recommended where such facility exists.

Acute non-lymphocytic leukaemia is less responsive to chemotherapy than is ALL. The three treatment phases delineated for ALL are less clear cut. Induction agents include cytosine arabinoside, 6-thioguanine and daunomycin. Many patients with acute non-lymphocytic leukaemia may present with hyperleucocytosis. Leucopheresis with or without hydroxyurea, if available, can bring dangerously high white cell counts to acceptable levels over a short time. Precautions recommended to avoid tumour lysis syndrome for BL should be followed.

The major causes of death in acute leukaemias are infection and haemorrhage. With the availability of platelet transfusion, haemorrhagic complications are less of a threat than was the case two decades ago, and infections remain the major cause of mortality.

Chronic leukaemias are on the whole very rare. The chronic lymphatic type is rarely seen and most cases are of chronic granulocytic type. Treatment is similar to adult cases and busulphan improves the quality of life. During the blast crisis or accelerated phase, treatment is as for acute myeloid leukaemia.

Wilms' tumour or nephroblastoma

Epidemiology

There appears to be no difference between tropical and temperate zones in the incidence of Wilms' tumour. The incidence rate is said to be fairly constant from country to country and even from continent to continent, irrespective of other ethnic group differences. Because of this it has been suggested that Wilms' tumour be used as an index tumour to gauge the completeness and accuracy of cancer registration.[20]

Clinical features

Wilms' tumour can occur at birth although the majority present between two and four years of age. The most common presenting symptom is abdominal swelling, often noted by the mother while washing the child. Other features include haematuria, vomiting and weight loss. The most useful investigation is intravenous pyelography which shows distortion of the pelvicalyceal pattern. Microscopic examination of urine may reveal an excess of red blood cells. The

Table 5.11.6 Staging of Wilms' tumour.

Stage	Characteristics
I	Tumour limited to the kidney and completely resected
II	Tumour extends to the pseudocapsule, para-aortic glands or renal vein, BUT completely resected
III	Residual non-haematogenous tumour confined to the abdomen
	Tumour left at operation or spillage at operation
IV	Haematogenous spread to lungs, liver, bone and brain
V	Bilateral renal involvement

differential diagnosis includes BL, neuroblastoma and polycystic disease. The staging system in use is that recommended by the American National Wilms' Tumour Study group or its modification (Table 5.11.6).

Treatment

Wilms' tumour is a curable childhood tumour. Any child suspected of having Wilms' tumour should, therefore, be transferred forthwith to a central hospital. Like BL, it should be treated with respect and as an emergency. Investigations should be performed and completed to enable surgery to be undertaken within 24–48 hours of diagnosis. Wilms' tumour is the oldest, and perhaps the classic example, of the successes achieved through a combined modality approach to management. Disease free survival at two years (often regarded as cure) has improved from <10 per cent when surgery was the only treatment offered in 1914–23 to now well over 90 per cent when all the modalities (surgery, radiotherapy and chemotherapy) are used. Surgery should be performed as soon as possible, caution being exercised to avoid spillage. Postoperative radiotherapy to the tumour bed is recommended, except for children under two years of age with localized early-stage tumour where routine postoperative radiotherapy is not necessary. The combination of actinomycin-D and vincristine is superior to either drug given alone. The dose of actinomycin-D is usually 15 μg/kg per day for five days (or the entire five days dose can be given as a single injection to avoid frequent needling). The dose of vincristine is usually 1.4 mg/m^2. Following the initial chemotherapy dose, continued cyclic therapy is given initially after six weeks and subsequently every three months up to 15 months.

The long-term complications of treatment include growth retardation due to radiotherapy and the development of second malignant neoplasms. The estimated cumulative risk at 20 years for second malignancy is about 12 per cent and the most common cancer is bone sarcoma.[21] It is not known whether this is due to prolonged survival or genetic predisposition.

Retinoblastoma

The frequency of retinoblastoma is similar to Wilms' tumour, accounting for about 7.5 per cent of childhood tumours in East Africa (Table 5.11.1). About 60 per cent of retinoblastomas are sporadic and 40 per cent are familial with the predisposition being transmitted in an autosomal dominant manner. However, not every person who inherits the predisposing mutation will develop retinoblastoma. Knudson suggested a 'two-hit' hypothesis. In hereditary cases one gene change ('first hit') is present in every cell of the body and a second change ('second hit') occurs in a somatic target cell, the retinoblast. In the sporadic form both 'hits' occur in the same retinoblast. Using appropriate probes (restriction fragment lengths and isoenzymic alleles of loci on chromosome 13) it is possible to predict among predisposed families with a fair degree of accuracy (94 per cent) who are likely to develop retinoblastoma.[22]

The initial phase of visual failure (amaurotic cat's eye) may be indicated by visual defect, strabismus and nystagmus. Walking children tend to bump into objects on the affected side. The majority of children in tropical regions present with extra-ocular spread, with the orbit destroyed and the tumour fungating and infected. For such advanced tumours, palliative enucleation may be attempted. In less advanced stages if facilities exist cryosurgery or light coagulation may be tried.

Neuroblastoma

In comparison with the incidence figures from England and Wales, available information in the tropics would suggest an almost 90 per cent deficiency of neuroblastoma and cerebral tumours. Whether this is due to diagnostic inaccuracy or racial factors is difficult to say.

Clinical features

Neuroblastomas can arise anywhere along the sympathetic chain from the neck to the pelvis. The majority (80 per cent) arise from the abdomen, usually the suprarenal gland. Abdominal tumours present with abdominal pain, mass, anorexia, nausea and vomiting. Thoracic tumours present with dyspnoea, cough

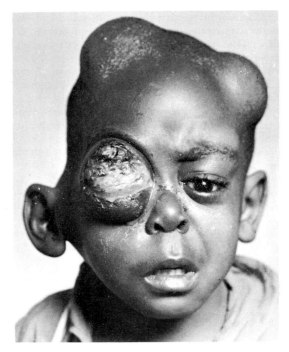

Fig. 5.11.6   Multiple bone secondaries from suprarenal neuro-blastoma (Uganda).

and evidence of superior mediastinal compression syndrome. Most patients (>60 per cent) in a tropical environment present with widespread metastases (Fig. 5.11.6) and up to 50 per cent have bone marrow infiltration. The differential diagnosis includes BL, Wilms' tumour and chloromatous infiltration in acute myelogenous leukaemia.

Oncogene amplification

Recent progress in this neoplasm is in the field of molecular biology. Amplification of N-*myc* oncogene has been identified in almost all human neuroblastoma cell lines tested. The clinical significance of this has been studies in untreated patients. Genomic amplification (3–300 copies) of N-*myc* was found in 38 per cent of 89 patients. Amplification correlated very significantly with disease stage and has now been shown to be a powerful prognostic indicator.[23]

The behaviour of this tumour is unpredictable and cases of spontaneous regression have been reported. The great strides made in molecular biology can only be equalled by the pathetic lack of progress in treatment. The goal of treatment is usually palliation. For early-stage disease, surgery should be offered. The role of postoperative radiotherapy has not been defined. Palliative radiotherapy for metastatic bone pains is recommended. Effective cytotoxic agents include cyclophosphamide, vincristine and dacarbazine. Studies of the role of vitamin B_{12}, which is thought to effect maturation, have given conflicting results. Good responses have been reported in infants; however, they do well irrespective of treatment.

Soft tissue sarcomas

In Western populations, soft tissue sarcomas ranks fifth in the incidence of malignant tumours in children under 15 years, and together with bone tumours account for about 10 per cent of childhood cancers. In the tropics, soft tissue sarcomas are apparently much more frequently observed and together with bone tumours account for over 15 per cent of paediatric neoplasms, being second only to malignant lymphomas (Table 5.11.1). This is probably because other commonly diagnosed childhood cancers in the temperate regions, notably leukaemias, primary brain tumours and neuroblastomas, are relatively rare in the tropics.

Rhabdomyosarcoma

The most common childhood soft tissue tumour is rhabdomyosarcoma. It accounts for well over 50 per cent of such tumours and is usually located in the head and neck region. Other less frequent sites of presentation are the vagina, vulva and urinary bladder. Rhabdomyosarcomas are high-grade tumours of striated muscle origin. They have a propensity to spread by local extension as well as via lymphatics and the bloodstream. The staging system widely used is that recommended by the Intergroup Rhabdomyosarcoma Study Group (IRSG) and this is summarized on Table 5.11.7. Historically, the primary treatment was wide

Table 5.11.7   Intergroup rhabdomyosarcoma staging.

Stage	Criteria
I	Localized disease completely resected
II	Microscopic residual disease following gross resection with or without regional nodes
III	Incomplete resection or biopsy with gross residual disease
IV	Metastatic disease

excision. However, surgical excision lost popularity because of the poor cosmetic and functional results. Mega-voltage irradiation was considered an alternative, but only for loco-regional control. The IRSG have tested several study protocols the results of which can be summarized as follows:

- The prognosis of rhabdomyosarcoma gets worse with increasing stage.
- For localized tumours amenable to complete resection (IRSG I), postoperative radiotherapy is not necessary if the patient is given vincristine, actinomycin-D and cyclophosphamide (VAC).
- For group II patients, the three-drug combination (VAC) failed to improve results obtained with the two drugs (vincristine and actinomycin-D). For such patients, postoperative radiation is necessary.
- The addition of doxorubicin to the three drugs provides no advantage in group III or group IV patients when radiotherapy is used in addition.
- Any recurrence, local or metastatic, is associated with poor prognosis.[24]

Kaposi's sarcoma

Kaposi's sarcoma is often classified with soft tissue sarcomas. In Western countries, the tumour is rare in childhood but in tropical Africa it is commonly diagnosed. The clinical picture is that of widespread lymphadenopathy. The lymph node areas commonly affected are those of the neck (Fig. 5.11.7a), axillae and mediastinum (Fig. 5.11.7b) and the differential diagnoses include tuberculosis and malignant lymphoma. Both of these can occur concurrently with Kaposi's sarcoma or complicate its treatment. In tropical Africa, Kaposi's sarcoma is endemic and the childhood form behaves aggressively, very similarly to the epidemic form seen in association with the acquired immunodeficiency syndrome (see pp. 600–4). Without treatment, patients with childhood Kaposi's sarcoma succumb within 6–12 months. Childhood Kaposi's sarcoma responds to combination chemotherapy consisting of actinomycin-D, vincristine and dacarbazine. The dosages used are as follows: actinomycin-D 0.42 mg/m^2 per day, daily for five days; vincristine 1.40 mg/m^2 with first course and dacarbazine 200 mg/m^2 daily for five days; all three drugs are given intravenously.

Bone sarcomas

The bone tumour seen in the tropics is osteosarcoma; it accounts for about 5 per cent of all childhood tumours. The age group most affected is 9–15 years. The

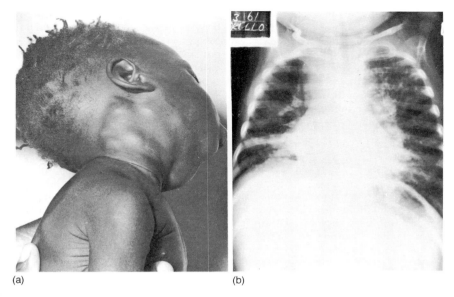

(a)   (b)

Fig. 5.11.7   (a) Kaposi's sarcoma, presenting as bilateral lymphadenopathy in an 18-month-old boy. (b) Same child showing bilateral hilar lymphadenopathy (Uganda).

majority (75 per cent) occur in the lower limbs, especially the distal femur. The prognosis is related to tumour bulk, location, extent of primary disease and histology. For instance, patients with detectable metastases at presentation almost invariably succumb to their disease. Those with axial skeleton involvement have an equally poor prognosis, presumably because adequate excision is not possibble.

Before 1972 the prognosis of patients with osteosarcoma was poor and their quality of life was compromised by amputation. The five-year survival reported was around 20 per cent. The demonstration of effectiveness of high-dose methotrexate and leucovorum rescue and doxorubicin against metastatic osteosarcoma, has greatly altered the outlook in this disease. Well-designed studies have demonstrated that chemotherapy can prolong the disease-free and overall survival rates in patients with non-metastatic osteosarcoma. Advances in other areas include limb-sparing procedures now performed in many centres and aggressive surgical resection of pulmonary metastases.

Ewing's sarcoma is extremely rare in the tropics. This rarity may be due to racial and/or ethnic differences. It is generally accepted that Ewing's sarcoma is rare among black races. In tropical Africa, bone involvement with BL often resembles Ewing's sarcoma.

Liver cancer

Hepatocellular carcinoma (HCC) is among the top ten malignancies affecting mankind. In the tropics and subtropics, it is probably the most common malignant tumour encountered. It affects predominantly young adult males, with a peak incidence observed in the third and fourth decades. In those areas of the world where HCC is endemic, it is not uncommon to find children aged 10–15 years dying of this malignancy.

Clinical, epidemiological and experimental evidence support the view that hepatitis B virus is causally related to HCC. Other important factors to be considered in the tropics are aflatoxin food contamination and malnutrition.

In the tropics and subtropics, HCC behaves aggressively, presenting with acute right upper quadrant pain and mass, weight loss, ascites and jaundice. Without treatment, patients with HCC will die within three months of diagnosis. The treatment is primarily palliative. Surgical resection, if feasible, is the only hope for cure. However, recurrence in the remaining lobe is the rule rather than the exception, especially in cirrhotic livers. Hepatic artery ligation or embolization are effective palliative procedures, especially for the relief of pain. Cytotoxic chemotherapy has so far been disappointing. Some responses are observed in up to 40 per cent of patients treated with doxorubicin at a dose of 60–75 mg/m^2 every three weeks. These responses tend to be short-lived.

The development and demonstration of effectiveness of hepatitis B vaccine provides some hope for the future. A vaccination programme has been initiated in the Gambia by the World Health Organization. A reduction in incidence of HCC in 20–30 years will indeed confirm the aetiological relationship between hepatitis B virus and HCC.

Hepatoblastomas occur primarily in infancy and childhood. The histological appearance is comparable to the fetal liver. Hepatoblastomas carry a high mortality rate. Generally, only patients with resectable disease have a chance for cure and, as with HCC, relapse rate tends to be high. The use of doxorubicin with or without cisplatin has been shown to be particularly effective with some complete responses. However, this drug combination is particularly toxic and should only be used in an appropriate centre under the close supervision of an oncologist.

References

1. Templeton AC. *Tumours in Tropical Countries*. Berlin, Springer, 1973.
2. Waterhouse J, Muir CS, Shanmugaratnam K, Powell J eds. *Cancer Incidence in Five Continents*, Vol. IV (IARC Scientific Publications, No. 42). Lyon, International Agency for Research on Cancer, 1982.
3. Parkin DM, Stjernsward J, Muir CS. Estimates of the worldwide frequency of twelve major cancers. *Bulletin of the World Health Organization*. 1984; **62**: 163–82.
4. WHO. *World Health Statistics Annual*. Geneva, WHO, 1977.
5. Hammond GD. The cure of childhood cancers. *Cancer*. 1986; **58**: 407–13.
6. Miller RW, McKay FW. Decline in US childhood cancer mortality. *JAMA*. 1984; **251**: 1567–70.
7. Elmes BGT, Baldwin RBT. Malignant disease in Nigeria: an analysis of a thousand tumours. *Annals of Tropical Medicine and Parasitology*. 1947; **41**: 321–8.
8. Edington GM, Maclean CMU. A cancer rate survey in Ibadan, Western Nigeria, 1960–1963. *British Journal of Cancer*. 1965; **19**: 471–81.
9. Burkitt DP. A sarcoma involving the jaws in African children. *British Journal of Surgery*. 1958; **197**: 218–23.
10. Geser A, Brubaker G. A preliminary report of epidemiological studies of Burkitt's lymphoma, Epstein Barr virus infection and malaria in North Mara, Tanzania. In: Lenoir G, O'Conor E, Olweny CLM eds. *Burkitt's Lymphoma: A Human Cancer Model* (IARC Scientific Publication, No. 60). Lyon, International Agency for Research on Cancer, 1985.
11. Nonoyama M, Pagano JS. Homology between Epstein–Barr virus DNA and viral-DNA from Burkitt's lymphoma and nasopharyngeal carcinoma determined by DNA–DNA re-association kinetics. *Nature*. 1973; **242**: 44–7.
12. de-The G, Geser A, Day NE *et al*. Epidemiological evidence for a causal relationship between Epstein–Barr virus and Burkitt's lymphoma: results of the Ugandan prospective study. *Nature*. 1978; **274**: 756–61.
13. Zech L, Haglund U, Nilsson K *et al*. Characteristic chromosomal abnormalities in biopsies and lymphoid cell lines from patients with Burkitt and non-Burkitt lymphomas. *International Journal of Cancer*. 1976; **17**: 47–56.
14. Ziegler JL, Magrath IT. Burkitt's lymphoma. *Pathobiology Annual*. 1974; **4**: 129–42.
15. Olweny CLM, Katongole-Mbidde E, Otim D, *et al*. Long-term experience with Burkitt's lymphoma. *International Journal of Cancer*. 1980; **26**: 261–6.
16. Olweny CLM, Katongole-Mbidde E, Kiire C, *et al*. Childhood Hodgkin's disease in Uganda: a ten year experience. *Cancer*. 1978; **42**: 787–92.
17. De Vita VT, Serpick AA, Carbone PP. Combination chemotherapy in the treatment of advanced Hodgkin's disease. *Annals of Internal Medicine*. 1970; **73**: 881–95.
18. Jiminez E. Lymphomas and leukaemias. 2. Tropical America. *Clinics in Haematology*. 1981; **10**: 894–915.
19. Sackmann-Muriel F, Svarch E, Eppinger-Helft M, *et al*. Evaluation of intensification and maintenance programmes in the treatment of acute lymphoblastic leukemia. *Cancer*. 1978; **42**: 1730–40.
20. Innis MD. Nephroblastoma: possible index cancer of childhood. *Medical Journal of Australia*. 1972; **1**: 18–20.
21. Meadows AT, D'Angio GF, Mike V, *et al*. Pattern of second malignant neoplasms in children. *Cancer*. 1977; **40**: 1903–11.
22. Cavenne WK, Murphree AL, Shull MM *et al*. Prediction of familial predisposition to retinoblastoma. *New England Journal of Medicine*. 1986; **314**: 1201–7.
23. Brodeur GM, Seeger RC, Sather H *et al*. Clinical implications of oncogene activation in human neuroblastomas. *Cancer*. 1986; **58**: 541–5.
24. Maurer HM. The Intergroup Rhabdomyosarcoma Study: Update, November 1978. *National Cancer Institute Monographs*. 1981; **56**: 61–8.

Paediatric surgery

S. D. Adeyemi

Although paediatric surgery is a relatively new speciality in the tropics, surgical diseases of children abound here just as much as anywhere in the world. The two clear differences between the tropics and the industrialized world as far as the practice of paediatric surgery is concerned are: (1) late presentation in treatment centres, and (2) inadequate facilities. Attempts are made in this chapter to emphasize these problems and provide practical solutions to them within the limits of the resources generally available in developing countries. The chapter is divided into two major areas, one dealing with surgical diseases of the newborn and the other with those of children outside this age.

Surgical diseases of the newborn

The care of the surgical neonate is challenging anywhere, particularly in the tropics. The reasons for this are two-fold: the delicate physiology and anatomy of the newborn, and the emergency nature of most of the conditions requiring surgical treatment in this period. Therefore, it is very important for the paediatrician or primary physician to make the diagnosis early and make appropriate referral. Some of the more common surgical conditions are described below.

Common surgical causes of respiratory distress

The common surgical causes of respiratory distress are: (1) abdominal distension, (2) neck masses compressing the trachea, (3) oesophageal atresia and tracheo-oesophageal fistula, and (4) congenital diaphragmatic hernia and eventration (Fig. 5.12.1). (See also pp. 229.)

Abdominal distension

Respiratory distress is caused by splinting of the diaphragm which is the muscle of respiration in the baby. The important causes of abdominal distension are dealt with later.

Neck masses

Neck masses may cause respiratory distress in the newborn by compressing the trachea thereby producing stridor, usually due to the size and weight of the mass. Common masses that can do this are large cystic hygromas (Fig. 5.12.2), congenital hyperplasia and teratoma of the thyroid. Cystic hygroma may be entirely cystic or may contain cystic and solid components. When this is the cause of respiratory distress, aspiration of the cyst may produce temporary

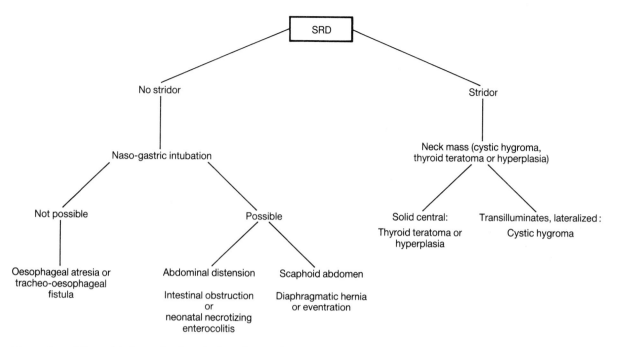

Fig. 5.12.1 Differential diagnosis of surgical respiratory distress (SRD).

relief but urgent arrangements for excision of the mass in a specialized centre should follow. Should aspiration fail to produce relief, intubation may be attempted if the expertise is available, but intubation is generally difficult as the trachea is invariably deviated. A neck radiograph showing the position of the trachea is always useful before intubation is attempted.

The term goitre encompasses thyroid hyperplasia and teratoma, which may be difficult to differentiate from one another clinically. A history indicating that the mother received antithyroid drugs or potassium iodide or suffered iodine deficiency or hypothyroidism, suggests thyroid hyperplasia. In either condition, the trachea may be compressed and distorted, making tracheal intubation difficult if not impossible. In this situation a careful but quick removal of the thyroid isthmus (isthmusectomy) under local anaesthesia is sure to effect relief and is perhaps safer than attempting to do a tracheostomy with no endotracheal tube in place. If this cannot be done the baby is transported to an appropriate centre in the prone position so that the neck mass hangs freely.

Oesophageal atresia with tracheo-oesophageal fistula

This is the most common cause, outside the abdomen,

of surgical respiratory distress in Nigeria. There are two mechanisms: aspiration of saliva which cannot be swallowed, and reflux of stomach juice into the lungs via the fistula. In many cases, the problem is compounded by attempts at feeding the baby out of ignorance of the existing abnormality. The result is severe pneumonitis and pneumonia. Early diagnosis is possible if foaming of saliva is observed and by routinely passing a fairly stiff naso-gastric tube (size 8 or 10) with radiopaque marking which is arrested in the neck if atresia is present. This is confirmed with a plain radiograph of the chest and abdomen which also shows gas in the abdomen suggesting a fistula between the distal oesophagus and the trachea.

The baby is nursed in an oxygenated incubator with head elevated at 60°, and a tube placed for aspirating saliva from the blind upper pouch. Intravenous fluids and broad-spectrum antibiotics are essential. Feeding by mouth is contra-indicated. Urgent transfer to a specialized unit for division of fistula and repair of the oesophagus is mandatory.

Congenital diaphragmatic hernia and eventration

These conditions presenting in the newborn constitute the most urgent emergency. When presentation is delayed outside this age, the symptoms are mild in the

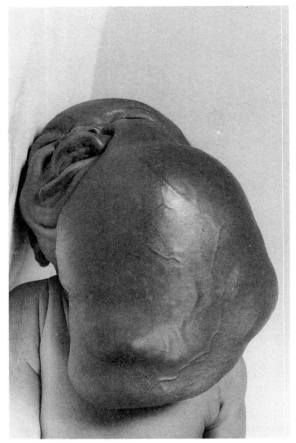

Fig. 5.12.2 Large cystic hygroma associated with respiratory distress from tracheal compression.

form of recurrent lung infections and treatment is elective. In developing countries, many babies with these conditions fail to make it to the treatment centre. The major symptoms of respiratory difficulty and cyanosis are caused by the space-occupying effect of abdominal viscera in the chest, resulting in hypoplasia of the ipsilateral lung and mediastinal shift to the contralateral side. Thus, the apex beat is shifted, and breath sounds are diminished on the affected side where bowel sounds can also be heard in the chest. No time should be wasted in transferring the baby to a specialized unit. This should be done in an oxygenated incubator with the baby lying on the affected side so that the good lung can ventilate freely. Intravenous fluids with added sodium bicarbonate should be administered. If the expertise is available, an endotracheal tube may be passed for supplying oxygen into the lungs.

Bagging via a face mask is dangerous as some of the air will end up in the stomach and compound the problem. Placement of a naso-gastric tube in the stomach helps to minimize distension of this organ.

Rarely, the hernia may be manually reduced through a laparotomy incision. The abdominal viscera are then covered with moist, sterile gauze and the baby transferred to a specialized unit to complete the surgical treatment. Congenital diaphragmatic hernia may be repaired through the abdomen or chest. Eventration is generally treated with plication of the diaphragm through a thoracotomy.

Intestinal obstruction

This is the most common cause of emergency operative treatment in the newborn. Abdominal distension is prominent and is due to gaseous distension of bowel proximal to the obstruction. The more distal the obstruction, the greater the distension and vice versa. In duodenal obstruction, organ distension is limited to the stomach and duodenum which present as epigastric fullness. Delay in treatment not only causes loss of fluids and electrolytes through vomiting and sequestration in the gut, but much required nutrients cannot be supplied to the baby effectively, particularly if facilities for parenteral nutrition are not available. It is possible to make the diagnosis of intestinal obstruction in the first 24 hours of life (Fig. 5.12.3) .

Proximal bowel obstruction

This refers to obstruction situated at or above the proximal jejunum and which is associated with mainly epigastric fullness. Often the babies suffering this type of obstruction have passed meconium, therefore a rigid adherence to the idea of constipation as indicating obstruction is misleading. Vomiting is invariable. What is variable is the colour, which may be clear if the obstruction is proximal to the ampulla of Vater or bile-stained if postampullary. Abdominal radiographs help in sorting out the various forms like duodenal atresia in which a double bubble is seen (Fig. 5.12.4) or jejunal atresia which demonstrates few distended loops of bowel with fluid levels.

Initial resuscitation with intravenous fluids, antibiotics and naso-gastric suction to prevent aspiration of vomitus is indicated. Corrective surgery, if performed in the first week of life, usually gives good results.

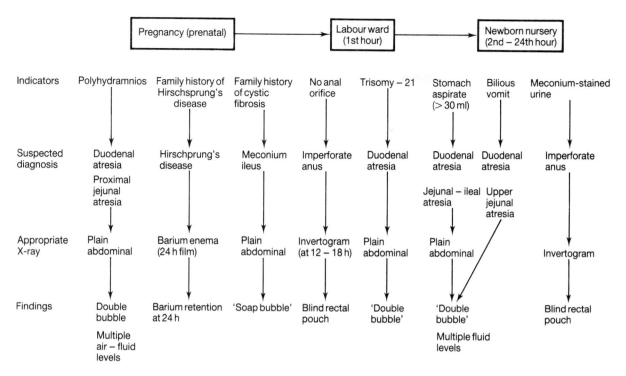

Fig. 5.12.3 Early indicators of intestinal obstruction and radiographic findings.

Distal bowel obstruction

This comprises distal jejunal, ileal, colonic and anorectal obstruction usually caused by atresia or Hirschsprung's disease. It is not always easy to differentiate these on plain abdominal radiograph and often the baby is too distressed because of late presentation to allow more detailed investigations, such as a barium enema. In these situations an urgent laparotomy to decompress the bowel is as life-saving as performing a tracheostomy for an obstructed airway. The diagnosis may then be ascertained at laparotomy and the appropriate treatment carried out. Resection is usually necessary for distal small bowel obstruction but a right transverse colostomy may be all that is needed at this emergency surgery for a poorly defined Hirschsprung's disease or imperforate anus. Further investigation may follow if the baby survives.

The proportion of Hirschsprung's disease that presents as neonatal bowel obstruction is increasing. As the disease is limited to the rectosigmoid in the majority, a right transverse colostomy usually succeeds in decompressing the bowel until the baby is ready for a pull-through procedure at about 8 to 12 months. Before

doing this it is mandatory to confirm the diagnosis with a rectal biopsy which shows absence of ganglia.

Imperforate anus is the most common cause of intestinal obstruction in the newborn, although obstruction is not invariable as some forms of imperforate anus (especially in girls) are decompressed through a fistula which is part of the pathology, e.g. anovestibular and recto-vaginal fistulae. It is crucial to decide correctly from the outset whether a baby with imperforate anus has a low or high lesion in relation to the puborectalis sling. This may be decided by clinical or radiological examination or both (Fig. 5.12.5). For example, an anovestibular fistula in a girl and a perineal fistula in a boy are indicative of low lesions. On the other hand, a single perineal opening of the cloacal type and a high recto-vaginal fistula in a girl or meconium-stained urine in a boy indicate high lesions. Generally, low lesions are treated definitively with anoplasty or proctoplasty at birth and the prognosis is good. A high lesion is treated with a decompressing right transverse colostomy, followed by an abdominal perineal pull-through in the first year. This distinction becomes irrelevant, at least temporarily, when a baby presents with abdominal distension and distress, and

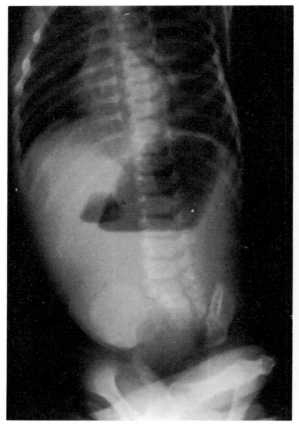

Fig. 5.12.4 Plain abdominal radiograph of a baby with duodenal atresia. Shows 'double bubble' in an otherwise gasless abdomen.

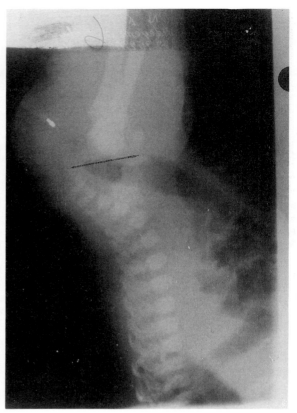

Fig. 5.12.5 An invertogram (upside-down lateral radiograph) of a baby with imperforate anus. The thick straight line between the pubic bone and the last sacral vertabra marks the position of the puborectalis sling. The rectum ends at about the line; therefore this baby was treated as a case of 'high' lesion.

the distinction cannot be made readily. A right transverse colostomy followed by appropriate investigations is the right step in such situations.

Necrotizing enterocolitis

This is unique in being the only major acquired cause of abdominal emergency in the newborn. It would appear to be a disease of sophistication, and is therefore much less common in rural areas of the tropics. It is seen mostly in urban centres where breast-feeding is less practised and the use of formula milk in vogue. Breast-milk contains IgA, an immunoglobulin with a protective function on bowel mucosa. Other factors that have been incriminated include umbilical vessel catheterization, respiratory distress syndrome, prematurity and infection; the common pathway being ischaemic infarction of the bowel and opportunistic bacterial invasion. Infection in the form of septicaemia or gastroenteritis is the major predisposing factor in the tropics. The disease is equally prevalent in preterm and full-term babies. Early signs are abdominal distension, vomiting, and occult blood in stool. In the tropics, some babies present late with rectal bleeding or bowel perforation. The diagnosis is confirmed if any of the above symptoms or signs are associated with pneumatosis intestinalis (intramural air) which is pathognomonic of the condition (Fig. 5.12.6). These babies are often too sick to survive surgery and, in any case, essential postoperative supporting measures like parenteral nutrition may not be available in most tropical countries. Extended medical treatment consists of nasogastric suction, intravenous fluids, fresh blood

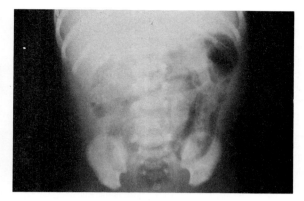

Fig. 5.12.6 Necrotizing enterocolitis. Straight X-ray of abdomen shows air in the intestinal wall (pneumatosis intestinalis).

transfusion and antibiotics which must include metronidazole, an anti-anaerobe. Surgical treatment should be reserved only for babies with perforation and unabating rectal bleeding. The principles of surgery are: (1) resection of all necrotic bowel, (2) exteriorizing the ends as ostomies, and (3) re-establishing bowel continuity after oedema and sepsis have subsided, usually not more than two weeks after the resection.

Anterior abdominal wall defects

These present mainly as exomphalos (omphalocoele), gastroschisis and ectopia vesicae. Exomphalos is the most common and is caused by failure of the abdominal viscera to return to the abdomen from the yolk sac at about the ninth week of fetal development. It presents as a mass protruding from the abdomen through a central defect and is covered by a sac derived from the peritoneum and yolk sac. The umbilical cord is located at the apex of this sac (Fig. 5.12.7). A useful and practical classification is one which takes into account the visceral content of the sac. A major exomphalos contains most of the small and large bowel and the liver and spleen; a medium one contains small and large bowel, and a small one contains only a few loops of small bowel.

Occasionally the sac is ruptured during a difficult labour or shortly after delivery if allowed to dry up. When this happens ruptured exomphalos may be confused with gastroschisis which is another congenital visceral herniation through an anterior wall defect not covered by a sac. Other differences between the two are shown in Table 5.12.1. In gastroschisis the bowel is

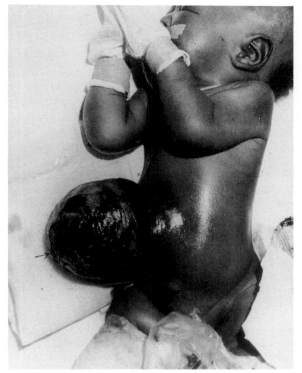

Fig. 5.12.7 Large exomphalos treated by painting sac with formalin. Arrow shows position of umbilical cord which has been excised.

oedematous, thickened dusky and foreshortened as a result of the chemical peritonitis caused by the amniotic fluid.

The initial measures in the management of these two problems are geared towards (1) ensuring that the sac of the exomphalos does not become dry and infected, (2) combating temperature and fluid loss from the exposed viscera in ruptured omphalocoele and gastroschisis. To

Table 5.12.1 Differences between ruptured exomphalos and gastroschisis.

Ruptured exomphalos	Gastroschisis
Torn sac attached	No sac
Central defect involving the umbilical cord	Lateral to umbilical cord (usually the right)
No peritonitis	Chemical peritonitis of viscera
Associated congenital abnormalities common	Associated abnormalities uncommon

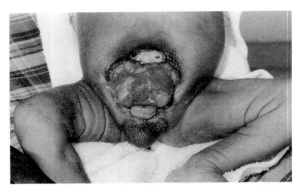

Fig. 5.12.8   Ectopia vesicae: bladder mucosa exposed. There is associated epispadias.

this end, the mass is wrapped in sterile, moist gauze dressing and the baby is nursed in an incubator or alternatively wrapped up in gamgee to keep it warm. Intravenous fluids and antibiotics are necessary if the viscera are exposed. Oral feeding is possible in uncomplicated exomphalos.

The definitive treatment of exomphalos may be conservative in which the sac is painted with sclerosant solutions, such as mercurochrome, formalin and alcohol, or surgical in which reduction and repair of the defect may be effected. In the absence of facilities for mechanical ventilation, only small omphalocoeles can be safely repaired without causing a significant rise in intra-abdominal pressure, respiratory embarrassment from splinting of the diaphragm, and cardiac failure from vena caval obstruction. The majority of omphalocoeles are best suited for conservative treatment in developing countries.

The treatment for gastroschisis and ruptured exomphalos can only be surgical in the absence of a sac. Whenever possible an artificial sac is created which allows the gradual reduction of the hernia followed by repair of the defect.

Ectopia vesicae is the result of failure of migration of mesoderm in the lower part of the abdomen. Consequently, the anterior wall of the bladder and the part of the rectus muscle anterior to it, are absent, exposing the mucosa of the posterior wall and the ureteric orifices (Fig. 5.12.8). The pubic symphysis is widely separated. In the male there is always an associated epispadias and in the female the clitoris is bifid.

Nursing care before surgical treatment should ensure that the surrounding skin remains healthy. This may be achieved by nursing the baby on a frame in a prone position which allows urine to drip straight into a collector and not come in contact with skin. Surgical repair may be undertaken with early closure of the bladder. The incidence of incontinence with this method is 90 per cent. Alternatively, the bladder may be excised and a ureterosigmoidostomy performed so that urine and faeces are passed through the anus, a situation which may not be acceptable in some communities.

Hydrocephalus

This refers to enlargement of the ventricles (hydrocephalus internus) or of the subarachnoid space (hydrocephalus externus) due to a disturbance in the flow of cerebrospinal fluid (see p. 234–5). The causes may be congenital, e.g. aqueduct stenosis or rarely stenosis of the foramen of Monro or foramina of Luschka and Magendie, and the Arnold–Chiari malformation found in association with myelomeningocoele; or acquired, e.g. postmeningitis adhesions, after intraventricular haemorrhage and following traumatic intracranial haemorrhage.

The clinical presentation is related to the enlarged head and the pressure effects on intracranial structures. Rarely, it may be a cause of difficult labour although head enlargement is unusual at birth. Other features include separation of the suture lines, wide anterior fontanelle, the 'cracked pot' sign on percussing the skull, downward displacement of the eyes ('setting-sun' sign) and a tense fontanelle. Convulsions, strabismus and increased muscle tone also occur.

Useful investigations include plain skull radiograph which reveals the widened sutures and the thinned skull bone ('beaten silver' appearance), and air encephalography which demonstrates the enlarged ventricles. Venticular puncture through the lateral angle of the anterior fontanelle is used to determine cerebrospinal fluid pressure (over 200 mm water in hydrocephalus) and to obtain fluid for chemical and bacteriological analysis. In the presence of a rapidly enlarging skull or increased intracranial pressure, treatment is surgical consisting of drainage of cerebrospinal fluid into the right atrium, peritoneal or pleural cavity, using a shunt and valve.

Postneonatal surgical diseases

Acute abdominal pain

In most cases acute abdominal pain indicates an acute abdomen. The common causes of acute abdominal pain in children living in the tropics and the sequential approach to diagnosis are shown in Fig. 5.12.9. If the

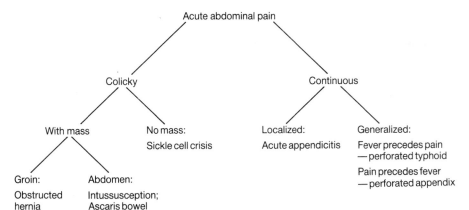

Acute abdominal pain

Colicky   Continuous

With mass   No mass: Localized: Generalized:

             Sickle cell crisis   Acute appendicitis   Fever precedes pain
                                                 —perforated typhoid

Groin: Abdomen: Pain precedes fever
Obstructed   Intussusception;   —perforated appendix
hernia   Ascaris bowel
           obstruction

Fig. 5.12.9 Differential diagnosis of acute abdominal pain.

pain is colicky in nature, the most likely causes are intussusception (between the ages of 3 and 18 months with a peak at 6 months), ascaris bowel obstruction (slightly older children), obstructed inguinal hernia (mainly infant), and sickle cell abdominal crisis (usually associated with previous episodes of sickle cell crises).

Intussusception is the most common cause and is associated with the highest mortality. Presentation is late and usually obstruction is established, thus precluding the use of therapeutic barium enema reduction. A sausage-shaped abdominal mass and red-currant jelly stool make the diagnosis highly likely. An early intussusception can be reduced at laparotomy; in late cases bowel resection is necessary. A barium enema will outline the intussuscepted part of the bowel and can be used as a non-operative method of reduction (Fig. 5.12.10).

Most children who present with bowel obstruction due to a mass of ascaris worms (Fig. 5.12.11) can be

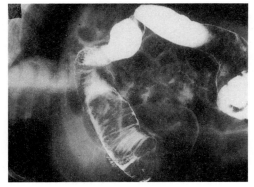

Fig. 5.12.10 An intussusception outlined by barium enema in a five month-old infant.

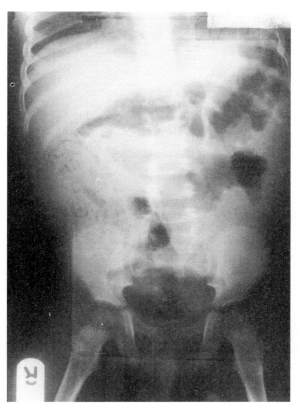

Fig. 5.12.11 Plain abdominal radiograph showing on the right a mass of ascaris worms causing intestinal obstruction.

treated conservatively with intravenous fluids and naso-gastric suction (see p. 638). Administration of an anthelmintic is better withheld until the worms disentangle, as it may have a negative effect on this process. If this fails, the next step is a laparatomy and manual dislodgement of the worms from the usual site of obstruction in the terminal ileum into the large bowel. Resection is only necessary if there has been bowel gangrene.

The most common complication of inguinal hernia seen in the tropics is obstruction. Rarely, the earlier complication of incarceration or the late one of strangulation are seen. Therefore, the majority of children with complicated inguinal herniae require groin exploration as they present late. If strangulation can be ruled out, an attempt at reducing the hernia may be made by sedating the child with pethidine 1–1.5 mg/kg body weight and lying him in the Trendelenberg position for 30 minutes. If this does not result in reduction, gentle pressure can be applied. Any

Table 5.12.2 Common abdominal masses.

Cause	Organs primarily involved	Age range (years)	Pathology	Clinical picture	Useful investigations	Treatment
Nephroblastoma (Wilm's tumour) (see pp. 883–4)	Kidney	3–6	Variety of tissue types. Very malignant. Metastases to liver, lungs common, 5% bilateral	Weight loss, haematuria (20%), hypertension (10%), liver involved (60%)	Intravenous urography (IVU)	Nephrectomy; actinomycin-D, vincristine; radiotherapy (>18 months)
Neuroblastoma (see pp. 884–5)	Adrenal	2–8	Arise from primitive dorsal neural crest. Metastasis has occurred in 80%	Abdominal mass, weight loss, bone pain, hypertension	IVU, VMA*, bone marrow biopsy	Excision; vincristine, cyclo-phosphamide; radiotherapy
Burkitt's lymphoma (see pp. 875–80)	Ovaries, retroperi-toneal lymph nodes, kidneys, liver, spleen (also jaw, thyroid)	5–14	Lymphocytic lymphoma associated with herpes virus	Abdominal masses, weight loss	Biopsy of suspected masses	Debulking Cyclophosphami-de Second-look laparotomy and resection indicated if there is residual mass following chemotherapy.
Schistosomiasis (see pp. 650–6)	Liver, spleen, colon, urinary bladder	5–14	Caused by larva of blood fluke (formation of granuloma, polyps in colorectum, portal and urinary systems)	Portal hypertension, gastro-intestinal bleeding, haematuria, bloody diarrhoea	Isolation of ova in urine, faeces; liver biopsy; splenoporto-graphy	Chemotherapy (antimony drugs); surgery
Hydatid disease (see pp. 738–9)	Liver, spleen, kidney (also lungs, brain)	3–15	Caused by larva of *Echinococcus granulosus*	Mass, pain, jaundice	Plain radiograph; Casoni's skin test; liver scan	Surgical resection or enucleation Albendazole
Sickle cell disease (see pp. 828–30)	Spleen	8–13	Hypersplenism	Severe anaemia with poor response to transfusion	Genotype, platelet count (low)	Splenectomy

* Vanilmandelic acid.

attempt less than 100 per cent successful is an indication for exploration. If successful, 48 hours is allowed for oedema to subside before herniotomy is done for technical ease.

Sickle cell abdominal crisis may mimic appendicitis but may be easily distinguished from it through a good history and physical examination which reveals stigmata of sickle cell disease such as anaemia, jaundice and hepatomegaly (see p. 829). Also the pain is not localized. Treatment is medical with intravenous fluids and gastric suction, antibiotics and analgesics. Transfusion with packed cells may be necessary.

Acute appendicitis is not as uncommon in the tropics as previously thought. The pathophysiology is related to luminal obstruction of the organ by faecolith, ascaris, lymphoid hyperplasia or *Yersinia enterocolitica* in some parts of the tropics. The peak age is 7–9 years and it presents as an initial central colic which becomes localized in the right iliac fossa as a continuous pain. Fever and vomiting, which are not generally prominent, may become so the younger the child is than five years. The treatment is emergency appendicectomy to prevent perforation which converts the situation to a more grave one with higher morbidity and mortality. When this occurs there is need for longer resuscitation with intravenous fluids and electrolytes before appendicectomy.

Another condition which presents with generalized peritonitis and fever is a perforated typhoid ulcer which may be indistinguishable from a perforated appendix (see p. 585). The children suffering from typhoid perforation are more toxic, may be jaundiced and often have had fever and diarrhoea preceding the abdominal pain. Happily, both conditions can be treated through a McBurney type of incision. An appendicectomy, suction of peritoneal fluid and drainage of the pelvis and abdomen are carried out for perforated appendix. Closure of the perforation, usually situated in the distal ileum, with evacuation of peritoneal fluid is the treatment for a typhoid ulcer. Chloramphenicol is the antibiotic of choice for typhoid and must be started pre-operatively and continued intra- and post-operatively. Ampicillin is regarded as a second-choice drug.

Periodic administration of anthelmintic preparations to children is a common practice in many homes in the tropics in an attempt to deworm them. Many of these preparations contain anticholinergic agents which cause abdominal distension from ileus, and pain which may mimic generalized peritonitis. A good history usually reveals the problem and treatment is simply intravenous fluids and naso-gastric suction until the effect of the drug wears off.

Abdominal masses

These are summarized in Table 5.12.2.

Scrotal swellings

The most common scrotal swelling in the tropics, as anywhere else, is inguino-scrotal hernia which is most common in infants. Complications of the hernia are also likely to occur in this age group; therefore, herniotomy should be performed as soon as possible. The major constraint here is anaesthesia, as local anaesthesia is not suitable for this operation. Ketamine, a short-acting general anaesthetic, may be used intramuscularly in doses of 6–8 mg/kg body weight.

The other common causes are epididymo-orchitis, torsion of the testis, testicular hydrocoele and testicular tumour such as teratoma. They can be differentiated as shown in Fig. 5.12.12. Scrotal hydrocoele is one of those lesions that demonstrate spontaneous regression, this usually happens in the first or second year of life. Therefore, surgical treatment is deferred until then if it persists. Torsion may be associated with maldescent and often there is a history of trauma. Urgent exploration of the scrotum through the groin and derotation of the torsion is indicated followed by orchidopexy. If gangrene of the testis has already taken place then orchidectomy should be performed and the testis replaced with a prosthesis at puberty.

Epididymo-orchitis is often associated with urinary tract infection and responds well to antibiotic ther-

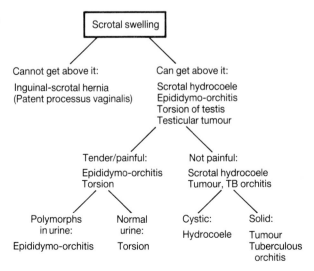

Fig. 5.12.12 Differential diagnosis of scrotal swelling.

apy and rest. An intravenous urogram is helpful in detecting any underlying urinary tract abnormality.

Testicular tumours are not common but are no less important differential of scrotal swellings. When suspected, a high orchidectomy is indicated and the testis is submitted for histopathological examination. Appropriate chemotherapy and/or radiotherapy will seem more suitable treatment than extensive retroperitoneal dissection, unless the facilities for the former are unavailable.

Tuberculous orchitis though more common in adults, may occur in children. A history of tuberculous chest infection is helpful. A positive Heaf or Tuberculin test may be followed by a trial of therapy with antituberculosis drugs.

Anterior abdominal wall hernias

The most common anterior abdominal wall hernias are umbilical, para-umbilical and epigastric in that order; Spigelian hernia is uncommon (Fig. 5.12.13). Umbilical hernia is highly prevalent in black children and in many cases does not require treatment. Surgical repair is indicated if there are complications, e.g. pain or obstruction. Cosmetic repair may be necessary where the hernia is a giant one or where the skin is redundant, even if the defect is small (less than 1 cm in diameter).

Para-umbilical hernia is less common but more likely to be associated with troublesome symptoms. It should be repaired when the diagnosis is made. Epigastric hernia is also troublesome and may mimic peptic ulcer symptomatically. It often requires surgical treatment. The sites and orientation of the defects of the various hernias are shown in Fig. 5.12.13.

Pyloric stenosis

This is an acquired condition of the neonatal period and is often seen in slightly older infants in the tropics who present anaemic and marasmic. The triad of projectile non-bilious vomiting, constipation and visible epigastric peristalsis should suggest the diagnosis. It is confirmed by palpating a peanut-sized mass (pyloric mass) above the umbilicus just to the right of the midline with the recti muscles relaxed by flexing the hips; it is most readily palpated during feeding and before vomiting. Barium meal should be reserved for the few occasions on which the mass is too small to be felt. The radiographic features are gastric distension, a double pyloric channel (rail roading) and a beak appearance at the proximal end of the pyloric canal. Resuscitation with correction of malnutrition, anae-

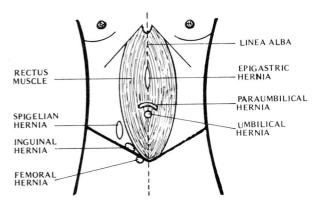

Fig. 5.12.13 Position, shape and orientation of defects in common external hernias.

mia, fluid and electrolyte deficits (hypochloraemic alkalosis) takes precedence over pyloromyotomy.

Surgical infections

Superficial infections are common, particularly in immunodepressed children due to measles or malnutrition. These skin abscesses are well localized and result from staphylococcal infection. Abscesses in the head and neck are more likely to follow a throat infection and have a greater tendency to be associated with cellulitis as indicated by erythema, as streptococcus plays a contributory role here. These superficial abscesses should be allowed to suppurate in order to facilitate surgical drainage. Antibiotics should not be used for localized infections, since they tend to delay suppuration. They are, however, indicated in the presence of cellulitis. Cloxacillin is the antibiotic of choice.

Paronychia This is infection around the fingernail, although it may spread some distance proximally. Infection involving only the base of the nail is referred to as an eponychia while that involving subungual tissues is called subonychia. Paronychia often presents as a painful, red, swelling which may contain pus. In the absence of an abscess, treatment consists of warm compresses followed by zinc oxide dressings, elevation of the hand and antibiotics, preferably cloxacillin. Surgical drainage, and in some cases, partial or total removal of the nail, is necessary if an abscess has formed. Chronic paronychia of the 'dish-washer' or 'washerman' type is uncommon in children. When encountered, fungal infection must be suspected. The fingers should be protected from water and appropriate antifungal chemotherapy administered. The consequent nail deformities often make nail avulsion necessary.

Pyomyositis, an infection of major groups of skeletal muscles, e.g. of the thigh, arm, abdominal wall or calf, usually follows a systemic infection which becomes localized in these bulky muscles. Symptoms include fever, anaemia and painful swelling which is tender and fluctuant. Doubtful cases may be aspirated, when pus should be encountered. The most frequent causative organism is staphylococcus followed by streptococcus. Many children with pyomyositis require blood transfusion before and after surgical treatment which entails drainage and debridement under general anaesthesia. Analgesia and rest of the limb are important and so is physiotherapy after healing has taken place.

Trauma

The common causes of trauma in childhood in the tropics are road traffic and home accidents. Sports injuries are less common than in industrialized countries. Boys are significantly more affected than girls by a ratio of two to one. The common home accidents are falls, cuts, insertion of foreign objects into body orifices and burns in order of frequency. Generally, home accidents are more frequent causes of trauma in the rural areas than are road accidents. The reverse is not necessarily true for urban centre but the proportion of trauma caused by road accidents is higher than in the rural areas. Blunt trauma in the form of head injury, liver or splenic injuries, and fractures are more common than penetrating wounds, although the latter are on the rise in urban centres. Therefore, injury to multiple organs is quite common. When this occurs the correct approach is to take care of the airway, maintain adequate circulation, and attend to head injury, urinary tract and gastro-intestinal injuries in order of priority.

Chest injury, particularly pneumothorax and traumatic diaphragmatic hernia, may occur without any apparent rib fracture because of the resilience of these bones in children. Tension pneumothorax should be suspected in blunt trauma in the presence of respiratory difficulty, shifted mediastinum, hypertympany of the affected side and diminished air entry. A diagnostic tap with a glass syringe and needle going through the second intercostal space, in the mid-clavicular line, will cause the plunger to rise on its own. A trocar may then be inserted at the same spot and used to thread in a rubber catheter for drainage. This procedure takes precedence over a chest radiograph which may be done later. A more permanent drainage with a chest tube preferably with underwater sealed drainage connected to suction should be effected when the facility is available.

Traumatic diaphragmatic hernia should be suspected in any blunt trauma to the chest and abdomen which is accompanied by dyspnoea, scaphoid abdomen and mediastinal shift. The diagnosis is easily confirmed with a chest radiograph following placement of a naso-gastric tube which is shown on X-ray to be in the chest as the stomach frequently is part of the hernia. Surgical reduction and repair through the abdomen or chest should be carried out promptly.

Trauma to the head may result in subdural or extradural haematoma or subarachnoid haemorrhage. The lucid interval is not a common feature in the extradural haematoma of childhood. Any of these injuries may be announced by drowsiness, vomiting and convulsion, indicating brain swelling. Time may be bought by giving mannitol intravenously, following which the child should be transferred to a specialized unit. In less severe cases, hydrocortisone may be used to combat brain oedema.

Splenic rupture is about the most common abdominal injury in blunt trauma. Efforts should be geared towards preserving splenic tissue as much as possible because of its major role against infections, particularly in children.

Fractures generally are treated conservatively in children by closed reduction and immobilization with plaster of Paris. Precise alignment and end-to-end apposition of the fragments are not necessary since these are compensated for as the child grows. Exceptions to this conservative approach to treatment of fractures in children: (1) fractures near joints, (2) fractures of bones in inaccessible locations, and (3) rotational malposition of fractures of the shaft. Operative correction is indicated in these.

Constipation

There are two major causes of chronic constipation in the majority of children in the tropics (see pp. 198–9, 401). One is congenital, Hirschsprung's disease, and the other acquired or 'habit constipation'. The former is caused by the congenital absence, as a result of arrest of migration, of both Auerbach's and Meisner's groups of ganglia. The latter is the result of a combination of diet, poor toilet training, bad toilet habit and to some extent emotional and psychogenic factors. The important clinical features which differentiate the two types are: (1) constipation from birth as typified by delay in passage of meconium for longer than 48 hours in Hirschsprung's disease, (2) soiling is absent in Hirschsprung's disease but is a regular feature in acquired constipation, and (3) the rectum in Hirschsprung's disease is empty whereas the column of faeces often extends close to the end of the rectum in the acquired type. Barium enema is best done before any wash-out. The classic appearance in Hirschsprung's of contracted rectosigmoid and dilated proximal colon contrasts with the uniform dilatation of the rectum down virtually to the anus that is usually seen in acquired constipation. Rectal biopsy should always be done if there is sufficient reason to suspect Hirschsprung's disease.

An abdominoperineal pull-through operation is usually necessary to treat Hirschsprung's disease after adequate bowel preparation. The treatment of acquired constipation consists of evacuation of faeces from the bowel digitally with the use of aperients and colonic wash-out, dietary advice and toilet training.

Acquired anorectal lesions

The most important of these is rectal prolapse. Fissure-in-ano may occasionally be the cause of constipation in the infant. Fistula-in-ano often results from inadequate treatment of perianal abscess, another lesion found in this area. In Nigeria these lesions, except rectal prolapse, are uncommon.

Rectal prolapse is one condition which brings the child promptly to hospital because of the fright the experience generates in many parents. Young children are predisposed to rectal prolapse because of two anatomical disadvantages: (1) the sacral lordosis which supports the rectum against gravity in adults is absent, and (2) the attachment of the rectum to the sacrum is relatively loose, thus allowing for the bowel to slide easily.

As not all children develop rectal prolapse, there must be factors that precipitate it. In tropical countries, these factors include malnutrition, gastroenteritis, measles, poliomyelitis and trichuriasis infection. Others include paraplegia (often associated with myelomeningocoele), posterior urethral valves and generally conditions associated with chronic increase in intra-abdominal pressure. The majority of prolapses seen in Nigeria are complete and have a high tendency to bleed easily. An important differential diagnosis is complete intussusception and must always be ruled out. Failure to make this distinction may be catastrophic. They may be differentiated by inserting the index finger between the anal canal and the protruding bowel. In rectal prolapse, a cul-de-sac is encountered as the finger is advanced cephalad. In intussusception there is no obstruction to the movement of the finger in this direction.

Some prolapses reduce spontaneously following the act of defaecation, some have to be helped in but there are a small minority which become obstructed, or irreducible. The procedure for reducing a rectal prolapse is similar to that for reducing an obstructed hernia. The child is sedated and placed in Trendelenberg position; ice packs may be placed over the prolapse. After about 30 minutes the prolapse may be reduced by gentle, steady pressure. A successful reduction should be followed by firm strapping together of the buttocks with adhesive tape, maintaining this position for about 24 hours. Then the child is encouraged to pass a stool with the underpants on and preferably in the erect position. This conservative management, coupled with identification and treatment of the precipitating factor, often gives good results. Otherwise, one of the very simple forms of surgical treatment of rectal prolapse, e.g. Thiersch stitch, should be carried out.

Genito-urinary problems

Hydronephrosis

This occurs following obstruction to urine flow at or distal to the pelvic-ureteric juction, with progressive

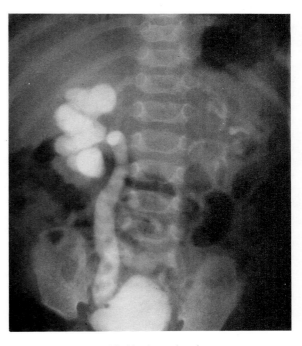

Fig. 5.12.14 Right sided hydronephrosis.

dilatation of the calyces and pelvis and pressure on the adjacent renal parenchyma. In the newborn, the obstruction is often a component of renal pedicle atresia. The result is a flank mass and secondary infection from stasis. Haematuria and pyuria are common presenting symptoms in older children. Diagnosis is aided with intravenous pyelography (Fig. 5.12.14) or, if the kidney is non-functioning, retrograde pyelogram. The nature of surgical treatment will depend on the pathology and may range from division of an obstructing band or artery to pyeloplasty or even nephrectomy (see pp. 784–805).

Posterior urethral valves

This is the most common cause of lower urinary tract obstruction in children and the most common cause of urinary retention in boys. It is uncommon in girls. It may be complicated by hydroureter and hydronephrosis. The severe form occurs in the newborn in whom there is extravasation of urine as urine peritonitis or urine-induced inflammation of suprapubic and perineal tissues. The baby is often stillborn. The moderate form also occurs in the newborn who present with urinary retention and poor urine stream but with no extravasation. The mild form is generally seen in the postneonatal period, sometimes in school-age children. It presents as dysuria (straining at micturition) and may be associated with rectal prolapse and inguinal hernias, which result from chronically raised intra-abdominal pressure. It may also present as failure to thrive, unexplained hypertension or as the incidental finding of an abdominal mass.

Pretreatment assessment of the upper urinary tract with determination of serum potassium and blood urea, and intravenous urography are useful in choosing the course of treatment. Staged treatment with high urinary diversion followed later by valvectomy is preferred for those in whom the upper tracts have been significantly damaged. Otherwise, excision of the membranous valves in the posterior urethra after confirming the diagnosis with an expression cystogram is the usual approach.

Undescended testis

This term is generally used when the testis is situated outside the scrotum, but strictly two groups of such testes should be excluded: those that can be brought down to touch the bottom of the scrotum (retractile) and the ectopic testes which are considered to have undergone normal descent, except that they fail to find their way into the scrotum. Many children are brought to hospital on detecting the condition at a preschool medical examination. Very few are detected in infancy. It is by far more common on the right than the left and bilaterality occurs in 5–10 per cent. A small fraction of cases are associated with hypospadias. Nearly all are associated with inguinal hernia, even if the latter is not symptomatic. Early surgical placement in the scrotum is advisable. An undescended testis may be complicated by torsion, trauma and an increased potential for malignancy. Spermatogenesis will be impaired if the testis is allowed to remain in the abdomen beyond the age of six years because of the higher temperature in this location. After this age orchidopexy may not correct this defect. Fortunately one normal testis will suffice for fertility. Orchidopexy has no effect on the possibility of malignancy but it enhances early detection should this occur.

Further reading

Adeyemi SD, da Rocha-Afodu JT, Olayiwola B. Outpatient herniotomy with ketamine: a prospective study of 50 herniotomized children and review of 219 herniotomies with ketamine. *West African Journal of Medicine*. 1985; **4**: 155–61.

Rickham PP, Soper RT, Stauffer UG eds. *Synopsis of Paediatric Surgery*. Chicago, Year Book Medical Publishers/Georg. Thieme Publishers, 1975.

Rickham PP, Hecker W. Ch, Prevot, J eds. *Paediatric Surgery in Tropical Countries. Progress in Paediatric Surgery*. Baltimore–Munich, Urban and Schwarzenberg, 1982.

CHAPTER 13

Diseases of the ears, nose and throat

Christopher Holborow

Ear, nose and throat diseases are common in tropical areas. They are a great source of worry to both general physicians and nurses since examination may appear to be difficult and some very serious life-threatening problems may develop which, if not dealt with correctly, may lead to considerable residual disability. The symptoms are relatively few in number and diagnosis is usually possible by careful examination, providing one has good illumination – an otoscope is essential, but so often the battery has been inactivated by heat or humidity or is simply unavailable. A concave head-mirror using reflected light (there is always sunlight) is a simple instrument too little used; both hands are left free to use instruments or control the child and the technique is not very difficult to acquire.

Much treatment must, of necessity, be left to nurses, dispensers and primary health care workers; ear, nose and throat doctors, so few in number in most tropical countries, have therefore a more than usually vital task in training their colleagues.

The ear

Pain

Earache is a very common complaint in childhood; those too young to complain may rub their ears or bang their heads.

Auricle

Trauma causing a haematoma (cauliflower ear) is obvious. The blood may be evacuated, but unless firm, even pressure is applied for some time it often reforms. Boils and furuncles are best not incised for fear of involving the cartilage and causing perichondritis. Magnesium sulphate paste on a wick will often draw the pus out and relieve the pain. Perichondritis may also follow ear-piercing, especially where there have been multiple perforations of the pinna with dirty wool or pieces of bamboo passed through the cartilage. Antibiotics may well be needed to prevent much cartilage destruction.

External meatus

Foreign bodies are a frequent cause of pain. Insects are best killed with alcohol or vegetable oil and then removed piecemeal. Seeds and nuts are often more difficult and should be removed with a wax hook (a paper clip may be bent to form a 2 mm horizontal hook) which can be passed behind the object, rotated 90° and withdrawn. Syringing causes vegetable foreign bodies to swell and forceps usually push them deeper, possibly through the eardrum.

Otitis externa is common in hot and humid climates. Bacterial or fungal infection, or a combination of both, causes swelling of the meatal skin which, being tightly attached to the cartilage, causes much pain. The drum may be invisible so otitis media or mastoiditis may be suspected. If there is pain on moving the pinna, it is likely that the condition is otitis externa and if a tuning fork test shows that air conduction is better than bone conduction (Rinne test positive) the diagnosis is firm. Fungal infection is especially painful. The treatment is to clean the meatus. Antibacterials used locally may cause sensitivity. Antifungals (Nystatin or Fungilin) are useful, but perhaps the best thing to do is to insert a gauze wick soaked in glycerine and ichthammol which reduces the meatal swelling and does not cause sensitivity.

Wax may cause pain and deafness, especially if it has swollen after water has entered the ear in swimming. It can be removed with the wax hook or by syringing, though if there is an underlying perforation the latter may initiate an infected discharge. It may have to be softened by the use of 5 per cent sodium bicarbonate ear drops which are much better, cheaper and more easily obtained than proprietary drops. Keratosis obturans is more difficult to manage. This occurs when desquamated epithelium and wax are combined to form a very resistent plug which blocks and may even erode the meatus. This condition is often associated with chronic bronchitis and bronchiectasis perhaps due to stimulation of the vagus nerve and reflex excessive production of wax. Otitis externa is very often associated with eczema or seborrhoeic dermatitis. Simple treatment following aural toilet is often satisfactory if local steroid drops are not available or too expensive.

Middle ear

In children, the most common cause of earache is acute otitis media. Following a cold or tonsillitis, infection spreads up the Eustachian tube, pus forms in the middle ear cleft, the drum bulges with great pain which is relieved when it finally ruptures; a purulent discharge follows. Decongestant nasal drops (0.5 per cent ephedrine in saline) may clear the tube sufficiently to allow natural drainage and healing, but antibiotics are required if the discharge persists for more than two days. The usual course is resolution and healing; only a small minority go on to chronic middle ear infection or scarring and conductive deafness. Rarely the pain of acute otitis continues, the discharge persists and acute mastoiditis develops. The infection will have spread to the mastoid air cells; it is then possible for it to extend into the sigmoid sinus with septicaemia, the temporal lobe or cerebellum with brain abscess or to the inner ear with labyrinthitis signalled by dizziness and vomiting.

At this stage, there is often swelling behind and immediately above the ear which may be pushed outwards. Pain is felt to pressure above and behind the meatus and the child will be deaf in that ear.

This dangerous condition requires effective doses of parenteral antibiotics. A subperiostal postaural abscess may be drained by incision; the facial nerve is superficial below the ear so a short incision is required. Cortical mastoidectomy is needed to drain the mastoid if antibiotics fail.

Discharge

In many societies where medical information is lacking, discharge from the ear is considered a normal condition and the frequency of its occurrence is thought to confirm this. The character of the fluid is a very valuable guide to the disease process.

Blood

A bloody discharge may be caused by trauma; it is easy to scratch the meatus when attempting to remove wax or relieve the irritation of otitis externa. The tympanic membrane may be perforated by foreign bodies and a drop of blood may precede the purulent discharge that follows rupture in acute otitis media. In cases of traumatic perforation, the ear should be kept absolutely dry and clean and the drum should heal. In head injuries, considerable bleeding may occur indicating that the fracture line runs through the temporal bone. This is a particularly important sign when a fracture is not visible radiologically.

Clear fluid

A clear serous fluid may arise from atopic otitis externa. Rarely, following a fracture as described above, a meningeal tear may allow loss of cerebrospinal fluid; this will contain glucose.

Muco-purulent discharge

The most common discharge in childhood is a profuse, inoffensive, yellow or whitish mucus. This is characteristic of tubo-tympanic otitis media due to infection ascending the Eustachian tube from the naso-pharynx. The perforation of the drum is usually inferior and the hearing is impaired to some degree. This is obvious disease, easy to recognize and safe; complications are very rare. Treatment is aural toilet and eradication of nasal infection.

Less often the discharge is scanty, fetid, often

brownish, but sometimes containing flecks of white epithelial debris. This indicates attic disease; the perforation in this case is small, marginal (implying bony erosion) and above, or above and behind the short process of the malleus. Hearing may not be much affected. This is a potentially dangerous disease but insidious and often overlooked unless serious spread to the labyrinth, temporal lobe or cerebellum occurs. In sub-Saharan African countries, attic disease is much less common than in the Indian subcontinent and South-east Asia.

In otitis externa the discharge is variable. The dry variety may show scales of epithelial debris, the wet variety, soft cheesey material, thick pus or sometimes black fungal threads and masses. The condition is often atopic with bacterial or fungal infection. The diagnosis must be made in many cases on other signs and symptoms, the character of the pain, and irritation which may be severe and lead to much trauma and further infection from scratching. Good hearing is always preserved.

Deafness

General

Deafness in children may be sensorineural where lesions of the labyrinth or central nervous system prevent the reception of sound stimuli, or conductive where there is an obstructive lesion in the outer or middle ear preventing sound from reaching the cochlea.

Sensorineural deafness may be very severe; conductive deafness is usually partial or moderate in degree. In assessing deafness, a very careful history is important and clinical tests are vital, and are nearly always sufficient to give a reasonable picture of the degree of handicap.

In practice, there is very little difference between an infant who is born deaf and one who develops a profound deafness before the development of speech. In either case, there is nearly always some hearing but speech will only develop if this residual hearing is used. It is usually of no real importance to decide whether the hearing defect was present at birth or developed soon after, but it is of critical importance to identify hearing loss as early in life as possible, so that training may start and speech develop. Sadly, in tropical developing countries there are few special schools available for deaf children. In the industrial world, the incidence of profound deafness is approximately one child in every 1000 births. In tropical countries, the figure is rather higher, sometimes up to two per 1000.

Sensorineural deafness

Infants who have a family history of deafness, maternal infections during pregnancy or perinatal problems, who are late to talk or walk, or who have other congenital defects must be considered as being at risk (Table 5.13.1). The frequency of sporadic cases of deafness makes testing of all babies important. The mothers' views should never be ignored and it is important to remember that a minor degree of conductive deafness may be an additional and significant handicap when the baseline is already low.

Genetic causes are especially common in societies where first-cousin marriage is traditional. Perinatal causes are important and preventable but the resultant deafness is less severe than that caused by infections such as rubella, meningitis and measles. Malnutrition, malaria and enteric disease play a considerable but as yet incompletely understood part.

Table 5.13.1   Causes of congenital/prelingual deafness (with approximate percentages in the developed world).

Genetic 30%
    Dominant (occurs from one generation to the next)
    Recessive (more sporadic)
    Many syndromes
Non-genetic 20%
    Prenatal: Rubella
             Cytomegalovirus
             Ototoxic drugs (streptomycin, salicylates)
             Syphilis
    Perinatal: Prematurity
             Anoxia
             Jaundice
             Birth trauma
    Postnatal: Meningitis (meningococcal, pneumococcal, viral)
             Measles
             Lassa fever virus
             Enteric disease
             Otitis media
             Ototoxic drugs
Unknown 30%
Specific defects of ear 20%

Conductive deafness

The main causes of conductive hearing loss are shown in Table 5.13.2. Deafness associated with a mucopurulent discharge due to chronic otitis media is very common in rural tropical areas. In some dry, dusty regions where children have been studied, a very large proportion have discharging ears; in humid areas infection also spreads from the naso-pharynx. Prevention of damage to the middle ear mechanism by

Table 5.13.2 Causes of conductive deafness.

Congenital lesions
  Atresia of external meatus and middle ear usually with
    microtia
  Atresia associated with other facial defects
  Middle ear deformities
  Many syndromes, e.g. Treacher Collins, cleft palate
External auditory meatus
  Wax
  Foreign bodies
  Otitis externa
Middle ear lesions
  Trauma: Ossicular disruption
             Perforated tympanic membrane
  Otitis media — acute or chronic
  Eustachian malfunction atelectasis
  Serous otitis

continued infection is essential to promote healing and conserve as much hearing as possible. In many areas where doctors are scarce, most of the children must be treated by health care workers with only minimal otological training and without special instruments for examination. At the end of this section on the ear, a chart is reproduced to assist in the early treatment of the ears (Fig. 5.13.1).

Serous otitis

Non-suppurative otitis media with fluid or mucus in the middle ear due to Eustachian tubal blockage is very common in Western countries, although much less so in tropical areas. The only symptom is deafness; this is often variable and usually of only moderate degree (20–25 db loss), but of significance to a child in a noisy classroom. The drum may be yellowish or dull. Myringotomy and aspiration of the fluid, with or without the insertion of a ventilation tube (grommet), restores the hearing. Adenoidectomy and treatment of nasal infection helps to clear the Eustachian tube.

Acoustic trauma

Deafness caused by noise is entirely preventable and totally untreatable. It is more common in the working population but children may be exposed to noise, for instance when assisting their parents in metal work such as hammering out old oil drums for further use. The high-frequency hearing loss is maximal at 4 000 and 6 000 cycles per second and can be detected early with an audiometer. Later, clinical speech tests show the typical loss involving difficulty in hearing in conditions of background noise, and an inability to hear the high-frequency, low-intensity consonants which makes speech appear indistinct.

Testing hearing

Most cases of deafness can be assessed without complicated and expensive equipment. Screening for infants should be universally employed to pick out the deaf at the earliest possible age so that education can be started with the greatest benefit. During the first six months of life, a sound (such as a hand clap) in the region of 90–100 db will evoke a 'startle response' or a blink (cochleo-palpebral response). False results are common and the tests may have to be repeated. At six months of life, a response is obtained to a female voice; pure tones are less effective. Most infants at six months respond to soft 'meaningful sounds' by turning their head. Spoon and cup sounds indicating food, rattles, the rustle of paper and mother's voice will elicit a response, while sounds without significance will be ignored after perhaps one initial response. The position of the sounds is critical, two to three feet at one side of the head at the level of the ears will be effective while sounds above the head will not. There are many pitfalls in testing and experience is required in avoiding visual hints. At three years of age, performance tests may be given using pure tones or voice, the child pointing to common objects named. The mouth of the tester must be covered to avoid lip reading.

The nose

In general, there are few nasal signs and symptoms. Children in any part of the world are remarkably phlegmatic about nasal troubles and nowhere more so than in the tropics where the young seem completely unconcerned about blocked noses running with thick muco-pus.

Discharge and obstruction

The origin of the discharge should be noted: whether it is unilateral or bilateral, from the whole mucosa or a sinus ostium, or whether it is principally anterior or posterior. The character of the discharge: clear and watery, clear and mucoid, purulent, fetid or blood-stained is also of great importance. Nasal discharge and obstruction go together. Their significance is largely aural, infection from the nose involving the Eustachian tube so that deafness and middle ear infection follow.

Unilateral discharge and obstruction may be present from birth due to choanal atresia, a rare condition

#	PATIENT'S COMPLAINT	PAIN	DISCHARGE	ITCHING	DEAFNESS	QUESTIONS?	TEST	PROBABLE DISEASE	FIRST TREATMENT WITHOUT SEEING EARDRUM	APPEARANCE of EARDRUM	ACTION to be TAKEN	MEDICAL OFFICER	E.N.T. CLINIC
1	PAIN	+	DROP OF BLOOD	−	(+)	AFTER INJURY?	*	TRAUMATIC PERFORATION	KEEP EAR DRY AND CLEAN	Some blood	KEEP EAR DRY AND CLEAN UNTIL HEALED	FAILURE TO HEAL IN 6 MONTHS	VERY FEW
2	PAIN	+	−/+ BLOOD THEN PUS	−	(+)	AFTER A COLD?	PRESSURE ABOVE & BEHIND EAR MAY HURT / DOES HURT & SWELLING	ACUTE OTITIS MEDIA / ACUTE MASTOIDITIS	ANTIBIOTIC (SYSTEMIC) AND EPHEDRINE NOSE DROPS	Drum swollen Red then Pus	CONTINUE TREATMENT IF NECESSARY	DRAIN SURGICALLY	SOME FOR SURGERY
3	PAIN	+	+/−	+	−	WITH ITCHING NOW OR EARLIER?	PAIN ON MOVING EAR	ACUTE OTITIS EXTERNA	CLEAN EAR - SYRINGE IF WET ANTIBIOTIC (SYSTEMIC) ANTIFUNGAL (LOCAL)	Meatal walls swollen	CONTINUE TREATMENT ESPECIALLY CLEANING	*	VERY FEW
4	PAIN / DISCHARGE	+	+	−	(+)	PAIN (DIZZYNESS) FOUL DISCHARGE	PRESSURE DOES HURT	ACUTE ON CHRONIC OTITIS MEDIA (ATTIC)	ANTIBIOTIC (SYSTEMIC)	Pus- Foul smelling	ANTIBIOTIC(S)	ALL SOON	PROBABLE EARLY SURGERY
5	DISCHARGE	−	+	−	(+)	FOUL DISCHARGE	*	CHRONIC OTITIS MEDIA (ATTIC)	SYRINGE GENTLY SPIRIT DROPS		CONTINUE TREATMENT	ALL IN DUE COURSE	POSSIBLE LATER SURGERY
6	DISCHARGE	−	+	−	(+)	VARIABLE DISCHARGE POSSIBLY FOUL		CHRONIC OTITIS MEDIA (INTERMEDIATE)	SYRINGE GENTLY SPIRIT DROPS		CONTINUE TREATMENT UNTIL DRY	THOSE THAT DISCHARGE AFTER 6 WEEKS	SOME FOR ASSESSMENT
7	DISCHARGE	−	+	−	(+)	MUCOID DISCHARGE	*	CHRONIC OTITIS MEDIA (MUCOID)	SYRINGE GENTLY SPIRIT DROPS CHILDREN: EPHEDRINE NOSE DROPS	or	CONTINUE TREATMENT & REPEAT TREATMENT UNTIL DRY	THOSE THAT DISCHARGE AFTER 12 WEEKS	VERY FEW
8	ITCHING	−	+	+	−	ITCHING AND DISCHARGE	POSSIBLE PAIN ON	OTITIS EXTERNA (WET)	SYRINGE GENTLY SPIRIT DROPS + FUNGICIDE	Wall swollen White/Yellow Debris	CONTINUE TREATMENT CLEANING IMPORTANT	THOSE THAT HAVE SYMPTOMS	VERY FEW
9	ITCHING	−	−	+	−	ITCHING	MOVING EAR	OTITIS EXTERNA (DRY)	KEEP DRY, CLEAN ANTIBIOTIC (LOCALLY) + FUNGICIDE	Perhaps black fungus threads	CONTINUE TREATMENT CLEANING IMPORTANT	AFTER 4 MONTHS	VERY FEW
10	DEAF	−	−	−	+	SUDDEN HEARING LOSS: ONE OR BOTH EARS	*	WAX	OIL FOR 4 DAYS SYRINGE FIRMLY	Black or brown mass	REPEAT IF NECESSARY	FAILURE TO CLEAR	VERY FEW

Fig. 5.13.1   Treatment of ear disease: a chart to assist primary health workers and health workers without otological training. (Reproduced with permission from *Tropical Doctor*, 1986; **Jan**: 33.)

where either posterior bony or membranous blockages prevent the normal mucous stream from reaching the pharynx. Bilateral choanal atresia, owing to the overriding tendency of the newborn to breathe through the nose, is fatal if unrecognized. Perforation of a membranous septum, if possible, is life-saving. The most common cause of unilateral discharge is a foreign body, often a seed, nut or bead pushed into the nose, or perhaps a piece of paper, wool or fibre used to alleviate the irritation of nasal allergy. Infection follows rapidly, sometimes with bleeding. Should a foreign body remain in the nasal cavity for a long time, a stone or rhinolith forms as calcium salts are deposited. If neglected, the stone may enlarge and erode the septum, blocking both nasal fossae, expanding the nose and requiring surgical removal. Foreign bodies are best removed with a hook rather than forceps.

Tumours are not common. Teratomata occasionally cause obstruction. Trauma may cause a septal haematoma, easily recognized as a reddish, soft swelling arising from the midline and blocking both anterior nasal fossae. This may resolve, but pressure may cause cartilage necrosis or a septal abscess with later nasal bridge collapse. An abscess is more tense and the nose is very tender; both may be evacuated.

Adenoid enlargement is probably the most common cause of bilateral nasal obstruction in childhood. These lymphoid masses usually regress at about 8–10 years, but may cause nearly complete obstruction in the young. Maxillary sinusitis may result from this obstruction often resolving as soon as adenoidectomy is undertaken. Nasal polyps, occurring in atopic individuals, are more commonly found in adults than in children. Obstruction and a thin watery discharge are signs of this. Nasal allergy was once said not to occur in the Negro races; this is not true.

A clear, watery discharge following a head injury suggests a fracture of the anterior cranial fossa with cerebrospinal fluid leak. The presence of sugar in the fluid is confirmatory.

A wide variety of pathogenic fungi and yeasts cause nasal infection and discharge in tropical environments (see pp. 624–32). Rhinosporidiosis predominantly affects the nasal mucosa where the characteristic lesion is a bleeding polyp containing the sporangium from which spores spread via the lymphatics. It chiefly affects children from Sri Lanka and India. Phycomycoses cause serious disease, often starting with granulomatous lesions in the nose and much mucoid discharge. *Aspergillus* infection, sometimes contracted from birds, is characterized by a watery, mouldy smelling discharge and a greyish membrane. *Candida albicans* commonly occurs in the mouth and occasionally in the nose in the

young and those in a poor state of general health. The white patches can be removed without bleeding. Diagnosis in all these cases is by identifying the fungus in scrapings or biopsy.

Finally one must bear in mind the common cold and the infectious fevers which may start with a clear discharge, as do both meningitis and poliomyelitis.

Bleeding

Epistaxis is common in young children in whom nasal catarrh and the habit of nose-picking both occur frequently. The site is nearly always 'Little's area', the vascular anastomosis on the antero-inferior part of the nasal septum. Unilateral bleeding implies a local cause, while bilateral bleeding is often the result of generalized disease. Traumatic causes include blows, fractures of the nose and those conditions already mentioned above. Nose studs or rings through the alae my contribute to crusting and minor trauma. Tumours are rare, but the angiofibroma of puberty bleeds with extraordinary vigour, and blood may gush out as if a tap were turned on.

Diseases of the blood and blood vessels are numerous but relatively rare. Haemophilia, leukaemia, deficiencies of vitamin C and K, and thrombocytopenia, all cause bleeding and are identified by the appropriate tests.

Pressure and cautery will control most cases of bleeding. A small balloon-tampon in the postnasal space and an anterior pack may be needed to stop generalized haemorrhage. Very rarely, arterial ligation is needed. As 90 per cent of the blood supply of the nose comes from the carotid system, the external carotid is the artery to tie.

Anosmia

Children rarely, if ever, complain of anosmia. It occurs in cases of nasal obstruction and in children where there is a fracture in the region of the cribriform plate or, sometimes by contre-coup injury from an occipital blow.

The throat

In general, the causes of sore throat may be elucidated by a careful history, examination in a good light and, if necessary, bacterial culture. Young children will easily show their throat by opening their mouth widely and putting their tongue out. The use of a tongue depressor is often resented. Wide Negro mouths are a joy to the paediatric ENT doctor! The cervical lymphatic glands must always be palpated in the examination.

Tonsillar disease

Acute tonsillitis is usually caused by the haemolytic streptococcus and is characterized by whitish spots of debris and pus in the crypts that stand out on red and swollen tonsils. The cervical glands are large and the temperature may be 38–40°C. A peritonsillar abscess or quinsy can present with an asymmetrical palatal swelling pushing the tonsil outwards and downwards. Trismus and dysphagia are marked; incision and drainage of the pus gives great relief.

Diphtheria is a severe infection requiring immediate treatment with penicillin and, of more importance, antitoxin (see pp. 505–8). The sore throat is less severe than in tonsillitis but the greyish or brownish adherent membrane and toxaemia should make European-trained doctors unfamiliar with this disease keep it in mind.

Infectious mononucleosis (glandular fever) should be considered if what seems to be a case of tonsillitis persists despite antibiotics. The tonsils have a 'glassy' appearance and generalized glandular and splenic enlargement assist diagnosis. The Paul–Bunnell test is positive during the first two to three weeks of the disease. Chronic tonsillitis is extremely rare in children.

Pharyngeal disease

Non-specific viral pharyngitis is common, and pharyngitis also occurs in the infectious fevers, the chronic granulomata and as part of the symptom pattern in many of the reticuloses. Examination of the blood or bone marrow may be important in cases of difficult diagnosis where sore throat is a symptom. Vitamin deficiency, especially of vitamins B and C, may be responsible for sore throats and ulceration of the mucosa. Malnutrition predisposes to many conditions, fungal mucosal infection such as 'thrush' (the white patches of candida on the oral mucosa) amongst others, the most severe being the destructive ulceration of mouth and pharynx in cancrum oris now seen only in grossly malnourished children.

Laryngeal disease

The great importance of laryngeal disease in the young is obstruction to the airway (see pp. 706–24). The principal sign of this is stridor or noisy respiration. It is important to note the noise in relation to the phase of respiration, inspiratory stridor indicating an obstruction above the level of the glottis, biphasic stridor at the glottis and expiratory stridor (asthma is an example) obstruction below the level of the glottis.

Congenital conditions include laryngeal cysts, webs, and haemangiomata which usually produce symptoms as the lesion canalizes at about six months of age. Most common of all is laryngo-malacia, causing the intermittent stridor of inspiratory laryngeal collapse. In this latter condition, stridor occurs when the child is excited or upset.

Foreign bodies are not uncommon causes of wheezy stridor. They rarely lodge in the larynx but pass on to the trachea or bronchi – usually on the right side – with incidents of choking and cyanosis. Vegetable foreign bodies are very irritant and lead to infective bronchitis. Any object may give rise to obstructive emphysema or pulmonary collapse and, as only a tiny number are coughed out spontaneously, their removal by bronchoscopy is a matter of some urgency. This may be very difficult and a thoracotomy may be required in some instances, especially in the presence of mucosal swelling.

Inflammatory disease includes most of the conditions mentioned above. Of great importance is acute epiglottitis. In this condition, the epiglottis is infected with *Haemophilus influenzae* which may cause sudden death in infants, as the swollen mass is drawn into and obstructs the larynx as a 'ball valve'. Diphtheria and acute laryngo-tracheo bronchitis may cause very severe obstruction.

Laryngeal paralysis in neurological conditions, poliomyelitis or coma following head injury cause obstruction by fluid overflow and abolition of the cough reflex. Much of the problem may be overcome by nursing the child in a lateral-supine or head-down tilted position so that gravity will do what the normal protective reflexes cannot.

The only common tumours in children are multiple papillomata. Akin to dermal warts and probably of viral origin, these multiple growths occur in poorly nourished children. They usually regress at puberty. They may block the larynx, recur when removed and seed on to raw areas and so are life-threatening; such patients often needing tracheostomy.

Some pharyngeal conditions cause obstruction to both respiration and swallowing. Infected tonsils are sometimes a cause, but are rarely large enough. A tonsillar sarcoma should be suspected in gross unilateral enlargement. Two posterior pharyngeal swellings must be differentiated; tuberculous abscess in a cervical vertebal body gives rise to a fluctuant midline swelling, while an abscess forming in a retropharyngeal gland is prevented by fascial attachments from extending across the midline.

A retropharyngeal abscess in a child is potentially a very serious matter and, if conservative measures are followed, careful observation of the patient is mandatory as laryngeal oedema and obstruction may develop very rapidly. Evacuation of the abscess by incision may lead to inhalation of pus and broncho-pneumonia but, in the head-down position and with adequate suction, it is the method of choice when the abscess is fluctuant. Impending obstruction warrants tracheostomy.

Tracheostomy

Tracheostomy, a life-saving procedure in many of the conditions mentioned above, is necessary to bypass obstructive lesions and useful in both reducing the respiratory dead-space and allowing easy suction of secretions in fluid obstruction of the lower respiratory tract. It is difficult to perform and fraught with danger in infancy, and a considerable problem in childhood, but unless the skill and equipment for laryngeal intuba-tion are available it may be the only immediate treatment. It is far better performed as an elective rather than an emergency measure so, if possible, a decision must be taken in good time. Suprasternal, xiphisternal and intercostal inspiratory recession at rest is a sign of severe respiratory obstruction and, if humidity, oxygen and medical treatment do not help, surgery is the next step. In infants and young children, a vertical incision is best and it is especially important to keep strictly to the midline as the soft trachea is difficult to palpate and may move laterally. The second, third and fourth tracheal ring should be incised and a window should not be made. Decannulation must be under-taken as soon as possible, especially in infants. Humidification of the inspired air and continual care is needed postoperatively with careful and atraumatic suction.

Further reading

Ballantyne J, Groves J eds. *Scott Brown's Diseases of Ear, Nose and Throat*. London, Butterworths, 1979.

Holborow C. Prevention of deafness in rural tropical areas. *Tropical Doctor*. 1985; **15**: 39–41.

Holborow C. Treatment of otitis media and ear infections. *Tropical Doctor*. 1986; **16**: 32–3.

Holborow C, McPherson B. Simple treatment for the infected ear. *Tropical Doctor*. 1986; **16**: 31–2.

Kameswaran S (ed.) *ENT Diseases in a Tropical Environment*. Madras, India, Higginbotham, 1975.

Northern J ed. *Hearing Disorders*. Bristol, Wright, 1985.

CHAPTER 14

Orthopaedic disorders

R.L. Huckstep

A very different pattern of orthopaedic conditions exists in children in the subtropics and tropics from that seen in Europe and North America. Bone and joint infections and poliomyelitis are still common and, in many cases, treatment is not sought for months, or even years, after the onset of disease. Deformities may be severe and sometimes difficult to treat. Calipers, wheelchairs, and other supports as designed and manufactured in economically rich countries are quite unrealistic in price and design for most developing countries. It is the purpose of this chapter not only to describe the common conditions seen, but also to discuss methods of treatment which are realistic in such conditions.

Congenital deformities

Foot deformities

Flat feet are common in normal young children and treatment is seldom necessary. Other foot deformities are uncommon in those who walk with bare feet. Occasionally spastic flat foot, or a rigid subtaloid joint, is associated with a calcaneo-navicular bar and this may require surgery. A cavus or claw foot deformity may be associated with a neurological disorder but is usually idiopathic. The wearing of tight shoes may cause a hallux valgus deformity of the big toe in those who already have a congenital predisposition.

Occasional clawing of the other toes is also seen, due to the same causes. Dorsal displacement of the fifth toe may occur, especially in those with a family history. Severe clawing of the toes or dorsal displacement of the little toe may require tenotomy of the extensor tendons, arthrodesis of the proximal interphalangeal joints or correction for tightness of the overlying skin.

Congenital talipes equinovarus

This is a true congenital deformity which may affect one or both feet (Fig. 5.14.1a) and is common. The deformity consists of equinus of the ankle, adduction of the forefoot and varus or inversion of the foot. The calf is thin, but muscle power initially is normal and sensation is unaffected.

The condition must be differentiated from an equinovarus due to an associated spina bifida in which

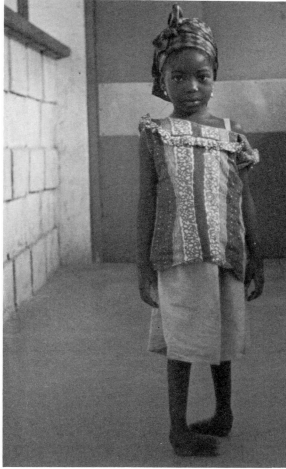

(a)

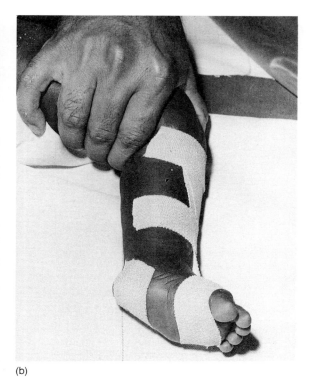

(b)

Fig. 5.14.1 (a) Severe uncorrected bilateral congenital talipes equinovarus in a 5 year old; (b) strapping; (c) wool and plaster.

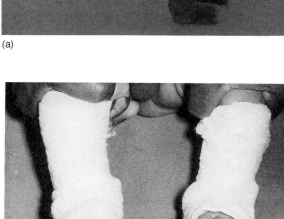

(c)

there is both sensory loss and motor weakness, and from poliomyelitis in which sensation is normal and muscle power alone is affected.

Treatment must be started at birth with manipulations, followed by serial plasters. Firm support of the ankle is important to avoid damage to the tibial epiphysis. Adduction of the forefoot is corrected first, followed by correction of varus and equinus deformities. Too much correction must not be attempted initially and the foot should be strapped (Fig. 5.14.1b) before padding the heel and foot with wool and applying below-knee plasters or splints (Fig. 5.14.1c). In mild cases, strapping alone may be adequate. In fat children, above-knee plasters with the knee at 90° may be required and the plasters must be changed initially once a week and thereafter every two or three weeks until an easily maintained position of at least 30° eversion and dorsiflexion is obtained. Denis Browne splints, as used in Europe and North America, require expert supervision, and this is not always available in developing countries.

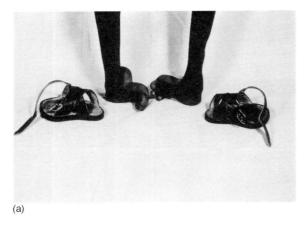

(a)

Fig. 5.14.2 (a) Severe congenital talipes equinovarus – untreated, (b) sandals for severe deformity.

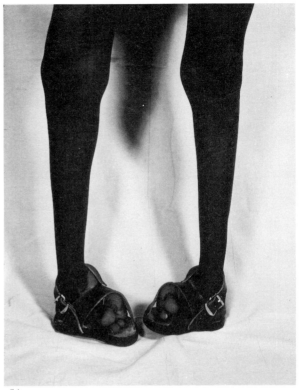

(b)

Adequate follow-up is essential and daily stretching must be continued for at least three years by parents, as recurrence is common. Ideally, lace-up boots with the right boot on the left foot and the left boot on the right foot, with a 6–9 mm raise on the outer side of the sole and heel, should be worn when the child starts to walk.

In children first seen when over six months old, manipulation under general anaesthetic is usually required and often extensive soft tissue release of fibrous tissue on the inner side of the foot is needed. This should *not* be delayed if conservative measures are unsuccessful. In untreated talipes in older children a wedge resection of the bones on the lateral side of the foot may also be indicated, after the age of four years.[1] Over the age of 12 or 14 years a triple arthrodesis of the subtaloid joints, plus tendon transfer will allow full and permanent correction. Occasionally simple sandals (Fig. 5.14.2a, b) or surgical boots, rather than operation, is all that is required in the untreated adult, but most patients will demand surgical correction.

Congenital talipes calcaneovalgus

This deformity is the opposite of equinovarus and is less common. It is due to intra-amniotic pressure on the fetus, rather than a true genetic abnormality. Treatment by manipulation and plasters in equinus leads to a rapid improvement in a few weeks. The occasional refractory case is usually due to a congenital vertical talus and may need operation.[2]

Congenital genu recurvatum

This is also due to intra-amniotic pressure, a high oestrogen level and lax ligaments. Immobilization in a padded plaster, in as much flexion as possible, for three weeks will usually effect a cure[3], in those cases without a true dislocation of the knee or fibrosis of the quadriceps. In these latter conditions operation may be necessary.

Congenital dislocation of the hip

This appears to be rare in Africa and in many other tropical countries. It is a true congenital dysplasia with delayed epiphyseal appearance of the head of the femur, anteversion of the femoral neck and a sloping acetabulum, in addition to a dislocation (see pp. 189–90). The African custom of babies being carried on their mothers' backs will abduct the hips and tend to reduce a dislocation. The custom of carrying babies in this way, however, is no longer so prevalent,

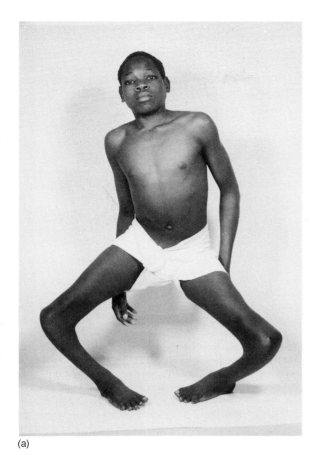

(a)

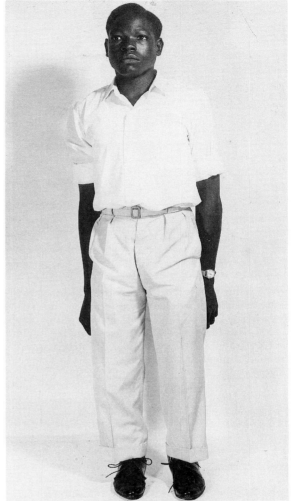

(b)

Fig. 5.14.3 (a) Severe genu varus (Blount's disease) in 14-year-old boy; (b) after correction by wedge resections to upper tibiae.

and many are born in hospitals where improving standards of postnatal examination should enable cases to be diagnosed.

In untreated babies there is a delayed appearance of the epiphyseal head of the femur, anteversion of the femoral neck and a sloping acetabulum, in addition to a subluxation or dislocation.

Girls are affected five times more often than boys and in one-third of cases both hips are affected.

Diagnosis by examining all babies at birth for a positive Ortolani click is essential, as treatment at this stage by a simple abduction splint is easy and usually effective. If this fails, abduction plasters or skelecasts may be necessary and sometimes operative correction. A missed dislocation will present later as telescoping of the hip, a high buttock fold, short leg, limitation of abduction in flexion, widening of the perineum and a positive X-ray. There will also be abnormality of the hip joint. It is much more difficult to treat and, apart from traction in abduction or plaster, may also necessitate operations such as open reduction, pelvic osteotomy and reconstruction of the acetabulum, plus rotation osteotomy of an anteverted femoral neck.

Genu varum and genu valgum

Knock knees and bow legs are common in childhood and are often familial. If unassociated with

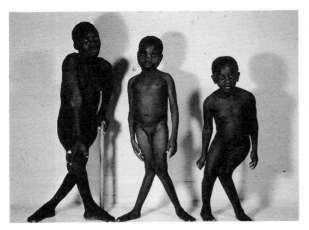

Fig. 5.14.4 Multiple lower-limb deformities: from left to right –
spastic, genu varum, TB hip and knee.

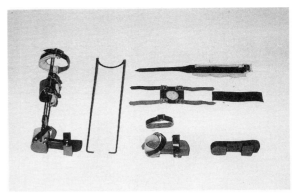

Fig. 5.14.5 Simple caliper and clog from galvanized wire and
local leather.

poliomyelitis, injury or bone disease, they usually
improve without treatment after the age of three years.
Occasionally, corrective osteotomy is required at the
ages of 12 or 14 years (Fig. 5.14.3a, b) and night splints
are used where there is more than 7.5 cm separation of
the medial malleoli at the age of three years in genu
valgum.

Other varus or valgus deformities of the knee may be
due to rickets, paralysis, injury to the epiphysis and
fractures or osteomyelitis destroying the growth plate of
the lower femur or upper tibia (Fig. 5.14.4).

Other congenital conditions

Drug-induced malformations are uncommon. Other
true congenital deformities, such as malformed limbs,
extra or absent digits, and trigger thumb in babies,
appear to be as common in the subtropics and tropics as
elsewhere. Amputation is rarely indicated for severe
limb deformities, but reconstruction may have a very
real place, provided the patient will be benefited
functionally as well as cosmetically. A useless extra
digit, however, should be amputated.

Poliomyelitis

Poliomyelitis is a paralytic disease which may destroy
the anterior horn cells of the spinal cord and cause
paralysis of limbs, trunk, respiration and swallowing

(see pp. 750–2). Some patients remain permanently
paralysed after the acute disease. The number of
children with untreated severe residual paralysis in the
tropics and subtropics is estimated at several million,
and 90 per cent of all acute cases still occur in those
under five years. Epidemics of paralytic poliomyelitis are still extremely common in India, South–east
Asia, Africa and South America. Programmes of
prevention of poliomyelitis are described on pp. 82,
750–2.

Muscle charting is a quick method of assessing the
power of paralysed muscles, and these are graded from
zero to five. A power of three indicates that the muscle
concerned can just lift the joint across which it acts
against gravity. If the power is greater than three there
is usually no necessity for external support. A power of
less than three in the dorsiflexors of the knee or ankle
usually means that the joint requires an external
support. A simplified above-knee caliper is shown in
(Figs. 5.14.5 and 5.14.6)[4, 5, 6] and this will support both
knee and ankle. If the knee extensors have adequate
power, however, the caliper need only extend from
below the knee. Crutches may be necessary as well,
but these will need strong arms, particularly triceps,
if both legs are also severely involved. A wheelchair
may be required for patients with severe paralysis[7]
involving arms as well as both legs. The requirement in developing countries is for simple appliances to be cheap, comfortable, effective and locally
made.[6]

A limb cannot be fitted with a caliper if there is severe
deformity, and an operation will be necessary to correct
it. This should only be performed if the patient will
thereby be enabled to walk, with crutches if necessary.

Manufacture of a simple caliper

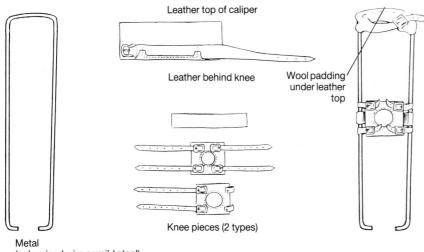

Leather top of caliper

Leather behind knee

Wool padding under leather top

Knee pieces (2 types)

Metal
(galvanised wire or mild steel)

Completed simple above and below knee calipers

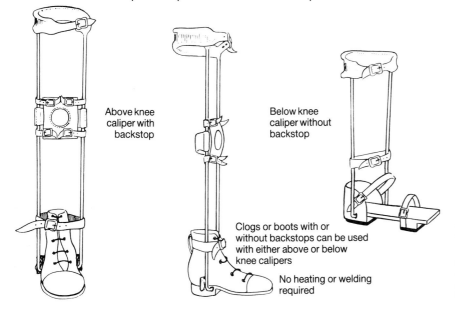

Above knee caliper with backstop

Below knee caliper without backstop

Clogs or boots with or without backstops can be used with either above or below knee calipers

No heating or welding required

Fig. 5.14.6 Manufacture of clog and caliper. (Reproduced with permission from Huckstep RL, *Poliomyelitis – A Guide for Developing Countries Including Appliances and Rehabilitation for the Disabled*, Edinburgh, Churchill Livingstone, 1975.)

Deformities are usually caused by imbalance between muscles acting across a joint and occasionally by other factors, such as gravity or weight-bearing, on weak limbs. The common deformities of the lower limb are flexion/abduction of the hip, flexion of the knee and equinus of the ankle (Figs. 5.14.7 and 5.14.8).

Deformities of the knee and hip can often be corrected by subcutaneous division of the ilio-tibial band combined with an open division of the biceps tendon.[5,6] This tight band is divided above the knee, in

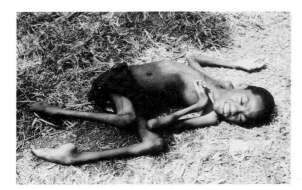

Fig. 5.14.7   Severe polio deformities in a 14-year-old boy.

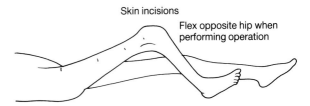

Skin incisions

Flex opposite hip when performing operation

Division of tensor fascia lata and tight structures anterior to hip

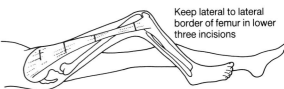

Keep lateral to lateral border of femur in lower three incisions

Care with popliteal vessels and lateral popliteal nerve

Care with femoral artery

Postoperative plaster

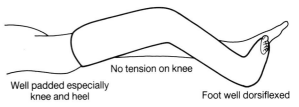

Well padded especially knee and heel

No tension on knee

Foot well dorsiflexed

Fig. 5.14.9   Operative correction of deformities – hip and knees. (Source as for Fig. 5.14.6.)

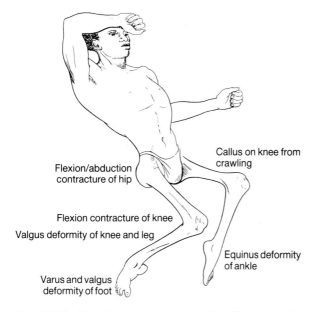

Flexion/abduction contracture of hip

Callus on knee from crawling

Flexion contracture of knee

Valgus deformity of knee and leg

Equinus deformity of ankle

Varus and valgus deformity of foot

Fig. 5.14.8   Typical contractures of polio. (Source as for Fig. 5.14.6.)

one or two areas of the mid-thigh and one finger's breadth below the anterior superior iliac spine with a tenotomy knife or old-style cataract knife (Fig. 5.14.9). Severe contractures of the hip may also require extensive division of all structures anteriorly and laterally in the hip. A contracture of more than 30° of the knee will necessitate open division of the biceps tendon, lateral intermuscular septum and ilio-tibial band in addition. The structures which must be carefully preserved in these operations are the popliteal vessels and popliteal nerves at the knee and the femoral

artery at the hip. Postoperatively, patients with mild knee deformities are treated by serial manipulations and plasters, while severe knee contractures require Russell traction.

An equinus ankle can be corrected easily and well by subcutaneous division of the tendo Achillis, with allowance for its rotation (Fig. 5.14.10)[3,6]. The posterior two-thirds in the upper part and medial two-thirds in the lower part will require subcutaneous division with a tenotomy knife. Care must be taken not to damage the posterior tibial vessels and nerve.

The severe lower limb deformities in a 14-year-old boy were partly corrected by these methods (Fig. 5.14.11a–d).

Tuberculosis of bone and joint

Tuberculosis of bone and joint is almost always due to bloodstream infection from elsewhere, often from a

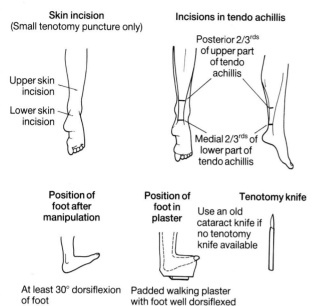

Skin incision
(Small tenotomy puncture only)

Upper skin incision

Lower skin incision

Incisions in tendo achillis

Posterior 2/3rds of upper part of tendo achillis

Medial 2/3rds of lower part of tendo achillis

Position of foot after manipulation

At least 30° dorsiflexion of foot

Position of foot in plaster

Padded walking plaster with foot well dorsiflexed

Tenotomy knife

Use an old cataract knife if no tenotomy knife available

Fig. 5.14.10 Subcutaneous correction of equinus ankle. (Source as for Fig. 5.14.6.)

primary focus in the lungs (see pp. 539–40). There may, however, be a delay of years between primary focus and secondary involvement of bone or joint. The spine, hip and knee are most frequently affected, but other joints may also be involved. The initial infection either starts as a synovitis or involves an epiphysis near the joint. In the acute stages there may be a low-grade pyrexia, with a patient unwell rather than toxic, as in pyogenic arthritis and osteomyelitis.

In the major joints the onset is usually insidious, with the warm, rather than the hot swelling of a pyogenic arthritis and slight rather than severe pain. If untreated, the synovitis progresses to a frank arthritis with joint destruction and finally a fibrous union in a deformed position. The initially clear yellow synovial fluid of a synovitis becomes cloudy and progresses to thick yellowish caseous fluid as the joint is destroyed. Abscesses may discharge through the skin in untreated patients, and these will then become secondarily infected with pyogenic organisms. The abscesses may also track some distance before pointing and a psoas abscess in the groin secondary to spinal caries is an example of this.

In the hip, there is pain and spasm with abduction and flexion in the early stages and this progresses to adduction and flexion as joint destruction occurs (Fig. 5.14.4).

In the knee, there is usually a flexion deformity with marked synovial thickening, slight tenderness and some effusion, which is in contrast to the early quadriceps wasting. This may progress to a marked deformity with fibrous ankylosis in the later stages.

In the spine there is often an angular kyphos, especially in the thoracic region and in the early stages there is tenderness associated with spasm of the spinal muscles. There may also be an abscess (Fig. 5.14.12) and signs of spinal cord compression – sensory, motor and bladder disturbances – must always be looked for. In cases involving several vertebrae, a severe kyphosis may develop, the ribs may be crowded together and the likelihood of secondary respiratory insufficiency or infection greatly increases.

Confirmation of tuberculosis includes a raised ESR with a normal white blood count, normal agglutination tests for brucella and salmonellae, a positive Heaf test and evidence of recent or old pulmonary tuberculosis on chest X-ray. More specific tests include aspiration of the joint or of an abscess. The finding of acid-fast bacilli on microscopy, a sterile culture for pyogenic organisms and a positive culture and guinea-pig inoculation for tuberculosis, all help to confirm the diagnosis. Occasionally, a gland biopsy with culture and histology may be helpful, as may a biopsy of the synovia of joints.

X-rays will show osteoporosis of the affected joints in the early stages followed by narrowing of joint spaces, frank destruction and disorganization in the later stages, with late fibrous ankylosis. In the spine, the disease starts at the adjacent margins of two adjoining vertebral bodies and even in early cases involves the intervertebral disc as well. An antero-posterior X-ray in tuberculosis of the thoracic spine will usually show an abscess.

Treatment

This includes resting the patient, resting the joint involved, and treating debility due to other diseases and malnutrition. Specific treatment with streptomycin, plus either INAH (isoniazid) or TB1 (thiacetazone), or both, must be carried out for at least three months and then followed by INAH plus TB1 alone (but see also pp. 544–5). A dose of not less than 0.25 g daily of streptomycin for a small child to 1 g per day after the age of 12 years, should be aimed at, for at least one month and preferably continued for three to six months. This should be combined with INAH (25 mg three times daily (tds) for a small child to 100 mg tds over the age of 12 years). In the convalescent or quiescent stages, oral chemotherapy with INAH in the above doses, plus TB1 (12.5–50 mg tds), should be continued for at least six to twelve months and

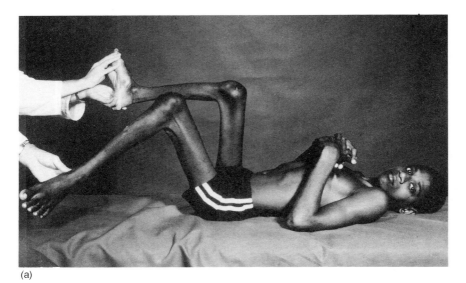

(a)

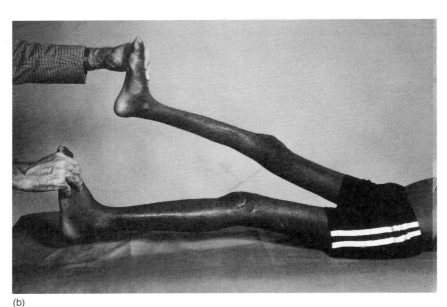

(b)

Fig. 5.14.11 (a) Severe polio deformities in 14-year-old boy; (b) soft tissue and bony correction; (c) walking with above-knee caliper (right); (d) back home, walking without support.

sometimes longer as an out-patient.[8] A recrudescence will necessitate re-admission to hospital or dispensary and further rest, plus streptomycin. PAS (*para-aminosalicylic acid*) in doses of 4–16 g per day often causes nausea and is seldom taken, especially by the out-patient.

Treatment may take many months, or even years and may involve surgery at an earlier stage in economi-cally poor countries, owing to lack of facilities and the difficulties of follow-up necessary in carrying out long-term conservative treatment. Where possible, however, bony operations on growing ends of bone (i.e. knee) should be deferred until 12–14 years of age, as resulting severe growth disturbances may occur with earlier operation.

Rifampicin has now become available as an effective

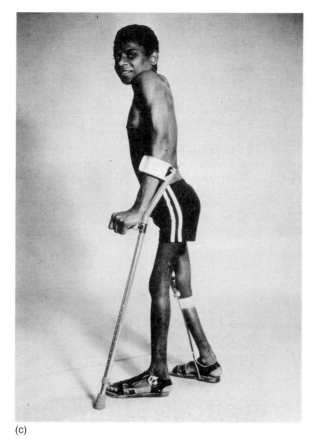

(c)

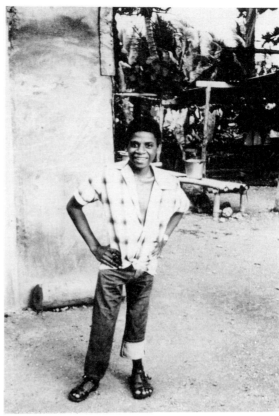

(d)

alternative antituberculous drug in a dose of 10 mg/kg daily, together with ethambutol, 15–20 mg/kg daily and INAH, 10–20 mg/kg daily, for six to nine months. Unfortunately, the first two are still very expensive for the long-term therapy required in bone infection. Rifampicin also has an occasional toxic effect on the liver. Other new drugs are also proving effective in tuberculosis. (See pp. 544–5.)

Hip In the early stages, tuberculosis of the hip can be cured by Russell traction and adequate chemotherapy. A hip spica may enable the patient to be treated at home or in a dispensary. Failure of conservative treatment, or severe joint destruction, will necessitate early arthrodesis.[9]

Knee The stage of synovitis and early arthritis can be cured by adequate treatment with Russell traction

followed a month or two later by rest in a cylinder plaster. Once gross destruction of bone and joint occurs, however, arthrodesis will be necessary.

Other joints Rest in plaster and chemotherapy may sometimes obviate the necessity for operation, provided gross destruction has not occurred.

Spine Tuberculosis of the cervical spine is best treated with a Minerva plaster for several months, until healing occurs. In the case of associated paralysis, cervical traction with a Glisson's sling is initially indicated, followed by a plaster bed with a head extension. Young children may not tolerate this and will require a Minerva plaster without preliminary traction, or a light-weight skelecast.[10]

Tuberculosis of the upper thoracic spine should be treated by a plaster jacket with a neck extension.

Tuberculosis of the mid- and lower thoracic spine, and of the lumbar spine, should be treated with a jacket spica extending to above the knee on one side with the hip in 30° of flexion or a skelecast.

Tuberculosis of the spine with paralysis will necessitate rest in a plaster bed or in a harness, followed by drainage of the abscess and sometimes decompression of the cord. In the thoracic spine this will entail a simple drainage operation (costotransversectomy) or a transthoracic decompression, freeing the cord and grafting the vertebrae. In cases of severe kyphosis, antero-lateral decompression[11] will be required. These operations will hasten the healing process in the thoracic spine, especially in older children. The cervical and lumbar spines, however, are best treated conservatively, except where complications such as paralysis and abscesses do not improve over a period of weeks on an adequate conservative regimen. The Medical Research Council Working Party (1985)[12] on tuberculosis of the spine, has guidelines for treatment in various countries.

Abscess pointing   An abscess which is either large or pointing (Fig. 5.14.12) should be aspirated and streptomycin (0.5–1.0 g) instilled. This procedure may have to be repeated. Occasional open drainage is required, but the wound must always be closed over suction drainage following this, to prevent secondary infection.

The abscess is usually cold or only slightly warm and non-tender (cf. pyogenic infections). The pus is yellowish and may contain necrotic bone and there is little or no odour as in pyogenic infections.

Acute osteomyelitis

Acute osteomyelitis is usually due to a bloodstream infection, but may be secondary to direct injury. It commonly occurs in sickle-cell anaemia.

Classically, the metaphyses of long bones are involved in bloodstream infections, but in sickle-cell anaemia the entire shafts of long bones, vertebrae and the hands and feet may be involved and multiple infections are common (Fig. 5.14.13). The staphylococcus is usually responsible, except in sickle-cell anaemia when it is commonly a salmonella. Infection with *Salmonella typhi* itself, however, is rare.[13,14] The onset is acute with a toxic, ill, pyrexial child, with severe pain, swelling and heat in the site of infection. There may be a fluctuant abscess and the regional glands are enlarged.

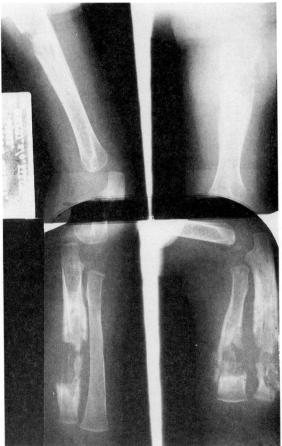
Fig. 5.14.13   Osteomyelitis of humerus, radius and ulna in sickle-cell anaemia with pathological fractures.

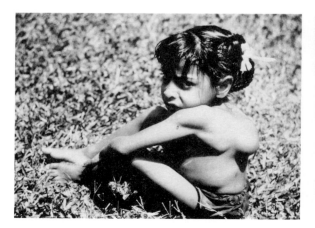
Fig. 5.14.12   TB thoracic spine – kyphosis and abscess.

Diagnosis is confirmed by a high white blood count with a polymorpholeucocytosis, a positive blood culture and by aspiration and culture of pus from an abscess. Blood should also be taken for sickling in endemic areas. X-rays, for the first one to two weeks, usually show nothing. In sickle-cell anaemia, however, there may be rarefaction and bone destruction within one week of infection (see pp. 822–34). The early stages of a sickle-cell crisis may often mimic an acute osteomyelitis, but the diagnosis can usually be confirmed clinically by aspiration of pus and culture of the responsible organism from the blood.

Treatment, to be effective, must be energetic and early. Aspiration of pus and replacement with penicillin, plus systemic treatment with large doses of penicillin and tetracycline are indicated, and this must not be delayed until the responsible organism is known. The dose of penicillin should be 125 000–500 000 units six hourly initially, and treatment must be continued for at least four weeks. In sickle-cell anaemia, gram-negative organisms, such as salmonella, may be involved. More effective antibiotics, such as cloxacillin, ampicillin, erythromycin and trimethoprim compound, should be used if necessary but the first two are expensive and all four may have side-effects. The sensitivity of the organism responsible must always be determined and the side-effects and cost of newer drugs weighed against possible therapeutic advantages.

The limb or limbs affected should be rested in well-padded splints or plaster back slabs and elevated. Repeated aspirations may be necessary and, occasionally, open drainage with drilling of the cortex of the bone. The periosteum should not be stripped and no more than one or two drill holes should be made. The wound should always be closed, if possible, following operation, with suction drainage.

Fractures of long bones are common in sickle-cell osteomyelitis, but respond well to conservative treatment, as do spinal infections. Recurrent attacks of infection, however, are common in sickle-cell anaemia. Secondary infection of epiphyses may lead to dislocation of joints, late osteoarthritis, contractures and growth disturbances. Untreated infections usually progress to sinus formation and chronic osteomyelitis.

Chronic osteomyelitis

Chronic osteomyelitis is usually secondary to acute osteomyelitis or to compound fractures, and is particularly common when treatment has been started late or has been inadequate. A resistant organism, or the continued presence of an avascular piece of bone (seques-trum), or a retained foreign body in a compound fracture will prevent healing.

Sometimes, infection may start as a chronic osteomyelitis with a cavity surrounded by sclerotic bone, with a small retained piece of bone (Brodie's abscess). On other occasions, the infection may be subacute or chronic initially, as in infections with brucella, *Salmonella typhi* and mycotic infections. A low-grade staphylococcal infection may also cause chronic osteomyelitis.

Sequestrectomy is usually indicated, provided that the bone surrounding the sequestrum (involucrum) is sufficiently developed to prevent a fracture occurring; otherwise surgery should be delayed in long bones lest a gap be left. Thick-walled cavities may have to be curetted and free drainage afforded to pus. In the presence of severe infection with skin loss, part of the wound should be left open and secondary closure attempted later, preceded by split skin grafting. In most cases, however, the skin should be closed if possible, but sutures should either be loose to allow drainage, or better still, suction drainage should be used. In severe infections, a polythene tube left down to the wound will allow six hourly local instillations of the appropriate antibiotic. Elimination of excessive dead-space by a pressure bandage and immobilization in a well-padded splint completes the treatment, which may take many months.

Arthritis

This is a generalized inflammatory or degenerative lesion of a joint and may involve one joint or several.

A pyogenic arthritis is usually caused by staphylococcus but other organisms, such as streptococcus and salmonella group, may be responsible in the tropics. The onset tends to be acute with the rapid formation of pus, a hot swollen joint, severe pain and spasm, and constitutional disturbance and pyrexia. Occasionally it may be subacute or chronic.

Spread may be direct from a penetrating wound, or secondary to bloodstream infection or an adjacent osteomyelitis.

Diagnosis is confirmed by aspiration and culture of pus from a joint and by a raised white blood count with a polymorpholeucocytosis and by a positive blood culture. X-ray images may show nothing specific for the first one to three weeks, but will be helpful in differentiating a bony injury or other unsuspected pathology. Delay in treatment may lead not only to joint destruction, but also to growth disturbances. The joint should be aspirated if possible and pus replaced by one million units of crystalline penicillin. In early

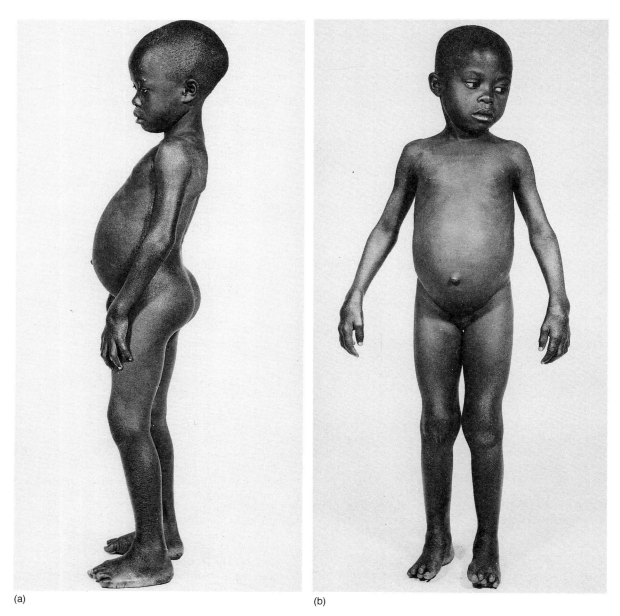

(a)   (b)

Fig. 5.14.14 Ugandan girl with Still's disease a) and b) from the front and side showing involvement of wrists, elbows, knees and ankles, c) and d) thickening of toes and fingers (spindling).

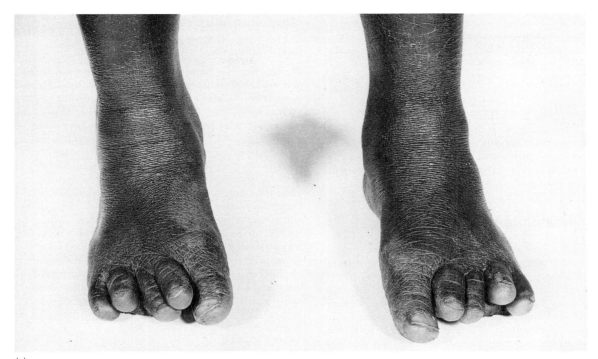

(c)

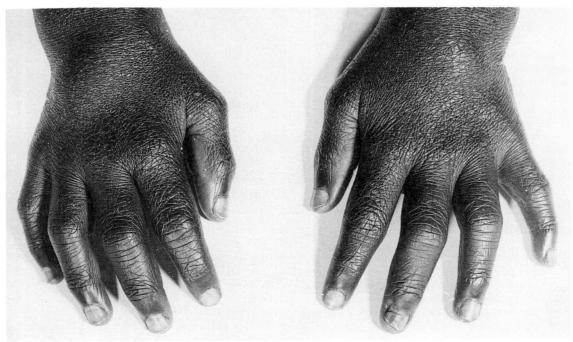

(d)

pyogenic arthritis involving the hip joint, immediate open aspiration and drainage is indicated, as complete destruction of the femoral head may occur. Rest by splinting or modified Russell traction,[10] is also indicated in the early stages. Systemic treatment should include large doses of penicillin initially and this should be changed to other antibiotics, such as cloxacillin or trimethoprim compound, if sensitivities indicate this, or if response is poor. Chemotherapy should be continued for at least six weeks; the patient must be kept non-weight-bearing and the joint rested until complete healing has occurred. Analgesics will also be required in the acute stages.

Rheumatoid arthritis

This is uncommon in many tropical countries, except at higher altitudes. It is a chronic non-bacterial inflammatory process which usually affects more than one joint and is of unknown aetiology. It is usually known as Still's disease in children and commonly affects the hands, wrists, elbows, knees and ankles and tends to be symmetrical (Fig. 5.14.14 a, b, c, d). Any other joints, including the hips, spine and sacroiliac joints, may also be involved. In children, the spleen and lymphatic glands are often enlarged and the ESR is raised. Examination of the joints affected shows synovial thickening with effusion and limitation of movements. X-rays show generalized rarefaction with narrowing of the joint space and, in the later stages, evidence of damage to the joint itself with secondary osteoarthritis. Treatment is symptomatic, with attention to inflammatory foci, improvement of general health and salicylates. Prednisone has a dramatic effect during acute exacerbations, but is only palliative and has side-effects. Local heat, wax baths, traction on joints and active exercises may all be of some benefit. There is no known cure at present, but there is a tendency for the disease to become quiescent after several years.

Other arthritides

Other joint conditions which may occur in children include degenerative osteoarthritis often due to previous injury, Perthe's disease or slipped epiphysis, haemophilia, congenital syphilis and rheumatic fever. Many febrile conditions may also cause joint pain without involving the joint directly.

Miscellaneous disorders

Bone tumours

Benign tumours include osteochondroma of long bones and enchondromata and ecchondromata of hands and feet. They seldom become malignant or require treatment. Giant cell tumours may be benign or malignant. The prognosis in osteosarcoma used to be almost hopeless (Fig. 5.14.15), even after amputation. In all suspected malignant tumours it is essential to confirm the diagnosis by biopsy before amputating the limb. A whole new era of management is opening up, however, with the use of adjuvant chemotherapeutic agents systemically, such as adriamycin, vincristine and methotrexate, and the prognosis is improving. The medication is usually extremely toxic and expensive, and treatment must often be continued for at least two years. The five-year survival rate even with adjuvant chemotherapy is probably less than 40 per cent in osteogenic sarcoma but may be better in Ewing's sarcoma and some other tumours (see pp. 885–6).

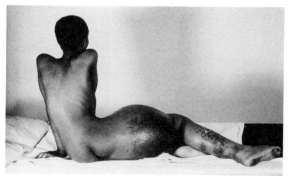

Fig. 5.14.15 Massive untreated osteogenic sarcoma in a 15-year-old girl.

Burkitt's tumour

This tumour of children is probably caused by a virus and has a geographical distribution.[15] It may involve the jaws and long bones as well as the abdomen and chest. It can present as a paraplegia with sensory, motor and bladder involvement, but seldom with vertebral involvement or a kyphos (cf. tuberculosis). Several dramatic and probable cures have been reported after limited doses of cytotoxic drugs (see p. 879). Newer methods of management have included large doses of chemotherapy followed by autogenous bone marrow transplantation.

Rickets

This condition is discussed on pp. 376–9. The long bones are bent and in crawling infants the arms tend to be bowed as well as the legs. Joints may be tender and X-rays show widened and cupped epiphyses. Osteotomy may be necessary to correct deformities.

Perthe's disease

This is a disease usually occurring in children between the ages of three and ten years and leads to avascular necrosis and softening of the head of the femur. It is caused by interruption of the blood supply to the capital epiphysis. It is sometimes secondary to trauma or sickle-cell anaemia, but is in many instances idiopathic. It appears to be less common in Africa than in Europe and North America. The onset is insidious with slight pain and limping. Movements of the hip are surprisingly good, except for external rotation and abduction (cf. slipped epiphysis). X-ray shows flattening of the femoral head with increased density and later fragmentation, an increased joint space on X-ray due to thickening of the cartilage, with no involvement of the acetabulum (cf. tuberculosis).

Treatment ideally is by Russell traction for one to two months until the pain has settled, followed by an abduction splint on both legs plus crutches for up to two years in severe cases until the head has revascularized. This long-term regimen is often impossible to carry out in developing countries. The alternative is to cover the fragmented head in severe cases with an osteotomy of the upper femur or of the acetabulum. Osteoarthritis is a late complication, even in well-treated cases, but cases vary considerably in prognosis.

Slipped epiphysis

Slipping of the femoral epiphysis which is often seen in Europe and North America between the ages of 10 and 15 years, appears to be less common in tropical and subtropical countries. Treatment should be early reduction and pinning of both the affected side and prophylactically on the opposite side.

Spastic monoplegia, hemiplegia, diplegia and quadriplegia

These conditions are due to damage to the cerebral cortex or basal nuclei in infancy and early childhood. Aetiological factors range from birth trauma, meningitis and Rhesus incompatibility to viral encephalitis, hypoglycaemia and cerebral malaria. The end result of these conditions is spasticity of one or more limbs, often associated with a degree of mental impairment, which is less than appears at first sight (see pp. 759–61).

In the case of a tight tendo Achillis, elongation is sometimes required but a complete subcutaneous tenotomy should be avoided. Occasionally an obturator neurectomy or adductor tenotomy for severe spasm of the adductors of the thigh is also required as well as other tenotomies and occasionally tendon transfers. Below-knee calipers with backstops are often helpful but *never above*-knee calipers. The best results are obtained by prolonged rehabilitation in special centres with specially trained physiotherapists. This is often difficult to achieve in economically poor countries. Prevention of the initial cause is the first priority, as the prognosis is only fair, even after prolonged treatment.

References

1. Evans D. Relapsed club foot. *Journal of Bone and Joint Surgery*. 1967; **49B**: 792–3.
2. Harrold AJ. Congenital vertical talus in infancy. *Journal of Bone and Joint Surgery*. 1967; **49B**: 634–43.
3. Huckstep RL. Orthopaedic problems in East Africa. *Journal of the Royal College of Surgeons of Edinburgh*. 1966; **11**: 206–23.
4. Huckstep RL. Calipers for the developing countries of the world. *Rehabilitation of the Disabled in Africa* 1964; **1**: 19–34.
5. Huckstep RL. Orthopaedic appliances for developing countries. *Tropical Doctor*. 1971; **1**: 64–8.
6. Huckstep RL. *Poliomyelitis – A Guide for Developing Countries Including Appliances and Rehabilitation for the Disabled*. Edinburgh, Churchill Livingstone, 1975: pp. 279.
7. Hunt SCM, Huckstep RL. Wheelchairs for developing countries. *East African Medical Journal*. 1967; **44**: 387–99.
8. Dickson JAS. Spinal tuberculosis in Nigerian children – a review of ambulant treatment. *Journal of Bone and Joint Surgery*. 1967; **49B**: 682–94.
9. Kirkaldy–Willis WH, Chaudri MR, Anderson RJD. Arthrodesis of the hip with staple fixation. *Journal of Bone and Joint Surgery*. 1958; **40A**: 114–20.
10. Huckstep RL. *A Simple Guide to Trauma*, 4th Edn. Edinburgh, Churchill Livingstone, 1986: pp. 397.
11. Caperner N. The evolution of lateral rhachotomy. *Journal of Bone and Joint Surgery*. 1954; **36B**: 173–9.
12. Medical Research Council. Working Party in Tuberculosis of the Spine. 1985.
13. Huckstep RL. Recent advances in the surgery of typhoid fever. *Annals of the Royal College of Surgeons of England*. 1960; **26**: 207–30.
14. Huckstep RL. Changed character of osteomyelitis. *British Medical Journal*. 1967; **iii**: 739.
15. Burkitt DP. A sarcoma involving the jaws in African children. *British Journal of Surgery*. 1958; **45**: 218–23.

CHAPTER 15

Diseases of the eye

D.D. Murray McGavin

This brief chapter on eye diseases can only highlight conditions presenting in a busy general clinic, which are significant either because they are common eye problems or because they have the potential of causing severe visual impairment or blindness. Early recognition of a disease process is important so that a decision may be made either to treat the child at the clinic or refer the child for specialist opinion.

Examination of a child's eyes

In diagnosis more is missed by not looking than by not knowing. An advantage in ophthalmology is that many conditions can be seen and so a diagnosis can be made. But this does not diminish the importance of obtaining a detailed and clear history. The complaint of the child or parents may refer to a number of abnormalities:

- a changed appearance, e.g. red eye or squint;
- pain, e.g. ocular discomfort or headache;
- reduced or disturbed vision, e.g. amblyopia ('lazy' eye), myopia or optic neuritis;
- watering or discharge, e.g. a blocked tear duct or conjunctivitis.

Clearly some of these signs and symptoms may coincide.

The 'technique' of examining a child is often dependent on a reassuring and understanding attitude by the medical practitioner for both the parent and the child. A few moments given to chatting with the child or together examining the torch or ophthalmoscope, perhaps shining the light into one's own eye, can avoid frustrating and sometimes impossible situations! In the smaller child, however, it may be necessary to wrap a blanket around the trunk with the arms pinned to the sides while a colleague or parent holds the head firmly between two hands. Even this can be done gently, if firmly.

Instruments for basic screening examinations of children should include:

- a test chart such as the Landolt's 'C' chart;
- a pin-hole disc to screen for refractive errors;
- a hand torch;
- a magnifying lens or loupe;
- a direct ophthalmoscope;
- fluorescein dye strips; local anaesthetic drops, e.g. amethocaine (1 per cent); a short-acting mydriatic, e.g. tropicamide (1 per cent) or cyclopentolate (1 per cent);
- lid retractors and lid speculum.

If it is assumed that specialist expertise is available, even if at some distance, only a few further items are needed for the routine treatment of conditions such as corneal abrasion, retained corneal or conjunctival foreign body, lid or peri-orbital injuries requiring sutures and various infective states of lids, lacrimal sac, orbit, cornea and conjunctiva. These items include:

- eye pads, adhesive tape and bandages;
- sterile hypodermic needles;
- fine suture material, needle-holding and plain forceps;
- cotton wool 'buds';
- scissors;
- antibiotics – systemic antibiotics, eye drops and ointment;
- corticosteroid eye drops and ointment.

Warning   One should always be careful in using topical corticosteroids and note that there are many combined antibiotic–corticosteroid preparations. In certain infectious conditions, for example Herpes simplex keratitis, the consequences of topical corticosteroids can be disastrous. If there is doubt regarding the diagnosis, avoid corticosteroids.

A clear history obtained, the child hopefully reassured by a gentle approach, the next step will be actual examination. This will have commenced as the child and parent appeared in the clinic. The general appearance of the child, any obvious physical abnormalities and also the relationship between parent and child will be noted. Indeed the likely complaint may immediately be evident – bilateral red eyes with purulent discharge (conjunctivitis), an obvious squint, an opaque cornea (corneal leucoma), are some examples. If a patient enters the clinic with obviously poor vision and yet apparently normal anterior segments of each eye, immediate consideration will be given to posterior segment eye disease such as optic atrophy or primary pigmentary retinal dystrophy (retinitis pigmentosa).

If each patient is examined systematically, eye defects can quickly be identified. Thus, the medical practitioner can concentrate on the particular eye complaint before weariness or distraction disturbs the young patient. It is a good principle to begin with the external appearance, followed by the anterior segments of both eyes and then progress posteriorly to the fundus of each eye.

Eye disorders

The orbit

The orbit is the bony cavity which contains the eye and extra-ocular structures, such as muscles, nerves, blood vessels and orbital fat. In children, the main presentations of orbital disease are inflammatory or due to tumours. Also, an orbital cyst will often have the characteristic clinical presentation of an orbital neoplasm.

Orbital cellulitis

Orbital cellulitis presents as a unilateral picture in an ill child who usually has fever. There is oedema of the peri-orbital region, particularly the eyelids which are hot and inflamed. The eye shows variable degrees of proptosis visualized, with some discomfort to the child, by separating the eyelids which are tense and closed over the eye. There is associated oedema of the conjunctiva (chemosis) with discharge. Complications of orbital cellulitis include intracranial inflammation which may be manifest as cavernous sinus thrombosis (a bilateral picture) and meningitis. Septicaemia may occur. These complications are of grave significance. An abscess may occasionally form which discharges spontaneously. However, immediate systemic broad-spectrum antibiotic therapy is required for all patients. An antibiotic ointment may be applied topically primarily as a protective lubricant for the anterior eye. Often orbital cellulitis is a consequence of sinus infection. The ethmoid sinuses situated medial to the orbit have very delicate walls demarcating each sinus from the orbit. Other causes include foci of infection in the nose, the peri-orbital tissues and within the eye itself (endophthalmitis).

Parasitic infections

These may cause orbital cellulitis, notably the *Loa loa* worm (Calabar swelling). Unlike acute bacterial orbital cellulitis, the picture is localized to the orbital region usually without the systemic features of fever and malaise and resolves in some days without residual damage. The blood picture helps differentiation – raised eosinophils associated with parasites.

Cystic lesions

A cystic lesion in the orbit will present with unilateral proptosis and may be parasitic, as in hydatid cyst, a dermoid cyst or possibly a mucocele. Expert opinion will be required in patients with unilateral proptosis and the treatment will generally be surgical.

Tumours

Unilateral proptosis of a quiet eye, which has progressed gradually, is the characteristic presentation of an orbital tumour. The degree of proptosis can be measured by comparing with the other eye, either with a proptometer (exophthalmometer) or by observing the difference in situation of each eye by looking from above. Note the direction of proptosis i.e. straight forward, with depression of the globe or lateral displacement. This will give some indication of the position of a tumour within the orbit. Refractive changes may occur due to pressure on the globe and retinal folds may be seen on ophthalmoscopy. Primary orbital tumours include haemangioma, glioma, neurofibroma and rhabdomyosarcoma (see pp. 873–87). Extension from surrounding structures may arise from intracranial tumours, sinuses and the naso-pharynx. Burkitt's lymphoma will often involve the orbit. Metastases may occur in leukaemia. Extension from the eye may occur in retinoblastoma. Surgical removal by orbitotomy will be required in most instances and malignant tumours may require exenteration (removal of all contents within the orbit). Protect the eye by lubrication with antibiotic ointment. Orbitotomy will have disappointing results if the cornea is scarred due to exposure.

Eyelids and lacrimal system

The eyelids and the formation of tears provide protective mechanisms for each eye.

Eyelids – congenital defects

Ptosis may be unilateral or bilateral and may produce a characteristic backward tilt of the head. Besides the most common congenital type, ptosis may be due to a variety of conditions: inflammatory, neuromuscular, traumatic or neoplastic – a careful history is always important and the origin of the problem investigated. In congenital ptosis, depending on the degree of disability, surgical repair may be indicated, particularly as the eye can develop amblyopia.

Another common congenital defect is epicanthus – a crescent-shaped fold of skin over the medial canthus which is characteristic of some Eastern races and which may mislead by giving the appearance of a squint (pseudostrabismus).

Eyelid inflammations

External hordoleum (stye) is a very common infection in the region of the eyelash follicle. Nearly always due to staphylococci it usually responds to topical antibiotic eye ointment and hot compresses.

Chalazion

Chalazion or meibomian lipogranuloma is a common granulomatous inflammation with localized swelling, originating in the meibomian glands of the tarsal plate. A vertical surgical incision through the conjunctival surface of the eyelid (incising 'away' from the eye) is required, following infiltration with local anaesthetic. A chalazion clamp effects eversion of the eyelid.

Blepharitis

Bacterial, viral and allergic inflammation may produce characteristically inflamed lid margins. In seborrhoeic blepharitis, crusts adhere between and at the base of eyelashes. Crusts should be removed with warm, moist, cotton wool swabs and antibiotic eye ointment applied. Combined antibiotic – corticosteroid eye ointment may be appropriate here, but be certain there is no viral infection involved. Viral infections which may cause blepharitis include *Herpes simplex*, molluscum contagiosum and the common wart (see pp. 614–6). Insect bites on the eyelid produce considerable oedema with inflammation (see pp. 960–1).

Other infective conditions which may cause inflammation and often much scarring and which will require treatment of the general infection in the first instance are cutaneous leishmaniasis, anthrax, actinomycosis and yaws. Cancrum may also produce scarring of the eyelid with possible cicatricial ectropion which may require surgical plastic repair.

Ectropion and entropion

The eyelid turning out (ectropion) in children may be due to the conditions noted above. It may also follow injury, including burns, or be a consequence of facial nerve paralysis. The eyelid turning in (entropion) will be less common but can occur in chronic trachomatous scarring, usually affecting older children. The treatment of ectropion and entropion is surgical – but the cornea must be protected as much as possible with lubricating antibiotic eye ointment.

Lacrimal system

The lacrimal gland is situated in the supero-temporal and anterior aspect of the orbit. Tears pass across the eye, drain into the inferior and superior lacrimal puncta, through the canaliculi to the lacrimal sac and into the naso-lacrimal duct which opens below the inferior turbinate within the nose. In very young children, tearing (epiphora) on one or both sides is common. Usually the cause is congenital stenosis of the tear passages which spontaneously improves with growth during the first year of life. Gentle probing of the ducts may be necessary – but this should be avoided if possible until the child is one-year-old – and must be carried out by a specialist.

Acute dacryocystitis

This is inflammation of the lacrimal sac which fills with pus or mucopus and is generally due to inadequate flow of tears through the naso-lacrimal duct. The area below and slightly nasal to the inner canthus becomes swollen and, in the acute stage, inflamed. It may be extremely tender but mucopus can often be expressed into the conjunctival sac. Treatment is with topical and systemic antibiotics. The parent may be taught how to express and clean away the extruded mucopus by gentle pressure on the lacrimal sac from the side of the nose towards the eye. Thereafter, topical antibiotic drops can be instilled three or four times daily for 2–3 weeks. (See Fig 5.15.1.)

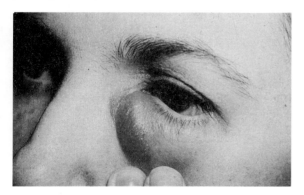

Fig. 5.15.1 Acute dacryocystitis. (Courtesy of Professor GJ Johnson.)

When the inflammation has entirely resolved and if epiphora persists and is unrelieved by expert irrigation of the tear ducts, a surgical procedure, usually dacryocystorhinostomy (DCR) is required. Occasionally, a persistent and recurrent inflammation of the lacrimal sac necessitates total removal of the sac (dacryocystectomy) which will resolve the inflammatory situation but often leaves a chronically watering eye.

Dacryo-adenitis

This is very much less common and can be associated with infections which may be viral (e.g. mumps), bacterial (e.g. tuberculosis and leprosy) or fungal (e.g. blastomycosis). Treatment will be appropriate to the underlying cause.

Squint, amblyopia and refractive errors

Squint (strabismus)

Squint is common in childhood. Early treatment is very important as a persistent squint can result in permanently reduced vision in the squinting eye (amblyopia; 'lazy' eye). A child with a suspected squint should be fully assessed without delay.

The six extra-ocular muscles of each eye act in concert with the fellow eye. Disturbance of vision affecting one or both eyes may result in a squint. This disturbance in clear vision may be due to a refractive error in one or both eyes, or disturbance of the pathway for vision (e.g. corneal opacity, cataract, intra-ocular inflammation, retinal disturbance and optic nerve disease).

A concomitant squint is the classical squint of childhood which can be convergent (esotropia), the most common type; divergent (exotropia); and vertical (hyper or hypotropia). A characteristic of these squints is the same angle of deviation in all directions of gaze. However, some squints 'alternate' where the fixing eye may at one time be one eye and at another time be the other eye. This reduces the likelihood of amblyopia which develops more often in an eye which is constantly deviated. Spectacle correction may fully or partially control some squints, but often surgery is required. Temporary occlusion of the dominant eye can reduce amblyopia pre-operatively.

A child with epicanthus may have the appearance of a squint (pseudostrabismus). Other types of true squint may be: (1) congenital – usually due to neural or muscular congenital defects; (2) traumatic; (3) due to intracranial inflammation or tumour; (4) due to neural or muscular disease. Any possible squint, real or imagined, whatever its likely cause, should be referred, without delay, to an ophthalmologist.

Refractive errors

The visual acuity of each eye, or an attempted assessment of vision in the younger child, is an essential part of the initial record in any eye examination. If a child is able to fix on the 'C' or 'E' test card with each eye, and the vision is reduced, a quick means of determining the presence of a refractive error is to use the pin-hole disc. Vision will improve, often dramatically, while looking through the tiny aperture of the disc.

Children generally begin life 'long-sighted' (hypermetropia) which gradually lessens as the child grows into the teenage years. In some children, at differing ages, the refractive state of the eye progresses on to 'short-sight' (myopia). Correction for hypermetropia is with plus spherical lenses and for myopia, minus spherical lenses. Myopia generally increases during the growing years becoming relatively static around 18–22 years. Hypermetropia is often associated with the concomitant strabismus of childhood and the squint may be wholly or partially controlled by corrective plus spherical lenses. Astigmatism most often indicates some asymmetry of the corneal curvature and this is corrected by plus or minus cylindrical lenses.

The red eye

Eye diseases in warmer climates which have the potential of going on to blindness, and which affect huge numbers of children, often present with a red eye. An approach to diagnosis is outlined in Fig 5.15.2. Here we shall consider the features of the common anterior segment eye inflammations presenting to the medical practitioner as conjunctivitis, keratitis or anterior uveitis (iridocyclitis).

Conjunctivitis and keratitis may occur together as part of the same disease process simply because of anatomical continuity, while anterior uveitis is a deeper inflammation with evidence of inflammation anteriorly around the limbus (corneoscleral margin), described as ciliary 'flush'.

Conjunctivitis is an extremely common and disagreeable condition which usually has bacterial, viral or allergic origins. In itself it is not a sight-threatening inflammation and vision is generally good although sometimes blurred by discharge on the cornea. However, the consequences of unresolved conjunctivitis may be dangerous to sight: (1) if the cornea becomes directly involved, and (2) if conjunctival scarring, as in trachoma, distorts the neat and uniform position of the eyelids causing eyelashes to scarify the cornea.

Bacterial conjunctivitis may be caused by a variety of organisms including staphylococci, gonococci, *Haemophilus influenzae*, *Pseudomonas* and pneumococci. *Moraxella lacunata* may induce a characteristic inflammation at the canthi – angular conjunctivitis. If it is possible to make some identification of the organism with a Gram-stain that is ideal. A broad-spectrum antibiotic eyedrop given intensively as required (perhaps hourly initially and reducing over 7–10 days) with the same antibiotic ointment at night generally provides adequate treatment. It is always wise to treat both eyes, although one may be predominantly affected, the second eye having

drops three or four times a day. It will be important to avoid inoculating the second eye by extreme care in cleanliness and instilling drops in the better eye first. Do not pad the eye in conjunctivitis.

Neonatal conjunctivitis (ophthalmia neonatorum) in its classical form is the consequence of infection of the female genital tract and the newborn child develops conjunctivitis within a few days of birth (see pp. 582–3). Organisms which commonly cause neonatal conjunctivitis are the gonococcus and *Chlamydia trachomatis*. Gonococci may induce a very acute form of bilateral conjunctivitis with tense, swollen and inflamed lids which on separation may discharge pus quite alarmingly. It is vital that intensive treatment is instituted immediately, as any secondary involvement of the infant's cornea can be a danger to sight. Not all gonococci are sensitive to penicillin (see p. 583). A suitable regime for gonococcal conjunctivitis is a single intramuscular injection of cefotaxime (100 mg/kg) or kanamycin (25 mg/kg) plus tetracycline (1 per cent) eye ointment or erythromycin (0.5 per cent) eye ointment intensively at first (hourly), then reducing to three times daily for 14 days. *Chlamydia trachomatis* will cause a milder form of conjunctivitis. These infants should be treated with erythromycin estolate orally as syrup (50 mg/kg per day for 14 days). It is very important that these organisms are identified if at all possible, as systemic therapy for both parents should be advised.

Viral conjunctivitis may be caused by many viruses which can induce a variety of symptoms and signs. Significant viruses include enterovirus 70 (acute haemorrhagic conjunctivitis or 'Apollo' conjunctivitis), adenoviruses 8 and 19 (epidemic kerato-conjunctivitis – and in association with fever and pharyngitis, pharnygo-conjunctival fever) measles virus and molluscum contagiosum (see pp. 600–23). There is no specific treatment for these listed, apart from molluscum contagiosum where any lid papilloma is cauterized or has curettage after local anaesthesia. Secondary bacterial infection may be controlled with topical antibiotics and it is important to monitor carefully the situation in a child ill with measles, considering the general nutritional state also. Corneal scarring following measles infection is common in many countries – all children with measles must be given vitamin A, 200 000 units orally (see later).

Allergic or hypersensitivity conjunctivitis is most commonly evident in warmer climates as vernal conjunctivitis or phlyctenular conjunctivitis.

Vernal conjunctivitis (spring catarrh) is a *Type I hypersensitivity* response particularly common in children (Fig 5.15.3). The child may complain of severe itching and irritation and there is some white discharge. Strings of mucus may be present. The conjunctiva is thickened

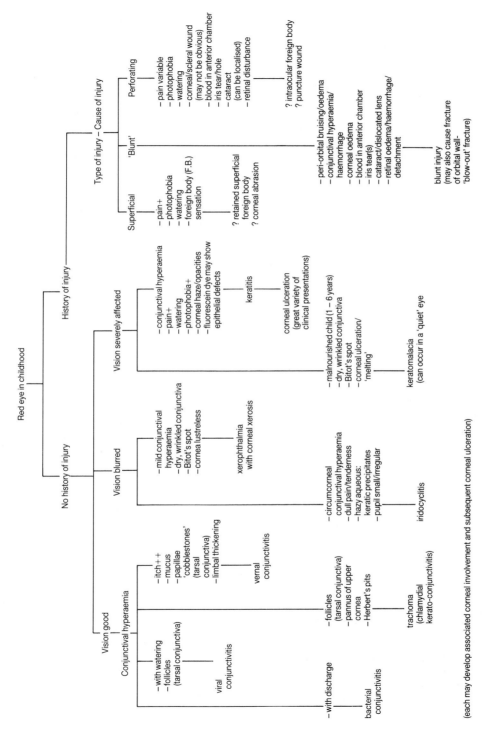

Fig. 5.15.2 Flow chart showing an approach to the diagnosis of red eye.

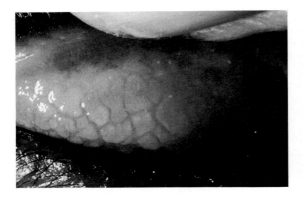

Fig. 5.15.3 Vernal conjunctivitis. Papillae ('cobblestones') of the tarsal conjunctiva. (Courtesy of Dr JDC Anderson.)

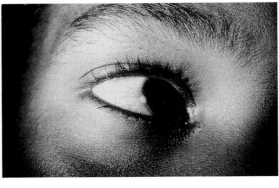

Fig. 5.15.4 Phlyctenular conjunctivitis. Phlycten at the limbus. (Courtesy of Dr JDC Anderson.)

and red, particularly the tarsal conjunctiva which may have quite dramatic papillae ('cobblestones') with fissures between. The limbal conjunctiva may be thickened and raised and the conjunctiva in general has a velvet-like appearance. The cornea may be involved and in some instances a characteristic ulcer with a plaque of adherent material is present in its base. The condition tends to improve in adult life. Treatment requires careful and expert control for one particular reason – the great danger of long-term, ill-advised topical corticosteroid therapy. This will provide welcome and fairly rapid improvement in most cases and may create a false sense that there is always a remedy for a recurrent problem. Secondary glaucoma can occur with topical corticosteroids and it is a great tragedy to see a young person beginning adult life blind, due to bilateral cupped optic nerve heads following long-term recurrent therapy with corticosteroids. An alternative is topical Opticrom (cromoglycate) which is less dramatic in its effect but is safe and can be use two to six times each day. If medical therapy is ineffective, refer to a specialist who may consider treating the excrescences with cryotherapy.

Phlyctenular conjunctivitis (Type IV hypersensitivity). A phlycten (Fig 5.15.4) is a micro-abscess which may occur on conjunctiva or cornea but is most often found on the limbal conjunctiva. It is evidence of a hypersensitivity reaction often associated with tuberculosis, although it may be due to other bacterial influence. Corneal phlyctens may cause extreme discomfort. Phlyctens respond readily to topical corticosteroids. A patient presenting with this condition requires investigation for tuberculosis.

Keratitis with the possible sequelae of corneal ulceration which may heal leaving a scar (corneal

leucoma) or go on to perforation with all the consequences of intra-ocular infection is sadly very common in hot climates. It is in this area so often that the need for immediate treatment is vital, as any disturbance of corneal clarity may have a significant effect on vision. Inflammation of the cornea may be superficial, which has greater potential for healing, or it may be deeply situated. The corneal epithelium will replace itself readily without scarring. Any loss of epithelium or the deeper structures of the cornea is recognized as a corneal ulcer. Corneal ulcers may be due to infection by many organisms, bacterial, viral or fungal and corneal epithelium which is devitalized for whatever reason e.g. injury, exposure, nutritional inadequacy, allows ready access to a pathogen. In bacterial corneal ulcers there is typically a focus of pus within the corneal substance with surrounding corneal oedema and conjunctival inflammation with discharge. Vision is usually profoundly reduced. In association, there may be pus in the anterior chamber (hypopyon) which forms its own fluid level. Treatment for a bacterial corneal ulcer requires intensive therapy with topical and subconjunctival antibiotics.

If the organism can be identified and sensitivities determined that will be advantageous – but a simple Gram-stain will often give an indication of appropriate therapy, the significance being the importance of immediate intensive treatment. Chloramphenicol (0.5 per cent) eye drops (every 30 minutes initially and then reducing) may be used in the first instance. Alternatives are fortified gentamicin 14 mg/ml or enriched tetracycline (1 per cent) (with polymyxin). Subconjunctival preparations which may be used are benzyl penicillin (500 000 units) if there are Gram-negative cocci or gentamicin (20 mg/0.5 ml) with methicillin

(100 mg/0.5 ml) which have a broad-spectrum of efficacy. Atropine (1 per cent) drops daily should be used for cycloplegia and mydriasis.

The most important virus affecting the cornea and one which is widespread throughout the world is the Herpes simplex virus. Herpes simplex keratitis is typically recurrent, beginning as primary epithelial involvement with fine punctate lesions but often progressing in recurrence to a distinctive pattern of superficial ulceration (dendritic ulcer) (Fig. 5.15.5). The condition may worsen with deeper, stromal keratitis (disciform keratitis) and possibly be complicated further as a kerato-uveitis. Treatment in primary Herpes simplex keratitis is with topical antiviral agents – idoxuridine (IDU) or adenine arabinoside (Ara-A) (see p. 616). If deeper complications are evident trifluorothymidine may be used, but most often acycloguanosine (acyclovir) has preference. In recurrent epithelial disease, the infected epithelium may be gently removed with a cotton wool bud after topical anaesthesia – then the antiviral drug of choice used locally for 10–14 days. Deeper, stromal keratitis indicates an immune process and local corticosteroids are appropriate, but only in combination with a topical antiviral agent preferably when the newly grown epithelium is intact. The balance between corticosteroid requirement and the danger of virus replication needs fine judgement.

Fungal infection of the cornea (mycotic keratitis) may develop in isolation, often when injury with vegetable matter is reported, or it may complicate other infections or inflammation, particularly where corticosteroids have been used. Where treatment for a presumed bacterial ulcer has failed to respond, consider a mycotic infection (see pp. 624–32). The classical picture is a slow-growing ulcer with irregular margins often with small 'satellite' foci associated. However, the

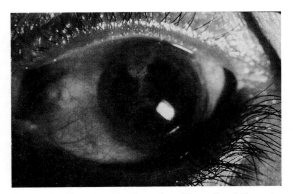

Fig. 5.15.5 Herpes simplex keratitis. Dendritic ulcer. (Courtesy of Dr JDC Anderson.)

clinical picture cannot provide a definite diagnosis. A Gram-stain is an important aid to diagnosis in differentiating bacterial or fungal infection. Fungal ulcers are common in hot, humid climates. Most commonly, *Aspergillus*, *Fusarium* and *Candida albicans* are implicated, but other fungi will also affect the eyelids and occasionally the eyeball itself. Fungicides are not always readily available and it may be necessary to use whatever can be obtained. Drugs which may be used include clotrimazole, miconazole and econazole, natamycin and amphotericin-B. Amphotericin-B is toxic to the cornea. Flucytosine given orally, (200 mg/kg per day), is effective in candida infection, but it should be given with one of the imidazoles (clotrimazole, miconazole and econazole) to prevent acquired resistance. A recent study from New Delhi suggests good results with silver sulphadiazine (1 per cent) ointment.

Anterior uveitis (iridocyclitis). Inflammation of the iris (iritis) and the ciliary body (cyclitis) often causes pain and blurring of vision. The eyeball is slightly red with circumcorneal injection (ciliary flush); examination with a focal light and magnification will reveal haziness of the aqueous in the anterior chamber (flare) and there may be cells circulating in the aqueous. These cells may adhere to the posterior cornea (KP; keratic precipitates). The pupil may be sluggish in reaction and show adhesions to the anterior lens face (posterior synechiae). In hot climates, anterior uveitis is often secondary to exogenous influences which produce deep corneal inflammation and ulceration. Examples of endogenous causes which may produce inflammation are onchocerciasis, leprosy, tuberculosis and syphilis. Another recognized association is juvenile arthritis (Still's disease) (see p. 924). However, the cause of the endogenous type is often not apparent, and careful systemic examination is necessary. Treatment of endogenous inflammation is with daily atropine (1 per cent) eye drops for mydriasis and cycloplegia and corticosteroid eye drops according to requirements (at least four times daily) to reduce inflammation. If the cause is determined, whether exogenous or endogenous, this will require appropriate therapy.

Retina, choroid, optic nerve

A genetically determined eye disease which is relatively common in different parts of the world is primary pigmentary retinal dystrophy (retinitis pigmentosa). Small accumulations of pigment, usually beginning in the equatorial retina, have a characteristic 'bone corpuscle' appearance. Night blindness may be described as a presenting symptom. There is progressive loss of visual field, attenuation of the retinal arterioles and eventual optic atrophy. Unfortunately, there is no effective treatment yet available.

Vascular retinopathies occurring in childhood are few but may indicate anaemia, leukaemia, and sickle-cell disease. Diabetic retinopathy and Eales' disease (perivasculitis retinae) are generally found in older age groups.

Inflammatory disorders predominantly begin in the choroid (posterior uveal tract) and subsequently involve the retina giving the picture of choroido-retinitis. In the active phase there is a hazy, whitish appearance with blurred margins often localized to an area of the fundus. The inactive phase reveals the area which has been involved as a demarcated white scar often with pigment at the periphery. An obvious localized visual field defect remains. This appearance is caused by many conditions including tuberculosis, syphilis, toxoplasmosis, toxocariasis and onchocerciasis.

Toxoplasmosis

Toxoplasma gondii may cause infection *in utero* and localization of infection may excite a retinitis with subsequent retino-choroiditis (see p. 170). Typically, the inflammation has settled by the time a diagnosis is made and very often is an incidental finding in later life. However, the characteristic scar of quiescent toxoplas-mosis (Fig 5.15.6) can involve the region of the macula or be adjacent to the optic nerve and a visual defect becomes apparent. In this context, it is important that a child presenting with a squint has careful examination of both fundi. In active disease, if sight is threatened by the position of the inflammation, consideration can be

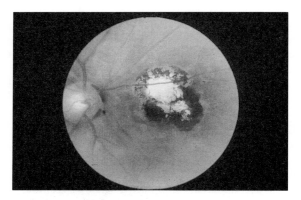

Fig. 5.15.6 Choroido-retinal scar of toxoplasmosis. Demar-cated lesion with pigment at the periphery. (Courtesy of Pro-fessor GJ Johnson.)

given to treatment with clindamycin, pyrimethamine and sulphadiazine, together with folinic acid in view of potential bone marrow depression. Such therapy requires to be carefully monitored. Corticosteroids may be used only in conjunction with antimicrobial therapy.

Toxocariasis

Toxocara canis and *Toxocara cati* may cause localized inflammation in the retina and choroid. There may also be severe pan-uveitis and endophthalmitis.

Avoidance of infection causing toxoplasmosis and toxocariasis requires careful hygiene for children in contact with cats and dogs.

White pupil

The differential diagnosis of the white pupil (leucocoria) is important in children, particularly in the early recognition of cataract and retinoblastoma. A white pupil may be due to:

- congenital cataract;
- retrolental fibroplasia (retinopathy of prema-turity) – where too much oxygen has been given to newborn premature babies;
- persistent hyperplastic primary vitreous – where hyperplasia occurs in the anterior vitreous associ-ated with persistent vascular patterns which should have regressed by the time of birth;
- toxocariasis;
- Coat's disease – a rare condition often affecting males in childhood and early teenage years, where exudative, or possibly haemorrhagic extravasation usually of the central retina becomes an organized mass of tissue;
- retinoblastoma.

Retinoblastoma

A retinoblastoma may present with a white pupil or a squint. It is a rare, malignant tumour of infancy which in the early stages appears as a white elevation of the retina (see p. 884). Other foci of tumour tissue in the retina are seen as the condition progresses. Spread occurs forward into the vitreous and deposits may be seen in the anterior segment of the eye. Extra-ocular extension occurs through the sclera, along the optic nerve to the brain and via the bloodstream. The prognosis by this time is very poor indeed. Various forms of irradiation may be used and for localized lesions photocoagulation or chemotherapy can destroy the tumour. Photocoagulation is applied around the small tumour. Chemotherapy over an extended period may supplement local treatment. Enucleation may be necessary with as much of the optic nerve removed with clean dissection in view of the recognized spread of the tumour posteriorly. The other eye must be thoroughly examined at regular intervals, as independent tumour formation may appear in the second eye in up to 30 per cent of patients.

Optic neuritis

Optic neuritis may affect the anterior nerve (papillitis) or the posterior part of the nerve (retro-bulbar neuritis). Comparison of the optic nerve heads in each eye often gives a measure of the degree of pallor of the affected nerve. Optic atrophy will not recover, but detection of the underlying cause is of paramount importance. There are varying degrees of optic atrophy which can be the consequence of a variety of 'insults' to the optic nerve whether due to inflammation (e.g. syphilis, onchocerciasis), trauma, pressure effects, drug toxicity (e.g. ethambutol, quinine), eating poorly prepared cassava, or demyelinating disease.

Major blinding diseases

Corneal ulceration and scarring

Much of the eye disease affecting children which may go on to blindness is due to gross disturbance of the cornea. Corneal ulceration, whether bacterial, viral, fungal or nutritional in origin may result in considerable scarring or possible perforation with disorganization of the anterior eye. Suppurative (bacterial and fungal) corneal ulceration, Herpes simplex keratitis and measles infection have been mentioned previously. Measles is a very common cause of corneal ulceration and scarring. The measles virus invades the conjunctival and corneal epithelium. Malnourished children who may have chronic diarrhoea and in whom resistance to infection is depressed are especially vulnerable. Associated vitamin A deficiency puts these children at risk of devastating corneal ulceration. All of these young patients require vitamin A (200 000 units) at least once, and if required, also on the second day and one to four weeks later. Secondary Herpes simplex keratitis may occur. The clinical picture may be further complicated by corneal exposure in a very ill child. Measles immunization should be given priority as an important measure in the prevention of blindness (see pp. 369–73, 496–502).

The notes following include other major causes of corneal scarring – trachoma, nutritional corneal ulcera-tion, injuries, onchocerciasis and leprosy. However, it should be understood that severe eye problems in onchocerciasis and leprosy occur mainly in adults. Early recognition of these conditions is important so that eye complications may be prevented if possible.

Trachoma (Chlamydial kerato-conjunctivitis)

Trachoma is an ancient disease which may affect about 350 million people in the world today. *Chlamydia trachomatis*, in active form is widespread in hot, dry and dusty climates and is directly related in its severe pathological effects to poor hygiene and poor living standards (see pp. 596–7). This organism is also described as the TRIC agent which may also be transmitted sexually. There are a number of different serotypes. In the classical eye disease it is transferred by personal contact and often by flies. After infection is established, the conjunctiva shows inflammation to varying degrees and follicles (lymphoid tissue) and papillae appear, noticably on the upper tarsal conjunctiva (Fig 5.15.7). A superficial keratitis may ensue which progresses to pannus formation, typically at the upper aspect of the cornea, with downgrowth of new vessels and corneal haze (active trachoma). Attempts at healing will take place. Scarring to varying extent will be seen on everting the upper lid and follicles which may have occurred at the corneal limbus regress leaving small (Herbert's) pits. In time, the fibrotic scar tissue may so distort the eyelids that the upper lid in particular is turned inwards (entropion) and eye-lashes, which themselves are deranged, rub against the cornea (trichiasis). This is extremely damaging to the corneal surface. The normal tear film is grossly disturbed by damage to conjunctival glands and the devitalized cornea is vulnerable to other pathogenic organisms which may cause corneal ulceration with all the conse-

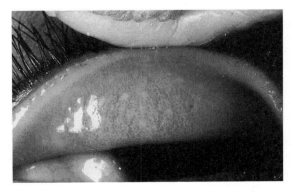

Fig. 5.15.7 Active trachoma. (Courtesy of Dr JDC Anderson.)

quent dangers in an unhealthy eye. The cycle of recurrent reinfection must be broken, by instruction in good hygiene – particularly regular face washing – and suitable medication. Treatment of trachoma is effected with a tetracycline eye ointment, twice daily for six weeks. Intermittent regimens can also be employed. *C. trachomatis* is also sensitive to sulphonamides and erythromycin. Scarring effects of trachoma affecting the eyelids require surgical repair. The great burden of this preventable infection, both for individuals and for communities may be alleviated by 'curative medicine' but can ultimately be prevented by education in hygiene and improving the conditions of those living in poverty.

A simple grading system for trachoma recognizes five signs:

- Trachomatous inflammation: follicles (TF) requires five or more follicles at least 0.5 mm in size on the flat surface of the upper tarsal conjunctiva.
- Trachomatous inflammation: intense (TI) presents diffuse inflammatory thickening of the upper tarsal conjunctiva obscuring more than half of the deep tarsal vessels.
- Trachomatous scarring (TS) of the tarsal conjunctiva is seen as white fibrotic lines or bands.
- Trachomatous trichiasis (TT) has at least one eyelash rubbing on the eyeball or evidence of ectopic eyelash removal.
- Corneal opacity (CO) where at least part of the pupil is blurred or obscured.

Xerophthalmia; keratomalacia

Vitamin A deficiency which affects at least half a million very young children (age one to six years) every year is one of the great tragedies of inadequate care where the knowledge exists to combat the disease (see pp. 367–73). The malnutrition that is evident may not be confined only to inadequate vitamin A intake but may be part of an associated picture of protein–energy malnutrition and the eye complications may be more severe because of intercurrent infection such as measles. Vitamin A is essential for the healthy state of epithelium and also for the formation of visual purple (rhodopsin) necessary for the normal functioning of the retina. The photochemical response of the retina to light requires an adequate supply of vitamin A to restore a cycle of normal function. An early feature of deficiency of the vitamin is night blindness. Epithelial disturbance induces characteristic primary signs which are classified as conjunctival xerosis (XIA), Bitot's spot with conjunctival xerosis (XIB), corneal xerosis (X2), corneal ulceration with xerosis (X3A) and

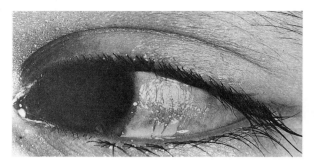

Fig. 5.15.8 Bitot's spots.

keratomalacia (X3B). Other signs are night blindness (XN), xerophthalmia fundus (XF) and xerophthalmia scars (XS). The conjunctiva loses its glistening lustre and becomes dry and wrinkled. Bitot's spots appear usually in the temporal interpalpebral region and have a foamy appearance (Fig. 5.15.8). The corneal epithelium may also become dry and lustreless. Ulceration of the cornea can develop in a relatively quiet eye and may progress to keratomalacia where the cornea 'melts' alarmingly (Fig. 5.15.9). These last two distinctive changes will result in various degrees of scarring and in severe cases may go on to corneal staphyloma (bulging cornea with uveal tissue adherent behind) or phthisis bulbi. A xerophthalmia fundus shows pale yellow spots. Treatment is urgent – Day 1: 200 000 units (110 mg) vitamin A orally (if a child is too ill to accept vitamin A orally, water-soluble vitamin A may be given by intramuscular injection (first dose)); Day 2: 200 000 units; one to four weeks later a further 200 000 units. (Half doses are given if a child is less than one year old). If bacterial infection is suspected then a topical or systemic antibiotic should be given. If Herpes

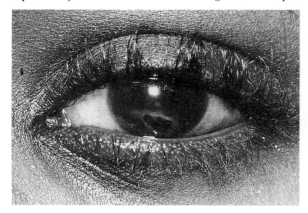

Fig. 5.15.9 Keratomalacia in a child with kwashiorkor treated with skimmed milk without a vitamin A supplement.

simplex infection is considered, topical IDU or acyclovir two hourly is required. Do not ignore the child's general nutritional condition. Prevention will always be the priority as a single dose of vitamin A every four to six months (100 000 iu) will preclude the disease. Most important is the education of communities that vitamin A is found in such foods as dark green leafy vegetables, carrots and fruits such as mangoes and papayas.

Injuries

Any injury to the eye requires prompt attention. In the particular case of a burn affecting the eye the treatment must be given immediately within seconds rather than minutes if that is possible.

A superficial corneal abrasion may be due to an object scraping the surface of the eye and occasionally it can be a troublesome recurrent problem. Fluorescein dye will outline any break in the corneal epithelium. The cornea is extremely sensitive and this injury is the cause of severe pain. In treatment, the principle is to 'splint' the eyelid against the eye by applying a pad and bandage for at least 24 hours (large abrasions will require rebandaging for some further hours) having instilled a short-acting cycloplegic eye drop, e.g. cyclopentolate (1 per cent) once, and an antibiotic drop or ointment. The antibiotic should be continued four times daily for at least five days.

A superficial foreign body (FB) may be removed with a cotton wool bud or a sterile hypodermic needle having first instilled a local anaesthetic drop, e.g. amethocaine (1 per cent). Remember to evert the upper lid to determine whether an FB is situated behind the eyelid on the tarsal conjunctiva – this procedure is effected by gently grasping the eyelashes of the upper lid and rotating the lid upwards against a spatula or similar instrument placed on the anterior surface of the eyelid above the tarsal plate. A metallic FB on the cornea may leave a ring of rust – some of this may be gently removed but do not be afraid to leave rust behind if it does not lift easily. The cornea is a thin structure approximately 0.5 mm thick at its centre and these procedures require magnification and a delicate touch. Following removal of the FB instil a short-acting cycloplegic, e.g. cyclopentolate (1 per cent) once, and antibiotic drops or ointment. Pad and bandage for 24 hours. Continue with the topical antibiotic for at least five days.

Burns of the eye require emergency irrigation with water – the irrigation continuing for some minutes until all the burning substance including particulate matter is washed away. Some of the particulate matter may need to be picked off with forceps. It is important also to irrigate into the conjunctival fornices behind the eyelids. This procedure can be effectively done using available tap water. A topical anaesthetic may be used. The most damaging substance to enter the eye is alkali, e.g. lime – potentially much more damaging than acid. With alkali burns there is a real danger of severe corneal scarring. After immediate intervention by irrigation, instil antibiotic ointment frequently each day (perhaps hourly for a day or two initially) and this can be supplemented with corticosteroid eye ointment which may reduce the possibility of adhesions between the lids and the eyeball (symblepharon). Try to avoid any adhesion by frequent use of ointment and regular and deliberate mobility of the eyelids and eyeball.

Blunt injury may cause considerable damage to the eye even without rupture of the globe – which may also occur. There may be peri-orbital injury with lacerations, oedema and bruising, fracture of the bony orbit (often the floor of the orbit – a blow-out fracture, which may cause adhesions of the inferior extra-ocular muscles), or damage to the eyeball with conjunctival haemorrhage, corneal abrasion and oedema, tears of the iris, blood in the anterior chamber (hyphaema), traumatic cataract and dislocated lens, retinal oedema or detachment. Later sequelae include raised intra-ocular pressure due to damage to the trabecular meshwork through which aqueous drains in the angle of the anterior chamber. The extent of any injury should be assessed. A total hyphaema requires emergency release of blood surgically. Severe damage will need specialist advice.

A perforating injury may be caused by an intra-ocular foreign body (IOFB) or possibly a sharp-pointed object such as scissors or a pencil. Again, the extent of injury should be determined, topical and systemic antibiotics given, the eye padded and the patient referred to an ophthalmic surgeon.

Injury to the eye may occur as a result of locally unique causes. In Africa 'spitting' snakes such as certain species of cobra can cause venom-induced kerato-conjunctivitis with blepharospasm (see p. 956). Irrigation with water is an immediate priority. Traditional eye medicines can cause severe visual impairment due to corneal ulceration and scarring. Irritant substances introduced into the eye are usually herbal in origin but may be mixed with human or animal urine. Solar retinopathy (eclipse blindness), which is the consequence of a solar-induced burn of the macula, classically occurs when viewing an eclipse of the sun and can cause marked loss of central vision. In one area of the subtropics, children sustain a macular burn when competing with each other to see who can gaze longest at the sun.

Cataract

Cataract may be found in children and usually presents as a congenital abnormality. Congenital cataract may be the consequence of maternal infection during pregnancy, most often rubella. Genetic factors also predispose to congenital cataract. Early surgery is indicated if the cataract is large, but it is suprising at times that relatively good vision may be obtained even with centrally placed lens opacities. Dilatation of the pupil may indicate if surgery would help in the case of a centrally situated cataract, both by allowing examination of the posterior eye and also by possible temporary improvement in vision. Specialist opinion is advisable. A traumatic cataract may be the outcome of severe trauma to the eye whether blunt injury or perforating injury.

Glaucoma

Glaucoma may occur in association with other eye conditions such as intra-ocular inflammation and tumours but the usual presentation in the child is congenital glaucoma (buphthalmos; ox eye). Congenital glaucoma may be unilateral or bilateral and is usually noticed in the young child because the eye is large in size due to stretching of the distensible walls of the globe. There are splits in Descemet's membrane deep in the cornea. The child experiences photophobia. The angle of the anterior chamber of the eye and associated structures may show a variety of features suggesting dysgenesis which will cause varying degrees of obstruction to aqueous outflow with consequent rise in intra-ocular pressure. Beware the situation where parents have described their child as having 'lovely big eyes' – it can be a prelude to heartache. Surgical intervention is usually sweeping division of abnormal tissue overlying the drainage angle (goniotomy) or possibly trabeculotomy or trabeculectomy.

Onchocerciasis

In some areas of the world 'river-blindness' will lead if untreated to possible visual handicap although this is rare before the age of 15 years (see pp. 686–9). Onchocerciasis is found in West and Central Africa and Central and South America. It is spread by the bite of various species of the 'black biting fly', *Simulium*. Onchocerciasis, a parasitic disease, is caused by the filarial worm *Onchocerca volvulus* and the signs and symptoms are caused by the microfilarial larvae in various concentrations in the body, but often affecting the skin and eyes. Subcutaneous nodules may occur,

dermatitis with scratch marks are characteristic and there may be skin atrophy, depigmentation, and associated lymphoedema. Eye changes include 'snowflake' opacities in the corneal stroma, and sclerosing keratitis primarily affecting the corneal periphery. An iridocyclitis may occur with the possibility of secondary glaucoma and cataract. Microfilariae may be visualized in the anterior chamber with magnification. Choroidoretinal degeneration and optic atrophy are relatively common and may have a profound effect on vision. Treatment of inflammation of the anterior eye will be similar to that described for anterior uveitis (iridocyclitis). Specialist advice should be requested. There is fresh hope in the treatment of onchocerciasis with a new drug ivermectin (Mectizan) which is described on p. 688.

Leprosy

While children are considered susceptible to infection by *Mycobacterium leprae* in view of close family contact, complications, including ocular problems, are more common in patients who have had leprosy for a long time (see pp. 553–76). Early diagnosis is important so that treatment can be instituted and long-term ocular complications reduced. These include, in predominantly tuberculoid leprosy, lagophthalmos due to facial nerve paralysis with paralytic ectropion and consequent epiphora. Exposure keratitis aggravated by fifth nerve involvement and corneal anaesthesia may ensue with the danger of corneal ulceration, hypopyon, endophthalmitis and phthisis bulbi. In predominantly lepromatous leprosy there may be loss of eyebrows and eyelashes (madarosis); nodules (lepromata) may be present at multiple sites – the limbus with keratitis, the episclera and sclera and the iris with an associated iridocyclitis. Acute iridocyclitis may lead to posterior synechiae and secondary glaucoma and will require energetic treatment with atropine (1 per cent) and topical corticosteroids. Chronic iridocyclitis may induce iris atrophy and evident miosis with secondary cataract. Vision will be considerably affected and mydriasis should be intermittently sustained with topical therapy such as phenylephrine (5 per cent). Management includes lubrication of the anterior eye, a regular and deliberate regime of blinking ten to fifteen times each day and consideration of lateral tarsorrhaphy as a further protective measure.

Much of the eye disease briefly discussed in this chapter is preventable. Our energies should be directed towards eradicating the tragedy of 'avoidable blindness', while continuing the care of those with existing disease and conveying encouragement to those whose visual impairment is sadly established – that they also might have hope and belief that their own contribution in life can be immensely worthwhile.

Further reading

Dawson CR, Jones BR, Tarizzo ML. *Guide to Trachoma Control.* Geneva, World Health Organization, 1981.

Foster A, Sommer A. Childhood blindness from corneal ulceration in Africa: causes, prevention and treatment. *Bulletin of the World Health Organization.* 1986; **64**(5): 619–3.

Klauss V. Newborn ophthalmia (ophthalmia neonatorum). *Community Eye Health.* 1988; **2**: 2–4.

Madan Mohan, Gupta SK, Kalra VK *et al.* Topical silver sulphadiazine: a new drug for ocular keratomycosis. *British Journal of Ophthalmology.* 1988; **72**: 192–5.

Sandford-Smith J. *Eye Diseases in Hot Climates.* Guildford, Butterworth Scientific, 2nd edition, 1990.

Sommer A. *Field Guide to the Detection and Control of Xerophthalmia.* Geneva, World Health Organization, 1982.

Thylefors B, Dawson CR, Jones BR *et al.* A simple system for the assessment of trachoma and its implications. *Bulletin of the World Health Organization.* 1987; **65**: 477–83.

WHO. *Methods of Assessment of Avoidable Blindness.* WHO offset publication No. 54. Geneva, WHO, 1980.

WHO. *Strategies for the Prevention of Blindness in National Programmes. A Primary Health Care Approach.* Geneva, WHO, 1984.

Wright E, Foster A. Suppurative keratitis: a blinding corneal infection. *Community Eye Health.* 1988; **2**: 5–7.

CHAPTER 16

Poisoning and accidents

Nimrod Bwibo

Accidents and poisoning are progressively assuming an important position as a health problem in the tropics and subtropics. They have hitherto comprised a small proportion of causes of hospital admission and death; being surpassed by nutritional, infectious and parasitic diseases.[1-4] In industrialized countries, accidents and poisoning are the first cause of death in children over the age of one year. Of children under five years of age one to two per cent are involved in poisoning incidents each year. The picture in developing countries is unknown. Retrospective studies, based on hospital admission, show that accidents and poisoning account for a small proportion of childhood deaths. The situation is changing, both in rural and urban areas, due to increasing hazards on the farms, in homes, in industries and on the roads.

The incidence of accidents and poisoning varies from country to country and even from region to region within a country. Falls and burns lead the list of causes of accidents, while kerosene, other household agents and drugs top the list of poisonings. There is a need for epidemiological surveys in developing countries to collect accurate statistics on accidents and poisoning, in order to structure preventive programmes.

POISONING

Factors causing poisoning

Multiple factors increase the risk of poisoning. They are grouped into those due to the host, the environment and the nature of the poisoning agents. The first and foremost factor relating to the host is young age. Curiosity is part of normal development; the preschool child is always exploring his environment and has a great tendency to put things in his mouth. A bad taste or foul smell is not a deterrent.

Accidental poisoning commonly occurs in young children; 80 per cent are less than five years of age. The incidence diminishes in normal children thereafter, while mentally retarded child remains at high risk of accidental poisoning in later childhood. Poisoning in teenagers raises the possibility of a suicidal gesture or attempt. Active, ill-disciplined and impulsive children are liable to repeated accidental poisoning. All types of accidental poisoning occur more often in boys than in girls (ratio 3:2).

Ninety per cent of childhood poisonings occur in the home and its immediate surroundings. Chemicals may be stored within reach of children in inappropriate containers such as old food and beverage bottles, and thus are easily mistaken as food. Children aged one to two years are able to reach chemicals and drugs left at low levels, while chemicals kept at a height can still be reached by three to five-year-olds by climbing. Apart from an abnormal physical environment, social factors within the family such as stress, or tiredness and hunger in the child are known to predispose to childhood accidents and poisoning in Western countries.[5] This is likely to be true also in developing countries. A mother who is ill, pregnant or recently delivered has a reduced capacity to supervise the children. Other factors include large family size, a deprived social setting and over-crowding. Increasing prescription of pyschotropic drugs increases the likelihood of poisoning in the home.

There are a growing number of poisoning agents in the form of chemicals in homes and farms and of dispensed drugs in homes. Some of the drugs are free samples given to health workers to take home. Many drugs dispensed to patients are left over after the illness has subsided. In some cases when patients return to hospital for a progress check up, they are given another supply of drugs instead of being instructed to continue with the previously supplied medicines or to destroy them. Many of the drugs are attractively coloured and may remind a child of sweets. Adults who take their medicines in the presence of young children, may make a child want to take medicine too.

Clinical features of poisoning

There may be a history of the child having been seen ingesting a known or unknown chemical. In many cases, however, no such history is available, as the child was unsupervised at the time of taking the poisoning agent. In such a situation, poisoning is suspected from the symptoms.

Not every case of suspected poisoning turns out to be so in practice. A panic-striken mother who finds her child with a bottle of medicine is likely to pick him up and rush to hospital before establishing that the medicine was ingested. Often the substance is taken in too small an amount to cause harm or is non-toxic and hence no symptoms occur. Energetic treatment of such cases is a waste of time and effort and may carry some risks.

A child who was previously known to be in good health and who suddenly develops curious symptoms should be suspected of having ingested a poison. The seriousness of the symptoms depends upon: the quantity and chemical nature of the poisoning agent; the time elapsed since ingestion; the nutritional status of the child; and the state of the stomach at the time of ingestion. If the stomach is empty, the chemical is likely to be absorbed rapidly and the symptoms present earlier than when the stomach contains food which may delay absorption by binding or diluting the chemical.

Symptoms of acute poisoning are usually general and non-specific. Characteristic signs indicating particular chemicals will be discussed later. The general symptoms may be gastro-intestinal, such as nausea, vomiting and diarrhoea. Breathing may be altered and central nervous system effects are fairly common, including excitability, drowsiness, convulsions and coma.

Clinical assessment

The patient should receive a thorough baseline assessment, noting if the child is in any danger from shock, respiratory arrest or cardiac failure. The state of consciousness (Table 5.16.1) and the pupillary reactions should be recorded. The type and rate of respiration are important to document. Be watchful for the development of the symptoms and signs of shock, by monitoring blood pressure and pulse. Urine production should also be assessed; catheterization may be necessary. Body temperature should be recorded.

Table 5.16.1 Grades of consciousness.

0 Conscious and alert
1 Drowsy but responding to vocal command
2 Unconscious but responding to minimal stimuli
3 Unconscious but responding only to maximal painful stimuli
4 Unconscious with no response whatsoever

Laboratory assessment

The laboratory is useful to a limited extent in confirming the diagnosis, determining biochemical derangement (glucose, urea, electrolytes, acid–base balance) and assessing the progress of treatment. For diagnosis, laboratory tests such as gas–liquid chromatography, if available, can be used to identify the chemical or drug in the serum or urine of the suspect. The blood levels of the poisoning agent, e.g. salicylates or iron, can be determined and used to monitor the progress of treatment.[6]

Management

Emergency and life-saving treatment procedures should precede the obtaining of a detailed history. Most lives are lost due to respiratory failure, hence respiratory care is of paramount importance. The comatose patient should be placed on his side, semi-prone and should have debris and vomitus suctioned from the mouth; an oro-tracheal tube may need to be inserted. A naso-gastric tube is introduced to aspirate the stomach contents. After establishing a clear airway, ventilation must be adequately maintained and oxygen administered if necessary.

Intravenous fluids are given to combat shock, maintain tissue perfusion and correct acid–base and electrolyte imbalances. Blood pressure and pulse are monitored to assess recovery from shock. While doing this the patient must be well wrapped to avoid hypothermia.

One of the initial values of the history is to indicate which specific antidote to give and to avoid certain treatment procedures, such as emesis in the case of ingestion of caustic agents, which would be contra-indicated. A detailed history consists of the age and sex of the child, the name of the agent ingested, if known, and how much of it is estimated to have been ingested. The container should be requested. It must be remembered that the missing contents do not necessarily represent the quantity ingested. Sometimes missing liquid has been spilled on to the floor; occasionally the missing quantity could have been shared with other children. The time of ingestion is estimated since this will be relevant to the point at which the onset of symptoms might be expected. Patients should not therefore be sent away too soon, only to develop symptoms later, as in the case of iron poisoning where symptoms are delayed; nor should over-zealous treatment be carried out when symptoms are not expected.

It is not unusual for a suspected patient, particularly a girl, to feed a young sibling with the chemical while she is playing the mother's role. In such a situation, the younger child may be severely sick and comatose, but left at home apparently asleep while the girl is rushed to hospital symptom-free, simply because she has been seen swallowing the agent or holding the bottle concerned. Caution should also be taken to avoid over-enthusiastic treatment of suspected patients without symptoms who have remained well for a long time.

Enquiry should be made as to whether the patient had eaten or not before ingestion, had vomited after ingestion, the type of first-aid that was provided and its effects, and the progress of the symptoms. One should ascertain that there has been no head injury.

The primary object is to remove the poisoning agent from the stomach. This is done as speedily and safely as possible. The removal of the poison is effected by inducing emesis (vomiting), or gastric wash-out (gastric lavage) or by catharsis.[7] Emptying the stomach is of doubtful value if attempted later than four hours after ingestion. However, a worthwhile recovery of salicylates can be achieved up to 24 hours after ingestion and of tricyclic antidepressants up to eight hours later. Emesis is contra-indicated after corrosive acid or alkali poisoning, or if petroleum products have been taken. It should also not be induced in patients who are drowsy or unconscious, unless the airway is protected to avoid inhalation by using a cuffed endotracheal tube.

Induced vomiting is accomplished by mechanical means or the use of drugs. The former involves simply gagging the back of the throat which elicits vomiting. The safest emetic to use is ipecacuanha syrup (ipecac). The dose is 10 ml for a child aged 6–18 months and 15 ml for older children. This is often followed by one to two cups of water and repeated after 20 minutes if necessary. Salt solutions, mustard and apomorphine can be dangerous and should not be used; the last is a respiratory depressant.

To carry out a gastric wash-out the patient lies on his left side with the head low. A large-bore naso-gastric tube is then inserted. When this is in the stomach the wash-out is best carried out using warm normal saline to avoid hyponatraemia or hypothermia. The procedure is carried out until the return fluid is clear. A sample of the wash-out material is kept for chemical analysis. It is advisable to leave some medication in the stomach after the wash-out to reduce any further absorption of the chemical. Desferrioxamine is used for iron poisoning and activated charcoal for aspirin poisoning. Emesis and lavage recover on average about 30 per cent of the stomach contents; if a long time has elapsed since accidental ingestion, neither is likely to be beneficial. Further absorption may be reduced with a cathartic, though they are not commonly used. This consists of magnesium sulphate (epsom salt) or sodium sulphate (glauber's salt) in a dose of 250 mg/kg given thrice daily. Magnesium should not be given to patients with renal failure.

In the case of poisons which are absorbed through the skin, such as organophosphate compounds, washing with plenty of water removes the chemical thus preventing further absorption. Similarly, eye contamination is removed by copious irrigation with normal saline.

There are several ways of actively enhancing the elimination of poisons from the body. These are: a forced diuresis, peritoneal dialysis, haemodialysis, exchange blood transfusion and the use of anti-dote. Meticulous conservative treatment with these specialized techniques increases the chance of survival, even in the most serious cases of poisoning.

Forced diuresis

This is utilized to assist the kidneys to excrete poisons such as long-acting barbiturates, salicylates and isoniazid. The procedure consists of increasing the amount of body fluid so as to enable the proximal renal tubules to excrete the poisoning agent. An infusion of 5–7 litres/M^2 of dextrose saline every 24 hours is given intravenously. A diuretic, such as Lasix (frusemide), may be added to speed up the urine flow. Another method is to increase the osmotic load using 15 per cent mannitol intravenously in a dosage of 1–2.5 g/kg over four or six hours. In the case of salicylate poisoning, sodium bicarbonate is added to the drip to alkalinize the urine and enhance its excretion. Alkalinization, however, interferes with calcium and magnesium metabolism which may need supplementation. It is advisable to determine serum electrolytes frequently to monitor for hyponatraemia or hypokalaemia which are most likely to occur in prolonged forced diuresis.

Peritoneal dialysis

This is technically easy to do and requires minimal equipment, but is least effective. This procedure is not useful for drugs which are highly bound to the tissues of the body, such as tranquillizers, antidepressants, hallucinogens and antihistamines. Osmolar fluid is used for this procedure and the addition of alkaline solution increases clearance of some drugs.

Haemodialysis

This is indicated in the following situations:

- if the poison is excreted primarily by the kidneys;
- if the patient is in coma or hyperactive due to dialysable drugs;
- hypotension that may threaten renal or hepatic failure;
- marked hyperosmolality;
- severe acid–base disturbance requiring rapid correction and not responding to conventional therapy;
- severe electrolyte disturbance which cannot be corrected by conventional therapy;
- marked hypothermia and hyperthermia.

Exchange blood transfusion

This is indicated for small children who have ingested drugs such as iron that are highly protein-bound, and which are likely to remain in the circulation for a long time or form toxic metabolites which accumulate in blood. The procedure is most helpful in massive poisoning. Electrolytes, acid–base balance and vital functions must be closely and carefully monitored. The procedure requires experienced personnel.

Specific antidotes

Specific antidotes are available for very few of the poisoning agents. They comprise the following:

- dimercaprol (BAL) and EDTA for heavy metals;
- desferrioxamine for iron;
- nalorphine for narcotics;
- methylene blue for nitrates and nitrites;
- diphenhydramine (Benadryl) for phenothiazides;
- pyridine-2-aldoxine methiodide (2 PAM) and atropine for phosphate ester insecticides.

Specific poisoning

The specific agents causing accidental poisoning are numerous and are usually classified into four broad groups:

- Medicaments – preparations prescribed for either internal or external use by medical personnel.
- Household agents – poisons used in homes and gardens, for example kerosene and organophosphate insecticides.
- Food agents – substances used as food or drink.
- Miscellaneous – substances that cannot be grouped in any of the above categories.

Table 5.16.2 shows the type and incidence of poisoning seen at Mulago Hospital in Uganda in a six-year period from January 1963 to December 1968,

Table 5.16.2 Type and incidence of poisoning, Uganda.

Group	No.	%
Medicaments	48	36.9
Household poisons	56	43.1
Kerosene	(34)	
Pesticides	(20)	
Others	(2)	
Food agents	24	18.5
Waragi (alcohol)	(15)	
Food poisoning	(4)	
Mushrooms	(1)	
Cooking oil	(1)	
Miscellaneous	2	1.5
Total	130	100

Reproduced with permission from Bwibo NO, *British Medical Journal*, 1969; **4**: 601–2.

according to the above four classifications. During that period only 130 children were admitted with accidental poisoning out of a total admission of 20 061; seven of the poisoned children died.[8] Examples of the common types of poisoning agents are described in detail hereafter.

Specific poisons

Organophosphates

Organophosphate compounds are toxic pesticides used in agriculture and public health. They are normally used as sprays to kill insects on farms or in homes. The lethal dose of these compounds varies tremendously as shown in Table 5.16.3.

Table 5.16.3 Organophosphate insecticides and their estimated oral lethal dose for man.

Compound	Lethal dose
Chlorothion	1 g
Diazinone	1 g
DFP	100 mg
ENP	250 mg
Metathion	1 g
Metacide	300 mg
OMPA	20 mg
Para-oson	100 mg
Protosan	1 g
Rogor	15 g
Systox	100 mg
TEPP	20 mg
Thio-TPP	40 mg

Diazinone is used in homes. It is absorbed in small amounts through the skin but its main route of entry into the body is by inhalation of dust and spray, causing cumulative toxicity.

Diazinone and the other organophosphate insecticides exert their toxic effects by inhibiting cholinesterase and pseudocholinesterase – the enzymes that hydrolyse acetylcholine. The enzyme inhibition is either effected directly or via an active metabolite which forms inactive stable phosphorylated enzyme complexes. The signs and symptoms of toxicity are a consequence of this enzyme inactivation and are manifested when the enzyme level is reduced to less than 20 per cent of normal activity. In children with malnutrition, who normally have low levels of plasma cholinesterase, only small amounts of organophosphate may be enough to cause symptoms. When the enzyme is inhibited, acetylcholine accumulates at both ganglionic and postganglionic synapses and at the motor end-plates with the resulting features of the poisoning. Acetylcholine is excitatory in low concentration and paralytic in high concentration, thus the clinical symptoms will vary.

Organophosphate compounds are lipid soluble and accumulate in adipose tissue. This leads to delayed elimination from the body and prolonged clinical features. The symptoms fall into three groups: nicotinic, muscarinic and general central nervous system effects. Nicotinic effects consist of: muscular fasciculation, twitching, tremors, incoordination, respiratory and skeletal muscle weakness, and in severe cases paralysis. Muscarinic effects consist of: anorexia, nausea, vomiting, diarrhoea, bronchospasm and increased bronchial secretions leading to pulmonary oedema and difficulty in breathing, salivation, increased lacrimation, constriction of pupils, palpitations, tachycardia and hypertension. In severe cases, bradycardia and heart block occur. General central nervous system effects are: drowsiness, mental confusion, anxiety, hyperexcitability, ataxia, coma and convulsions. Paralysis of the respiratory centre and depression of phrenic nerve activity occur in severe cases. In an individual patient these features may be mixed and sometimes atypical. For example, the pupils may be of normal size or dilated; a low-grade fever may occur and glycosuria without ketones may be noticed when urine is examined.

Treatment

Early effective treatment prevents development of the late severe features. The mouth and throat are usually full of secretions which should be suctioned first to keep the airway clear and prevent aspiration. Gastric lavage is then carried out as quickly as possible to remove unabsorbed quantities of the poison. Bicarbonate solution (1–2 litres at 5 per cent) is recommended for the gastric wash-out, but any other available fluid can be used.

Atropine sulphate and pyridine-2-aldoxime methiodide (2 PAM) are the antidotes for organophosphate compounds. Atropine is given as 0.5–1.0 mg i.m. or i.v. every 15–30 minutes until atropinization is achieved, i.e. flushed face, dry mouth and dilated pupils. A total of 12 mg of atropine in 24 hours is advised. In moderately severe cases, 6–8 mg have been found to be effective. Atropinization should be maintained by further administration in severe cases. Atropine counteracts the consequences of acetylcholine but does not affect the neuromuscular sequelae; nor does it reactivate the inactivated cholinesterase enzyme for which 2 PAM is needed in a dose of 50 mg/kg intravenously at 12 hourly intervals. The combination of atropine and 2 PAM is very effective. Supportive therapy must also be given. Oxygen is administered when there is dyspnoea and coma, and intubation may be necessary. Intravenous fluids are useful in correcting dehydration through diuresis, and in feeding the patient in coma. Drugs that usually lower cholinesterase level, such as morphine, phenothiazide derivatives and barbiturates, should be avoided as they will enhance the symptoms of the poison. Death occurs from respiratory failure due to pulmonary oedema and paralysis of the respiratory centre, and from cardiac failure.

There are various other pesticides on the market. Warfarin, a rodenticide, is commonly used to kill rats. It causes poisoning by inhibiting prothrombin and hence presents with bleeding. Vitamin K corrects the hypothrombinaemia. Blood transfusions may be used in very severe cases. Naphthalene found in moth balls and repellant cakes when ingested, presents with abdominal cramps, nausea, vomiting, diarrhoea, confusion, sweating and convulsions. Its treatment is on the general lines of supportive therapy. Other pesticides that may be encountered are: cyanide, copper sulphate, nitrite-thiosulphate, thalium, DDT, gammexane and chlorinated hydrocarbons.

Kerosene (Paraffin)

Kerosene is the single most common cause of poisoning in childhood in any community in Africa, and many parts of the developing world. It is available in most homes, where it is used as cooking fuel and for lighting. The danger arises from it being stored in the wrong way. It is normally bought and kept in food bottles, especially fruit and soda bottles, which attract children who think that they are drinking their usual beverage. It accounted for 34 (26 per cent) of the 130 poisoned children at Mulago Hospital in Uganda.[8]

Kerosene is a volatile hydrocarbon and is inhaled into the lungs as the child is drinking it and during vomiting. When ingested it is readily absorbed from the stomach and excreted by the lungs. Inhalation into and excretion from the lungs produces a chemical pneumonitis and pulmonary oedema. The degree of symptoms depends not only upon the quantity drunk but also upon the proportion of impurities present. These include naphthanic and aromatic hydrocarbons; their quantities vary with the source of the crude oil.

Concerning clinical features, there may be no symptoms when the quantities ingested are small. The symptoms are nausea and vomiting due to stomach irritation; attempted first-aid treatment at home may also induce vomiting. The main symptoms involve to the respiratory system; they include cough, and difficult, rapid breathing. There may be confusion and drowsiness, and even coma due to depression of the central nervous system. Examination reveals varying degrees of dyspnoea with retraction and cyanosis in severe cases. On auscultation there are usually coarse crepitations with rhonchi in lung fields, an indication of chemical pneumonia. Radiologically, the lung fields show hyperexpansion with patchy consolidation.

Treatment

Caution should be taken to avoid further inhalation. Induced vomiting is contra-indicated; this avoids further inhalation and the risk of aspiration. There is controversy regarding gastric wash-out: some authorities suggest that instead the stomach contents should be aspirated gently, avoiding causing vomiting.

Further management is basically symptomatic and supportive. Oxygen is administered where dyspnoea is marked; increased humidity is considered beneficial. Intravenous fluids help in the correction of dehydration and also in diuresis. The role of antibiotics for pneumonia is unclear, since the pneumonia is of chemical origin, although they may be important later on when secondary bacterial pneumonia is a possibility. Corticosteroids have been claimed to reduce pneumonitis and pulmonary oedema.

Iron

Iron in the form of ferrous sulphate is a common drug found in homes, having been prescribed for the treatment of iron-deficiency anaemia. Other forms of iron medication, like gluconate, are also available. Iron tablets are coloured and attractive to children who may ingest a large quantity. Ingested iron in toxic doses causes shock which may occur immediately or may be delayed for a few hours or as long as 24 hours. Toxicity depends upon the amount of iron ingested. Amounts greater than the total iron-binding capacity (TIBC) of tissue proteins cause severe symptoms arising from gastric erosions and necrosis and haemorrhagic necrosis of the liver. The patient presents with vomiting, bloody diarrhoea, gastro-intestinal haemorrhage, dehydration from severe vomiting, shock, jaundice, drowsiness, convulsions and coma. Patients with no shock or coma recover.

Treatment

Treatment of iron poisoning consists of induced vomiting and gastric lavage in hospital. Gastric lavage is done using sodium bicarbonate which gives insoluble ferrous carbonate. Desferrioxamine, an iron-chelating agent, can be left in the stomach in a dose of 5–10 mg of desferrioxamine in 200 ml of water to bind any remaining iron. Patients in shock and coma should receive desferrioxamine (10 mg/kg per hour not exceeding 80 mg/kg per 24 hours) intravenously for 12–24 hours. BAL or EDTA can be used but are slow to act. Peritoneal dialysis may be life saving. Shock should be treated promptly by blood transfusion or intravenous fluids. Late complications of iron poisoning are cirrhosis of the liver, liver failure and pyloric stenosis. The last needs surgical treatment.

Aspirin (Salicylate)

Aspirin is the most common drug causing poisoning in children. The poisoning usually occurs accidentally but may also occur during therapeutic use when large doses are administered to a child repeatedly leading to accumulating amounts that eventually reach toxic levels. Aspirin is the most common available drug in the home and in many shops, even in the most remote parts of tropical countries. It is commonly bought and administered for pains and aches and fever for both adults and children.

Most aspirin containers sold in many tropical countries can be opened easily by children. Following ingestion, aspirin is readily absorbed reaching high blood levels within a few hours of ingestion. It is eliminated from the body through the kidneys as unchanged aspirin or its metabolites. Toxicity depends upon the amount ingested; more than 0.5 g/kg body weight is lethal.

Aspirin produces an initial respiratory alkalosis, particularly in children above four years of age; this is due to hyperventilation secondary to central nervous stimulation. The body compensates by excreting base via the kidneys. A metabolic acidosis ensues due to accumulation of acetoacetic acid as a result of an increased metabolic rate and vomiting. Dehydration occurs due to hyperventilation, hyperpyrexia and vomiting. An increased metabolic rate is responsible for an elevated body temperature. Carbohydrate and lipid metabolism is disturbed. Hypoglycaemia occurs due to increased carbohydrate metabolism but hyperglycaemia may occur due to decreased synthesis and increased breakdown of glycogen. Gastric irritation may result in bleeding which may also occur due to deranged platelet function. The fact that aspirin inhibits the formation of prothrombin in the liver may also contribute to a bleeding diathesis.

The clinical features of aspirin poisoning thus include hyperventilation, nausea and vomiting, hyperpyrexia, profuse sweating and flushed skin. Severe cases may develop circulatory collapse, oliguria, confusion, delirium, convulsions and coma. The severity of the symptoms correlates with the serum levels and the time following ingestion. If it is not possible to determine serum salicylate levels, a simple practical laboratory method for confirmation of aspirin poisoning is the ferric chloride urine test.

Lead

Lead causes acute or chronic poisoning. It is found in paints, batteries and waterpipes although it is now used less than before. It can be absorbed from the skin and in India where lead cosmetic is applied traditionally to the eyes and forehead in children, it has been known to cause toxic symptoms. Acute lead poisoning causes vomiting, abdominal pain and melaena stools. In its chronic form, it is associated with muscle weakness, poor appetite, occasional vomiting, failure to thrive, pallor, lethargy or irritability and mental retardation. Convulsions and coma may occur. A characteristic blue line may be seen on the gums. X-rays of long bones show lead lines as transverse bands of increased density. The urine usually contains large amounts of coproporphyrin and glucose; the blood lead is more than 60 mg/100 ml. There is basophilic stippling of the red blood cells. Therapy of lead poisoning centres on maintaining a good urinary flow while giving an initial injection of BAL (dimercaprol) (4 mg/kg) followed after four hours by a combination of BAL (4 mg/kg) and Ca EDTA (calcium sodium edetate) (12.5 mg/kg) intramuscularly four hourly for five days.

Mercury

Mercury is an ingredient of pesticides and cattle dips. It is also found in lightening creams commonly sold in many countries in Africa. Mercury is absorbed through the skin and may reach toxic serum levels to cause symptoms similar to those described in acrodynia in the days when mercury was used in teething powder. A report of 111 cases of mercury poisoning in children 1–12 years of age from a rural agricultural area gives examples of the various clinical features.[9] They include a skin rash, profuse sweating, pink palms and soles of the feet associated with mutilation of the toes and fingers, loss of teeth, anorexia, diarrhoea, rectal prolapse, tachycardia and hypertension; mental retardation also occurs. These children had high levels of mercury in urine and serum. Their siblings, who did not have symptoms, also had elevated mercury levels in urine and serum indicating that these symptoms arise as an idiosyncrasy. Mercury poisoning is treated by BAL which eliminates mercury rapidly. EDTA or penicillamine are also effective in reducing serum levels of mercury. Sedation is required when intense itching is a problem.

Barbiturates

Ingestion of toxic amounts of barbiturates, most commonly as phenobarbitone, leads to impaired consciousness, hypotension and respiratory depression. Treatment is by:

- lavage to reduce further absorption;
- forced alkaline diuresis in severe cases;
- maintaining respiration and body temperature;
- circulatory support;
- correction of electrolyte imbalance.

Phenothiazine derivatives

These compounds are used to stop vomiting and therapeutic poisoning can occur. The drugs in this group include prochlomperazine, chlorpromazine and thioridazine. The patients present with extrapyramidal symptoms such as incoordinated dystonic movements of the limbs, torticollis, opisthotonos, trismus, oculogyric crises, rigidity, tremors and if large amounts of the drug have been taken, convulsions and coma. Treatment is by lavage, and diazepam (Valium), in a dose of 1–5 mg/kg, given slowly intravenously. Dystonic reactions are rapidly abolished by an injection of orphenadine hydrochloride (20–40 mg) or procyclidine hydrochloride (5–10 mg).

Lye

As industrialization increases tropical countries, several strong alkalis are being used in households for cleansing purposes. Lye, a colourless material, is such a cleansing material used in homes to make soap. These chemicals causes severe corrosion of skin and mucous membrane on direct contact; they cause poisoning in the two to four year old age group. The incidence of the poisoning in Cairo University's Hospital, Munira, averages 300–500 a year.

Burning oropharyngeal and retrosternal pain occurs immediately on ingestion, thus limiting the quantities ingested. Severe cases are associated with shock, pallor, anxiety and excessive salivation. In cases of ingestion of small quantities, the symptoms may be mild. As the corrosion heals it forms strictures in the oesophagus and rarely in the stomach with increasing dysphagia and malnutrition. Occasionally, severe injury may occur to the larynx causing asphyxia, hoarseness of the voice and narrowing of the airways. Perforation of the oesophagus may occur leading to mediastinitis, pneumothorax, pyopneumothorax or para-oesophageal abscess.

Cases reaching the hospital early should be managed immediately using weak acids and demulcents to neutralize the alkalis. Milk, citrus fruit juice, dilute vinegar, white of egg, butter, or olive oil are useful treatment agents. Causing emesis or passing a naso-gastric tube are contra-indicated. Severe airway obstruction should be treated by tracheostomy. Late cases with established oesophageal strictures need radiological confirmation and thereafter repeated dilation under general anaesthesia. In impossible strictures, gastrostomy feeding is indicated.

Favism

This is caused by eating broad beans (*Vicia fava*) or inhaling the pollen of their flowers; the individuals at risk have glucose 6-phosphate dehydrogenase (G6PD) deficiency in their red blood cells. Favism is commonly seen in areas near the Mediterranean Sea and also in parts of Asia, Africa and among the North American blacks (see pp. 223–8, 440, 827–8).

G6PD deficiency is a sex-linked recessive condition, hence the majority of cases of favism are boys. G6PD is concerned with the aerobic pentose shunt pathway providing reduced triphosphopyridine nucleotide (TPN). This in turn is the coenzyme for the reduction of glutathione by glutathione reductase. Reduced glutathione is essential for the protection of haemoglobin from oxidative injury by agents like fava beans.

The clinical features of acute favism arise from acute haemolysis and include severe sudden pallor, fever and tachycardia occurring within two hours of ingestion. Red discoloration of urine due to haemoglobinuria is followed by jaudice and splenomegaly. Death occurs within 24–38 hours in severe cases. Recovery is gradual in the survivors taking 4–6 weeks for the blood indices to return to normal.

Supportive therapy with transfusion of normal red cells should be carried out. When anuria occurs, dialysis is necessary. In communities where this condition occurs, such individuals should avoid exposure to the bean and its pollen.

Fluorosis

Fluorosis is endemic in India, China, Japan, the Persian Gulf, South–west America and parts of Kenya. In such countries the fluoride content of water is very high. Fluoride water content of up to 8 parts per million may not be associated with pathological changes (see p. 383). However, other factors such as hormonal dysfunction, protein–energy malnutrition, low calcium and magnesium intake and vitamin C deficiency may act to potentiate the effect of high levels of fluoride. Fluorosis occurs in two forms: chronic endemic dental fluorosis and skeletal fluorosis. Fluoride is deposited in bone and enamel; it is likely that fluoride absorption by osseous tissues is an uptake process, whereas enamel deposit is a simple ion-exchange phenomenon. Fluoride is probably exchanged for hydroxide radicals producing fluorapatite-like compounds – those which derange osteoid mucopolysaccharides.

Dental fluorosis affects the permanent dentition especially the central incisors and first molars. In exceptional circumstances deciduous teeth are affected. There are various grades of involvement: initially the enamel becomes opaque and chalky white then brownish black with irregular patches and transverse bands as time goes on. Subsequently, teeth become eroded with irregular pits and they may easily chip off; there is usually no associated dental caries.

Susceptibility to dental fluorosis seems to be restricted to the age group 8–16 years, because the damage takes place while the crowns of the permanent teeth are calcifying. The disease may start even in infancy in babies of fluoride-intoxicated mothers who are breast-fed, such that as the teeth erupt fluorosis becomes recognized.

Skeletal fluorosis takes time to occur and hence it is not a disease of children. In this form, sclerosis occurs in bones, ligaments, tendons and interosseous membranes. The characteristic clinical features include backache, spinal deformities, fixation of the thoracic cage in inspiration and neurological symptoms. The last may be a result of narrowing of the spinal canal consequent upon fluoride deposits in the vertebral column.

Cyanide

Cyanide poisoning occurs in many tropical countries in acute or chronic forms following eating of foodstuffs that contain cyanogenetic glycosides, such as cassava (*Manihot utilissima*) and lima beans (*Phaseolus lunatius*) and various cereals such as maize, sorghum and millet. In cassava they are contained in the leaves, stems and tuberous roots, being chiefly concentrated in the outer coat of the roots, possibly as a protection against pests. The bitter variety of cassava has more cyanogenetic glycosides than the sweet variety.

Cyanide causes poisoning by paralysing cellular respiration. The cyanide radical combines with cytochrome oxidase, an enzyme responsible for transfer of oxygen in cellular respiration, making the enzyme unavailable for oxygen transfer. This results in cytotoxic hypoxia and death.

Acute cyanide poisoning may occur in children who dig up and eat cassava or other foodstuffs that contain cyanogenetic glycosides. A whole family may be affected after a meal of cassava – more so during scarcity of food when cassava is harvested before it has matured and cooked before it has been prepared properly. Normally the poison is removed from the cassava through fermentation or washing.

The clinical features are characterized by asphyxia and cyanosis, and a characteristic odour in the breath of the poisoned individual. The patient presents with vomiting, drowsiness, weakness, cyanosis and dilated pupils.

The treatment is based on the fact that high concentrations of methaemoglobin compete with cytochrome oxidase for cyanide ion. Sodium nitrite is given as 3 per cent solution intravenously at the rate of 2.5–5.0 ml per minute for three to four minutes. The nitrite then causes methaemoglobinaemia which releases cyanide from the enzyme. The released cyanide is mopped up with sodium thiosulphate solution (25 per cent) given intravenously at the rate of 2.5–5.0 ml/minute. All tissues contain the enzyme rhodanase, which facilitates the transfer of sulphur from thiosulphate to bind cyanide ions forming thiocyanate. These are the major pathways for detoxication of cyanide.

Chronic cyanide poisoning is characterized by three neurological disorders: tropical ambylopia, nerve deafness and ataxic neuropathy.[10]

In tropical ambylopia, there is a gradual onset of bilateral visual blurring in children 5–15 years of age. In tropical nerve deafness there is tinnitus, a buzzing in the ears that goes on for weeks or months and may give rise to partial deafness in the end.

Tropical ataxic neuropathy occurs in older children and adults, and is characterized by pain and paraesthesiae in the legs and feet followed by unsteadiness in gait. Ataxia, like nerve deafness, is irreversible.

Ambylopia, and to a lesser extent ataxia, is associated with mucocutaneous lesions: angular stomatitis, glossitis, blepharitis and scroto-inguinal dermatitis which respond rapidly to brewers' yeast or vitamin B complex. Prevention of cyanide poisoning consists of soaking cassava and discarding the water or fermenting cassava, then drying before grinding or pounding to make flour. Children should be instructed to avoid eating unfamiliar vegetables and uncooked cassava.

Prevention of accidental poisoning

Many adults are not aware that medicines which are perfectly safe to them in normal dosages are poisonous to children either in small or large amounts. Awareness of this can go a long way in assisting to implement preventive measures. The subject should be included in the training of community health workers, teachers, pastors and shop-keepers. The most effective preventive measure for poisoning is the safe storage of those medicines and any chemical agents. There has been a rapid increase of household chemicals as well as farm chemicals in tropical countries; they should be stored or locked away – keeping them at a height is no solution as many children would still climb and reach them. Many poor families have no space in their homes where such chemicals and medicines can be locked, thus they are stored under the bed. Once the parents know the dangers of these agents they will take the trouble to keep them out of reach of the children. Storing chemicals such as kerosene in containers that normally contain food and beverage (such as soda bottles) is extremely dangerous. Children are attracted to drink the contents in such bottles, mistaking them for food; different types of bottles should be used instead. Toxic substances should not be stored with or near food.

Small children should be under constant supervision from older siblings or parents; this must be remembered, especially in times of stress and jubilation within the family. Many medicinal tablets are sugar-coated and coloured; these attractive features mislead children who then eat them as sweets. This danger is made worse when children are coaxed to take their medicine as sweets. It is desirable to discard safely unwanted chemicals and unused or outdated medicines, since their accumulation in the household just increases the danger of their ingestion by children. Dropping these chemicals and drugs in latrines is a safe way of disposal. Children imitate adults as part of their learning mechanism; if adults take medicines in their presence, the children are more likely to imitate and may take a dangerous amount of the drugs. Adults should therefore be discouraged from the habit of taking their medicines in front of children. The recent develop-

ment of encouraging older children to understand the part they can play in improving the health of their younger siblings, the co-called 'child-to-child' approach[11] is very appropriate in the case of accidents. The informed and more mature older child can make a considerable contribution in shielding brothers and sisters from the risks of accidents of all sorts.

Another measure which reduces childhood accidental poisoning due to drugs is for doctors to prescribe small amounts of drugs at any one time so as to lessen the accumulation of large quantities in homes. This has its disadvantages in the case of drugs that need to be taken for a long time, especially if patients cannot afford the transport to return to the clinic frequently for further supplies.

Chemicals in common use in the homes and on farms should be labelled and their constituents indicated. This facilitates the identification of the poisoning agent and provision of antidote where it is possible. Labelling should be enforced by the government; legislation should be introduced requiring production of safe packing and containers by the manufacturers. Children one to three years of age are unable to open plastic containers with the press-and-turn type of cap similar to car radiator caps. Various safety caps in common use in North America and Europe have markedly reduced the incidence of poisoning in those countries. There is the possibility that introducing them will increase the cost of drugs.

Poisoning centres are playing a significant role in reducing the incidence and severity of poisoning in Western countries by providing health education, first-aid information and information on the general management of poisoned individuals. The public are therefore aware what to do to save life and are informed about the methods of prevention of poisoning. The introduction of poisoning centres in the tropics and subtropics would serve some useful functions. The complex issue of prevention of ingesting poison as a suicidal activity requires the expert understanding of the social, cultural and psychological factors involved in suicide. This issue also needs to be addressed, as it is on the increase in the tropics (see p. 397).

References

1. Sinette CH. The pattern of childhood accidents in South-Western Nigeria. *Bulletin of the World Health Organization*. 1969; **41**: 905–14.
2. Seriki O. Accidental poisoning in children. *Postgraduate Doctor*. 1983; **5**: 142–7.
3. Mahdi AH, Al-Rifai MR. Epidemiology of accidental home poisoning in Riyadh (Saudi Arabia). *Journal of*

Epidemiology and Community Health. 1983; **37** (4): 291-5.

4. Korb FA, Young MH. The epidemiology of accidental poisoning in children. *South African Medical Journal*. 1985; **68** (4): 225-8.

5. Sibert R. Stress in families of children who ingested poison. *British Medical Journal*. 1975; **3**: 87-9.

6. Padmore GRA, Webb SF. The laboratory, the clinician and the poisoned patient. *Practitioner*. 1980; **224**: 81-4.

7. Matthew H, Lawson AHH. *Treatment of Common Acute Poisoning*. Edinburgh, E and S Livingstone, 1970.

8. Bwibo NO. Accidental poisoning in children in Uganda. *British Medical Journal*. 1969; **4**: 601-2.

9. Meme JS, Brown JC, Kagia J *et al*. Mercury poisoning as a cause of acrodynia in children, a preliminary report. *East African Medical Journal*. 1981; **58**: 641-9.

10. Monekosso GL. Endemic neuropathies in the Epe District of Southern Nigeria. *West African Medical Journal*. 1958; **7**: 58-62.

11. Aarons A, Hawes H, Gayton J. *Child to Child*. UK, Macmillan, 1979.

ACCIDENTS

There are many gaps in our knowledge regarding the predisposing causes and types of accidents, the circumstances leading to them, their severity and their outcome. The common aetiological factors of accidents are road traffic, burns, falls and drowning. There are several others factors, such as animal bites, insect stings, snake bites, sharp wood and thorns that cause accidents in tropical countries. The types or nature of accidental injuries vary. They include: fractures, head injuries, bruises, dislocation, subluxation, cuts, puncture wounds, burns, scalds, drowning, bites and goring by cows; severity varies. For mild injuries parents do not seek medical treatment. Severe injuries that occur far away from health institutions do not reach hospitals due to transport difficulties. Hence, many accidents are not recorded or reported in tropical countries. The outcome of the accidents depends upon their management; where there is delayed treatment or no treatment at all, complications are likely to arise.

Accidents should be reported or registered according to age groups: 1-4, 5-9 and 10-14 years. This provides comparable data from different countries. The nature of accidents differs between these age groups. Children in the one to four year age group, are exploring and learning about their environment at home and suffer accidents which are not reported in the 10-14 year age group. Adolescents with their tendency to experiment have accidents in circumstances to which young children would not be exposed. Thus the age and developmental characteristics of the victim are important in the causation, nature and severity of

accidents. The sex of the victim is also an important factor: boys are usually far more affected by accidents than girls, except for burns which affect girls more than boys.

Most of the accidents involving young children occur at home or near home, with or without the presence of the adults. Childhood accidents outside the home occur in the playground, on the road, in public places or in leisure places while swimming or climbing. In each of the areas where accidents take place, there is a host of precipitating circumstances. These environmental factors must be recognized in order to prevent accidents.

Children may sustain burns, cuts or bruises from abuse by their parents or guardians in tropical countries.

As a part of primary health care, the communities should be involved in the prevention of accidents. First and foremost, people should be aware of the type of accidents that take place in their community. Local health workers, teachers, and school-leavers can all participate in community surveys for collection of data which can be analysed to provide the basic information on the type, frequency and severity of the accidents, who is the involved victim, when and where they are involved and the possible circumstances. The community should also be involved in formulating methods of prevention. The World Health Organization is currently working out questionnaires which can be tested for use in the developing countries for this type of exercise.

As in the case of accidental poisoning, community health workers and other influential members of the community need to be aware of the various forms of accidents and their consequences. This information can be given in a number of ways: on news media, newspapers, radios and television. Newspapers in the vernacular would be the most effective method of dissemination of this knowledge.

Road traffic accidents

Road traffic accidents (RTA) have become a major public health problem, affecting both adults and children. These accidents are beginning to fall in number in most developed countries but they are rapidly rising in most of the developing tropical countries as transportation is developed in urban and rural areas. In many tropical countries, road traffic accidents occur in excess of the vehicle density; for instance, the accident rates per 100 million vehicles miles in developing countries are over twenty times higher than those of USA where the vehicle density is very high. Fatality rates from RTA in developing countries are 10–20 times those of developed countries. Children are involved in accidents as passengers in their parents' vehicles or buses, as pedestrians, or while at play near busy streets in urban areas.

Several factors collectively or singly facilitate or precipitate RTA. They include factors operating at several levels:

- road factors;
- characteristics of the victim;
- characteristics of the driver;
- features of the vehicle;
- miscellaneous factors.

Roads may have defects in construction in a poor state of repair with many pot-holes or slippery, or pass through a busy urban or rural market area, or may have few or confusing traffic signs. Streets may be poorly lit and roads in rural areas may have corners, or hills or bushes which obscure vision. Children may be careless in crossing the roads, or play alongside roads oblivious to the possible dangers from vehicles. They may be passengers sitting in seats without seat belts, or may be newcomers to towns and not know how to cross the streets. Generally, children below the age of nine years cannot safely cross streets unaccompanied. School crossings may be unavailable in urban streets for schoolchildren to use.

Drivers may be tired from driving trucks or buses for long distances without rest or may be under the influence of alcohol or drugs. They may be poorly trained, and hence, unskilled. Drivers of commercial trucks have the habit of driving in the middle of the roads and at great speeds with no regard to drivers of small vehicles. Such drivers often cause accidents during the day, but especially at night. Vehicles may be in a poor state of maintenance with no brakes, headlights or horns. There are many such unroadworthy vehicles on the roads in developing countries.

Stray goats or cows may roam onto the roads and streets in town. Motor cycles, bicycles, rickshaws and carts all share the roads and are commonly involved in accidents. In wet seasons, fog and rain interfere with visibility, thus contributing to the occurrence of accidents. Night travel, vehicles broken down and left on the road at night, or slow-moving vehicles commonly increase the risk of accidents.

Studies from Europe show that the age group 6–14 years has the highest risk from road traffic accidents and that boys are more affected than girls. Studies in developing countries are awaited to provide this information. Boys cycling in a busy tropical urban area

are known to be involved frequently in RTA. A recent police release in Kenya reported that 1 691 people died from traffic accidents in 1985: 754 passengers, 713 pedestrians and 224 drivers. A total of 12 459 people were injured in that year, of whom 17 per cent were children compared with 14 per cent in 1984. This increased trend in occurring in other developing countries.

Injuries resulting from RTA include fractures, joint dislocations, wounds, internal injuries to organs and structures, cuts and bruises. Fractures which normally involve the femur, tibia, humerus, radius and ulna may be compound fractures with big open wounds and bleeding vessels. The internal organs commonly injured are the spleen, liver, intestines and urinary bladder. Chest injuries involving tears of the lung and head injuries with concussion and tentorial tears are also common. Injuries are usually multiple.

Initial management at the site of the accident is usually by non-medical personnel. At the hospital, junior doctors are the first line of medical staff to attend to such injuries, hence in their training they should be instructed in the correct procedures of managing injuries. Casualty management should consist of first seeing that the patient is breathing and that the airway is clear; many lives are lost from respiratory failure. Any bleeding should be stopped by application of clean cotton wool and bandages. The patient should be asked where the pain is and analgesics given to relieve that pain. The patient should be in a safe and comfortable position to stop further injuries. Evidence of shock should be looked for and, if present, should be corrected by intravenous fluids and/or blood transfusion. The patient should be thoroughly assessed for head and spinal injuries. A system-by-system check is done so as not to miss any injuries. Rib fractures and long bone and skull fractures are determined or excluded by x-ray investigations (but see pp. 1023–4).

Injuries on the road, like injuries on the farm, may be complicated by tetanus. The patient should therefore be given tetanus toxoid at monthly intervals – three doses altogether.

Patients who are unable to reach health institutions are liable to develop wound infections and their unreduced fractures heal with limb deformities or shortening, which handicaps the subsequent life of child. Those surviving with head injuries may have mental retardation crippling them for life. Treatment of some of the RTA injuries usually take a long time and is costly to the state or the family. During treatment, the child may miss many days of schooling. These social and economic costs add to the misery of the child and anxiety of the family. Mortality depends upon the initial life support. This calls for members of the community to know first-aid and apply it, rather than shy away or stand by at the site of accident just waiting for the police to come, while the victim is in real danger.

Prevention

Prevention of road traffic accidents involves proper construction and maintenance of roads and proper street lighting. Dangerous junctions should be avoided and zebra crossings constructed in appropriate places. Legislature should be enforced to curb reckless driving and driving under the influence of alcohol. Seat belts in vehicles should be used. Children should be instructed in the proper use of road signs as a practical example in a specially designed area with traffic signs. Theoretical instruction can also be done at school. There should be school crossing areas manned during the time the children come to and leave school. Youths should wear head helmets while riding motor cycles and a speed limit enforced. Vehicles should not be overloaded. Vehicles travelling at night should have rear reflectors, so that if one breaks down and is abandoned on the highway it can be seen by an approaching driver. All vehicles should undergo regular checks to ensure that they are fit to be on the road. There is a need to review the instructions in driving by driving schools. Any flaws during tests should be curbed, particularly the possibilities of new drivers bribing the driving test officials to give licences before they acquire driving skills.

Falls

Falls commonly occurs in children of all ages. The actual causes of falls differ in different settings. In rural areas, children fall from trees which they climb for adventure or in pursuit of fruits. They also fall from steep slopes, buildings, rugged paths and on the poorly constructed floors of latrines; they may fall into wells. In urban areas, children fall from staircases, balconies, open concrete drains, worn-out street pavements, unfilled construction holes, discarded old vehicles, or from moving motor cycles, bicycles or vehicles. Small children are known to fall from open bedroom windows on to the pavement outside. Young children often fall at home while the older children are playing outside the home. Boys are more often involved in falls than girls.

Various injuries arise from falls. They include simple and compound fractures of limbs, bruises, cuts, head injuries and internal injuries involving rupture of spleen or liver. Severe injuries result in death, and head injuries may involve the brain. Facial injuries usually result in broken or lost teeth, injuries to the gums, lips or tongue. Treatment of injuries should be done immediately along the lines described in RTA. It is unusual to see deformities and infected wounds resulting from neglected and untreated fractures due to falls.

Prevention

Falls can be reduced by improving housing construction with safety standards. Busy pavements should be repaired regularly and whenever pot-holes develop. Drainage in urban areas should be well protected and construction pits should be filled. Trees along streets should be trimmed regularly to avoid branches falling on pedestrians and playing children. In rural areas, where the falls are mainly due to climbing trees, children should be instructed about climbing, while inexperienced small children should be stopped from climbing; here again the 'child-to-child' approach is useful.

Burns

Burns occur frequently in children all over the world. As in RTA, one should consider the causes, the victim, the circumstances leading to burns, the nature of the injuries and their treatment. Most occur in the home. The victim usually a young child, may pull a table cloth and spill kerosene from a lamp sitting on the table, starting a fire. Similarly, a candle left on the table with a table cloth can be pulled over by the child causing burns. Hot tea or soup may cause scalding in children in this way. Children may be left sleeping in locked houses which catch fire and burn them severely or to death. This is a particular risk during the dry season. In some tropical countries, lightning may strike a house or a school with children in the classrooms and start a fire. Kerosene and charcoal cooking-stoves are often used in the tropics and are a common cause of burns. With increasing industries in the tropical countries, children are sometimes burned by chemical disasters. Electric burns occur but rarely in the urban areas.

Cooking is often done on three stones on the ground, thus the crawling infant or toddler is at high risk of the burns or scalds from falling into such fires. A young child with no experience in the dangers of open fires, likes to experiment by putting his fingers in the fire. Such children have been known even to sit on the burning charcoal of a stove. Girls are more often involved in burning accidents than boys as they help with cooking. Children with epilepsy may fall into a fire while suffering a fit.

The extent of the injury is measured by the percentage of skin surface burnt. An estimate of the surface area of the burn may be derived from the rule of 9 for children over 12 years old; that is the head, arms, one-quarter of the trunk and one-half of each leg are each taken to represent 9 per cent of the body surface area. For each year under 12 years, the proportion of the head is 1 per cent greater and each lower extremity 0.5 per cent less. Burns exceeding 10 per cent body surface need resuscitation and urgent treatment. Moderately severe burns involve 10–30 per cent body surface while those above 30 per cent are severe and often fatal. Burns are also expressed in terms of depth of skin involved. Superficial burns are first-degree burns; these give rise to painful erythema. Second-degree burns involve partial thickness of the skin and are characterized by blisters. Third-degree burns involve the full thickness of the skin. Such deep burns expose the muscles, bones or ligaments and cannot heal without surgical intervention with skin grafting.

Many children with minor burns are never taken to hospitals; severely burnt children usually do go if the hospital is accessible. There are many such burnt patients in tropical hospitals. Some hospitals have established burns units so as to give specialized care. First-aid treatment at home with various oils, ghee, butter and herbal medicines may increase the risk of infection. Septicaemia and tetanus are not unusual in burnt patients in the tropics. Early hospital treatment aims at preventing infection by covering the burnt area with a clean sterile gauze.

Open treatment of burnt wounds is preferred to closed treatment. Analgesics are given for pain. Substantial fluid loss occurs; shock requires aggressive treatment with intravenous fluids including plasma. Surgical intervention is usually necessary. Sepsis is anticipated and treated as it arises; tetanus toxoid is advised. Burns involving skin around joints are notoriously known to cause contactures, particularly if neglected. Burns on the face interfere with the child's appearance causing embarrassment to child and family. Keloid formation is common in Africans, again affecting the appearance of the child.

Prevention

Raising the cooking place is effective in keeping the toddlers away from open fires or hot liquids. Similarly, kerosene stoves should be kept out of reach of children. Electrical fixtures should be repaired regularly in urban houses to avoid loose connections causing short circuits and fires. Protecting houses from lightning should be enforced in areas where this is a menace; the use of wire conductors would be quite effective. Most traditional grass-thatched houses in Africa have a long top-stick on the roof. This is normally in contact with a central post in the middle of the hut and it is possible that it functions as an earthing conductor. As tropical countries have increasing cloth manufacturing industries, legislature should prohibit manufacture of dangerous inflammable clothes.

Neighbours should participate in looking after children in urban slums when a mother goes out to the market, rather than leaving the children locked up only to burn to death if the house happens to catch fire.

Drowning

Toddlers and small children are at great risk of drowning in lakes, rivers, canals, wells or puddles of water. Fortunately, hypothermia is not so great a problem in the tropics. During the rainy season, unfilled construction holes and old quarries get filled with water and attract small children to swim. Torrential rains cause flash floods in which children may be the first to drown.

Prevention

Teaching children to swim is very effective in reducing drowning. The public should participate in draining unnecessary collections of water. Construction companies should be required to fill the big open holes from which they scoop soil while constructing buildings or roads. Such holes are common in tropical cities, along highways and in quarries.

SNAKE BITE

Martin Brueton

Identification and diagnosis
Clinical features
Treatment

Antivenin
Prevention
Further reading

It is estimated that there are about 3000 species of snakes in the world and these are found predominantly in the tropical regions of the continents of Asia, Africa and America. At least 400 of these species belong to the four families Colubridae, Elapidae, Viperidae and Hydrophidae which are usually regarded as venomous. The distinction between venomous and non-venomous snakes is so ill-defined that any snake bites should be regarded as potentially serious. They are largely a problem in the rural tropics, thus reliable data for incidence, mortality and morbidity are scarce. In India, the annual mortality has been reported to exceed 20 000 and in Brazil 2000.

Venom is the secretion of modified salivary glands connected by ducts to the poison fangs situated in the upper jaw either at the front or at the back. It is a complex mixture of enzymes and proteins with different activities, and its composition and toxicity may vary with the age and physical state of the snake and the environmental conditions.

Some useful medical generalizations about venom effects can be made by considering the four major snake families concerned.

Colubridae

The poisonous species have fangs at the rear of the upper jaw. Because of the situation of the fangs, only large snakes can inflict a dangerous bite to human beings. In certain regions of Africa the boomslang is the most dangerous snake of this family. The venom is highly haemolytic in action.

Elapidae

This family has fixed poison fangs in the front of the upper jaw. Cobras, kraits (*Bungarus*), mambas, and all the poisonous snakes in Australia, and the coral snakes belong to this family. The majority of the poisonous species produce a neurotoxin.

Viperidae

Vipers have large poison fangs in the upper jaw lying posteriorly against the palate in a sheath of mucous membrane when relaxed, but these become straight at the time of bite. Usually, reserve fangs are found on either side of the main fangs. The head is usually covered with small scales. In some species large scales may be found. The puff adder (*Bitis*), Russell's viper and *Echis carinatus* belong to this family. Members of the subfamily Crotalinae are distinguished by the presence of a sense organ located between the eye and the nostril. The mocassin and copperheads of North America, the pit viper of Asia, the bushmaster (*Lachesis muta*), and the rattlesnakes all belong to this family. The venom has a potent anticoagulant effect.

Hydrophidae

Sea snakes are found in warm waters of tropical areas. They have valvular openings on the top of the snout and vertically flattened tails. All the species belonging to this family are reported to be poisonous but are rarely aggressive.

Identification and diagnosis

In this short section it is not possible to give details of methods of identifying poisonous species in the tropical regions of the world. It is of the greatest importance that the medical practitioner is acquainted with the identifying characteristics of poisonous snakes likely to be encountered in the area where he or she practises. In most countries it will be possible to obtain charts giving salient features for distinguishing poisonous from non-poisonous snakes. The diagnosis of a snake bite case can be simplified materially if the snake has been captured. Unfortunately, the living or dead snake is seldom brought for inspection and, if so, the battered, mutilated body of the snake often presents difficulties in identification. The description by the patient or relatives is usually vague.

Clinical manifestations will indicate whether a patient has been bitten by a poisonous snake or by a non-poisonous one, and the medical officer will have to rely more on clinical judgement, based on local and general signs and symptoms, to decide whether a patient requires specific therapy or not.

The coagulability of the child's blood may be helpful diagnostically. Russell's viper and *Echis* bites can be ruled out, provided the test is done 30 minutes or later after the bite, if the blood from a finger collected on a clean watch glass coagulates in less than 10 minutes. By this simple means and in the absence of neurotoxic symptoms, it is surprising how many cases can be discharged without using antivenin. In addition, the microscopic examination of the urine for red cells is not infrequently of diagnostic value.

Poisoning as a result of Elapidae (cobra and krait) bites is characterized by the rapid onset of typical central nervous system signs. These do not always follow the same sequence or pattern. Variation will depend upon numerous factors, including the dose of venom injected, the size of the snake and in children the age and weight of the patient. Young children, therefore, have the highest mortality.

Clinical features

These include local cytotoxic changes and general effects with signs of neuro-, cardio- or nephrotoxicity, reduced blood coagulability and venom hypersensitivity reactions.

Local

The bites by Elapidae (kraits, mambas), coral snakes and sea snakes do not produce any local swelling. Cobra bites may produce local reactions which vary from place to place. A burning sensation at the site of the bite followed by numbness or shooting pain along the axis of the limb may develop. Bites by Viperidae and Crotalidae usually produce marked oedema, oozing from the wound, petechiae, or local discoloration. The extent of the swelling will indicate the severity of envenomation.

A tight tourniquet, applied just above the area of the bite and not loosened at 15–20 minutes intervals to allow brief circulatory reflow, invariably produces severe oedema in the area of the bite. This makes it difficult for the attending physician to determine whether the swelling is due to poison or due to the blocking of the circulation.

Fang marks may not always be easy to locate. If they are located, the distance between the fang marks can give an indication as to the size of the snake.

Bites by non-poisonous snakes as a rule do not give rise to intense pain and local swelling is minimal.

General

Elapidae If the symptoms are of the nature of ptosis, strabismus, slurred speech, dysphagia, and drooling of saliva, along with vomiting, giddiness, muscular weakness and drowsiness, it may be taken as the bite by a member of the Elapidae family (or sea snake group – see later). The patient may complain of a sensation of weight on the chest. There may be laboured respiration and the temperature of the patient may be normal or subnormal. Little local reaction may be seen in these bites but pain radiating from the bite may begin within an hour or more. In the case of krait and coral snake bites, sometimes there may be violent abdominal pain, but in the case of cobra bites there may be considerable local pain and swelling, occasionally followed by necrosis.

Viperidae In cases of Viperidae bites, the pain is so severe in character that the victim feels as if a hot coal has been placed on his skin. There is marked oedema, often with local serum-filled blebs, ecchymosis, an increased clotting time and persistent oozing of blood from the site of the puncture, proportionately more profuse relative to the depth of the wound inflicted. A fall in blood pressure with a small volume, thready pulse, nausea, vomiting and collapse may occur. Pupils are widely dilated but are sensitive to light. Haemoptysis and epistaxis are quite common and haematuria is present in varying degrees. Petechiae are often extensive and subconjunctival haemorrhages may be present. Severe abdominal pain may occur due to extravasation of blood into the peritoneal cavity. In severe poisoning, unless promptly treated with specific antivenin, convulsions follow and death often ensues from cardiac failure. Even if death does not supervene, extensive local sloughing, suppuration or gangrene may develop in the bitten limb.

Hydrophidae Sea snake bites show little or no local symptoms. Symptoms may appear after a latent period of 30 minutes to a few hours. There may be muscular pain, stiffness and progressive weakness. Ptosis and incoordination of muscles may be seen. In cases of severe envenomation, blurring of vision, thirst, vomiting and difficulty in breathing occur. The urine of such patients contains myoglobin, albumin and erythrocytes. Tubular necrosis may be followed by acute renal failure.

Treatment

Delayed or inadequate treatment may result in disaster. It is essential that the nature of poisoning be determined before initiating specific antivenin therapy. Treatment to be effective must:

- arrest further absorption of the venom at the site of the bite;
- destroy as much venom as possible from the wound locally;
- neutralize the systemic absorbed venom by specific antivenin therapy;
- counteract the systemic reactions produced by the venom;
- be prepared for the untoward hypersensitive reactions due to foreign proteins in the antivenin;
- provide for follow-up watchfulness and care for secondary reactions including infection.

Most patients and relatives are terrified and require reassurance. The limbs should be immobilized using a splint or sling. Analgesics should be given, avoiding salicylates which can exacerbate gastric bleeding; persistent vomiting should be treated with chlorpromazine. Close attention must be paid to general supportive measures, such as maintaining an airway in the presence of jaw or tongue paralysis and vomiting.

Adjustment of fluid and electrolyte balance is indicated in the presence of shock, severe vomiting, haematuria and albuminuria. The onset of anaphylaxis requires treatment with steroids and antihistamines. In the neurotoxic syndrome, oxygen is helpful to overcome hypoxia and respiratory impairment. In the event of respiratory failure, prolonged artificial respiration should be resorted to, particularly in Elapidae envenomation.

The presence of necrotic tissue, interference with local blood supply, and the toxic action of venom on leucocytes and other phagocytic cells increase the hazard of secondary bacterial infection which may necessitate antimicrobial therapy. Tetanus prophylaxis with toxoid or antitoxin is advisable. Gas-gangrene antitoxin is not recommended as a regular measure. Some authorities recommend the use of EDTA if tissue necrosis is due to snake venom.

Intramuscular injections should be avoided since they can lead to large haematomas.

A tourniquet is commonly applied, using a handkerchief or piece of cloth, a few centimetres proximal to the fang marks to occlude the venoms and lymphatic flow from the bitten area; although there is no good evidence of benefit from human studies. It is important not to increase local ischaemia or cause local oedema which might be mistaken for the effects of a bite from an innocuous snake. The ligature should be released for 60 seconds after every 15 minutes and may be moved proximally as the swelling increases; it should be removed only after specific antivenin therapy is started. Unless an incision is carried out within a few minutes of the bite, most authorities agree that late incision and suction of blood may do more harm than good, by introducing infection and causing persistent bleeding.

The bitten part and the surrounding skin should be washed with a mild antiseptic, such as a weak solution of potassium permanganate, to inactivate the unabsorbed venom. (For 'splitting' cobra eye injury see p. 937.)

Antivenin

In cases of snake venom poisoning, specific antivenin is the only effective remedy in saving the life of a patient. Antivenins are usually prepared from horse serum by approximately 30 laboratories in various parts of the world. Most are intended for treatment of bites from the important venomous snakes of that particular geographical area. In India, the antivenin produced is polyvalent, and is effective against the venoms of the four most common, potentially lethal species (cobra, krait, Russell's viper and *Echis*) present in that country.

Most commercial antivenins are now purified immunoglobulins, and they carry a lesser risk of serum reactions. Antivenin is indicated if there is severe systemic envenomation, as evidenced by hypotension or other signs of cardiotoxicity, neurotoxicity, impaired consciousness, spontaneous bleeding or impaired coagulation. Supporting evidence includes a peripheral leucocytosis, ECG abnormalities, rising serum enzymes, haematuria, myoglobinuria, uraemia, oliguria and severe anaemia.

Preliminary intradermal skin testing should be carried out – if it is positive, pretreatment with epinephrine and antihistamines may be partially effective in preventing reactions. The best results are obtained if the full quantity of antiserum in all severe cases of envenomation is injected intravenously diluted in glucose saline immediately the diagnosis is made. The dose of antivenin in children should not be less than that recommended by the manufacturer for adults, as the concentration of venom in children is more than that in adults. An aqueous solution of adrenaline should be kept ready in case of any adverse reaction. It is advantageous to infiltrate the area around the fang marks with antivenin in cases of viperine poisoning if these are seen shortly after being bitten. This will help to detoxify the venom locally to some extent and prevent necrotic changes in the area which is one of the features of viperine venom.

Non-poisonous snake bites generally require no treatment, unless the snake was a python or other large species. Precautions against bacterial infection should be taken. The snake's teeth frequently break off in the wound and should be removed.

Prevention

Most snakes are timid and nervous, attempting to escape and seek cover when disturbed. Particularly dangerous activities are collecting firewood, poking sticks into burrows, holes and crevices and climbing rocks and trees covered in dense foliage. Snakes are nocturnal for the most part, sheltering in dark places during the day. Unlit paths and roads are particularly dangerous after heavy rain. The likelihood of snakes remaining in the vicinity of dwellings can be reduced by eliminating the rodent population, by keeping the surroundings clean and the grass short. Children should be prevented from playing in disused buildings, rubble, and areas overgrown with grass.

Further reading

Smith HM, Smith RB, Saurin HL. A summary of snake classification (Reptilia Serpentes). *Journal of Herpetology.* 1977; **11**: 115–21.

Warrell DA, Snakes. In: Strickland GT ed. *Hunter's Tropical Medicine.* 6th edn. Philadelphia, Saunders, 1984. pp. 800–12.

Warrell DA. Davidson NM, Greenwood BM *et al.* Poisoning by bites of the saw-scaled or carpet viper (*Echis carinatus*) in Nigeria. *Quarterly Journal of Medicine.* 1977; **46**: 33–62.

WHO. Progress in the characterization of venoms and standardization of antivenoms. WHO Offset Publication No. 58. Geneva, World Health Organization, 1981.

ARTHROPOD-PRODUCED DISEASES
A. Miller

Myiasis	Blood-sucking arthropods
Ectoparasites	Stinging insects
Pediculosis	Urticating caterpillars
Fleas	Vesicating beetles
Ticks	Venomous arthropods
Chiggers or 'red bugs'	Allergy
Other mites	Diagnostic and protective meaasures
Scabies	Further reading
Bites and stings	

Myiasis

The worm-like larval forms of various insects occasionally infest children through outdoor exposure, close association with animals, or ingestion of contaminated food. Flies (Diptera) of various kinds are almost always responsible for such parasitism, which is then known as myiasis, and is diagnosed by finding living fly maggots in various parts of the human body. Typical larvae are cylindrical, whitish, segmented, legless and headless, ranging in length from 1 to 30 mm.

Cutaneous myiasis

Myiasis may begin in healthy skin and produce furunculoid or migratory lesions, or it may arise in abrasions and wounds in which flies deposit eggs or larvae. Only one or a few larvae are usually present in the former types of lesions, while many, sometimes of several species, commonly occur in the latter event.

Papular or furunculoid lesions, eventually opening at the summit through which the larva breathes and may be detected, are characteristic of the human or tropical bot, *Dermatobia hominis*, in the American tropics, and of the tumbu fly, *Cordylobia anthropophaga*, in Africa. Boil-like lesions may be occasionally caused by the primary screw-worm, *Cochliomyia hominivorax (americana)*, throughout the New World; by cattle warbles, *Hypoderma* spp., which are world-wide although not indigenous in Africa; by flesh flies, *Wohlfahrtia* spp., and by various species of bot flies that normally infest wild animals in temperate as well as tropical regions of the world.

Dermatobia glues its eggs to mosquitoes, flies, or ticks and the larvae drop to the skin of man when these carriers alight on it. *Cordylobia* deposits eggs on soil, clothing, or bedding and the larvae penetrate the skin after contacting the host. *Cochliomyia* deposits eggs directly on the skin, and *Hypoderma* on body hair.

The lesions produced after the larvae penetrate are usually, but not necessarily, on exposed parts of the body, and are single, grouped, or widely separated. They commonly contain one larva, but sometimes several. Symptoms progress from minor itching and pain to local tenderness and severe pain as the lesions increase in size (to 20 mm or more) over a period of usually several weeks. Open lesions may produce a serous discharge, but there is little pus unless secondary bacterial infection and abscess formation occur after death or escape of the larva. The larvae when fully grown (15–30 mm) leave the host to pupate in the ground.

The larvae may be removed by slightly widening the already-present opening under local anaesthetic, and then gently squeezing out the maggot. Cleansing and the use of local antiseptics and antibiotics are indicated to combat secondary infection.

Migratory lesions, which occur infrequently, are of two types: itching serpentine superficial red tunnels (one form of creeping eruption) caused by the young larvae of horse bots, *Gasterophilus* spp., which are world-wide in distribution; and painful subcutaneous evanescent cysts due to the deeply wandering larvae of cattle warbles, *Hypoderma* spp., which are found all over the world, except in Africa where they have occurred only in imported cattle.

The lesion of creeping eruption, commonly on the arms, contains a single minute larva about 1 mm long with transverse rows of spines, which may advance 1 or 2 cm a day. The larvae are acquired either from handling horses bearing the eggs on their hair or from eggs deposited by the fly directly on the hairs of the patient's skin. The infestation terminates spontaneously, but may be treated by local freezing or by removal of the larva with a needle after applying machine oil to make the skin more transparent.

Infestation of man by cattle warbles results from exposure to the adult flies outdoors in association with cattle, or possibly from handling cattle which have eggs on their hairs. Individual larvae up to 2.5 cm (1 inch) in length have been excised from subdermal sites or cysts.

Traumatic cutaneous myiasis, originating in wounds upon which flies deposit eggs or larvae, may be caused by over 50 different species of flies. A few of these, such as the Old World screw-worm, *Chrysomya bezziana*, of Asia and Africa, are obligate parasites developing only in living tissues. The others, collectively of world-wide distribution, are facultative parasites that ordinarily breed in decaying organic matter, so that adults may be attracted by the odours or exudates of wounds or soiled skin and the larvae invade both necrotic and normal tissues. The effect of such infestation depends upon the nature and number of larvae, the extent and site of damage, and the advent of secondary infection. While the presence of scavenger species of larvae may promote healing of the wound, other types of larvae may cause permanent injury or death. Infestation may occur in bandaged as well as exposed wounds and begin in small abrasions as well as larger cutaneous lesions of any kind. Usually, a number of larvae are present burrowing in the tissues, sometimes several hundred of one or more species. They eventually leave the wound to pupate elsewhere, but the period of infestation may continue for weeks, especially if reinfestation is not prevented. Treatment consists of the manual removal of the larvae, and cleaning and dressing of the wound. Application of chloroform (5 per cent in a light vegetable oil) for 30 minutes by douching and wet-dressing aids the removal of larvae. There are no medications which will dislodge maggots. Chemical insults tend to make them retract making it more difficult to find or remove them.

Myiasis of orifices and cavities

Myiasis of the nose, mouth, ear, sinuses, anus, rectum or vagina, like the foregoing, may be caused by various species of larvae that are introduced by flies attracted to lesions or odorous discharges. Either facultative or obligate parasites may be involved and the degree of injury and systemic effects vary with the species, number and site.

Infestation of the nasal passages and sinuses is accompanied by severe headache, fever, swelling, and purulent bloody discharges (*peenach* of India, *bicheiro* of tropical America). Heavy infestations with screw-worms may result in erosion of cartilage or bone of the head, and even death. The sheep bot, *Oestrus ovis*, causes *tamné* or *thim'ni* in North Africa, particularly in shepherds, by depositing larvae in the nose or ear which penetrate the nasal cavities, sinuses and mouth, causing severe headache, pain, sleeplessness and inflammation.

Treatment consists essentially of the manual removal of larvae or dislodgement by various forms of irrigation, including ephedrine solution or a milk–chloroform emulsion.

Other forms of myiasis

Ocular and urinary myiasis occur rarely, but enteric myiasis may be occasionally encountered or suspected in children. More than 40 species of fly larvae have been reported as accidental parasites of the stomach or intestines. Heavy and prolonged infestations may produce enteritic and neurological symptoms of varying degrees of severity. The presence of maggots in stool specimens is inconclusive unless possible contamination from flies or soiled containers is precluded. Treatment consists of purging or the use of anthelmintic. An unusual type of maggot in Africa, the Congo floor maggot, pricks the skin to suck blood of persons sleeping on the floors of native huts.

The pentastomes, linguatulids, or 'tongue worms' are degenerate arachnids. In various tropical regions, especially in Central Africa, *Porocephalus armillatus* may infect children, and these long (male 3–5 cm, female 9–12 cm), cylindrical annulated parasites have been found singly or in numbers in the intestine, mesentery, lungs, beneath the conjunctiva and elsewhere. There is no specific treatment, except surgical removal.

Ectoparasites

Pediculosis

Infestation with lice is of common occurrence where hygienic standards are low. It may also be found, despite cleanliness, in children who acquire it from associates. Since human lice are restricted to man and animal lice do not infest him, pediculosis arises only from contact with other infested individuals or with objects bearing dislodged parasites.

Lice are segmented, flattened, pale or greyish in colour, and have a single clasping claw on each of the six legs. They live on or next to the skin, sucking blood several times a day, and can survive off the host no longer than one week. The eggs or 'nits' are glued to the base of hairs or in the inner seams and folds of clothing. They are whitish, ovoid, and 1 mm long, hatch in five to seven days on the body, and survive about a month at room temperature. The young lice mature in one to two weeks, and adults live about a month.

Head lice (*Pediculus humanus capitis*) and body lice (*P.h. humanus*) are elongate and attain a length of 3–4 mm. They cause small red pruritic papules, excoriation, and sometimes urticaria and secondary impetiginous infection.

Pubic or crab lice (*Phthirus pubis*) are short, broad, up to 2 mm long, and are less active that *Pediculus*. Although in adults they are most common on the pubic and peri-anal hair and also infest body hair and beard, in infants they occur on the scalp, and in older children on the eyelashes. The bites cause blue itching spots and eyelash infestation may cause blepharitis. Lice can transmit typhus, relapsing fever, and probably skin infections.

The treatments of choice are malathion and carbaryl, benzyl benzoate has been used traditionally but is more irritant to the skin. Lindane is no longer recommended because of the emergence of resistant strains. The most effective application is as a lotion which should be applied all over the body and to dry hair, allowed to dry and removed by washing after 12 hours. Lice and nits should be removed by fine-tooth combing. Family contacts should be treated and the powder preparations used to disinfect clothing and bedding.

Fleas

Fleas have a vertically compressed, segmented body and six legs; they are dark in colour and are active jumpers. Some that live on other animals, especially those on dogs, cats, rats, and pigs, also attack man to suck blood but usually do not stay on the skin. However, the sticktight flea (*Echidnophaga gallinacea*), and the chigoe or jigger flea (*Tunga penetrans*) remain attached for days. The eggs drop to the ground, floor, or into the nests and bedding of animals and here the larvae and pupae develop to adults. Rodent fleas transmit plague and murine typhus.

The sticktight flea infests poultry, wild birds, rats and domestic animals in warm regions, and children may be exposed to them in and around homes where the animal hosts are present. The fleas attach firmly to the skin, causing irritation and sometimes ulceration.

The chigoe occurs in tropical America, Africa and the West Indies, commonly parasitizing both animals and man. The female burrows into the skin, especially on the toes, feet and legs, grows to the size of a pea, and produces intense itching, inflammation, swelling and ulceration which may lead to severe secondary infection or tetanus. Multiple infestation sometimes produces a honeycomb appearance on the affected skin.

The fleas should be removed with a sterile needle or fine-pointed knife and the wounds treated and dressed. Shoes and insect repellents may be used prophylactically, and control around premises can occasionally be attempted by excluding or disinfesting animals, and by cleaning and treating floors and ground with insecticidal sprays or dusts, such as those containing, benzene hexachloride or malathion. Pet dogs and cats can be disinfested by flea powders or collars.

Ticks

Hard (ixodid) ticks attach firmly to the skin and have an unsegmented brown or grey body which is flat or swollen with blood and bears eight legs (six when young). They parasitize domestic and wild animals, lay their eggs on the ground, cling to vegetation to await a host, and attach to suck blood and remain fixed on the skin for a week or longer. Their presence may be unnoticed; when unfed they may appear to be moles, or they may be hidden in skin folds or under hair. The bite may cause only local erythema and irritation, rarely tumefaction or fever; potentially it may transmit tick typhus, spotted fever, plague, tularaemia, Lyme disease and other tick-borne diseases.

Especially in children, the bite of a single female tick which has been attached anywhere on the body for several days may very rarely cause a sudden onset of tick paralysis. An ascending, usually bilateral flaccid paralysis of Landry's type begins with incoordination, is complete in 12–24 hours, and may end fatally. Recovery usually occurs rapidly if the tick is removed before signs of bulbar paralysis appear. Tick paralysis occurs more frequently in girls than in boys, perhaps because ticks are more effectively hidden in long hair. Ticks should be removed by means of forceps, aided if necessary by applying petrolatum, ether, or heat, such as with a cigarette or hot match head, to induce withdrawal of the toothed anchoring mouthparts. Forceful removal may leave these imbedded and necessitate excision. Ticks in or around the home can be controlled by spraying or dusting with benzene hexachloride or other insecticides and applying similar dusts to dogs. Some protection from ticks outdoors is achieved by wearing boots and clothing that overlap upwards and by using repellents.

Soft (argasid) ticks may be domiciliary pests, living concealed in crevices or soil and emerging to suck blood for 15 to 30 minutes as the occupant sleeps or rests. Their bites may be irritating or painful, and can transmit relapsing fever, but they are not associated with tick paralysis.

Chiggers or 'red bugs'

Chiggers (not to be confused with chigoe fleas), also known as harvest mites and by various local names, are minute, red, six-legged larval mites (*Trombicula* spp.) which attach themselves to the skin by their mouthparts to feed for several days as parasites on small animals, birds and man. They develop in soil under vegetation and are encountered in grassy or wooded countryside. The bite produces an intensely itching red papule which becomes haemorrhagic and indurated and may persist for a week or more. The lesions, usually multiple, occur most frequently below the waist. Antipruritics and local anaesthetics must be re-applied frequently; topical collodion, with or without benzocaine, is effective for longer periods. Prompt bathing after exposure, with several applications of thick lather, will remove or kill chiggers and minimize the bites. Protection against attack is provided by insect repellents, such as diethyltoluamate, applied to bare arms and legs, and to edges and openings of clothing, or the use of permethrin-treated clothing. Liberal use of sulphur dust within clothing is also fairly effective. In India, South-east Asia and Japan some species of chiggers transmit scrub typhus (see p. 598).

Other mites

In addition to the scabies itch mite, parasitic rat and bird mites, non-parasitic mites infesting dry plant products and food may cause pruritic skin lesions. The food-infesting species may also be passed in stools, urine or sputum but are rarely pathogenic. Eradication measures should be aimed at the source of infestation. Blood-sucking rat and mouse mites can transmit rickettsial pox.

Scabies

This sarcoptid mite is discussed on p. 849.

Bites and stings

Blood-sucking arthropods

Insects, ticks and mites which pierce the skin to suck blood inject salivary toxins that cause varying reactions which depend upon the species of arthropod and the sensitivity of the individual. Mosquitoes, sandflies, biting gnats, bed-bugs, fleas, lice and mites typically produce pruritic macules, wheals or papules, but the degree of irritation and the progression, extent and duration of the lesions are affected by the individual's innate or acquired tolerance and the site of the 'bite'. Antipruritics, emollients and antiseptics relieve the itching and guard against secondary infection, while the immediate application of an antihistamine cream may decrease the reaction. The primary reactions may be more intense in young children than in adults, and children show a higher incidence of insect dermatoses. Hypersensitization may very occasionally result in local and systemic phenomena, extreme swelling, urticaria and other allergic manifestations seasonally over a period of years.

Papular urticaria (lichen urticatus) may result from sensitivity to fleas, bed-bugs, chiggers and mosquitoes, responding to protection from exposure by change of residence or the use of insecticides in the home. Soft ticks, 'kissing bugs' (triatomids), tsetses, and other bugs and flies inflict painful bites which may or may not produce local swelling and protracted effects in accordance with individual sensitivity. Avoidance, repellents, bed nets, screens and environmental control with insecticides may be variously enlisted to cope with the problem. Indoors, insecticidal sprays containing pyrethrins and chlorinated hydrocarbons will kill flying insects, while properly applied residual sprays provide long-lasting control against mosquitoes, bugs and fleas.

Stinging insects

Bees, wasps and some ants inject venom by means of a caudal sting, usually in self-defence or to protect nearby nests. The species vary in aggressiveness; various bees, hornets, yellow jackets, velvet 'ants' (wasps) and various ants are frequent offenders. The effect of the sting varies with species, site and sensitivity of the victim.

The initial sharp pain of bee and wasp stings is followed by local swelling and throbbing pain which gradually subside within a few hours. Numerous stings have cumulative, more prolonged, and sometimes systemic effects, but are rarely fatal. However, death from anaphylactic shock may occur within an hour following a single sting in hypersensitive individuals who have been sensitized by similar stings at some earlier time. Some tropical and subtropical bethylid wasps, which occasionally invade houses, inflict relatively mild stings but may produce short-lived systemic effects, such as numbness, itching, diarrhoea, and wheezing. The sting of the honeybee is armed with recurved teeth and the poison apparatus may remain attached to the skin after the bee is brushed away. It should be scraped off with finger nail or knife blade to prevent continued injection of venom. Prompt administration of topical or oral antihistamines, ice packs, soda, ammonia, or other palliatives and, if necessary, infiltration of 2 per cent procaine will relieve pain and swelling. For hypersensitive individuals, emergency treatment is imperative, using subcutaneous adrenaline or oral ephedrine sulphate together with antihistamines topically, orally or intravenously. If necessary, an intravenous infusion of procaine hydrochloride (0.1 per cent; 250–500 ml) may be considered. Desensitization may later be accomplished by a graded series of injections of bee venom.

Stinging ants include species varying from 1 to 25 mm in length. They usually attack in large numbers when the nest is disturbed, but some tropical species are spontaneously aggressive when foraging on the ground or on vegetation. Small fire ants (*Solenopsis* spp., South and Central America, southern USA) cause vesicular, pustular and indurated lesions which are initially painful and may have extensive and severe effects in children. The large *tucandeiras* (*Paraponera clavata*, Central and South America) cause agonizing burning pain and severe systemic symptoms for several hours, and by mass attack are capable of stinging a victim to death. Many species of ants do not sting but bite with their mandibles, causing pain and fright by the mechanical effects which are sometimes aggravated by venom or irritating secretions ejected on the wound. No specific antidotes for ant stings are known; local anaesthetics and sedatives may relieve acute distress until the pain eventually subsides. Ants around the home may be killed by chlordane sprays and poison baits, but for lasting control the colony must be destroyed by treating the nest with chlordane dust or fumigants (carbon bisulphide, DDVP, or cyanide, stored and used with proper precautions to avoid accidental poisoning of children and domestic animals).

Urticating caterpillars

'Stinging' by the larvae of certain moths and butterflies results from contact with poisonous body hairs or spines which release an irritating fluid when the tips are broken off. Such hairs or spines, either exposed or hidden, are possessed by relatively few species in certain groups of Lepidoptera of world-wide distribution; most caterpillars are harmless. Contact is made with urticating species by accidental brushing or pressing against the larvae. Epidemic dermatitis, irritation of oral and respiratory mucosa, and sometimes even asthma may be caused by wind-blown poison-hairs from cast skins when a species is abundant. A few species of adult moths also have irritating properties and cause outbreaks of dermatitis when, attracted by lights, they settle on exposed skin.

The effect varies with species, degree of contact and individual sensitivity, ranging from a minor stinging sensation to extensive rashes, swelling, intense local pain, malaise and prostration. Children may rarely be severely affected, developing fever, nausea, vomiting and paralytic symptoms that may continue for several days. The contact site should be promptly cleaned with soap and water or alcohol, and a palliative such as calamine lotion applied. Pain and systemic effects may require sedation with phenobarbitone, analgesics and bed rest or hospitalization. Oral antihistamines and corticosteroids are said to have been beneficial for acute cases in South America.

Vesicating beetles

Blister beetles (Meloidae) of world-wide distribution, and some tropical staphylinid beetles (*Paederus* spp.) contain cantharidin or other irritating substances in their body fluids. They are encountered on plants or around lights, and, when crushed on the skin, they cause a burning sensation, erythema and blisters which heal in a few days but may leave a scar. Washing and calamine lotion are palliative. Contact may sometimes produce acute conjunctivitis, fever, headache and arthralgia, and accidental swallowing can cause severe intoxication and irritation of the urinary system.

Venomous arthropods

The bites of centipedes, soft ticks and some bugs sometimes cause local pain and swelling with varying systemic effects, but the symptoms are self-limited if uncomplicated by secondary infection and are not fatal. Hard ticks may cause a fatal paralysis, as mentioned earlier.

Spiders

Although most spiders are harmless, the bites of certain species may cause severe injury. Poison is injected by a pair of anterior fangs. Local pain and swelling result from the bites of American tarantulas. Extensive necrotic, slow-healing lesions, gangrenous sloughing and systemic effects are caused by some South American ground spiders and the house-inhabiting *Loxosceles laeta* of Chile and Uruguay and localized necrotic ulcers by *L. reclusa* of South-eastern and Central United States. Severe systemic symptoms and sometimes death, especially in young children, are caused by the black widow (*Latrodectus mactans*; Canada to Chile) and related spiders (*L. tredecimguttatus*, *L. geometricus*, and other varieties occurring variously in the Mediterranean area, Africa, Asia, Australia, Philippines, Hawaii and West Indies). *L. mactans*, which attains a body length of 13 mm and a leg spread of 40 mm, is black with a red, typically hourglass-shaped, ventral spot, and variable additional red spots on the abdomen. It usually occurs on or near the ground or in outhouses, but may be encountered elsewhere. The female bites on chance contact but is aggressive only when guarding eggs in the web. Sharp pain at the site of the bite (two punctures) is followed quickly by spreading pain, muscular aches and spasms, cramps, abdominal rigidity, motor disturbances, anxiety, hyperactive reflexes, convulsions and shock; nausea, dyspnoea, cold sweats and leucocytosis may occur. The symptoms may simulate appendicitis or other acute abdominal conditions, including, in Negro children, a sickle-cell crisis. Death may result in 18–36 hours, but usually the acute symptoms abate after 24 hours and subside in three or four days, although a long convalescence may ensue.

While ligature and application of an ice bag immediately after the bite may minimize the effects, serious cases require bed rest, sedation and the use of specific antivenin (Lyovac, 2.5–5 ml), if available. The pain may be somewhat relieved by slow intravenous or intramuscular injection of 10 per cent calcium gluconate (0.05–0.1 ml/kg, repeated as necessary) or intravenous injection of a muscle relaxant (e.g. methocarbamol), prolonged hot baths, and subcutaneous morphine sulphate alone or with intramuscular phenobarbitone. For localized pain, infiltration with procaine is effective. Cortisone therapy has been found helpful in both systemic and necrotic arachnidism. Dapsone (50 mg twice daily) has been shown to be effective in treating the necrotic effects of brown recluse spider venom (*L. reclusa*). Spiders around the home may be controlled by crushing, burning or spraying them with chlordane.

Scorpions

These inject venom by means of a caudal sting (single puncture). Only some species produce neurotoxic systemic effects; others cause only intracutaneous local haemorrhage and bee sting-like pain and swelling that subsides in a few hours or a day or two. The noxious species may cause death, particularly in children under seven years of age (case fatality rates up to 60 per cent in some areas). Intense local pain (but no swelling at site), and sometimes regional lymphangitis and lymphadenitis are quickly followed by generalized numbness, weakness, muscular spasm, epigastric pain, excessive salivation and rhinorrhoea, rapid breathing and dyspnoea, speech impairment, fever, excitement and convulsions (precipitated by a touch or noise), drowsiness and prostration. The symptoms may gradually subside, or death may occur from respiratory paralysis. Prompt application of a tourniquet and an ice pack may slow the spread of venom from the site of injection. Local infiltration of 2 per cent procaine solution to relieve the pain and sedation with short-acting barbiturates are of value. Supportive treatment and group-specific antivenin, if available, should be administered. Scorpions are susceptible to DDT and chlordane.

Allergy

Atopic hypersensitivity to arthropods or their products may occur as idiosyncrasies in children more often than in adults. It may be manifested as exaggerated immediate or delayed reactions, or anaphylactic shock following bites or stings, as indicated above; as periodic or chronic urticaria, eczema, oedema or asthma from arthropod debris in house dust or regional atmospheres; or as digestive, dermal or respiratory symptoms after the ingestion of shellfish or honey. Ubiquitous floor or dust mites (*Dermatophagoides* spp. and others) are the source of potent allergens in house dust.

Diagnostic and protective measures

Diagnosis of arthropod injury, infestation or allergy involves awareness of possible aetiology, circumstantial history of exposure, specific knowledge of the habits and pathogenicity of suspect arthropods, and their identification from available specimens or the patient's description. Signs and symptoms may or may not be specific, and require differential diagnosis from a wide range of other pathologies, including entomophobia. The nature, location and chronology of lesions or systemic effects and the milieu and activities of the patient should be considered. Protective measures are defined by the nature of the arthropod. Avoidance of exposure of children to attack or infestation may variously include good hygiene, sanitation or disinfestation of premises, the use of bed nets, screens or protective clothing, and the application of repellents to skin or clothing. Children should be cautioned and taught to avoid contact with spiders, scorpions and caterpillars as a general safeguard.

Further reading

Bariga O. Immune reactions to arthropods. In: *Immunology of Parasitic Infections.* Baltimore, University Park Press, 1981. pp. 283–317.

Bücherl W, Buckley E eds. *Venomous Animals and their Venoms,* Vol. III. *Venomous Invertebrates.* New York, Academic Press, 1971.

Nelson WA, Bell JF, Clifford CM *et al.* Interaction of ectoparasites and their hosts. *Journal of Medical Entomology.* 1977; **13**: 389–428.

Pennell TC, Babu SS, Meredith JW. The management of snake and spider bites in the south eastern United States. *American Surgery.* 1987; **53**: 198–204.

Yunginger JW. Advances in the diagnosis and treatment of stinging insect allergy. *Pediatrics.* 1981; **67**: 325–8.

SECTION 6

Practical Aids

Tony Waterston

CHAPTER 1

Introduction

Tony Waterston

The doctor working in an isolated environment in a developing country needs practical help from supporting services in both diagnosing and treating the awkward problems which have a habit of presenting at inconvenient times of the day or night. This section is designed to be a guide to the 'back-up' services, which (if they are available) are not always used in the most effective way. In developed and developing countries alike, laboratory technicians find that requests are made for investigations which are inappropriate. This is the first meaning of the term 'appropriate' which appears throughout this section: 'well-fitted to the need'. Thus in the investigation of anaemia, we learn from Dr. Hughes (pp. 974–84) which tests are appropriate.

A broader meaning of the term 'appropriate' appears on pp. 968–92. Here consideration is given to the need not just of the individual patient, but also of the country and the setting in which he or she lives. This public health responsibility must be taken seriously in view of doctors' access to a large slice of national resources. Yet if equipment and drugs are used profligately (with the best of motives) they will only be available to the favoured few and supplies will not last long. Hence our technology (of investigation, hospital care and follow-up treatment) should be appropriate—and this does not mean second best. Appropriate technology is just as important a concept for industrialized countries as it is for the less-developed: in most Northern States, the costs of health care are rapidly outstripping the funds allocated. Costs can be reduced, often with additional benefit of individual patients, by a careful assessment of which tests and which drugs are both appropriate and cost-effective.

The last two chapters (Clements and Seaman) aim to give assistance in difficult situations—with regard to sick children as individuals and in a group. Sadly there are few paediatricians who may not at some time be faced with the problems of planning the care of displaced children 'en masse'. It is here that teamwork is of the essence, since paediatricians must work with agriculturalists, aid officials and politicians to mitigate the grave effects of such a disaster. Here too, the emphasis should be on the response which is most appropriate to the situation.

CHAPTER 2

The appropriate use of drugs

Nigel Speight

The importance of drugs

Safe, cheap and effective drugs are a vital part of any strategy to improve the health of children in the Third World. These drugs must be distributed widely and in large quantities to meet the needs of whole populations, most of whom live in rural areas. Unfortunately, so many factors operate to prevent this that it remains a distant prospect in most countries. Instead, most district hospitals, health centres and dispensaries are in permanently short supply of most essential drugs. Their staff, however well-trained, are therefore helpless to combat the majority of common treatable conditions. This inevitably undermines their prestige in the eyes of the local population and handicaps their efforts in other important areas such as health education and preventive medicine.

One problem is philosophical. In the controversy between the proponents of preventive and curative medicine, drugs have been seen as very much a part of the latter and have suffered accordingly. However, the preventive versus curative debate is increasingly a non-issue, in that both approaches are seen as important in their own right, and are complementary rather than alternatives. In any case, drugs frequently play a vital role in preventive strategies. For instance, part of any antituberculosis campaign involves the curative drug treatment of established cases. Similarly, any strategy to prevent rheumatic heart disease in children must provide the entire child population with easy and early access to penicillin. Vaccines and oral contraceptives are examples of drugs which are purely preventive.

In addition, much of the promotional activity of drug firms is rightly seen to be inappropriate and therefore to be resisted. However, this issue (which is explored further later) should not be allowed to inhibit wide usage of effective drugs prescribed rationally. Opponents of inappropriate Western technology should not discourage the search for an appropriate technology of drugs.

Problems of drug availability

Supply and distribution

Most drugs have to be imported using scarce foreign exchange. While most countries are attempting to reduce this dependency by establishing local pharmaceutical industries, it is unlikely that they will be able to become self-reliant in this field of high technology in the short-term future. The main question is how to get the best value for money from what foreign exchange is available. A ruthless policy of cost-effectiveness is vital to ensure maximum benefit to the whole population.

The question of cost-effective drug policies is examined in greater detail later. Assuming these have been implemented, there still remains the problem of supply and distribution. Most countries have problems in directing doctors to rural areas, and drugs have a natural tendency to follow doctors. Thus, national teaching hospitals usually have a large number of doctors who have relatively easy access to extremely expensive drugs. There is then a gradation down through regional and district hospitals, and at the bottom are health centres and dispensaries staffed by paramedics with very few essential drugs at their disposal.

The only solution to this gross imbalance is to limit the availability of expensive drugs in teaching hospitals, and to use the freed resources to increase the quantity of drugs flowing to the periphery. This is essentially a political problem and the strength of the vested interests involved should not be underestimated. Doctors at the national teaching hospitals form a powerful lobby, especially when they number most of the leading politicians and their families among their patients!

Cost-effectiveness and drug prescribing

The practice of medicine in the developing world has been strongly influenced by Western medicine in the past and this continues to be the case. While much of this influence has been beneficial, one area where this is not so is in the approach to prescribing drugs. Western doctors have been able to indulge in extravagant prescribing policies, confident that the state, the insurance company or the patient will foot the bill. Therapeutics are largely taught in isolation from questions of cost, so that doctors are free to luxuriate in the philosophy of the best drug for the patient regardless of cost. The pharmaceutical industry has been only too happy to exploit this, producing a stream of new drugs with claims that they are superior to their predecessors. Advertising pressure persuades doctors to prescribe new drugs while older drugs are pushed into premature obsolescence as their patents expire and they become less profitable. This is unnecessarily wasteful even in the context of relatively wealthy countries and highly inappropriate when it occurs in the Third World.

The mass of pharmaceuticals available can, in general, be subdivided into two main groups which for the purpose of discussion are labelled types A and B.

Characteristics of a type A drug

- invented more than 15 years ago;
- safe and effective and has withstood the test of time;
- widely used since development;
- cheap because of wide usage, expiry of patent and subsequent price competition;
- available as generic name preparation;
- not advertised and in danger of becoming obsolete;

Characteristics of a type B drug

- developed within last 10–15 years and therefore:
- still on patent and therefore:
- only available under brand name;
- heavily advertised under brand name;
- extremely expensive relative to type A alternative;
- some advantage claimed in efficacy, safety or convenience relative to type A alternative (this seldom justifies the increased cost).

Relative to the health care budget of any developing country, it is economically impossible to provide type B drugs for the whole population.[1] Every time a type B drug is used it wastes resources that could have been spent on more type A drugs for more people. The cost differential between most type A and type B drugs is not merely 10–20 per cent; many type B drugs are 50–100 times as expensive as type A equivalents. The whole therapeutic emphasis in developing countries should therefore be placed on type A drugs.

In developing such a strategy, the most effective approach is to prohibit the import of type B drugs in the first place. Simply to rely on cajoling doctors to prescribe economically is unlikely to be effective. WHO has developed a limited list of 200 drugs for use in the Third World.[2] Governments should draw strength from this WHO policy in their battles to develop a type A policy.

The role of multinational drug companies

Multinational drug companies direct most of their attention to developing and promoting drugs to market in developed countries. The Third World market being much smaller is only of peripheral interest to them. In their activities in the Third World, multinationals tend to behave much as they do in the West, i.e. promoting type B drugs. In this they rely more on direct contact with doctors by drug representatives than on journal advertising. In the mid-1970s in Tanzania, it was calculated that there were four drug representatives for every doctor in the country.

If Third World governments decide to adopt type A

drug policies, this will completely undercut the promotional efforts of the drug companies. Governments should then ask the drug companies to redirect their efforts towards the true health needs of their countries: the provision of large quantities of type A drugs, and further research to produce cheap and effective drugs for specific Third World needs.

Doctors' attitudes to limited list/type A drugs

Most doctors will initially be extremely resistant to the restriction of their freedom to prescribe type B drugs. This resistance will usually be strongest in doctors in teaching hospital and those who have received training in the West. (These doctors are of course those who are most likely to be asked to sit on committees developing drug policies!) However, the economic situation in most countries has deteriorated so much over the last 10 years, that most teaching hospital doctors have had to face economic reality in the form of shortages of essential drugs in their own hospitals. Accordingly, they are becoming increasingly sensitive to the inappropriateness of their previous prescribing practices. However, such attitudes die hard and it is only fair to recognize that much of their basis is a praiseworthy desire to do the best for one's individual patients.

Safety and side-effects of drugs

The attitude of Western-trained doctors to the questions of safety of type A drugs is often inappropriate in a Third World context. No one likes settling for second best but the reality is that Third World countries cannot hope to match Western standards in health care. The following examples show how unrealistic Western attitudes can harm the interests of Third World patients.

A large consignment of drugs from America was imported into an East African country. It was found that most of them had 'time-expired' since manufacture. An expatriate physician rejected the entire consignment out of hand. It is quite possible that most of the drugs were safe and at least 90 per cent effective. For the prospective patients, they would probably have been considerably better than nothing (which was the likely alternative).

An English neurologist wrote to the *British Medical Journal* opposing the recommendation of phenobarbitone for use in the Third World, despite it being on the WHO list of 200 essential drugs. His reasoning was that because supplies might be erratic, patients might suffer rebound status epilepticus if they ran out of tablets. He failed to suggest an alternative drug, although the most likely alternatives (carbamazepine and sodium valproate) are far more expensive. The economic reality is that the choice for most epileptics in the Third World is phenobarbitone or nothing.

Other areas where Western standards of drug safety are not appropriate for export include chloramphenicol, aspirin and bronchodilators. Chloramphenicol is now widely acknowledged to be justified on grounds of cheapness, broad-spectrum and efficacy in treating life-threatening infections. Aspirin was recently withdrawn for use on children under the age of 12 years in the UK. This is because of a small statistical association with Reye's syndrome which is a very rare condition anyway. This decision is utterly irrelevant to Third World paediatrics.

The causes of the epidemic of asthma deaths in the West in the 1960s are still inadequately understood. One theory is that they were a result of over use of isoprenaline inhalers, leading to cardiac arrhythmias. Many patients were found dead, clutching their inhalers, and this was taken as support for the theory. However, it is now generally accepted that most patients died from lack of additional treatment (steroids and hospitalization) and that it may have been the very efficacy of the isoprenaline inhalers in providing symptomatic relief that discouraged patients from seeking additional treatment. Despite this new understanding, the older bronchodilators have been pushed into obsolescence in the West and replaced by the supposedly safer and more selective bronchodilators, salbutamol and terbutaline.

Type A bronchodilators include: isoprenaline (sublingual and inhaled); ephedrine (oral); adrenaline (subcutaneous); and aminophylline (i.v. and oral). Salbutamol and terbutaline are type B drugs. The bronchodilator controversy is of very little relevance in the Third World and total reliance on a strategy using type A drugs is justified.

Rational prescribing

Even if a country adopts a strict type A drug policy and ensures generous distribution of these drugs so that they are accessible to the entire population, there is no guarantee that the drugs will be effective. For drugs to be effective they must be prescribed rationally. Irrational prescribing takes many forms and is extremely common in Western medical practice as well as the Third World. Common examples in a Third World context include:

- Treating gastroenteritis with antibiotics and anti-diarrhoeal agents rather than oral rehydration and explanation.
- Treating upper respiratory tract viral infections with antibiotics and/or antimalarials.
- Giving iron therapy to children with sickle cell anaemia or thalassaemia.
- Giving anabolic steroids to children with malnutrition.
- Giving multivitamin preparations as general tonics/placebos.
- Giving a two-week supply of iron for iron-deficiency anaemia and telling the parent to come back for more when it is finished (rather than explaining that four to six months treatment is needed to replenish iron stores and prescribing accordingly).
- Using injections rather than the oral route to impress parents. Injectable drugs are always more expensive than oral equivalents. They are also more painful.
- Treating helminth infections 'because they are there' in conditions where early re-infection is likely.

Placebo prescribing

Osler said that the main characteristic which differentiates man from animals is his desire to take medicines. Doctors world-wide have been only too willing to indulge this weakness with the result that many prescriptions are medically unnecessary. While placebos are harmless *per se*, placebo prescribing should be strongly opposed on the grounds that it is wasteful, gets in the way of rational management and explanation, and encourages the patients/parents to return for more. For instance if parents receive a placebo prescription on the first occasion they bring their child with a viral upper respiratory tract infection, they will keep coming to the clinic every time one of their children gets a cold. If on the other hand they receive an honest explanation about the lack of available treatment and good prognosis in virus infections, and are not given a placebo, they will be less likely to return unnecessarily.

Similarly, correct explanation and advice concerning oral rehydration in the first attack of gastroenteritis will mean that the parents can be self-reliant in all future attacks and will make no future demands for drug 'treatment'.

I once visited a mission clinic where it was the policy that every patient attending should receive an injection of vitamin B to keep them satisfied. Even if one

conceded the desirability of such a strategy, something useful, such as tetanus toxoid, would be preferable.

Prescribing philosophy

'Restrictionist prescribing or encouraging self-reliance

Underlying much Western medical practice is a philosophy which can best be called 'restrictionist' whereby only the doctor can diagnose illness and prescribe treatment. This encourages total dependence on the medical profession and does not matter too much in countries with easy access to doctors, although it is not ideal. This restrictionist philosophy is even less appropriate in the Third World where patients/parents may have great difficulty in getting to a doctor/paramedical worker. It should be replaced by a philosophy whereby parents are encouraged to become more self-reliant and to understand and manage illness episodes.

Thus, parents should be given drugs in advance for relapsing conditions (e.g. asthma), with indications on when and how to use them. They should be given large supplies of drugs for long-term treatment, e.g. antituberculous drugs, antiepileptics, oral iron. It is pointless and wasteful to tell parents to keep coming back for further supplies evey four weeks. If you cannot persuade the parents of the logic of giving six months of oral iron on the first occasion, then telling them to come back every four weeks is unlikely to succeed either. They should be encouraged to manage minor illnesses themselves and to recognize when they should seek advice or treatment through teaching and explanation of appropriate at-risk symptoms and signs.

More time should be spent explaining the nature and purpose of important treatment and less time prescribing unnecessary or irrational treatments. Pessimism about the ability of parents to behave sensibly becomes a self-fulfilling prophecy. One should only 'blame the parents' as a last resort, when all attempts at explanation and persuasion have been tried. Parents want the best for their children otherwise they would not have brought them for medical attention in the first place.

Diagnosis before treatment

Another strongly held Western medical belief is that 'Diagnosis must precede treatment'. While there is much virtue in this motto, it also has many disadvantages, especially for acute and serious illness in the

Third World. Purity of diagnosis is no consolation for the parent if the child dies.

Accurate diagnosis is often difficult because of lack of access to laboratory facilities or because of the nature of the illness, e.g. primary tuberculosis. Accordingly it is often justifiable to reverse the motto and say 'Treatment may precede diagnosis', especially when that treatment is inherently safe and where the possible diagnoses include life-threatening illness.

Another way in which delay in diagnosis leads to delay in treatment is when the child has to be referred on to a large centre for diagnosis and management. It is justifiable to decentralize emergency life-saving treatment to the smallest possible health station. For instance, a febrile comatose child could/should be given chloramphenicol (for meningitis) and i.m. chloroquine (for cerebral malaria) before transporting to the larger centre. This may save the child's life and will not do any harm, even if the diagnosis turns out to be a viral encephalitis.

Practical examples of therapy for common conditions

Hookworm anaemia

This is a condition where a pragmatic preventive approach is worth considering, pending the ideal development of total latrine usage in the population (see also p. 646). Since the iron-deficiency anaemia is the main problem, it might be prevented in an endemic area by a strategy whereby all children are given three months of oral iron a year. This policy proved effective in a study in Malawi where hookworm anaemia was eradicated in a population of 20 000 children. Since oral iron is extremely cheap, such a policy could be justified as cost-effective compared with hospital care for severe cases. It also enables one to stop worrying about having to treat the hookworms. A case could equally be made for mass treatment of hookworm in a six-monthly, single-dose schedule. Comparative research is needed to determine which strategy might be more effective.

Streptococcal infections

Here again a preventive approach aimed at the whole child population is needed (see also p. 514). Streptococcal tonsillitis is a common and unpleasant illness, and no child deserves to suffer repeated attacks. Its complication, rheumatic heart disease, is an important cause of morbidity and mortality in the Third World. Its disappearance in the West is almost

certainly due to entire populations having easy access to treatment with penicillin. Such a situation is unlikely in the Third World for several decades and an alternative strategy is needed. This might consist of twice daily prophylactic phenoxymethylpenicillin for the entire preschool population and the provision of generous quantities of the same drug throughout health centres and dispensaries for prompt treatment of older children. The cost of such a strategy would be less than that of developing cardiac surgery services or paying for future cases of rheumatic heart disease to go overseas for cardiac surgery.

Febrile convulsions and epilepsy

In Western paediatrics, it is now realized that instructing parents in how to take antipyretic measures during febrile episodes is more effective in the prophylaxis of further convulsions than long-term anticonvulsant medication (see also p. 756). In addition, the efficacy of rectal diazepam as an emergency treatment administered by parents to shorten any convulsions which may occur is well-established and could, with benefit, be used widely in Third World paediatrics, both for febrile convulsions and epilepsy.

In the long-term treatment of childhood epilepsy, phenobarbitone should be regarded as the drug of first choice for grand mal epilepsy on grounds of both efficacy and cost. It should be prescribed in large quantities to reduce the chance of cessation of treatment, especially in families living long distances from health centres.

Asthma

Asthma probably affects 10–15 per cent of children in the Third World, similar to European populations (see also p. 722). With such a common condition, only a strategy that relies almost totally on type A drugs has any chance of meeting the needs of the majority of asthmatic children. The following are suggested as front-line bronchodilator drugs:

- Oral ephedrine – stock supplied to families for future use in episodic asthma and maintenance treatment in perennial asthma.
- Subcutaneous adrenaline and intravenous aminophylline – for emergency use in health centres/hospitals.
- Oral prednisolone – for use as crash courses for inpatient care and also as out-patient treatment initiated by parents of an established asthmatic child

after suitable instruction. Also for long term, low-dose therapy in severe perennial asthma under good medical supervision.

- Salbutamol, terbutaline, cromoglycate (Intal), beclomethazone (Becotide) – although these are very good drugs used widely in the West, they are all type B and too expensive to be considered for widespread use. If any spare resources exist once the majority of patients are satisfactorily treated, these resources would be best spent on beclomethazone.

References

1. Speight ANP. Cost-effectiveness and drug prescribing. *Tropical Doctor*. 1975; **5**(2): 89–92.
2. WHO. The selection of essential drugs. *Technical Report Series*. 1979; **641**.

CHAPTER 3

Appropriate use of the laboratory

Andrew Hughes

The laboratory tests that are available in tropical areas vary enormously in range and complexity. This chapter looks at types of laboratory test that could be made available at different levels of health care. Appropriate use of laboratory facilities is illustrated using a number of common conditions.

Types of laboratory

Primary health care centres/rural dispensaries

Laboratories in primary health care centres or rural dispensaries offer a basic range of tests appropriate to the most common diseases, e.g. haemoglobin (Hb) estimation, sputum examination for mycobacteria, thick blood films for parasites, and stool microscopy for ova and parasites. The laboratory may be run by a locally trained, full-time laboratory attendant or by local clinic staff who have been trained locally in performing a limited number of relevant laboratory tests. Larger centres may have a permanent doctor on site; smaller centres almost certainly will not, though one may visit from time to time.

Small hospitals

In small hospitals (up to 100 beds), laboratories are usually staffed by one or two locally trained, full-time laboratory workers. Additional tests offered may include simple blood chemistry (e.g. blood urea and glucose) and a modest blood transfusion service.

District/regional hospitals

In district/regional hospitals (up to 500 beds) a reasonable range of tests in haematology, clinical chemistry, microbiology and parasitology are usually available. A blood bank and histopathology and cytology facilities are often present. Staff usually include a variable number of laboratory technologists, trained overseas, plus locally trained laboratory assistants and attendants. The laboratory may be headed by a pathologist, so that postmortem facilities may be available.

Major hospitals

Such hospitals (more than 500 beds) include large referral and teaching hospitals, where laboratory facilities approximate to those available in more developed countries.

As most medicine practiced in the tropics is not associated with teaching hospital facilities, only laboratories up to and including district/regional hospital level are considered. Available facilities are often dictated by the supply of water and electricity, financial resources for equipment, reagents and materials (particularly foreign exchange) and the experience and expertise of the laboratory staff.

Types of laboratory test

Tests offered may be grouped as follows:

- *Screening tests* of clinically well subjects, for example Hb and urine tests on antenatal patients, Hb and syphilis testing on blood donors and screening of contacts in diarrhoea outbreaks. Screening for HIV infection is also now mandatory for blood donors.
- *Confirmatory tests* used to confirm a diagnosis already made on clinical grounds, for example thick blood films for malaria, cerebrospinal fluid (CSF) examination in meningitis and sputum in pneumonia. These tests can also give useful additional information, such as antibiotic susceptibility patterns or parasite densities.
- *Diagnostic tests* used when a firm clinical diagnosis has not been made, or to differentiate between possible diagnoses. For example, red cell morphology in anaemia, stool samples for microscopy and culture in diarrhoea, and liver function tests in jaundice.
- *Follow-up tests* to monitor the effectiveness of treatment. For example, Hb in anaemia, sputum in tuberculosis (TB) and urine glucose in diabetes.
- *Tests in research and/or survey work.* These will depend on the type of work being carried out and the local laboratory facilities and expertise available. They may be directed towards a patient population, normal subjects or a geographical area.

The tests that should be available in the different types of laboratory are described below.

Primary health care centre laboratories

Laboratory tests in this situation should be technically simple and inexpensive, as independent of regular electricity as possible and relevant to the prevalent diseases in the area. (See Table 6.3.1.)

Hb estimation carried out using a colorimetric method has distinct advantages in terms of accuracy. Suitable colorimeters for measuring haemoglobin include, the Corning 252, Walden Precision Apparatus CO700D, and the BMS CYANOX I haemoglobinometer*.

All three instruments require dilution of the blood sample before measurement; capillary or venous blood

Table 6.3.1 Laboratory tests in primary health care centres

Haematology
Haemoglobin
Blood film for malaria parasites
Thin blood film for:
Red cell morphology
White cell differential count
Sickle cell screening test
Emergency blood transfusion
Chemistry
Urine analysis (protein; glucose; ketones)
Microbiology/parasitology
Gram stain
Ziehl–Neelsen stain
Urine and stool microscopy
VDRL tests

samples may be used. The Corning 252 and CO700D Colorimeter can be operated from mains electricity or a 12 V car battery. The CYANOX I haemoglobinometer is battery-operated and has the advantage that it is a direct-readout machine. An alternative, although less accurate, piece of equipment is the BMS and manual (model 10–1010) haemoglobinometer. This has the advantage that the blood does not need to be prediluted and results are highly reproducible. It can be operated from batteries or from the mains electricity using a transformer. The Lovibond comparator requires predilution of blood and is less accurate than the instruments just described. It is suggested that patients could initially be screened for paleness of their mucous membranes and *only* those that appear pale should undergo Hb estimation. Hb estimation is a relatively easy skill to learn, and can be taught to non-medical staff. It is unusual to miss severe anaemia with the clinical screening test.

Thick films are essential in malarious areas, and films may be satisfactorily stained with Giemsa or Field's stains.

Thin blood films, examined for red cell morphology and abnormalities in the number and types of white cells, can be very helpful even at this level, though it can be a difficult skill to acquire. Most usefully the recognition of severely hypochromic red cells, especially if associated with microcytosis, can indicate iron deficiency. The recognition of macrocytic red cells and hypersegmented polymorphs, suggesting folate deficiency, is more difficult for laboratory workers at this level. Examination of white cells can be useful in

---

*Corning 252 Colorimeter: Ciba Corning Diagnostics Ltd, Halstead, Essex C09 2DX, UK. WPA Medical Digital Colorimeter: Walden Precision Apparatus Ltd, The Old Station, Linton, Cambridge CB1 6NW, UK. BMS CYANOX I and manual haemoglobinometer: Buffalo Medical Specialities M & G Inc, PO Box 17247, Clearwater, Fl 34622-7247, USA.

indicating bacterial, viral or parasitic infection, and is more useful than a simple total white cell count. Thin films may be stained with either Leishman's or Field's stain, after fixation with methanol.

A sickle cell screening test, using the sodium metabisulphite slide test, can be useful in areas where sickle cell disease is prevalent. A positive test associated with sickled and nucleated red cells on the thin blood film and a low Hb is typical of sickle cell disease, while a positive test with no sickled cells on the thin film and a normal or slightly low Hb indicates sickle cell trait.

If possible, *a blood transfusion service* should be available, if only to transfuse severely anaemic patients as an emergency. The lack of regular electricity or gas supplies usually makes the establishment of a blood bank impossible. A kerosene refrigerator for vaccines is usually available, and it is suggested that blood grouping antisera could be stored there and possibly blood stored overnight (if the temperature is 2–8°C). Patients and prospective donors can be ABO and Rhesus grouped and either the same group or group O blood be given after a simple cross-match to exclude ABO incompatibility. Red cells from the donor can be mixed with serum from the recipient in a small glass tube and left at room temperature for 30–40 minutes and then the sedimented red cells examined microscopically for agglutination. This serves as a check on compatibility within the ABO system, but will not detect incompatibilities of the Rhesus or other blood group systems. Comprehensive cross-matching can be difficult to carry out since a dry block or waterbath set at 35–37°C is required. This is most easily obtained using mains electricity but a thermos flask can be used. A small supply of blood collection bags should be kept available, as well as blood-giving sets.

Chemistry facilities are usually limited to urinalysis, although the Corning 252 and the WPA CO700D colorimeter with the appropriate filters can be used for essential blood chemistry assays. Although convenient, the multiple reagent strip tests are usually too expensive for regular use. The sulphosalicylic acid technique is recommended for detection of protein and either Clinitest tablets or Benedict's reagent for sugar. Inexpensive reagent strips for detecting protein, glucose and ketones are helpful and may be cut into two lengthwise for economy.

Ziehl-Neelsen staining for the acid-fast bacilli of TB is straightforward, though the appropriate samples in children are often difficult to obtain. Gram staining for other bacteria is also easily carried out and may help in the diagnosis of infection, particularly suspected meningitis, though this does depend on the ability of the local staff to undertake lumbar puncture. With meningitis, Gram staining of CSF can be difficult to interpret. A simple white cell count in a chamber can be helpful if the laboratory staff are able to do it. In general though, at this level of care, Gram and Ziehl–Neelsen stains are more useful in the diagnosis of disease in adults.

Direct microscopy of urine and faeces is straightforward and useful in detecting parasitic and bacterial infections. Microscopy of faeces is of limited value in the investigation of acute diarrhoea, but can be valuable if diarrhoea is persistent in looking for *Giardia, Strongyloides, E. histolytica* and *Trichuris trichiura*, or large numbers of pus cells. It can also be especially useful in looking for hookworm in children with suspected iron-deficiency anaemia. Urine microscopy is useful in detecting or confirming haematuria, particularly when investigating urinary schistosomiasis. Reagent strip tests for blood are usually too expensive for regular use. Leucocytes may also be looked for, their presence suggesting urinary tract infection. Non-centrifuged specimens should be examined unless schistosome eggs are being looked for, when the deposit from a centrifuged specimen or urine left to sediment for an hour should be examined.

Because of the continuing prevalence of syphilis in the tropics it is convenient to have the Venereal Diseases Research Laboratory (VDRL) tests available locally to screen antenatal patients. It is technically straightforward and requires only one reagent, though this needs to be kept in a refrigerator. Minimal equipment is needed and the test is read macroscopically.

Small hospital laboratories

Basic services such as electricity and water may be more reliable in small hospitals, and laboratory staff more highly trained. This may permit a wider range of laboratory tests to be carried out, particularly in blood chemistry. The Corning 252 or the WPA CO700D colorimeter can be used. The CO700D colorimeter is a recently developed digital colorimeter with nine built-in filters. It is also cheaper than the Corning 252. The most valuable assays are outlined in Table 6.3.2. Urine testing should be expanded to include tests for bilirubin and urobilinogen. Chemical methods are recommended, rather than reagent strips, due to the expense of the latter. Strip tests for bilirubin and urobilinogen are less stable than the standard chemical tests.

Urine bilirubin and urobilinogen and serum assays of total and conjugated bilirubin, total protein and albumin allow most problems of jaundice to be adequately diagnosed (see later). If serum assays are to

Table 6.3.2. Laboratory tests in small hospitals

Haematology
    Haemoglobin (colorimetric)
    Total white cell count (manual)
    Differential white cell count
    Blood film for parasites
    Red cell morphology (thin film)
    Reticulocyte count
    Sickle cell screening test
Blood transfusion
    Blood grouping
    Cross-matching
    Maintenance of blood bank
Chemistry
    Serum assays for urea, glucose, total and conjugated
      bilirubin, total protein and albumin
    Urine tests for protein, glucose, ketones, bilirubin and
      urobilinogen
    CSF protein and glucose
Microbiology/parasitology
    Ziehl–Neelsen for sputum and skin smears
    Gram stain of pus and CSF
    Microscopy of urine or faeces
    VDRL tests
    ? Bacterial culture/antigens

be undertaken, an electrically operated centrifuge is desirable, as is a waterbath.

Reticulocyte counts are technically easy and can be helpful in assessing anaemia and early response to treatment.

If there is a reasonably reliable electricity or gas supply or a generator with a regular supply of fuel, a blood bank can be established, with a small stock of blood being stored in a specially designed blood bank refrigerator maintained within the strict limits of 2–8°C with the ideal being 4°C. It is necessary to check and chart the temperature of the refrigerator once a day and to avoid opening the door unnecessarily. Electricity also allows a proper cross-match to be carried out easily by the saline and albumin methods at 37°C in a waterbath or dry block. The ability to store blood is clearly an advantage if there is a regular surgical commitment. Storage of blood for up to 35 days is possible if the temperature of the blood bank can be held consistently between 2 and 8°C. Blood showing signs of haemolysis must never be transfused.

Bacterial culture facilities provide more exacting microbiological diagnoses and permit antibiotic susceptibility testing. This is usually not possible as good facilities are required to store, make up and autoclave culture media, with excessive contamination a constant problem. There are, however, an increasing number of commercially available antisera for detecting bacterial antigens, especially the organisms commonly responsible for meningitis (*Meningococcus*, *Haemophilus* and *Pneumococcus*). The technique provides a rapid result and is technically relatively simple. The antisera need to be stored in a refrigerator and are expensive.

District/regional hospital laboratories

In these laboratories, staff are usually better trained, electricity and water supplies are constant and thus a more comprehensive range of tests are possible. The limiting factor is usually financial, in terms of the materials and reagents that can be made available regularly (see Table 6.3.3).

In haematological investigations the haematocrit can be a useful addition to the Hb in the investigation of

Table 6.3.3 Laboratory tests in district/regional hospitals

Haematology
    Haemoglobin/haematocrit
    Total white cell count
    Differential white cell count
    Blood film for parasites
    Red cell morphology
    Platelet count
    Reticulocyte count
    Sickle cell test
    Hb electrophoresis
    Coagulation tests
    Bone marrow aspiration
    Direct Coomb's test
    Blood bank
Chemistry
    Urea/creatinine
    Electrolytes
    Glucose
    Total protein/albumin
    Total and conjugated bilirubin
    Calcium/phosphate
    Iron
    Alkaline phosphatase
    CSF glucose/protein
    Urine for protein, glucose, bilirubin, urobilinogen, ketones
Microbiology/parasitology
    Ziehl–Neelsen and Gram stains
    Stool and urine microscopy
    Bacterial culture
    Antibiotic sensitivity
    VDRL tests
    Widal and brucella serology
    ? Bacterial antigens
Histology/cytology
    Surgical/postmortem
    Aspirates
    Cervical smears
    Sputum

anaemia, as it allows the mean cell haemoglobin concentration (MCHC) to be calculated. A value of less than 30 per cent suggests iron deficiency. A well made and stained thin blood film examined by an experienced observer is, however, the most useful investigation in anaemia.

A range of simple coagulation tests may also be available (see p. 835). A simple 'screen' for patients with suspected bleeding disorders should include a bleeding time, a platelet count, a prothrombin time (PT) and a partial thromboplastin time with kaolin (PTTK). Haemophiliacs will typically have a normal PT with a prolonged PTTK that corrects to normal on the addition of normal plasma. Acquired clotting disorders occurring with liver disease or disseminated intravascular coagulation (DIC) usually have a prolonged PT and PTTK and in DIC a low platelet count. Bleeding associated with a low platelet count requires a bone marrow aspiration to exclude diseases like leukaemia and hypoplastic anaemia. A normal marrow suggests immune platelet destruction (as in immune thrombocytopaenia, ITP). The most common symptom is nose bleed, and most patients have a local reason for bleeding and not a bleeding disorder.

At this level, the best screening test for abnormal haemoglobins is the tube solubility test, which enables rapid identification of normals, sickle trait and sickle cell disease. This can usually be backed up by Hb electrophoresis on cellulose acetate at alkaline pH which readily separates haemoglobins A, F, S and C.

A more comprehensive blood transfusion service is usually available with facilities for blood storage and full cross-matching. It is often possible for fresh plasma to be prepared, and sometimes stored as fresh frozen plasma (FFP). This is helpful in the treatment of bleeding disorders due to coagulation factor deficiency, although not as effective in haemophilia as giving specific factor preparations. Occasionally it is possible to make cryoprecipitate (Factor VIII) locally for haemophiliacs and platelet concentrates for bleeding due to thrombocytopaenia associated with bone marrow disease. It is usually not possible to hold stocks of freeze-dried concentrates of Factors VIII and IX, as they are very expensive. It is often possible to prepare plasma-reduced blood or to divide an adult donation into two or three smaller bags. This can be valuable in paediatric transfusion where volume can be a limiting factor.

A major problem in blood transfusion is the shortage of blood, as requests exceed donations. Medical staff should encourage relatives of patients who require transfusion to donate blood to the blood bank pool and thus help to keep stocks at a reasonable level. All blood should be suspected of being HIV positive, and transfusion restricted if screening is not possible.

Some investigations can usually be done in the event of suspected transfusion reactions, though antibody identification in the patient's plasma is limited by the expense and short shelf-life of the necessary test red cells. A direct Coomb's test may be available, which can be helpful in the investigation of suspected immune-mediated haemolysis (e.g. haemolytic disease of the newborn) and tests to exclude infected blood should be performed.

In clinical chemistry, a wider range of serum assays is usually available, including electrolyte measurement. It is unlikely that estimations of chloride or bicarbonate will be done, and blood gas analysis is best restricted to large teaching hospitals.

Laboratories will vary in their ability to perform enzyme assays. It is perfectly possible to investigate jaundice satisfactorily without aminotransferase or alkaline phosphatase measurements. The latter, however, can be useful if calcium and phosphate levels are available. In areas where glucose-6-phosphate-dehydrogenase (G6PD) deficiency is common it can be helpful to have an enzyme assay capability, or at least a screening test (the fluorescence test is probably the easiest).

Microbiology laboratories in district/regional hospitals will usually have a reasonable range of bacterial culture facilities for the more detailed identification of organisms involved in infection. This is often associated with antibiotic susceptibility testing. There is often a greater range of serological investigations, including syphilis, typhoid, brucella and HIV infection. Some laboratories may have antisera for bacterial antigen identification, which is especially useful in meningitis where prior treatment with antibiotics may suppress bacterial growth in the laboratory. It may also provide rapid and specific confirmation of the diagnosis. Antisera are, however, expensive and this often limits the extent of serological diagnostic techniques that are available.

Tuberculosis diagnosis usually depends on the identification of acid-fast bacilli (AFB) in patient samples like sputum (see pp. 519–52). This is not easy to obtain from children and the diagnosis is often made on clinical grounds with a chest X-ray and a Mantoux test. Some, but not all, laboratories may have TB culture facilities, but growth of mycobacteria may take several weeks. TB meningitis can be difficult to diagnose. AFB are rarely seen in CSF and the diagnosis usually depends on clinical suspicion and CSF findings of an increased number of lymphocytes with raised protein and moderately reduced glucose. TB culture, if available, is useful, and a chest X-ray may be abnormal.

Most laboratories will not have trained staff or facilities for diagnostic virology due to the high capital cost of equipment and recurrent expenditure involved.

To make the best use of the available microbiological facilities it is important, where possible, to send the relevant samples to the laboratory before antibiotics have been started. If the patient is already on antibiotics, the laboratory should be informed. In some circumstances, for example where the diagnosis remains in doubt or treatment appears to be unsuccessful, it is worth considering stopping all antibiotics for 12–24 hours and then reculturing the relevant specimens. New doctors should visit the microbiology laboratory to find out what facilities exist, how specimens should be collected and what significant antibiotic resistance occurs locally.

Histology services vary greatly. The processing of biopsy and surgical specimens may be done locally and reported by the pathologist, especially if he/she is a histopathologist. If facilities are limited or a referral service within the country does not exist there is a UK-based postal service available*. Specimens can be sent either processed in a paraffin block or unprocessed in formalin. Postal results are usually available within 2–4 weeks of sending.

Fine-needle aspiration cytology can be very useful provided the limitations regarding exact diagnosis, especially with lymph node aspirates, are borne in mind. As long as there is someone available locally to examine the slides, this can be a rapid and cheap way of obtaining a diagnosis if the lesion or organ is readily accessible.

Postmortems will usually be carried out at district/regional level, and may be done by the pathologist or other medical and surgical staff. Permission is not often sought or readily given by relatives for elective postmortems, though in selected cases this would be very valuable. It is, however, usually acceptable and useful to take postmortem needle biopsy samples. It is advisable to find out what the local procedure is regarding postmortems.

Suggested investigation of some common conditions

Fever

Blanket investigation should be avoided. It is not only bad clinical practice but also wasteful of laboratory

*Postal histology: Dr S. Lucas, Department of Morbid Anatomy, School of Medicine, University College London, University Street, London WC1E 6JJ, UK.

time. There is no substitute for a clinical history, where possible, and careful, repeated clinical examination. Regular measurement of the patient's temperature and accurate recording are also helpful.

Laboratory tests for the febrile patient are of two types: screening tests and specific tests.

Screening tests

The two most useful screening tests are a thick blood film for malaria parasites and *Borreliae* (if relapsing fever is prevalent), and a total and differential white blood cell count. Both these can be made available at all levels of health care where there is a laboratory, and can be of use in the diagnosis of both acute and chronic (more than two weeks duration) fever (see Figs. 6.3.1. and 6.3.2). (See also p. 664.)

Malaria is usually associated with a positive blood film for parasites. However, in holoendemic malaria areas, positive blood films may not be related to the cause of the fever. There is normally a lymphocytosis, with 'reactive' changes in the lymphoid cells. Malaria pigment may be seen in lymphocytes or monocytes. However, in the very early stages of malaria there can be a polymorphonuclear leucocytosis (PMNL). Associated anaemia and splenomegaly strongly suggest malaria.

A PMNL suggests a bacterial or pyogenic infection, particularly if associated with a negative B/F. Its absence suggests typhoid while an actual lymphocytosis, particularly if associated with 'reactive' changes in the lymphocytes, suggests a viral infection.

While malaria should be suspected in a febrile patient with anaemia, it should not be forgotten that infections can occur in patients with pre-existing anaemia such as sickle cell disease, thalassaemia or G6PD deficiency. Sickle cell crises may cause fever without evidence of a precipitating infection but, unlike malaria, splenomegaly is not a feature. Sickled and nucleated red cells should be seen in the thin blood film, the latter often being responsible for a falsely raised total white cell count. Infection associated with G6PD deficiency is usually associated with jaundice due to haemolysis.

Fever associated with tumours or lymphomas can have a variable WBC differential count. While lymphoma cells are rarely seen in blood films, the presence of 'blast' cells strongly suggests acute leukaemia.

Figures 6.3.1 and 6.3.2 are not exhaustive, and conditions with obvious and diagnostic physical signs have been left out.

A urine sample may be included as part of the screening tests, as urinary tract infections in children

B/F and WBC differential count

B/F + PMNL −	B/F + PMNL +	B/F − PMNL +	B/F − Reticulocytosis Sickled and nucleated RBCs	B/F − PMNL −
Malaria	**Bacterial infection (Malaria)**	**Bacterial infection Pus**	**Sickle cell disease**	**Viral infection Typhoid**

Fig. 6.3.1   Thick blood film (B/F) and white cell differential count (WBC diff.) in acute fever.
B/F +(−) = malaria parasites present (absent); PMNL +(−) = polymorphonuclear leucocytosis present (absent).

may cause fever with no specific symptoms. In peripheral laboratories a non-centrifuged sample of urine can be microscoped for pus cells and bacteria, while in laboratories with proper microbiological facilities the sample can also be cultured. The collection of clean urine samples from children, especially in a tropical environment, is not easy and this has to be borne in mind when assessing the results obtained. (See pp. 1010–11 for techniques of urine collection).

Specific tests

The specific tests listed in Table 6.3.4 are usually only possible in district or regional hospitals, and what is done will be dictated by the clinical findings. In fever alone, cultures of urine and blood are useful. The value of blood culture is increased by taking samples when the patient has fever, observing an aseptic technique (to decrease the isolation of unwanted and potentially confusing contaminants) and taking at least 5 to 10 ml of blood. It is important, if bacterial culture is to be of maximum use, to take the relevant specimens before the patient is put on antibiotics. Once antibiotics have

Table 6.3.4   Specific laboratory tests for patients with fever

Bacterial culture	Serology	Histology
Pus	VDRL	biopsies of:
Swabs	Widal/brucella	Liver
Urine	Bacterial	Pleura
CSF	antigens	Peritoneum
Blood		Lymph node
Stool		Spleen (if leish-
Aspirates		maniasis
		suspected)

been started, microbiological investigations are often unrewarding. Re-investigation of treatment failure may best be achieved by stopping the antibiotics, if possible, and reculturing relevant samples after 24 hours.

The range of serological diagnostic techniques varies from laboratory to laboratory, and local availability should be checked on. Most useful is the Widal test for typhoid and, where available, detection of bacterial antigens. This test provides a rapid and reliable diagnosis of bacterial meningitis, even if the patient has already received antibiotics.

Histology can be helpful, especially in the diagnosis of TB and lymphoma, though in many places results may only be available retrospectively, but even this can be valuable. 'Dab' preparations from unfixed biopsy material or fine-needle aspirates may permit a rapid diagnosis to be made while waiting for histological confirmation.

Meningitis

The diagnosis of bacterial meningitis rarely presents problems (see also p. 745). It is often clinically apparent, and in situations where a sample of CSF can be obtained the specimen is usually turbid. Laboratory investigations require a reasonably well trained

WBC diff.

Polymorpho- nuclear leucocytosis	Neutropenia	Eosinophilia	Normal
Pus	Malaria Disseminated TB Visceral leishmaniasis Brucellosis	Parasitic infection	Localized TB Brucellosis Toxoplasmosis Endocarditis Trypanosomiasis

Fig. 6.3.2   White cell differential count (WBC diff.) in chronic fever.

CSF

Appearance	Clear	Turbid	Slightly turbid or clear	Slightly turbid or clear
Cell count	Nil (Occasionally L)	Raised + + (mainly PM)	Raised + (mainly L)	Raised + (mainly L, occasionally PM)
Bacterial stains	Negative	Positive Gram	Negative	Negative Gram Positive Ziehl–Neelsen + / −
Protein (g/l)	0.15–0.4	Raised + / + +	Raised + / −	Raised + / + + +
Glucose (mmol/1)	2.2–3.3	Decreased + +	Normal	Decreased +
Culture	Negative	Usually positive	Negative	Occasionally positive
Bacterial antigens	Negative	Positive	Negative	Negative
Diagnosis	**Normal**	**Bacterial meningitis**	**Viral meningitis**	**Tuberculous meningitis**

Fig. 6.3.3 CSF findings in suspected meningitis. PM = polymorphs; L = lymphocytes.

laboratory worker but it is possible, even in peripheral laboratories, for a cell count and a Gram stain to be done. The former is usually raised and, with care, organisms may readily be seen on the latter.

Tuberculous meningitis, on the other hand, remains a considerable problem both in clinical and laboratory diagnosis, even when laboratory facilities are reasonably sophisticated. Laboratory findings are summarized in Fig. 6.3.3. (See also p. 536.)

The findings in bacterial meningitis are fairly clear-cut. The only problem may be with a child who has been partially treated before being seen. This can alter the CSF findings, which may look like a viral meningitis. In this situation, the ability to look for bacterial antigens is most useful.

Brain abscesses may produce any of the above findings, and encephalitis is likely to most closely resemble viral meningitis.

TB meningitis remains a problem as CSF findings are often equivocal, though a modest lymphocytosis associated with a raised protein and moderately decreased glucose are suggestive findings, especially if there is headache, vomiting and cranial nerve palsies (see p. 537). Mycobacteria may not be seen in a Ziehl–Neelsen stained preparation and culture may take several weeks. In atypical cases of meningitis, TB should always be considered, as should rare causes like fungi and cryptococcus that may produce similar findings to either TB or viral meningitis, especially with associated HIV infection.

Chronic diarrhoea

Unlike acute diarrhoea, where there is often a bacterial or viral aetiology, chronic diarrhoea is more often associated with parasites or worms in the gastro-intestinal tract (see p. 477). Thus, microscopy of saline and iodine stool preparations, which is possible at all laboratory levels, is the most useful initial investigation in these patients (Table 6.3.5). AIDS should also be suspected.

Cryptosporidium is best looked for in a preparation stained by a modified Ziehl–Neelsen technique.

Table 6.3.5 Gastro-intestinal parasites causing chronic diarrhoea

Entamoeba histolytica
Strongyloides stercoralis
Schistosoma mansoni
Cryptosporidium
Giardia lamblia
Trichuris trichiura
Balantidium coli
Isospora belli

Stool culture is unrewarding and is usually restricted to laboratories in district/regional hospitals. Acute diarrhoeas may lead to chronic states due to acquired lactase deficiency, with diarrhoea due to the lactose load in the colon. Testing stools for sugar, using either a Clinitest tablet or Benedict's reagent, is a useful screening test and should be positive in these circumstances. This is a simple test that can be available at all laboratory levels. If available, the test can be repeated with a Clinistix test strip. This is specific for glucose, and should therefore be negative.

Laboratory tests for the diarrhoea of malabsorption are not considered in this chapter.

Jaundice

The most common causes of jaundice in neonates, infants and children are given in Table 6.3.6. In investigating jaundice, the initial tests should aim to categorize the jaundice as either unconjugated or conjugated (Table 6.3.7). Subsequent tests should aim to identify the cause of the jaundice (see p. 224).

The serum assays are usually only possible in district/regional hospital laboratories, although they can sometimes be done in small hospital laboratories. The urine tests could be done at all laboratory levels using either reagent strips (expensive), tablets (Ictotest for bilirubin) or chemicals (Fouchet's reagent for bilirubin and Ehrlich's reagent for urobilinogen). A simple test that can be done anywhere is to shake vigorously a sample of urine and observe the colour of the froth. Yellow froth indicates that bilirubin is present in the urine, white froth its absence. This may at least help in distinguishing the two major groups, haemolytic and hepatic jaundice. Enzyme assays (transaminases and alkaline phosphatase) may help in differentiating between the various types of jaundice but are not considered absolutely necessary as they are expensive and not always available, even in large hospital laboratories.

If haemolytic disease of the newborn (HDN) is suspected, the tests in Table 6.3.8 should be requested (see also p. 224). They are usually only available in a regional/district hospital laboratory but ABO and Rhesus grouping and an Hb estimation may be available in a peripheral laboratory if it holds blood grouping antisera. The perspex colour comparison strip (icterometer) is a valuable screening test for moderate to severe jaundice in neonates, applied either to the nose or gum.

HDN can be seen with either a Rhesus-negative mother and Rhesus-positive baby or with a group O mother and a group A, B or AB baby. The DCT is

Table 6.3.6 Common causes of jaundice in neonates (N), infants (I) and children (C)

Haemolysis
    Haemolytic disease of newborn (N)
    Glucose-6-phosphate dehydrogenase deficiency (N/I/C)
    Sickle cell disease (I/C)
    Thalassaemia (I/C)
    Malaria (I/C)
Physiological (N)
Hepatic
    Congenital infections (N): syphilis; toxoplasma; rubella;
        cytomegalovirus; herpes
    Hepatitis (N/I/C)
    Septicaemia (N/I/C)
    Urinary tract infections (N/I/C)
Obstructive (rare)
    e.g. Biliary atresia (N)

usually positive with Rhesus incompatibility but only weakly positive or negative with ABO incompatibility. The Hb and bilirubin help to assess the severity of the anaemia and hyperbilirubinaemia, respectively.

Where the initial tests indicate haemolysis, but HDN is not suspected, then the tests in Table 6.3.9 should be considered. Peripheral laboratories may only be able to provide a blood film for malaria parasites, a sickle screening test and a thin blood film to look for sickle cells and the hypochromia and target cells of thalassaemia. In more sophisticated centres, Hb electrophoresis and a G6PD screen or assay are often available. A reticulocyte count can be useful in helping to confirm that the anaemia is a haemolytic one.

In neonatal jaundice the tests in Tables 6.3.8 and 6.3.9 may be requested together.

In hepatic jaundice the suggested investigations are listed in Table 6.3.10. The WBC differential count may help in detecting a bacterial or viral infection, while urine and blood cultures are more specific. VDRL testing for syphilis is usually the only significant serological test that can be done. It is likely that only a white count and differential and VDRL would be available in peripheral laboratories, though it is possible to microscope urine for signs of infection.

Anaemia

The most common causes of childhood anaemia are listed in Table 6.3.11. (See also p. 822.) Once anaemia is suspected by finding pale mucous membranes, the following initial tests, which can be done at all laboratory levels, should be requested:

- Hb to confirm the presence of anaemia and to assess its severity;

Table 6.3.7 Initial laboratory investigations in the jaundiced patient

Urine – Bn :	Negative	Negative	Positive	Positive
– UBn:	Excess	Normal	Normal	Normal
Serum – CB :	Normal	Normal	Increased	Increased
– UCB:	Increased	Increased	Increased	Normal or slightly increased
Diagnosis :	**Haemolysis**	**Physiological**	**Hepatic**	**Obstructive**

Bn = bilirubin; UBn = urobilinogen; CB = conjugated bilirubin; UCB = unconjugated bilirubin.

Table 6.3.8 Laboratory investigations in suspected haemolytic disease of the newborn (HDN)

Baby
  ABO and Rhesus blood group
  Hb
  Bilirubin
  Direct Coomb's test (DCT)
Mother
  ABO and Rhesus blood group

Table 6.3.9 Laboratory investigations in suspected non-immune haemolysis

Hb and reticulocyte count
Thick blood film for malaria parasites
Thin blood film for RBC morphology
Screening sickle test
Hb electrophoresis
G6PD screen/assay

Table 6.3.10 Suggested laboratory investigations in hepatic jaundice

Total WBC count and differential
Urine culture
Blood culture
VDRL tests

Table 6.3.11 Common causes of anaemia in childhood

Iron deficiency (malnutrition or hookworm infestation)
Folic acid deficiency
Malaria
Sickle cell disease
Thalassaemia
Infections

Thin film findings

Hypo-chromia	Hypo-chromia	Macro-cytosis	Sickle cells	Blast cells
Micro-cytosis	Micro-cytosis	Hyperseg-mented Polymorphs	Nucleated RBCs	
	Target cells		Reticulo-cytosis	
	Nucleated RBCs			
Iron deficiency	**Thalass-aemia**	**Folate deficiency**	**Sickle cell anaemia**	**Leukae-mia**

Fig. 6.3.4 Thin blood film test for red cell morphology.

- a thick blood film for malaria parasites (and trypanosomes if appropriate);
- a thin blood film for red cell morphology (see Fig. 6.3.4).

With suspected iron deficiency, a stool should be examined for the presence of hookworm. Thalassaemia and sickle cell disease can be confirmed by Hb electrophoresis, if this is available. Suspected leukaemia should be confirmed by a bone marrow aspirate.

If the diagnosis is still not clear, then the tests listed in Table 6.3.12 should be requested, though these will probably only be available in hospital laboratories. Bone marrow aspirates can confirm suspected megaloblastic changes associated with folate deficiency and can be stained for iron to assess body iron stores. It can help in the diagnosis of visceral leishmaniasis and may reveal malignant cell infiltration or suggest hypoplasia as a cause for the anaemia.

A raised reticulocyte count, especially if associated with an unconjugated hyperbilirubinaemia and excess urobilinogen in the urine, suggests haemolytic anaemia and the tests listed in Table 6.3.13 can be done (see also Tables 6.3.8 and 6.3.9).

The last three tests in Table 6.3.13 will probably only be available in larger hospital laboratories. Hb electrophoresis may confirm either suspected sickle cell disease or thalassaemia. A positive Coomb's test indicates immune-mediated haemolysis, although this is not common. The G6PD screen/assay may be normal if done during or immediately following a bout of haemolysis as all the deficient cells will have been

Table 6.3.12 Supplementary laboratory investigations in anaemia

---

Bone marrow aspirate
Reticulocyte count
Serum bilirubin
Urine urobilinogen
Blood urea

Table 6.3.13 Laboratory investigations in suspected haemolytic anaemias

---

Thick blood film for malaria parasites
Sickle cell screening test
Hb electrophoresis
G6PD screen or assay
Direct Coomb's test

---

haemolysed. The test is best done several weeks later when the patient has recovered.

In investigating anaemia it is unlikely that assays for iron, total iron-binding capacity, ferritin, folic acid and vitamin B_{12} will be available. Much can be achieved, however, by careful examination of a thin blood film.

Conclusion

The scope and complexity of laboratory investigations in the tropics is very variable, and often dictated by the local availability of trained staff, regular water and electricity supplies, and financial resources. However, much useful information can be gained by the judicious use of a few key investigations, many of which can be made available even in small health centre laboratories. In general, one should find out what the local facilities are (including what can be sent elsewhere) and use them in consultation with the pathologist or the laboratory technologist. There must be adequate quality assurance for all laboratory work, to ensure reliability of results. Safety precautions must be taken to protect patients, relatives and staff – especially in the era of AIDS.

Further reading

Cheesbrough M. *Medical Laboratory Manual for Tropical Countries: Vol. I, Clinical Chemistry and Parasitology, Laboratory Equipment*, 2nd Edn. Tropical Health Technology/Butterworths, 1987.

Cheesbrough M. *Medical Laboratory Manual for Tropical Countries: Vol. II, Microbiology*, 1st Edn. Tropical Health Technology/Butterworths, 1984.

Dacie JV, Lewis SM. *Practical Haematology*, 6th Edn. London, Churchill Livingstone, 1984.

Evatt BL, Lewis SM, Lothe F, McArthur JR. *Anaemia: Fundamental Diagnostic Haematology*. Atlanta/Geneva, US Dept Health and Human Services/WHO, 1983.

WHO. *Manual of Basic Techniques for a Health Laboratory*. Geneva, WHO, 1980.

CHAPTER 4

Appropriate technology for health

Katherine Elliott

What is technology?

There is considerable mystique attached to the word 'technology'. This mystique suggests that technology is the product of special experts, working in expensively equipped laboratories to devise new ways of solving problems. The average person is a little nervous about technology, although often appreciative of its benefits. There is a non-human dimension to much of the modern, sophisticated technology which explains this mixture of feelings. People like to feel that they still have some control over what is happening in their lives, and that choices remain for them. But very few want to give up all the advances that modern technological expertise has made possible. The question is how to use this expertise wisely and more equitably, especially in the provision of health care in a world where such gross discrepancies in health status and health care services exist.

In thinking about technology for health, it is perhaps important to look again at the word 'technology' and strip away some of the mystique. All that the word really means is 'the systematic application of knowledge to practical tasks', in other words, a way to carry out a task, using a tool and/or a technique, together with the necessary skills and knowledge. For example, breast-feeding could be called a technology, although no hardware is involved. It answers the problem of how to feed the newborn. Success in breast-feeding is a

technique, an art as old as the human race, which is passed on by the more experienced to new mothers throughout the world. Breast-feeding is equally appropriate in both developing and developed countries. Research has shown that mothers' milk is formulated in such a way as to precisely meet the physiological requirements of the infant.

Modern technology has made it possible for well-meaning people to tamper with this age-old art without fully understanding all the implications of their actions for mothers and babies who live in very different socio-economic circumstances, without access to safe water or the money to buy breast-milk substitutes in sufficient quantities. Bottle-feeding has saved many infants, but it has killed many millions more than it has saved. Reversing the trend is difficult, expensive and time-consuming. Technology transfer therefore needs careful consideration before implementation where the well-being of people is likely to be affected.

Useful knowledge

In 1975, Dr Maurice King suggested that 'In our age, the greatest challenge before world medicine is to see that the most useful parts of the knowledge we already have are brought to all those who need it'. Many years later, in the tropics and subtropics, there seems still to be to long away to go before this challenge is fully met and the most useful parts of the child health knowledge we possess reach all families.

Seven particular areas have been highlighted by UNICEFs Child Survival Programme: growth monitoring, oral rehydration therapy, immunization, breast-feeding, food supplementation, family spacing, and female education. Even on their own, these measures, using simple and appropriate technologies, would have an enormous, and in some cases immediate, impact on child mortality and morbidity in vast areas of the world.

In the long-term, only socioeconomic progress and environmental improvements can lead to better child health, but how long is 'long-term' likely to be? The situation which currently exists, where so many children are at risk of death or impaired development from basic diseases in an era which also witnesses births resulting from *in vitro* fertilization procedures and heart/lung transplants in small children, is no longer considered acceptable. If technology can facilitate these wonders, what is stopping technology from solving the seemingly simpler everyday child health problems in the developing countries?

The answer might be found by asking more questions and finding effective answers to these.

Technology for whom?

There are a number of simple measures and interventions which have already been recognized as having the potential to reduce child health problems considerably in all the less privileged parts of the world. These are not being applied widely or effectively enough, for lack of a basic health care infrastructure. Some form of basic health care at community level is essential, both to deal with illness and also as an entry point for preventive health care programmes and health education. The shape of health care at community level is going to vary considerably from one area to another, according to the resources that can be made available and the needs to be met. What is clear, however, is that with limited resources it cannot follow the Western model of high-cost, high-technology, hospital-based medical care, supplied by highly trained health professionals. Nor would this type of care necessarily be the correct answer to the problems which cause so much of the ill-health, for which some kind of behaviour change and introduction of basic facilities are often essential. Even among prosperous and more sophisticated societies, the real value of this type of health care is now being seriously questioned, as new health problems replace the older ones, and resources available for curative health care are being stretched.

The answer is now seen almost everywhere as the development of what is being called primary health care. This is day-to-day curative and preventive care, including health education, with participation at community and family level, backed up by referral possibilities to district hospitals and special medical centres for problems that are beyond the scope of the primary health care service. Primary health care can be given by a wide variety of health workers, provided that they are given appropriate training, professional back-up and supervision – and supplied with the right kind of tools with which to carry out their tasks.

In the training, supervision and support and, above all, in the daily work of primary health care workers, there is a crucial role for appropriate technology – both hardware and software and a mixture of both: educational technologies, communication technologies of all kinds, equipment, record-keeping, supplies, and administration. Where the conditions for delivery of primary health care are most difficult, the technology needs to be most carefully selected for its appropriateness.

What makes technology appropriate?

'Appropriate' generally means 'suited to' or 'in keeping with' particular circumstances or situations. Bearing in mind then that its place is usually to be at primary health care level, to be appropriate a technology should meet all or most of the following criteria:

- effective;
- culturally acceptable and valuable;
- affordable;
- sustainable locally;
- measurable;
- environmentally accountable;
- possessive of an evolutionary capacity;
- politically responsible.

Effective

This means that, above all, it must work. It must fulfil its purpose in the circumstances in which it needs to be used. For example, specially built incubators are fine for low-birth-weight babies in places that can afford to buy them and have reliable electricity supplies. But wrapping the baby up closely with its mother, 'the kangaroo technique', in a warm, humid atmosphere may serve the purpose almost as well in most situations and is an appropriate, alternative technology for perinatal care.

Culturally acceptable and valuable

Technology must fit into the hands, minds and lives of its users without disrupting a social fabric which may already be fragile. For example, it may be wiser to enlist traditional birth attendants in the detection of high-risk pregnancies and provide them with some training and appropriate equipment, rather than to damage their status by suggesting that they are not capable of taking good care of expectant mothers.

Affordable

This does not mean that to be appropriate a technology must always be cheap. The trade-offs between cost and effectiveness should always be carefully considered and the choice should be an informed one, made only after full consideration of all the resources that can be made available and the urgency and importance of the need to be met. Solar-powered refrigerators may turn out to be a useful example. The initial cost may be higher than the cost of a conventionally powered refrigerator for vaccine storage. But lower running and maintenance costs may justify the bigger investment, especially where there is no electricity and it is difficult to be sure of keeping up regular supplies of kerosene or bottled gas.

Sustainable locally

Any technology that is appropriate ought not to be overdependent on imported skills or scarce supplies of spare parts for its continuing functioning, maintenance and repair.

Measurable

The impact and performance of any technology needs continuing and proper evalution if it is going to be widely recommended. A good deal of naive thinking still bedevils the 'appropriate technology' world and does its cause no good. Mistakes must be publicized rather than conveniently overlooked.

Environmentally accountable

The technology should be environmentally harmless or, at least, minimally harmful. The indiscriminate use of insecticides and pesticides is a case in point. Clear instructions in local languages comprehensible to semi-literate local people should be included as part of the technology package. In this context, it could be useful also to consider the indiscriminate use of antibiotics, and the wrong use of drugs in general, as problems of resistance begin to cause anxiety in some areas.

Evolutionary capacity

This is not always possible but it adds to the appropriateness if the introduction and acceptance of a technology can pave the way towards further health benefits. For example, community-level training programmes in oral rehydration therapy are an excellent way to promote local interest and cooperation in improving water supplies, sanitation, food hygiene and nutrition.

Politically responsible

In introducing new ways to provide health care, it may not be a good idea to alter an existing balance in a manner that may prove counter-productive. For example, to encourage minimally trained health care workers to take on new tasks and initiatives and use appropriate technologies without first gaining the support of influential medical leaders in the area for this increased delegation of medical responsibility, may wreck a system that is already useful and prevent the successful introduction of a new element to the system.

Does appropriate mean second best?

Techniques and equipment appropriate to conditions in developing countries must never be classed as second rate just because they may not be generally used among the industrialized nations. All countries need to look carefully at the appropriateness of the technologies used in health care. It is equally essential that available resources are used wisely and most effectively in the developed countries – to examine for example the appropriateness of intensive neonatal care against the 'kangaroo method'. Similarly, the use of oral rehydration therapy for dehydration caused by diarrhoea is as appropriate for management of acute diarrhoea in the developed as in the developing countries. It is safe, effective and cheap. Unfortunately, routine use of intravenous therapy and hospitalization of young children with dehydration is common practice in most developed countries (unnecessarily so) and physicians could learn a great deal from their counterparts in the Third World about appropriate technologies for management of dehydrating diarrhoea.

Certain technologies may no longer be widely used in the developed countries for a variety of reasons. Disease patterns have changed, circumstances have altered, and in some cases shortages of some types of trained health care personnel have encouraged the introduction of greater automation, based on advanced technology. Not everyone is happy, for example, about the widespread use of fetal monitoring by machine. The fetal stethoscope remains an appropriate fetal monitoring device in trained hands in any situation – and training in its use and the correct interpretation of the observations made is a skill that needs to be extended to birth attendants everywhere.

On the other hand, there should be no romanticism about the innate appropriateness of local technologies. A handmade pottery jar looks picturesque on a mother's head as she makes her way to collect water for her family's needs. A plastic bucket is, however, much lighter to carry, much easier to clean and will not break. It may well be that the most economical and effective solutions for problems that typically occur in the developing countries can best be found in the adaptation of advanced technologies to a low-resource environment. The work of PATH (Program for Appropriate Technology in Health) on the use of complicated polymers as vaccine and sterilization safety markers and in the whole field of diagnostic techniques, the possibility of more robust one-shot vaccine 'cocktails', the use of two-way radio communication links powered by solar panels – these are all good examples of appropriate application of sophisticated science and technology to meet special needs.

Traditional technologies

Traditional technologies – for example, acupuncture, rice or other cereal-based oral rehydration solutions to prevent or treat dehydration due to diarrhoea, an upright position for the mother during childbirth, herbal remedies of various kinds – all of these and more are now considered worthy of scientific investigation with a view to their wider applicability, including their appropriateness in developed countries. Technology transfer should never be viewed as simply a one-way process.

There are perhaps three important decisions to be made about any indigenous technology. Is it scientifically sound and beneficial; neither harmful nor beneficial; or harmful? It may be appropriate even if it falls into the second category because it carries some local significance. Unnecessary meddling with people's lives wastes time and energy that could be used better for other purposes. Harmful technologies must obviously be discouraged and it is sometimes useful to offer a 'similar' but safer alternative. For example, where it is common practice to put some substance on

the cut surface of the umbilical cord, such as cow dung or other potential source of infection, it is more appropriate to continue the practice of dressing the cut cord but to provide a safe (and exciting looking) alternative for this purpose, such as gentian violet or acriflavine. Compromise almost certainly has a part to play in the promotion of appropriate technology for health.

Appropriate technology – whose responsibility?

Appropriate technology presents a vital challenge to many different disciplines and interests. It is no longer a question of gadgets and gimmicks. It is a key aspect of the much needed rapid implementation of primary health care. As such, it is in no way a simple matter but something which ought to attract the best brains in all sciences and industries.

A mistake that has been made in the past is the inadequacy of communication between the people with the problems and the people who might already have, or could develop, answers to the problems. This is where the romanticism about 'appropriate technology' may sometimes have played a dangerous role. It may be a waste of effort for well-meaning 'technologists', living and working in an advanced setting, to try to decide what might be helpful in a less advanced setting. Without the facts and actual experience of the realities, their answers may not meet the real needs and could cause disillusionment all round.

On the other hand, the health workers at the grass-roots level may not be able to imagine that technological expertise, if properly informed, might be in a position to provide them with more reliable and easier ways to deal with their problems. They know that record-keeping at community level is a burdensome chore. They may know about and may even possess a pocket calculator. They have, however, no access to the computer industries to ask for the development of record-keeping devices for use at community level, preferably solar-powered and totally robust, but still at an affordable price. In promoting the development of appropriate technologies for health, there is the 'go-between' gap, which is only gradually being filled. Far more emphasis is needed on technology 'software' – strategies for more effective communication, management, community organization, training and methods for developing information, education and communications to reach and involve communities and families.

Chance and serendipity have sometimes made

important contributions. The history of the PATH vaccine safety marker is one good example. Everyone concerned with immunization programmes realized that the 'cold chain' was crucial and wished that there could be an easy way to pick out any supplies of vaccine (especially measles) that had been exposed, somewhere along the line of the cold chain, to too high a temperature for too long. If only, they said, there could be some simple marker that changed colour when the vaccine was no longer effective to use. It so happened that representatives of PATH were meeting with people from a large chemical industry and this 'if only' came up in conversation. It transpired that the industry had, some years previously, developed a complex polymer which changed colour with a combination of time and temperature and had stored their discovery away as having no obvious use. The polymer was unearthed, developed and field-tested; it is now available as a safety marker for individual vaccine vials all the way to the periphery of the cold chain.

While chance can play a part, appropriate technology is too important to be left to chance. Dr E. F. Schumacher, whose book *Small is Beautiful* considerably influenced the fresh approach to the role of technology in development, spoke in 1977, just before his untimely death, about the need to involve the A–B–C–D combination.

'**A**dministration – people from government, the tax gatherers and spenders.

Business – the private sector, which has the capacity to make things viable and durable. Without this know-how, the best of ideas can wither away and valuable time be wasted.

Communicators – the people of the word, both written and spoken. Their help needs to be enlisted at all levels and in all societies.

Democratic social organizations – all kinds of social and interest groups everywhere: unions and trade guilds, church groups, clubs (especially those which involve women). Women, both within their families and through their formal and informal organizations, play a particularly critical role in the adaptation and application of appropriate technologies which relate to primary health care. In many communities, certain women have traditionally acquired skills and experience as birth attendants and as advisors on maternal and child health matters. It is clear that, if appropriate technologies for primary health care are to be applied successfully at family and community levels, women need to be involved in decision-making and their critical community role needs to be recognized.'

Clearly, appropriate technology always requires the interest and support of all the sections of Schumacher's A–B–C–D combination: those who plan, manage and pay for health care; the world of science and industry where technologies are invented, developed and marketed; the communication people who pass information and knowledge wherever it needs to go; and society in general with its varying groupings and interests.

An intersectoral approach

There are many dimensions to health since it is concerned with all aspects of life. An intersectoral approach is important in thinking about appropriate technology for health, and those working in the health sector must therefore look beyond the health sector. Technologies to do with housing construction and materials, food supplies, storage and preparation, diversification and productivity in agriculture, energy supplies, transport and every type of communication – all of these sectors outside the direct health field, and more, nevertheless can affect the health of the people and appropriateness must always be a consideration.

To take a single example, better cooking stove designs save fuel and produce less smoke. Promoting their use will reduce respiratory and eye diseases, save either expense or valuable maternal time and energy in obtaining scarce fuel supplies, reduce the danger to children of accidental burns, protect against soil erosion through loss of trees for firewood, improve nutrition in general and weaning practices in particular, and increase the chances of unsafe drinking water being boiled before being given to children. Interest in appropriate technology ought to be used to promote intersectoral cooperation in any area and to encourage different ministries to work together at a government level. It is also a useful way for non-government or voluntary organizations and programmes to work constructively together, rather than in isolation as can sometimes happen and which may prove to be wasteful.

Local and international support

It follows from the above considerations that responsibility for providing appropriate technology for health must be accepted at all levels because this is an interpersonal as well as an interdisciplinary and intersectoral activity. It is too important to be left to a few enthusiasts at either local or international level. The interface must be made as broad as possible. Communications play a central role because transfer of technology requires good methods of passing on information in a practical and acceptable way, not only from, to and at community level, but also nationally and internationally. The wheel should not need to be reinvented too many times if a health-appropriate technology information network can be established and gradually strengthened. This needs better intelligence systems, decision-making mechanisms and improved linkages between the appropriate technology field and those responsible for overall health care strategies. For all of this, appropriate political and social technologies are required. One very real danger is of 'appropriate technology' becoming a catchword, the simple answer to all the problems. It is not at all simple and those involved need to be aware of this and should never become complacent about what they are trying to achieve.

One of the most important tasks of all is that of the 'honest broker' and many more of these are needed. The 'honest broker' knows about the whole range of possibilities that exist, or could perhaps be invented in a certain health-related area, for example diagnostic technologies at health centre and small hospital level. This includes both the tangible things – the hardware – and the techniques and information known as software. The broker is in a position to set out the choices that are, or could be made, available in a way that can be readily understood both at international and local level. Not only choices must be on offer, but also advisors to facilitate making the choices and to teach about the best way to use technologies. But all choices on offer must be reliable ones – well tried and tested – because in the end it is the local people who have to live with the choice, use it to meet their needs, help to pay for it and become responsible for its maintenance and repair. In this context it is crucial that strong links are developed and maintained between relevant personnel in both developing and developed countries, and between the countries concerned, to ensure that exchange of information, experiences and expertise takes place. This transfer of knowledge can take place through a variety of channels: international agencies; regional and country-based workshops and training and refresher programmes; information dissemination, on a global, national and local scale; networking between voluntary organizations and non-governmental organizations, for example the work of AHRTAG*. The media have an important role to play, and improvements in communications

*The Appropriate Health Resources and Technologies Action Group, founded in 1977 by the author, has developed an extensive resource and information centre and collaborates with similar centres overseas. It also produces several international newsletters on topics of major significance for maternal and child health at primary health care level. Address: 1 London Bridge Street, London SE1 9SG, UK.

technologies may well facilitate internationalization of knowledge about developments in appropriate technology.

Therefore, the maximum amount of relevant expertise is required of those who assemble the technological choices, work out effective adaptations according to local circumstances and carry out stringent testing and evaluation. Providing this expertise calls also for appropriate funding to support information activities, training, the establishment of lists of 'best buys' in appropriate technology for health, together with an appropriate advisory service for the consumers.

Applications of appropriate technology

Other chapters in this book have outlined many areas where appropriate technology can contribute to better child health care. Hospital-based technologies may require less adaptation of existing equipment than those needed for community use. Nevertheless, even in the hospital setting, there will be environmental factors to consider such as heat, dust and humidity, as well as reliability or otherwise of power supplies. Human factors are just as important in relation to both operating and maintenance skills. And cost is always a factor from every angle.

A good example of the right kind of collaborative investment by health care experts together with industry is the recent development of a small, rugged X-ray machine (see pp. 1019–20). This will take care of straightforward diagnostic needs, is not unduly sensitive to the fluctuations of local electricity supplies and an operator can learn to use it with a few weeks of training, for which an appropriate manual is supplied. Here the 'package' has been developed with the help of a wide range of appropriate in-puts and has been thoroughly field-tested before being put on the market. The end-product is an important and reasonably priced contribution to appropriate technology for diagnosis in the developing world.

Towards the end of 1985, UNICEF, WHO and the Aga Khan Foundation organized and sponsored a significant workshop. Its members considered how to move towards more effective use of primary health care technologies at the family and community level. Discussions centred around four crucial areas in child health: delivery care technologies, immunization technologies, nutrition-related technologies and communication technologies. The workshop report describes technologies that can be recommended and identifies some of the many gaps that remain to be filled. Ways to overcome some of these are known to be on their way; bridging some of the others remains much more problematical. One crucial gap is the need for better training, monitoring and evaluation materials. Another is for better ways to procure community involvement in the delivery of child health care and nowhere is this need more clearly seen than in our ever-growing concern about the AIDS problem.

Conclusion

There must be broad-based support for the whole process of appropriate health-related technology development and transfer. It needs to be legitimated at all levels. The possible value of some indigenous technologies must not be overlooked. Appropriate technology for health must be the concern of all who work in the health field, both nationally and internationally, and in all other sectors which relate in any way to health.

In some situations, this will require a fundamental reorientation of both the health system and of decision-makers to recognize the importance of the adaptation of and transfer of appropriate technologies for health and to ensure their effective application at levels where their use will have the greatest impact.

Spreading the word about what needs to be developed in appropriate technology for health and about what is already available is the responsibility of all who care about equity in child health care throughout the world.

Appendix: Basic guidelines for the district level hospital physician

- Assessment of most serious local health problems.
- Analysis of data collected.
- Setting goals and priorities for action.
- Decisions about intervention strategy: curative and preventive, based on availability of resources, costs and benefits.
- Decisions about most appropriate hard technologies.
- Decisions about most appropriate soft technologies.

Examples

Area	More appropriate	Less appropriate
Investigation	BRS (X-ray)	Whole-body scanner
Neonatal intensive care	Kangaroo method	Incubator
Records	Parent-based chart	Clinic-based chart
Treatment of mild dehydration	Oral rehydration therapy	Intravenous therapy
Assessment of the newborn	Simplified diagnostic score (Sigtuna) based on heartbeat and breathing	APGAR score
Parasitic infections	Improvements to water and sanitation facilities and health education	Drug therapy
Malnutrition	Small-scale gardening and animal rearing	Food supplementation programmes
Cold chain technology	Cold boxes/solar refrigerators	Kerosene-/electric-powered refrigerators
Neonatal/perinatal care	Training traditional birth attendants	Training and introducing midwives to new areas
Acute respiratory infection	Home care without drugs	Drug therapy with antibiotics
Hospital treatment	Admit children with parents for care while in hospital	Use of nurses and medical auxiliaries for hospital care
Growth monitoring	MUAC measurement with old X-ray film	Weighing scales
	Parent-/home-based growth charts	Clinic-based growth charts
Ventilation in hospital	Architecture/materials proper ventilation	Air-conditioning

Considerations

Most appropriate epidemiological approach

- costs involved;
- personnel available;
- levels of literacy;
- timescale;
- facilities for analysing data;
- cultural factors;
- number of people within the district area.

Appropriate goals and priorities

- most serious child health problems;
- aetiological causes of morbidity and mortality;
- feasibility of achieving goals within constraints of resources available.

Strategy

- curative approach vs preventive approach;
- allocation of resources to these approaches;
- likely benefits of strategy *vis-à-vis* health problems in relation to costs.

Hard technologies: appropriateness

- geographical circumstances;
- costs;
- supply lines and logistics;
- access to repair and maintenance;
- access to regular power supplies;
- cultural factors.

Soft technologies: appropriateness

- development of training materials;
- management structures;
- community awareness and participation;
- manpower availability;
- resources available to develop training programmes;
- record-keeping systems;
- health education materials;
- supervision of health-workers.

Further reading

Directions. Newsletters published by Program for Appropriate Technology in Health (PATH), 4, Nickerson Street, Seattle, Washington 98109, Seattle, USA.

Elliott K. *Auxiliaries in Primary Health Care: An Annotated Bibliography*. London, Intermediate Technology Publications, 1979.

Jequier N. Appropriate technology: the challenge of the second generation. In: Tyrrell DAJ, Henderson W, Elliott K eds. *More Technologies for Rural Health*. London, Royal Society, 1980.

McRobie G. *Small is Possible*. London, Jonathan Cape, 1981.

Primary Health Care Technologies at the Family and Community Level. Report of a workshop sponsored by the United Nations Children's Fund, the Aga Khan Foundation and the World Health Organization. Aga Khan Foundation, PO Box 435, 1211 Geneva 6, Switzerland, 1986.

Schumacher EF. *Small is Beautiful*. London, Blond and Briggs, 1973.

Werner D. *Where There Is No Doctor*. Hesperian Foundation, PO Box 1692, Palo Alto, CA 94302, USA, 1977.

Werner D, Bower B. *Helping Health Workers Learn*. Hesperian Foundation, PO Box 1692, Palo Alto, CA 94302, USA, 1982.

CHAPTER 5

Child-care in refugee situations

John Seaman

The emergencies which have a profound effect upon the health of populations and a disproportionate effect on the health and welfare of children are those which share two characteristics. These are the displacement of a population away from its home area and more importantly, its concentration into a camp for the provision of relief (Fig. 6.5.1). Because of the poor siting and lack of services which characterize most new camp sites and the increase in population density, disease and malnutrition may rapidly become epidemic, particularly among children under five years of age. Recent population movements in Africa have led to crude mortalities in such populations of the order of 2/1000 per day; rates which have sometimes been sustained for periods of weeks or months.

In theory, major population movements might be caused by a wide range of events, including earthquakes and other natural disasters. In practice they have chiefly resulted from war, political repression and famine. In recent times, such movements have occurred on a vast scale, not only in the well-publicized cases such as the recent events in the Horn of Africa, but also in many countries of Central and South America, West and Southern Africa, Asia and Australasia. Fortunately the effects of population movement are, like those of other emergencies, largely predictable. The best approaches to the provision of relief are well understood; even if they are not always effectively implemented.

The health problems of displaced populations are qualitatively very similar to those of poor settled populations. They differ only in scale, and in the fact that the highest rates of mortality and morbidity occur in the period immediately after displacement, precisely at the time when levels of organization of services are least.

The techniques which are used in the management of displaced populations are essentially the same as those applied under more normal conditions. The difference lies in the priority accorded to different actions and in the speed with which these must be implemented. In time, morbidity and mortality will fall. After a few months, the health problems of a displaced population will be very similar to those of any urban slum, with the exception that a displaced population will usually remain dependent upon external supplies of food.

The approach to the provision of emergency services is therefore based upon two principles. First, an understanding of the health problems which can be foreseen in a newly displaced population, and which can therefore be prevented or minimized in effect. Second, the active collection of information to recognize, quantify and monitor other problems as they arise. Emergency services are directed towards priority health problems, and are designed in such a way that there is coverage of defined population groups.

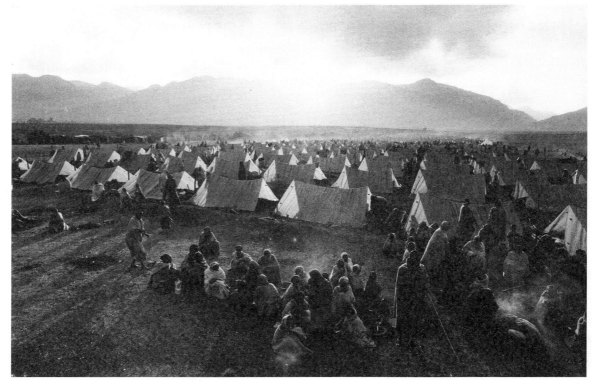

Fig. 6.5.1   Korem Camp, Ethiopia, 1985.

Health problems of displaced populations

The health problems of displaced populations can be most easily understood in terms of the health conditions of a population prior to movement; the reasons for and the effects on health of the movement itself; and lastly the changes in the epidemiology of disease and malnutrition which follow the concentration of a population into a camp or temporary settlement. Not all of these effects may be expected in every case. They are summarized in Table 6.5.1.

Health conditions before movement

The health problems of rural populations in the developing countries are described at greater length elsewhere in this book. However, in the context of emergencies, they set the scene for the creation of other problems and the major relevant features are summarized here.

In demographic terms, such populations tend to be youthful: 10–15 per cent of a rural population is likely to be under five years of age: 40–50 per cent under 15 years of age. Both adults and children will be lighter and smaller at a given age or height, and the population may usually be expected to contain a small proportion of frankly malnourished children. It is probable that their diet has been, at least seasonally, deficient in vitamin A, and that body stores of this vitamin are low. Intakes of vitamin C and some B vitamins may also have been low. A variable but sometimes large proportion of the children will not have been immunized against measles, pertussis or other diseases; and they will be subject to malaria, trachoma and a range of intestinal parasites and other pathogens. In many cases their experience of organized medical services will be minimal.

Effects of movement

Wholesale population movement is rare. In most cases only part of a population will move, sometimes with marked effect on population structure. At the extremes, a displaced population may be composed almost

Table 6.5.1 The origins of the health problems of displaced populations

Original population
  High proportion of children <5 years of age
  Pre-existing malnutrition
  Low vitamin A reserves
  Low immunization coverage
Movement
  Possible increase in proportion of children <5 years of age
  Reduced food intake
  Environmental exposure
  Possible introduction of or exposure to new diseases
'Concentration'
  Poor sanitation and increase in diarrhoea
  High risk of measles epidemic
  Increase in scabies, conjunctivitis
  Poor food supply, shortage of fuel, utensils, lack of shelter
    causing increase in malnutrition
  Increase in vitamin A deficiency
  Possible increase in vector-borne disease

entirely of young men or of women and children.

Political repression often selectively affects the better-off and better educated, and may lead to an exodus of young men and women from urban areas. Poor rural farmers who are affected by food shortages do not stay to starve in their villages, but will migrate in search of food. The patterns of migration which result are complex, and as variable as the economic alternatives available in any place, but tend often to demand the division of the family. Adult men, for example, may seek agricultural work at a distance: women and children may move to urban areas to seek work or to beg. In some cases, men in the economically active age groups may remain to guard livestock and other property.

Population movement itself may cause a marked deterioration in the health of children. Movement is usually on foot and may be over considerable distances. The combined effects of fatigue, exposure, food shortage, a deterioration in dietary quality and the obvious difficulty of providing adequate child-care under these conditions may reduce nutritional status and increase the prevalence of malnutrition.

The movement of population may also cause the movement of disease, eg. typhus and relapsing fever with Ethiopian refugees to the Sudan; or the exposure of a population to a new disease at the point of arrival. Many deaths from malaria amongst Kampuchean refugees in Thailand occurred for this reason.

Effects of concentration

It has been rare for the movement of a population to be foreseen in sufficient time for adequate arrangements to

be made for their reception. Typically, and particularly where movement is across a national border, there is difficulty in locating a suitable site for a camp. Few countries have suitable well-drained sites with access to potable water which are not already settled or farmed. Issues of land tenure may arise, as may differences in some countries between regional and central governments, or between government and relief agencies as to their respective responsibilities. People may arrive and settle spontaneously at the nearest convenient location. Where movement follows famine this is often within or next to a town, as people seek opportunities for employment.

Two main health problems will arise, chiefly affecting children. First, there will be an increase in the incidence of communicable disease. Little imagination is required to foresee the conditions which arise when 100 000 people are concentrated on a small site without latrines. Diarrhoeal disease, often including epidemic bacterial dysentery, will increase because of gross insanitation and the contamination of water supplies. Measles may rapidly become epidemic as a large group of susceptible children are brought together, as will scabies and other skin diseases, and conjunctivitis.

Second, there will be an increase in rates of malnutrition. Food supplies are often inadequate in both quantity and quality. In the short run, only grain may be available for distribution. Household utensils and fuel may also be in short supply. In some cases, where populations have moved to highland areas, food shortage may be compounded by environmental exposure. This, and the effects of communicable disease may cause a rapid deterioration in nutritional status. In most instances this is most marked in the under five years age group. In the worst cases, 50 percent or more of this age group have been below 80 per cent of Harvard reference values for weight-for-length.

Vitamin deficiencies may also be a serious problem. Where rations are deficient in vitamin A, an increase in rates of deficiency may be expected in displaced populations in most developing countries. Vitamin B deficiencies have rarely caused major health problems, although beriberi does regularly occur in some refugee populations in South-east Asia where the diet is based on polished rice. Scurvy is unpredictable in occurrence. Outbreaks of scurvy have occurred in camps in Sudan and Somalia. In Sudan this was associated with a diet containing very little vitamin C: in Somalia it followed the closure of markets in which refugees had been exchanging vitamin C–deficient rations for other foods. However, scurvy has not been observed in many populations whose intakes of vitamin C were at least as low as in these cases.

The approach to relief

Relief for displaced populations should aim at prevention, it should take account of the variation in problems which may occur under specific conditions and it should allow for the continuous modification of services as health conditions change and improve.

As the greatest burden of morbidity and mortality will occur during the early period in the life of a camp, this requires a reordering of conventional approaches to the provision of health care. Training, habit and instinct may lead the medical practitioner, when confronted with a disorganized population numbering many tens of thousands with apparently overwhelming health problems, to open a clinic or hospital. However, efforts should be directed away from clinical care towards the more pressing problems of the prevention of disease and the organization of systems through which services can be delivered to the whole population or to selected population groups.

This approach is described under three main headings. First, immediate actions which must always be taken to minimize mortality and morbidity; second, the period of recovery, when services are being developed; third, the problem of modifying and phasing out services in the long-term. These are summarized in Table 6.5.2. In each period, the collection of information is a high priority.

Immediate actions

Immunization

The concentration of a large population of non-immune children will inevitably lead to an epidemic of measles. This will cause high mortality. Moreover, the care of sick children will occupy and distract medical staff from other activities. Measles immunization should therefore be carried out at the earliest possible opportunity, and ideally as children arrive at the camp. Except where the population is small, other immunizations should be delayed until levels of organization are sufficient to ensure that a useful coverage can also be obtained with second and third doses. In some situations immunization against yellow fever may also be a priority.

Vitamin A

High-dose vitamin A capsules or liquid should be administered to all children, ideally as they arrive at the camp.

Water and sanitation

The provision of adequate supplies of water for drinking and washing and attention to the problem of sanitation are an obvious priority. Neither problem

Table 6.5.2   Steps in the development of health programmes for displaced populations

Information required	Use of information	Action
Immediate • map • census • anthropometric survey	• size and location of population • number of children • prevalence of PEM • requirement for supplementary feeding • number and location of feeding centres	• measles immunization • vitamin A distribution • simple improvements in sanitation • louse control • simple out-patient/day care services • home visiting programme
Recovery • mortality • out-patient morbidity data • repeat anthropometric survey • feeding centre attendance	• monitoring changes in disease • estimating coverage of supplementary feeding • changes in prevalence of PEM	• supplementary feeding programmes • development of community based health programmes • development of MCH/antenatal services • pertussis, polio and other immunizations
Long-term • surveys of specific diseases, e.g. tuberculosis • anthropometric surveys • continued collection of morbidity/mortality data	• planning control programmes • nutrition and disease surveillance	• development of community based PHC • reduction of trained staff to appropriate affordable levels • possible introduction of services for local population.

PEM = protein–energy malnutrition; MCH = mother and child health care; PHC = primary health care.

may be easy to solve. Under many conditions, the provision of adequate quantities of good quality water will require specialized engineering assistance and equipment. The construction of pit latrines, although often recommended, is less easy than it may appear at first sight. To supply a latrine to each family of a population of 10 000 people may require the construction of upwards of a thousand latrines. People may be unimpressed with the need for latrines and even less so about providing the labour for construction, particularly when there are few adult men in the population. Communal latrines are more quickly and easily constructed but are rarely successful in use since they are soon fouled and people are usually reluctant to clean them.

In practice it may be possible to quickly improvise improvements in water supply and sanitation. Where water is obtained from a river or other open source, contamination may be reduced by simple expedients such as building a fence or by employing guards to restrict the access of the population to a few supervised collection points. An improvement in sanitation may be quickly secured by establishing defaecation areas well away from, and where they will not drain into, water sources: if a road grader or bulldozer can be obtained these areas may be periodically scraped to reduce smell and to diminish the breeding of flies.

Vector control

This, like the provision of water is a specialized topic. The control of body and head lice is a priority in areas where typhus and relapsing fever occur. Pyrethrin-based dusting powders are of low toxicity and are probably the most suitable agents for use in large populations. Where supplies are difficult to obtain or access to the population is restricted, residual preparations may be more appropriate. Flies may breed in vast numbers in some camps and be a serious nuisance and health hazard. These can be controlled by cyclical 'ultra low volume' insecticide spraying although this is expensive. The chemical control of mosquitoes in camps is rarely justified and should not be considered without expert appraisal.

Collection of information

Some health problems of children, and specifically malnutrition, can be assumed to be important in most displaced populations. To plan and manage services for these, information will be required to quantify the problems, monitor changes and to assess the coverage and effectiveness of the services which have been organized. The following information is the minimum which is required.

- *A map.* Camps may cover a considerable area and a map is essential as a basis for the collection of other information, the siting of services, and at a later date to provide specific 'addresses' for the follow-up of patients. This is of special importance if a tuberculosis control programme is to be organized. Initially a simple sketch map will suffice, which can be elaborated later to show sections of the camp, services, and when the camp is settled, even individual houses.

- *A census* is required as the basis for almost any other information collection or health activity. Small populations may be completely enumerated. An estimate of larger populations is usually more easily and accurately obtained from a house count multiplied by an estimate of house occupancy obtained by sample or systematic survey. A rough age and sex breakdown may be obtained in the same way.

- *An anthropometric survey* should be done as soon as is reasonably possible to estimate the prevalence of malnutrition in children under about five years of age. The anthropometric index which is most widely used is weight-for-length. A random cluster survey of the weight-for-length of children under five years of age allows an estimate to be made of the proportion of children below a specified 'cut-off' level, usually 80 per cent of reference values. Children with oedema are counted separately. This, taken with population data, provides an estimate of the number of malnourished children in the population, from which the need for supplementary feeding services may be decided. A survey also gives a baseline with which future survey results may be compared and progress monitored.

- Efforts should be made to obtain reliable and regular data on *mortality*, ideally by age group. This can be difficult, unless there is a definite burial ground or a single system for the disposal of the dead.

Recovery phase

The objective of child health and nutrition programmes in displaced populations must be to obtain the greatest benefit for the maximum number, not a high standard of service for a few. If this is to be achieved quickly for a large population where there are few skilled personnel two principles must be observed. First, the main effort must be directed away from the direct provision of clinical services. Second, work must be delegated at an early stage to less-skilled people: if this is not done, coverage of the population cannot be achieved.

Health services

A practical order for the development of health services is to establish an out-patient service capable of coping efficiently with large numbers of children suffering from diarrhoea, dehydration, respiratory tract and other serious but relatively easily diagnosed infections. This may be used as the basis for the organization of a community health programme to achieve greater population coverage of services.

Out-patient services The considerable demand which may exist for medical services, the lack of experience of some parts of the population in their use and the self-selecting nature of the patients make static clinics an inefficient approach to the solution of general health problems. Very large numbers of patients may attend for treatment: many of these may have only trivial complaints. For this reason patients should be selected and sorted on arrival. More serious cases may be selected in the waiting area and given tickets for priority admission. All patients should first be seen by paramedical staff and should only be seen by qualified staff when referred. Buildings may be simple in construction, but should be laid out to control patient flow and to give space for demonstrations, eg. oral rehydration, health education. Sometimes trained staff may be recruited locally. If not, they must be trained.

Drugs Drugs should be restricted to a limited number of appropriate generic preparations. A drug store with an adequate stock control system should be organized as a priority.

Hospital services The temptation to organize a field hospital should be resisted. The value of a hospital lies in the provision of nursing care, investigation and more complex treatment than can be provided at home. In most camps these possibilities do not, at least in the short run, exist. Hospitals tend rapidly to fill with the undiagnosable and chronically ill and impose impossible demands on the skilled nursing which is available. Day-care facilities for rehydration or a few beds for overnight observation are usually sufficient. Children should be accepted for treatment only if accompanied by their mother or an older relative.

Community based health services These provide the key to the efficient delivery of services. Community health workers (CHW) are usually literate people drawn from

or selected by the displaced population. With a short training and some organization the CHW can take responsibility for a defined section of the population. Within this they can locate and motivate the ill and malnourished to attend services; communicate with the population where programmes are planned, eg. immunization, and maintain records on patients requiring follow-up visits and of mortality. With further training the CHW may also give health education and provide oral rehydration and other simple remedies. If, as conditions improve, a tuberculosis control programme is organized, the CHW can assist with case-identification and follow-up.

Immunization As soon as levels of organization are sufficient to ensure high levels of coverage, immunization should be extended to include diphtheria, pertussis, tetanus, poliomyelitis and BCG. If only poor coverage was obtained with the initial measles immunization, this should be repeated.

Records of *attendances and diagnoses* made at clinical facilities may provide, with intelligent interpretation, a crude estimate of the incidence of disease in the general population. Sharp rises in attendances for specific conditions, eg. dysenteries and measles, may stimulate further investigation, as may the observation of even single 'sentinel' cases of particular diseases.

The treatment and control of malnutrition

Two types of service are usually organized: 'supplementary' centres which are intended for the treatment and sometimes the prevention of less-severe malnutrition and 'therapeutic' centres for severely malnourished children (see also pp. 358, 493).

Supplementary feeding centres These are intended to provide an additional cooked supplement of food to moderately malnourished children to speed their recovery. In general, children of from 70–79 per cent of Western reference values for weight-for-length are included in this category. The diets vary with the foods available but are usually 'high-energy' mixtures of cereal/legume/oil · or dried skimmed milk (DSM)/ oil/sugar. The quantity given to each child per day as a supplement is typically in the range 2—4 MJ (500–1000 kcal). Where food supplies and time permit, it may be possible to prepare these foods in ways familiar to the population concerned (see pp. 335–57, 358–66).

Ideally, centres should be distributed within the camp area for easy access and should accommodate no more than 200 children, although centres for more than 10 000 children have been successfully run. Supplementary centres may also be an efficient way to provide other services, eg. de-worming, vitamin A distribution and the treatment of scabies.

When the rations distributed to a displaced population are grossly inadequate in quantity, 'supplementary' centres may also provide a means of maintaining a higher food intake for children, pregnant women and sometimes other specific groups. A larger ration is given. In extreme cases where no general ration is available at all, this may be the full food requirement for a large part of a camp population. In one camp in Ethiopia up to 60 000 prepared meals were supplied each day. Large and highly organized kitchens are required.

Therapeutic feeding centres   These may be run on a day-care or (usually better) 24-hour basis to allow for night feeds. The children admitted are usually below 70 per cent of Western weight-for-length reference values. Many will also be suffering from a range of infections and will require close medical supervision. The feeding regimens are those used routinely under more normal

conditions. In general, DSM/oil/sugar mixes are used because of availability and convenience. These are mixed in the ratio 80:50:40 by weight (which if tied in a plastic bag may be kept for several days): 170 g of this mixture dissolved in one litre of water provides approximately 30 g protein and 3.7 MJ (900 kcal). Suitable diets with a similar protein–energy content may also be made from other mixtures of foods.

Records should be kept of *attendances at feeding centres*, which, taken with the results of an anthropometric survey, gives an estimate of the coverage of the service.

Vitamin deficiencies   Ideally, vitamin deficiencies should be controlled by an improvement in the general ration. Where this is impractical because of lack of supplies or cost, it may be necessary to consider the distribution of vitamins. In practice, this has been required only for vitamin A and C. Occasional cases of other vitamin deficiencies are probably best treated individually. The specific vitamin should be used in each case: there is no case for the routine use of 'multivitamin' tablets (see pp. 367–79).

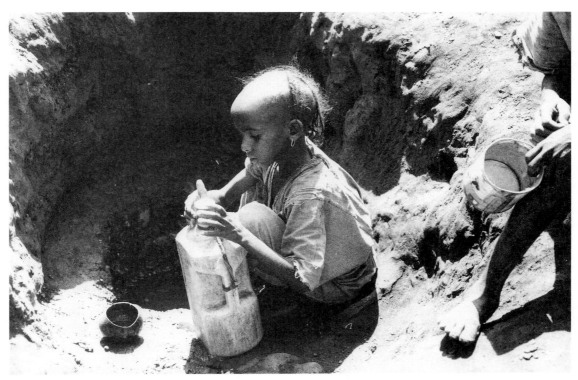

Fig. 6.5.2   Inadequate water supply, Wad Kowli Camp, Sudan, 1985.

Water supply and sanitation   Consideration should be given to organizing permanent solutions to these problems. The provision of adequate supplies of water, particularly in remote or dry areas may require quite complex engineering works (Fig. 6.5.2). In many situations it may be difficult, for reasons which have already been given, to supply latrines to each family in a large population. Where it is practical to supply family latrines it is important to use a design which will improve sanitary conditions. Roughly built pit latrines may allow flies and mosquitoes to breed and be a bigger risk to health than no latrines at all. In dry climates, carefully located defaecation areas may represent the best option for health.

The long term

Long-term actions involve modifying and phasing out services with changing health needs.

The high rates of mortality and morbidity which characterize many displaced populations are rarely sustained for longer than a few weeks or months. The combined effects of successful health programmes, spontaneous social reorganization and improved food supplies will lead to an improvement in the health of children. Often, mortality will fall to, or even below, the levels typical of rural populations in the developing countries. As mortality and morbidity from diarrhoea, malnutrition and other diseases fall, it is possible to phase out feeding centres and other emergency measures and to consider the introduction of other health programmes. If a community health programme has been organized it is often simple and inexpensive to introduce programmes for the control of tuberculosis and trachoma.

It is important not to use the opportunity to elaborate clinical services to a level of complexity which is above the level of services available to the surrounding population and which is too expensive to be maintained in the long term. It is usually most appropriate to develop community health services to a higher level of organization and to reduce clinical services and the numbers of trained medical staff to a level which can be maintained. Many displaced populations remain in camps for periods of years. There are cases where the successful development of such services for displaced populations has been the stimulus to the development of similar services for the surrounding rural population.

Further reading

Seaman J (Ed) Medical care in refugee camps. Disasters. *The International Journal of Disaster Studies and Practice*. Vol 5 No 3 1981.

Simmonds S, Vaughan P, Gunn SW. *Refugee community health care*. Oxford, Oxford University Press. 1983.

United Nations High Commissioner for Refugees. *Handbook for emergencies*. Geneva, UNHCR, 1981.

CHAPTER 6

Practical procedures

C. J. Clements

The procedures described here have been used many times, and work satisfactorily. The methods are both practical and practicable. The minimum of trained help is needed.

The tropical paediatrician must be both jack of all trades and master of as many as possible. He will need to become skilled in a number of difficult but frequently life-saving procedures, often carried out in disadvantageous conditions. He will have to obtain samples of body fluid which in an adult would be difficult, but in a child appears well nigh impossible! Techniques can soon be learned, however, and the impossible performed daily.

The majority of procedures are made more difficult in paediatrics by an uncooperative patient who presents an evermoving, diminutive target. Suitable instruments may be scarce, though the advent of scalp vein needles has simplified many procedures considerably. These have 'wings' of plastic, giving them their trade name of Butterfly Needles. In the last few years more disposable instruments, catheters, and tubes designed for paediatric use have been manufactured, but they may not be readily available in smaller tropical hospitals. Good improvisation is still necessary.

Many practical procedures are frightening to the patient. Gentle reassurance helps to calm younger children. Sedation is rarely necessary, but older children need a certain amount of explanation, as do their mothers. A masterly infusion is of no avail if it is taken down by a relative who does not much care for the look of it.

The operator should seek the maximum chance of success in a procedure by first assembling everything required. If an assistant is available this will help to secure the patient. The way the baby is restrained in a blanket should be studied carefully (Fig. 6.6.1).

The mother/father should be invited to be present during the procedure, which should be explained to

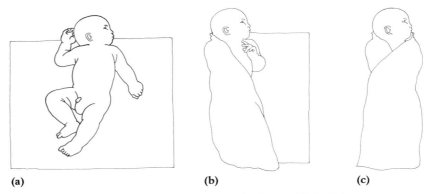

(a)   **(b)**   **(c)**

Fig. 6.6.1   Restraining the infant. (All drawings in this chapter by J. Gardner and R. Smith.)

them. All practical procedures in paediatrics can be potentially messy. Without due care, body fluids will end up being spread around everything, including the nurse and the paediatrician! Remember that all body fluids should be regarded as potentially infectious. If you work on this premise, you will safeguard yourself against hepatitis B, human immunodeficiency virus and a variety of other pathogens. Avoid getting body fluids on your skin, and if there is contact, wash the fluid off at once.

Venous infusions

This is probably the most important procedure to be mastered. The site selected varies with the age of the patient and the urgency with which therapy is required. The smaller peripheral veins are the safest and the most commonly used. The scalp veins may be large enough to use until four or five years of age. Of the other peripheral veins the dorsum of the hand or foot provides large vessels which may be easily entered. When there are veins visible the choice is personal and usually depends on how easy it is to fix the needle in place (Fig. 6.6.2).

In a collapsed child the choice of sites may be restricted to the larger veins, the most commonly used being the long saphenous, the femoral and the subclavian veins. The use of the umbilical vein is restricted to the first few days of life, and is then reserved for certain specific procedures only.

Scalp vein infusions

Indications

Scalp veins are an excellent route for infusions in the

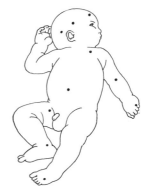

Fig. 6.6.2   Sites for intravenous infusion.

first two years of life, when they are relatively large. The needle is easily secured and allows virtually full movement of the child, to the extent that he can be picked up and nursed in the parent's arms. There are sufficient veins to choose from so that, by careful rotation of the needle around available sites, intravenous therapy can be continued almost indefinitely.

Method

Several veins are relatively constant and suitable for use. They include the vein on the forehead in the midline, in my experience the best one to choose as it allows maximum change of position of the head. Also suitable are the postauricular vein and the branches of the temporal vein running in front of the pinna and close to the more tortuous artery. The infant should be secured in a blanket as shown in Fig. 6.6.1. If available, an assistant should also steady the head. A generous area of scalp around the selected area is shaved with a

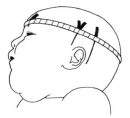

Fig. 6.6.3 Scalp vein infusion.

safety razor and the skin is cleaned with spirit. An elastic band around the head (Fig. 6.6.3) will act well as a tourniquet, or if preferred, the assistant's thumb may occlude the vein.

A 21 or 23 gauge needle will usually be suitable, although premature infants may need a 25. If Butterfly Needles are not available, the same procedure can be carried out with a standard hypodermic needle. It is possible to make a serviceable alternative to a Butterfly Needle from a 21 gauge needle. The bevel must be filed to a less acute angle and the plastic removed from the other end. A fine polythene catheter is then forced over the end of the needle and the apparatus is sterilized before use. The needle is flushed with saline or other clear fluid to avoid an airlock later. Blood can be gently 'milked' into the vein in a similar manner to venipuncture, and the vein fixed by pulling the skin taut with the free hand. The needle, bevel upwards, is introduced through the skin at an angle of 30° (Fig. 6.6.4) in the line of the vein. The experienced operator will recognize a 'plop' when the vein is entered, and this will be confirmed by a rush of blood up the tubing. Enough fluid is then syringed through the needle to clear it of blood and if a Butterfly Needle is used, the syringe can be left on until the job of securing is completed. Plaster of paris cut from a roll to approximately 2 × 5 cm pieces is ideal, dipped in hot water, and placed round the

needle. The original angle of the needle should be maintained at 30° by packing sufficient plaster underneath it. When the plaster is hard, the infusion set can be connected.

Special precautions

Blood, electrolyte replacement fluid, drugs, and food can all be given by scalp vein. If, however, caustic drugs such as calcium gluconate, Aminosol, or 50 per cent dextrose are given in this way, the infusion site must be carefully watched to ensure that the fluid is not infiltrating the tissues. Unpleasant sloughing of the scalp can occur, requiring grafting at a later date. Occasionally an artery will be cannulated by mistake; it is reasonable to leave the needle *in situ* and establish an infusion if there is no obvious alternative vessel and if the circumstances are desperate enough. Hypertonic solutions or drugs likely to produce an intimal reaction should not be given.

Peripheral vein infusions

Hand When a suitable vein can be seen on the dorsum, cannulation should present no problem. In a plump or oedematous child where no vein is visible, it may be necessary to use anatomical landmarks. The venae comitantes of the fifth digital artery are relatively large in the infant, draining into the vein between the fourth and fifth metacarpals. This vein is usually straight (Fig. 6.6.5) and lies in the middle of the space between the fourth and fifth metacarpals.[1]

Method

The limb must be secured on a splint before the needle is introduced. A well-equipped hospital may have a

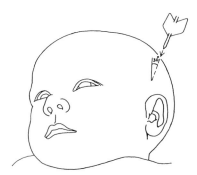

Fig. 6.6.4 Scalp vein infusion.

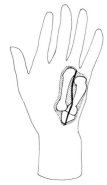

Fig. 6.6.5 Fifth metacarpal vein.

variety of aluminium splints precut to size. Tailor-made splints can rapidly be fashioned from a double layer of cardboard from the infusion set box, covered with tape over the sharp edges and with a gauze lining. The fingers should be secured over the edge of the splint with some gauze packing under the wrist. This maintains the wrist in a slightly flexed position and suitably displays the dorsum of the hand. It is always best to secure the arm in the splint with bandages and then pin the splint to the sheet or tie it to part of the bed. Restraints round the wrist are avoided as they tend to restrict the blood supply and damage skin.

An assistant's grasp around the forearm above the splint will steady the limb and act as a tourniquet. The dorsum of the hand is cleaned and the vein is made to stand out by gently tapping it. A Butterfly Needle (gauge 21 or 23) is attached to a syringe and flushed through with normal saline.

The operator passes the needle through the skin and should pause a moment until the wriggling has stopped. The tip of the needle, bevel up, is advanced and blood will flow into the Butterfly tubing as soon as venipuncture is accomplished. The tourniquet is released and the Butterfly secured before connecting the infusion set.

Antecubital fossa The veins here are larger and therefore more easily seen or palpated. A similar technique is used to the hand.

Particular attention must be paid to splinting the elbow firmly in extension. If the splint is loose enough to allow the elbow to flex, the needle will soon cut out of the vein. The splint needs to be firmly anchored if the patient is restless. An in-dwelling cannula is much better than a needle in this situation, but it requires a larger vessel.

Small intravenous cannulae While intravenous infusion through a peripherally sited needle is adequate for the majority of occasions, there are circumstances where large volumes of fluid must be administered rapidly, or when maintenance of a dependable infusion is an absolute necessity. The use of a small intravenous plastic cannula is ideal in these circumstances.

Method

Any vein of adequate size and length can be used. Because the portal of entry is larger than with a Butterfly Needle, it is worth anaesthetizing the skin at the selected site with an intradermal bleb of 1 per cent lidocaine.

Use a 16 gauge needle as a trochar to pierce the skin through the bleb. The skin might otherwise be tough enough to damage the cannula. Remove the trochar needle. Select an appropriate sized cannula-needle-stylet. The cannula-needle-stylet device is usually advanced bevel up. Gently introduce its tip into the entry point already prepared by the trochar needle. Advance the device under the skin until the vein is entered. This point is indicated by the feel of a 'plop' or by the entry of blood into the hub of the device.

Do not remove the inner stylet yet. Slip the cannula lying over the needle-stylet along and over the tip of the device and into the lumen of the vein. If the vein is large enough it may be easier to advance the needle-stylet 2 to 3 mm further into the vein lumen, and withdraw the needle-stylet 5 mm back down the cannula before advancing the cannula further up the vein. The stylet is then removed and the cannula hub attached to the intravenous infusion. Secure the cannula in position.

Complications

If the stylet is withdrawn so that its tip has been within the cannula, it must not be advanced again without checking with great care that the stylet has not sliced off a piece of the plastic wall of the cannula. This could create a serious complication if it resulted in a free intravascular embolus of plastic.

Aseptic technique should be observed for insertion of the cannula. Phlebitis, bacterial contamination and septicaemia are known complications of cannulation. The infusion site must be checked several times a day for such evidence and the cannula removed at once if there are any signs of complications.

Umbilical vein catheterization

Indications

This route may be used for any condition requiring the giving of intravenous fluids in the newborn period. The vessel is large and easily catheterized. It is chosen in the absence of suitable peripheral veins, or for speed, and is particularly useful in exchange transfusions. The procedure becomes difficult after seven days of age. During resuscitation of the newborn, drugs may be administered directly into the umbilical vein with needle and syringe (see p. 226).

Method

Scrupulous care must be taken to ensure a sterile technique. It is rarely necessary to restrain the infant, as it is not a distressing procedure. The cord and clamp are thoroughly cleaned with antiseptic solution along with a generous area of surrounding abdomen. The area is draped with sterile towels, allowing access to the umbilicus. The cord is then cut cleanly across with a scalpel blade leaving 1–2 cm of umbilical stump clear of the abdominal wall. A decisive cut must be made as the cord can easily slip aside. Bleeding from the cut vessels at this point may be profuse and can be stopped by gripping the cord with toothed forceps. The cord is wiped clean of Wharton's jelly and blood, allowing the three vessels to be distinguished. The vessels are in no fixed position but the two arteries are easily differentiated from the vein by the way the cut ends stand out from the jelly with their walls contracted. The vein tends to be wider and gaping. The wall of the vein is picked up with forceps and the lumen inspected. Any clot visible should be removed with fine forceps. Rarely, a metal sound is needed to open the vein slightly. The umbilical catheter is held a few centimetres from its tip with forceps and gently guided into the vein. The catheter is advanced down the lumen and should progress easily. Undue force at this point can create a false passage through Wharton's jelly outside the vein wall. It is important to remember that the vessels follow a spiral course within the cord and then turn sharply towards the liver after entry into the abdomen. The tip is encouraged to follow the correct course by rolling the catheter between finger and thumb – half a revolution to the left and then to the right. The catheter has been passed far enough when blood flows freely back (normally 5–7 cm). Blood is then allowed to flow back to fill the entire catheter before it is attached to the prepared infusion set. It is advisable to secure the ·catheter in place with a silk purse-string suture tied around the cord stump. A loop of suture material around the cord tends to slide off. This also prevents blood leaking back past the catheter. A small dry gauze dressing is then applied.

Complications

This procedure has a sufficient number of serious complications to make it desirable to use peripheral veins if possible. There are few alternatives to using the umbilicus in premature infants, and it remains the route of choice for exchange transfusions. Extreme care must be taken with aseptic technique. Some centres advocate prophylactic antibiotics and these would be especially indicated with a 'dirty' cord.

On removal of the catheter it is wise to send the tip to the laboratory for bacteriological studies. The catheter tip may be a focus for embolus formation as well as for infection. If the tip of the catheter comes to lie in the femoral vein, the right atrium, or one branch of the

portal vein, specific dangers arise. Femoral vein thrombosis, cardiac arrhythmias, and necrosis of one lobe of the liver following perfusion with a hypertonic solution such as 10 per cent dextrose have all been reported. Mesenteric vessel thrombosis is well recognized.

Umbilical artery catheterization

Only large centres running neonatal special care units are likely to require this procedure which is primarily to enable measurement of blood pressure and blood gases in the ill newborn. To minimize risks associated with the procedure, it is essential that correct placement of the catheter tip be confirmed by radiography. It does not have general application in tropical paediatrics, although it should be said that some practitioners accustomed to the procedure prefer it to using the umbilical vein for exchange transfusion.

Cut-down

Indications

If all peripheral veins are unsuitable and an emergency arises where intravenous therapy is urgent, it may be necessary to cut-down on to a large vein. The long saphenous vein is commonly chosen for its large size and constant anatomical relationships. In practised hands this procedure can be done very rapidly.

Method

The long saphenous vein passes anterior to the medial malleolus. In the conscious patient local anaesthetic is infiltrated into the skin (Fig. 6.6.6a), and an incision is made through the full thickness of the skin at right angles to the vein (Fig. 6.6.6b). Once through the skin, blunt mosquito forceps are used to dissect and expose the vein. An instrument is passed behind the vein and brought back grasping a loop of catgut (Fig. 6.6.6c). This is brought in a loop above and in front of the vein and gentle traction is applied (Fig. 6.6.6d). A hole is cut in the vein wall with fine dissecting scissors below the catgut and the cut edge of the wall is picked up with forceps (Fig. 6.6.6e). It is important to make this cut deep enough or a false passage may be created between the layers of the vein wall. A short bevelled catheter filled with fluid may then be introduced and the tension on the catgut released. This allows the catheter to be passed up the vein. If introduction is difficult, a metal sound may be used to open the vein. Leaking back is prevented by tying the loop of catgut around the vein

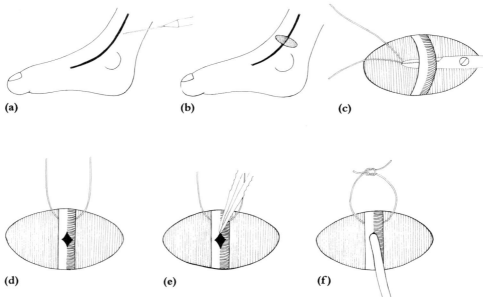

(a)   (b)   (c)

(d)   (e)   (f)

Fig. 6.6.6a–f.   Cut-down.

containing the catheter (Fig. 6.6.6f). It is unnecessary to ligate the vein distal to the catheter as there is then a chance of subsequent recannulization.

Silk sutures are used to close the skin incision and a sterile dressing is applied. It is as well to loop the catheter back up the leg under the dressing to avoid direct traction on the cut-down site.

Precautions

This is a minor operation and full sterile precautions must be taken to avoid introducing infection. A cut-down in the neonate entails catheterization of a very small vein and great care must be taken to identify the vessel. Many useless minutes can be spent attempting to cannulate the venae comitantes that run close by. They are too small to be of value; the long saphenous vein lies beneath them.

Subclavian infusion

Uses

This technique is ideal for emergency situations where no peripheral sites are available due to vasomotor collapse. This will usually be due to severe dehydration, and speed is often life-saving. Because of the difficulty of securing the infusion, this procedure cannot usually be maintained for more than an hour or two. But after initial rehydration by this route a more conventional method can be used. The subclavian infusion has the advantage of using one of the largest veins in the body, and one with fixed anatomical relationships. The main disadvantage is that like the internal jugular venipuncture, it is a 'blind' procedure. It is better carried out on the right subclavian vein, there being a danger of damaging the thoracic duct on the left.[2]

Method

The anatomical relationships of the right subclavian vein are shown in Fig. 6.6.7. The artery and brachial plexus lie above and behind the vein and the oesophagus and trachea lie medially. The apex of the lung is posterior to all these structures. In the diagrammatic view (Fig. 6.6.8) it can be seen that the needle must be inserted flat to the skin, as in a normal venipuncture. Taking a point half-way along the clavicle and a quarter of an inch below it, the skin is pierced. Keeping the needle close to the undersurface of the clavicle, it is pushed medially, aiming the end of the needle point at the upper margin of the sternoclavicular joint. During its course in this direction, the needle will penetrate the subclavian vein tangentially and blood will flow back down the needle.

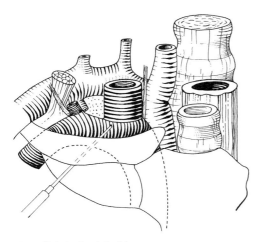

Fig. 6.6.7 Subclavian infusion.

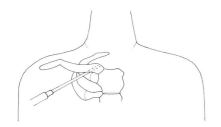

Fig. 6.6.8 Subclavian infusion.

Complications

If the needle passes directly through the vein and into the artery, bright blood will spurt back. The needle can be withdrawn a little and the vein re-entered. If the needle pierces the trachea, air will enter the syringe and the needle can be withdrawn with little risk of surgical emphysema.

Needle

The choice of needle clearly depends on what is available. Hypodermic and lumbar puncture (LP) needles have the disadvantage that a sharp point is left behind in the vein, so a short bevel is essential. A suitable choice is a modern plastic intravenous cannula which leaves only the soft outer polythene sheath in the vein once the stilette has been withdrawn (e.g. Bardic Intracath No. 18). In children under 18 months, a 3-inch 14 gauge needle can be used with a 1.65 mm (outer diameter) Portex catheter threaded up to the needle tip. As soon as the needle enters the vein, the catheter can be pushed gently into the lumen and the needle withdrawn.

Precautions

The procedure may be helped if the child is sedated with paraldehyde, for example, which is safe. The end of the catheter or needle should be firmly strapped to the chest wall and the child observed, perhaps by his mother, for as long as the infusion is running.

Intraperitoneal infusion

Indications

This is a convenient and safe way to give moderately large volumes of blood or fluid in a short space of time, and is thus suitable as an out-patient procedure. The fluid is not, however, given into the intravascular compartment, and some time may elapse before the blood volume has been restored or anaemia corrected. As such it is not recommended in the treatment of a severely dehydrated child whose blood volume must be re-expanded quickly. In most cases of mild – moderate dehydration, the use of oral rehydration solution (see p. 479) is likely to be equally effective and safer.

Method

A no. 21 needle (1.5 inches) is connected to an infusion set containing the appropriate fluid. The skin is prepared with spirit and the needle is introduced into the skin midway between the umbilicus and the xiphisternum. The infusion set is turned full on and the needle is advanced through the anterior abdominal wall. Fluid will flow freely as soon as the peritoneal cavity is entered. The needle should be taped in position so that it does not advance further. The required volume can then be run in over 10 to 15 minutes.

Special precautions

It is possible to transfuse too quickly. The abdomen becomes tense and the diaphragm is displaced upwards, embarrassing respiration. There is a theoretical risk of perforating a viscus with the needle, but this is very unusual, presumably because the gut is moved aside by the needle and the flow of fluid. The procedure is more dangerous when the gut is fixed by adhesions, and is unsafe when tuberculous enteritis has been diagnosed. Intraperitoneal bleeding must occur now and again but is almost never significant.

Amount of intraperitoneal fluid

In the treatment of mild dehydration, it should not be necessary to give more than half the normal fluid requirement for 24 hours by this route. A suggested maximum volume would be 75 ml/kg body weight given as a bolus over 10 minutes. Any signs of distress or breathing difficulties are indications for discontinuing the infusion. If there is a medical indication for a greater volume of fluid replacement, another route should be considered. Whole blood is usually given in amounts up to 20 ml/kg body weight and should not be a problem in terms of volume.

Venipuncture

A large number of laboratory investigations require a sample of venous blood. The site selected for venipuncture should always be the safest possible one (Fig. 6.6.9).

Many children will have suitable veins on the dorsum of the hand or in the antecubital fossa, and even in the neonate it may not be necessary to use a major vessel.

Jugular puncture

Indication

The neck is a clean area and the veins are of adequate size, making this site high on the list of preferences when performing venipuncture. Both internal and external jugular puncture can be simple if the child is held correctly, impossible if the patient moves and wriggles.

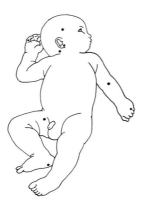

Fig. 6.6.9 Sites for venipuncture.

Method for external jugular vein

This vein is nearly always large, but in a few children it may be so small as to be of no practical value. If present it will stand out clearly as it courses towards the clavicle in the supraclavicular fossa. The child is secured as in Fig. 6.6.1, and held so that the head is turned to one side and is slightly lower than the body. The vein will fill from below in this position if the child is encouraged to cry. To occlude the vein distally actually makes the procedure more difficult. Using a No. 21 disposable needle or a Butterfly attached to a syringe, the skin is pierced over the course of the vein, in the direction of the clavicle. With a short but firm movement the needle enters the vein.

Method for internal jugular vein

If, after attempting both external veins, no blood has been collected, or worse, haematomas have developed from nicked vessels, the internal vein may be used. This vessel lies on the deep surface of the sternomastoid and joins the subclavian vein to form the innominate vein behind the sternoclavicular joint. The child is restrained as in Fig. 6.6.1 with the shoulders on a flat surface, the neck a little extended and turned to one side. After cleaning the skin, the needle is inserted behind the sternomastoid muscle at the junction of its upper and middle thirds, directing the needle at the suprasternal notch and advancing it until the vein is entered. A little suction is kept on the syringe throughout, and if no blood results the needle is withdrawn while still aspirating. It is better to avoid the left side of the neck with its thoracic duct. There is a slight danger of penetrating the carotid artery which lies deep and medial to the vein.

Special precautions

If extravascular bleeding is encountered, the needle is withdrawn and firm pressure is applied to the puncture site with the child in the upright position. Crying increases the tendency to bleed, so the child is picked up and soothed while the pressure is maintained.

Femoral vein venipuncture

Indications

This method is useful for obtaining a blood sample from any age of patient, but especially the infant. It has the advantage that a large amount of blood for several investigations can easily be obtained from one venipuncture.

Method

The infant is restrained (as in Fig. 6.6.1) leaving the legs free. The selected leg is abducted and held at the lower end of the femur while the other leg is held out of the way with the assistant's other hand. As will be seen in Fig. 6.6.10 the femoral artery is palpable as it emerges below the inguinal ligament in the middle of the femoral triangle. The femoral nerve runs lateral to it while the vein runs medial to the artery. The skin is cleaned with spirit and the position of the pulsating artery is checked. The needle is then introduced at 90° to the skin, aiming just to miss the artery medially a short distance below the inguinal ligament. A firm movement of the needle will transfix the vein. The needle is then withdrawn very slowly, applying a negative pressure to the syringe all the while. Venous blood will flow back as soon as the needle tip is lying in the lumen of the vein. It is then a simple matter to withdraw as much blood as is required.

Special difficulties

It is possible to nick the artery during the procedure. The blood supply to most of the lower limb will be impaired from either spasm of the vessel or pressure from the ensuing haematoma. On withdrawal of the needle, arterial blood may ooze from the puncture site. Firm pressure for two or three minutes will prevent a haematoma forming. The puncture site must always be inspected afterwards to ensure bleeding has stopped. As this is a particularly unclean area, it is as well to cover the wound with a waterproof plaster for an hour or two. Uncommonly, infection of the bone may follow penetration of the periosteum by the needle, and

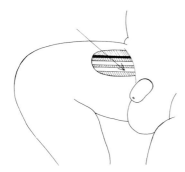

Fig. 6.6.10 Femoral vein site for venipuncture.

sloughing of the femoral head has been reported. Although there are several potentially alarming complications of this procedure, femoral puncture is an extremely useful technique and one well worth mastering.

Needle

A no. 21 or 23 gauge needle is satisfactory for most infants. A particularly elegant method is to use a Butterfly Needle, avoiding the problem of keeping the syringe steady while withdrawing blood.

Heel stab

This method of collecting blood samples is used extensively in the newborn period when it is often difficult or undesirable to perform repeated venipuncture. It is ideal for serum bilirubin and blood sugar estimations.

Method

The infant may be placed face down in his cot, or conveniently on the lap. When the peripheral circulation is poor the heel is first warmed by immersing the foot in a bowl of warm water. The heel is cleaned with spirit and allowed to dry. Some operators prefer to grease the skin with petroleum jelly, as this causes the blood to escape in globules making collection easier. The heel is grasped by encircling it with the thumb and first finger of the left hand. A disposable stilette or pointed scalpel blade is then used to stab the heel pad. There is a surprising amount of tissue to penetrate even on a premature infant and the beginner will tend to 'understab', thereby requiring several attempts before an adequate blood flow is obtained. Ideally, free-flowing whole blood can then be collected drop by drop, but in practice it is often necessary to squeeze the heel pad slightly and collect the drop of blood that emerges before releasing the pressure, then squeezing again. If microestimation is available, a plain glass capillary tube will be used for collection. In most instances, however, a plain glass container will suffice. The blood which collects on the heel pad is touched against the same spot on the neck of the container until sufficient blood has been collected. Unclotted blood may be collected in heparinized capillary tubes.

   Mixing with the heparin is effected by introducing a small metal pellet into the tube, sealing both ends with plasticine and then drawing a magnet backwards and forwards along the length of the tube. If blood gases are to be estimated care must be taken to warm the heel first. The results obtained will then be for capillary blood, being close to arterial values.

Precautions

A fresh stilette must be used for every patient. If the skin is not cleaned properly first, it is possible to produce a troublesome infection such as a subfascial abscess or osteomyelitis. Bleeding is stopped after the procedure by covering the wound with a wisp of cotton wool and applying gentle pressure for a few seconds. Small patches of plaster are not recommended as the skin rapidly becomes sodden underneath.

Finger prick

This technique is similar to the heel stab and can be used on much older children. It can however be extremely painful. Either the finger pulp or the ear lobe can be used instead of the heel.

Marrow aspiration

Uses

This procedure is essential in the diagnosis and management of childhood leukaemia and the diagnosis of other haematological disorders. Various sites are available depending on the age of the child.

Method

The simplest site for most children over two years of age is the anterior superior iliac crest. The skin is prepared with iodine and the surrounding area is draped with sterile towels. In conscious patients a small amount of local anaesthetic is infiltrated through the skin as far as the periosteum. The skin is nicked cleanly with the point of a scalpel blade just below the anterior superior iliac crest. The tip of a trocar and cannula can then be introduced easily through the skin at right angles. Any small trocar is usually suitable. Almost at once the surface of the bone is encountered and a reasonable amount of pressure is needed to introduce the trocar and cannula into the marrow cavity. There is a sudden lack of resistance when it has been passed far enough, and the trocar can then be removed. This leaves the cannula firmly embedded in the outer table of bone with its tip in the marrow cavity. A 10 ml syringe is then connected to the cannula, and marrow withdrawn. Often considerable suction is needed to obtain a specimen of marrow, which looks like thick bright red blood, and an inexperienced operator may give up too early on a correctly placed cannula. This part of the procedure may be extremely painful for the patient.

If no marrow is obtained, the cannula can be advanced a short distance. The drops of marrow are immediately placed on a glass slide and spread in a similar manner to a blood film. On removing the cannula at the end of the procedure, firm pressure with a sterile gauze stops any bleeding and a dry dressing should then be applied. The toddler below two years of age may have marrow aspirated from the shaft of the tibia. This is a useful site which is readily penetrated, and easily immobilized. The site of entry is the upper third of the medial aspect of the shaft well below the condyle. The method is otherwise identical with that for the pelvis. Some operators preferred to tap the sternal marrow at a point in the midline of the sternum between the second and third ribs, while others select a vertebral body.

Precautions

As a pathway is going to be created from the exterior into the marrow, maximum sterile precautions must be taken throughout the procedure, including masks, gowns, and surgical gloves. If repeated aspirations are planned on the same child, it is often kinder to give a general anaesthetic. However, it is possible to sedate a small child with diazepam or even give a short-acting anaesthetic agent such as ketamine hydrochloride.

Urine collection

Urinalysis is a common paediatric investigation. For many tests a clean sample is adequate. Bacteriological studies however, may require suprapubic aspiration (see also p. 784ff.).

Clean urine sample

The 'clean catch' or 'mid-stream' method is preferred when possible. The perineum and prepuce are washed with soap and water, drawing back the prepuce in the older child. In infants micturition may be induced by placing a cold hand on the abdomen, stroking the back along the spinal column, or momentary inattention. Older children can cooperate and may be able to interrupt their stream, but the difficulty of 'catching' the sample should not be underestimated. A wide-necked sterile container is needed, and a girl may be more comfortable seated.

Less satisfactory methods include taping a sterile test-tube or collecting bottle of suitable dimensions over the penis, having previously cleaned the skin. The bottle can be fastened to the abdominal wall with adhesive tape. Excellent proprietry urine-collecting bags are available for boys and girls which have a built-in adhesive edge to them. These can be applied over the cleaned genitalia of infants. They have the disadvantage of being easily contaminated by faeces.

Urethral catheterization

Catheterization carries the risk of introducing infection and therefore has largely been replaced by suprapubic puncture when a specimen free of possible contaminants is required. It is still necessary for introducing radio-opaque dye, emptying a distended bladder to facilitate abdominal examination, or as a prelude to a variety of surgical procedures.

Method

In the older child it may be possible to pass one of the smallest standard urethral catheters. However, infants will require a much finer tube than is usually available, and various substitutes may be found on the paediatric ward. Umbilical catheters and feeding tubes both make excellent alternatives. The perineum should be thoroughly washed with soap and water and in boys particular attention should be paid to the prepuce. If retractile, it can be drawn back, but no force should be used for this. One end of the catheter is placed in the sterile receptacle ready to catch the urine. Using maximum sterile precautions, one hand is used to part the labia or steady the penis, the other to grasp the free end of the catheter. The tip of the catheter can be dipped in sterile lubricant before being passed into the urethra. No force must be used at this stage but gentle pressure will allow the tip of the catheter to pass into the bladder.

Precautions

The urethral opening is difficult to find in small girls, and it is important not to pass the catheter vaginally, realize the error, and then attempt urethral catheterization with the contaminated tip. A fresh sterile catheter will be needed.

Suprapubic aspiration

Indications

Suprapubic aspiration of urine has the advantage of avoiding contamination and does not require the cooperation of the child to obtain the specimen. It may be particularly useful in a busy out-patient clinic, as the technique is easily learned, and has a high success rate. It is slightly easier in infants because the bladder is largely extrapelvic.[3]

Method

A disposable 21 gauge needle (1.5 inches) and a 10 ml syringe are used. The child is restrained and laid on a flat surface. The skin is thoroughly cleaned with soap and water, and finally with spirit. The needle is held at right angles to the skin in the midline 2 cm above the pubic symphysis, and passed through the anterior abdominal wall into the bladder in one movement. A sample of urine is then aspirated. The procedure should not be carried out unless a full bladder can be percussed. Keep a sterile container ready, as the infant may void during the preparation process.

Precautions

The bladder presents a larger target when it is full. There is a greater chance of a full bladder soon after a feed, and older children can be given a large drink of water half an hour before the manoeuvre. To prevent the nuisance of spontaneous voiding, a penile clamp can be made from a suitable weakened paper clip covered in rubber. For girls, a pad may be placed against the vulva and the thighs pressed firmly together. A contra-indication is local skin sepsis.

Lumbar puncture

Indications

The majority of lumbar punctures will be performed to confirm clinically suspected meningitis or encephalitis. Occasionally, cytotoxic and antibiotic drugs may be given by this route.

Method

The child must be positioned properly, and this is without doubt more important and more difficult to achieve than the actual lumbar puncture. The patient must be lying on the left side on a hard flat surface with the back flexed, and the plane of the back as vertical as possible. An assistant is needed to flex the neck on to the chest and draw the knees up towards the chin. In larger children this can be done with the crook of one of the assistant's elbows over the back of the neck and the other behind the knees. The infant can be tucked into this position by the use of the assistant's hands alone. A balance must be struck between restraining the child so completely that he is bursting to free himself and that of poor restraint where he is wriggling free. The position of the anatomical landmarks is checked and the skin is cleaned with spirit around the proposed site of puncture. Sterile towels are used to drape the surrounding skin. The posterior superior iliac crest is approximately opposite the interspace between the fourth and fifth lumbar vertebrae. In larger children it is kinder to infiltrate the skin with 1 per cent lignocaine local anaesthetic, but with smaller children this is undesirable as the landmarks may be lost. It is helpful to keep the thumb of the gloved left hand on the spine of L_4 vertebra while introducing the lumbar puncture needle in the L_4/L_5 interspace.

The skin should be pierced in one quick action and the needle poised with the tip just under the skin. It is only natural that the child squirms at the moment the skin is punctured, making passage of the needle between the spines difficult. It is now possible, using the thumb on L_4 spine as a marker, to advance the needle in the correct direction between the spines, passing it in a horizontal plane and in a slightly cephalic direction, aiming approximately for the umbilicus. The needle will pass fairly easily until it encounters the ligamentum flavum where slightly more pressure is needed. Immediately after this, the needle is felt to 'plop' as it penetrates the dura. The stilette can be removed and cerebrospinal fluid will drip out into sterile collecting bottles. If the child is screaming or is held too tightly, this may be under pressure. If no cerebrospinal fluid is obtained the stilette can be reinserted and the needle advanced slightly. Sufficient time must be allowed for the cerebrospinal fluid to flow back, especially if it is under low pressure as in a dehydrated baby. Under no circumstances must a syringe be attached and suction applied to try and withdraw the fluid even if no drops have emerged. Once collection is complete (usually less than 1 ml), the needle is withdrawn and collodion on a cotton wool swab is applied to the skin. It is rarely of value to measure the pressure of cerebrospinal fluid in children.

An alternative to the prone position is to have the child seated upright with a pillow on his lap or with his arms over a bed table, and an assistant holding his arms and legs out in front of him. The lumbar puncture can then be performed on his lumbar spine in the same way. The needle used should be 20 to 22 gauge with a stilette, the length of the shank depending on the size of the child. In neonates, the easiest and least traumatic needle is a No. 23 Butterfly, but there have been reports of dermoid tumour induction using needles without stilettes.

Precautions

Full sterile technique must be used to avoid introducing infection into the cerebrospinal fluid. Under no circum-

stances must a lumbar puncture be performed if there is evidence of raised intracranial pressure. This may result in 'coning' where the brain stem herniates through the foramen magnum. Hence, fundoscopy should always be performed first. If in doubt over whether the intracranial pressure is raised it is better to treat for meningitis on suspicion without doing a lumbar puncture.

Problems

Older children may complain of headaches afterwards and they should be encouraged to lie flat for several hours. Occasionally frank blood will flow back when the stilette is withdrawn, indicating a vein has been punctured. The needle should be withdrawn and reinserted one interspace higher or lower.

Subdural tap in infancy

Indication

When a subdural haematoma or effusion is suspected, a diagnostic and therapeutic tap should be performed. The exact time of suture closure varies tremendously between individuals, but this is primarily a procedure on neonates, and is rarely undertaken beyond the first year of life.

Method

The infant is wrapped as shown in Fig. 6.6.1. The two lateral angles of the anterior fontanelle are located and the area over them is shaved. The skin is then cleaned with spirit. With a hand on either side to steady it, the assistant, who will hold the head throughout, lowers the infant's head on to two sterile towels. The outside edges of the upper towel are brought up over the assistant's hands and gathered together with a towel clip in the midline, encircling the head except for the area around the anterior fontanelle. With full sterile technique, a needle and stilette are introduced at right angles to the scalp over the most lateral point of the fontanelle (Fig. 6.6.11). The needle needs firm pressure to pass through the skin, but extreme caution is necessary once the needle is passing more easily. It must be advanced a small amount at a time, awaiting the tell-tale 'plop' as it passes through the dura. Once through, the stilette is removed and drops of the effusion will flow back. These should be collected in a sterile bottle for analysis. On withdrawal of the needle, gentle pressure and a piece of cotton wool soaked in collodion will seal the puncture.

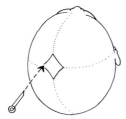

Fig. 6.6.11 Subdural tap.

The same procedure may be undertaken on the other side of the fontanelle.

Special precautions

Too large a needle will tear the dura excessively. A short bevel No. 21 lumbar puncture needle is quite big enough. An overenthusiastic exploration may result in the needle being pushed into the substance of the brain. Extreme care, then, must be exercised once the needle is through the skin. If in doubt as to the depth of the needle, the stilette should be withdrawn repeatedly while exploring for fluid. On no account must a syringe be used to apply suction. The manoeuvre is not to be undertaken lightly for it may result in subdural haematoma formation, and there is a real risk that infection may be introduced into the brain or cerebrospinal fluid.

Thoracocentesis

Indications

For diagnostic reasons or to remove an unduly large quantity of fluid.

Technique

If the fluid is loculated, fluoroscopy may be needed. If it is not loculated, the child sits, either on his bed and leaning on a bed table or, if small, on the assistant's knee. Sometimes it helps to immobilize an apprehensive child, and this is accomplished by sitting him on an assistant's lap, facing the side of his bed, and having a second assistant lean across the bed and seize the child's outstretched hands. The two assistants can hold the patient in a satisfactory position, but the operator has to kneel in relative discomfort. The procedure is carried out under full sterile precautions, the skin being well cleaned and the operator gloved. Local anaesthetic is used to infiltrate the skin and intercostal muscle. The gauge of the aspiratory needle is determined by the underlying fluid, pus obviously needing a wider needle, and the critical point is the choice of a needle with a short bevel. If much fluid is present a three-way tap between needle and syringe minimizes the risk of inducing a pneumothorax. (Removing a full syringe from the needle and covering the needle butt with the thumb while the syringe is emptied is not safe, and is a bad and unacceptable habit).

The needle should be introduced at the lower border of an interspace, to avoid the intercostal bundle. When fluid is obtained, artery forceps are clamped to the needle, level with the skin, to prevent any accidental change of position. As much fluid as seems sensible is removed. A huge exudate is normally drained in stages on separate days.

Complications

Thick pus may be difficult to aspirate but sterile saline injected into the pleural cavity dilutes the pus and allows removal. Pneumothorax and haemothorax from lung damage can occur, and if the child begins to cough the needle must be removed. Infection may be introduced if aseptic technique is not followed scrupulously.

The most usual technical error is to forget, or to fail to realize, that the diaphragm may be elevated, and to insert the needle below the pleural cavity. The most frequent error of judgement is the failure to appreciate how tiring to the child a long procedure may be. A really ill child is better lying on the side, over a pillow.

Abdominal paracentesis

Indications

To remove excessive fluid, rarely for diagnostic purposes.

Technique

The child lies or sits in the position of maximum comfort. If a small volume is required a short bevel needle is chosen; if a large volume, a trochar and cannula of suitable size. Full sterile precautions are used and the skin is infiltrated with local anaesthetic. The site chosen depends upon the position of the patient – a point at the lower quadrant, or in the midline halfway between umbilicus and pubic symphysis is usually suitable. A needle is inserted obliquely, to prevent leak back of fluid. If a trochar is used it is held at right angles to the skin and advanced with care, avoiding any sudden forward thrust. It is easier if the skin is first nicked with a scalpel blade. When sufficient fluid has been drained, or aspirated, the wound is sealed with collodion. Occasionally a skin suture is needed to prevent leakage.

Complications

The bladder may be punctured, particularly if the midline site is chosen, and the child should always micturate before the procedure. Haemorrhage is rare, but one school of thought believes a many-tail bandage should be applied to maintain intra-abdominal pressure after draining a large effusion. The risk of haemorrhage from portal vessels is said to be reduced. More practical advice, perhaps, is to drain such an effusion slowly, maybe over several consecutive days. If much ascitic fluid is removed the child may become hypoprotei-naemic.

Liver biopsy

This technique is not to be described here. It is probably the most hazardous manoeuvre carried out as a 'practical procedure' – not because of any intrinsic difficulty but because of possible subsequent complications. It is not of direct therapeutic value, but it is a diagnostic test. For it to be safely performed, the platelet count and prothrombin time should be checked, blood must be available for transfusion, and a surgeon capable of carrying out a laparotomy must be at hand. If this situation exists then the technique of needle biopsy is likely to be known, and there should be someone available with first-hand experience who can demonstrate it. The inexperienced are well advised to practise in the autopsy room. Different needles require quite different methods, and absolute familiarity with the instrument is essential.

Pericardial tap

Indications

For diagnosis or treatment, e.g. of purulent pericarditis or of pericardial haemorrhage.

Technique

Various puncture sites are favoured, but the easiest is probably a point some 2 cm within the apex of the heart shadow as judged on X-ray – or the left outer edge as judged by percussion – in the 5th left interspace. The child should sit, resting comfortably against pillows. With strict sterile technique the skin is infiltrated with local anaesthetic, and a suitable short bevel aspirating needle attached to a three-way tap and a syringe is introduced. Pus needs a larger needle than blood or serous fluid. The needle is advanced posteriorly, towards the spine, until the pericardium is punctured and fluid is obtained. If the myocardium is touched the needle will oscillate with the heart beat. As in performing thoracocentesis it is easier if arterial forceps are clamped to the needle, when in position, to act as a stop against the skin and to prevent accidental displacement. Air can be deliberately introduced to allow contrast radiography.

Should aspiration at that site fail, or be unacceptable for any other reason, the best alternative is perhaps a point 1 cm to either side of the xiphoid process. The needle is introduced at 45° to the skin and advanced upwards and slightly posteriorly.

Complications

Not common. If the myocardium is damaged or punctured, bleeding can occur. A pneumothorax may be caused by poor technique. Major trauma to the heart is difficult to achieve and fear of this procedure, on the operator's part, is largely emotive. It may soothe both patient and the operator if the child is sedated.

Gastric and duodenal intubation

A tube may need to be passed into the stomach or duodenum for a number of reasons. Some infants need feeding by a tube into the stomach, and it has recently been recognized that there are advantages in transpyloric feeding requiring intubation of the duodenum. Diagnostic procedures include aspiration of stomach contents to examine for the swallowed tubercle bacillus, and of intestinal secretions to examine for enzymes or bacterial microflora. Special capsules have been developed for obtaining biopsy material from the small bowel. Obstruction of the intestines will require repeated aspiration of the stomach as part of a therapeutic regimen, and ingestion of poison may require gastric lavage to be performed.

Intragastric feeding

Indication

Babies with poorly developed suck and swallow reflexes are candidates for intragastric feeding. These may include premature infants, babies with respiratory or cardiovascular problems who become distressed during a feed, and babies who are ill and do not feed well. Cases of neonatal tetanus, where the stimulation of feeding is to be avoided, are further examples.

Method

Usually a No. 5 Argyl feeding tube is suitable for premature babies. This is 38 cm long and has a sentinal line which is radio-opaque. The naso-gastric tube is measured against the patient and passed an equivalent distance from the ear lobe past the tip of the nose to the xiphisternum. Argyl tubes provide markers on the side for this. The baby is then wrapped in a blanket (Fig. 6.6.1) and the end of the tube is lubricated. Sterile water is usually sufficient, but some centres use glycerine for lubrication. The tip of the tube is passed directly back into one nostril and the soft plastic easily passes into the oropharynx and thence into the stomach. When the measured amount of tube has been passed, a small amount of stomach content is aspirated into a syringe. The aspirate, usually in the form of mucus, is then dropped on to blue litmus paper. If the mucus has originated from the stomach it will have a high acid content and will turn the litmus paper pink. If no aspirate is obtained a small amount of air is blown down the tube with a syringe, and can be heard bubbling into the stomach with a stethoscope placed over the abdomen. This air should be re-aspirated once it is certain the tube is correctly placed.

If the trachea has been intubated, the mucus is scanty and alkaline, the cry is abnormal, and the infant is distressed. The tube is taped to the face as it emerges from the nostril (Fig. 6.6.12). A 20 ml syringe is then attached to the free end with the plunger removed. The baby is nursed in arms if he is well enough, or if not, in the incubator with his head raised slightly. The feed is poured into the barrel of the syringe and allowed to flow

in by gravity. Occasionally, mucus in the tube obstructs free flow, and gentle patting with the palm of the hand over the open end of the syringe is sufficient to clear the tube. On no account should the plunger be replaced and the fluid forced into the stomach.

Special precautions

The tube can safely be left down several days, although the position of its tip must be checked with the litmus test before every feed. Commonly the tube becomes blocked or is pulled out after several days and needs replacing. If the baby goes cyanosed during feeding, the procedure must be stopped at once and the position of the tube checked. It may be that in very small infants a tube in one nostril is seriously obstructing the passage of air into the lungs. If only occasional tube feeds are required, it is possible to pass the tube orally and withdraw it afterwards, in which case a slightly larger tube can be used (e.g. No. 8 Argyl). Continuous intragastric feeding has not been considered here. The principle is the same but the hazards are greater.

Intubation of the upper small bowel

This procedure is similar to intubation of the stomach but requires more tube, real patience and is helped by encouraging the child to lie on his right side. Fluoroscopic examination using a radio-opaque tube is ideal but rarely possible. A less elegant but more practical method is to pass the tube at night, tape it firmly in position, restrain the child's hands and wait until morning. A tube reluctant to pass through the pylorus is often coiled upon itself and should be withdrawn a little and passed again. If this manoeuvre is not successful, the child's position should be changed from the right lateral to the dorsal or ventral, and helped by an intravenous injection of metoclopramide (Maxolon). Success in crossing the pylorus is shown by spontaneous drainage of duodenal juices, which are alkaline to litmus. The exact position can only be located by X-ray.

Gastric aspiration

The swallowed tubercle bacillus can be recovered from the stomachs of children who do not cooperate in providing sputum specimens. The tube is usually passed through the mouth. The approximate length of tube to be passed is estimated by measuring the distance from the bridge of the patient's nose to the xiphisternum and adding 2 cm. The tube is marked and passed up to this point. This should be done reasonably

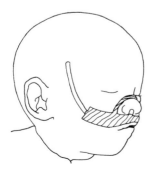

Fig. 6.6.12 Naso-gastric intubation.

accurately or excess tubing may curl up and the tip lie in the cardia. Mucus is aspirated from the stomach to check for acidity, and once it is certain that the tube is correctly positioned, 10 ml of sterile water are syringed down the tube. After a brief pause, aspiration of the syringe will produce a sample of gastric 'washing' which may be sent to the laboratory for examination. The tube is then withdrawn.

Gastric lavage

Indications

Children are notorious for 'tasting' anything which comes within their gaze and reach; this varies from mother's pills to household bleach or poisonous fruits. Children are unreliable about the quantity of poison taken or the timing of ingestion, and will modify their answers to questioning in a way they hope will appease the questioner and stave off punishment! Gastric lavage is not without hazards and some judgement will need to be exercised in assessing whether the quantity of poison involved justifies the procedure. The use of an emetic drug such as ipecacuanha may be a preferable alternative to lavage.

Technique

An unconscious child needs intubation with a cuffed endotracheal tube to protect the lungs before starting. The child is secured in a blanket in such a way that he cannot interfere with the procedure. He is placed on his side on a couch or table with his feet raised and his head lower than his stomach. A gag may be needed to open the mouth, and this will also prevent the tube from being bitten. A rubber tube of suitable size is well lubricated and passed into the oropharynx. The approximate distance needed to pass the tube can be estimated by measuring against the patient the distance from the bridge of the nose to the xiphisternum. If the child will cooperate he should be asked to swallow as the tube is passed further down into the stomach. Suction apparatus to clear the pharynx should be available in case of vomiting. Before lavage, the child should be checked to ensure his upper airway is adequate.

The operator need not be concerned that the trachea of a conscious patient has been intubated by mistake. If a tube has passed easily it may be safely assumed to be correctly positioned. A funnel is attached to the tubing and 100 ml of warm tap water are then poured into it. A very small child may require half this amount. The funnel is then lowered, allowing water and gastric content to drain out. Failure to drain freely may be due

to a blockage of the tube with solid material from the stomach. If it does not clear with repositioning and introduction of more water the tube will have to be removed and another passed. A further 100 ml of water are poured down the tube and this process is repeated five or six times or more if stomach content is still being washed out.

Complications

If laryngeal spasm is induced the tube must be withdrawn and not passed again, as there is a danger of gastric content spilling into the lungs.[4] If it is felt that aspiration has occurred, steroids and antibiotics should be given and bronchoscopic suction performed. Correct positioning of the patient will avoid these complications. After gastric aspiration conjunctival haemorrhages are often seen, and petechiae may be noted on the head and neck. Although they are harmless they testify that this is a savage assault on a child. The psychological trauma cannot be overestimated, and however guilt-ridden and distressed the parents may be they should be encouraged to stand by their child whilst the procedure is carried out.

Eye drops

Indications

Any purulent discharge of the eye should be treated with antibiotics, but a swab must be taken for culture first.

Method

The infant may be swaddled (see Fig. 6.6.1) and placed on his back. Larger children will also need restraining. The eye is cleaned of discharge by wiping once with a sterile swab soaked in sterile water from the nasal side outwards. The swab is then discarded and if discharge still remains, a second swab should be used. The eye which is less affected is treated first. The eyelids may be slippery, and a clean swab may help to pull the lower lid down. It is very much easier if an assistant opens the lids leaving the operator free to insert the drops. These are placed on the conjunctiva between the eyelids and the eyeballs. Ointment is sometimes preferred to drops and this too should be placed on the conjunctiva of the lower lid.

Precautions

Great care is taken not to touch any part of the patient with the dropper. The bottle must be checked carefully before the drops are instilled. The administration of the wrong drug into the eye could cause irreversible damage. It is important to check for cloudiness in the liquid, to ensure that they are the correct drops, and to verify the date of expiry. If the preparation comes in a metal tube, small slivers of metal from the nozzle can contaminate the ointment. If these are seen the eye must be washed with sterile water to flush the slivers away and the tube must be discarded.

Intradermal injection

Indications

This procedure is required for the administration of small volumes of fluid, as in BCG immunization.

Method

The skin is cleansed and the arm or leg firmly grasped from behind, pulling the skin taut. With the syringe almost flat along the skin, the needle is slid under the epidermis with a short 'scooping' action. The needle tip is then in the correct plane and can easily be advanced a little, sufficient to cover the bevel completely. When the injection has been given correctly there will be a well-circumcised bleb in which the hair follicles are obvious. If the bleb subsides rapidly the injection is partly subcutaneous. On withdrawal of the needle, the skin can be wiped with a sterile swab from the site of the needle puncture towards the 'bleb'. This will prevent leak-back down the needle track.

Complications

Intradermal injection may need a little pressure on the syringe plunger to produce an adequate bleb. If the bevel is not completely intradermal, fluid will escape, perhaps as a jet or spray. The operator's eye should not be close to the injection site, for most substances given intradermally are irritant or dangerous to the eye.

Temperature taking

Indications

If temperatures are to be recorded, and that is a matter of constant debate, they need to be accurate and the procedure safe.

Method

The actual site selected for measuring temperatures varies with the age of the child. All observations are preceded by shaking the mercury to the zero mark with a flick of the wrist.

Up to one year The infant can be placed face downwards across the lap. It is a simple matter to insert the bulb of a rectal thermometer by first lubricating it with a small amount of petroleum jelly. It is passed into the rectum until the bulb is covered. An ordinary thermometer should not be used as it is more fragile and less accurate. Two hands can be used to restrain the infant gently, one across the back and one on the buttocks. It is better not to hold the end of the thermometer or a sudden movement by the infant may snap off the stem. Similarly when a baby is in an incubator the legs should be lifted into the air to prevent any sudden movement that could break the stem. The thermometer is left in place for 30 seconds and read. An ordinary thermometer does not record below 35°C, and when the mercury does not rise above 36°C it is absolutely vital that a special low-range thermometer is used which will register down to 29°C.

One year upwards The thermometer is placed under the axilla with the bulb covered. The side nearest the observer is used and the child's arm is folded across the chest and held there. The temperature is read after 3 minutes.

Seven years onwards Those children who can be trusted to cooperate may have their temperatures recorded by placing the bulb under the tongue then closing the lips. Firm instructions must be given not to bite on the glass! The thermometer is read after one minute. A recent hot or cold drink will of course upset the reading.

Special points

There is always a danger of the glass shattering. If this happens, the pieces must be carefully removed. Mercury swallowed is harmless and no special treatment is needed.

Stool collection

Local custom and ingenuity determine the most appropriate container for bringing stool specimens to the hospital laboratory from out-patients. A match-box or a discarded pill-box appropriately labelled are often the simplest.

But much more important information can be gleaned from fresh stools, and it may be desirable to collect a specimen from the child either in the ward or in the out-patient department without his cooperation. A gloved finger in the infant's rectum will usually stimulate defaecation, but a more refined method is to use a length (about 10 cm) cut from an ordinary drinking straw. For diagnostic use in the global eradication of poliomyelitis, the Expanded Programme on Immunization of the World Health Organization is developing a special plastic cannula. The end is first greased with lubricating jelly and then passed into the rectum. If loose stool is present, it will begin to flow down the straw, which when withdrawn contains the required specimen. If formed stool is present, and the straw is rotated slightly, a specimen of stool may be recovered as a core inside the tip of the straw.

References

1. Hanid TK. Intravenous injections and infusions in infants. *Paediatrics*. 1975; **56**, 1080.
2. Matthews TS. Difficult transfusions. *East African Medical Journal*. 1966; **43**, 464.
3. Matthews TS. Suprapubic aspiration in the outpatients department. *East African Medical Journal*. 1968; **45**, 144.
4. Wingate DL. *British Journal of Hospital Medicine*. 1969; **2**, 775.

CHAPTER 7

Appropriate imaging techniques

P. E. S. Palmer

In any small or large hospital in the developing world about one-third of the diagnostic imaging will be of patients under the age of 15 years. An X-ray of the chest will be needed most frequently, closely followed by X-rays for skeletal injury, mainly of the limbs. Varying with locality, skills and the particular interests of the physicians, other examinations will include the abdomen (particularly for intestinal obstruction), the urinary tract, and the gall-bladder of children wherever there is ascaris. The paranasal sinuses and the skull are requested, often unnecessarily. The pattern of X-ray examinations will only be slightly modified if there is also an ultrasound unit available in the hospital.

Imaging equipment

The World Health Organization has provided specifications for imaging at each level of patient care. The guidelines are simple:

- For small hospitals or clinics, without a radiologist or trained radiographer: the WHO Basic Radiological System (BRS) with a BRS operator.[1] If the work increases, add a trained radiographer to the BRS.
- For provincial or district hospitals where there are trained radiographers (and perhaps a radiologist): the WHO General Purpose X-ray Unit, supplemented by the BRS for additional rooms. If funds

are available, the WHO General Purpose Ultrasound Unit.
- In the large university or referral hospital: in addition to the above, the WHO Special Purpose X-ray Units and Special Purpose Ultrasound Units. If funds permit: a General Purpose computerised tomography (CT) Unit (and Special Purpose CT units wherever there are specialized clinical departments).[2] In this last category of hospital there must be radiologists, radiographers and highly trained specialist clinicians.

WHO basic radiological system (WHO-BRS)

By far the most important of all the specified units is the WHO-BRS (Fig. 6.7.1), which will produce excellent radiographs of well over 90 per cent of all the requirements of any busy, non-specialist hospital and over 80 per cent of the requirements of provincial or university hospitals. The BRS does not provide fluoroscopy because WHO believes that this has an unacceptable diagnostic error rate, an increased risk of radiation and a material increase in capital and maintenance costs. (Fluoroscopy is provided by the WHO General Purpose X-Ray Unit.)

The WHO-BRS can be installed in any room larger than 4 × 5 m: the walls seldom need additional radiation protection. In the developing world, the battery-

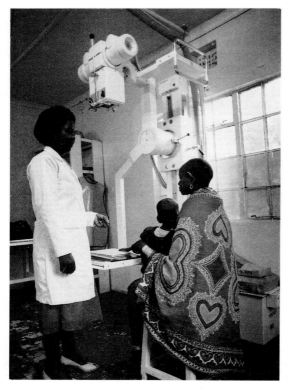

Fig. 6.7.1 Imaging.

proven by extensive WHO-supervised field trials in Latin America and Africa. The radiographic results are excellent. The University of Lund in Sweden has shown that the film quality equals that of the most expensive generators available. This high quality can be duplicated in developing countries by relatively inexperienced operators who are not trained radiographers. The use of the WHO Manual of Radiographic Technique is an inherent part of the Basic Radiological System.[4] The BRS can be used with any type of X-ray film or chemical. The skin radiation dose to patients X-rayed with the BRS is 60 per cent or less than that from a standard X-ray generator, due to its very sophisticated design, which nonetheless makes it very easy to maintain and operate. While not referring only to children, there is a WHO Manual of Radiographic Interpretation for General Practitioners which is also part of the system.[5]

A word of caution is necessary. Sales representatives will claim that their equipment, often designed as a mobile or ward unit, or a simple X-ray machine with a table, can perform all the examinations and is much less expensive than the BRS. WHO tests of such equipment have disproved these claims and show that the radiation dose per examination can be much higher, both to patient and operator. Nor can such units be easily used by unskilled operators to produce high quality and versatile results. Certainly they are cheaper, but they cause many more problems in maintenance, installation and quality control. The worst product of all is the gift of equipment which has become 'redundant'. This should usually be refused (politely!).

Ultrasound

It is tempting to purchase an ultrasound unit first when money is scarce, because it is about half the cost of a WHO-BRS. Unfortunately, it is really useful only for the abdomen and the neonatal skull. It cannot image the two most common needs, the chest and the skeleton. It is of great advantage for the liver, and the abdomen generally, but it should always be purchased as the second item of imaging equipment, not the first: only in a hospital totally restricted to obstetrics should it take preference over an X-ray unit. The specifications of the WHO General Purpose Ultrasound Unit will provide every examination which is likely to be needed in any small or even quite large hospital. This has been confirmed by tests in a university hospital in a developing country, where a small real-time portable ultrasound unit satisfactorily imaged 95 per cent of the problems of patients of all ages.[6] Battery-operated ultrasound units are now becoming available.

powered X-ray generator is strongly recommended: it will work from any 5 A wall outlet at any voltage, will continue for several weeks if the main power supply fails and can be recharged whenever there is electricity available. It is not affected by voltage or any power fluctuation: the batteries will not need attention for three to five years. The alternative BRS unit, powered from the mains, requires at least 60–70 A, 220 V and is very sensitive to mains and line voltage fluctuations. The darkroom, which must be more than 2 × 3 m, needs a water supply and drainage but, except in very cold countries will not require special water heating (or cooling). If less than 12–15 patients per day are examined, film processing should be by hand (full details are available in the WHO Manual of Darkroom Technique, available in many languages).[3] However, with experienced staff the WHO-BRS can examine 40 patients per day, but a small automatic film processor will then be desirable: again, WHO can make recommendations.

Can the BRS X-ray children and, where ultrasound is not available, obstetrical problems? This has been

Recording the ultrasound image is still somewhat of a problem, because it can be expensive. It must be remembered that ultrasound will require physician time: while it is easy to train operators to take good X-ray films which can then be examined by the doctor, this is seldom true of ultrasound, which almost always needs the personal attention of the physician. It takes a great deal of experience and training for a technician to produce satisfactory images which a physician can interpret. A very careful review should be made of the needs and the available physician time before the purchase of ultrasound is contemplated, and X-ray equipment should always be available first.

Which images to request

Guidance in paediatric imaging can be obtained from the WHO Technical Report Series 757 which ought to be read wherever there is paediatric imaging anywhere in the world.[7] An international panel of experts in paediatric imaging have laid down clearly what examinations are clinically reliable, radiation- and cost-effective, when and how they should be used and when to choose ultrasound first. There is a similar report for General Diagnostic Imaging.[8] For too long paediatricians (and their colleagues concerned with adults) have added additional projections and complex examinations without carefully surveying the results and discarding those which are not really productive. The WHO guidelines (which many have considered too conservative) are of extreme importance to the children of the developing world.[6] They advocate cost- and radiation-effective imaging.

Appropriate use of imaging

Diagnostic imaging can play a major role in suggesting or confirming the diagnosis and assessing the results of treatment. In four active parasitic infections (ascariasis, trichuriasis, cerebral cysticercosis and urinary schistosomiasis) the definitive diagnosis can reliably be made by imaging alone (see p. 653). In many other instances the parasite can be recognized, but by that time it is usually dead and seldom of practical importance.[9]

It is not possible to list here all the appropriate uses for diagnostic imaging in tropical diseases, but it must be emphasized that there is often a marked difference in the reaction of a Western patient to a parasite or infection when compared with an indigenous inhabitant of the tropics whose body has become familiarized by recurrent exposure. The images of the local people will also vary between those who are continuously infected compared with those with intermittent

exposure. There are geographical variations to the same parasite or bacterial infection which can only be learned by experience in any particular locality.[10] For example, tuberculosis in babies in the tropics may resemble staphylococcal infections in the Western child: a lung abscess in the tropics may be amoebic without any other evidence of the infection. An acute osteomyelitis can be due to tuberculosis, an orbital tumour can be a hydatid cyst or lymphoma. The most common cause of intestinal obstruction may be ascaris, which is also in some places one of the most common causes of jaundice in children: an acute arthritis may be due to guinea-worm. A knowledge of the patient's background is of the utmost importance when interpreting the image.

Sequence of investigation

Assuming that X-ray imaging (other than fluoroscopy) and ultrasound are both available, the pattern of investigation is straightforward. (See Table 6.7.1.)

Abdomen

Ultrasound should be used first for all suspected liver, gall-bladder, pancreatic and pelvic disease. It is excellent for the demonstration of intra-abdominal hydatid cysts wherever they may be (p. 738), and reliable for the investigation of the uterus and adnexia. A pleural effusion resulting from a liver abscess can also usually be found with ultrasound; it can be used to demonstrate thickened ureters and bladder walls in schistosomiasis and to assess treatment. It can demonstrate renal morphology but not physiology.[11] It is particularly useful in suspected urinary tract obstruction, and can demonstrate urinary calculi, but is not always reliable if the examination is negative. Ultrasound can recognize ascariasis as a case of intestinal or biliary obstruction. It is less reliable in the retro-peritoneal tissues, but if CT is not available may give useful information.

X-rays of the abdomen are useful for suspected intestinal obstruction and for gut perforation (an erect film is essential for both) and for urinary calculi (with or without contrast). Abdominal films are seldom of help in the differential diagnosis of chronic abdominal pain and will not be useful in acute appendicitis, or ruptured ectopic pregnancy. Many foreign bodies can be demonstrated, but not all.

Excessive diarrhoea and vomiting in children may cause electrolyte disturbances, which can produce an adynamic bowel with distention and fluid levels in the erect film and closely mimic obstruction.

As user experience increases, ultrasound can reliably

Table 6.7.1   Imaging: in order of preference

	Clinical diagnosis	Method of imaging
Liver	Abscess	1. U/S; if negative repeat in 24 and 48 h 2. X/R of chest for pleural fluid and raised diaphragm
	Cyst (e.g. hydatid)	1. U/S 2. X/R for calcification: X-ray chest for other cysts
	Tumour	1. U/S; add chest X-ray for metastases
Gall-bladder	Jaundice and pain	1. U/S 2. X/R, plain and with contrast (IV for biliary ducts)
Pancreas	Cyst Pancreatitis	1. U/S 2. X/R is unlikely to show cyst but may show calcification or local ileus
Oesophagus and stomach	Foreign body	1. U/S
	Pyloric obstruction	1. U/S (X-ray not used without fluoroscopy)
	Ascaris	1. U/S 2. Plain X-ray
Bowel	Obstruction or ileus Intussusception	1. X/R (supine and erect) 2. U/S to locate stricture or intussusception or mass (beware of electrolyte imbalance causing pseudo-obstruction)
	Perforation	1. X/R: erect

Abdomen	Appendix abscess
	   Caecal abscess
	   Helminthoma
		1. U/S
		2. X/R may show localized ileus or small bowel obstruction

	Abdominal hydatid disease	1. U/S 2. X/R may show calcified cysts but can be normal
	Peritonitis/ascites	1. U/S to show fluid 2. X/R to show perforation or ileus (erect)
	Typhoid and other dysenteries	Nil – X/R may show perforation in typhoid (erect film)
	Psoas abscess	1. X/R to show spine and soft tissues 2. U/S to show retroperitoneum
	Pregnancy	1. U/S whenever available X/R never to be used if U/S available X/R in last four weeks of pregnancy only Indications: A. For position of fetus – PA film B. For size, shape or development of fetus – PA oblique C. Multiple pregnancy – PA D. Obstructed pregnancy – erect, lateral
Pelvis	Inflammatory disease/abscess	1. U/S X/R nil
	Ovarian or adnexal cyst	1. U/S X/R nil
	Ectopic pregnancy	1. U/S X/R nil
	Acute appendix or amoebic abscess	1. U/S (may show mass) X/R nil

Kidney	Chronic inflammation
	   Hydronephrosis
	   Tumour
	   Calculus
		1. U/S
		2. X/R, plain and contrast urography

Ureters	Schistosomiasis
	   Obstructed
	   Calculus
		1. U/S
		2. X/R with contrast – always use X/R if U/S negative or incomplete information obtained

Bladder	Chronic inflammation
	   Calcification
	   Calculus
		1. U/S
		2. X/R with contrast – always use contrast if U/S negative or incomplete information obtained

Table 6.7.1 Continued

	Clinical diagnosis	Method of imaging
Skeleton	Trauma	1. X/R (U/S nil), AP–lateral – review films, if any doubt, other projections: opposite limb to show normal No injury seen but clinically still doubtful (e.g. scaphoid) repeat in 10 days
	Infection	1. Radionuclide scan if available 2. If not, X/R. If normal, treat if clinically indicated Repeat in 10 days: serial films every two weeks as indicated
	Infected arthritis (very small child or infant)	1. U/S. If negative repeat in seven days
	All other children	1. X/R, if negative repeat in seven days
Skull	Trauma	Nil except tangential X/R for suspected depressed fracture
	Raised intracranial pressure:	
	Hydrocephalus	1. U/S if fontanelles open 2. X/R: single lateral skull
	Meningitis	1. U/S if fontanelles open
	Sinuses	Nil
Chest	Any indication	1. X/R AP or PA – review – further films if needed U/S not helpful except for small pleural effusions

U/S = ultrasound; X/R = radiography; 1 = use this method first (where available); Nil = do not image, use clinical judgment.

demonstrate the hypertrophied pylorus in infantile pyloric obstruction or the sausage tumour of intussusception. In the neonate it can show congenital bowel strictures, annular pancreas, choledochal cysts and can be useful in meconium ileus. It can differentiate the cause of a swollen testicle (torsion-vs-tumour) and can locate a non-descended testicle.

Obstetrics

If ultrasound is not available, X-rays of the pregnant abdomen are justified only in the last four weeks and should never be used to diagnose early pregnancy. The indications for radiography are for malposition, multiple pregnancy, fetal abnormalities and disproportion in the last four weeks of pregnancy. The patient must always have an empty bladder before obstetrical radiography.

- If disproportion is suspected, a single erect lateral view of the pelvis should be taken.
- If fetal abnormality or maturity is the indication, a single prone oblique projection is needed.
- If the fetal presentation is the problem, a single prone (not an oblique) film is needed.[12]

Ultrasound can monitor fetal growth, position, placental location, multiple pregnancy and with experience, many other parameters, particularly neural developmental abnormalities, fetal cardiac rhythm, etc.

Chest

Provided a good-quality film is available, only a frontal projection (PA or AP depending on the child's age) is needed and should be reviewed first before requesting any lateral projection. All additional views (e.g. apical, lordotic, etc.) are dependent only on the findings of the first film. The indications for chest X-rays (and skeletal examinations) do not differ for children in the tropics and subtropics but, because of the prevalence of parasitic infections, there are additional reasons. There are many misleading findings; to quote only a few, any case of lobar pneumonia (however high the fever, however quick the response to antibiotics) which does not clear radiologically in four weeks or in which there is obvious lymphadenopathy, should be suspected as being tuberculous until proved otherwise. Heavy lung markings bilaterally, and sometimes with mild lymphadenopathy can be due to ascariasis or other worms, or to the initial stage of schistosomiasis (the Katayama syndrome – p. 651).

Skeleton

In the vast majority of injuries only an AP and lateral projection of the injured part are needed and should then be reviewed. It should never be a routine to X-ray the opposite (normal) limb or joint until the film of the injured side has been reviewed and doubt occurs. Similarly, there is no indication for routine oblique views of the spine, or any part of the skeleton. Only occasionally will they be needed when the original films have been checked.

Skull

Pathological findings on imaging of the skull are rare. Ultrasound should be used in the neonate and young infant with open fontanelles for suspected hydrocephalus, haematoma or developmental neuro-abnormality (e.g. agenesis of the corpus callosum). With experience imaging is extremely useful in monitoring bacterial meningitis for the early recognition of complications and the assessment of treatment and prognosis. Plain skull radiography is seldom of use, except when a single lateral projection to observe skull thinning, marrow hyperplasia and widening of the sutures may be indicated. In the absence of well-localized neurological findings, X-rays of the skull are likely to be non-contributory: in most cases clinical examination or laboratory tests provide the same information. Skull X-rays are seldom of any use in skull trauma at any age, but particularly in the paediatric age groups. In children, opacification of the paranasal sinuses does not necessarily imply significant pathology and can occur in the healthy patient. The indications for X-rays in sinusitis and upper airway infections in children are limited and usually only required where there are suspected complications or failure of treatment. Ultrasound can be used to assess fluid within the sinuses but the accuracy of this technique has not yet been decided. X-rays of the mastoids are seldom of any significance in young children and are very difficult to interpret in older children and adults.

Skeletal tumours and infections

X-rays may be negative in the early stages of both traumas and infection. The differential diagnosis can be extremely difficult in children (as can the histology) and careful clinical correlation is essential. A normal radiograph in a suspected case of osteomyelitis is an indication for treatment and re-X-ray in about two weeks. Radionuclide scanning, if available, will provide earlier information. Even if treatment is clinically successful, the bony, often destructive changes will continue in spite of appropriate therapy. Healing as seen radiologically takes a long time.

Ultrasound can be useful for congenital dislocation of the hip and in young children may aid in the recognition of infective arthritis. Ultrasound may show soft tissue oedema in early osteomyelitis.

Both examinations require skill and patience to be successful.

Errors

Fifty per cent of radiographic diagnostic errors occur from the poor quality of radiography or films taken in non-standard positions or incorrect exposures. Fifty per cent of the errors with ultrasound are due to lack of proper training and experience, inadequate time spent upon the examination or failure to repeat a negative examination (e.g. in the liver) 24 hours later. It should be remembered that regular checks are necessary for ultrasound equipment to maintain technical quality. The units do not yet go on forever without attention and can slowly deteriorate. In all imaging, closer attention to technical detail, be it film processing, positioning or ultrasound techniques and equipment will not only increase the yield but, more importantly, significantly decrease the error rate.

References

1. *Technical Specifications for the X-Ray Apparatus to be used in a Basic Radiological System* (unpublished WHO document RAD. 85. 1) Geneva, WHO, 1985.
2. *The Future Use of New Imaging Technologies in Developing Countries*. WHO Technical Report Series 723. Geneva, WHO, 1985.
3. Palmer PES. *The WHO Basic Radiological System: Manual of Darkroom Technique*. Geneva, WHO, 1985.
4. Holm T, Palmer PES, Lehtinen E. *The WHO-BRS: Manual of Radiographic Technique*. Geneva, WHO, 1986.
5. Palmer PES, Cockshott WP, Hegedus V *et al. The WHO Basic Radiological System: Manual of Radiographic Interpretation for General Practitioners*. Geneva, WHO, 1985.
6. Wachira MW, Palmer PES. *The Capability of Small Real Time Ultrasound Scanner and the Physician Training Required To Use It* (unpublished WHO report). Geneva, WHO, 1982.
7. *Rational use of Diagnostic Imaging in Paediatrics*. WHO Technical Report Series 757. Geneva, WHO, 1987.
8. *A Rational Approach to Radiodiagnostic Investigations*. Report of a WHO Scientific Group on the Indications for and Limitations of Major X-Ray Diagnostic Investigations. WHO Technical Report Series 689. Geneva, WHO, 1983.
9. Palmer PES. Diagnostic imaging in parasitic infections. *Pediatric Clinics of North America*. 1985; **32**(4): 1019–40.
10. Reeder MM, Palmer PES. The differential diagnosis index of tropical diseases and the geography of infectious and parasitic diseases. In: *The Radiology of Tropical Diseases*. Baltimore, Williams and Wilkins, 1981: xv–xx.
11. Palmer PES. Ultrasound and CT scanning. *East African Medical Journal*. 1986; **63**(2): 140–4.
12. Palmer PES, Cockshott WP, Hegedus V *et al.* Obstetric X-rays. In: *The WHO-BRS Manual of Radiographic Interpretation for General Practitioners*. WHO, Geneva, 1985. pp. 81–6.

Index